Surgical Pathology of the Liver

Surgical Pathology of the Liver

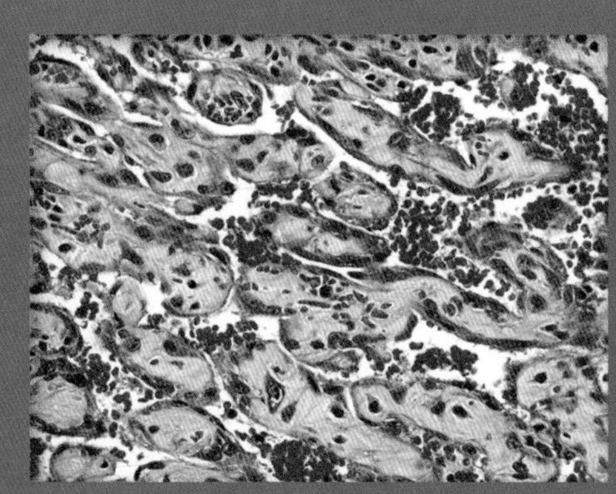
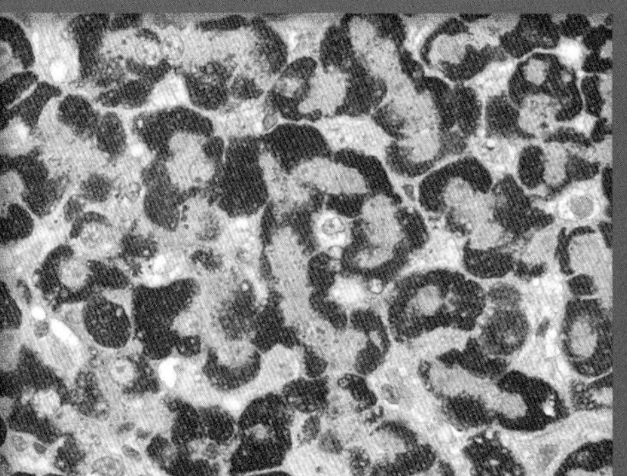
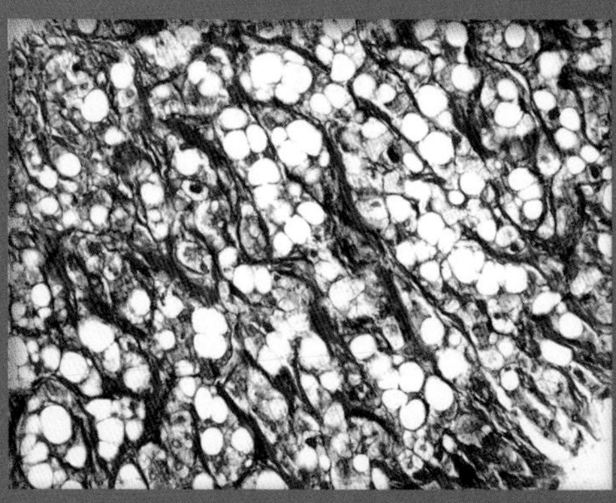

Michael S. Torbenson, MD
Professor of Pathology
Department of Laboratory Medicine and Pathology
Mayo Clinic
Rochester, Minnesota

Lizhi Zhang, MD
Associate Professor of Pathology
Department of Laboratory Medicine and Pathology
Mayo Clinic
Rochester, Minnesota

Roger K. Moreira, MD
Assistant Professor of Pathology
Department of Laboratory Medicine and Pathology
Mayo Clinic
Rochester, Minnesota

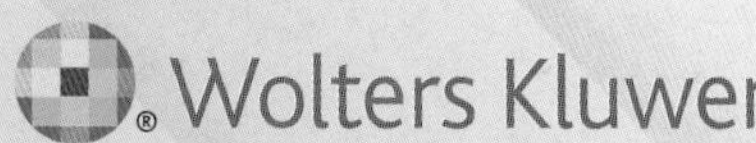

Philadelphia • Baltimore • New York • London
Buenos Aires • Hong Kong • Sydney • Tokyo

Senior Acquisitions Editor: Ryan Shaw
Supervising Development Editor: Kristina Oberle
Editorial Coordinator: Jennifer DiRicco
Editorial Assistant: Amy Masgay
Marketing Manager: Dan Dressler
Production Project Manager: David Saltzberg
Design Coordinator: Stephen Druding
Manufacturing Coordinator: Beth Welsh
Prepress Vendor: S4Carlisle Publishing Services

9 8 7 6 5 4 3 2 1

Printed in China

Library of Congress Cataloging-in-Publication Data

Names: Torbenson, Michael S., author. | Zhang, Lizhi, MD, author. | Moreira, Roger K., author.
Title: Surgical pathology of the liver / Michael S. Torbenson, Lizhi Zhang, Roger K. Moreira.
Description: Philadelphia: Wolters Kluwer Health, [2018] | Includes bibliographical references and index.
Identifiers: LCCN 2017042915 | ISBN 9781496365798
Subjects: | MESH: Liver—pathology | Liver Diseases—pathology | Specimen Handling
Classification: LCC RC846.9 | NLM WI 700 | DDC 616.3/62071—dc23 LC record available at https://lccn.loc.gov/2017042915

LWW.com

RRS1709

CONTRIBUTORS

Vishal S. Chandan, MD
Associate Professor of Laboratory Medicine and Pathology
Mayo Clinic
Rochester, Minnesota

Andrew L. Folpe, MD
Professor of Laboratory Medicine and Pathology
Mayo Clinic
Rochester, Minnesota

Rondell P. Graham, MBBS
Assistant Professor
Department of Laboratory Medicine, Anatomic Pathology, and Genomics Laboratory
Mayo Clinic
Rochester, Minnesota

Yajue Huang, MD, PhD
Associate Professor
Department of Laboratory Medicine and Pathology
Mayo Clinic
Rochester, Minnesota

Andrea Jones, MD
Department of Laboratory Medicine and Pathology
Mayo Clinic
Rochester, Minnesota

Murli Krishna, MD
Associate Professor of Laboratory Medicine and Pathology
Mayo Clinic Florida
Jacksonville, Florida

Dora Lam-Himlin, MD
Associate Professor
Department of Laboratory Medicine and Pathology
Mayo Clinic
Scottsdale, Arizona

Jason Lewis, MD
Associate Professor of Laboratory Medicine and Pathology
Mayo Clinic
Jacksonville, Florida

Ellen D. McPhail, MD
Associate Professor of Laboratory Medicine and Pathology
Mayo Clinic
Rochester, Minnesota

Roger K. Moreira, MD
Assistant Professor of Pathology
Department of Laboratory Medicine and Pathology
Mayo Clinic
Rochester, Minnesota

Taofic Mounajjed, MD
Assistant Professor
Department of Laboratory Medicine and Pathology
Mayo Clinic
Rochester, Minnesota

Rish K. Pai, MD, PhD
Associate Professor of Pathology and Laboratory Medicine
Mayo Clinic
Scottsdale, Arizona

Bobbi S. Pritt, MD, MSc
Professor of Laboratory Medicine and Pathology
Division of Clinical Microbiology
Mayo Clinic
Rochester, Minnesota

Michael Rivera, MD
Assistant Professor
Department of Laboratory Medicine and Pathology
Mayo Clinic
Rochester, Minnesota

Samar Said, MD
Assistant Professor
Department of Laboratory Medicine and Pathology
Mayo Clinic
Rochester, Minnesota

Marcela Salomao, MD
Assistant Professor of Laboratory Medicine and Anatomic Pathology
Mayo Clinic
Scottsdale, Arizona

Douglas A. Simonetto, MD
Assistant Professor of Medicine
Division of Gastroenterology and Hepatology
Mayo Clinic
Rochester, Minnesota

Maxwell L. Smith, MD
Associate Professor of Laboratory Medicine and Pathology
Mayo Clinic
Scottsdale, Arizona

Michael S. Torbenson, MD
Professor of Pathology
Department of Laboratory Medicine and Pathology
Mayo Clinic
Rochester, Minnesota

Sudhakar K. Venkatesh, MD
Professor of Radiology
Department of Radiology
Mayo Clinic
Rochester, Minnesota

Michael L. Wells, MD
Senior Associate Consultant
Department of Radiology
Mayo Clinic
Rochester, Minnesota

Tsung-Teh Wu, MD, PhD
Professor of Laboratory Medicine and Pathology
Mayo Clinic
Rochester, Minnesota

Saba Yasir, MBBS
Assistant Professor
Department of Laboratory Medicine and Pathology
Mayo Clinic
Rochester, Minnesota

Lizhi Zhang, MD
Associate Professor of Pathology
Division of Anatomic Pathology
Mayo Clinic
Rochester, Minnesota

PREFACE

This book is written by surgical pathologists for surgical pathologists. All of the authors are practicing GI/liver pathologists or radiologists at the Mayo Clinic who see lots of cases. The chapters thus reflect both the literature and the extensive personal experience of the authors. The goal of the book is to focus on diagnostic histopathology, including those laboratory and clinical findings that readers are most likely to find directly useful when evaluating liver histology for clinical care.

In addition to a comprehensive coverage of general liver pathology, this book also includes a number of chapters that are uncommonly included in liver pathology text books, but chapters we believe the readers will find useful: definition of liver pathology terms, use of immunohistochemistry and special stains in medical liver pathology, electron microscopy, cytopathology, molecular pathology, and hematopathology. All of the chapters integrate the use of immunohistochemical stains and other supporting studies into the morphological findings and focus on providing practical differential diagnoses, ones that are prioritized by likelihood and hopefully avoid being a mere laundry list of potential associations. The book is extensively illustrated and the images have been chosen with care, both for their stand-alone education value and to be an integrated extension of the information conveyed in the text.

Our efforts in writing this book were strengthened by the outstanding administrative support of Alison Smarzyk, which we gratefully acknowledge.

Finally, we welcome any feedback on what you the reader found useful and what was less useful—as in the end, the only real way to judge a book is by its cover, with those books having pristine and perfect covers so much less beautiful than the raggedy, scuffed, covers of a well-used book. We hope this book will be the latter.

CONTENTS

1 The normal liver

Samar Said, MD

1.1 GROSS ANATOMY

The liver is located in the right upper quadrant of the abdomen, under the diaphragm. It has a smooth surface and is red-brown in color. The liver consists of a larger right lobe, left lobe, caudate lobe, and quadrate lobe. The right and left lobes are separated by the falciform ligament. The liver weighs 840-2,580 g in adult men and 780-2,400 g in adult women.[1,2]

The normal gross anatomy is reviewed in more detail in Chapter 2, but the Couinaud classification divides the liver into eight segments, which are defined by the vascular supply and biliary drainage, where each segment has its own vascular pedicle and biliary drainage.[3] In this classification, the middle hepatic vein divides the liver into right and left hemilivers—this plane corresponds to a line extending from the left side of the sulcus for the inferior vena cava superiorly to the middle of the fossa for the gallbladder inferiorly; the right hepatic vein divides the right hemiliver into anterior and posterior segments; the left hepatic vein divides the left hemiliver into medial and lateral parts; and the portal vein divides the liver into upper and lower segments. The segments are numbered in a clockwise manner. The eight segments are: segment 1: caudate lobe; segment 2: lateral superior segment of left hemiliver; segment 3: lateral inferior segment of left hemiliver; segment 4a: medial superior segment of left hemiliver; segment 4b: medial inferior segment of left hemiliver; segment 5: anterior inferior segment of right hemiliver; segment 6: posterior inferior segment of right hemiliver; segment 7: posterior superior segment of right hemiliver; and segment 8: anterior superior segment of right hemiliver. The Couinaud classification works best with radiology images but can be hard to use with resection specimens.

1.2 VASCULAR SUPPLY

The liver has a dual blood supply from the hepatic portal vein and hepatic artery. Approximately two-thirds of the blood supply of the liver comes from the portal vein, which drains the spleen and the intestine before reaching the liver. The portal system blood enters into the liver via the portal vein, which quickly divides into the left and right branches of the portal vein. The blood then moves along this route: portal vein branches (located in portal tracts), venules, periportal sinusoids, hepatic sinusoids, central veins, hepatic veins, inferior vena cava, and finally the right heart. The remaining one-third of the liver's blood supply comes from the hepatic artery, which carries more richly oxygenated blood and follows one of three routes: a plexus around the portal vein branches, a plexus around the bile ducts, or terminal hepatic arterioles, which move blood from the portal tracts into the sinusoids.[4]

1.3 LYMPHATICS

The hepatic lymph comes primarily from the sinusoids and enters into the space of Disse. After that, it flows to the channels traversing the limiting plate and enters the interstitial space of either the portal tract (parallel to the bile flow and opposite to the blood flow), sublobular veins, or the hepatic capsule. It is thought that 80% or more of the hepatic lymph drains through lymphatic channels located in the portal tracts.[5] Most of the lymphatics drain into hepatic nodes located along the hepatic artery and then into celiac lymph nodes. Other efferent routes include parasternal lymph nodes, posterior mediastinal lymph nodes, and left gastric lymph nodes.[6,7]

1.4 BILE FLOW

Bile canaliculi represent the beginning of the bile drainage system in the liver. The bile canaliculus is an intercellular space between two adjacent hepatocytes, separated from the rest of the intercellular space by tight junctions. Bile canaliculi can only be seen when they are distended because of cholestasis; they are invisible by light microscopy in normal livers. They drain into the canals of Hering (lined by hepatocytes and biliary epithelium), which are connected to small bile ductules in the portal tracts. Both the canals of Hering and the bile ductules are also invisible in the normal liver, but various injuries can elicit a bile ductular reaction, in which case the bile ductules are visible at the periphery of the portal tract. The ductules drain into the interlobular bile ducts, which merge to form septal/trabecular bile ducts and ultimately become the common hepatic duct.[8]

1.5 NORMAL HISTOLOGY

Portal tracts

The normal portal tract contains at least one profile of three luminal structures: an interlobular bile duct, portal vein, and hepatic arteriole (Fig. 1.1). On

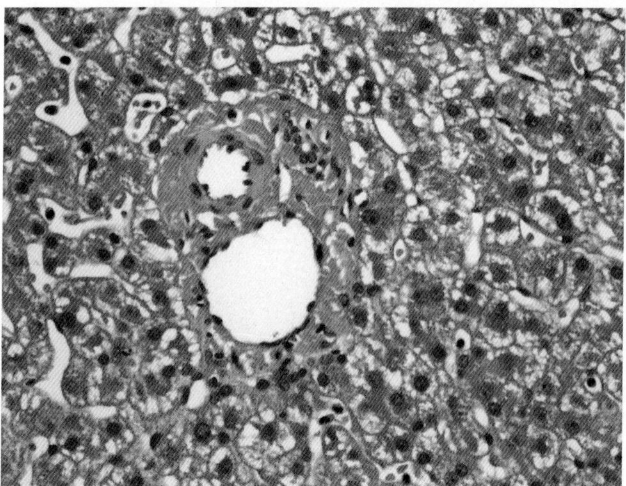

Figure 1.1 Normal portal tract. This portal tract is normal and shows a bile duct, hepatic arteriole, and portal vein, with minimal inflammatory cells.

average, the portal tracts have two interlobular bile duct profiles, two hepatic artery profiles, and one portal vein profile. These structures are surrounded by connective tissue composed of mainly type I collagen. Depending on the angle of sectioning, one of these structures might not be seen in few portal tracts.[9] The portal tracts undergo successive branching, where they divide and get smaller as they move to the periphery. The degree of connective tissue present in a particular portal tract correlates with the size of the portal tract, with larger portal tracts containing more connective tissue than do smaller ones.

The bile ducts and the hepatic arterioles are usually of similar caliber and are located close to each other. This can be used as guidance when looking for the bile ducts in inflamed portal tracts or other conditions where bile ducts are difficult to see, such as in ductopenia. Bile ductules can be seen in response to biliary tract disease or other forms of liver injury, but should not be confused with the bile ducts. Bile ductular proliferations are located at the periphery of the portal tracts and are not paired with arterioles.

A minimal amount of chronic inflammation is present in the portal tracts, typically composed of small lymphocytes with rare mast cells. This is needed for normal liver hemostasis and function.[10] The portal tracts also contain lymphatics, fibroblasts, and nerves. The latter are seen on hematoxylin and eosin stain (H&E), only in the largest branches of the portal tracts. The hepatocytes located next to the portal tract form the limiting plate. With age, the number of inflammatory cells increases slightly and the collagen fibers of the portal tracts become denser.

Bile ducts

The interlobular bile ducts have cuboidal to low columnar epithelium with a centrally located nucleus, whereas the lining epithelium of the larger septal ducts is tall columnar with basally located nuclei. The biliary epithelial cells are well demarcated with uniform, round nuclei that do not overlap. The larger bile ducts are surrounded by Periodic acid-Schiff (PAS)-positive, diastase-resistant basement membrane. In normal liver, no inflammatory cells are seen inside the basement membrane of the bile ducts.

Hepatic lobules

The hepatic lobules contain polygonal-shaped hepatocytes with well-defined cell borders, eosinophilic cytoplasm, centrally located round nuclei, and visible nucleoli. Hepatocytes lack basement membranes, and most of them contain one nucleus; however, it is not uncommon to see a few cells with two nuclei. The number of binucleated hepatocytes increases with age, as does nuclear variability, with occasional large irregular and hyperchromatic nuclei. Glycogen-rich cytoplasm can herniate into the nuclei and form glycogenated nuclei, which may be seen in a few hepatocytes in healthy individuals. The hepatocyte cytoplasm has abundant glycogen and multiple organelles, including mitochondria, smooth and rough endoplasmic reticulum, lysosomes, peroxisomes, Golgi complexes, and organized cytoskeleton. Hepatocytes also produce albumin and many enzymes. Endoplasmic reticulum appears as basophilic granules or fibers, which may become more prominent in association with some medications. Mitochondria are not visible in most hepatocytes, but megamitochondria can be seen occasionally in hepatocytes in normal livers and more frequently in diseased livers.

Hepatocytes are arranged in plates separated by the sinusoidal labyrinth. The plates are one cell thick, but a few might appear thicker, depending on the angle of sectioning. This unique structure of the liver plates allows for direct contact between hepatocytes and the blood. In children less than 6 years old, however, the liver cell plates tend to be two cells thick. In normal liver biopsy and resection specimens, the sinusoids are either empty or may contain a few red blood cells and rarely white blood cells. Circulating megakaryocytes can also be occasionally seen. In neonates, the sinusoids may contain hematopoietic foci.

Hepatocytes frequently contain lipofuscin in the normal liver. Lipofuscin pigments are fine, gold-brown, retractile granules that orient along the canalicular domain of hepatocytes and are found mainly in zone 3 (pericentral vein). Lipofuscin consists of insoluble, highly oxidized fatty acids and misfolded proteins that are not degradable by the proteasome system or lysosomal enzymes. This "wear-and-tear pigment" tends to increase with age.

Hepatocytes exhibit functional heterogeneity.[11–17] The hepatocytes located near the portal tracts have the highest metabolic activity. They are exposed to blood with highest content of oxygen, insulin, glucagon, and amino acids, and they are the main site of protein synthesis, gluconeogenesis, glycolysis, and fatty acid metabolism. In addition, most enzymes (such as transaminase, glutamyltranspeptidase, and alcohol dehydrogenase) are located mainly in periportal hepatocytes, with the exception of glutamine synthetase and carbamoyl phosphate synthetase I, which are found predominantly in pericentral vein hepatocytes that have a higher capacity for detoxification of various molecules. Hepatocytes are also the storage site for copper[18,19] and a key site for storage of iron.

The space located between the hepatocytes and the sinusoidal endothelium is called the space of Disse. It contains hepatic stellate cells, nerve fibers, reticulin fibers (which consist mostly of type III collagen), and other components of the extracellular matrix. Neither stellate cells nor the space of Disse are visible in normal livers. Central veins are lined by endothelial cells. The smallest central vein branches have minimal or no collagen around them in the normal liver, although larger ones will have a thin collar of collagen.

Other cell types

Stellate cells contain small droplets of fat that are rich in vitamin A. It is thought that stellate cells have a role in vitamin A storage, sinusoidal blood flow regulation, hepatic regeneration, maintenance of the normal liver matrix, and development of hepatic fibrosis. They can also elaborate enzymes needed to degrade matrix components. Stellate cells also function as antigen-presenting cells. In animal models, they stain for vimentin, desmin, and glial fibrillary acidic protein, but there are no reliable immunostains to identify stellate cells in surgical pathology specimens. Activated stellate cells stain for α-smooth muscle actin.[20–27]

Kupffer cells rest on the sinusoidal wall. It may be difficult to differentiate them from endothelial cells, but they tend to have more irregular and plumper nuclei. Kupffer cells contain multiple enzymes and low concentration of α-1-antitrypsin. They can be highlighted by CD68 immunostains or by PAS stain after diastase digestion (PAS-D) when they are activated and are functioning as macrophages, scavenging various macromolecules and products of injured/dead cells. They also play a role in the host defense mechanisms against microorganisms and endotoxin.[28,29]

In addition, cytokines released by activated Kupffer cells can help modulate microvascular responses and the functions of hepatocytes and stellate cells.[30]

The liver is also particularly enriched for cells of innate immune system, such as pit cells, which have a granular cytoplasm, and are present on the endothelial lining.[31] Pit cells are liver-specific natural killers that play a vital role in defense against viral infections and metastasis.[32] Pit cells require special stains for their identification.

The hepatic sinusoidal endothelial cells are different from endothelial cells lining larger blood vessels and capillaries at other organ sites because of fenestration and lack of intact basement membrane. They play a critical role in maintaining the overall homeostasis of liver.

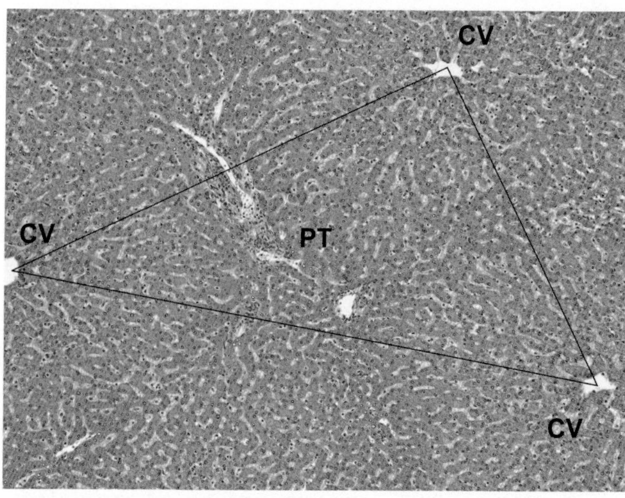

Figure 1.3 Liver structural units (microanatomy)—Mall model. The portal triangular lobule outlined by black lines with PT at the center of the lobule and three CVs at the periphery.

1.6 ORGANIZATION AND STRUCTURAL UNIT OF THE LIVER (MICROANATOMY)

The smallest structural and functional unit of the liver has been proven challenging to define. Multiple models have been proposed, but none appear to adequately explain all the pathologic and physiologic processes in the liver, reflecting the functional complexity of the liver. In the Kiernan model (the classical hexagonal lobule),[33] the terminal hepatic venule (central vein) is located at the center of the hexagonal lobule and the portal tracts are present at the corners of the hexagon (Fig. 1.2). True hexagonal organization is generally not seen in human livers, but the basic notion is still useful. In the Mall model,[34] which is defined by the biliary drainage, the portal tract is located at the center of the lobule and the central veins are at the periphery (Fig. 1.3). In the Rappaport hepatic acinus model,[35] the classical hexagonal lobule is divided into isosceles triangles where the portal tract is at one point of the base of the triangle and the central vein is at the apex (Fig. 1.4). Each triangle represents an acinus where the portal venule traverses the base of the triangle. In this formulation, zone 1 is the ellipsoid highly oxygenated area around the base of the triangle and zone 3 is the area away from the portal venule and more close to the central vein (apex of the triangle). Zone 2 is in between zone 1 and zone 3. In the Matsumoto module,[36] the hexagonal

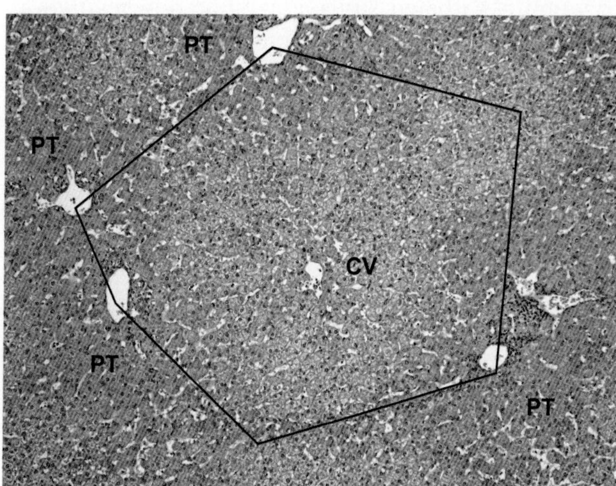

Figure 1.2 Liver structural units (microanatomy)—Kiernan model. The classical hexagonal lobule outlined by black lines with the central vein (CV) at the center and the portal tracts (PT) at the corners of the hexagon. A perfect hexagon is rarely seen in human liver.

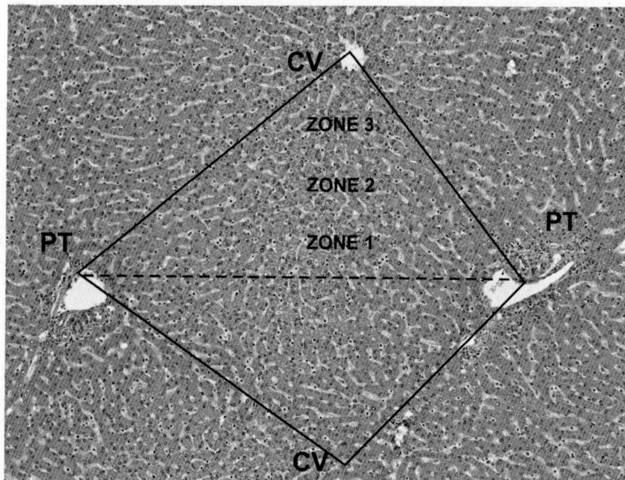

Figure 1.4 Liver structural units (microanatomy)—Rappaport hepatic acinus model. The diamond-shaped acinus outlined by black lines is composed of two triangles with the base axis between two PTs and the acinus divided into zones 1, 2, and 3.

lobule of Kiernan represents the secondary lobule, which consists of 6 to 8 primary lobules.

For the practical purposes of surgical pathology, the liver microanatomy is divided into zone 1 hepatocytes (the several rings of hepatocytes that are adjacent to the portal tract), zone 2 hepatocytes (those cells between zone 1 and zone 3), and zone 3 hepatocytes (those cells around the central vein).

1.7 STAINS IN NORMAL LIVER

Cytokeratins

CK8 and CK18 stain normal hepatocytes and intrahepatic bile ducts.[37] CKAE1/3, CK7, and CK19 stain intrahepatic bile ducts, whereas CK7 also stains intermediate hepatocytes.[37] There should be no significant bile ductular proliferation or intermediate hepatocytes in the normal liver. CK7 is a useful stain to use when biliary tract disease is suspected because it can be used to look for bile duct loss, ductular proliferation, and intermediate hepatocytes. However, full expression of CK7 in intrahepatic bile ducts is not seen until about 1 month of age.[38] Hepatocytes are positive for CAM5.2.

Glutamine synthetase

Glutamine synthetase strongly stains zone 3 (pericentral vein) hepatocytes. It is most commonly used to confirm the H&E impression of focal nodular hyperplasia, where it shows a distinctive "map-like" staining pattern. Glutamine synthetase is also used in subtyping hepatic adenomas, where a strong diffuse pattern suggests β-catenin activation and an increased risk for malignant transformation. Glutamine synthetase can also be used in medical liver biopsies to identify zonation (Fig. 1.5).

Polyclonal carcinoembryonic antigen

Polyclonal carcinoembryonic antigen (pCEA) stains bile canaliculi, showing a branching pattern. pCEA was historically used to identify hepatic differentiation when suspecting hepatocellular carcinoma. Hepatocellular carcinoma can have canalicular, cytoplasmic, and/or membranous pattern of staining, but only the canalicular pattern is specific for hepatocellular carcinoma (Fig. 1.6).

CD10

The immunostain CD10 highlights the bile canaliculi in normal liver, similar to pCEA. However, children less than 24 months of age physiologically lack expression of CD10 in the bile canaliculi (Fig. 1.7).[39]

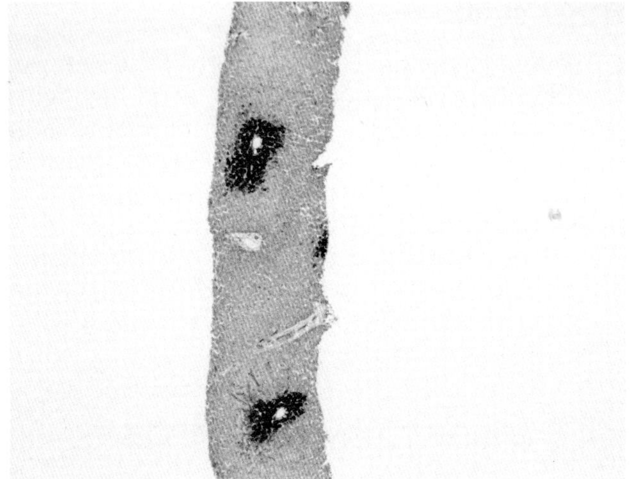

Figure 1.5 Normal glutamine synthetase stain. The zone 3 hepatocytes are positive.

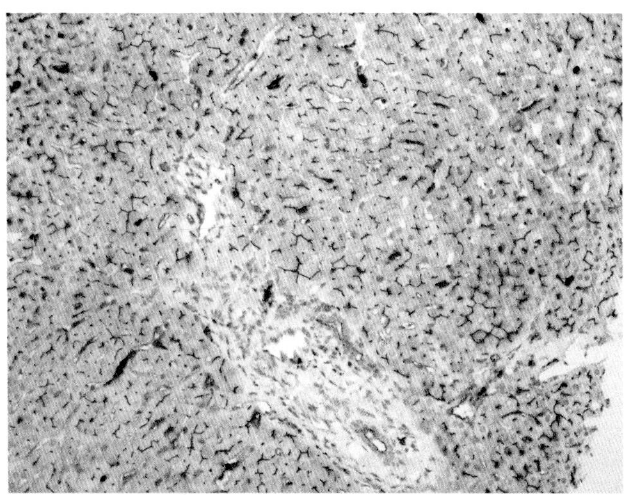

Figure 1.6 Normal polyclonal CEA stain. A typical canalicular staining pattern is seen.

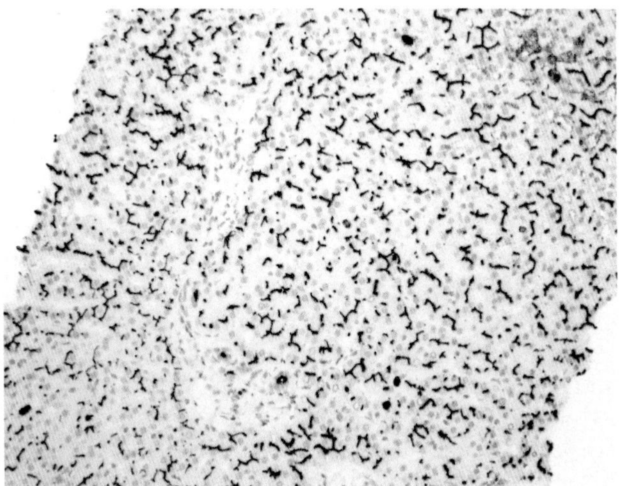

Figure 1.7 Normal CD10 stain. A typical canalicular staining pattern is seen.

Other stains

CD56 and CD57 can highlight pit cells. CD68 will stain Kupffer cells. Smooth muscle actin highlights activated stellate cells. Lipofuscin pigments stain with Ziehl-Neelson, glypican 3, and Fontana-Masson. Megamitochondria stain with phosphotungstic acid hematoxylin stain (PTAH). Normal hepatocytes stain with HepPar1, arginase, and albumin in situ hybridization. PAS-D stain is useful for highlighting the intracytoplasmic globules in α-1-antitrypsin deficiency.

1.8 LABORATORY LIVER TESTS

The main liver tests that should be reviewed when examining a liver biopsy include alanine transaminase (ALT, previously known as SGPT), aspartate transaminase (AST, previously known as SGOT), alkaline phosphatase, γ-glutamyl transferase, serum bilirubin, serum albumin, and prothrombin time/international normalized ratio. Depending on the pattern of liver injury, some of these tests will be affected more than the others.

Predominant elevations in transaminases (AST and ALT) indicate hepatocellular injury. Predominant elevations in alkaline phosphates, γ-glutamyl transferase, and serum bilirubin are seen in bile outflow impairment and cholestatic diseases. Decreased serum albumin levels and prolonged prothrombin time both point toward impaired liver synthesis. These tests, however, are not entirely specific for liver disease. ALT is more specific for liver disease than AST, which can also be elevated in nonliver diseases. Alkaline phosphatase has mainly liver and bone isoenzymes, but there are other isoenzymes as well. Alkaline phosphatase can be elevated in bone disease, in hyperparathyroidism, in pregnancy, and during growth spurts in children and adolescents. γ-glutamyl transferase, although not specific, can be helpful in these situations, with elevations favoring biliary tract disease.[40,41]

Additional tests can be performed depending on the clinical and histologic differential diagnosis. To evaluate for the possibility of Wilson disease, helpful testing includes serum ceruloplasmin, serum copper, 24-hour urine copper levels, and quantitative hepatic copper level. When evaluating for possible iron-overload disease, helpful tests include ferritin, iron saturation, quantitative hepatic iron level and iron index, and genetic testing for hemochromatosis when suspecting hereditary hemochromatosis. Serum α-1-antitrypsin levels and α-1-antitrypsin phenotyping are useful tests for α-1-antitrypsin deficiency. Autoimmune serology and immunoglobulin G (IgG) levels are helpful when considering autoimmune hepatitis, while antimitochondria antibody testing and serum immunoglobulin M (IgM) levels are helpful when considering primary biliary cirrhosis.

1.9 CHANGES RELATED TO AGE

There are several changes in the normal liver that are age related, the most important of which are listed below:

- Hepatic hematopoiesis is normal within the first few weeks after birth.
- Full expression of CK7 in intrahepatic bile ducts is not seen until about 1 month of age.
- The liver cell plates tend to be two cells thick in children less than 6 years of age.
- Children less than 24 months of age often lack physiologic expression of CD10 in the bile canaliculi.
- Serum alkaline phosphatase is elevated in children and adolescents and during pregnancy.
- With age, the number of inflammatory cells in the portal tracts increases, though the inflammatory cells are still typically minimal on H&E. The collagen fibers of the portal tract also become denser, though age per se does not lead to portal expansion (portal fibrosis).
- The amount of lipofuscin pigments in hepatocytes tends to increase with age.
- The number of binucleated hepatocytes increases with age as well as hepatocyte nuclear variability, with occasional large, irregular, and hyperchromatic nuclei.
- With age, the hepatic artery may show changes of arteriosclerosis similar to the aorta.

1.10 POTENTIAL PITFALLS

Normal anatomic variations can sometimes become diagnostic pitfalls, the most important of which are listed below:

- Large portal tracts normally contain more fibrous tissue than do small ones. This should not be interpreted as abnormal fibrosis.
- Minimal portal inflammation composed predominantly of lymphocytes can still be within the spectrum of normal for older patients.
- Depending on the angle of sectioning, some normal portal tracts might not show bile ducts. Thus, ductopenia is defined as absence of bile ducts in more than 50% of the portal tracts.
- PAS-D-positive globules can be seen in Kupffer cells of patients with elevated globulin levels; these do not indicate α-1-antitrypsin deficiency.
- Few hepatocytes can contain lipid droplets. This should not be considered as steatosis or fatty change.

REFERENCES

1. Molina DK, DiMaio VJ. Normal organ weights in men. Part II: the brain, lungs, liver, spleen, and kidneys. *Am J Forensic Med Pathol.* 2012;33(4):368–372.
2. Molina DK, DiMaio VJ. Normal organ weights in women. Part II: the brain, lungs, liver, spleen, and kidneys. *Am J Forensic Med Pathol.* 2015;36(3):182–187.
3. Couinaud C. *Le foie: etudes anatomiques et chirurgicales.* Paris: Masson, 1957.
4. Takasaki S, Hano H. Three-dimensional observations of the human hepatic artery (Arterial system in the liver). *J Hepatol.* 2001;34(3):455–466.
5. Ohtani O, Ohtani Y. Lymph circulation in the liver. *Anat Rec (Hoboken).* 2008;291(6):643–652. doi:10.1002/ar.20681.
6. Comparini L, Bastianini A. Graphic reconstructions in the morphological study of the hepatic lymph vessels. *Angiologica.* 1965;2(2):81–95.
7. Comparini L. Lymph vessels of the liver in man. Microscopic morphology and histotopography. *Angiologica.* 1969;6(5):262–274.
8. Ludwig J, Ritman EL, LaRusso NF, et al. Anatomy of the human biliary system studied by quantitative computer-aided three-dimensional imaging techniques. *Hepatology.* 1998;27(4):893–899.
9. Crawford AR, Lin XZ, Crawford JM. The normal adult human liver biopsy: aquantitative reference standard. *Hepatology.* 1998;28(2):323–331.
10. Robinson MW, Harmon C, O'Farrelly C. Liver immunology and its role in inflammation and homeostasis. *Cell Mol Immunol.* 2016;13(3):267–276.
11. Tosh D, Alberti GM, Agius L. Glucagon regulation of gluconeogenesis and ketogenesis in periportal and perivenous rat hepatocytes. Heterogeneity of hormone action and of the mitochondrial redox state. *Biochem J.* 1988;256(1):197–204.
12. Braeuning A, Ittrich C, Köhle C, et al. Differential gene expression in periportal and perivenous mouse hepatocytes. *FEBS J.* 2006;273(22):5051–5061.
13. Jungermann K. Metabolic zonation of liver parenchyma. *Semin Liver Dis.* 1988;8(4):329–341.
14. Baier PK, Hempel S, Waldvogel B, et al. Zonation of hepatic bile salt transporters. *Dig Dis Sci.* 2006;51(3):587–593.
15. Torre C, Perret C, Colnot S. Molecular determinants of liver zonation. *Prog Mol Biol Transl Sci.* 2010;97:127–150.
16. Burke ZD, Reed KR, Phesse TJ, et al. Liver zonation occurs through a beta-catenin-dependent, c-Myc-independent mechanism. *Gastroenterology.* 2009;136(7):2316–2324.e1–e3.
17. Sekine S, Ogawa R, Mcmanus MT, et al. Dicer is required for proper liver zonation. *J Pathol.* 2009;219(3):365–372.
18. Tao TY, Gitlin JD. Hepatic copper metabolism: insights from genetic disease. *Hepatology.* 2003;37(6):1241–1247.
19. Roberts EA, Sarkar B. Liver as a key organ in the supply, storage, and excretion of copper. *Am J Clin Nutr.* 2008;88(3):851S–854S.
20. Housset C, Rockey DC, Bissell DM. Endothelin receptors in rat liver: lipocytes as a contractile target for endothelin 1. *Proc Natl Acad Sci USA.* 1993;90(20):9266–9270.
21. Bouwens L, Baekeland M, Wisse E. Cytokinetic analysis of the expanding Kupffer-cell population in rat liver. *Cell Tissue Kinet.* 1986;19(2):217–226.
22. Viñas O, Bataller R, Sancho-Bru P, et al. Human hepatic stellate cells show features of antigen-presenting cells and stimulate lymphocyte proliferation. *Hepatology.* 2003;38(4):919–929.
23. Senoo H. Structure and function of hepatic stellate cells. *Med Electron Microsc.* 2004;37(1):3–15.
24. Balabaud C, Bioulac-Sage P, Desmoulière A. The role of hepatic stellate cells in liver regeneration. *J Hepatol.* 2004;40(6):1023–1026.
25. Friedman SL. Hepatic stellate cells: protean, multifunctional, and enigmatic cells of the liver. *Physiol Rev.* 2008;88(1):125–172.
26. Nagy NE, Holven KB, Roos N, et al. Storage of vitamin A in extrahepatic stellate cells in normal rats. *J Lipid Res.* 1997;38(4):645–658.
27. Schirmacher P, Geerts A, Pietrangelo A, et al. Hepatocyte growth factor/hepatopoietin A is expressed in fat-storing cells from rat liver but not myofibroblast-like cells derived from fat-storing cells. *Hepatology.* 1992;15(1):5–11.
28. Rogoff TM, Lipsky PE. Role of the Kupffer cells in local and systemic immune responses. *Gastroenterology.* 1981;80(4):854–860.
29. Rifai A, Mannik M. Clearance of circulating IgA immune complexes is mediated by a specific receptor on Kupffer cells in mice. *J Exp Med.* 1984;160(1):125–137.
30. Andus T, Bauer J, Gerok W. Effects of cytokines on the liver. *Hepatology.* 1991;13(2):364–375.
31. Gao B, Jeong WI, Tian Z. Liver: an organ with predominant innate immunity. *Hepatology.* 2008;47(2):729–736.
32. Bouwens L, Remels L, Baekeland M, et al. Large granular lymphocytes or "pit cells" from rat liver: isolation, ultrastructural characterization and natural killer activity. *Eur J Immunol.* 1987;17(1):37–42.
33. Kiernan F. The Anatomy and Physiology of the Liver. *Philos Trans R Soc Lond (1776-1886).* 1833;123:711–770.
34. Mall FP. A study of the structural unit of the liver. *Am J Anat.* 1906;5:227–308.

35. Rappaport AM, Borowy ZJ, Lougheed WM, et al. Subdivision of hexagonal liver lobules into a structural and functional unit; role in hepatic physiology and pathology. *Anat Rec.* 1954;119(1):11–33.
36. Matsumoto T, Komori R, Magara T, et al. A study of the normal structure of the human liver, with special reference to its angioarchitecture. *Jikeikai Med J.* 1979;26:1–40.
37. Van Eyken P, Sciot R, Callea F, et al. The development of the intrahepatic bile ducts in man: a keratin-immunohistochemical study. *Hepatology.* 1988;8(6):1586–1595.
38. Crawford JM. Development of the intrahepatic biliary tree. *Semin Liver Dis.* 2002;22(3):213–226.
39. Byrne JA, Meara NJ, Rayner AC, et al. Lack of hepatocellularCD10 along bile canaliculi is physiologic in early childhood and persistent in Alagille syndrome. *Lab Invest.* 2007;87(11):1138–1148.
40. Tygstrup N. Assessment of liver function: principles and practice. *J Gastroenterol Hepatol.* 1990;5(4):468–482.
41. Chopra S, Griffin PH. Laboratory tests and diagnostic procedures in evaluation of liver disease. *Am J Med.* 1985;79(2):221–230.

2 Gross processing of liver specimens

Roger K. Moreira, MD

2.1 GROSS ANATOMY

Weight

The normal human liver varies significantly in size, with an average weight of approximately 1,500 g (ranging between 838 and 2,584 g in a recent large autopsy study of normal healthy adults postaccidental death). The liver weight tends to be higher with increasing body weight and body mass index, but the overall correlation is poor.[1]

Surface anatomy

The normal surface of the liver is smooth, glistening, and uniform. The relatively translucent normal Glisson's capsule allows visualiziation of the normal, homogeneous tan-brown color of the underlying parenchyma. The liver edge (anteroinferiorly) normally forms a somewhat acute angle (which can become rounded in pathologic states leading to hepatomegaly). Anteriorly, four ligaments are present—the coronary, triangular, falciform, and round. Of these, the falciform ligament is of greater pathologic importance because it represents the landmark between the anatomic right and left lobes (discussed below). Posteroinferiorly, an area of peritoneal reflexion—the bare (i.e., not covered by the Glisson's capsule) area of the liver is visible within the triangular ligament, adjacent to which the inferior vena cava enters the liver. The hepatic hilum, gallbladder, round ligament, and part of the falciform ligament are also seen (Figs. 2.1, 2.2, and 2.3).

Hepatic lobes and segmental anatomy

Anatomically, the liver is divided into right and left lobes by the falciform ligament (Fig. 2.1). The right lobe is further divided in its medial portion into the caudate lobe (posteriorly) and quadrate lobe (anteriorly). This anatomic approach is the most commonly used by pathologists on routine examination of the liver (tumors, focal lesions, etc). Functionally, however, the liver is divided into right and left lobes (and eight segments) based on vascular supply, with the plane dividing the right and left lobes passing along a line between the gallbladder and the inferior vena cava (Fig. 2.4).

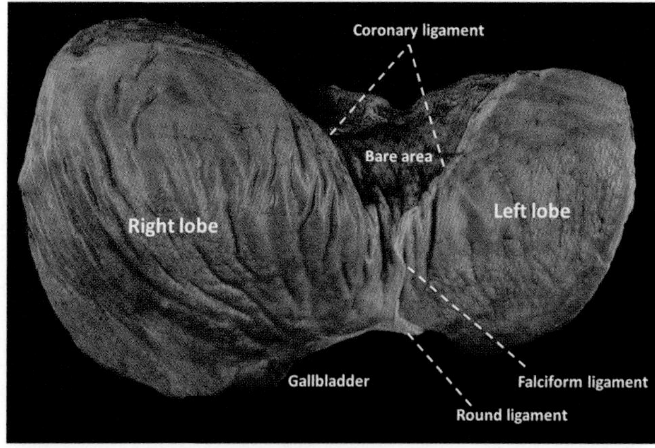

Figure 2.1 Gross appearance of a normal liver (postfixation), anterior view.

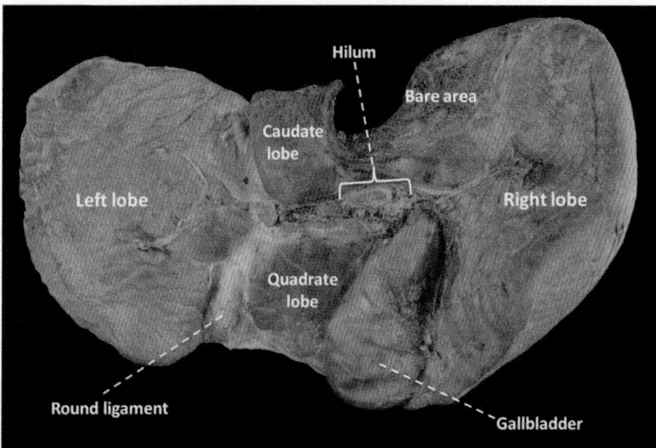

Figure 2.2 Gross appearance of a normal liver (postfixation), posteroinferior view.

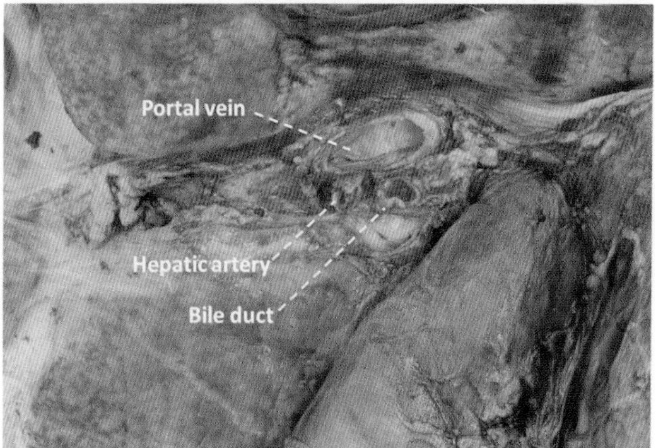

Figure 2.3 Gross image of hepatic hilar structures.

This functional segmentation is widely used by surgeons and radiologists, so it is important for pathologists to be able to recognize the pertinent anatomic landmarks for the purposes of surgical/radilogic–pathologic correlation.

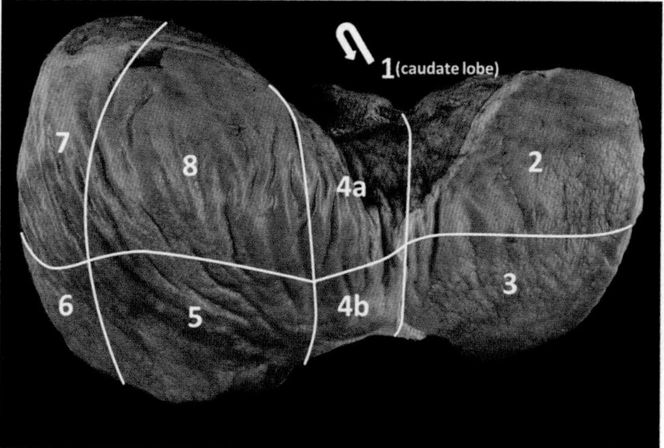

Figure 2.4 Segmental anatomy of the liver. The liver is subdivided into eight segments (further subdivided into subsegments) based on the vascular supply.

2.2 INITIAL SPECIMEN HANDLING

Regardless of the type of liver specimen received (see discussion about specific specimen types below), the initial step in the gross evaluation is to assure proper specimen identification, labeling, and fixation. Review of the available medical records should also be done routinely in order to obtain data about the indication of the procedure and identify potential need for especial processing techniques. Radiologic correlation is also extremely helpful during specimen grossing, especially in complex focal lesions and multifocal tumors because valuable information about the number and location of lesions as well as their relationship with adjacent structures can be obtained. For routine histopathologic examination, the tissue must be placed in the appropriate fixative (most commonly, formalin), but in cases in which a metabolic disease or lymphoma are suspected, a portion of fresh tissue should be placed in glutaraldehyde (for possible electron microscopy) or saline/RPMI medium (for possible flow cytometry). For larger specimens such as large wedges, lobectomies, and total hepatectomies, there should be a sufficient volume of fixative (ideally 25 to 50× the volume of the specimen, but 10× at a minimum),[2] and tissue should be allowed to fix for an appropriate amount of time in order to penetrate into the middle of the specimen. Tissue penetration rate varies depending on the type of tissue, fixative used, temperature, among other factors, and can be calculated using the following equation: $d = K\sqrt{t}$, where d is the penetration distance (mm), K is the diffusion constant (according to the type of fixative), and t is time (hours). For 10% formalin solution, tissue penetration is less than 1 mm/hour, and approximately 25 hours are needed to completely fix a 1-cm-thick specimen (i.e., 5 mm of penetration from each side) (Fig. 2.5). Specimen sectioning prior to fixation (sliced

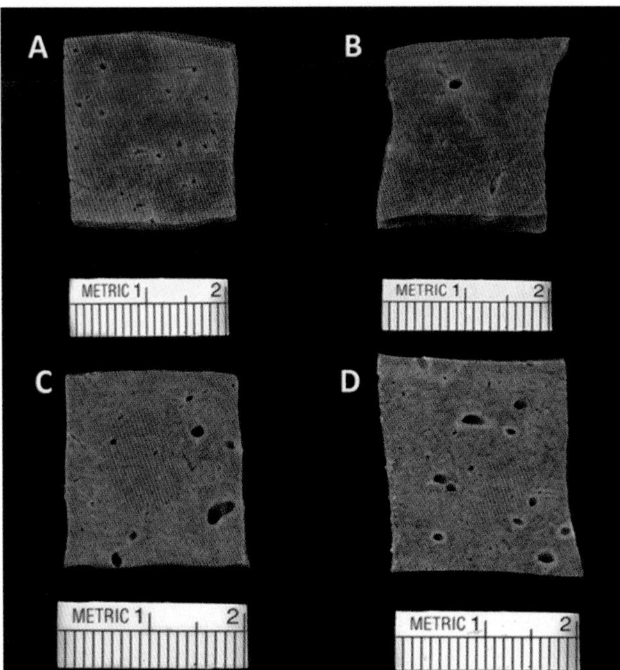

Figure 2.5 Formalin fixation of liver tissue. This panel shows a 2.5-cm cube of liver tissue sectioned at various times during the fixation process. **(A)** one hour, **(B)** 3 hours, **(C)** 12 hours, and **(D)** 20 hours. The fixation process was not complete for over 24 hours.

at 1-cm intervals) and perfusion with fixative solution are alternatives for large liver specimens in order to expedite tissue fixation. Finally, gross photographs are becoming a routine practice in most laboratories (Fig. 2.6), and gross images of the fresh, whole specimen as well as postfixation sections should be obtained. These images can be very useful diagnostically (i.e., gross correlation during slide review) and represent an invaluable educational resource.

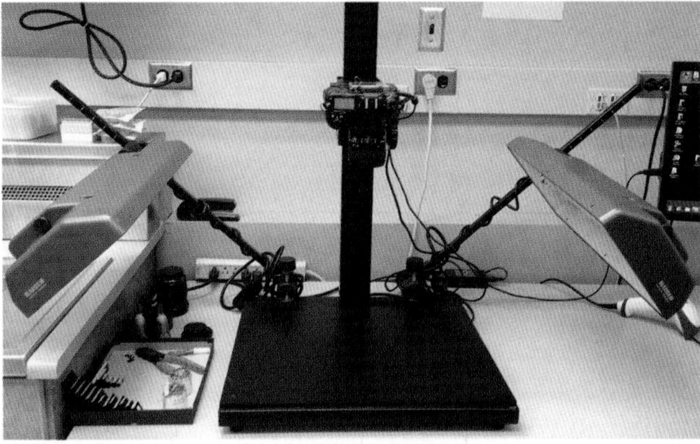

Figure 2.6 Gross photography station. Key elements include a gross specimen stage, digital camera with high-resolution capability, adjustable illumination, and lens with focal length that will allow both adequate focus and specimen handling.

2.3 LIVER SPECIMENS RECEIVED IN THE GROSS LAB

Core biopsies

Needle core biopsies are slender fragments of tissue obtained either percutaneously or transvenously for evaluation of medical or neoplastic diseases of the liver. The fragments vary significantly in length and width depending on the type and gauge of needle utilized. Needles are classified as large when their external diameter is greater than 1.0 mm (approximately 2 mm in 14G needles, 1.6 mm in 16G needles, 1.2 mm in 18G needles) and as thin when it is less than 1.0 mm (>20G).[3,4] Different types of needles are also used, including cutting needles (e.g., Tru-Cut) and suction needles (e.g., Menghini), with the latter having a tendency to produce more fragmented speciments.[5,6] When received in the gross lab, these specimens should be handled carefully to avoid crush and forceps artifact (Fig. 2.7) as well as further tissue fragmentation. The cores should also routinely be wrapped in lens paper to prevent loss of smaller fragments (Fig. 2.8). The length, diameter, color, and degree of integrity of the cores should be described. A standard panel of stains and levels is generally adopted by most centers for "medical liver" samples. At our institution, we generally perform two hematoxylin and eosin stain (H&E) levels, trichrome, reticulin, iron, and Periodic acid-Schiff diastase (PASD) stains for nontransplant medical livers and H&E levels and a trichrome for transplant biopsies.

Wedge biopsies

These represent specimens that contain a portion of the capsular surface of the liver at its base, with a varying amount of subcapsular liver parenchyma. Liver wedges are generally taken during open or laparoscopic surgery, for either superficial mass/mass-like lesions or for suspected nonneoplastic diseases. The most common scenarios for wedge

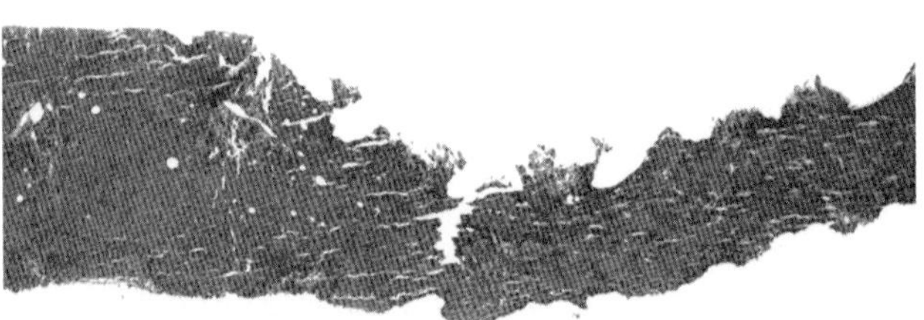

Figure 2.7 Crush artifact. In this example, a liver core biopsy shows multiple indentations with tissue crushing (mid and right parts of the core) caused by inappropriate handling during gross examination.

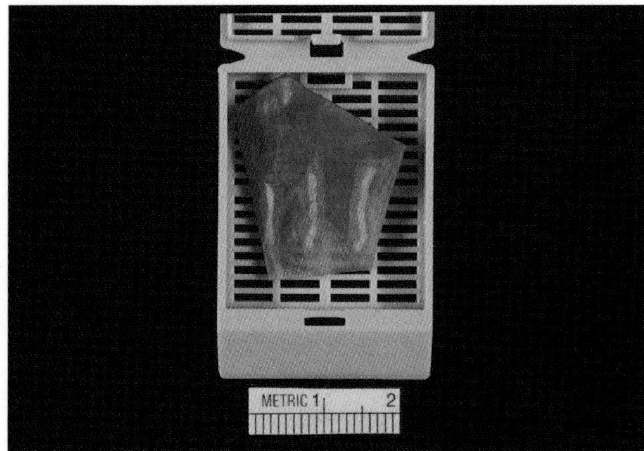

Figure 2.8 Core biopsy handling. Three liver cores are properly wrapped in lens paper and placed in a plastic cassette for paraffin embedding.

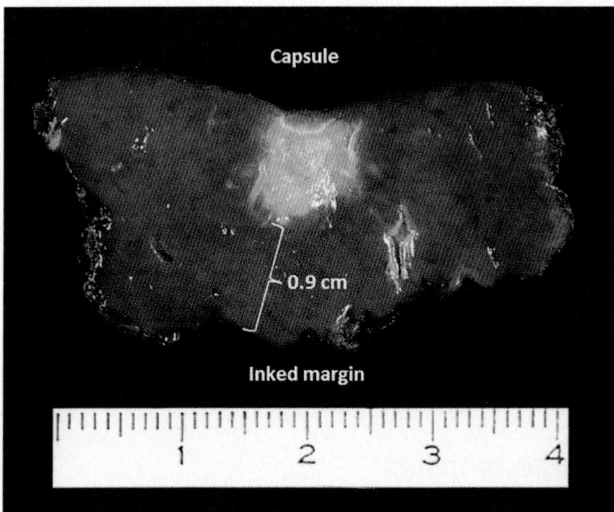

Figure 2.9 Liver wedge specimen. Proper grossing of a liver wedge sample performed for excision of a small subcapsular nodule. The parenchymal margins (inferior and lateral aspects) are inked black while the capsular surface (superior aspect) is not inked. Sections should be taken perpendicular to the capsule.

biopsies nowadays are (1) small subcapsular nodules found during oncologic surgery (e.g., Whipple's procedure, gastrectomies etc) and (2) bariatric surgery for grading/staging of fatty liver disease. In spite of its larger size compared to needle biopsies, wedges are generally less desirable specimens from a medical liver standpoint, because the majority of the tissue is subcapsular, and therefore subject to various artifacts and staging limitations associated with this location. When performed for a nodule/tumor, the noncapsular (cut surface) should be properly inked and considered a surgical margin (Fig. 2.9).

Lobectomy and segmentectomy (partial hepatectomy) specimens

Partial hepatectomies are generally performed for focal liver lesions. The gross specimen will show a smooth, glistening capsular surface around much of its external aspect but at least one facet will be rough, irregular, and generally with recognizable cautery effect, representing the parenchymal surgical margin (which should be inked). Orientation of the specimen and recognition of vascular structures and bile ducts may be difficult depending on the case, particularly if these structures are small, and discussion with the surgeon may be necessary if this evaluation is warranted. After description, measurement, and proper inking, the specimen should be serially sectioned at approximately 0.5 cm intervals, preferably on a plane perpendicular to the surgical margin, in order to facilitate evaluation of the distance between the inked margin and the lesion(s) of interest (Fig. 2.10). The liver capsule should be inspected for texture, appearance, translucency, as well as for any evidence of puckering, thickening, rupture, or nodularity. Upon sectioning, the characteristic of any focal lesion, inclusing size, location, number, color, consistency, circumscription, as well as any evidence of necrosis, hemorrhage, or scaring should be recorded, as should the distance between all lesions and the surgical margin. Hepatic vessels and bile ducts should be carefully inspected for any evidence of blood clot, tumors, or strictures. Sections of bile duct and hepatic vessels at the margin should also be taken if possible. Lastly, the appearance of the nonneoplastic liver is also important, but description and sectioning of the "uninvolved" parenchyma should focus on areas away from the tumor, which most reliably reflect the background

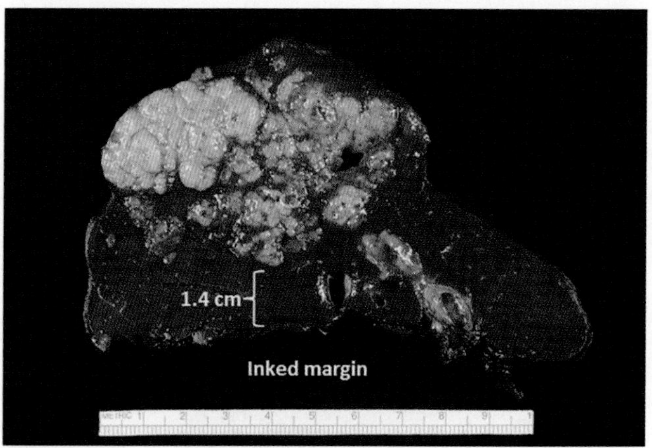

Figure 2.10 Lobectomy specimen. Similar to wedge samples, lobectomies will have one rough, cauterized aspect representing the parenchymal margin (inked black in this example). In addition to the parenchymal margin, vascular and bile duct margins can also usually be identified in lobectomy specimens.

liver (rather than abnormalities related to tumor compression). When dealing with liver tumors, the general rule is to submit approximately one section per centimeter of tumor (i.e., its maximal diameter). Sections from the periphery of the tumor (including capsule, if present) are most informative, especially when dealing with hepatocellular carcinomas, because peripheral sections will show tumor circumscription and most foci of small vessel invasion are located in this area. A larger number of sections is often necessary to identify possible areas of viable tumor in lesions with large areas of necrosis. It is our practice to submit the entire nodule (if feasible) before a diagnosis of a completely necrotic tumor histologically. For most types of tumor, especially if previously treated, the approximate percentage of necrosis should be recorded. Finally, vascular thrombi and embolization material can often be identified in previously treated tumors and their presence should be noted.

Explant liver specimens

Whole livers specimens are encountered in centers where orthotopic liver transplantation procedures are performed. The main purpose of examining these specimens are (1) to either confirm or identify the cause of liver failure and (2) characterize any tumors or focal lesions and the status of surgical margins. Again, clinical and radiologic correlation can greatly facilitate grossing of these specimens because specific concerns can be appropriately addressed and previously identified focal lesions at known locations can be properly sampled. This review will also alert the grossing pathologist or pathologist assistant about the presence of any intrahepatic biliary stents (Fig. 2.11) or vascular shunts, which may interfere with sectioning

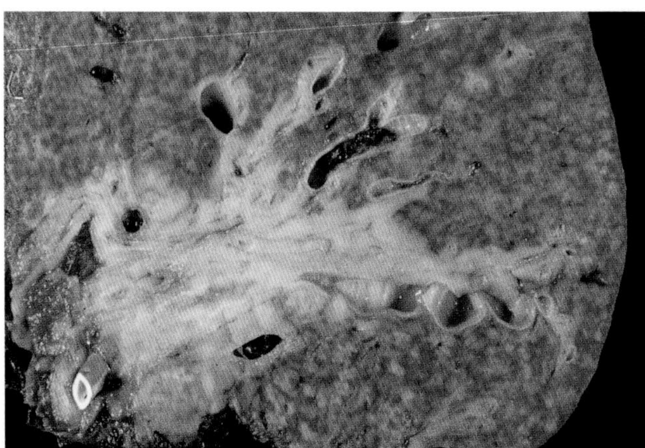

Figure 2.11 Stent. A hilar-type cholangiocarcinoma is illustrated in this image. A stent is present within an obliterated bile duct in the middle of the tumor. Stents may represent a significant hazard during handling and sectioning.

and represent an important hazard as a perforating/cutting object due to its metallic components.

At our institution, whole livers are perfused with formalin prior to sectioning. To accomplish this, the liver is injected with 10% buffered formalin through the portal vein, utilizing a nozzle with plastic tubing attached to a formalin pump. Depending on the length of the portal vein, the nozzle may need to be inserted into the left and right hepatic veins separately. There will be noticeable distension of the organ upon successful perfusion. Hemostats are used to immediately seal off the portal vein (or left and right portal veins), and the liver is immersed in formalin for several days prior to sectioning.

Once properly fixed, the examination should start by weighing and measuring the specimen and describing the surface appearance of the liver capsule. Any areas of capsular thickening, defects, or puckering should be noted. Next, the hepatic hilum and its structures (hepatic artery, portal vein, and bile duct) should be identified and a cross-section of this area (hilar margin) submitted for histology. Hilar vessels are usually clipped by the surgeon, helping their identification. Upon sectioning, any intravascular thrombi (blood clot or tumor) should be recorded. All lymph nodes in the porta hepatis area should also be sampled. Next, the gallbladder should be dissected from the liver bed and grossed as a routine cholecystectomy specimen. Once the porta hepatis and the gallbladder have been addressed, the final step is to carefully section the liver, ideally at 0.5 to 1.0-cm intervals. Although some institutions prefer to section the liver fresh, a thoroughly fixed whole liver is ideal for obtaining thin, uniform slices. Sectioning can be performed manually, using a long, sharp cutting blade or knife, or utilizing cutting devices. At our institution, we utilize a meat slicer for this purpose (Figs. 2.12, and 2.13). The main advantage of this unorthodox approach is that the entire specimen is sectioned at thin, contiguous, uniform slices at 0.5-cm intervals (which are very difficult to obtain with manual sectioning), ensuring optimal evaluation for small nodules or other focal lesions. The slices are then placed in an organized and contiguous fashion on a designated cutting board/platter with formalin pads.

Once sections are obtained, the liver parenchyma should be described and any fibrosis, nodularity, areas of necrosis or hemorrhage recorded. Most commonly, the liver will show a cirrhotic morphology, and the pattern of nodularity and range of size of regenerative nodules should be recorded. Any nodules that "stand out" from others due to size, color, or any other feature should be sampled. If the entire surface is relatively homogeneous, at least two to three sections from the right and left lobes and one from the caudate and quadrate lobes should be obtained (Fig. 2.14).

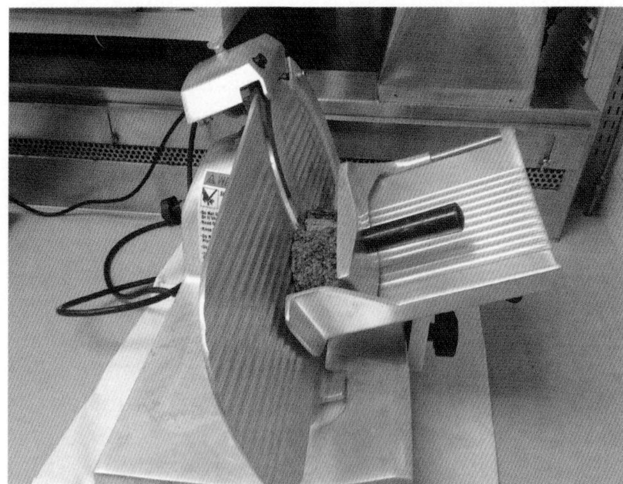

Figure 2.12 Meat slicer. Gross sectioning of whole liver/explant specimens can be greatly facilitated with the utilization of slicing devices, resulting in thin, contiguous, uniform sections with smooth, clean-cut surfaces.

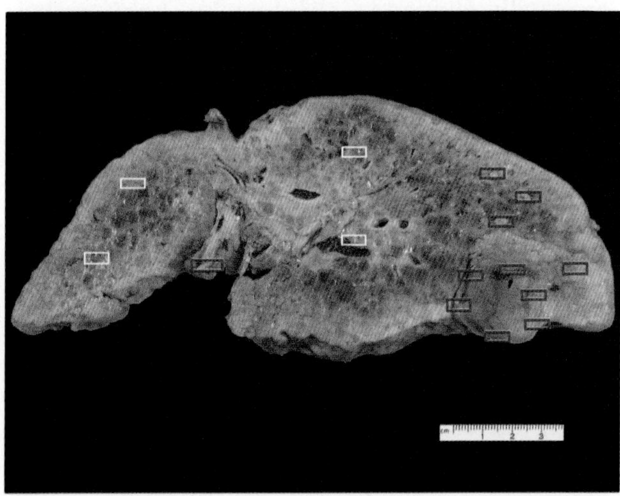

Figure 2.14 Routine sampling of explant specimens. A cirrhotic liver with a hepatocellular carcinoma (right inferior aspect of the specimen) is shown here. Tumor-related sections (*red rectangles*) include a) tumor (preferentially around the capsule), b) any suspicious smaller nodules (three suspected satellite nodules are sampled above the tumor due to their distinctive color compared to the surrounding cirrhotic nodules), and c) the hilar margin (*red rectangle* on the left of the image). Sampling of the nonneoplastic liver (*white rectangles*) should include at least a couple of sections per lobe **(right, left, caudate, and quadrate)**. An area consistent with treatment-related parenchymal necrosis (right-superior aspect of the peritumoral tissue) is also sampled.

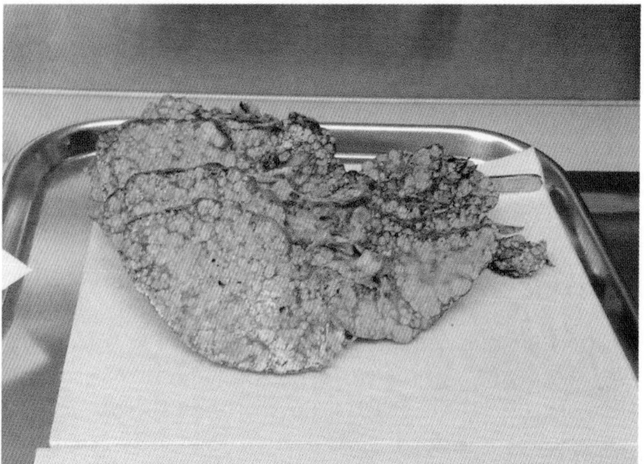

Figure 2.13 Meat slicer sections. Explant liver sections (uniformly measuring 0.5 cm in thickness) are organized in an orderly manner for gross examination by the pathology team.

REFERENCES

1. Molina DK, DiMaio VJM. Normal organ weights in men. *Am J Forensic Med Pathol*. 2012;33(4):368–372. doi:10.1097/PAF.0b013e31823d29ad.
2. Thavarajah R, Mudimbaimannar VK, Elizabeth J, et al. Chemical and physical basics of routine formaldehyde fixation. *J Oral Maxillofac Pathol*. 2012;16(3):400–405. doi:10.4103/0973-029X.102496.
3. Grant A, Neuberger J. Guidelines on the use of liver biopsy in clinical practice. British Society of Gastroenterology. *Gut*. 1999;45 Suppl 4(suppl 4):IV1–IV11. doi:10.1136/GUT.45.2008.IV1.
4. Cholongitas E, Shusang V, Papatheodoridis GV, et al. Risk factors for recurrence of primary sclerosing cholangitis after liver transplantation. *Liver Transpl*. 2008;14(2):138–143. doi:10.1002/lt.21260.
5. Piccinino F, Sagnelli E, Pasquale G, et al. Complications following percutaneous liver biopsy. A multicentre retrospective study on 68,276 biopsies. *J Hepatol*. 1986;2(2):165–173. http://www.ncbi.nlm.nih.gov/pubmed/3958472. Accessed September 25, 2016.
6. Gilmore IT, Burroughs A, Murray-Lyon IM, et al. Indications, methods, and outcomes of percutaneous liver biopsy in England and Wales: an audit by the British Society of Gastroenterology and the Royal College of Physicians of London. *Gut*. 1995;36(3):437–441. http://www.ncbi.nlm.nih.gov/pubmed/7698705. Accessed September 25, 2016.

3 The language of liver pathology: definitions of key terms

Michael S. Torbenson, MD

3.1 INTRODUCTION

Like all medical disciplines, liver pathology has its own vocabulary used to describe histological findings. Many of these terms are broadly used in general surgical pathology and will not be covered here. However, there are a number of terms used in liver pathology that are either specific to the discipline or commonly encountered. For some of these terms, finding definitions can be a challenge. Definitions from internet sources can be helpful but are often incomplete and are sometimes completely wrong. Because definition sources are sparse, the meaning of a given term can "drift," as one author uses a term in what is thought to be an accurate and authoritative way, whereas another author uses the same term somewhat differently, but also feels their approach is both accurate and authoritative. In some cases, regionally distinct usage of terms can develop when an influential liver pathologist trains residents and fellows in the vicinity and sees consult material from the region.

The goal of this chapter is to provide a reasonable reference for many of the important terms used in liver pathology, with illustrations as it seems appropriate. Not all of these definitions will satisfy all pathologists, but perhaps that is unavoidable given the varying usages by different authors. In addition, this chapter is not intended to be heavy-handed, insisting that terms can only be used in ways consistent with how they are defined herein. Indeed, different usages for these terms are also noted. Instead, this chapter is written in the hope of providing a reasonable understanding of what most authors intend when they use a specific term. These terms are important building blocks in describing liver pathology; understanding their specific meaning will substantially increase your enjoyment and understanding of the liver pathology literature.

These definitions are primarily focused on words used to describe microscopic findings, though many words used in gross description are also included. Definitions for different diseases and liver tumors are available in the relevant chapters.

Synonyms for various terms are also described, as appropriate. Of note, some synonyms are essentially interchangeable. As one example, scattered dead hepatocytes can reasonably be described as "acidophil bodies" or "spotty necrosis" or "hepatocyte apoptosis." In contrast, there are terms that are technically synonyms, at least to some degree, but should be avoided because they tend to undermine

- Cholestasis
- Chronic active hepatitis
- Chronic hepatitis
- Chronic persistent hepatitis
- Cirrhosis
- Confluent necrosis
- Councilman body
- Ductal plate malformation
- Ductopenia
- Elastosis
- Emperipolesis
- Fatty change
- Feathery degeneration
- Fibrin ring granuloma
- Fibro-obliterative duct lesion
- Fibrous cap
- Fibrous septa
- Florid duct lesion
- Foam cell arteriopathy
- Foamy degeneration
- Focal biliary cirrhosis
- Giant cell change/giant cell transformation
- Glycogen storing foci
- Glycogenated nuclei
- Granuloma
- Ground glass inclusions/ ground glass change Halo sign
- Hepatic plate thickening
- Hepatoportal sclerosis
- Hyaline body
- Impaired liver regeneration
- Incomplete septal fibrosis
- Induced hepatocyte
- Interface activity/interface hepatitis
- Intermediate hepatocyte
- Iron free foci
- Lamellar fibrosis
- Large cell change
- Limiting plate
- Lipofuscin
- Lobular collapse
- Lobule

clarity of communication. These "best avoided" synonyms include terms that are easily misinterpreted by clinical colleagues, such as *microgranulomas*, and terms that are obsolete such as *pericholangitis* and *chronic persistent hepatitis*.

3.2 BRIEF DEFINITIONS OF LIVER PATHOLOGY TERMS

Aberrant artery/arteriole

Technically, this term could refer to any nonnormal artery, but in common usage this term refers to an artery located in the hepatic lobule, instead of their normal location in the portal tract (Fig. 3.1). Aberrant arteries are a common feature of neoplasms, including hepatic adenomas and hepatocellular carcinomas. However, abnormal lobular arteries can also be found in reactive conditions such as focal nodular hyperplasia and in medical, nonmass forming liver disease. Examples of abnormal lobular arteries in medical liver disease include livers with vascular flow abnormalities, such as portal vein thrombi, and steatohepatitis with fibrosis.
Synonym: Unpaired artery, "naked" artery

Acidophil body

A single dead cell is referred to as an acidophil body (Fig. 3.2). In liver pathology, this term is used most commonly for single, scattered dead hepatocytes. Acidophil bodies have dense, eosinophilic cytoplasm and are typically smaller than the adjacent hepatocytes. The nucleus is usually absent or small and shriveled. Acidophil bodies can be seen in a wide variety of hepatic injuries. When prominent lobular acidophil bodies are the only pattern of injury, unaccompanied by inflammation or cholestasis or fatty change, then the differential is primarily drug effect, acute viral infection, and low-grade/transient ischemia.
Synonym: Apoptotic body, spotty necrosis, Councilman body

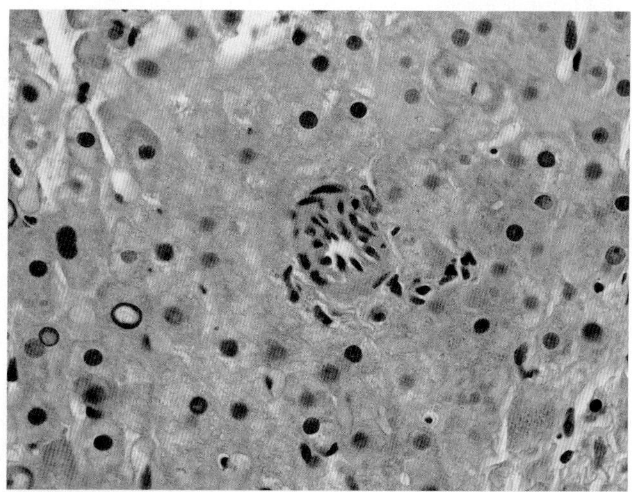

Figure 3.1 Aberrant artery. This artery is not in a portal tract, and so is "aberrant."

macronodular cirrhosis
Macrotrabecular
Mallory hyaline
Megamitochondria
Microabscess
Microgranuloma
Micronodular cirrhosis/
Microvesicular steatosis
Mucinous carcinoma
Multicystic
Multilocular
Nodular regenerative hyperplasia
Onion-skin fibrosis
Pale body
Panacinar necrosis
Pancreatic acinar cell metaplasia
Partial nodular transformation
Pericellular fibrosis
Pericholangitis
Periportal fibrosis
Periportal hepatitis
Phospholipidosis
Piecemeal necrosis
Pipestem fibrosis
Portal hepatitis
Portal vein herniation
Poulsen lesion/poulsen cristoffersen's lesions
Pseudoacinar
Pseudoground glass inclusions
Pseudorosettes
Pseudoxanthomatous change
Reticulin loss
Rhaboid morphology
Riedel lobe
Sanded glass nuclei
Small cell change
Spotty necrosis
Steatosis
Stellate cell
Triaditis
Von Meyenburg complex
Zones 1, 2, 3

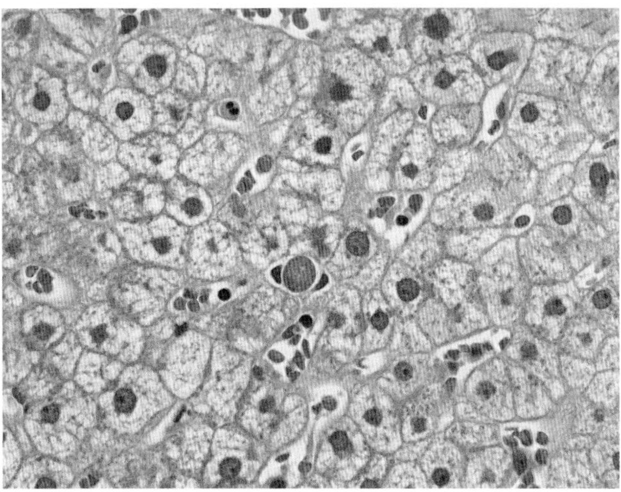

Figure 3.2 Acidophil body. A single dead hepatocyte is seen. The hepatocyte has lost its nucleus, is smaller, and more pink than its neighbors.

Accessory lobe

Accessory lobes affect approximately 10% of livers. They can be mistaken for mass lesions and can sometimes have tumors develop within them.[1–3] They are also at risk for torsion.[4] The most common accessory lobe is called a Riedel lobe (see separate definition entry). Most accessory lobes are connected to the liver by a thick pedicle and have a normal microscopic organization. Less commonly, accessory lobes are connected to the liver by a thin fibrovascular core containing blood vessels and connective tissue, bile ducts (often), and thin wisps or scattered islands of hepatocytes (occasionally). The accessory lobe itself might lack normal bile ducts and portal veins and can sometimes show nodular regenerative hyperplasia like changes. In contrast to an accessory lobe, ectopic hepatic tissue will have no connection to the liver.

Acinus

The hepatic acinus is the functional unit of the liver and is usually illustrated as an elliptical or diamond shaped structure with ends in the portal tract and a bulging middle extending from central vein to central vein. Although the acinus itself cannot be readily seen on histology, the acinus forms the basis for microscopic liver zones, which can be seen histologically, with zone 1 referring to hepatocytes near the portal tracts, zone 3 referring to hepatocytes near the central vein, and zone 2 referring to those hepatocytes in between. See also the entry for lobule.

Acute hepatitis

This term is commonly used to refer to any abrupt presentation of liver disease. There are formal clinical definitions for acute hepatitis, but formal definitions are rarely followed strictly outside of research studies. Although the formal definitions vary a bit, one common approach is to define acute hepatitis as an abrupt onset hepatitis that is less than 6 months in duration.

In cases presenting clinically as acute hepatitis, the histological findings will vary considerably depending on the type of injury, but can be predominately hepatitic, cholestatic, biliary, congested, fatty, or bland necrosis. The extent of injury in any of these patterns can range from minimal to marked. Of these injury patterns, a markedly active lobular hepatitis (Fig. 3.3) is almost always an acute hepatitis, as marked lobular inflammation is too injurious to be seen as a chronic pattern. Likewise, substantial hepatocyte necrosis indicates an acute injury for the same reason. Other than in these settings, there are no histological findings that can differentiate an acute hepatitis from a chronic hepatitis, so the term is typically avoided as a pathology diagnosis.

Of note, histological fibrosis indicates a chronic hepatitis, but the converse is not true, as the lack of fibrosis does not indicate an acute hepatitis. If there is a clinical history of an abrupt onset of the clinical disease, but definite fibrosis on the biopsy, then the findings suggest a flare of a chronic liver disease or a superimposed injury on top of an underlying chronic liver disease. In these settings, the term *acute on chronic* hepatitis is often used.

Acute yellow atrophy of the liver

This term is used in gross pathology. Although it is largely obsolete, occasionally the term is still encountered. In the setting of acute liver failure from extensive necrosis, the liver is often atrophic on gross examination and the surviving hepatocytes can show fatty change and cholestasis, all of which contribute to the liver looking small and yellow. This general pattern of injury can be seen in numerous causes of extensive liver necrosis, ranging from acute viral infection (Fig. 3.4) to drug injury.

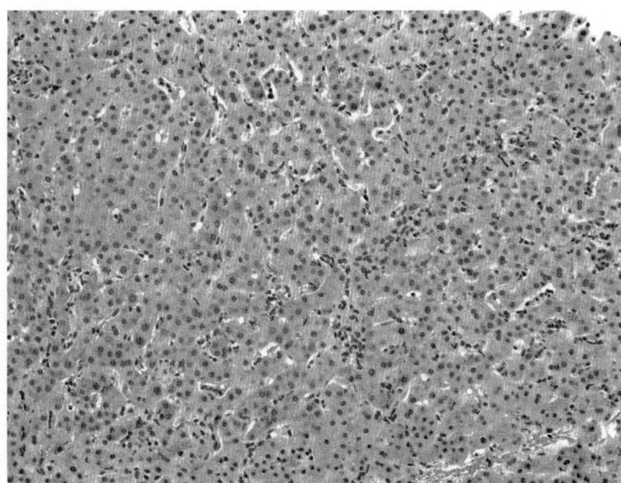

Figure 3.3 Moderate lobular hepatitis. This person presented with acute hepatitis and the lobules show moderate inflammation.

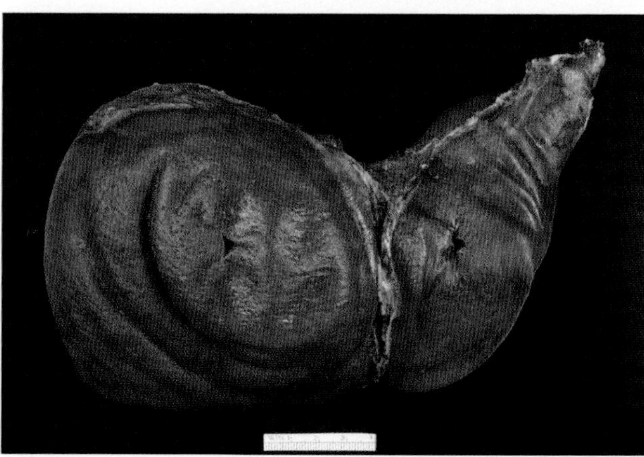

Figure 3.4 Acute yellow atrophy of the liver. The liver is markedly shrunken after acute hepatitis A, leading to a small and yellow liver. The yellow color was even more striking on the sectioned liver.

Alcoholic foamy degeneration

Individuals with alcoholic hepatitis can rarely (less than 1%) have a pattern of diffuse microvesicular steatosis (Fig. 3.5).[5] The explanation for this pattern of liver injury is not clear, but neither the amount nor the duration of alcohol intake appears to be causal factors.[5]

Synonym: Acute foamy degeneration

Apoptosis/apoptotic body

As formally defined, an apoptotic body results when a cell undergoes programmed cell death. In practical pathology usage, an apoptotic body is a single dead cell and can refer to dead hepatocytes, dead bile duct cells, dead lymphocytes, dead tumor cells, or any cell population with scattered single dead cells. Apoptotic bodies can have accompanying inflammation, depending on the cause of the injury.

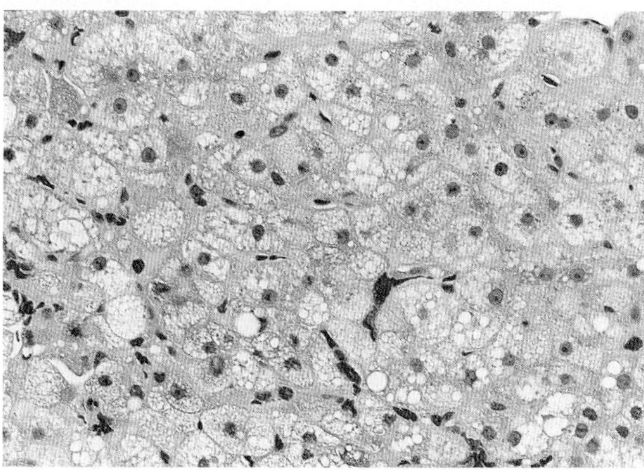

Figure 3.5 Alcoholic foamy degeneration. The hepatocytes show diffuse microvesicular steatosis.

Synonym: Acidophil body, spotty necrosis, Councilman body. However, all of these synonyms are reserved for apoptotic hepatocytes.

Ascending cholangitis

Ascending cholangitis refers to an infection of the extrahepatic biliary tree that has "ascended" up the biliary tree into the liver, typically manifesting as bile ducts that are dilated, lined by attenuated epithelium, and filled with neutrophils (Fig. 3.6).
Synonym: Suppurative cholangitis

Balloon cell/balloon cell change

Ballooned hepatocytes are enlarged, have rarified cytoplasm, and may contain Mallory bodies. They do not have fatty change, lacking both microvesicular and macrovesicular steatosis. They are best identified using lower power magnification, such as 4× or 10×, where they should truly stand out as being larger and more swollen than the adjacent hepatocytes, typically at least 50% bigger than their neighbors (Fig. 3.7). Ballooned hepatocytes are most commonly seen in fatty liver disease, where they can help make a diagnosis of steatohepatitis. However, balloon cells can be seen in a wide variety of other diseases, in particular with chronic cholestasis. In these other settings, balloon cells in isolation do not indicate an additional component of fatty liver disease.

Also of note, ballooned hepatocytes can be easy to over diagnose if you spend too much time at 40× or 60×, as there are many cells that are a bit bigger than their neighbor and have a hint of cytoplasmic clearing; overall, it's best to avoid calling these ballooned hepatocytes. You will certainly encounter hepatocytes with findings intermediate between those of classic ballooned hepatocytes and normal hepatocytes, but their diagnostic value is limited (Fig. 3.8). However, finding equivocal balloon cells should prompt continued examination for true balloon cells, as they can co-occur. Classic ballooned hepatocytes, and a subset of equivocal ones, will lose their normal expression of CK8/18.[6,7] However, these immunostains are not routinely employed in current diagnostic pathology to identify ballooned hepatocytes.
Synonym: Ballooning degeneration

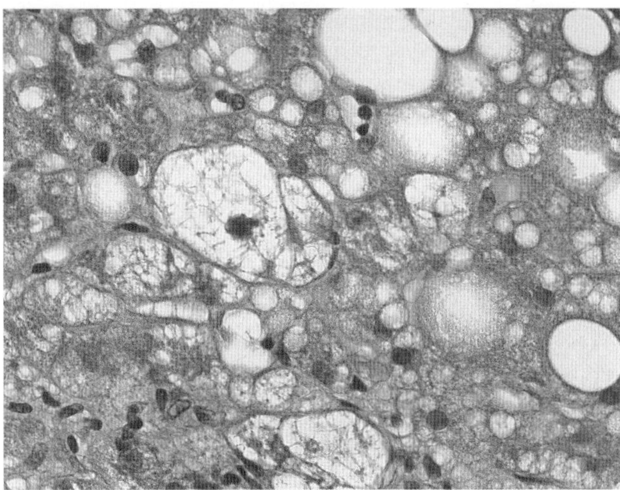

Figure 3.7 Ballooned hepatocyte. Ballooned hepatocytes are significantly bigger than the adjacent hepatocytes, show clear but flocculent cytoplasm, and have no fat.

Ballooning degeneration

Hepatocytes with ballooning degeneration are enlarged, rounded, and have rarified cytoplasm. Many will have Mallory hyaline. The term *ballooning degeneration* is

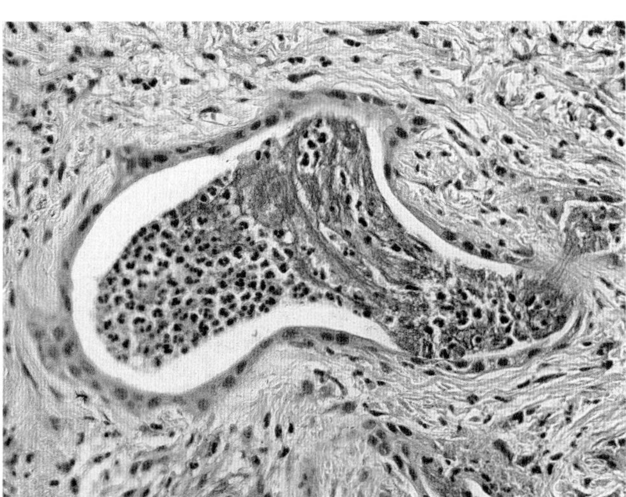

Figure 3.6 Ascending cholangitis. The bile duct is dilated, has attenuated epithelium, and is filled with neutrophils.

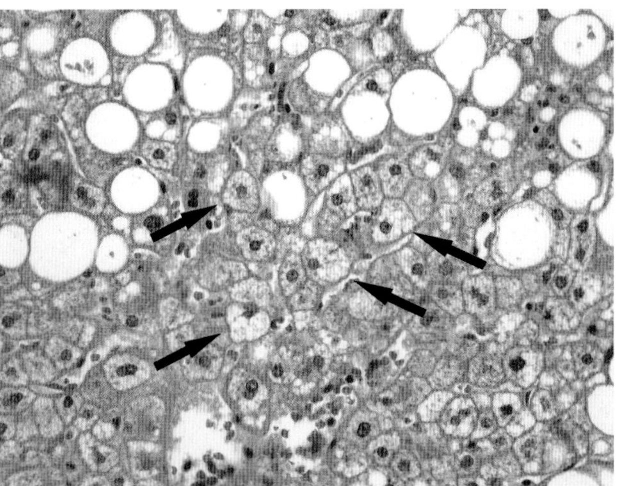

Figure 3.8 Equivocally ballooned hepatocyte. A cluster of equivocal ballooned hepatocytes (*arrows*). They have some features of a ballooned hepatocyte, but are they good enough?

used in two settings primarily. First, the term can describe scattered, typically single, injured hepatocytes in the setting of steatohepatitis. Secondly, the term can describe broad swaths of injured hepatocytes in the context of marked hepatitis or in the setting of cholestasis, where ballooning degeneration can be part of the pattern of cholate stasis. Some authors prefer the term *balloon cell* in the setting of steatohepatitis and ballooning degeneration for other situations, but there is no strong consensus on term usage.
Synonym: Balloon cell

Bile ductule

The bile duct is a tubular structure located in the portal tract that is lined by a simple cuboidal to low-columnar epithelium, which is composed of cholangiocytes. The bile duct is usually located in close proximity to the hepatic artery. In a normal portal tract, the bile duct and artery will be about the same size (Fig. 3.9). In severe chronic cholestatic liver disease, this may not be true, as the arteries can become more prominent.

Even in the normal liver, a bile duct may not be visible in up to 20% of the portal tracts. Of note, however, this absence of bile ducts is seen only in the smallest portal tracts and all normal medium-sized and larger portal tracts will have a bile duct. The bile duct should not be confused with bile ductules, which are quite different biologically, despite their similar names.

Bile duct duplication

Bile duct duplication is associated with chronic obstructive biliary tract disease, such as primary sclerosing cholangitis or other stricturing processes.

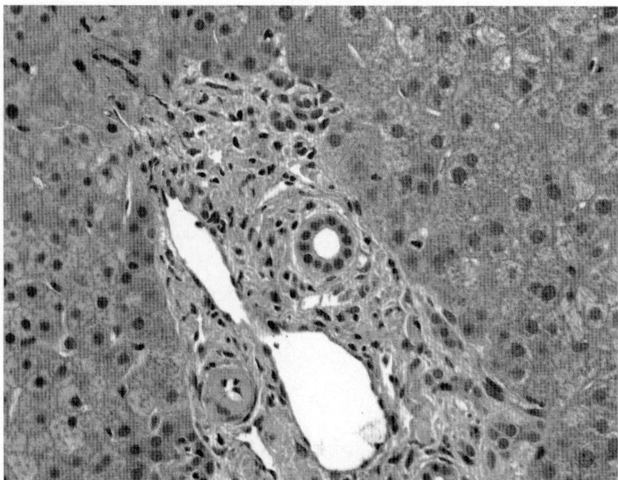

Figure 3.9 Bile duct. A bile duct is seen in the center of the portal tract. The bile duct is typically about the same diameter as the nearby hepatic artery.

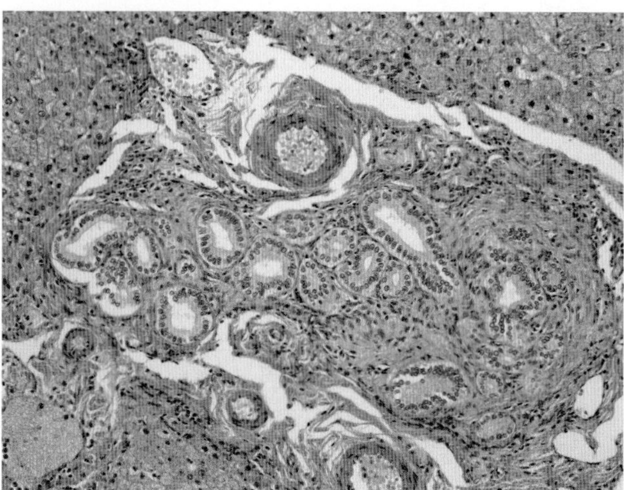

Figure 3.10 Bile duct duplication. This portal tract has too many bile ducts in the center.

Instead of the normal single bile duct, a portal tract with bile duct duplication will have a small cluster of bile ducts in the center of the portal tract (Fig. 3.10). This change is not the same as proliferating bile ductules, where the ductules are located at the periphery of the portal tract.

Bile duct metaplasia

Bile ducts can undergo metaplasia, usually in the setting of chronic biliary tract disease.[8] The metaplasia can take various forms, most commonly intestinal metaplasia (Fig. 3.11) or pyloric gland metaplasia, and very rarely hepatic metaplasia (Fig. 3.12). Intestinal metaplasia is also associated with an increase in the number of neuroendocrine cells within the biliary epithelium. Paneth cells can also be found. Rare cases of clear cell metaplasia have also been reported.[9]

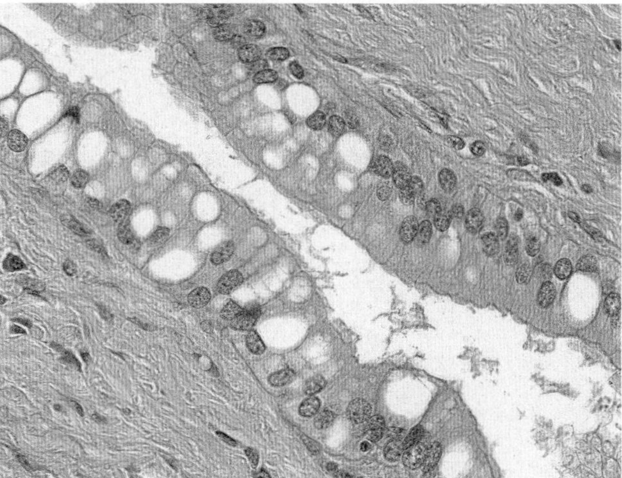

Figure 3.11 Bile duct with intestinal metaplasia. Goblet type cells are seen.

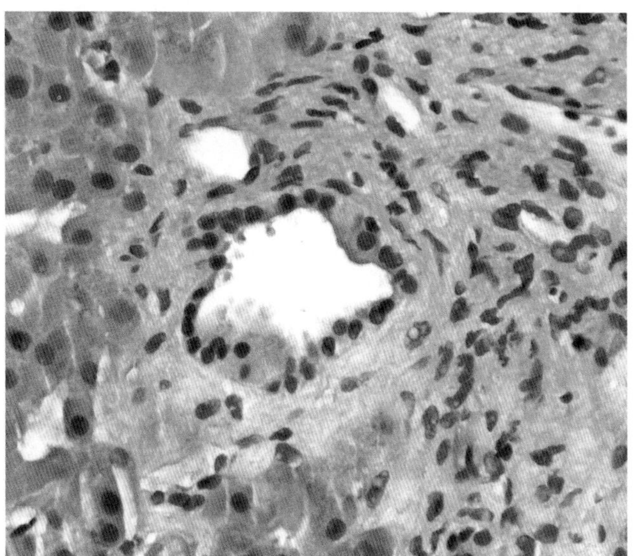

Figure 3.12 Bile duct with hepatic metaplasia. Areas of hepatic metaplasia will also stain positive with HepPar1 and Arginase 1.

In primary biliary cirrhosis, the bile duct cells can sometimes have increased mitochondrial mass,[10] giving them a densely eosinophilic appearance on light microscopy, a finding called "oncocytic metaplasia." Oncocytic bile duct metaplasia can occasionally be found in other conditions, in particular with chronic liver disease and advanced fibrosis.

Bile duct hamartoma

Bile duct hamartomas are composed of benign duct-like structures, usually with open lumens and bile deposits (Fig. 3.13). The duct-like structures interanastamose and can have a serpiginous appearance. They are found in the smaller branches of the portal tracts. The hamartomas can be small and microscopic, or can be larger grossly visible lesions. Most are less than 5 mm and almost all are less than 15 mm. The larger lesions typically have a background of dense fibrosis. They can be single or multiple and are often subcapsular.
Synonym: Ductal plate malformation, von Meyenburg complex

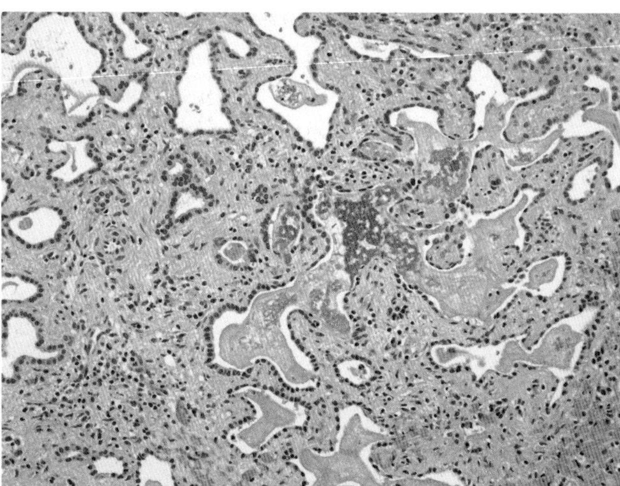

Figure 3.13 Bile duct hamartoma. This lesion is composed of interanastomosing bile ducts with gaping lumens and inspissated bile secretions. The stroma has dense collagen deposition but inflammation is usually negligible.

Bile duct lymphocytosis

This descriptive term is used to report lymphocytes within the bile duct epithelium, a finding that is often associated with bile duct injury (Fig. 3.14). Bile duct lymphocytosis is a key part of the pattern of injury seen in acute cellular rejection, but is also seen in many other conditions, including drug reactions, chronic viral hepatitis, autoimmune hepatitis, and primary biliary cirrhosis. Its presence in many diverse diseases shouldn't dissuade anyone from its potential diagnostic usefulness, remembering that the focus should be on determining whether the bile ducts are targeted by the inflammation or whether the finding represents a bystander effect, with focal mild lymphocytosis in the setting of a more generalized moderate or marked portal inflammation.
Synonym: Lymphocytic cholangitis

Bile infarct

A bile infarct can be seen with high grade, often acute, obstruction of the biliary tree or with long standing cholestasis. There will be a small circumscribed collection of bile stained and dead hepatocytes (Fig. 3.15). The center of the lesion commonly has extravasated bile. Most often, bile infarcts are located right next

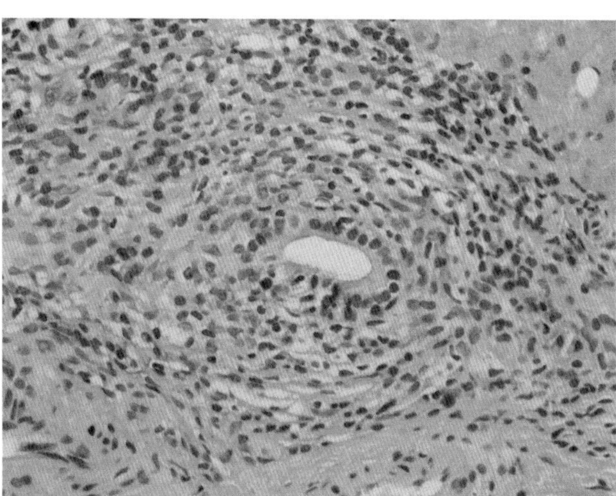

Figure 3.14 Bile duct lymphocytosis. A case of primary biliary cirrhosis shows a bile duct that is infiltrated by lymphocytes.

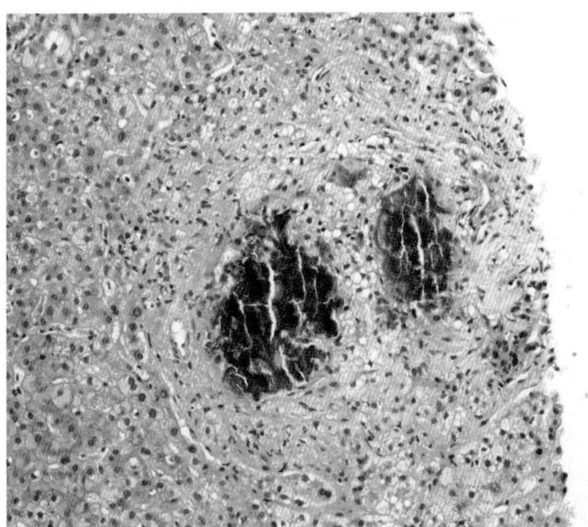

Figure 3.15 Bile infarct. A focus of extravasated bile is seen in the lobules, resulting from a high-grade bile duct stricture.

to a portal tract. A giant cell histiocytic reaction to the bile can also be seen.

Bile ductile

Bile ductules are different than the centrally located bile duct. Bile ductules are small, epithelial, tubular structures located at the periphery of the portal tracts (Fig. 3.16). Bile ductules are composed entirely of cholangiocytes and most often do not have a visible lumen, except for when the lumens have bile plugs. Bile ductules are a response to liver injury and can be seen in a wide variety of disease conditions, often being most prominent in the setting of obstructive biliary tract disease. The cell of origin for the bile ductules has been a major research interest for many years. At this time, the data suggests bile ductules most commonly originate from cells with stem cell–like features, but less commonly can originate from hepatocytes that undergo metaplasia. Bile ductules connect the canals of Hering to the bile duct.[11]

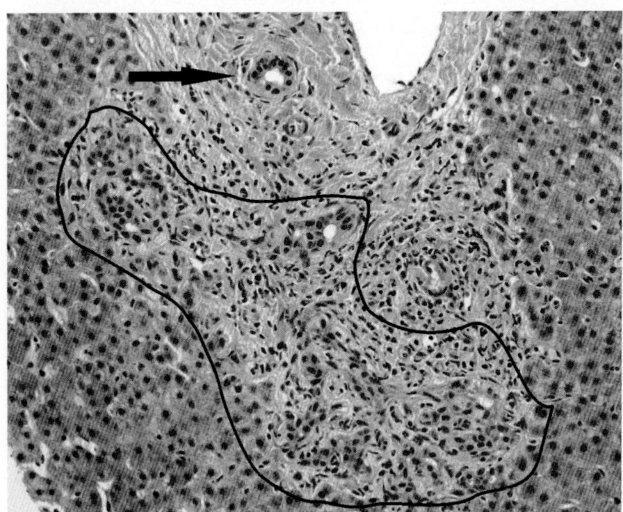

Figure 3.16 Bile ductule. The bile duct (*arrow*) is in the middle portion of the portal tract, next to the hepatic artery and portal vein, whereas the bile ductules (*circled*) are located at the interface between the portal tract and the lobule.

Bile ductular cholestasis

Bile ductules will occasionally be distended by bile plugs (Fig. 3.17). This can occur both in the setting of more generalized, profound lobular cholestasis and when the lobules show little or no cholestasis. In the former setting, the cholestasis is a nonspecific finding that reflects the overall severe cholestatic injury. In the latter case, the finding is most often idiopathic. There is older literature, largely based on autopsy studies, that associated bile ductular cholestasis with sepsis. However, in surgical pathology specimens most cases are not sepsis related and remain idiopathic. When a potential cause is identified, more definite confirmation of the cause is often difficult because patients tend to have debilitating illnesses and are on numerous medications, making it almost impossible to isolate a specific etiology. Nonetheless, associations have been made with total parenteral nutrition therapy, congestive heart failure, and alcoholic hepatitis. In the setting of severe alcoholic hepatitis, a bile ductular pattern of cholestasis is associated with an increased risk of subsequently developing clinical sepsis,[12] though the reason(s) are unclear.

Synonym: Cholangiolar cholestasis, cholangitis lenta

Bile ductular metaplasia

Experimental evidence suggests that liver injury can cause a reparative response where mature hepatocytes transform into bile ductules, a process called bile ductular metaplasia.

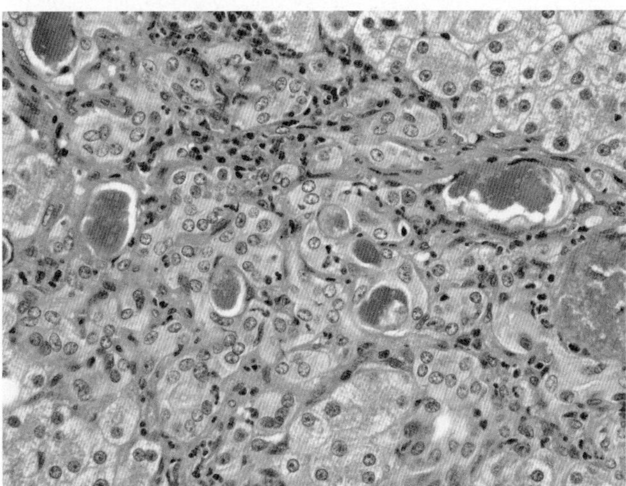

Figure 3.17 Bile ductule cholestasis. The proliferating bile ductules are dilated by bile plugs. The patient was not septic.

Bile ductular reaction

A bile ductular reaction is defined as increased numbers of ductules at the periphery of the portal tract (Fig. 3.18). In the normal liver, the portal tracts have few or no visible bile ductules. However, in response to liver injury, there can be a ductular proliferation, as the bile ductules are a source of liver progenitor cells and proliferate in response to injury. In many cases of mild liver injury, the bile ductular proliferation is mild and inconspicuous on hematoxylin and eosin stain (H&E), though it can be highlighted with special stains, such as cytokeratin 7. As the lobular injury becomes more severe, the ductular proliferation becomes increasingly visible on H&E. In other cases, the ductular reaction is the major pattern of injury and there is little or no lobular injury. This latter pattern can be accompanied by neutrophils and sometimes by portal tract edema and suggests biliary obstruction.

Many times a bile ductular reaction shows admixed neutrophils (Fig. 3.19). The admixed neutrophils should be in the stroma associated with the proliferating ductules and not in the lumen of the bile duct proper. Neutrophils in the main duct of the portal tract suggest ascending cholangitis, especially if the bile duct is dilated and the lining epithelium is attenuated (Fig. 3.6).

The ductular reaction is one of the key injury patterns in the liver. Historically, Popper and colleagues[13] were one of the first users of the term *ductular reaction*. They further subdivided ductular reactions into three types[14]: type I, associated with biliary obstruction; type II, associated with significantly active hepatitis; type III, associated with massive liver necrosis. This terminology of types I, II, and III is no longer used, but serves as a useful reminder of the major types of injury that can lead to a ductular reaction.

Synonym: Bile ductular proliferation, pericholangitis (obsolete)

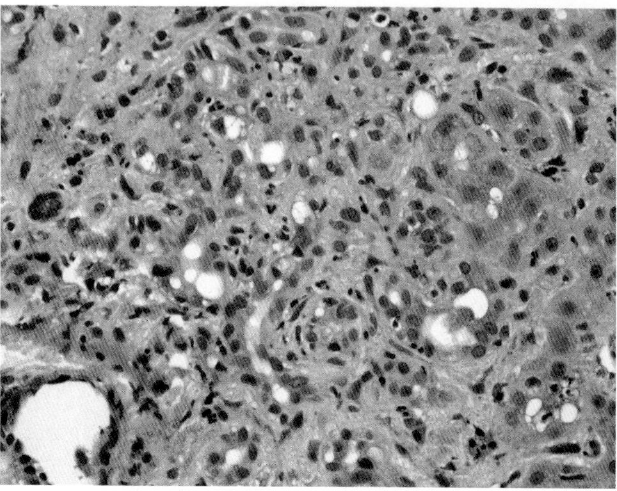

Figure 3.19 Bile ductular reaction, admixed inflammation. These proliferating bile ductules are associated with mild neutrophilic and lymphocytic inflammation.

Bridging fibrosis

The term *bridging fibrosis* is used when fibrous bands extend from either one portal tract to another portal tract (Fig. 3.20) or from a portal tract to a central vein. Synonyms are septal fibrosis and fibrous septa. Of note, however, there is nonuniform usage of these latter terms, especially the term *fibrous septa*. Although most authors use fibrous septa as a synonym for bridging fibrosis, occasional authors use the term *fibrous septa* to describe short fibrous extensions

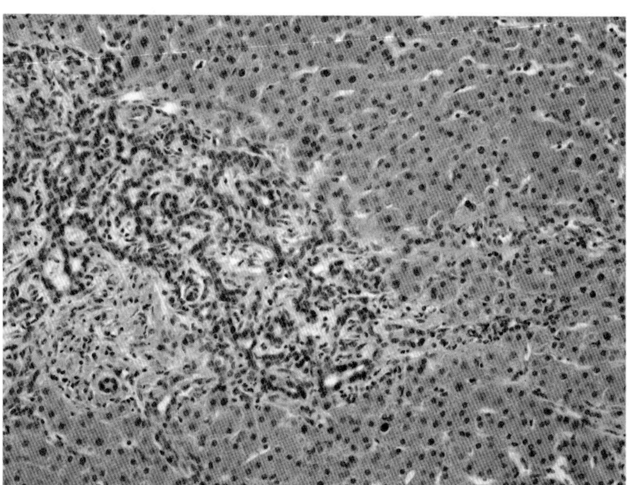

Figure 3.18 Bile ductular reaction. The portal tract shows marked ductular proliferation in this liver biopsy from a case with biliary obstruction.

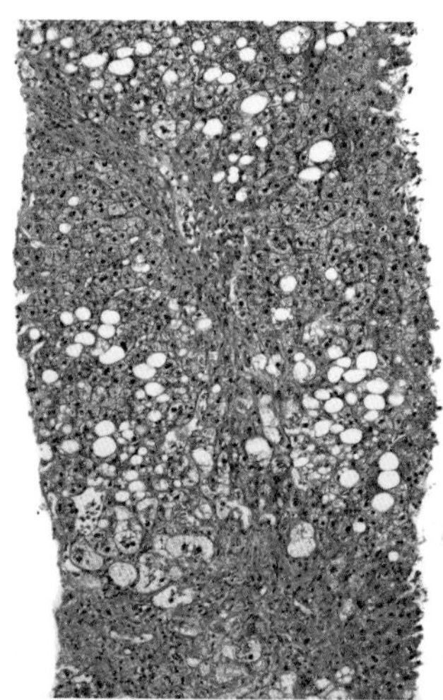

Figure 3.20 Bridging fibrosis, trichrome stain. Bridging fibrosis in a case of steatohepatitis.

from the portal tracts that do not actually connect two portal tracts, and thus would not be the same as bridging fibrosis.
Synonym: Septal fibrosis, fibrous septa (inconsistently used)

Bridging necrosis

With bridging necrosis, the lobules show an irregular band of dead hepatocytes that extends from central vein to central vein, central vein to portal tract, or less commonly from portal tract to portal tract. In the band of necrosis, the tissue often shows collapse and variable inflammation. This pattern is not specific for an etiology, but does indicate a severe liver injury. This pattern is most commonly seen in the setting of markedly active hepatitis or toxin exposure.

Canal of hering

The canal of Hering connects the lobules to the biliary tree. Canals of Hering are formed partly by cholangiocytes and partly by hepatocytes. They are not visible on H&E stains, but with keratin immunostains can be seen as thin, linear structures that are formed by cuboidal cells and extend from the portal tracts into zone 1 of the hepatic lobules. The canals of Hering often go in and out of the plane of section, so they may appear discontinuous on a single slide, but serial sections show a continuous line of cells extending from lobules into the portal tracts.

Cholangiocyte

Cholangiocytes are the epithelial cells that line the bile ducts and bile ductules. The canals of Hering are lined partly by hepatocytes and partly by cholangiocytes.
Synonym: Biliary epithelial cell

Cholate stasis

Cholate stasis is defined as swollen, pale hepatocytes located in zone 1 (periportal), resulting from injury because of chronic exposure to bile acids (Fig. 3.21). Cholate stasis results from chronic cholestasis. The hepatocytes in cholate stasis are sometimes confused for ballooned hepatocytes. Although there are some general similarities resulting from cell swelling, they are quite different. In cholate stasis, larger groups of often contiguous periportal hepatocytes are pale and swollen, whereas ballooned hepatocytes tend to be found as single, enlarged cells. As noted previously, cholate stasis affects the zone 1 hepatocytes, in contrast to the balloon cells in steatohepatitis, which are found mostly as scattered single cells, often in zone 3. The background changes are also distinct, as cholate

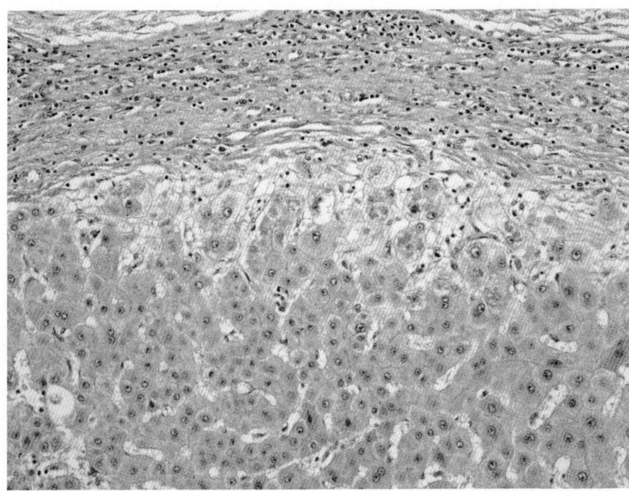

Figure 3.21 Cholate stasis. In this case of biliary cirrhosis, the hepatocytes at the edges of the cirrhotic nodules show swelling and Mallory bodies.

stasis is seen in the setting of chronic cholestasis, whereas ballooned hepatocytes primarily occur in the setting of steatohepatitis. Mallory hyaline can be found in both cholate stasis and ballooned hepatocytes. Copper stains typically show scattered, though often sparse, granules of copper in cholate stasis. A CK7 is also positive for intermediate hepatocytes in cholate stasis, but does not stain balloon cells in fatty liver disease.
Synonym: Feathery degeneration, psueodoxanthomatous changes (obsolete)

Cholestasis

Histological cholestasis is defined by the presence of bile in the liver, visible on H&E stains. The location of the bile varies in different cases and in most cases can be seen in multiple different compartments, with hepatocellular cholestasis the most common, followed in descending order of frequency by cholestasis involving the bile canaliculi, the proliferating ductules, and the bile duct proper. In general, the nonhepatocellular forms of cholestasis take longer to develop and are associated with more severe cholestasis. Outside of this general correlation with the severity and length of cholestasis, there is little or no additional diagnostic information contained in identifying bile in the hepatocytes versus nonhepatocyte location. The ductular cholestasis pattern has been linked to sepsis,[15,16] but is actually seen in many other severely cholestatic conditions and has little or no diagnostic specificity for sepsis. Furthermore, the major pattern of injury in sepsis is actually a nonspecific hepatitis and fatty change.[16]
Synonym: Bilirubinostasis

Chronic hepatitis

Chronic hepatitis is often used somewhat informally by pathologists to describe any lymphocytic inflammation in the liver, but such usage should be discouraged, as the term *chronic hepatitis* does have a distinct clinical implication, where it is commonly defined as elevated serum enzyme levels for greater than 6 months. The best histological finding that can support a diagnosis of chronic hepatitis is convincing fibrosis, though the opposite is not true, as many cases of chronic hepatitis can take years to decades to start fibrosing.

Chronic active hepatitis

This term is no longer used, but is of interest for historical reasons.[17] A major clinical question, one that persists to this day, is why some individuals with chronic hepatitis (viral, autoimmune, etc.) progress to cirrhosis whereas others do not. One of the earliest attempts to better understand this question focused on histology, dividing cases into chronic active hepatitis versus chronic persistent hepatitis. Chronic active hepatitis was thought to have the greatest risk for fibrosis progression and was defined by the presence of piecemeal necrosis (now called interface activity) and either periportal or septal fibrosis. In contrast, chronic persistent hepatitis (also see entry below) had a good prognosis and was defined by having absent or slight piecemeal necrosis and either no fibrosis or portal fibrosis. This approach deeply influenced the thinking of the pathology community but eventually had to be abandoned when data showed it did not predict disease progression. However, the notion of piecemeal necrosis (interface activity) still has clinical relevance and is part of essentially all modern grading systems for chronic hepatitis. The duality of portal fibrosis versus periportal fibrosis has also persisted in some staging systems, but perhaps more because of inertia than biological relevance, as mostly they are about the same thing.
Synonym: Chronic aggressive hepatitis (also obsolete)

Chronic persistent hepatitis

This term is obsolete but of historical interest. Early efforts to understand risk factors for fibrosis progression divided cases of chronic into one of two broad histological patterns: chronic active hepatitis versus chronic persistent hepatitis. In this duality, chronic persistent hepatitis had a better prognosis and was defined as having absent or "slight" piecemeal necrosis and either no fibrosis or mild portal fibrosis. See also the entry for "chronic active hepatitis."

Cirrhosis

Cirrhosis is a diffuse fibrosis of the liver leading to parenchymal nodularity. Rene Laennec (1781 to 1826), a distinguished French physician who invented the stethoscope, is often given credit for the first description of a cirrhotic liver, which he named after "kirrhos," the Greek word for "tawny." As is often the case in history, Laennec thought he was the first, but he was not, as cirrhosis was described more accurately and earlier by two British pathologists, John Browne (1642 to 1700) and Matthew Baillie (1761 to 1823). Nonetheless, Sir William Osler (1849 to 1919), a prominent and dominant North American physician, one of the four founders of Johns Hopkins Hospital, gave Laennec the credit for describing cirrhosis in his very influential English language medical text books, and this seems to have stuck.[18]

Confluent necrosis

If the necrosis pattern in a liver specimen is seen as scattered, single cells, then "spotty necrosis" or similar terms are used. However, if the apoptosis/necrosis involves multiple adjacent hepatocytes, then the term *confluent necrosis* is used. Confluent necrosis indicates a more severe pattern of hepatic injury. Confluent necrosis most commonly affects zone 3 hepatocytes, but with severe necrosis can extend to other zones of hepatocytes. The distinction between single cell necrosis and confluent necrosis in clinical practice should be made using common sense and with the goal in mind of conveying the overall findings in the biopsy. For example, if a biopsy specimen shows predominately spotty necrosis, but by carefully searching you also find a single area with 3 adjacent dead hepatocytes, the best descriptor for the overall pattern of injury is still spotty necrosis. In cases with severe confluent necrosis, bridging necrosis is also commonly found.

Councilman body

Councilman body is no longer a commonly used term, being replaced in the current literature by the terms *apoptotic body* or *acidophil body*. However, the term is of historic interest and is occasionally encountered in modern literature. Councilman bodies are named after the American pathologist William Councilman (1854 to 1933), who described apoptotic hepatocytes as a dominant finding in the pathology of yellow fever.
Synonym: Councilman hyaline body, acidophil body, apoptotic body, spotty necrosis

Ductal plate malformation

Ductal plate malformations can be diffuse in the setting of inherited polycystic liver and kidney disease or in the setting of congenital hepatic fibrosis, being found in most of the portal tracts. However, similar lesions can also be acquired, being found as single or small numbers of lesions, seen more commonly in cirrhotic than in noncirrhotic livers.

Ductal plate malformations are composed of elongated, interanastomosing bile ducts. They can encircle the portal tract in syndromic settings such as congenital hepatic fibrosis (Fig. 3.22). In other cases, particularly the sporadic lesions, they can form small nodules at the edges of portal tracts. Larger lesions can be grossly visible. The ducts typically have open lumens and bile plugs and are growing in a dense fibrotic background. Sporadic lesions are also commonly called von Meyenburg complexes.

Synonym: von Meyenburg complex (used mostly in nonsyndromic cases), bile duct hamartoma (used mostly in nonsyndromic cases)

Ductopenia

Ductopenia is defined as a reduction in the number of bile ducts. When ductopenia is well established, it's not that hard to recognize, if you think to look for it. However, early ductopenia can be very challenging to diagnose because in normal liver tissue some of the smaller portal tracts will not have bile ducts, potentially leaving you to wonder if your case is within normal limits or shows very early duct loss.

As a general rule, a biopsy is considered to be within normal limits if up to 20% of the smaller-sized portal tracts do not have bile ducts evident on H&E. With a keratin stain, rare portal tracts may still not have evident bile ducts, but fewer than on the H&E.

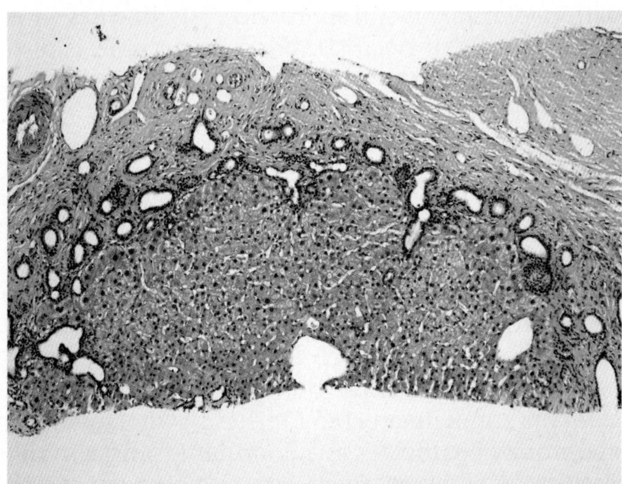

Figure 3.22 Bile duct plate malformation. This biopsy is from a person with congenital hepatic fibrosis.

Chronic inflammation in the portal tracts can obscure bile ducts and an immunostain should be used to confirm bile duct loss. Also of note, ductopenia can be accompanied by patchy bile ductular proliferation, so make sure you assess the bile ducts proper and not the bile ductules. One useful clue can be to look for portal tracts with hepatic arteries that are "unpaired" because they do not have a nearby bile duct.[19] When using this approach, be aware of this potential pitfall: scarred central veins can recruit hepatic arteries[20] and by doing so can mimic a portal tract with an unpaired hepatic artery.

To avoid over-diagnosis of ductopenia, a commonly used guideline is (1) the biopsy should be adequate, having at least 10 portal tracts; and (2) 50% or more of the smaller-sized portal tracts should be without bile ducts. Using a cytokeratin stain, such as CK7, CK19, or CK AE1/3 is strongly recommended. A 50% cutoff makes the diagnosis more specific, but not as sensitive. Thus, if you believe there are a reduced number of bile ducts, the possibility of early ductopenia can still be raised in the pathology report, even if duct loss falls between 50% and 20%. It is good practice to not diagnose ductopenia without knowing the serum alkaline phosphatase levels, as a normal or minimally elevated alkaline phosphatase level would be very unlikely with true ductopenia.

Occasionally a biopsy will be too small to comfortably use the 50% rule, but there will be a medium-sized or larger portal tract that is definitely without a bile duct. This finding is abnormal and almost always indicates ductopenia. Remember to correlate with the serum alkaline phosphatase levels.

Overall, the most common cause of ductopenia is chronic biliary tract disease, such as primary biliary cirrhosis or primary sclerosing cholangitis. Other important conditions associated with duct loss include drug effects and paraneoplastic syndromes, whereas some cases remain idiopathic despite full clinical and histological evaluation.

Elastosis

Focal injuries to the liver can sometimes lead to deposits of extracellular material that is rich in elastic fibers (Fig. 3.23). The extracellular deposits typically have other material in addition to the elastic fibers, principally reticulin.

Emperipolesis

Emperipolesis literally means the findings of one intact cell inside another intact cell. Emperipolesis, where lymphocytes are found within hepatocytes, has been proposed as a helpful microscopic criterion in making the diagnosis of autoimmune hepatitis.

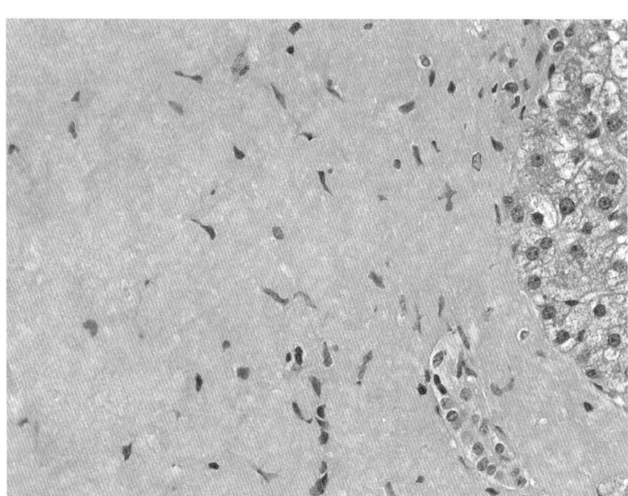

Figure 3.23 Elastosis. This image is from a case of nodular elastosis and shows broad areas of extracellular elastotic matrix deposition.

Emperipolesis may be diagnostically helpful if you can find it, though it seems most pathologists routinely cannot, myself included. After a long time of searching, I found a single case that probably shows emperipolesis, which I have photographed from numerous different angles to use in book chapters, as I am unsure if I will ever find it again (Fig. 3.24).

Fatty change

Fatty change, also called steatosis, indicates the presence of lipid droplets in hepatocytes, seen on H&E as small round empty spaces in the cytoplasm of hepatocytes. The vacuoles held fat, though the fat was removed by routine tissue processing. The fat is further divided into microvesicular fatty change and macrovesicular fatty change. A diffuse pattern of predominately microvesicular steatosis results from mitochondrial injury or inherited metabolic defects. In contrast, macrovesicular fatty change is seen in the metabolic syndrome, alcohol-related liver disease, drug effects, among many others. Of note, the macrovesicular pattern of fat essentially always is admixed with smaller droplets of fat, which is not too surprising as the larger droplets of fat have to come from somewhere. There is no good reason to call this finding "mixed micro and macrovesicular steatosis," as it is the expected pattern found in macrovesicular steatosis.

Synonym: Steatosis, fatty degeneration

Feathery degeneration

The term *feathery degeneration* refers to hepatocytes that are enlarged, swollen with pale flocculent cytoplasm, typically in proximity to a portal tract or fibrous band, in a liver with chronic cholestasis. Some authors use feathery degeneration more loosely, as a term to describe any swollen hepatocyte or groups of hepatocytes regardless of context, for example as a synonym for balloon cell. However, in the setting of fatty liver disease, ballooned hepatocyte is the preferred term.

Synonym: Cholate stasis, psueodoxanthomatous changes (obsolete)

Fibrin ring granuloma

Fibrin ring granulomas are composed of a well circumscribed cluster of macrophages with a central lipid droplet, with the central lipid droplet surrounded by a thin, eosinophilic "fibrin" ring (Fig. 3.25). In most cases, numerous granulomas are found and the fibrin ring granulomas will vary somewhat in their

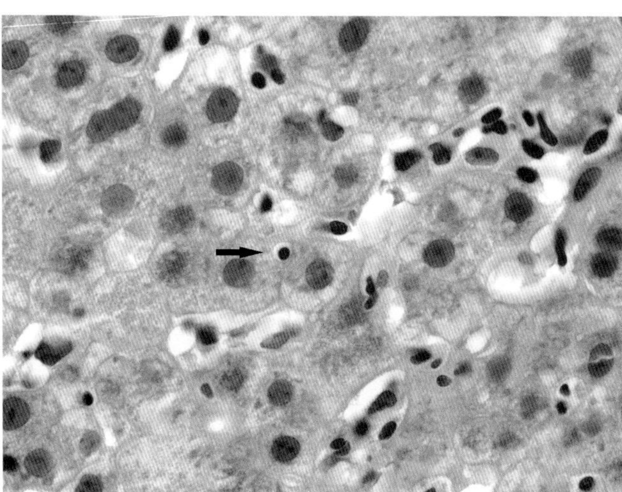

Figure 3.24 Emperipolesis. A lymphocyte (*arrow*) appears to be within the cytoplasm of a hepatocyte.

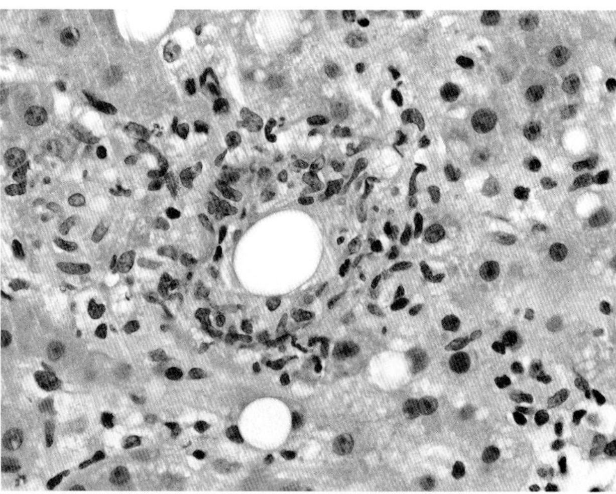

Figure 3.25 Fibrin ring granuloma. This granuloma in a patient with acute EBV hepatitis has a central droplet of fat with a thin rim of fibrin, surrounded by epithelioid histiocytes.

appearance. In addition to classic ones, there will be some granulomas that have less evident lipid droplets and others that have less evident fibrin rings. Fibrin ring granulomas are typically medium in size and are always noncaseating. The background liver typically shows fatty change. Their most famous association is with Q-fever, but they can be seen in many other conditions, including drug reactions, Epstein-Barr virus (EBV) and other infections, and Hodgkin's disease.
Synonym (not widely used): Doughnut hole granuloma or doughnut granuloma

Fibrous cap

Sometimes biopsies from cirrhotic livers can be badly fragmented and some of the fragments may have a rim of blue on the trichrome stain, suggesting a fragment of cirrhotic nodule. This finding is called a fibrous cap. When the fibrous caps are thick and surround much/most of the nodule, then advanced fibrosis is likely, but when caps are thin and incomplete, then this finding doesn't suggest much of anything.

Fibrous septa

The term *fibrous septa* is commonly used as a synonym for bridging fibrosis. However, *fibrous septa* lacks the clarity of meaning of the term *bridging fibrosis*, as many authors have used "fibrous septa" to describe portal tracts that have irregular fibrous extensions that do not reach the level of bridging fibrosis. The intent of the author can often, but not always, be deduced by the overall context of the sentence/paragraph. In diagnostic reports, the term *bridging fibrosis* has the advantage of an unambiguous meaning.
Synonym (inconsistencies in usage make this an imperfect synonym): Bridging fibrosis

Fibro-obliterative duct lesion

Fibro-obliterative duct lesions are round to oval scars that replace a bile duct (Fig. 3.26). Microscopically, fibro-obliterative duct lesions most commonly affect the medium-sized bile ducts,[21] but also can involve the larger bile ducts and appear to be the histological correlate of the "pruning" of the biliary tree seen by cholangiogram.[22] The precursor lesions to fibro-obliterative duct lesions are periductal or "onion skin" fibrosis. All of these changes result from chronic obstructive biliary tract disease and both can be found with any long-term obstruction/stricturing disease, for example primary sclerosing cholangitis. Overall, fibro-obliterative duct lesions are found in less than 10% of biopsy specimens with primary sclerosing cholangitis, with the frequency depending on the duration of the disease. A much higher frequency, about 40%, is found in explanted livers showing cirrhosis from primary sclerosing cholangitis. Fibro-obliterative duct lesions are not diagnostic of primary sclerosing cholangitis, despite what you might read in other places. They are known to occur in other settings, including chronic strictures of the biliary tree, for example with anastomotic strictures after liver transplant, and with *MDR3/ABCB4* gene mutations.[23]

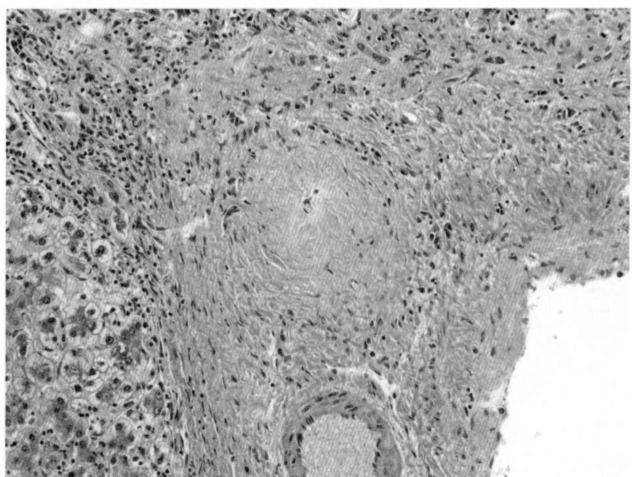

Figure 3.26 Fibro-obliterative duct lesion. The bile duct is gone, replaced by a fibrous scar.

Florid duct lesion

A florid duct lesion is defined as a bile duct that is surrounded and injured by lymphohistiocytic inflammation. The inflammation will be predominantly lymphocytic with ill-defined aggregates of histiocytes (Fig. 3.27). Less commonly, true epithelioid granulomas may be present. The main targets are the

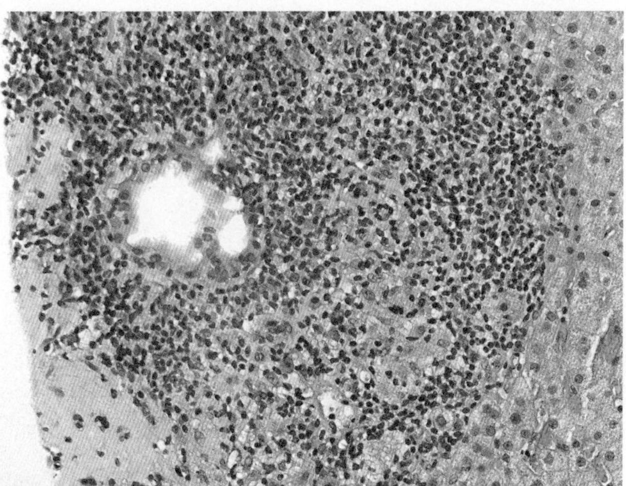

Figure 3.27 Florid duct lesion. The bile duct is surrounded by a dense lymphoplasmacytic infiltrate that also has clusters of histiocytes. The bile duct shows lymphocytic inflammation and injury.

medium-sized bile ducts, also called septal-sized bile ducts, whereas the small terminal bile ducts and the larger bile ducts are spared. Florid bile duct lesions are seen in primary biliary cirrhosis but also occur (albeit rarely) in drug effects.[24]
Synonym: Florid bile duct lesion

Foam cell arteriopathy

Foam cell arteriopathy is seen in medium and larger arteries as part of the pathology of chronic rejection. The vessel lumen is narrowed, often substantially, by thickened walls filled with foamy macrophages (Fig. 3.28). The sizes of vessels affected by this pattern of injury are only rarely sampled by peripheral liver biopsies, so this change is most commonly found in failed allografts. Portal veins rarely show the same change, a finding called foam cell venopathy.[25]
Synonym: Foam cell arteritis, foam cell endoarteritis, transplant arteriopathy

Foamy degeneration

The term *foamy degeneration* describes hepatocytes with microvesciular steatosis and is most commonly used as part of the longer term of *acute foamy degeneration of the liver*, a rare form of alcohol-related liver disease.[1] Note that some authors have used this term as a synonym for balloon cell change, but it is not. Likewise, some authors use the term *foamy degeneration* when they really mean cholate stasis, mostly in the nonpathology literature.

Focal biliary cirrhosis

Focal biliary cirrhosis is a term used almost exclusively in the literature on cystic fibrosis, where it conveys the observation that fibrosis can be very patchy, with focal areas that have the histological findings of cirrhosis, juxtaposed with other areas that show no or mild fibrosis. The areas that are "focally cirrhotic" also tend to show more chronic inflammation of the portal tracts along with bile ductular proliferation and often have inspissated secretions in the bile ducts and ductules. Nonetheless, the term is not used consistently, as some authors have used the term to indicate any degree of patchy fibrosis, inflammation, and ductular proliferation seen microscopically, even if there are no areas that suggest cirrhosis. In addition, the images provided in some papers to illustrate "focal biliary cirrhosis" suggest that nodular regenerative hyperplasia, which can also be seen in cystic fibrosis, was incorrectly interpreted as cirrhotic nodules.

Giant cell change/giant cell transformation

Hepatocytes with giant cell change or giant cell transformation have abundant cytoplasm and three or more nuclei (Fig. 3.29). This nonspecific reactive change can be seen in a variety of conditions, most commonly ones that are cholestatic. Less commonly, biliary epithelial cells can also have giant cell transformation, though the significance of this rare finding is uncertain (Fig. 3.30).

Glycogen storing foci

Glycogen storing foci are circumscribed aggregates of hepatocytes that have clear cytoplasm because of glycogen accumulation (Fig. 3.31). They stand out from the background liver at low power. The significance of these foci is not well understood, but often they are incidental findings in surgical resection specimens

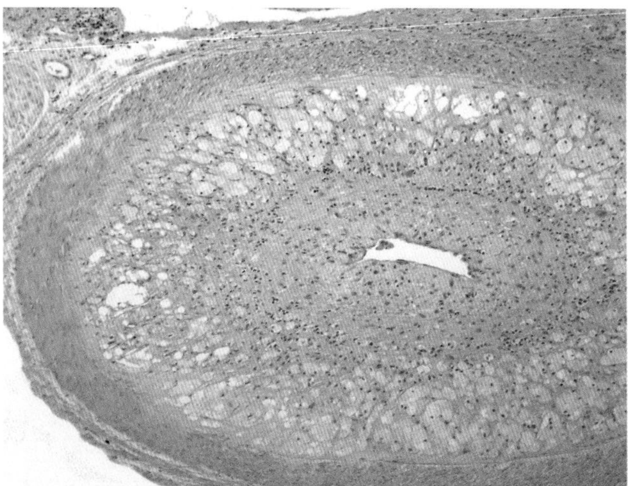

Figure 3.28 Foam cell arteriopathy. The artery lumen is markedly narrowed because of thick walls filled with foamy macrophages.

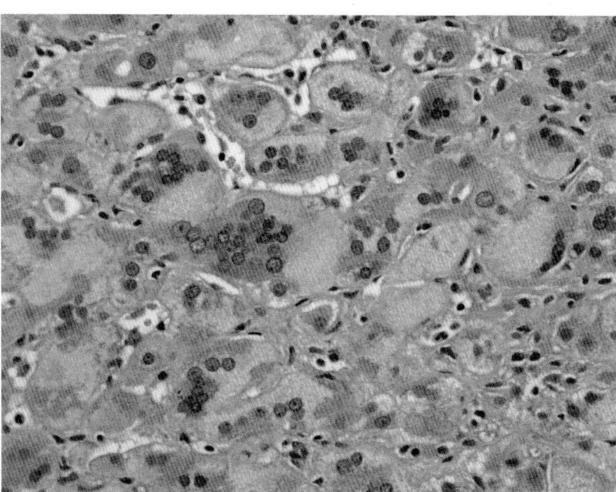

Figure 3.29 Giant cell change, hepatocytes. Giant cell change is seen in a case of idiopathic adult giant cell hepatitis.

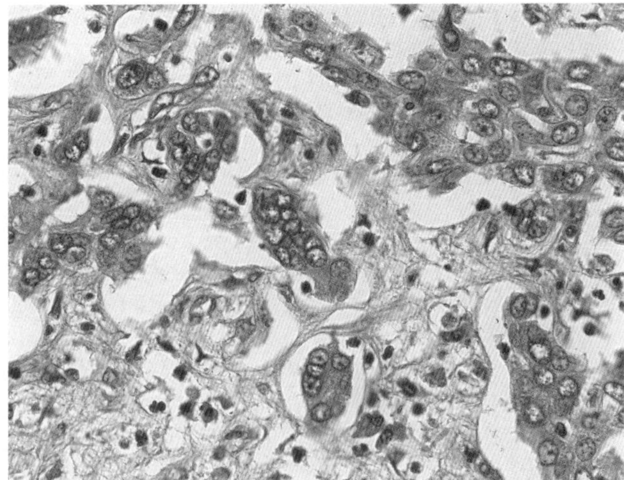
Figure 3.30 Giant cell change, bile ductules. The proliferation bile ductules show multinucleation, a rare finding of unclear significance.

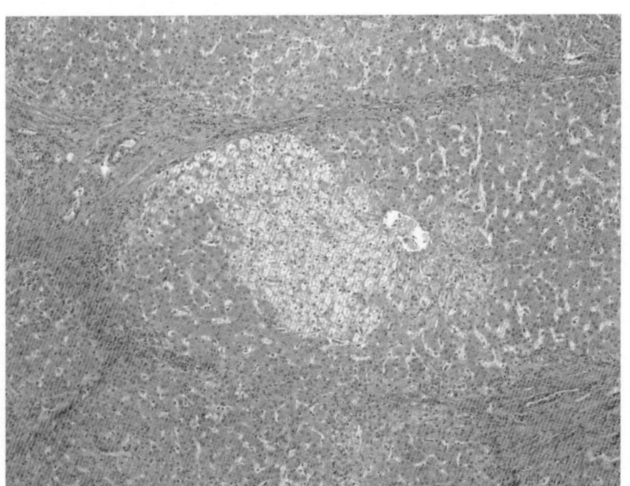
Figure 3.31 Glycogen storing foci. A discrete focus is seen of hepatocytes with clear cytoplasm.

for both primary and metastatic carcinoma and can be seen in both cirrhotic and noncirrhotic livers.

Glycogenated nuclei

Glycogenated nuclei have clear or white vacuoles that typically fill up most of the nuclei, leaving only a small rim of chromatin at the edges (Fig. 3.32). The inclusions may be more eosinophilic in some cases, depending on the stain. Glycogenated nuclei often cluster into small discrete patches. They can be found anywhere in the lobules, but overall are somewhat more common in zone 1 hepatocytes. Glycogenated nuclei are a common finding and are not very useful diagnostically. In most cases, there is no important clinical association. However, there is a modest association with diabetes mellitus.[26] They can also be found

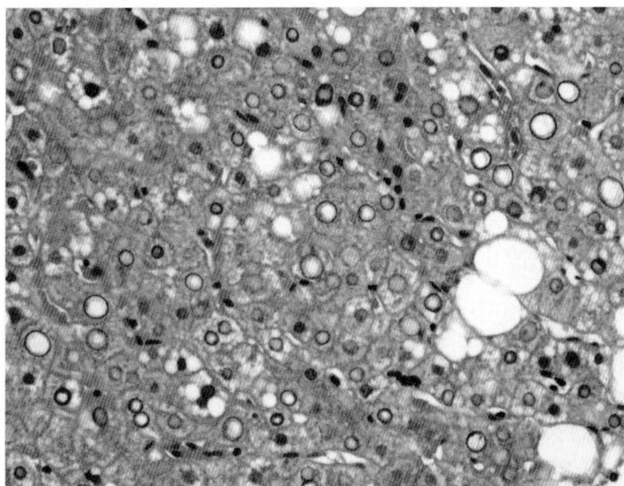
Figure 3.32 Glycogenated nuclei. A cluster of hepatocytes show glycogenated nuclei.

in drug effects, glycogen storage diseases, glycogenic hepatopathy, and Wilson's disease.

Synonym (rarely used): Glycogen nuclei

Granuloma

The most basic definition of a granuloma is a discrete collection of histiocytes; the histiocytes are tightly clustered into a ball and are typically epithelioid and not foamy (Fig. 3.33). In addition to the histiocytes, granulomas typically have varying degrees of admixed lymphocytes or other inflammatory cells. The question is sometimes raised as to what is the minimum number of histiocytes needed to qualify for a granuloma. There is little data on which to base a solid answer and most authors do not provide a formal definition

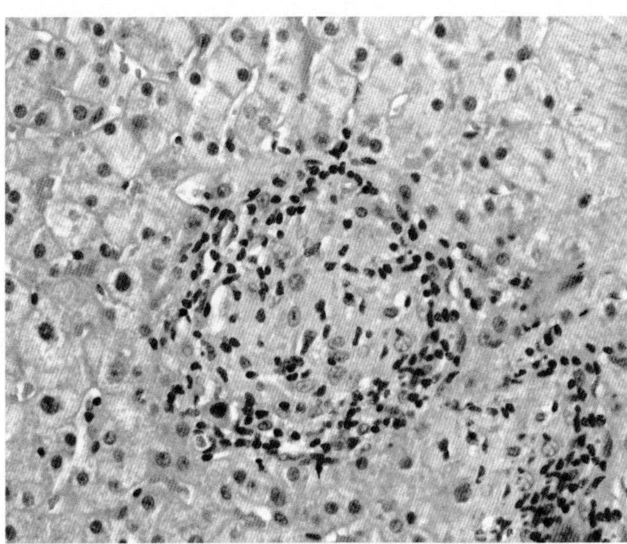
Figure 3.33 Granuloma. An epithelioid, noncaseating granuloma is seen in a case of primary biliary cirrhosis.

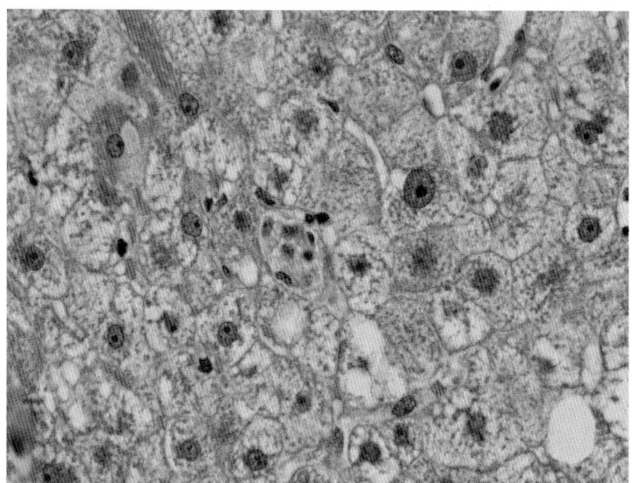

Figure 3.34 Microgranuloma. A small microgranuloma is seen in a case or resolving acute hepatitis.

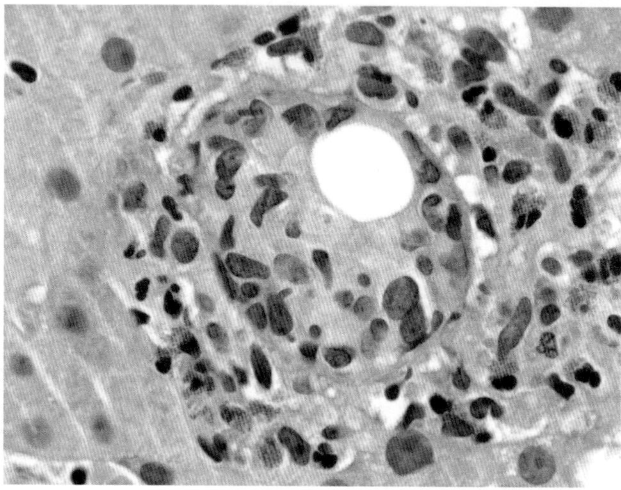

Figure 3.36 Granuloma, fibrin ring. A liver biopsy in a patient presenting with fevers showed fibrin ring granulomas.

for their studies. Smaller lobular aggregates of histiocytes are often called microgranulomas (Fig. 3.34), a very nonspecific finding that does not carry the same significance as the term *granuloma*, and various authors have suggested guidelines that about 3 to 7 histiocytes are needed to qualify for a microgranuloma. Thankfully, in most cases it is reasonably clear if a cluster of histiocytes qualifies for the term *granuloma*. In fact, if you ever feel the urge to count the number of histiocytes, then that's a pretty good indicator that the lesion is not quite a granuloma.

Granulomas can be further subdivided into caseating granulomas (Fig. 3.35), noncaseating granulomas, fibrin ring granulomas (Fig. 3.36), lipid granulomas (Fig. 3.37), fibrotic granulomas (Fig. 3.38), and foreign body granulomas (Fig. 3.39). Granulomas can be found in the portal tracts and the lobules and are commonly seen in both. In general, their location in the portal

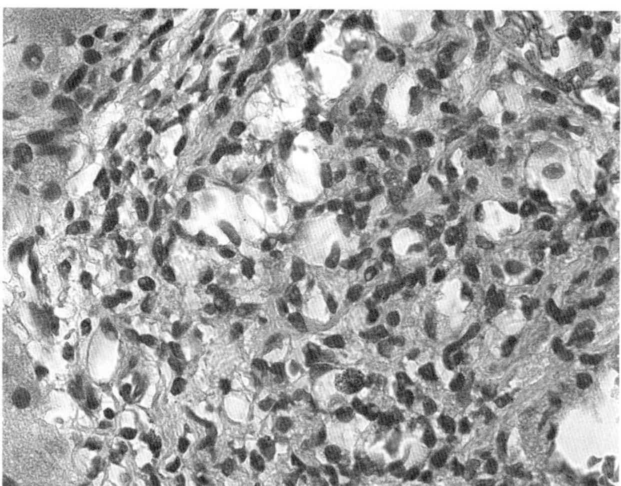

Figure 3.37 Granuloma, lipid. This lipid granuloma is composed of lipid laden macrophages and a bit of fibrosis. Lipid granulomas often contain mineral oil, a common food additive.

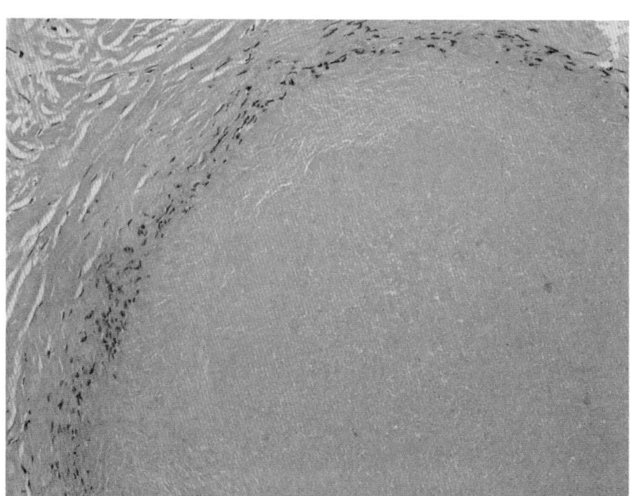

Figure 3.35 Granuloma, caseating. This large granuloma shows extensive central necrosis.

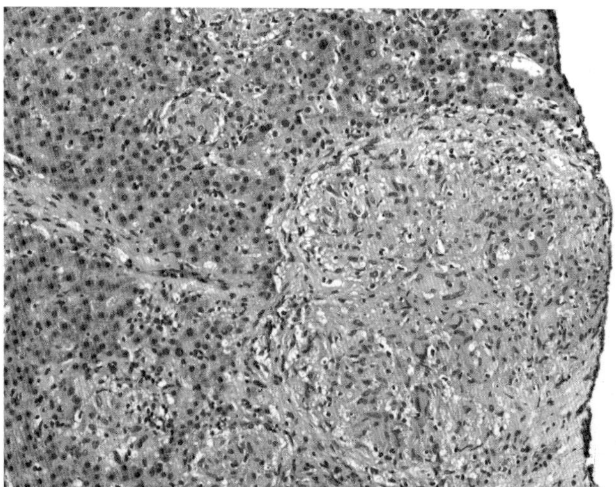

Figure 3.38 Granuloma, fibrotic. Extensively fibrotic granulomas are most commonly seen with sarcoidosis.

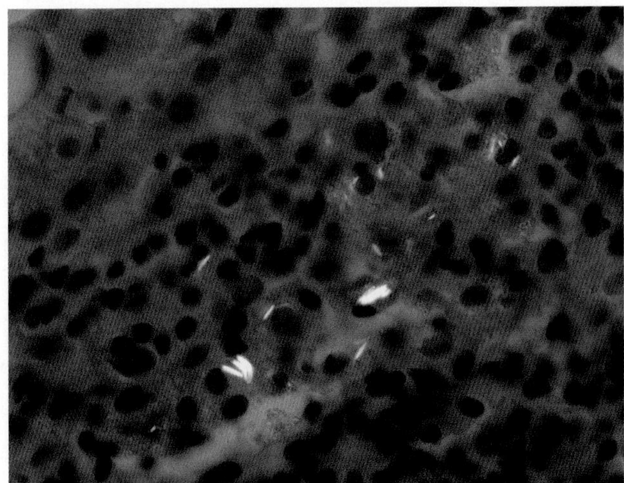

Figure 3.39 Granuloma, foreign body (polarized light). Polarizable material was evident in this granuloma, found in the portal tracts of a patient with a history of injection drug use.

tracts versus the lobules does not provide any strong etiological clues. The term *poorly formed granuloma* is used in cases where the histiocytes are not tightly aggregated and there are lots of other admixed inflammatory cells.

Ground glass inclusions/ground glass change

Ground glass inclusions occur in a subset of individuals with long-term chronic hepatitis B infection. The hepatocytes develop large, amphophilic, circumscribed inclusions that fill up the cytoplasm (Fig. 3.40). Affected hepatocytes have a single inclusion. When the cytoplasm shows less well-defined inclusions, the term *ground glass change* is often used. These findings represent the accumulation of viral particles in the smooth endoplasmic reticulum, typically badly mutated viruses that are unable to be secreted. Of note, other diseases can have inclusions that closely mimic ground glass inclusions, so immunostains are needed to prove chronic hepatitis B infection.

Halo sign

In livers that are cirrhotic because of chronic biliary tract disease and have ongoing cholestasis, the cirrhotic nodules at low-power magnification are often surrounded by a thin rim of edema and cholate stasis that give the impression of a halo surrounding the nodule (Fig. 3.41). The term *halo sign* is also used by radiologists for different purposes, to describe a number of different findings which share in common a central lesion or anatomical structure surrounded by a halo of low-signal intensity.

Hepatic plate thickening

In the normal liver, hepatocytes are organized into plates or cords that are one or two cells in thickness. The hepatic plates can be three to four cells in thickness when the liver is actively regenerating, but plates that are much thicker than that suggest a neoplastic process or malignant transformation. The thickness of the plates is determined by examining the reticulin stain (see also entry for reticulin loss).

Hepatoportal sclerosis

Portal veins can become atrophic and fibrotic in certain diseases, a finding called hepatoportal sclerosis. The walls can show smooth muscle hypertrophy early

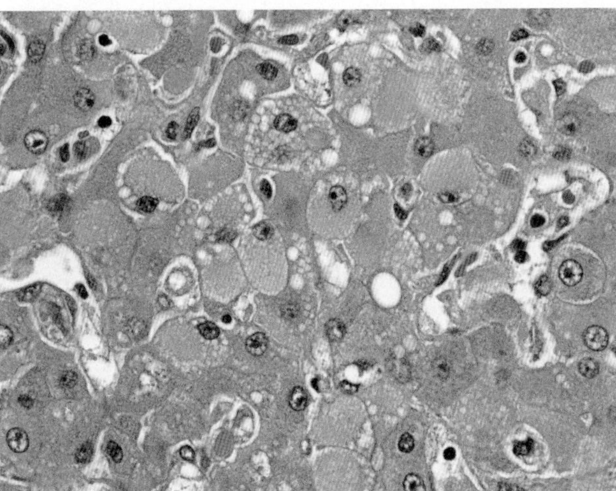

Figure 3.40 Ground glass hepatocytes. In this case of chronic hepatitis B, the hepatocytes show round, light gray–colored inclusions that fill the cytoplasm.

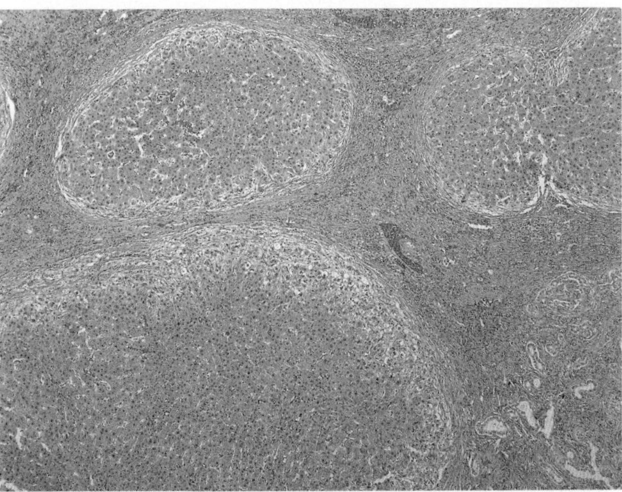

Figure 3.41 Halo sign. In this case of primary biliary cirrhosis, the cirrhotic nodules are surrounded by a rim of pale edematous tissue.

on, followed by atrophy, and fibrosis. Hepatoportal sclerosis is often accompanied by nodular regenerative hyperplasia.

Hyaline body

A hyaline body is a densely eosinophilic inclusion seen in the hepatocyte cytoplasm (Fig. 3.42). They are composed of various proteins, but stain for p62 and commonly for ubiquitin. They can be found in malignant hepatocytes and rarely in neoplastic cholangiocytes.

Impaired liver regeneration

The criteria for this diagnosis have not been well developed, either clinically or histologically, but the basic notion is that some patients, usually the elderly, have a liver insult that most individuals would readily recover from, but the patient does not. In these cases, the biopsy can show various patterns and degrees of injury, depending on the insult, but the Ki-67 shows a discordantly low proliferative rate for the degree of hepatocyte injury.

Incomplete septal fibrosis

Incomplete septal fibrosis is a morphological term used to describe livers with thin delicate fibrous bands that are often fragmented or incomplete, not fully extending from one structure to another, but with one end that ends as a blind ending. This gives the liver parenchyma a vague nodularity, with a macronodular pattern, but one that has too much fibrosis for a diagnosis of nodular regenerative hyperplasia, and not enough fibrosis and well-defined nodularity for a diagnosis of cirrhosis. The diagnosis is best made on wedge biopsies or resection specimens. On needle biopsy or fine needle aspirate, an accurate diagnosis of incomplete septal cirrhosis is challenging to make and the diagnosis is prone to error.

At a practical diagnostic level, incomplete septal cirrhosis can have overlapping clinical and histological findings with both nodular regenerative hyperplasia and partial nodular transformation. One reasonable approach is to classify a case as incomplete septal cirrhosis if there clearly are thin delicate fibrous bands accompanying the nodularity. If there is no fibrosis, then the best diagnosis is nodular regenerative hyperplasia. If there are thin bands of fibrosis and vague nodularity, but the changes are limited to sections from near the liver hilum, with normal histology or atrophic parenchyma in the peripheral sections, then consider a diagnosis of partial nodular transformation.

In some cases, incomplete septal cirrhosis appears to represent cirrhosis undergoing regression.[27,28] In other cases, it can be associated with longstanding idiopathic hepatoportal sclerosis (noncirrhotic portal hypertension).

Induced hepatocyte

In response to some medications, the smooth endoplasmic reticulum in hepatocytes proliferates, giving the cytoplasm a smooth amphophilic color (Fig. 3.43). In some cases, the induced change will affect only a part of the cytoplasm, resulting in a distinctive "two-tone" appearance. Chronic hepatitis B should be ruled out, as ground glass change can appear very similar.
Synonym: Hepatocyte adaptation

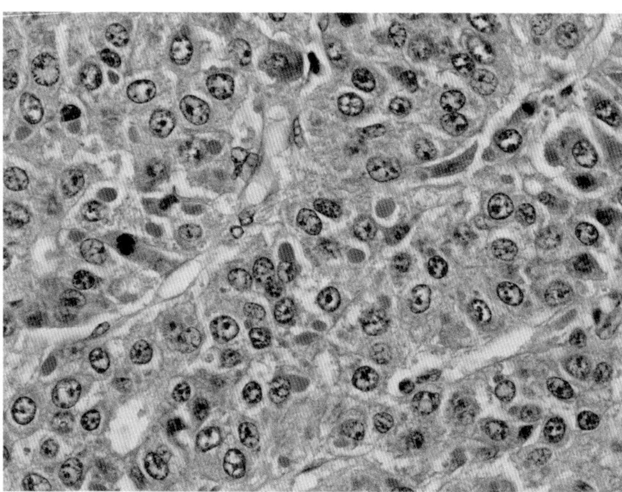

Figure 3.42 Hyaline body. This hepatocellular carcinoma has numerous hyaline bodies.

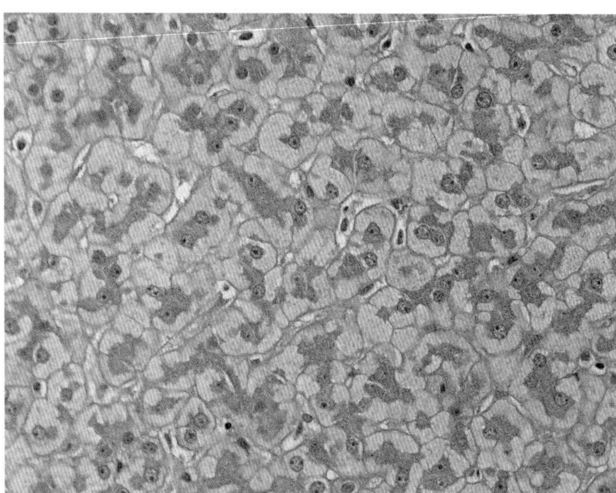

Figure 3.43 Induced hepatocyte. The hepatocytes show a distinctive amphophilic change to their cytoplasm, resulting from smooth endoplasmic reticulum hyperplasia in response to medication.

Interface activity/interface hepatitis

Interface activity describes inflammation and injury to hepatocytes that are immediately adjacent to the portal tract (Fig. 3.44). Interface activity is not specific for any disease and tends to track with the overall degree of portal inflammation, and to a lesser extent with the degree of lobular inflammation. Interface activity has found most renown in the setting of autoimmune hepatitis, but is equally common in acute and chronic hepatitis from many different causes. In fact, interface activity is commonly given its own score when using a formal grading system for chronic viral hepatitis.

Some pathologists believe they can distinguish interface activity from lymphocytes that have harmlessly "spilled-over" from the portal tract into zone 1, based on whether the inflammation at the interface is accompanied by hepatocyte damage. This belief is rather harmless, though it probably makes it challenging to grade inflammatory activity with formal grading schemas. *Synonym: Piecemeal necrosis (obsolete), periportal hepatitis (obsolete)*

Intermediate hepatocyte

Intermediate hepatocytes are CK7 positive hepatocytes, located primarily in zone 1 (Fig. 3.45). Intermediate hepatocytes are not present in normal liver, but are found with chronic cholestatic liver disease. Intermediate hepatocytes often look pretty similar to normal hepatocytes on H&E, so the CK7 stain is needed for their confident identification.

Iron free foci

When there is marked iron deposition in a cirrhotic liver, the iron tends to be diffuse, affecting most of the cirrhotic nodules to some degree. Premalignant and malignant hepatocyte proliferations can have less iron deposition, causing them to stand out grossly and on iron stains. These foci should be targeted when sectioning resection specimens and closely examined histologically to evaluate for hepatocellular carcinoma or cholangiocarcinoma.

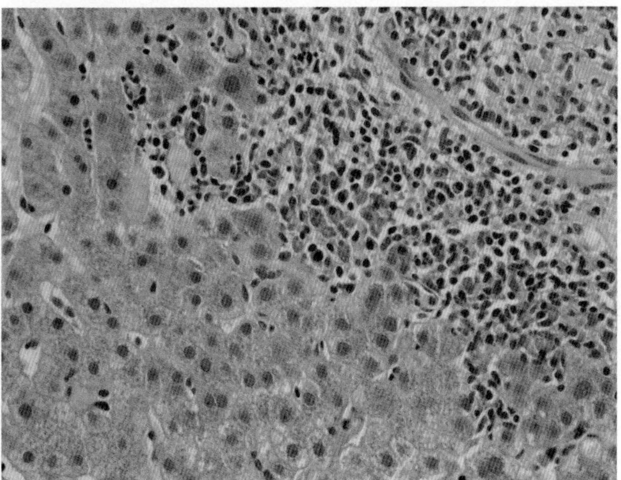

Figure 3.44 Interface activity. The hepatocytes at the edge of the lobule are infiltrated by inflammatory cells, giving the portal tract an irregular edge.

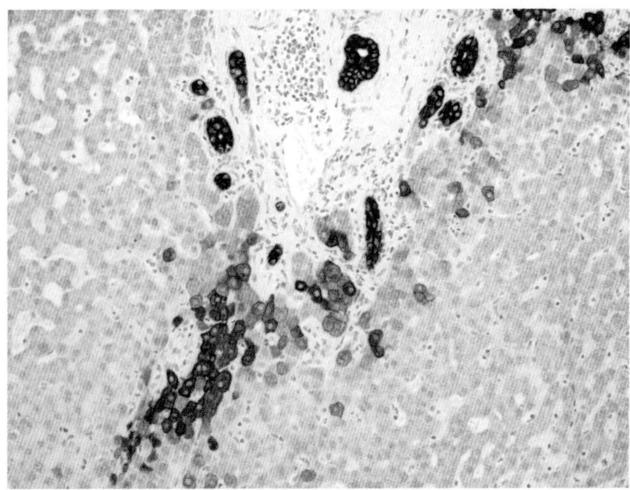

Figure 3.45 Intermediate hepatocyte. A CK7 immunostain highlights both the normal bile duct and the hepatocytes at the edges of the portal tracts. When hepatocytes express CK7, they are called intermediate hepatocytes.

Lamellar fibrosis

Lamellar fibrosis is used to describe intratumoral fibrosis that tends to align in parallel bands. Lamellar fibrosis is most commonly observed in fibrolamellar hepatocellular carcinoma, but can also be found, at least focally, in a subset of conventional hepatocellular carcinomas. The reason(s) for this unusual fibrosis pattern is not known.

Large cell change

Large cell change is used to describe hepatocytes that have both increased nuclear size and increased cytoplasm, resulting in a big cell with a normal to near-normal nuclear:cytoplasmic ratio. The nuclei tend to stand out at low power, as they are enlarged, hyperchromatic, and sometimes binucleated (Fig. 3.46).

Large cell change is seen most commonly in cirrhotic livers, in particular with chronic hepatitis B. In noncirrhotic livers, large cell change is rare, but also most commonly found with chronic hepatitis B infection, or in individuals with advanced age. The biological explanations for large cell changes remain controversial. In one model, large cell change results from senescent changes associated with wide spread but low-level DNA damage in hepatocytes,

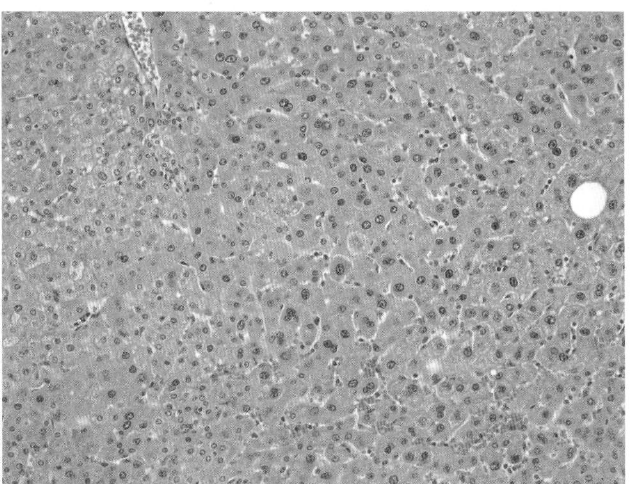

Figure 3.46 Large cell change. The hepatocytes in the middle of the image show large cell change. Compare to normal hepatocytes in the upper left.

thus eliminating hepatocytes at risk for malignant transformation. In this model large cell change serves as an indirect marker of increased risk for hepatocellular carcinoma. Alternative models suggest large cell change may be a direct precursor to malignancy itself.

Limiting plate

This term refers to the single layer of hepatocytes immediately adjacent to a portal tract.

Lipofuscin

Lipofuscin is a granular, brown, cytoplasmic pigment (Fig. 3.47). Lipofuscin in hepatocytes has a strong zone 3 distribution, or a zone 3 predominance when pigment is more widespread. Lipofuscin is composed of insoluble, highly oxidized fatty acids and misfolded proteins that are not degradable by the proteasome system or lysosomal enzymes.[29] Lipofuscin deposits correlate to some degree with age, leading to the moniker "wear and tear pigment." It is true that lipofuscin is more abundant in liver biopsies of the elderly,[30] but there is a wide variation between lipofuscin density in hepatocytes and the age of the person. This is because lipfoscin accumulation depends not only on oxidative damage (which increases with age), but also on the mitochondrial and protein repair mechanisms, as well as the effectiveness of the lysosomal systems, all of which have polymorphisms that can affect their functionality.[29]

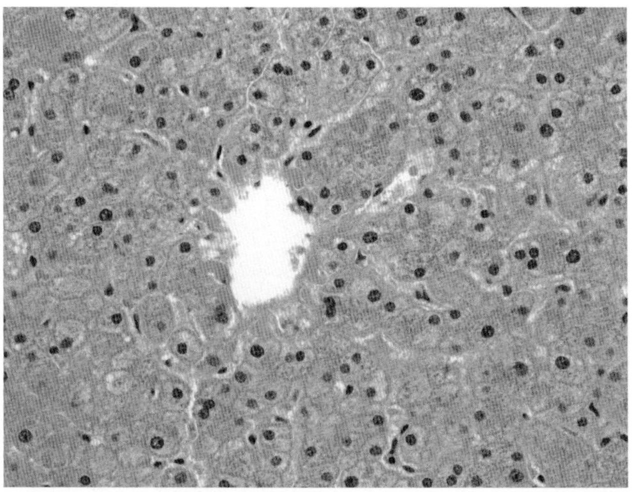

Figure 3.47 Lipofuscin. The zone 3 hepatocytes show a golden brown granular pigment.

The significance of lipofuscin in biopsies is currently limited to essentially that of a diagnostic pitfall, as lipofuscin can be mistaken for iron or bile or copper on H&E stains. The true nature of the pigment can be readily sorted out by doing iron or copper stains and by checking the serum bilirubin levels. If needed, a Fontana–Masson stain can be performed, as the lipofuscin stains with a granular black pattern. Glypican 3 immunostain also stains lipofuscin, an important pitfall when working up a tumor for possible hepatocellular carcinoma.

In liver pathology, the terms *ceroid pigment* and *lipofuscin* are essentially interchangeable, though some authors prefer the term *ceroid pigment* to describe pigment accumulation as part of a pathological process, primarily in macrophages, whereas lipofuscin is an age-related phenomenon. In addition, there are subtle differences between the two lipopigments in their autofluorescence spectra and their chemical composition, but these differences are largely inscrutable to most of us. Fortunately, however, to date there are no differences that reach diagnostic relevance.
Synonym: Ceroid pigment

Lobule

In common diagnostic pathology terminology, the hepatocytes are in the lobules and there is not much more to it than that. However, in anatomic terminology, a lobule is the "smallest unit" of the liver that has portal tracts, hepatocytes, and central veins. These anatomic lobules can also be diagrammed in three main ways. The lobules are often illustrated as "classic" lobules, a hexagonal shaped structure with a portal tract at each of the six corners and the central vein in the middle. The lobule can also be drawn as a "hepatic acinus," shaped like a short and fat diamond, with a top and bottom edge on portal tracts, whereas the larger middle edges extend from central vein to central vein. The hepatic acinus maps with blood flow and gives rise to the notion of hepatic zones, with zone 1 (periportal) getting the best oxygenated blood and zone 3 (around the central vein) the least oxygenated blood. Finally, another way to think of the liver is the "portal lobule," which is a triangle with a central vein at each edge and a single portal tract in the middle. The portal lobule maps best to bile flow.

Lobular collapse

Substantial liver injury can lead to parenchymal collapse, where the hepatocytes in large areas drop out. Early on, the dead hepatocytes may still be seen on the H&E, but in time the hepatocytes disappear and are replaced by a robust ductular proliferation with admixed inflammation. The native portal tracts can often still be seen, more closely approximated than in normal livers.

Macrotrabecular

This term is used to describe growth patterns in both hepatoblastomas and in hepatocellular carcinomas, where a tumor has a trabecular growth pattern and the individual trabeculae are especially thick. A common definition is trabeculae that are at least 10 cells thick, though 20 cells thickness has also been suggested as a cutoff. In both hepatoblastomas and hepatocellular carcinomas, the macrotrabecular pattern can be either a pure pattern or mixed with multiple other growth patterns. A CD34 stain will nicely highlight the macrotrabeculae.

Mallory hyaline

Mallory hyaline is seen on H&E stains as eosinophilic clumps and irregular aggregates of cytoplasmic proteins in hepatocytes, mostly commonly in ballooned hepatocytes (Fig. 3.48). Mallory hyaline is an indicator of cellular injury and is most commonly encountered with active steatohepatitis from any cause, or in the setting of chronic cholestasis or some drug reactions, such as with amiodarone. Mallory hyaline is not a required criteria for any diagnosis, but instead serves as a marker of active hepatic injury. In steatohepatitis, Mallory hyaline is found principally in a subset of ballooned hepatocytes, but it is the ballooned hepatocytes and not the Mallory hyaline that are used to evaluate the degree of active injury.

Mallory hyaline results from the aggregation of damaged and ubiquitinated cytoskeleton proteins. Although stains are not necessary, Mallory hyaline is positive for ubiquitin, p62, and cytokeratins 8 and 18.[31–33] There is good consensus on H&E when Mallory hyaline has classic morphology and is found in ballooned hepatocytes. However, hepatocytes can also show subtle cytoplasmic changes on H&E stains that are good enough to diagnose Mallory hyaline for some pathologists, but are insufficient for other pathologists. For this reason, the literature has recorded considerable variation in the frequency of Mallory hyaline in different diseases. The good news is that this doesn't matter much for clinical care, as there really are no diagnoses that depend on positive identification of Mallory hyaline.

Synonym: Mallory–Denk body

Microabscess

A microabscess is a small cluster of neutrophils in the sinusoids (Fig. 3.49). In nontransplanted liver biopsies, a specific cause is infrequently identified, but the differential includes drug effect and infection. In transplanted livers, microabscesses have been linked to cytomegalovirus (CMV) infection when they are numerous.[34] For example, one study found that >9

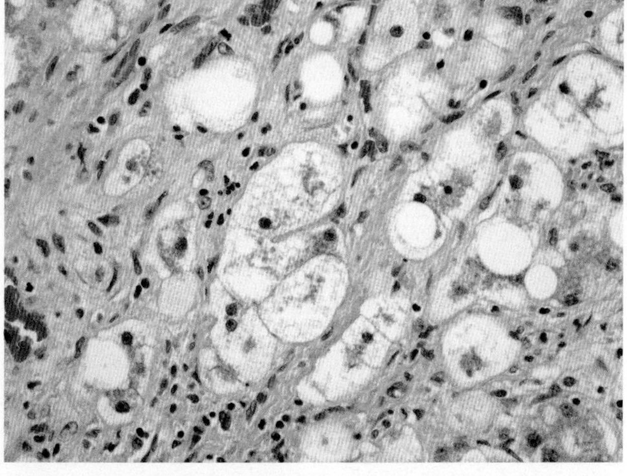

Figure 3.48 Mallory hyaline. The hepatocytes show extensive ballooning with pink cytoplasmic condensations of Mallory hyaline.

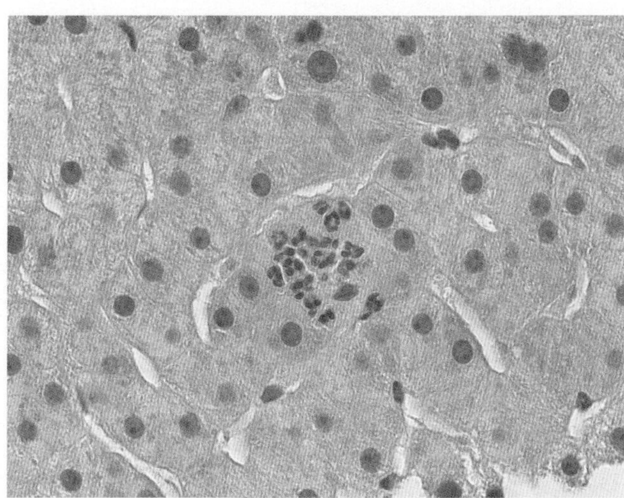

Figure 3.49 Microabscess. A small sinusoidal cluster of neutrophils is seen in a post-transplant liver biopsy. An immunostain for CMV was negative.

microabscesses in a biopsy was associated with CMV infection.[35] In contrast, microabscesses do not strongly suggest CMV when they are an isolated finding, and in most cases a specific cause is not identified. Nonetheless, allograft biopsies with smaller numbers of microabscesses are commonly further evaluated with an immunostain for CMV.

Microgranuloma

A microgranuloma is defined as a small collection of histiocytes (typically 3 to 7), usually in the lobules, in most cases indicating a site of recent hepatocyte death and drop out. They are typically few in number, may show slight pigment accumulation (Fig. 3.50), and are most commonly seen in the setting of a resolving hepatitis. They often stand out nicely on a periodic acid–Schiff diastase (PASD) stain as small clusters of positive cells against a background of paler staining hepatocytes. If microgranulomas are numerous, present in nearly every field, then the differential diagnosis is principally that of resolving infection or resolving drug effect. Overall, microgranulomas do not have the same differential as true granulomas. In addition, the term *microgranuloma* can be easily confused by clinical teams and is probably best avoided in clinical reports.

Micronodular cirrhosis/macronodular cirrhosis

Historically, the etiologies of most cases of cirrhosis were unknown, so they were described based on the morphology of the cirrhotic nodules. A micronodular pattern of cirrhosis showed small nodules, most of which were less than 3 mm in diameter, whereas macronodular cirrhosis had nodules that were greater than 3 mm in diameter. A category of mixed micro and macronodular cirrhosis was also used when no pattern seemed predominate. As time went on and specific etiologies of liver cirrhosis were discovered, authors commonly went back and correlated a new disease with its typical morphological pattern of cirrhosis. These studies generally showed that a micronodular pattern of cirrhosis correlated with etiologies of alcohol, α-1 antitrypsin deficiency, Wilson's disease, and hemochromatosis. Macronodular cirrhosis correlated in general with chronic viral hepatitis and autoimmune hepatitis. However, it was also clear that there were too many exceptions to use these patterns for disease categorization and that cirrhotic liver should be classified by the underlying cause of liver disease. Studies of patients with a known disease also revealed that micronodular cirrhotic livers could transform to macronodular cirrhosis over time, especially if the injury abated.[36]

Synonym: Micronodular cirrhosis: Laennec cirrhosis (obsolete), portal cirrhosis (obsolete)

Synonym: Macronodular cirrhosis: Post necrotic cirrhosis (partial synonym).

Microvesicular steatosis

Microvesicular steatosis refers to very small droplets of fat that diffusely fill the cytoplasm of hepatocytes as a result of a mitochondrial injury (Fig. 3.51). For practical purposes, this should be the predominant pattern of injury for a diagnosis of microvesicular steatosis, though scattered droplets of macrovesicular steatosis are not uncommon. Also of note, a diagnosis of microvesicular steatosis should be made with the

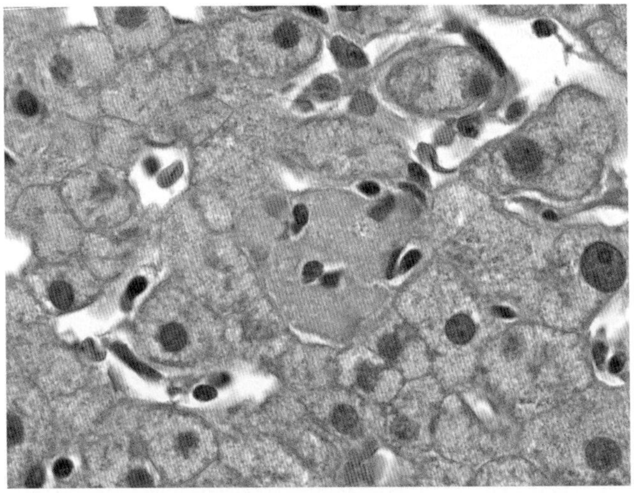

Figure 3.50 Microgranuloma, pigmented. A small pigmented microgranuloma is seen in the lobule.

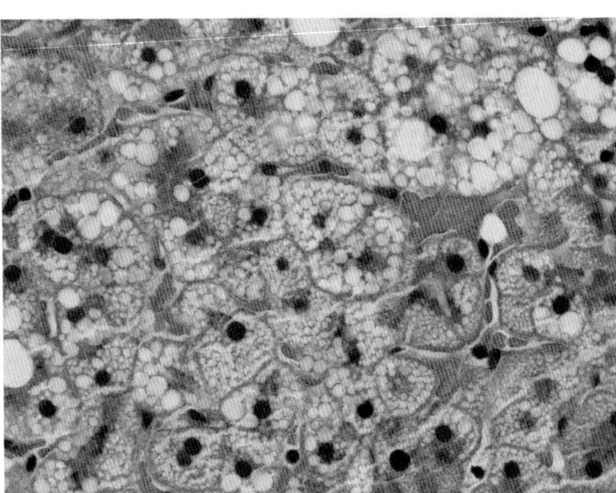

Figure 3.51 Microvesicular steatosis. The hepatocyte cytoplasm is diffusely filled with small droplets of fat. The nuclei are centrally located. Rare larger droplets of fat are also seen in the upper right.

H&E stain and not solely on Oil red O stains. Oil red O stains are more often confusing than they are helpful because they often show extensive small droplet staining in normal livers and in many different liver diseases, ones that are unrelated to microvesicular steatosis pathology.[37]

Megamitochondria

Megamitochondria are round to oval to needle shaped eosinophilic structures in the hepatocyte cytoplasm that represent injured and enlarged mitochondria (Fig. 3.52). They have been associated with fatty liver disease, both alcoholic and nonalcoholic, but they are found in a wide range of liver conditions. Megamitochondria can be seen anywhere within the hepatic lobules. When found in a periportal location, they can mimic α-1-antitrysin globules. When needed, histochemical stains will distinguish these two entities, with α-1-antitrysin globules staining positive for PASD, whereas megamitochondria are positive for phosphotungstic acid hematoxylin (PTAH) stain. Megamitochondria don't have any particular diagnostic significance. In fatty liver disease, they are not associated with the percent of fat or with ballooned hepatocytes.[38]

Mucinous carcinoma

Formally defined, a mucinous carcinoma should have 50% or greater extracellular mucin. On biopsy specimens, this term is often used somewhat more loosely to indicate "abundant" extracellular mucin, even if the mucin doesn't quite reach 50%. Mucinous carcinomas involving the liver most commonly originate from the colon, but can also arise from a large number of other sites. Rarely, cholangiocarcinomas also have a mucinous morphology.

Multilocular

The term *multilocular* is used when a single large cystic structure has internal septations. As an example, a grape fruit, when cut in half, shows thin membranous septations that divide the pulp into segments. In contrast, an aggregate of closely approximated but unilocular cysts is called multicystic.

Multicystic

A multicystic lesion is composed of an aggregate of individually unilocular cysts that are clustered together. As an example, a cluster of grapes can be thought of as "multicystic," with each grape representing a single cyst.

Nodular regenerative hyperplasia

Nodular regenerative hyperplasia is a reactive parenchymal nodularity that can be seen in a variety of conditions, in many cases owing to irregular blood flow within the liver. The liver has a nodular appearance on low power (Fig. 3.53) that results most often from atrophy of zone 3 hepatocytes, alternating with areas of normal-sized or even somewhat enlarged zone 1 hepatocytes. By definition, there should be either no or minimal fibrosis. The parenchymal nodularity is often very subtle and can be easily overlooked in biopsy. The nodularity can be enhanced by a reticulin stain, but the changes often remain subtle even then. At this point, studies have not identified other useful stains, though better stains would be much appreciated by most of us.

Onion skin fibrosis

In the setting of chronic downstream biliary tract obstruction, the medium and large-sized bile ducts can develop a striking collar of dense fibrosis, termed

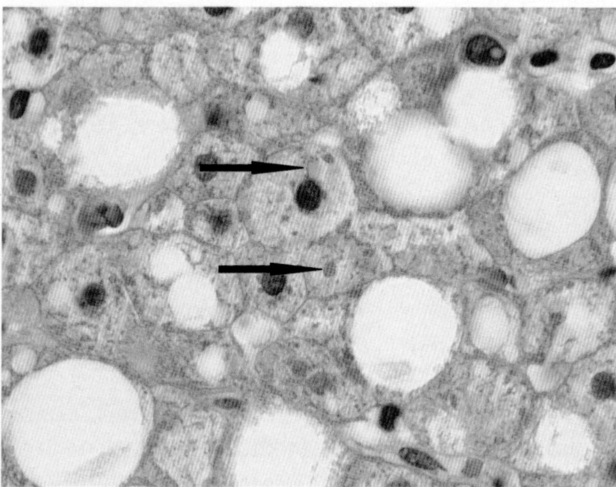

Figure 3.52 Megamitochondria. Several megamitochondria are present (*arrows*).

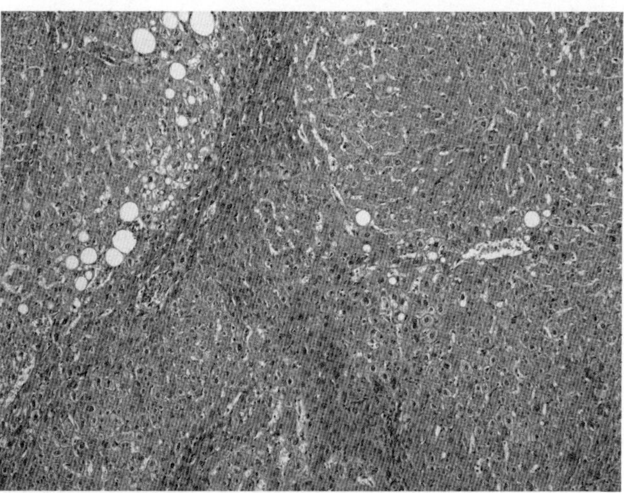

Figure 3.53 Nodular regenerative hyperplasia. The liver shows distinctive nodularity but no fibrosis.

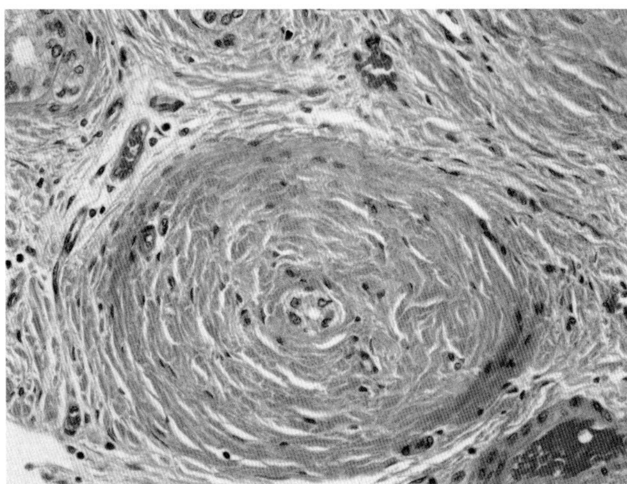

Figure 3.54 Onion skin fibrosis. The bile duct is small and atrophic, cuffed by dense laminated fibrosis.

onion skinning fibrosis. The fibrosis has a concentric, laminated, and sometimes edematous appearance (Fig. 3.54). In time, onion skinning fibrosis leads to fibro-obliterative duct lesions. Onion skinning fibrosis is an important histological finding, but be aware that the medium and larger-sized bile ducts in normal livers can have a bit of a collar of dense collagen, a finding that should not be over interpreted as onion skinning fibrosis. Onion skin fibrosis is not specific for primary sclerosing cholangitis. Nor is it sensitive, being found in only about 40% of livers explanted for primary sclerosing cholangitis.
Synonym: Periductal fibrosis

Pale body

The pale body is a single large cytoplasmic inclusion that is gray in color (Fig. 3.55). Their composition and origin is not clear, but they stain variably for fibrinogen, p62, and a number of other proteins. Pale bodies are found in many fibrolamellar carcinomas and a smaller number of conventional hepatocellular carcinomas.

Panacinar necrosis

Panacinar necrosis results from severe injury that leads to areas of confluent necrosis, with the loss of entire hepatic lobules, often leading to close approximation of the portal tracts. The void left by the dead hepatocytes is often filled with a brisk ductular reaction and inflammatory cells, including pigment laden macrophages.

Pancreatic acinar cell metaplasia

The soft tissue surrounding the bile ducts of the hilum and the connective tissue around the largest branches of the intrahepatic bile ducts can have small clusters of glands with acinar cell differentiation, resembling normal pancreas acini (Fig. 3.56). Pancreatic acinar cell metaplasia is commonly admixed with other benign peribiliary glands. This finding is seen in about 4% of explants and autopsy livers and can be found in both cirrhotic and noncirrhotic livers.[39,40] There is some debate as to whether pancreatic acinar cell metaplasia represents true metaplasia or heterotopia. There is evidence that supports both positions and, in the end, perhaps both have a component of truth.

Partial nodular transformation

Partial nodular transformation is a diagnosis made principally in autopsy specimens or in liver explants. The livers show a distinct nodularity in the hilum

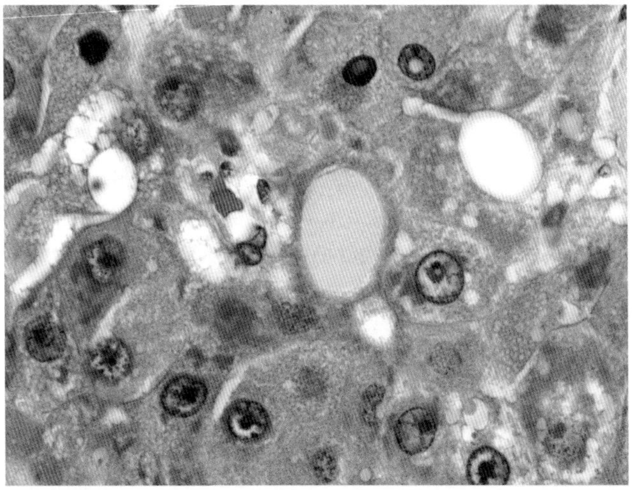

Figure 3.55 Pale body. This pale body is seen in a case of fibrolamellar carcinoma.

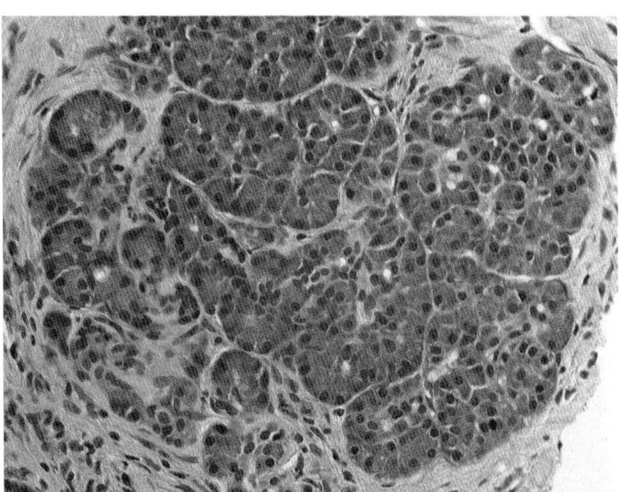

Figure 3.56 Pancreatic acinar cell metaplasia. A cluster of acinar cells were found in the hilum of this transplanted liver.

and often atrophy in the periphery. The nodularity results from an exuberant form of nodular regenerative hyperplasia resulting from a portal vein thrombosis or other blood flow abnormalities.

Pericellular fibrosis

Pericellular fibrosis is a pattern of fibrosis where an irregular mesh like network of fibrosis surrounds hepatocytes (Fig. 3.57). Pericellular fibrosis is typical of fatty liver disease but can also be seen with drug effects, as well as many other conditions. In most cases, pericellular fibrosis is predominately found in zone 3 and often is accompanied by fibrosis of the central vein. However, in some uncommon conditions, such as fibrosing cholestatic hepatitis C, the pericellular fibrosis can affect zone 1. Sometimes an over-stained trichrome stain can show sinusoidal staining, but the blue tends to not be as crisp as seen with true fibrosis and the staining is much more regular than the irregular staining of true pericellular fibrosis. Another diagnostic pitfall is that Kupffer cells become hyperplastic in the setting of chronic cholestasis and often stain blue on trichrome.
Synonym: Perisinsoidal fibrosis, chicken wire fibrosis (obsolete)

Pericholangitis

Pericholangitis is largely an obsolete term, though there are still some users. Pericholangitis is a bile ductular reaction that has admixed neutrophils. Historically, this term was used before primary sclerosing cholangitis was recognized as a distinct clinicopathological entity, being used to describe the histological changes in the livers of patients with ulcerative colitis and biliary tract disease. Unfortunately, this term has stuck around long after primary sclerosing cholangitis became the accepted term of choice. Even more unfortunately, those who continue to use this term do not appear to agree on what the term means, as evidenced by inconsistent usage. Some authors use it as a synonym for a ductular reaction and others using it as a synonym for small duct primary sclerosing cholangitis. Because of this confusion, the term is probably best avoided entirely.[41]

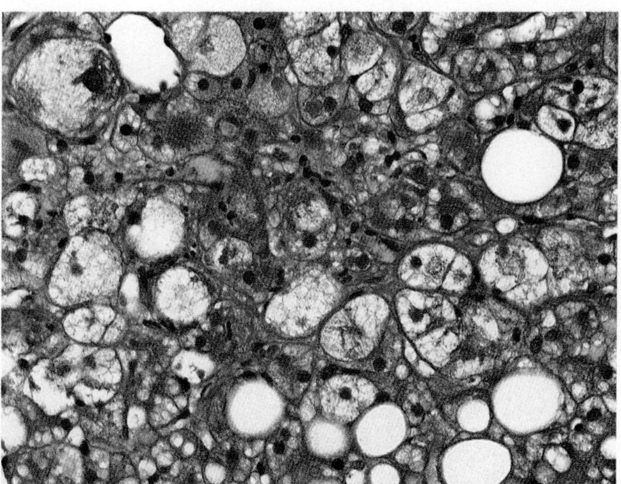

Figure 3.57 Pericellular fibrosis. A trichrome stain shows an irregular network of fibrosis.

Periportal fibrosis

The term *periportal fibrosis* is used inconsistently in both pathology reports and the literature. In older literature, authors attempted to separate chronic hepatitis into the categories of chronic active hepatitis versus chronic persistent hepatitis. In this setting, periportal fibrosis was thought to correlate with chronic active hepatitis and portal fibrosis with chronic persistent hepatitis. The notion of chronic active versus chronic persistent hepatitis has been abandoned, but the use of the terms portal fibrosis versus periportal fibrosis are still used by some pathologists, an interesting relic of the past.

In modern usage, some authors use these terms in a manner reminiscent of the historical literature, with portal fibrosis indicating portal tracts that are expanded by fibrosis, but have smooth borders, whereas periportal fibrosis has irregular borders. When used in this fashion, many illustrated examples of periportal fibrosis appear to represent ordinary portal fibrosis with somewhat brisk interface activity (reflecting the old notion of chronic active hepatitis). Overall, however, periportal fibrosis tends to be used essentially as a synonym for portal fibrosis, with individuals favoring one over the other based on the term used at their training center. Finally, "periportal fibrosis" has a slightly different meaning in the Batts–Ludwig staging system,[42] being defined as portal tracts that have thin, irregular fibrous extensions, or portal tracts with bridging fibrosis, as long as the bridges are rare and thin.

Periportal hepatitis

This term is largely obsolete but was used to describe inflammation at the portal tract-lobule interface, a finding now called interface activity or interface hepatitis. Piecemeal necrosis is another obsolete term for this same histological finding.
Synonym: Interface activity, interface hepatitis, piecemeal necrosis (historical, not in current usage)

Piecemeal necrosis

Piecemeal necrosis is an older and largely obsolete term, replaced by the term *interface activity* or *interface hepatitis*, which describes inflammation involving

the hepatocytes at the limiting plate, immediately adjacent to the portal tracts.
Synonym: Periportal hepatitis, interface activity (preferred), interface hepatitis

Pipestem fibrosis

This term has been used to describe portal-based fibrosis seen with schistosomiasis, where the portal veins become fibrotic and sometimes granulomatous. The portal vein walls become hyalinized, fibrotic, and torturous. In time, the portal veins become completely scarred down and are often accompanied by a reactive proliferation of the hepatic arteries. The entire portal tract can also become fibrotic, with round bulky portal tracts.
Synonym: Symmer's fibrosis, Symmer's pipestem fibrosis, Symmer's clay pipestem fibrosis

Phospholipidosis

Over 50 drugs can cause accumulation of phospholipids in the lysosomes of the liver and other organs, most commonly antidepressants, antimalarial, antianginal, and cholesterol-lowering agents.[43] The Kupffer cells of the liver show abundant foamy cytoplasm (Fig. 3.58). Electron microscopy shows lamellar inclusions within the lysosomes. Phospholipidosis is often accompanied by hepatic steatosis.

Portal hepatitis

Portal hepatitis refers to inflammation within the portal tracts, typically lymphocytic or lymphoplasmacytic. The synonym of portal chronic inflammation is more widely used.
Synonym: Portal chronic inflammation, triaditis

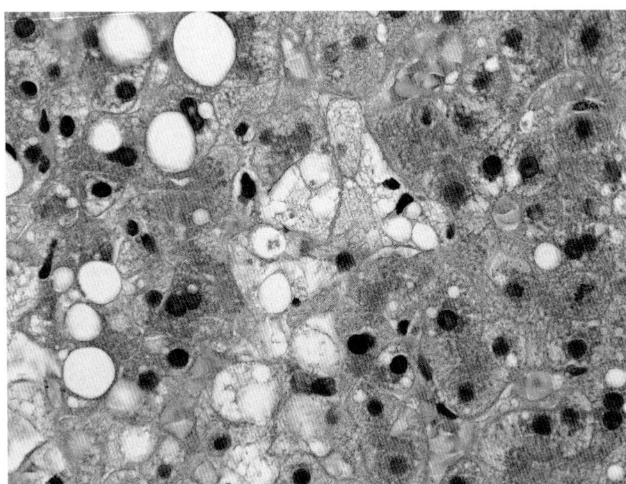

Figure 3.58 Phospholipidosis. The Kupffer cells in the center of the image are very large and foamy.

Portal vein herniation

Normal portal veins are located in the center of the portal tract. However, with noncirrhotic portal hypertension they can extend out of the portal tract into the lobules (Fig. 3.59). This finding can be very subtle and is not entirely specific, but suggests a diagnosis of hepatoportal sclerosis when well developed.

Poulsen lesion/Poulsen–Christoffersen's lesions

This term is hardly ever used anymore, but refers to bile duct lymphocytosis and reactive changes in the bile duct epithelium, seen in either chronic hepatitis C or B, but more commonly in hepatitis C. Classic Poulsen lesions are also associated with a lymphoid aggregate. Similar findings can be seen in wide variety of acute and chronic inflammatory diseases of the liver, where the degree of duct lymphocytosis and injury correlates with the amount of portal inflammation. There is no strong diagnostic or prognostic significance to this finding.

Pseudoacinar

This term is used to describe a growth pattern in hepatic neoplasms, mostly hepatocellular carcinomas. The neoplastic hepatocytes form a circular structure around a centrally dilated lumen. The sizes of pseudoacinar structures vary considerably (Figs. 3.60 and 3.61), from small structures that are similar to pseudorosettes, to large structures resembling glands, to very large structures approaching the size of thyroid follicles.
Synonym: Pseudogland

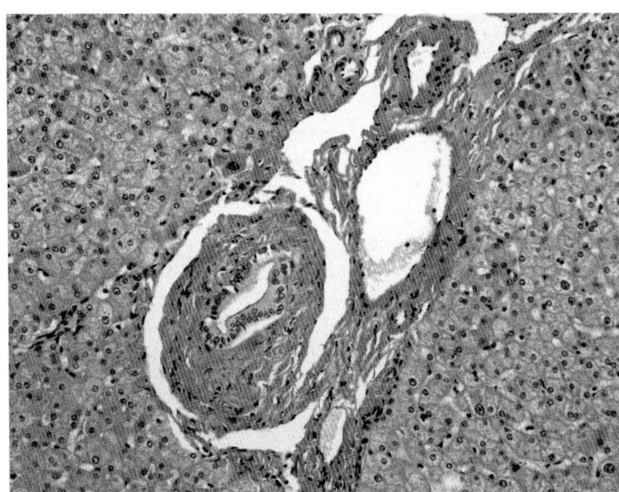

Figure 3.59 Portal vein herniation. The portal vein extends outside the portal tract in this case of noncirrhotic portal hypertension.

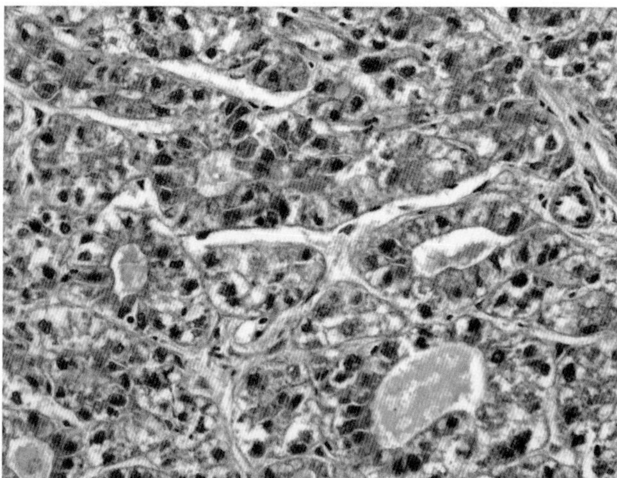

Figure 3.60 Pseudoglands. Small psuedoglands are seen in this hepatocellular carcinoma.

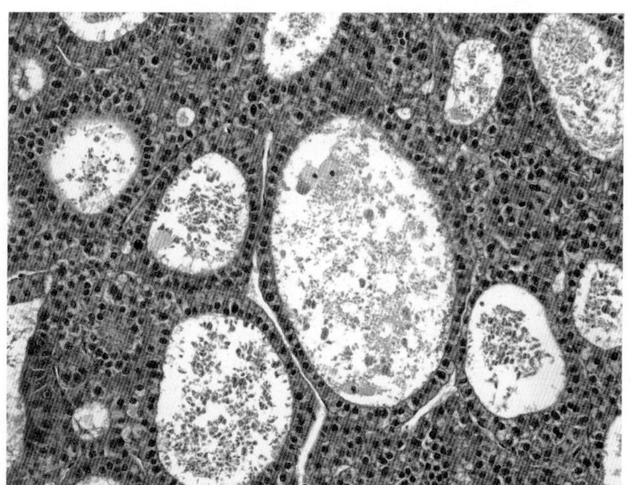

Figure 3.61 Pseudoacini. Large psuedoglands are seen in this hepatocellular carcinoma. Sometimes this pattern is called "follicular-like."

Pseudoground glass inclusions

Large amphophilic cytoplasmic inclusions in hepatocytes are called pseudoground glass when they are negative for hepatitis B surface antigen. The pseudoground glass change is composed of smooth endoplasmic reticulum proliferation and glycogen accumulation and develops in most cases as response to medications. The histological findings in glycogen pseudoground glass are essentially indistinguishable from hepatitis B–related ground glass inclusions on H&E (Fig. 3.62), but are readily distinguished with a HBsAg immunostain.

Synonym: Polyglucosan-like inclusions (polyglucosan body disease is an inherited primarily neurodegenerative disease, so the term "polyglucosan-like inclusions" has perhaps a slight risk of causing confusion)

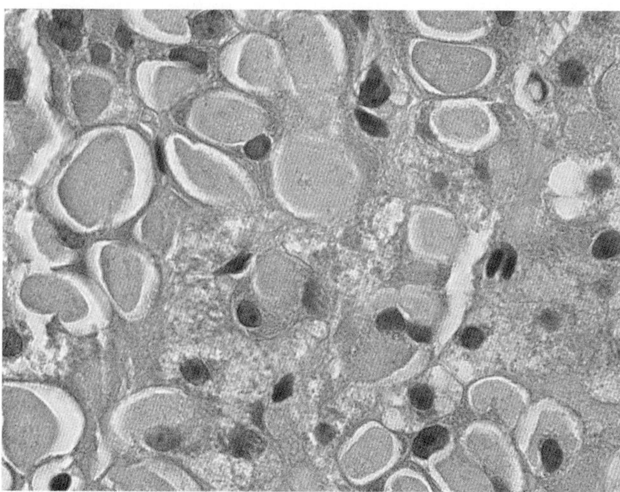

Figure 3.62 Pseudoground glass inclusions. This change was found in the liver of an immunosuppressed patient on many medications.

Pseudorosettes

This term is used to describe small groups of hepatocytes that have formed a circular structure (Fig. 3.63). This finding is thought to represent a regenerative change and is seen most commonly in the setting of either bland cholestasis or a cholestatic hepatitis. The pseudorosettes typically have a small central dilated canalicular structure resembling a lumen.

Pseudoxanthomatous change

Pseudoxanthomatous changes are most commonly seen with chronic cholestasis when hepatocytes, typically in zone 1, develop pale foamy cytoplasm. The swollen cytoplasm of the hepatocytes has some resemblance to lipid laden (xanthomatous) macrophages, thus the

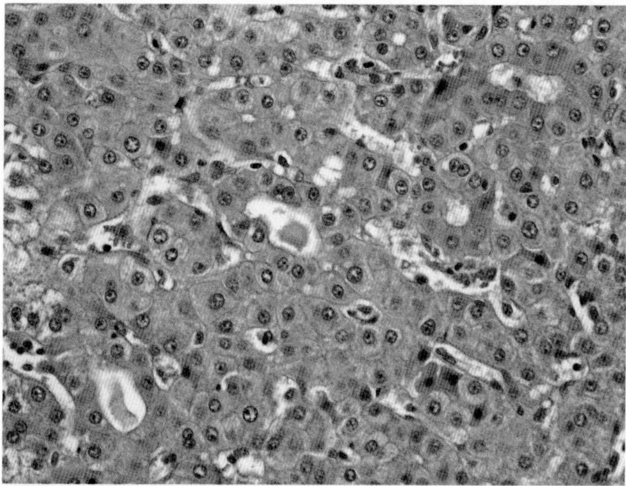

Figure 3.63 Pseudorosettes. Pseudorosettes can develop in the lobules with rapid liver regeneration or with cholestasis, as seen in this case.

term *pseudoxanthomatous*. Although not quite exactly synonyms, the terms pseudoxanthomatous change, feathery degeneration, and cholate stasis are often used interchangeably.

Reticulin loss

Reticulin stains play a key role in separating benign hepatocellular proliferations from hepatocellular carcinoma. In a normal liver, the hepatic cords or plates are thin, with a width of 1 to 3 cells, and essentially every hepatocyte will be touching reticulin on at least one of its borders. In contrast, the hepatic architecture is abnormal in hepatocellular carcinomas and there are large numbers of hepatocytes or discrete foci of hepatocytes that have no associated reticulin (Fig. 3.64). Although the reticulin stain has proven to be a very diagnostically powerful tool, there are rare hepatocellular carcinomas (<1%) that do not have reticulin loss and the diagnosis has to be made using other features. On the other hand, benign liver tissue with fatty change can show focal reticulin loss that can mimic hepatocellular carcinoma.[44] Thus, like with all special stains, the reticulin stain has to be interpreted in the context of the morphology.
Synonym: Reticulin reduction

Rhaboid morphology

The classic definition of a rhabdoid cell is a cell that shows abundant, densely eosinophilic cytoplasm, an amphophilic inclusion in the cytoplasm, and an eccentrically located nucleus with a prominent nucleolus. In many cases, this term is applied even if the cytoplasmic inclusions are not evident (Fig. 3.65).

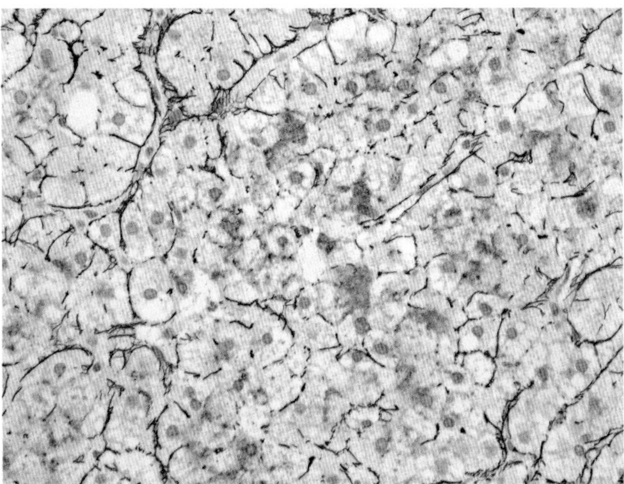

Figure 3.64 Reticulin loss. This hepatocellular carcinoma shows reticulin fragmentation and loss.

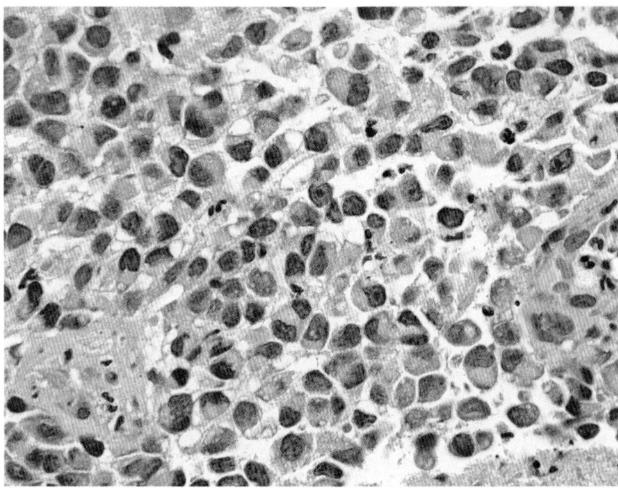

Figure 3.65 Rhabdoid morphology. This rhabdoid tumor of the liver has cells with abundant, eosinophilic, and eccentrically located cytoplasm.

Rhabdoid tumors of the liver show loss of INI1 nuclear expression.
Synonym: Rhabdoid change

Riedel lobe

A Riedel lobe is a gross anatomic term that describes a projection of the anterior right lobe of the liver that extends inferiorly, typically with the gallbladder along its left border, into the right flank and/or iliac fossa. Grossly, the lobe can be either tongue-like or like an upside down pyramid, with its top pointing down. The lobe can either lie anteriorly to the hepatic flexure or can displace the hepatic flexure. A Riedel lobe is a fairly common anatomic variant, with a prevalence of about 9%, and is overall more common in women.[4] A Riedel lobe is classified by some but not all authors as an accessory lobe. Clinically, it can sometimes be mistaken for a mass lesion.

Sanded glass nuclei

If nuclei in hepatocytes are found to have finely granular eosinophilic inclusions, they are called sanded glass nuclei. The inclusions largely fill the nucleus (Fig. 3.66). Sanded glass nuclei can be seen in liver specimens with chronic hepatitis B, where the inclusions represent accumulation of HBcAg. However, sanded glass nuclei are not sensitive for hepatitis B infection, being found only in a subset of individuals, usually with very high viral loads. Nor are sanded glass nuclei specific for chronic hepatitis B, being found occasionally in other diseases, including drug effects and hepatitis delta.

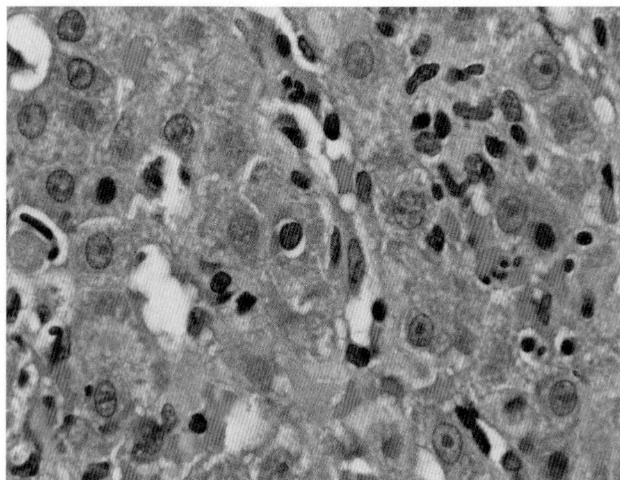

Figure 3.66 Sanded glass nuclei. The nucleus in the hepatocyte in the center of the image shows a homogenous glassy change.

Small cell change

Small cell change can be a precursor for hepatocellular carcinoma. This term describes small discrete aggregates of hepatocytes with reduced amounts of cytoplasm and slightly enlarged nuclei, leading to an increased N:C ratio. There is often mild nuclear hyperchromasia, but the foci is otherwise without significant nuclear atypia (Fig. 3.67). These foci tend to have higher proliferative rates but there should be no loss of reticulin. Molecular studies have shown chromosomal damage and other DNA changes consistent with a precursor to hepatocellular carcinoma. *Synonym: Small cell dysplasia*

Spotty necrosis

Spotty necrosis describes scattered single acidophil bodies in the hepatic lobules. These spotty foci of necrosis can be associated with a few inflammatory cells and/or Kupffer cells. In fact, in some cases all you see are small foci of a few lymphocytes and Kupffer cells, without the actual acidophil bodies being visible, a finding also referred to as "tombstones" because they mark the sites of hepatocyte death.

Steatosis

The synonyms steatosis and fatty change can be used interchangeably, though the term *steatosis* is more commonly used than the term *fatty change* in microscopic descriptions ("fat" retains its English roots, whereas "steatosis" is a new Latin term, with Greek roots). Steatosis is further divided into microvesicular steatosis or macrovesicular steatosis. In microvesicular steatosis, hepatocytes are normal in size, but their cytoplasm is diffusely filled by numerous small droplets of fat, which sometimes can be barely visible at the resolution of light microscopy. The hepatocyte nuclei are centrally located. In contrast, hepatocytes with macrovesicular steatosis have a single large droplet of fat that fills the entire cell cytoplasm, displacing the nucleus to the side (Fig. 3.68).

Of note, in most diseases with macrovesicular steatosis, there is a full range of fat droplet sizes, from tiny to medium to large (Fig. 3.69), but the histological focus should be the predominant pattern. For this reason, statements such as "mixed micro and macrovesicular steatosis" are almost always accurate but are almost never helpful, other than helping the pathologists to feel good about documenting everything, but at the expense of creating potential confusion among clinicians and patients, who can be left wondering how the changes are different than ordinary fatty liver disease. Of course pathologists know they are

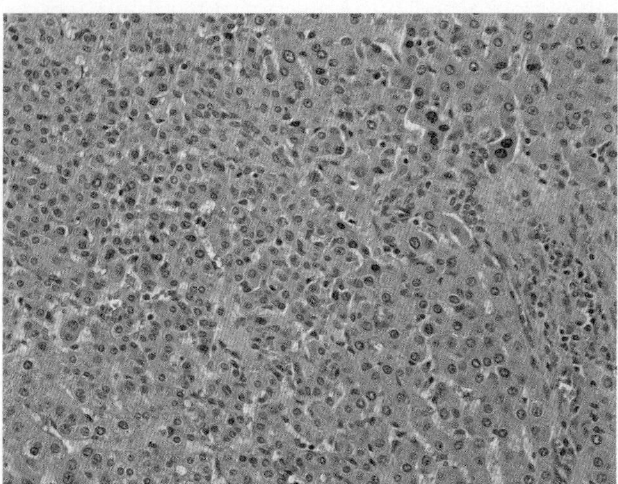

Figure 3.67 Small cell change. The hepatocytes are small, giving an increased N:C ratio, but show no significant cytological atypia.

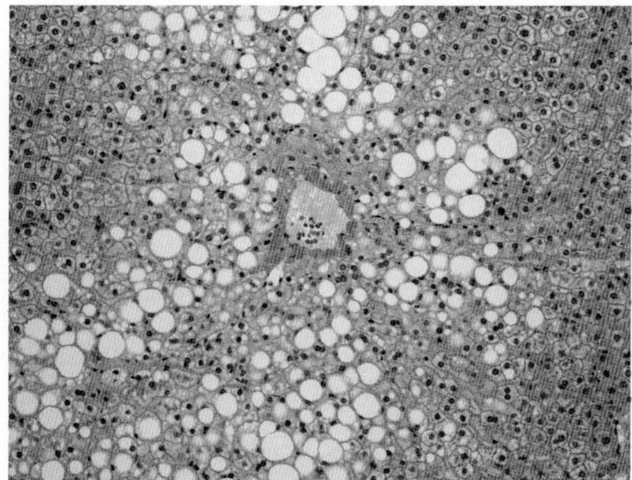

Figure 3.68 Macrovesicular steatosis. The macrovesicular steatosis involves zone 3 in this case of metabolic syndrome associated fatty liver disease.

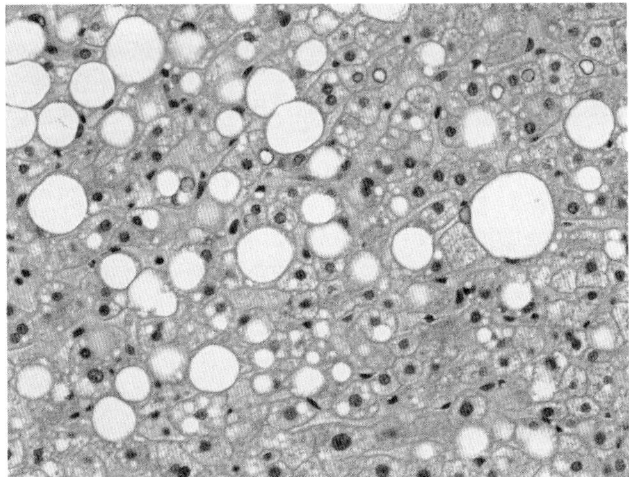

Figure 3.69 Macrovesicular steatosis. The hepatocytes show steatosis with varying-sized droplets.

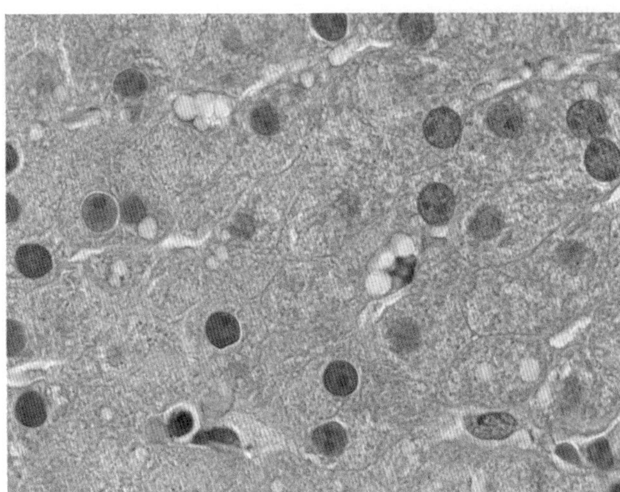

Figure 3.70 Stellate cell hyperplasia. In this case of hypervitaminosis A, the stellate cells have multiple tiny vacuoles in their cytoplasm.

not, as the big droplets of fat have to come from somewhere and they come from smaller droplets of fat, an observation often less clear to nonpathologists.
Synonym: Fatty change

Stellate cell

Stellate cells are pericytes found in the space of Disse. They have dendritic processes that extend around the liver sinusoids. Normally they store vitamin A, and probably have many other functions we are not aware of, but when activated they are thought to be major drivers of fibrosis. Stellate cells were previously called Ito cells, named after Toshio Ito, a Japanese Professor of Anatomy, who described them and differentiated them from Kupffer cells in 1951. Hepatic stellate cells were first described by von Kupffer in 1898, but he believed they were phagocytic cells.[45] Stellate cells are not visible in the normal liver, but can be seen with hypervitaminosis A as small sinusoidal cells with multiple tiny vacuoles that indent the nucleus (Fig. 3.70). When activated, they become more spindled shape, lose their lipids, and express smooth muscle actin.
Synonym (historical): Ito cell

Triaditis

This term is somewhat dated but refers generically to inflammation in the portal tract.
Synonym: Portal chronic inflammation

von Meyenburg complex

A von Meyenburg complex is a hamartomatous tangle of bile ducts, affecting the smaller branches of the biliary tree. Named after a Swiss pathologist Hanns von Meyenburg (1887 to 1971), chair of pathology at Zurich, this benign lesion can be sporadic or associated with polycystic kidney/liver disease. See also entries for bile duct plate malformation and bile duct hamartoma.
Synonym: Bile duct plate malformation, bile duct hamartoma

Zones 1, 2, 3

The area of the lobules that surround the portal tracts is called zone 1, whereas the lobular areas around the central veins are called zone 3. The area in between is called zone 2. The width of the zones is not precisely defined, but generally is assumed to divide the space from the portal tract to the central vein into three approximately equal zones.
Synonym: Rappaport zones

REFERENCES

1. Koga C, Murakami M, Shimizu J, et al. A case of extrahepatic hepatocellular cancer discovered during gynecological laparoscopic surgery. *Gan To Kagaku Ryoho*. 2015;42(12):1866–1868.
2. Leone N, De Paolis P, Carrera M, et al. Ectopic liver and hepatocarcinogenesis: report of three cases with four years' follow-up. *Eur J Gastroenterol Hepatol*. 2004;16(8):731–735.
3. Arakawa M, Kimura Y, Sakata K, et al. Propensity of ectopic liver to hepatocarcinogenesis: case reports and a review of the literature. *Hepatology*. 1999;29(1):57–61.
4. Glenisson M, Salloum C, Lim C, et al. Accessory liver lobes: anatomical description and clinical implications. *J Visc Surg*. 2014;151(6):451–455.

5. Uchida T, Kao H, Quispe-Sjogren M, et al. Alcoholic foamy degeneration--a pattern of acute alcoholic injury of the liver. *Gastroenterology*. 1983;84(4):683–692.
6. Lackner C, Gogg-Kamerer M, Zatloukal K, et al. Ballooned hepatocytes in steatohepatitis: the value of keratin immunohistochemistry for diagnosis. *J Hepatol*. 2008;48(5):821–828.
7. Guy CD, Suzuki A, Burchette JL, et al. Costaining for keratins 8/18 plus ubiquitin improves detection of hepatocyte injury in nonalcoholic fatty liver disease. *Hum Pathol*. 2012;43(6):790–800.
8. Kurumaya H, Terada T, Nakanuma Y. "Metaplastic lesions" in intrahepatic bile ducts in hepatolithiasis: a histochemical and immunohistochemical study. *J Gastroenterol Hepatol*. 1990;5(5):530–536.
9. Wu TT, Levy M, Correa AM, et al. Biliary intraepithelial neoplasia in patients without chronic biliary disease: analysis of liver explants with alcoholic cirrhosis, hepatitis C infection, and noncirrhotic liver diseases. *Cancer*. 2009;115(19):4564–4575.
10. Tobe K. Electron microscopy of liver lesions in primary biliary cirrhosis. I. Intrahepatic bile duct oncocytes. *Acta Pathol Jpn*. 1982;32(1):57–70.
11. Roskams TA, Theise ND, Balabaud C, et al. Nomenclature of the finer branches of the biliary tree: canals, ductules, and ductular reactions in human livers. *Hepatology*. 2004;39(6):1739–1745.
12. Altamirano J, Miquel R, Katoonizadeh A, et al. A histologic scoring system for prognosis of patients with alcoholic hepatitis. *Gastroenterology*. 2014;146(5):1231–1239.e1-6.
13. Popper H, Kent G, Stein R. Ductular cell reaction in the liver in hepatic injury. *J Mt Sinai Hosp N Y*. 1957;24(5):551–556.
14. Popper H. The relation of mesenchymal cell products to hepatic epithelial systems. *Prog Liver Dis*. 1990;9:27–38.
15. Lefkowitch JH. Bile ductular cholestasis: an ominous histopathologic sign related to sepsis and "cholangitis lenta". *Hum Pathol*. 1982;13(1):19–24.
16. Koskinas J, Gomatos IP, Tiniakos DG, et al. Liver histology in ICU patients dying from sepsis: a clinico-pathological study. *World J Gastroenterol*. 2008;14(9):1389–1393.
17. De Groote J, Gerber M, Hoofnagle JH, et al. A classification of chronic hepatitis. *Lancet*. 1968;2(7568):626–628.
18. Duffin JM. Why does cirrhosis belong to Laennec? *CMAJ*. 1987;137(5):393–396.
19. Moreira RK, Chopp W, Washington MK. The concept of hepatic artery-bile duct parallelism in the diagnosis of ductopenia in liver biopsy samples. *Am J Surg Pathol*. 2011;35(3):392–403.
20. Gill RM, Belt P, Wilson L, et al. Centrizonal arteries and microvessels in nonalcoholic steatohepatitis. *Am J Surg Pathol*. 2011;35(9):1400–1404.
21. Harrison RF, Hubscher SG. The spectrum of bile duct lesions in end-stage primary sclerosing cholangitis. *Histopathology*. 1991;19(4):321–327.
22. Ludwig J, MacCarty RL, LaRusso NF, et al. Intrahepatic cholangiectases and large-duct obliteration in primary sclerosing cholangitis. *Hepatology*. 1986;6(4):560–568.
23. Wendum D, Barbu V, Rosmorduc O, et al. Aspects of liver pathology in adult patients with MDR3/ABCB4 gene mutations. *Virchows Arch*. 2012;460(3):291–298.
24. Nakanuma Y, Ohta G, Takeshita H, et al. Florid duct lesions and extensive bile duct loss of the intrahepatic biliary tree in chronic liver diseases other than primary biliary cirrhosis. *Acta Pathol Jpn*. 1983;33(6):1095–1104.
25. Jain D, Robert ME, Navarro V, et al. Total fibrous obliteration of main portal vein and portal foam cell venopathy in chronic hepatic allograft rejection. *Arch Pathol Lab Med*. 2004;128(1):64–67.
26. Abraham S, Furth EE. Receiver operating characteristic analysis of glycogenated nuclei in liver biopsy specimens: quantitative evaluation of their relationship with diabetes and obesity. *Hum Pathol*. 1994;25(10):1063–1068.
27. Wanless IR, Nakashima E, Sherman M. Regression of human cirrhosis. Morphologic features and the genesis of incomplete septal cirrhosis. *Arch Pathol Lab Med*. 2000;124(11):1599–1607.
28. Schinoni MI, Andrade Z, de Freitas LA, et al. Incomplete septal cirrhosis: an enigmatic disease. *Liver Int*. 2004;24(5):452–456.
29. Jung T, Bader N, Grune T. Lipofuscin: formation, distribution, and metabolic consequences. *Ann N Y Acad Sci*. 2007;1119:97–111.
30. Schmucker DL. Age-related changes in liver structure and function: implications for disease? *Exp Gerontol*. 2005;40(8–9):650–659.
31. Schirmacher P, Dienes HP, Moll R. De novo expression of nonhepatocellular cytokeratins in Mallory body formation. *Virchows Arch*. 1998;432(2):143–152.
32. Stumptner C, Fuchsbichler A, Zatloukal K, et al. In vitro production of Mallory bodies and intracellular hyaline bodies: the central role of sequestosome 1/p62. *Hepatology*. 2007;46(3):851–860.
33. Lowe J, Blanchard A, Morrell K, et al. Ubiquitin is a common factor in intermediate filament inclusion bodies of diverse type in man, including those of Parkinson's disease, Pick's disease, and Alzheimer's disease, as well as Rosenthal fibres in cerebellar astrocytomas, cytoplasmic bodies in muscle, and

mallory bodies in alcoholic liver disease. *J Pathol.* 1988;155(1):9–15.
34. Lautenschlager I, Halme L, Höckerstedt K, et al. Cytomegalovirus infection of the liver transplant: virological, histological, immunological, and clinical observations. *Transpl Infect Dis.* 2006;8(1):21–30.
35. Lamps LW, Pinson CW, Raiford DS, et al. The significance of microabscesses in liver transplant biopsies: a clinicopathological study. *Hepatology.* 1998;28(6):1532–1537.
36. Fauerholdt L, Schlichting P, Christensen E, et al. Conversion of micronodular cirrhosis into macronodular cirrhosis. *Hepatology.* 1983;3(6):928–931.
37. Fraser JL, Antonioli DA, Chopra S, et al. Prevalence and nonspecificity of microvesicular fatty change in the liver. *Mod Pathol.* 1995;8(1):65–70.
38. Le TH, Caldwell SH, Redick JA, et al. The zonal distribution of megamitochondria with crystalline inclusions in nonalcoholic steatohepatitis. *Hepatology.* 2004;39(5):1423–1429.
39. Kuo FY, Swanson PE, Yeh MM. Pancreatic acinar tissue in liver explants: a morphologic and immunohistochemical study. *Am J Surg Pathol.* 2009;33(1):66–71.
40. Terada T, Nakanuma Y, Kakita A. Pathologic observations of intrahepatic peribiliary glands in 1000 consecutive autopsy livers. Heterotopic pancreas in the liver. *Gastroenterology.* 1990;98(5 Pt 1):1333–1337.
41. Ludwig J. Small-duct primary sclerosing cholangitis. *Semin Liver Dis.* 1991;11(1):11–17.
42. Batts KP, Ludwig J. Chronic hepatitis. An update on terminology and reporting. *Am J Surg Pathol.* 1995;19(12):1409–1417.
43. Donato MT, Gomez-Lechon MJ. Drug-induced liver steatosis and phospholipidosis: cell-based assays for early screening of drug candidates. *Curr Drug Metab.* 2012;13(8):1160–1173.
44. Singhi AD, Jain D, Kakar S, et al. Reticulin loss in benign fatty liver: an important diagnostic pitfall when considering a diagnosis of hepatocellular carcinoma. *Am J Surg Pathol.* 2012;36(5):710–715.
45. Suematsu M, Aiso S. Professor Toshio Ito: a clairvoyant in pericyte biology. *Keio J Med.* 2001;50(2):66–71.

4

Immunohistochemistry and special stains in liver pathology

Michael S. Torbenson, MD

4.1 OVERVIEW

This chapter considers special stains used in medical liver specimens and is organized into the following sections: up-front stains, stains used to work up injury patterns, and miscellaneous stains used in the practice of medical liver pathology. Of course, stains are very important in tumor evaluation too, and they are covered in detail in their respective chapters.

4.2 UP-FRONT STAINS

There is little or no data on the stains that should be ordered up-front on every medical liver biopsy. In general, different pathologists use different up-front stains based on their training and the local practices. The up-front stains can range from a very limited panel of one hematoxylin and eosin stain (H&E) and a trichrome stain, to a comprehensive panel of multiple H&Es, trichrome, iron, periodic acid Schiff without diastase (PAS), periodic acid Schiff with diastase (PASD), copper, and reticulin stains. Which end is better? Perhaps neither is perfect as a routine up-front panel. One reasonable approach is shown in Table 4.1.

H&E stains are critical and should be ordered on every case. Empiric experience provides compelling evidence that two H&E stains are better than one. Almost all pathologists can recall cases where a critical lesion was only identified on one of the H&Es.

Table 4.1 Routine up-front stains in medical liver pathology

Stain	Use in routine practice
H&E × 2	Every case
Trichrome (or similar)	Every case
Iron	Baseline biopsy, others as needed
PASD	Baseline biopsy, others as needed
Reticulin	As needed based on H&E findings
PAS	As needed based on H&E findings

Trichrome stain overview

Trichrome stains, or similar connective tissue stains such as Sirous Red, are critical for evaluating fibrosis. In resource-limited environments, a reasonable alternative approach is to cut additional blanks when the H&E is cut so that a trichrome stain can be ordered if needed. Cutting additional blanks at the same time as the blank for the H&E is cut is important, because there can be substantial tissue lost each time the block is faced in histology. There are a few situations where a trichrome stain is not necessary. First, if the H&E clearly shows established cirrhosis, then the trichrome stain is unnecessary. Second, follow-up biopsies performed soon after an initial biopsy may not need a trichrome. This situation arises most clearly in the transplant setting, where some centers will perform a follow-up biopsy to evaluate for response to therapy within days to weeks after an initial biopsy that showed acute cellular rejection. In this setting, a trichrome stain on the follow-up biopsy is rarely needed.

Iron stain overview

Iron stains are critical tools to look for iron overload. The Perls iron stain is fairly sensitive and very specific for detecting hemosiderin. It is the most widely used stain for iron evaluation, and most centers perform this stain on every medical liver biopsy. The Perls iron stain can also highlight ferritin as a light blue cytoplasmic blush, but this can be ignored and attention is focused on the granular deposits of hemosiderin.

In resource-limited environments, it would not be unreasonable to examine the H&E carefully and then order an iron stain if there is visible pigment on the H&E that suggests iron, if the serum ferritin is significantly elevated (>1,000), transferrin saturation is 45% or greater, or there are other clinical reasons to be concerned about iron overload disease. This approach admittedly would miss almost all biopsies with minimal iron accumulation and many biopsies with mild iron accumulation. However, minimal to mild iron accumulation in most cases has no clinical significance.

For clinical purposes, the amount of iron can be reported either descriptively (minimal, mild, moderate, marked) or by using a numerical system (0, 1+, 2+, 3+, 4+). In 1962, Scheuer proposed one of the first grading systems for evaluating hepatic iron using the Perls iron stain. Many additional iron grading systems have been proposed over the years, all providing largely similar semiquantitative data. The different systems vary in their approach, with some systems scoring the iron stain by the zonation of hemosiderin distribution, some systems scoring by the lowest magnification that discernable granules of hemosiderin can be seen, and some by the percent of hepatocytes positive for hemosiderin. Is one system clearly the best for clinical care? Not really, as they all seem to work fine. After all, hemosiderin accumulation has the greatest clinical relevance when it is moderate or marked, levels that are captured well by all grading systems. A numerical system is important in research studies, so the authors can do statistical analysis and generate a figure for the paper. However, for routine clinical care, a numerical grade is not necessary and your report will be perfectly fine using descriptors ("mild," "moderate," etc.) and the iron location (hepatocellular vs. Kupffer cell). Nonetheless, there are many reasonable grading systems to choose from if you prefer.

Reticulin stain overview

In medical liver biopsies, reticulin stains are most helpful in identifying nodular regenerative hyperplasia (Fig. 4.1). Nodular regenerative hyperplasia represents a continuum of changes, easy to diagnose when well developed, and equally easy to over diagnose when not. If there isn't clear nodularity on the H&E, make a diagnosis of nodular regenerative hyperplasia with caution. By definition, there should be no significant fibrosis, in particular bridging or worse. Some mild portal fibrosis can be seen in occasional cases. It's also worth checking the liver enzymes, looking for a disproportional elevation in alkaline phosphatase levels, a pattern typically found with nodular regenerative hyperplasia.

Some pathologists also find reticulin stains helpful in separating bridging necrosis from bridging fibrosis, with bridging necrosis showing reticulin fibers, which result from the collapsed and compressed reticulin meshwork normally present in the lobules. In contrast, fibrosis will have less reticulin deposits. However, most pathologists use the H&E and the trichrome to make this distinction. In the workup of well-differentiated hepatocellular neoplasms, reticulin stains play a critical role in separating benign from malignant hepatocellular proliferations.

Periodic acid Schiff without diastase overview

A PAS stain without diastase highlights glycogen but is not very helpful for most diagnostic purposes. Some individuals find the stain helpful to identify foci of lobular necrosis, which will stand out against the PAS-positive hepatocytes (Fig. 4.2). Another use is in the workup for ground-glass-type changes in the hepatocytes, where a negative PAS stain suggests fibrinogen storage disease.

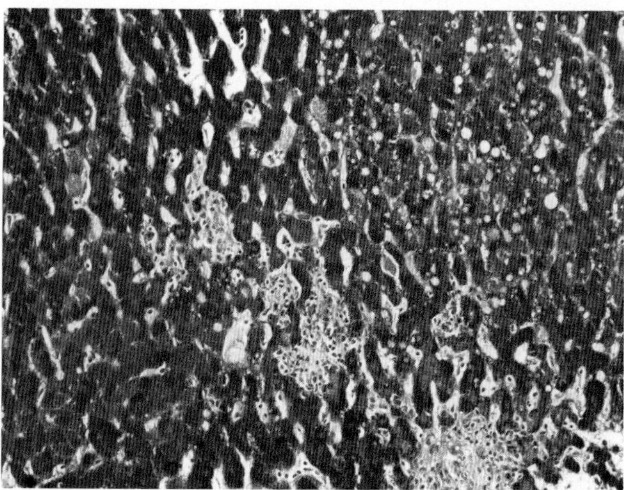

Figure 4.2 PAS stain. Scattered foci of lobular inflammation stand out against the PAS stain.

Periodic acid Schiff with diastase overview

PASD stains are helpful in identifying the intrahepatic globules of α-1-antitrypsin deficiency (Fig. 4.3). The globules can be easily overlooked on H&E, but are nicely highlighted on a PASD stain. They typically have a periportal distribution in noncirrhotic livers, but can be patchy, so the entire slide should be examined. Although not necessary, PASD stains also nicely highlight macrophages in areas of lobular inflammation (Fig. 4.4). Finally, PASD stains can highlight small Kupffer cell globules composed of

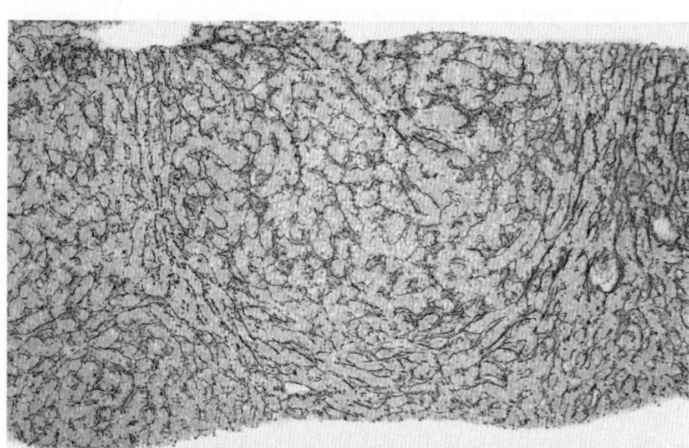

Figure 4.1 Reticulin stain. Nodular regenerative hyperplasia. The nodularity results from zones of atrophic hepatocytes juxtaposed with those that are normal in size and form ill-defined nodules.

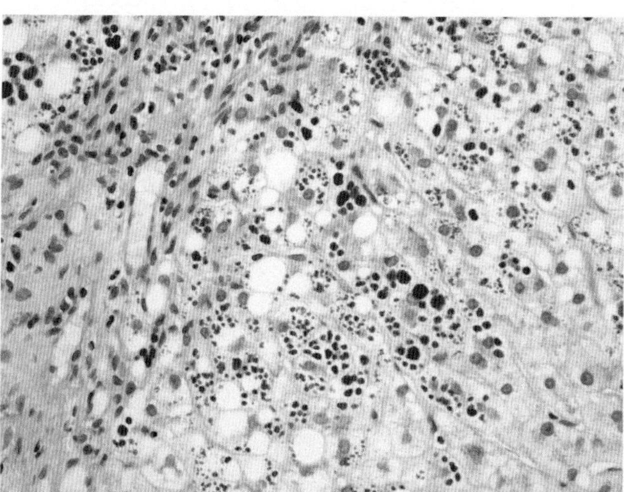

Figure 4.3 PASD stain. Numerous globules of α-1-antitrypsin are seen in this case; most biopsies don't have so many globules.

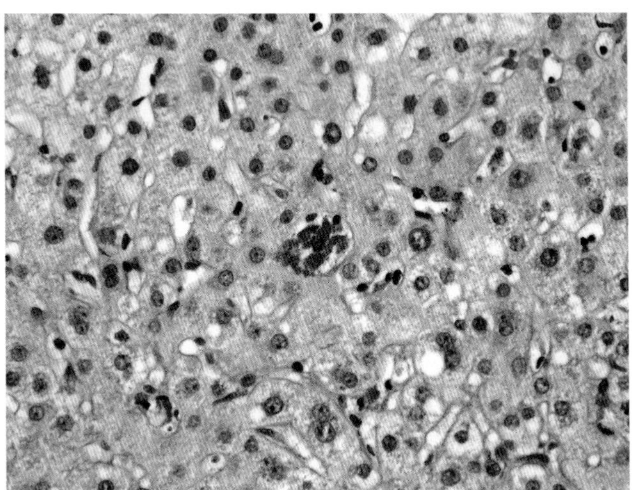

Figure 4.4 PASD stain. Scattered foci of lobular macrophages are highlighted.

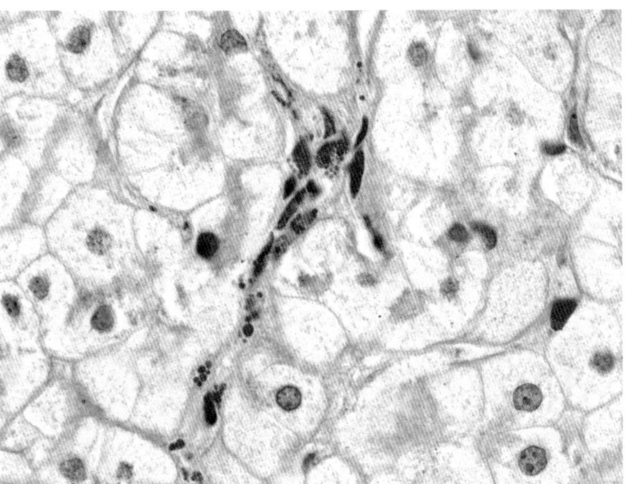

Figure 4.5 PASD stain. Small globules composed of immunoglobulins are seen in the Kupffer cell cytoplasm of this biopsy, which also showed autoimmune hepatitis.

immunoglobulin in the setting of autoimmune hepatitis (Fig. 4.5), primary biliary cirrhosis, or other diseases with hypergammaglobulinemia.

4.3 STAINS USED TO EVALUATE INJURY PATTERNS

Chronic cholestatic liver disease

Ductopenia

Bile duct loss is best assessed using a keratin stain. As a stand-alone stain, CK AE 1/3 works well, but CK7 works just as well for bile duct loss and also highlights intermediate hepatocytes, a typical feature found with ductopenia. As a general rule of thumb, at least 50% of the portal tracts should lack bile ducts to confidently diagnose ductopenia. The alkaline phosphatase will be disproportionately elevated, a useful additional piece of information before making a diagnosis of ductopenia.

Chronic cholestasis

There are two primary stains used to support a diagnosis of chronic cholestatic liver disease: the rhodanine copper stain and the CK7 immunostain. Both are useful in noncirrhotic livers, but in cirrhotic livers these stains are not specific for biliary tract disease.

Copper is normally excreted in the bile. With chronic cholestasis, copper accumulates in the lysosomes of periportal hepatocytes and can be detected with a copper stain (Fig. 4.6). The staining can be very focal, so the stain has to be examined carefully. CK7 is the second stain used to support a diagnosis of chronic cholestasis. CK7 normally stains the bile ducts and bile ductules, but the hepatocytes will be negative. However, in the setting of chronic cholestatic liver disease, CK7 stains the periportal hepatocytes (Fig. 4.7). These positive staining hepatocytes are called intermediate hepatocytes. Often, CK7-positive intermediate hepatocytes are evident on liver biopsies before copper accumulation is found. However, specimens can be negative for CK7 but positive for copper in long-standing, low-grade chronic cholestasis. CK7 and copper stains are often best used together and should always be interpreted in conjunction with the H&E findings. Finally, in congestive hepatopathy, the CK7 positivity in hepatocytes can show a zone 3 distribution (Fig. 4.8).[1]

Inherited chronic cholestatic liver diseases include the progressive familial intrahepatic cholestasis diseases, types 1, 2, and 3. Type 2 is caused by mutation in the *ABCB11* gene, which encodes the bile salt export pump (BSEP) protein. Immunostains for BSEP are not

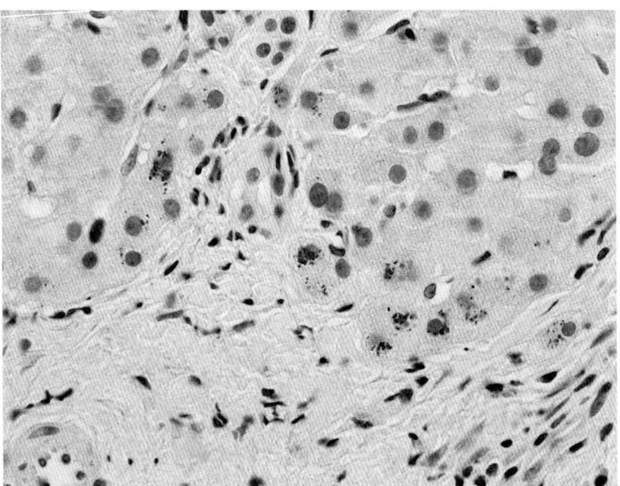

Figure 4.6 Rhodanine. Focal copper deposition is seen in the periportal hepatocytes in this case of primary sclerosing cholangitis.

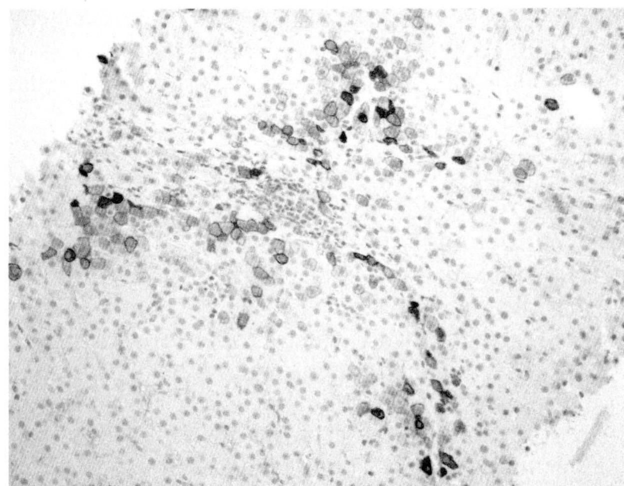

Figure 4.7 CK7 immunostain. Periportal hepatocytes (intermediate hepatocytes) are positive in this case of chronic cholestatic liver disease.

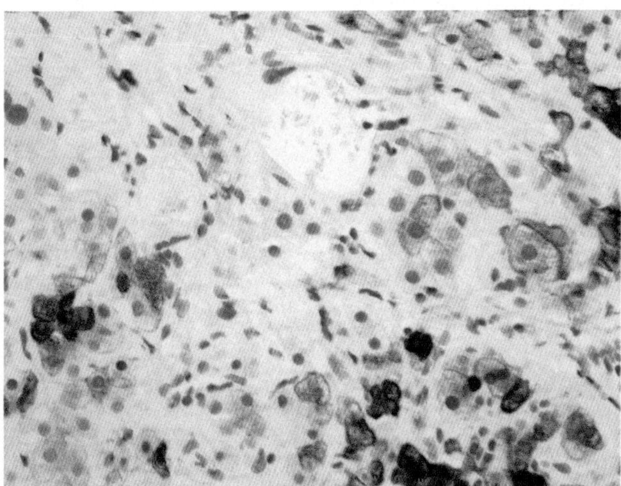

Figure 4.8 CK7 immunostain. The zone 3 hepatocytes are positive in this case of congestive hepatopathy.

widely available, but loss of the normal canalicular staining suggests *ABCB11* mutations. However, loss of staining is not very sensitive or specific, so must be confirmed by sequencing studies.[2–4] Likewise, PFIC3 is caused by mutations in the *ABCB4* gene, which encodes the multiple drug resistance 3 protein. The MDR3 immunostain is also not very sensitive or specific, but loss of canalicular staining suggests *ABCB4* mutations, which can then be confirmed by sequencing studies.

Autoimmune conditions of the liver

Autoimmune hepatitis

The plasma cells in autoimmune hepatitis are primarily immunoglobulin G (IgG)-positive, with much fewer numbers of immunoglobulin G (IgM)-positive plasm cells. In contrast, the portal tracts in primary biliary cirrhosis have equal or greater numbers of IgM-positive plasma cells, compared to IgG.[5] In overlap syndromes, the IgG and IgM levels are generally similar, so immunophenotyping of the plasma cells is not helpful in separating primary biliary cirrhosis alone from an overlap syndrome. PASD stains can highlight small round globules in the Kupffer cells.

Primary biliary cirrhosis

The histological findings in early primary biliary cirrhosis can be very patchy, so additional H&E sections are often very helpful if the initial H&E findings are either almost normal or show only mild, nonspecific changes. Copper stains and CK7 stains are also very helpful in identifying evidence of chronic cholestasis and can be positive even when the H&E findings are almost normal.

As noted above, the portal tracts in primary biliary cirrhosis have equal or greater numbers of IgM-positive plasma cells, compared to IgG. This finding correlates very well with serum findings, where primary biliary cirrhosis is also characterized by elevated serum IgM and IgG levels, whereas autoimmune hepatitis is characterized by elevated serum IgG levels. Immunostains for CD1a (Figs. 4.9 and 4.10) can also be helpful in some cases of primary biliary cirrhosis, because dendritic cells in the inflamed bile ducts can be positive.[6] PASD stains can also highlight small round globules in the Kupffer cells (See Fig. 4.5).

IgG4 disease

Immunostains for IgG4 can be very helpful in diagnosing IgG4 disease involving the liver (Fig. 4.11). However, IgG4-positive plasma cells are not specific

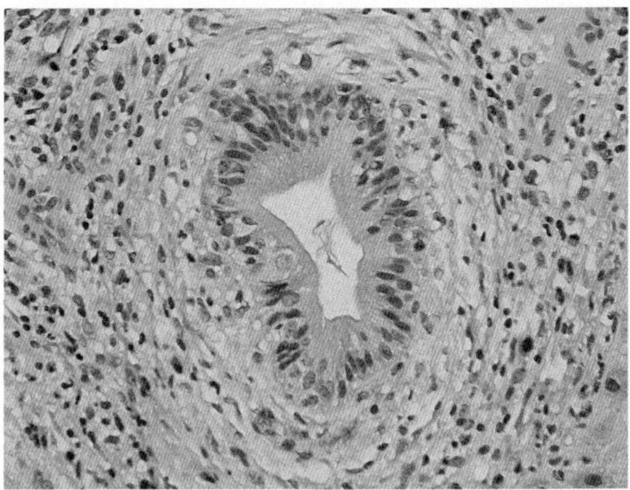

Figure 4.9 Primary biliary cirrhosis. The bile duct shows lymphocytosis and injury (see next picture).

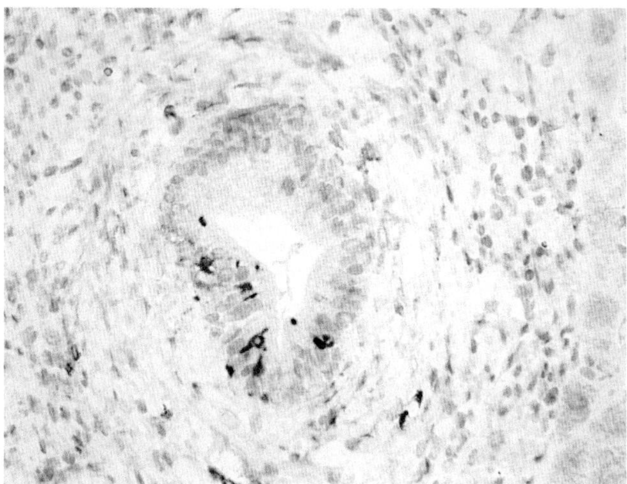

Figure 4.10 CD1a immunostain. Focal staining is seen within a medium-sized bile duct in this case of primary biliary cirrhosis. Same case as previous picture.

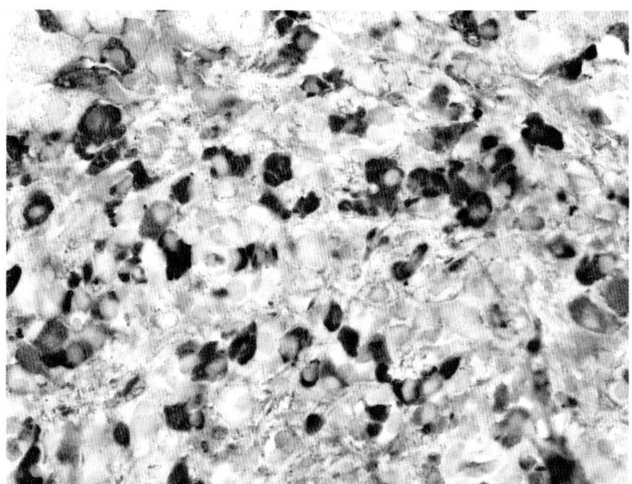

Figure 4.11 IgG4 immunostain. The immunostain shows numerous positive plasma cells in this case of IgG4 disease involving the liver.

for liver involvement by IgG4 disease. A common cutoff is 10 or more positive plasma cells per 40× field, but this approach has to be used with the H&E findings and some common sense. In fact, up to 20% of liver explants with primary sclerosing cholangitis will have IgG4 positivity, with many of them focally showing numbers similar to that seen in IgG4 disease, but with no other features to suggest IgG4 disease.[7]

α-1-antitrpsin deficiency

The PASD stain highlights the globules of α-1-antitrpsin deficiency (Fig. 4.3). The Z allele (MZ or ZZ) is the most common Pi-type associated with accumulation of hepatocyte globules, but the S allele (MS or SS) can develop globules occasionally,[8–11] especially when there is an additional source of liver disease.

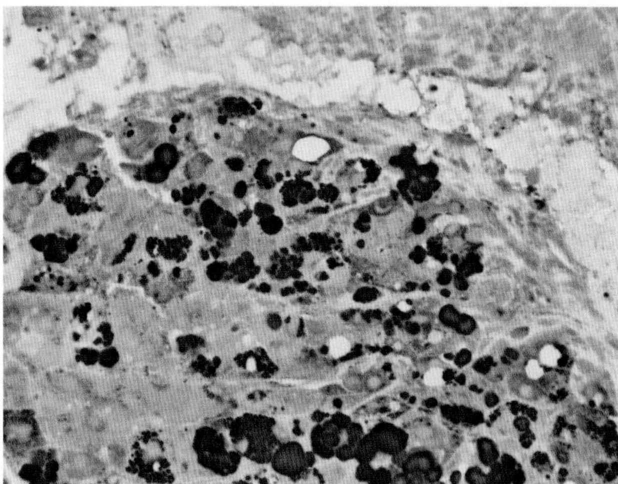

Figure 4.12 Alpha-1-antitrypsin deficiency, immunostain. The globules are nicely highlighted on this immunostain. Same case as Figure 4-3.

The globules can vary in size from very small to large. The globules are most prominent in the zone 1 hepatocytes, but can be found further out in the lobules. Affected hepatocytes will have multiple globules in their cytoplasm. In cases where the globules have unusual morphology or an unusual pattern of distribution, immunostains for α-1-antitrpsin deficiency can be helpful (Fig. 4.12). Of note, infants less than 3 years of ages with α-1-antitrpsin deficiency commonly do not have globules in their hepatocytes. Instead, the liver biopsies often show a cholestatic hepatitis or neonatal giant cell hepatitis pattern. Immunostains can be of some help in this situation, but Pi typing is needed to secure the diagnosis.

Amyloidosis

The Congo red stain is the most important stain for diagnosing amyloid in liver specimens (Figs. 4.13 and 4.14).

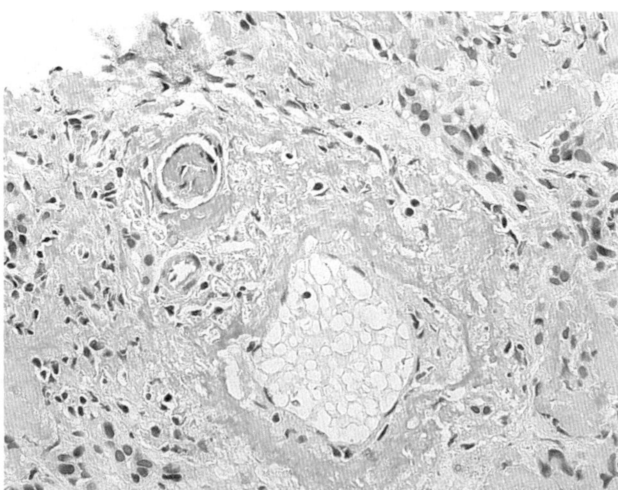

Figure 4.13 Congo red stain. The typical "salmon pink" color is seen in this case of amyloidis.

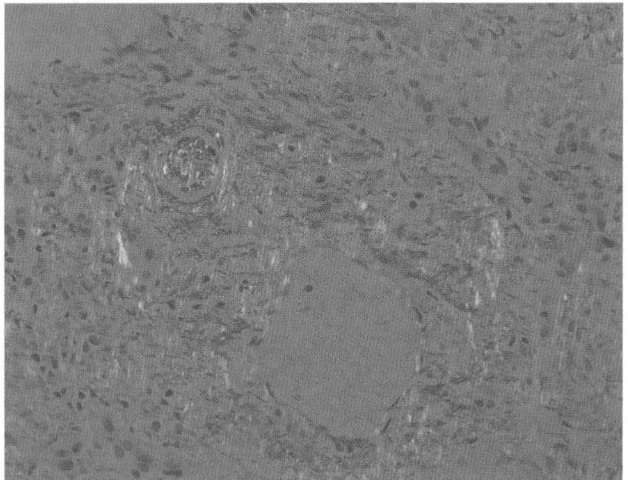

Figure 4.14 Congo red stain. Apple green birefringence is seen with polarization.

Other stains can be used to subtype the amyloid, such as kappa and lambda, but they are challenging to reliably interpret because of extensive background staining. Overall, mass spectrophotometry is the best method for subtyping amyloid.[12] However, immunostains for Lect 2 (Fig. 4.15) can confirm a diagnosis of globular amyloid.[13]

Infections

Fungal stains

Gomori methenamine silver (GMS) stains are important for evaluating granulomas, granulomatous inflammation, and abscesses. Although the GMS stain is performed primarily for identifying fungi, bacteria can also be positive (Fig. 4.16). The stain is always a bit dirty, so needs to be examined carefully. Some pathologists also find the PAS helpful when looking for fungi.

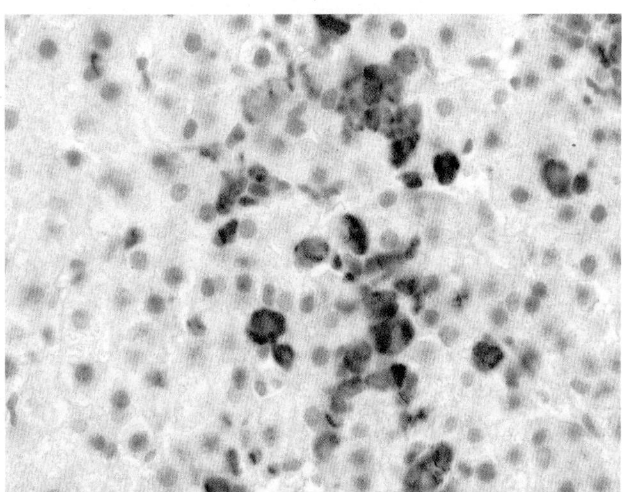

Figure 4.15 LECT 2 immunostain. The stain is strongly positive in this case of LECT amyloidosis (also called globular amyloid).

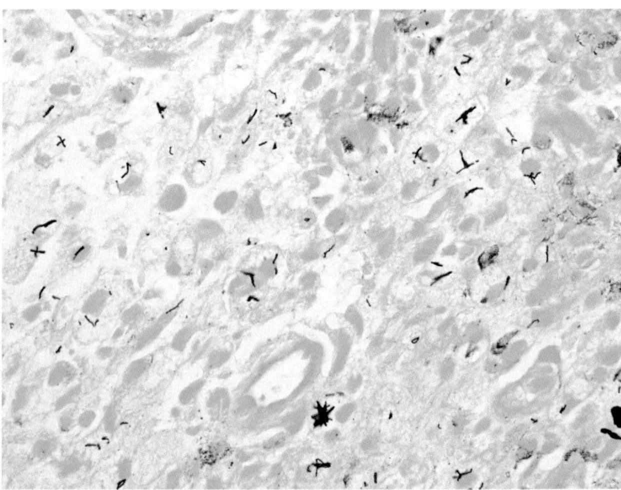

Figure 4.16 GMS stain. The stain is negative for fungi, but highlights bacteria.

Bacterial stains

Acid fast bacilli (AFB) stains are important for evaluating granulomas, especially if they are caseating. The most commonly used stain is the Ziehl–Neelsen stain (organisms red, background blue), but the Kinyoun stain is also widely used (organisms red, background green). The auramine-based stains are reportedly more sensitive than AFB stains but are not in common use.[14] Their major drawback is the need for a fluorescence microscope. The organisms are typically sparse, so the AFB stain should be examined carefully. If there is strong clinical suspicion, a repeat stain can be helpful if the first one is negative. Polymerase chain reaction (PCR) detection is also available in some centers, but there are sensitivity issues and the AFB stains should still be performed. A Fite stain is a type of acid fast stain (Fig. 4.17), used most commonly to detect *Mycobacterium leprae* (leprosy), *Nocardia*, and *Rhodococcus*.

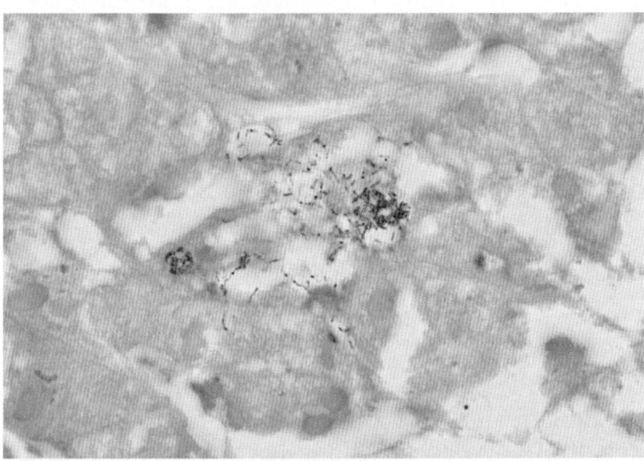

Figure 4.17. Fite stain. The stain is positive in a case of leprosy.

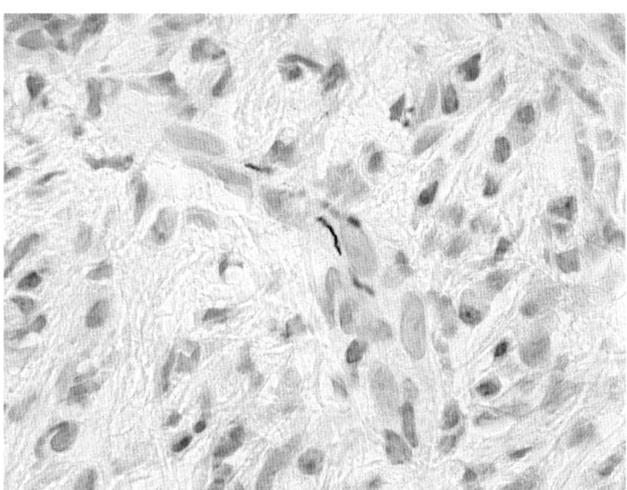

Figure 4.18 *T. pallidum*, immunostain. Organisms are seen within the endothelial cells. This case presented as a pseudotumor of the liver.

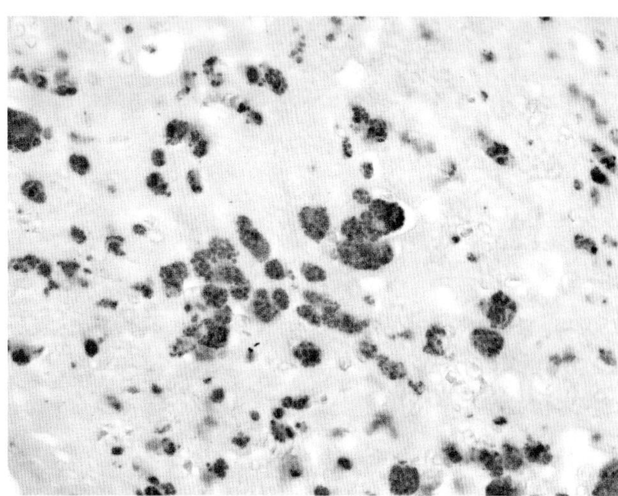

Figure 4.20 Whipples disease. An immunostain is positive (duodenal biopsy).

Syphilis can involve the liver, usually as a pseudotumor.[15] Silver stains such as Warthin–Starry have historically been an important stain in evaluating for the possibility of syphilis. However, silver stains are usually dirty, making them hard to read. They also are not very sensitive. Immunostains for *Treponema pallidum* are much more user friendly and much more sensitive (Fig. 4.18), but can also nonspecifically stain other bacteria, so positive stains need to be followed up by serology. The Warthin–Starry stain is also used to detect *Bartonella henselae*, the organism that causes cat-scratch disease and bacterial peliosis in the liver.

Gram stains and other general bacterial stains can be helpful for evaluating abscesses (Fig. 4.19). The most common organisms found in liver abscesses are streptococcal and Pseudomonas species but mixed bacterial and fungal abscess are not uncommon, so both bacterial and fungal stains are helpful. *Tropheryma whipplei* infections cause Whipple's disease. Liver biopsies in this setting are rare, but PAS stains highlight infected foamy macrophage, located in the portal tracts and lobules. Immunohistochemistry is available at some centers (Fig. 4.20).

Viral stains

There are a number of stains that can detect viral infections. For hepatitis B infection, the hepatitis B surface antigen (HBsAg) and hepatitis B core antigen (HBcAg) immunostains work very well. HBsAg is a cytoplasmic stain that can show various patterns, including scattered single cells, large solid blocks of cells, and in rare cases a membranous staining pattern (Figs. 4.21, 4.22, and 4.23). The immunostain for

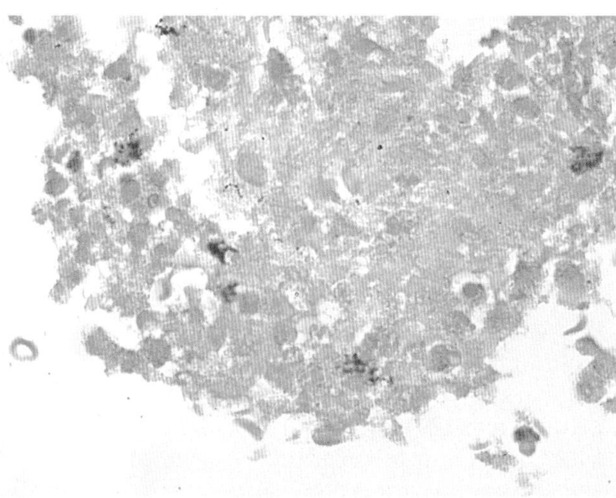

Figure 4.19 Gram–Weigart stain. Gram-positive organism are present in this liver abscess.

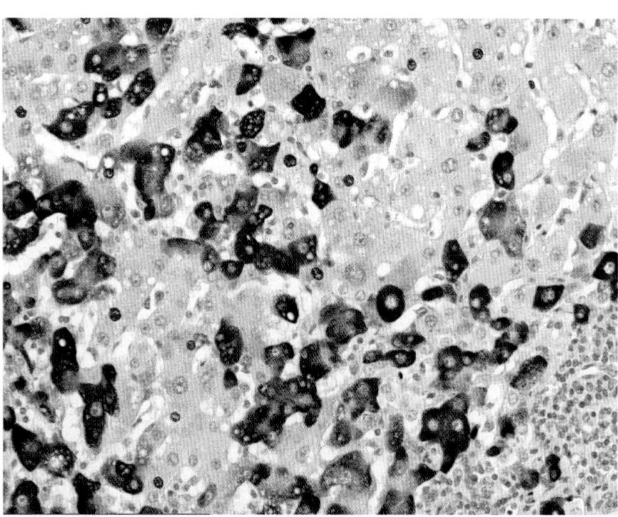

Figure 4.21 HBsAg. Scattered single cells are positive.

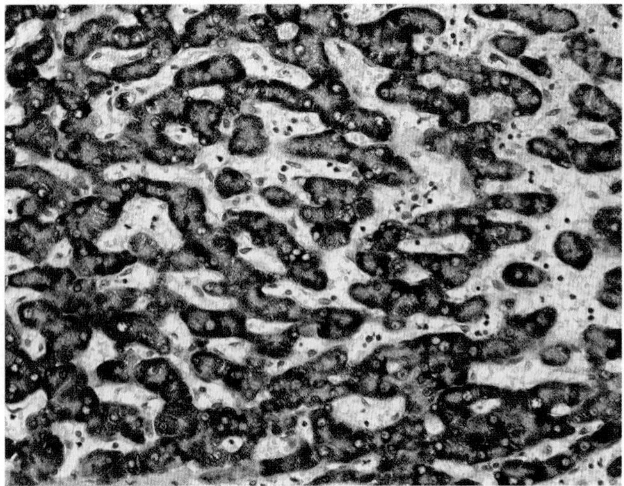

Figure 4.22 HBsAg. A large contiguous block of cells are positive.

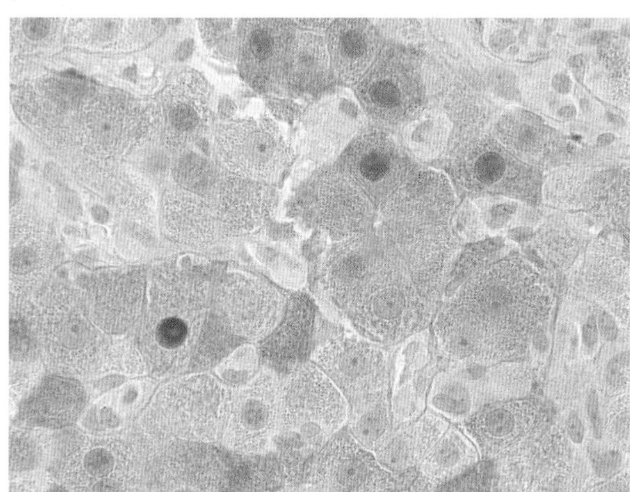

Figure 4.24 HBcAg. Both nuclear and cytoplasmic staining is seen.

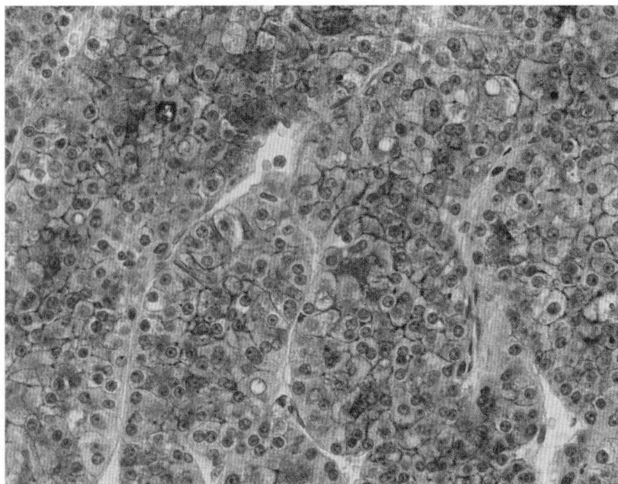

Figure 4.23 HBsAg. Membranous staining can also be seen.

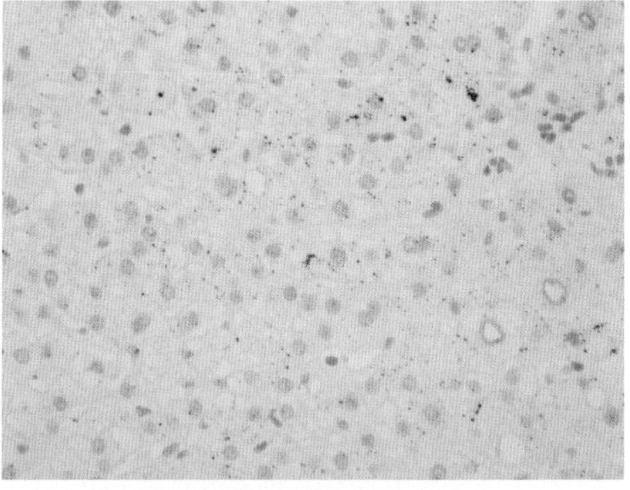

Figure 4.25 In situ hybridization for HEV. This liver transplant patient had a low-grade chronic hepatitis.

HBcAg is a nuclear stain mostly, but can also have cytoplasmic staining, most commonly in children or when there is a high viral load (Fig. 4.24). These immunostains are seldom needed for clinical care, as the presence of a chronic hepatitis B infection is generally known. However, they are still very useful, especially for evaluation of hepatocytes with ground glass change, and there continues to be rare clinically unknown chronic hepatitis B infections that are first diagnosed by liver pathologists. Immunostains and in situ hybridization stains have been developed for chronic hepatitis C and hepatitis E (Fig. 4.25) but are not widely available. For acute viral infections, the most commonly used viral stain in liver pathology is cytomegalovirus (CMV), but depending on the histology, immunostains for herpes simplex virus (HSV), adenovirus, varicella zoster virus (VZV), Epstein–Barr virus (EBER), parvovirus, and human herpesvirus 8 (HHV8) can all be useful.

Hepatocyte ground-glass-type inclusions

Ground glass inclusions in hepatocytes are large amphophilic cytoplasmic inclusions. The differential includes hepatitis B ground glass change and all cases benefit from HBsAg immunostains. Most of the hepatitis B virus (HBV)-negative cases are psuedoground glass inclusions that result from medication effect. All of these are PAS-positive. Most are also diastase sensitive, though the digestion can be incomplete in many cases. Other PAS-positive ground glass changes include rare conditions such as uremia from renal failure and glycogen storage disease type IV. Finally, fibrinogen inclusions, found in individuals with dysfibrinogenemia or afibrinogenemia, can look very similar, but are PAS-negative, phosphotungstic acid-hematoxylin stain (PTAH)-positive, and fibrinogen immunostain-positive.

Mallory hyaline

In general, the H&E findings are sufficient to recognize Mallory hyaline (also known as Mallory–Denk bodies) and stains are not needed for diagnostic purposes. However, Mallory hyaline can be stained quite nicely with ubiquitin, p62, and CK8/18 (Fig. 4.26). Other keratins can also sometimes be positive, such as CK19.[16] Mallory hyaline is most often found in ballooned hepatocytes and these ballooned hepatocytes will also lose their generalized cytoplasmic staining for CK8/18.[17]

4.4 SPECIFIC STAINS—HISTOCHEMICAL

Fontana–Masson

Lipofuschin is stained black on the Fontana–Masson stain (Fig. 4.27). Glypican 3 also beautifully stains most cases of lipofuschin.

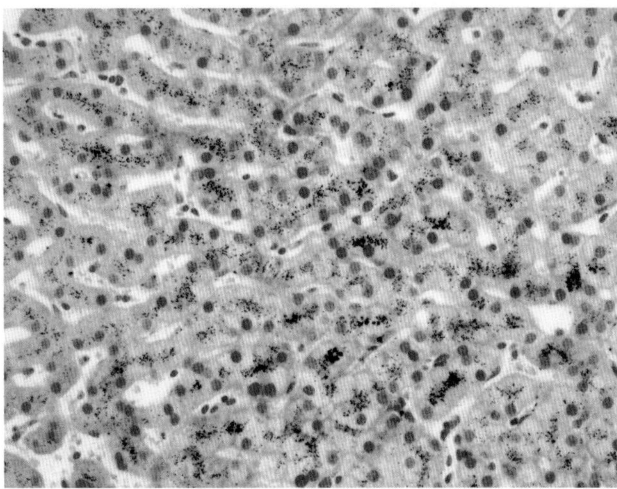

Figure 4.27 Fontana–Masson stain. The lipofuschin stains brown/black.

Hall's bile stain

This stain is also called Hall's bilirubin stain and will stain bile a dark green color (Fig. 4.28). This stain is rarely used in liver pathology because the histological appearance of bile on H&E stains is sufficiently distinct in most cases. A check of the laboratory results for recent serum bilirubin levels can also be helpful if there is uncertainty.

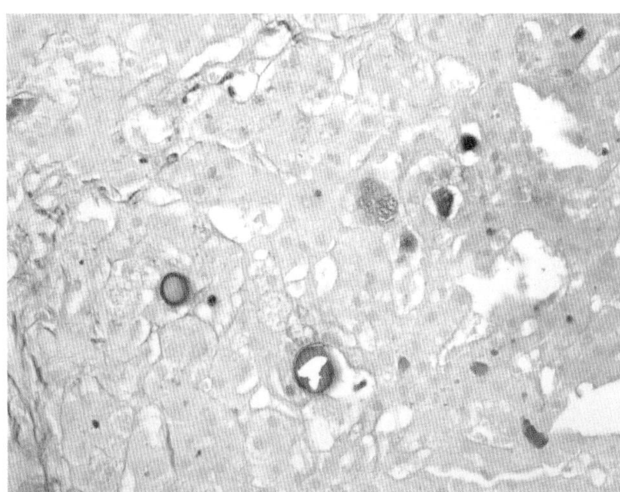

Figure 4.28 Hall's bile stain. The bile stains a distinctive green.

Oil Red O stain

This stain requires frozen tissue. It tends to be somewhat dirty, but brightly stains neutral fat (Figs. 4.29 and 4.30). Some centers use this stain to evaluate the degree of fat in donor liver biopsy specimens. Experience

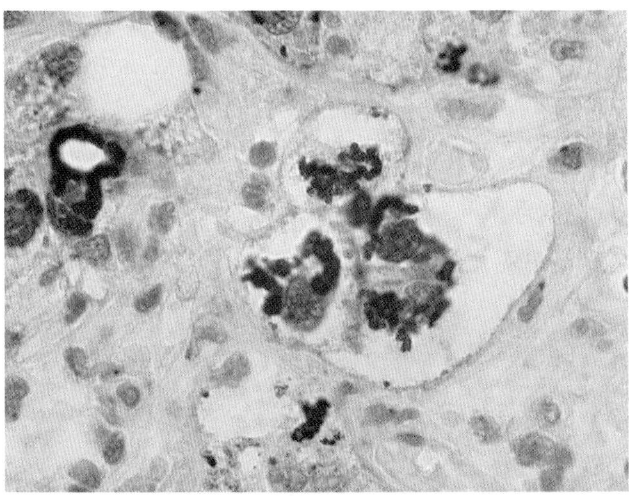

Figure 4.26 Mallory hyaline, p62. The Mallory hyaline is strongly positive.

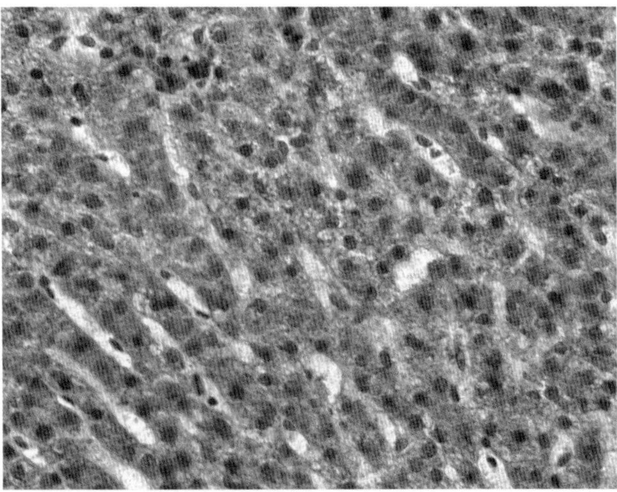

Figure 4.29 Normal liver, H&E. No fat is seen (see next picture).

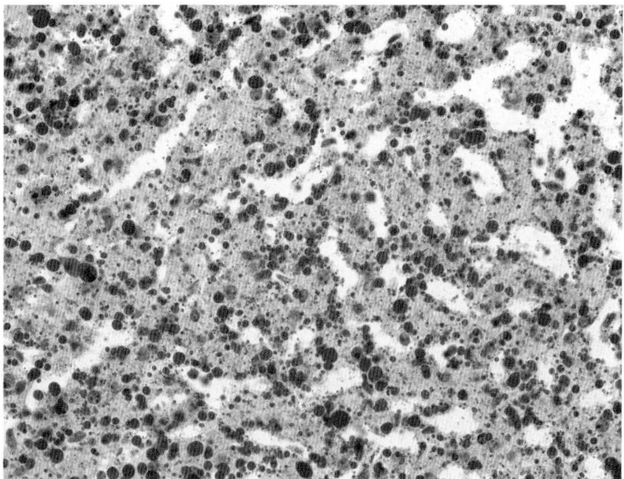

Figure 4.30 Oil Red O. The fat in this histologically normal liver is highlighted.

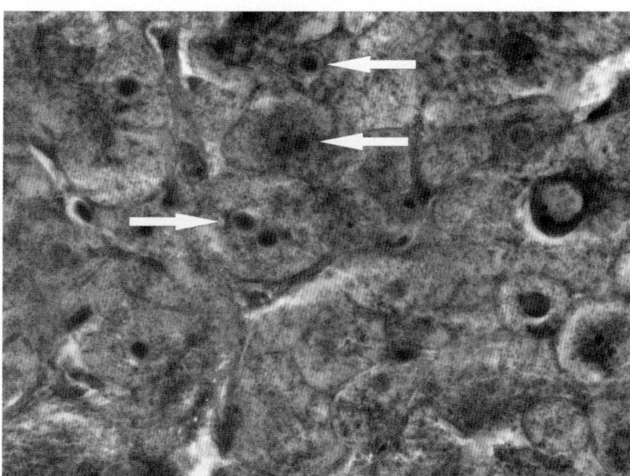

Figure 4.31 Phosphotungstic acid-hematoxylin stain. The megamitochondria are positive (*arrows*).

with the stain is required to avoid overestimating the amount of fat because hepatocytes in normal livers can have a fair amount of fat by Oil Red O stain. Interestingly, this same dye is also used to generate the red-color smoke found in some pyrotechnics, which is probably a better all-around use for this stain than in diagnostic liver pathology.

Orcein

The orcein stain highlights the ground glass inclusions in chronic hepatitis B, which stain a dark brown, but this role has been largely supplanted by immunostains for HBsAg. The orcein stain also highlights elastic fibers. Copper-binding proteins are also positive, but the rhodanine stain has replaced the orcein stain in most centers for evaluation of copper in the liver. The Victorian Blue also has these same staining characteristics (hepatitis B surface antigen, elastic fibers, copper-binding protein), but, like the orcein stain, is rarely used anymore.

Phosphotungstic acid-hematoxylin stain

The PTAH stain can be used to demonstrate megamitochondria in hepatocytes (Fig. 4.31). In most cases, the H&E appearance of megamitochondria is sufficient to make the diagnosis, but in rare cases there can be questions about the nature of the small, round to ovoid cytoplasmic structures. PTAH is also positive in the pseudoground glass inclusions in many cases of fibrinogen storage disease.

Sudan black

This stain is very similar to Oil Red O in almost all respects, including the need for frozen tissue.

Rhodanine

This stain is used to detect copper in the liver. However, it only detects copper deposited in lysosomes, not copper in the cytosol. For this reason, the rhodanine stain can be negative in some cases of Wilson's disease. In fact, if there is strong clinical suspicion for Wilson's disease, quantitative copper analysis is warranted, even with a negative copper stain.

Copper accumulation can be helpful in noncirrhotic livers to suggest chronic cholestatic liver disease. The copper deposits are found in the zone 1 hepatocytes and typically have a focal to patchy distribution. In a cirrhotic liver, mild copper accumulation is nonspecific and does not have the same diagnostic utility.

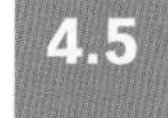

4.5 SPECIFIC STAINS—IMMUNOSTAINS

C4d

This stain is used when evaluating for antibody mediated rejection. In addition, a subset of cases with glycogen pseudoground glass are C4d-positive. Interestingly, dead (apoptotic) hepatocytes are often C4d-positive.

CD68

This stain can be used to highlight Kupffer cells. The KP1 clone also stains lysosomes and is positive in essentially all fibrolamellar carcinomas and a subset of conventional hepatocellular carcinomas.

CD10

This stain should highlight the canaliculi in normal liver lobules (Fig. 4.32). This normal pattern of staining

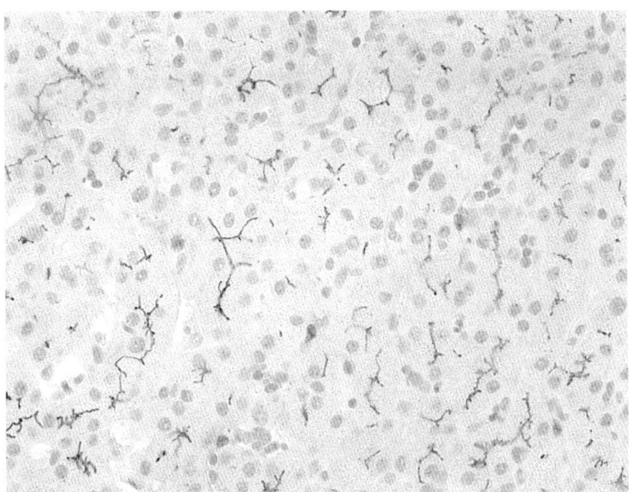

Figure 4.32 CD10, normal liver. The distinctive branching canalicular staining pattern is seen.

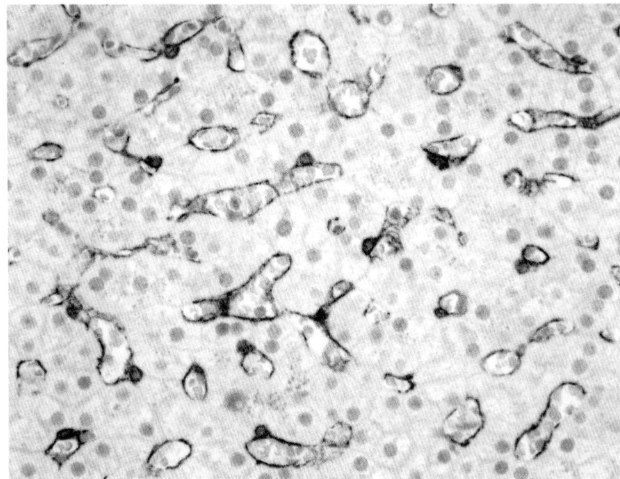

Figure 4.33 Smooth muscle actin. The lobules show diffuse staining in this case of vitamin A toxicity.

can be lost with the Alagille syndrome in liver biopsies from children who are greater than 2 years of age.[18] In areas of extensive ischemic or toxic necrosis, the hepatocytes can also lose their CD10 canalicular staining, often before the hepatocytes become obviously necrotic.

CD34

CD34 stains the sinusoids in zone 1 of the normal liver. With abnormally high arterial blood flow to the liver, there can be more diffuse staining of the sinusoids.

Ki-67

This stain is used to identify cells that are proliferating. In medical liver biopsies, Ki-67 stains can be useful when the biopsy is histologically almost normal, but the aspartate transaminase (AST) and alanine transaminase (ALT) are elevated. In the normal quiescent liver, less than 1% of hepatocytes are Ki-67-positive. In contrast, a significantly increased Ki-67 indicates active regeneration of the hepatocytes and suggests a recent or ongoing injury, even if the biopsy is otherwise almost normal. The Ki-67 stain can also be used in the opposite setting, where there is a known liver injury, with obvious histological injury. If the Ki-67 proliferative rate in the hepatocytes is minimal or absent, this indicates impaired regeneration of the liver, a phenomenon most commonly seen in the elderly.

Smooth muscle actin

Smooth muscle actin can be used to identify stellate cell activation (Fig. 4.33). Normally, the liver sinusoids are essentially negative, but with activation, from a variety of different causes, the stellate cells will express smooth muscle actin.

REFERENCES

1. Pai RK, Hart JA. Aberrant expression of cytokeratin 7 in perivenular hepatocytes correlates with a cholestatic chemistry profile in patients with heart failure. *Mod Pathol.* 2010;23(12):1650–1656.
2. El-Guindi MA, Sira MM, Hussein MH, et al. Hepatic immunohistochemistry of bile transporters in progressive familial intrahepatic cholestasis. *Ann Hepatol.* 2016;15(2):222–229.
3. Wendum D, Barbu V, Rosmorduc O, et al. Aspects of liver pathology in adult patients with MDR3/ABCB4 gene mutations. *Virchows Arch.* 2012;460(3):291–298.
4. Evason K, Bove KE, Finegold MJ, et al. Morphologic findings in progressive familial intrahepatic cholestasis 2 (PFIC2): correlation with genetic and immunohistochemical studies. *Am J Surg Pathol.* 2011;35(5):687–696.
5. Daniels JA, Torbenson M, Anders RA, et al. Immunostaining of plasma cells in primary biliary cirrhosis. *Am J Clin Pathol.* 2009;131(2):243–249.
6. Graham RP, Smyrk TC, Zhang L. Evaluation of langerhans cell infiltrate by CD1a immunostain in liver biopsy for the diagnosis of primary biliary cirrhosis. *Am J Surg Pathol.* 2012;36(5):732–736.
7. Zhang L, Lewis JT, Abraham SC, et al. IgG4+ plasma cell infiltrates in liver explants with primary sclerosing cholangitis. *Am J Surg Pathol.* 2010;34(1):88–94.
8. Hodges JR, Millward-Sadler GH, Barbatis C, et al. Heterozygous MZ alpha-1-antitrypsin deficiency in

adults with chronic active hepatitis and cryptogenic cirrhosis. *N Engl J Med*. 1981;304(10):557–560.

9. Gourley MF, Gourley GR, Gilbert EF, et al. Alpha-1-antitrypsin deficiency and the PiMS phenotype: case report and literature review. *J Pediatr Gastroenterol Nutr*. 1989;8(1):116–121.
10. Kelly JK, Taylor TV, Milford-Ward A. Alpha-1-antitrypsin Pi S phenotype and liver cell inclusion bodies in alcoholic hepatitis. *J Clin Pathol*. 1979;32(7):706–709.
11. Millward-Sadler GH. Alpha-1-antitrypsin deficiency and liver disease. *Acta Med Port*. 1981(Suppl 2):91–102.
12. Vrana JA, Gamez JD, Madden BJ, et al. Classification of amyloidosis by laser microdissection and mass spectrometry-based proteomic analysis in clinical biopsy specimens. *Blood*. 2009;114(24):4957–4959.
13. Chandan VS, Shah SS, Lam-Himlin DM, et al. Globular hepatic amyloid is highly sensitive and specific for LECT2 amyloidosis. *Am J Surg Pathol*. 2015; 39(4):558–564
14. Greenwood N, Fox H. A comparison of methods for staining tubercle bacilli in histological sections. *J Clin Pathol*. 1973;26(4):253–257.
15. Hagen CE, Kamionek M, McKinsey DS, et al. Syphilis presenting as inflammatory tumors of the liver in HIV-positive homosexual men. *Am J Surg Pathol*. 2014;38(12):1636–1643.
16. Pei RJ, Danbara N, Tsujita-Kyutoku M, et al. Immunohistochemical profiles of Mallory body by a panel of anti-cytokeratin antibodies. *Med Electron Microsc*. 2004;37(2):114–118.
17. Guy CD, Suzuki A, Burchette JL, et al. Costaining for keratins 8/18 plus ubiquitin improves detection of hepatocyte injury in nonalcoholic fatty liver disease. *Hum Pathol*. 2012;43(6):790–800.
18. Byrne JA, Meara NJ, Rayner AC, et al. Lack of hepatocellular CD10 along bile canaliculi is physiologic in early childhood and persistent in Alagille syndrome. *Lab Invest*. 2007;87(11):1138–1148.

5

Electron microscopy

Taofic Mounajjed, MD

5.1 INTRODUCTION

The rise of immunohistochemical, molecular, and serologic techniques in pathology over the past decades has somewhat sidelined certain diagnostic uses of the more traditional ultrastructural pathology[1–3]; however, electron microscopy remains a powerful tool in the evaluation of liver disease, both for research and for diagnosis. This chapter considers clinical conditions where ultrastructural analysis is particularly useful. It also briefly reviews correct retrieval and processing methods for electron microscopy, focuses on the ultrastructural features of nonneoplastic liver conditions most commonly evaluated by electron microscopy, and when relevant, discusses their differential diagnoses. Of course, this brief chapter cannot be all-inclusive to the vast field of ultrastructural liver pathology, but attempts to cover the most clinically relevant issues to the practicing surgical pathologist.

5.2 FIXATION METHODS FOR ELECTRON MICROSCOPY

Electron microscopy images are the outcome of a complicated and time-consuming processing of liver tissue. Interpretation of electron microscopy images requires, in addition to knowledge of the hepatic ultrastructure, experience with potential artifacts of fixation, embedding, sectioning, contrast staining, and microscopic imaging. If the clinician or pathologist has deemed that a liver biopsy might require ultrastructural evaluation, adequate tissue submission and processing is essential at the time of the biopsy. Small specimens (no larger than 1 mm^3 for optimal fixative penetration) should be submitted separately for electron microscopy.

Fixation

Fixation arrests cell metabolism and stops autolytic processes that start within minutes or even seconds following specimen retrieval.[4] Fixation also leads to crosslinking of organelles and substructures, which preserves them. For these reasons, fixation of tissue intended for electron microscopy use should be done as immediately as possible in order to achieve better visualization of ultrastructural detail, avoid artifacts, and prevent poor preservation or injury to organelles, which could

Table 5.1 Ultrastructural features that can be used to judge the quality of tissue preservation

Good fixation quality	Poor fixation quality
Open sinusoids	Sinusoids collapsed or destroyed
Sinusoids do not contain significant amounts of plasma or blood	Sinusoids filled with plasma or blood
Similar cell types should show similar appearance (e.g., staining/brightness)	Dark and light cells occur next to each other
Endothelial fenestration present	Absent endothelial fenestra
Open bile canaliculi (especially periportal)	Collapsed bile canaliculi
Nuclei of hepatocytes are round	Hepatocytes with irregularly shaped nuclei

mimic true pathology. Fixatives should be isotonic and isothermic to the cells[4]; although different labs have their own preferences, 1.5% to 2.5% buffered gluteraldehyde is universally accepted.

Although perfusion fixation methods have proven optimal for electron microscopy studies, this method is somewhat difficult to accomplish in needle biopsies, which generally undergo immersion fixation and have results of sufficiently good quality for diagnosis.[4–7] In the case of needle biopsies, two 3 mm × 1 mm cylinders of tissue are cut from the end of the tissue core, immersed immediately in fixative, then cut into pieces measuring no more than 1 mm in greatest dimension each. The small tissue fragments should be placed in glutaraldehyde fixative (for at least 1 to 2 hours) at room temperature. Tissue can be refrigerated but should not be frozen. The quality of tissue fixation can be inferred from certain ultrastructural features (Table 5.1)[4,6,8,9]; these features should be evaluated in each clinical case in order to avoid misinterpretation of fixation artifacts. In poorly fixed tissues, common artifacts include nuclei with serrated uneven edges, ballooned mitochondria, myelin-like whorls in mitochondria, and dense deposits in mitochondrial matrix.

Processing after fixation

After glutaraldehyde fixation, specimens are subjected to a washing buffer, osmium postfixation, ethanol dehydration, and embedding. Samples then undergo drying via critical point drying (routinely used) or hexamethyldisilazane-drying and are then mounted on stubs and sputter coated with 10 nm gold for scanning electron microscopy.[10,11] For transmission electron microscopy, thick sections (0.5 to 1 μm) are produced, stained with Toluidine Blue, and examined for optimal tissue selection. Then, 40 to 100 nm sections (ultrathin sections) are produced from Epon-embedded tissue, spread on mesh copper grids and stained with a uranyl acetate and lead citrate solution for ultrastructural evaluation.

Visualization

Toluidine Blue-stained thick sections provide a useful histological introduction to further detailed study by transmission electron microscopy. They allow examination of relatively large areas of tissue to determine the quality of fixation and to identify areas that are the most representative or have the most pronounced pathology for further trimming. In general, it is best to focus the study of immersion fixed needle biopsies on the outer and middles zones of the tissue, which are the best fixed.

Scanning electron microscopy offers more details about the endothelial lining (fenestrae) and the space of Disse. Therefore, scanning electron microscopy preparations are very useful for judging the condition of sinusoids,[12] though they do not allow for detailed evaluation of intracellular structures. Transmission electron microscopy, on the other hand, allows detailed examination of the fine structure of the various cell types present in the liver, and is therefore the primary tool used for diagnostic purposes in ultrastructural pathology; it can allow magnifications of up to 1,000,000×, with a resolution of about 5 nm. Transmission electron microscopy sections are surveyed first at low magnification (as low as 50×), which functions as a bridge between Toluidine Blue light microscopy and high-power transmission electron microscopy examinations. This survey provides information about the quality and content of the sections and allows for preselection of interesting areas for further examination.

Electron microscopy in formalin fixed paraffin electron microscopy bedded tissue

Formalin fixation results in poor tissue preservation; it leads to tissue extraction, especially affecting lipids, glycogen, ribosomes, membranous structures, and other cellular and intercellular matrix materials. Tissue preservation can be especially poor in tissue fixed by Bouin fixative.[13] Paraffin electron microscopy bedding per se, on the other hand, has little effect on the ultrastructure. Several factors can improve fine structure of paraffin electron microscopy bedded tissues, such as careful thin slicing and judicious selection.

Although preservation of fine structures in formalin fixed paraffin electron microscopy bedded tissue is generally imperfect, compactly organized cells with abundant cytoplasmic contents, such as hepatocytes, are usually better preserved than other tissue types. In comparison with glutaraldehyde fixation, formalin fixation leads to the following ultrastructural alterations[13]:

- The tissue becomes less homogenous in electron density (exaggerated contrast).
- The tissue has a pale and extracted appearance.
- Details are compromised at higher magnification, resulting from the uneven loss of phospholipids, membranous structures, matrix, and ribosomes.
- The cell membranes of discohesive cells, such as Kupffer cells, frequently show discontinuities at high magnification.
- There is loss of mitochondrial detail. The mitochondria appear contracted or distended and partly disintegrated. The cristae are poorly preserved.

- Among cytoplasmic contents, lipid, glycogen, and ribosomes are poorly preserved.
- Among organelles, the smooth endoplasmic reticulum and Golgi apparatus are poorly preserved.
- The cytoplasm shows irregular rarefactions representing lost liposomes, glycogen, endoplasmic reticulum, Golgi apparatus, and vesicles.
- Lipofuscin shows moderate alterations.
- Cell nuclei show peripheral condensation of their chromatin, with incomplete preservation of the nuclear membranes. The nuclear pores are difficult to identify.

The following structures show the least amount of alterations[13]:

- Cellular borders, including cilia and microvilli, are well defined.
- Intercellular junctions, such as desmosomes are well preserved.
- Closely packed rough endoplasmic reticulum is well preserved.
- Lysosomes, including large secondary lysosomes with phagocytized material, are usually well preserved.
- Collagen and basement membranes are well delineated.
- Microfilaments, such as seen in the pericanalicular region, are relatively well preserved.

Although many authors believe that transmission electron microscopy is a futile exercise in formalin fixed paraffin electron microscopy bedded tissue, others have found surprisingly well-preserved fine structure and others have even been able to identify viruses and other microorganisms by transmission electron microscopy.[13–18] In fact, transmission electron microscopy can be useful if separately submitted tissue in glutaraldehyde is not available. In such instances, the use of formalin fixed paraffin electron microscopy bedded tissue for transmission electron microscopy can provide the benefit of a more integrated approach, linking the light microscopic and ultrastructural findings. In our experience, transmission electron microscopy can be useful diagnostically in liver pathology, especially in conditions involving identification of abnormally accumulated materials (e.g., glycogen storage disease, lysosomal storage disorders, amyloid, and identification of hepatocellular inclusions). Abnormalities that require detailed examination of the delicate structure of small organelles (e.g., mitochondrial cytopathies), on the other hand, can be more difficult to ascertain in formalin fixed paraffin electron microscopy bedded tissues.

Artifacts

Artifacts can result at any step (from operative to photography) and should always be kept in mind when examining electron microscopy images. It can be very difficult to distinguish between genuine structures and artifacts.[4] Common artifacts include large endothelial gaps, cell shrinkage, widening of the space of Disse, changes in cell and/or nuclear shape, mitochondrial swelling, blebbing of membranes, and vesicle formation in intercellular spaces.[6]

5.3 THE NORMAL LIVER

In order to understand ultrastructural liver pathology, knowledge of the normal structures is essential. The next section provides a brief description of the fine structure of the different cell types seen in the liver.

The hepatocyte

The hepatocyte is the predominant cell type in the liver, accounting for approximately 60% of the total cell population[19,20] and approximately 80% of the liver volume.[21] Ultrastructurally, the hepatocyte has a polyhedral appearance, with quadrangular to hexagonal shapes in cut sections. The average hepatocyte diameter is 25 µm.[20] Approximately 55% of the hepatocellular cytoplasmic volume is cytosol.[20,21] The cytoplasm of the hepatocyte is remarkable and unique for being essentially packed with numerous organelles (Fig. 5.1), including mitochondria, peroxisomes, Golgi apparatus, smooth endoplasmic reticulum, rough endoplasmic reticulum, lysosomes, microtubules, microfilaments, and intermediate filaments. Glycogen abounds in the cytoplasm of normal hepatocytes and is predominantly in rosette (rather than monoparticulate) form, and distributed diffusely, but has an association with the smooth endoplasmic reticulum.[22,23] Lipid droplets can be found in small numbers under normal conditions within the cytosol (Fig. 5.2), especially near the sinusoids; lipid has a rounded, electron dense, and overall homogeneous appearance. Lipofuscin and hemosiderin pigment are also not uncommon (Figs. 5.3 and 5.4).

Polarity

The normal hepatocytes do not rest on a basement membrane, but they do have polarity (Fig. 5.5), featuring sinusoidal, lateral, and canalicular regions. The sinusoidal pole (Fig. 5.6), comprising approximately 40% of the hepatocellular surface, is in contact with the space of Disse and is covered by microvilli. Owing

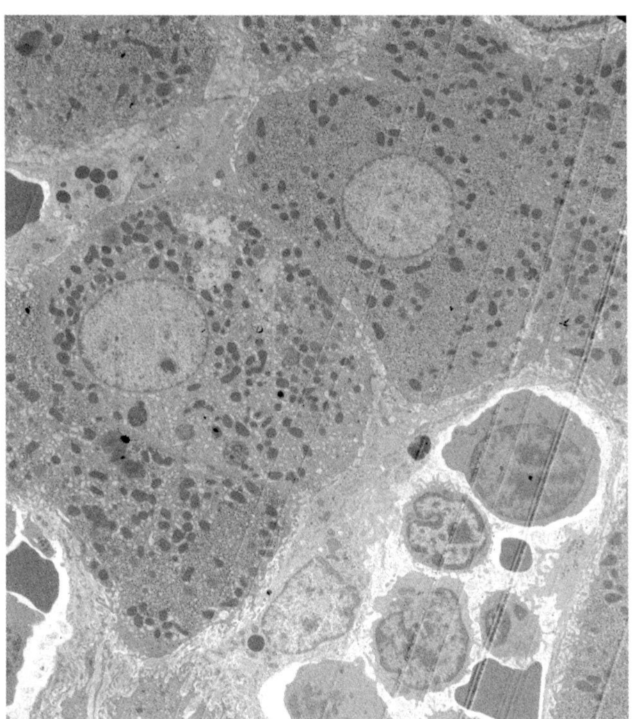

Figure 5.1 The normal hepatocyte. Normal hepatocytes (**upper** center) have a polyhedral appearance, with voluminous cytoplasm, abundant glycogen contents and numerous organelles.

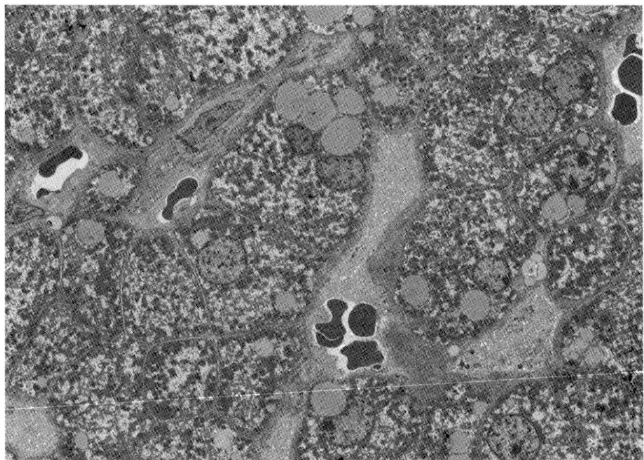

Figure 5.2 The normal hepatocyte. Lipid droplets can be found in small numbers within the cytoplasm of hepatocytes under normal conditions.

to the high level of endocytosis on this surface, the underlying cytoplasm contains many pinocytotic vesicles.

The lateral pole (Fig. 5.7), which is opposed to a neighboring hepatocyte, is straight and lacks microvilli. It contains various types of intercellular junctions (saccular unions, gap junctions, desmosomes, and intermediate junctions),[20,24–28] which provide

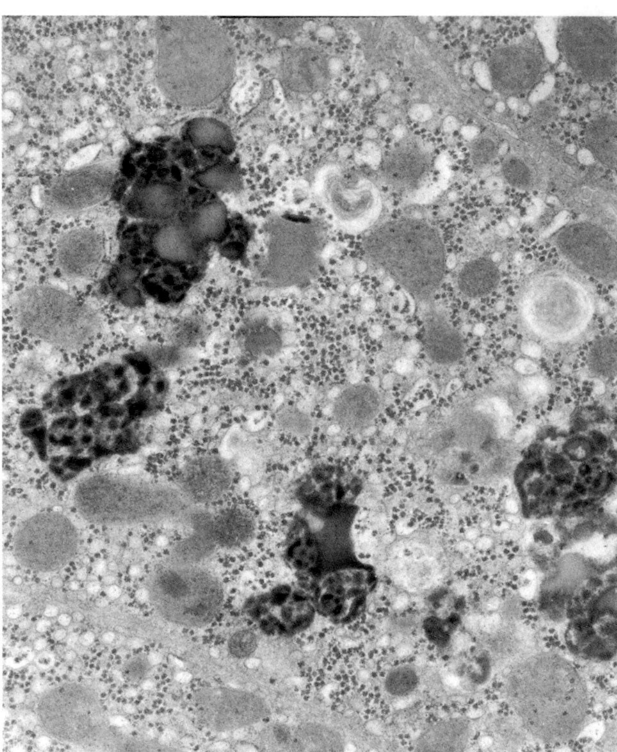

Figure 5.3 The normal hepatocyte. Lipofuscin consists of coarse, electron-dense granules, lipid droplets, and a heterogeneous matrix.

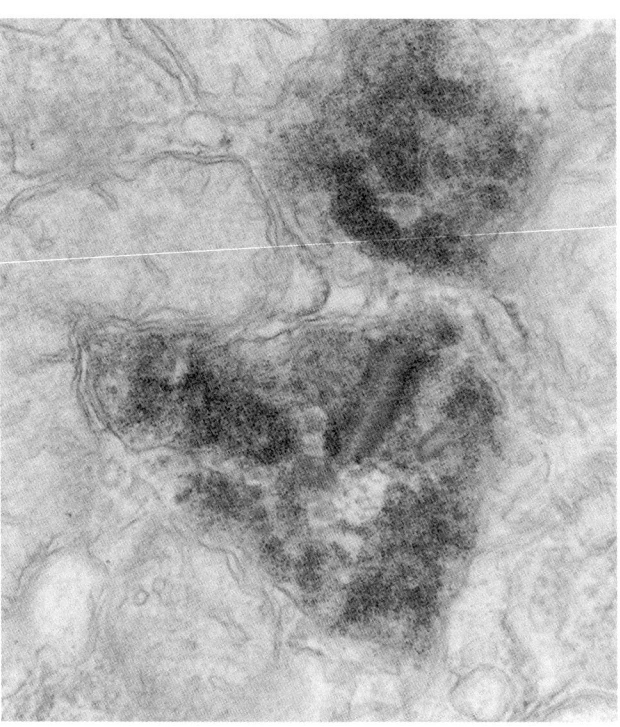

Figure 5.4 The normal hepatocyte. Hemosiderin consists of lysosomal aggregates of finely granular electron-dense material.

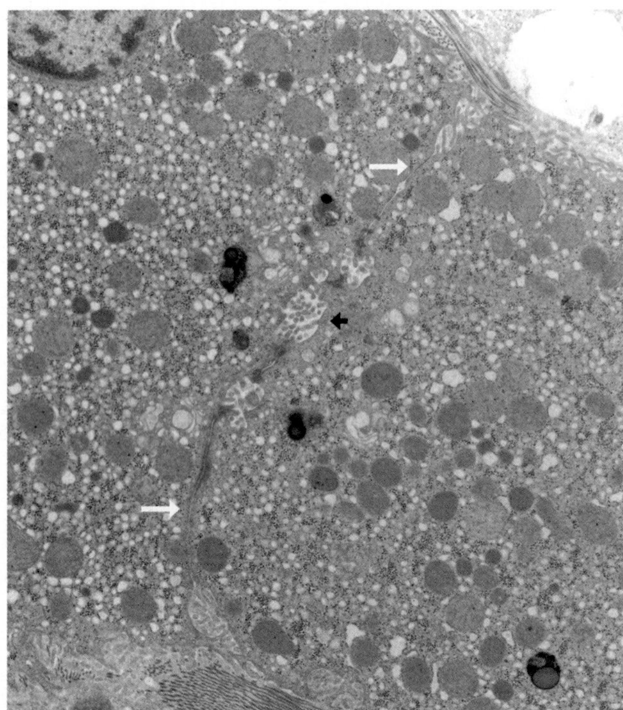

Figure 5.5 The normal hepatocyte: hepatocellular poles. Hepatocytes have three poles: the sinusoidal pole (upper right corner), the lateral poles (long white arrows), and the canalicular pole (short black arrow).

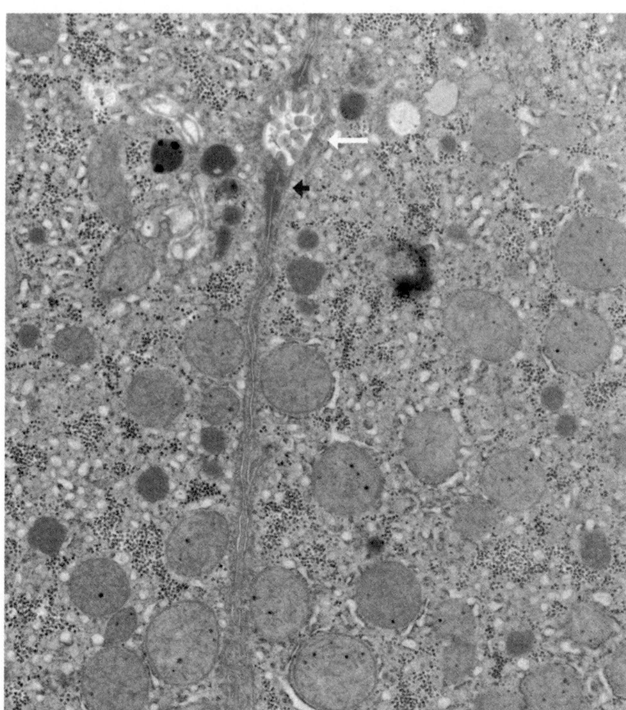

Figure 5.7 The normal hepatocyte: lateral pole. The lateral pole separates two neighboring hepatocytes. This pole is straight and lacks microvilli. Tight junctions (*short black arrow*) seal the bile canaliculus (*white arrow*) and separate it from the lateral pole

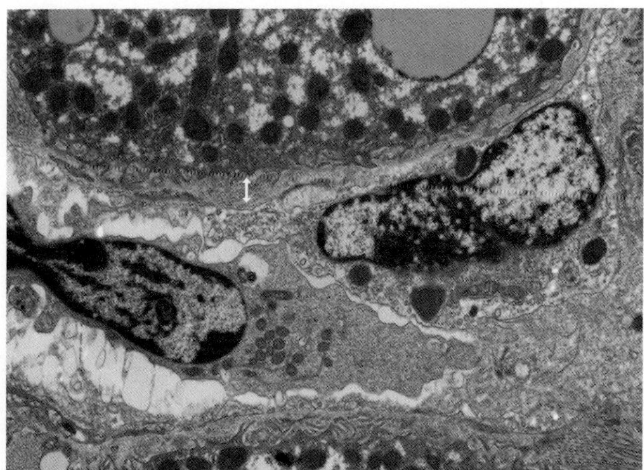

Figure 5.6 The normal hepatocyte: sinusoidal pole. This hepatic sinusoid is occupied by two Kupffer cells (center and center/bottom). Two hepatocytes (**upper lower** and **lower**) have numerous microvilli projecting into the space of Disse (*double-sided arrow*).

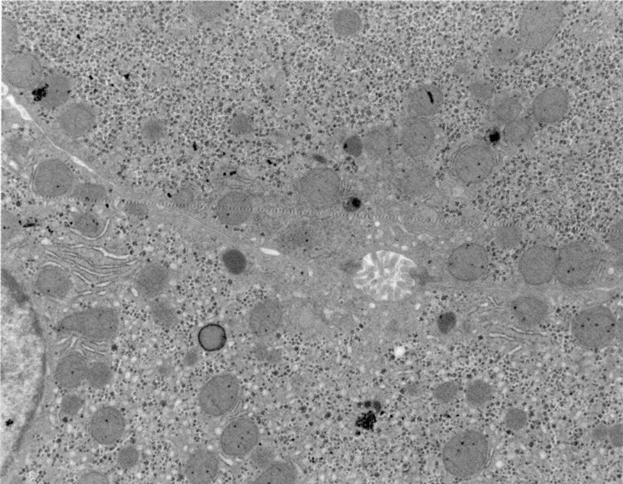

Figure 5.8 The normal hepatocyte: canalicular pole. The bile canaliculus (center **right**) is sealed on both sides by tight junctions, delineating it from the lateral pole. It contains microvilli and is surrounded by a rim organelle-free cytoplasmic zone.

cell-to-cell communication,[29,30] and tight junctions that seal the bile canaliculi.

The canalicular pole (Fig. 5.8) is sealed on both sides by tight junctions, delineating it from the lateral pole. The canalicular pole constitutes approximately 15% of the hepatocellular surface and, like the sinusoidal pole, contains microvilli. The pericanalicular ectoplasm, an organelle-free cytoplasmic zone that surrounds the bile canaliculus, is rich in microfilaments, which facilitate canalicular bile motility.[31,32]

Mitochondria

Mitochondria are the most numerous organelles in the hepatocyte (Fig. 5.9), accounting for approximately 18% of the hepatocyte volume.[20,33] They are bound by a double membrane with many shelf-like projections protruding from the inner membrane, known as "cristae" (Fig. 5.10). The lumen of mitochondria contains a "matrix" that is slightly more electron dense than the hepatocellular cytosol in normal hepatocytes. Matrical dense granules are commonly seen in normal mitochondria. Mitochondrial functions are numerous and involve cell respiration, oxidative phosphorylation, electron transport, ATP synthetase activity, urea cycle, fatty acid oxidation, and the citric acid cycle.[20]

The endoplasmic reticulum

The endoplasmic reticulum, a convoluted network of continuous membrane-bound cisterns, tubules, and saccules, constitutes approximately 15% of the hepatocellular volume.[21] It consists of the rough endoplasmic reticulum (60%, studded with ribosomes) and smooth endoplasmic reticulum (40%), which are in continuity with one another. Rough endoplasmic reticulum (Fig. 5.11) forms parallel stacks usually located around the nucleus, toward the vascular and biliary poles of the hepatocyte.

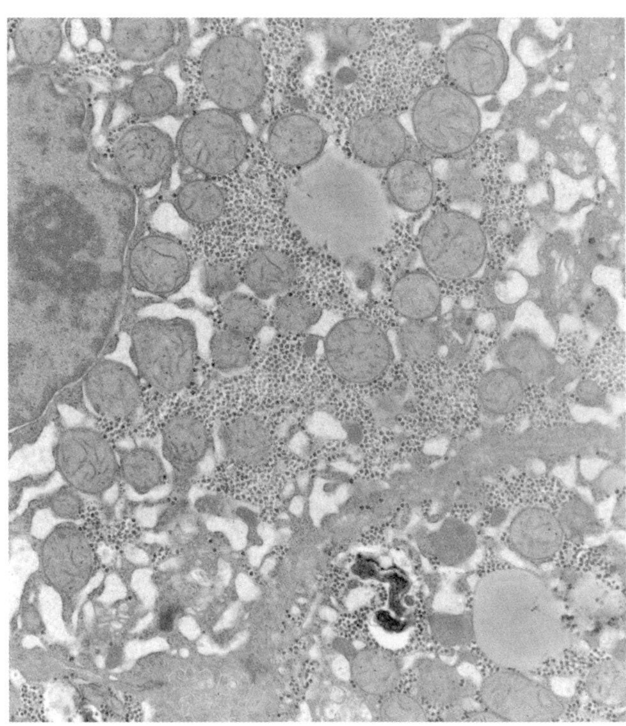

Figure 5.10 The normal hepatocyte: mitochondria. Mitochondria are bound by a double membrane with many cristae (shelf-like projections protruding from the inner membrane). The lumen of mitochondria contains a "matrix" that is slightly more electron dense than the hepatocellular cytosol. Small matrical dense granules are also present.

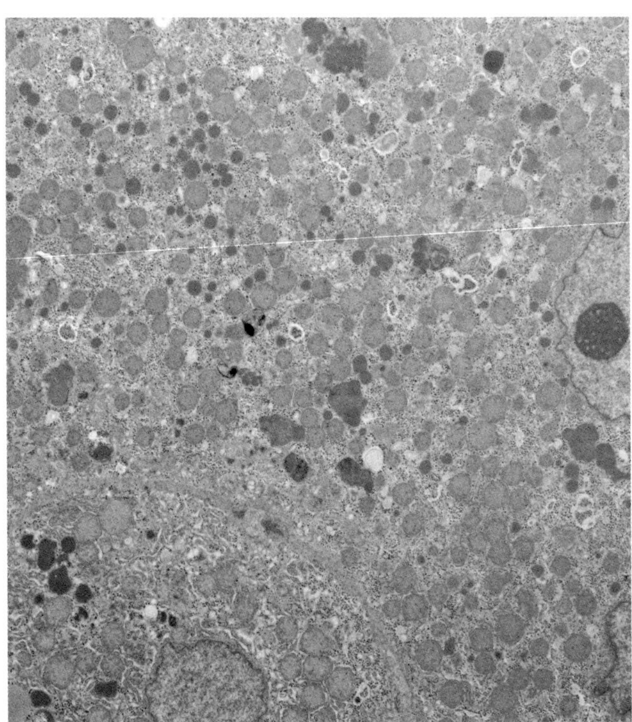

Figure 5.9 The normal hepatocyte: mitochondria. Hepatocytes are normally rich in mitochondria.

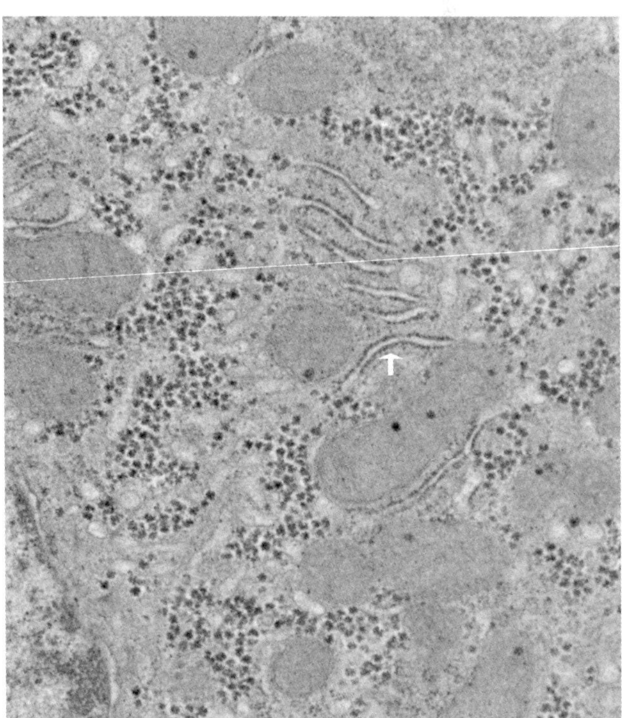

Figure 5.11 The normal hepatocyte: rough endoplasmic reticulum. The rough endoplasmic reticulum is a network of continuous membranes and tubules. It is characteristically studded by ribosomes (finely granular deposits along the membranes, arrow).

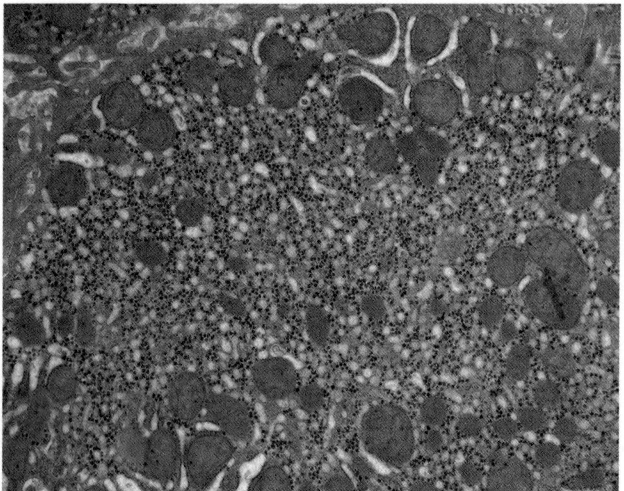

Figure 5.12 The normal hepatocyte: smooth endoplasmic reticulum. The tubules of the smooth endoplasmic reticulum are devoid of ribosomes and are associated with rich collections of glycogen (*rosettes*).

The rough endoplasmic reticulum is the site of protein synthesis, especially proteins for secretion.[34] The tubules of the smooth endoplasmic reticulum (Fig. 5.12) are devoid of ribosomes, and are located more toward the periphery of the hepatocyte; smooth endoplasmic reticulum is usually associated with rich collections of glycogen.[20,35–37] The smooth endoplasmic reticulum is the site of remarkable metabolic activity, including cytochrome P450 (located in endoplasmic reticulum membranes)[20]; its functions include lipid synthesis, glycogen and glycoprotein metabolism, bile acid synthesis, and drug detoxification. The latter function is reflected ultrastructurally by the expansion and shrinkage of the smooth endoplasmic reticulum in response to administration and withdrawal, respectively, of certain medications.[20,35,38–41]

The Golgi apparatus

The Golgi apparatus is a group of layered (4 or more layers) parallel, curved, and flattened saccules, with dilated peripheral rims associated with clusters of vesicles. The Golgi apparatus's main function is to modify secretory molecules arising from the smooth endoplasmic reticulum and rough endoplasmic reticulum (by processes such as glycosylation and sulfation) and sort them into individual chemically distinct vesicles, and then release them for delivery and fusion with target membranes.[20,42] The concave (aka trans) region of the Golgi apparatus is rich in very low-density lipoprotein vesicles and lysosomes.[43,44]

Lysosomes

Lysosomes are derived from the Golgi apparatus. They are membrane-bound organelles containing pleomorphic electron-dense material (Fig. 5.13). The pericanalicular region of the hepatocyte is the richest region in lysosomes.[20,44,45] The main lysosomal function is removal of cellular waste; they contain numerous enzymes that degrade the material within them; enzyme deficiencies result in various lysosomal storage disorders.[46] Such abnormal accumulations within lysosomes often allow at least broad categorization into a metabolic disease group based on the ultrastructural appearance of the deposits (e.g., phospholipidosis); but further classification often requires additional clinical and molecular characterization. Lysosomes are seen in hepatocytes under normal conditions; they represent normal cell turnover. Lipofuscin granules are lysosomes containing coarse, electron-dense granules, lipid droplets, and a heterogeneous matrix; they increase in hepatocytes with increased patient age.

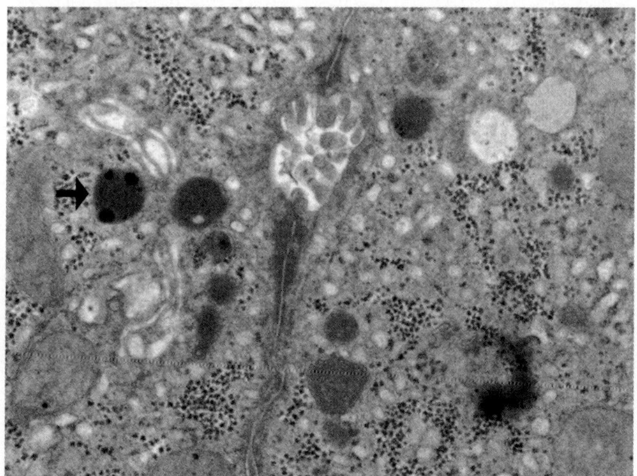

Figure 5.13 The normal hepatocyte: lysosomes. Lysosomes (*arrow*) are membrane-bound organelles containing pleomorphic electron dense material. They are often seen in normal hepatocytes in a pericanalicular distribution.

Peroxisomes

Peroxisomes (Fig. 5.14), whose functions include hydrogen peroxide metabolism and oxidation of long chain fatty acids,[47] occupy approximately 2% of the total hepatocellular cytoplasmic volume.[20] Peroxisomes are bound by a single membrane and have a finely granular and homogeneous matrix. They are seen usually in association with smooth endoplasmic reticulum, but can also have random localization

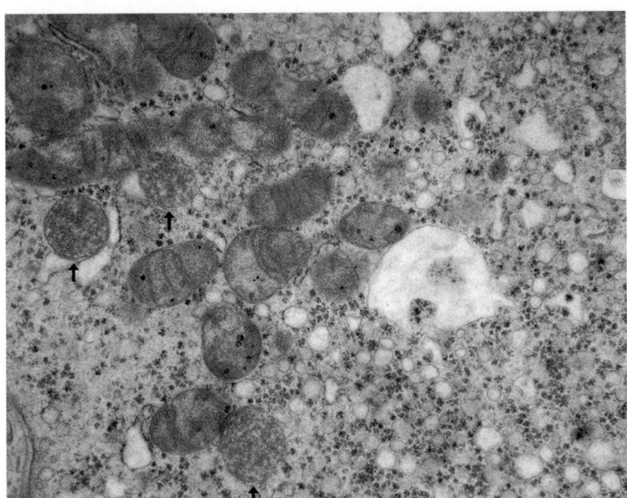

Figure 5.14 The normal hepatocyte: peroxisomes. Peroxisomes (arrows) are bound by a single membrane and have a finely granular and homogeneous matrix. In comparison to mitochondria, peroxisomes lack the double membrane and cristae and have a more granular matrix.

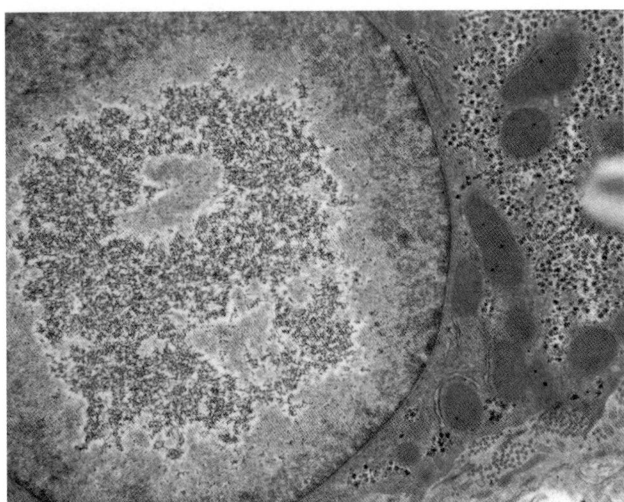

Figure 5.15 The normal hepatocyte: nuclear inclusions. Nuclear inclusions such as glycogen inclusions are often seen in pathologic conditions, but can occasionally be seen in normal hepatocytes.

within the cytoplasm.[48] They are more numerous in Zone 3 hepatocytes. It is essential to examine electron microscopy images methodically for the presence of peroxisomes within hepatocytes in every case; the absence of peroxisomes, characteristic of Zellweger syndrome, can be otherwise easily missed.

The nucleus

Nuclear abnormalities are seldom of diagnostic importance in the current practice of liver ultrastructural pathology; however, a brief description is provided of the hepatocellular nuclear fine structure. The hepatocellular nucleus is large, round, and is surrounded by two membranes separated by "the perinuclear cisterna." The membranes meet periodically, creating many nuclear pores (3,000 to 4,000 per cell).[20] The outer membrane is continuous with the rough endoplasmic reticulum; the perinuclear cisterna is also in continuity with the cisterna of the rough endoplasmic reticulum.[49] The nucleus has one or more 8 to 10 µm nucleolus; the mean number of nucleoli per hepatocyte is 2.7.[20] Nuclear inclusions such as glycogen inclusions and lipid inclusions (Figs. 5.15 and 5.16) can be seen in pathologic conditions, but can occasionally be seen in normal hepatocytes as well.[20] In addition to being occasionally seen in normal hepatocytes, nuclear glycogenosis can be seen in various conditions including diabetes mellitus, Wilson disease, Gilbert syndrome, Rotor syndrome, glycogen storage disease, and total parenteral nutrition.

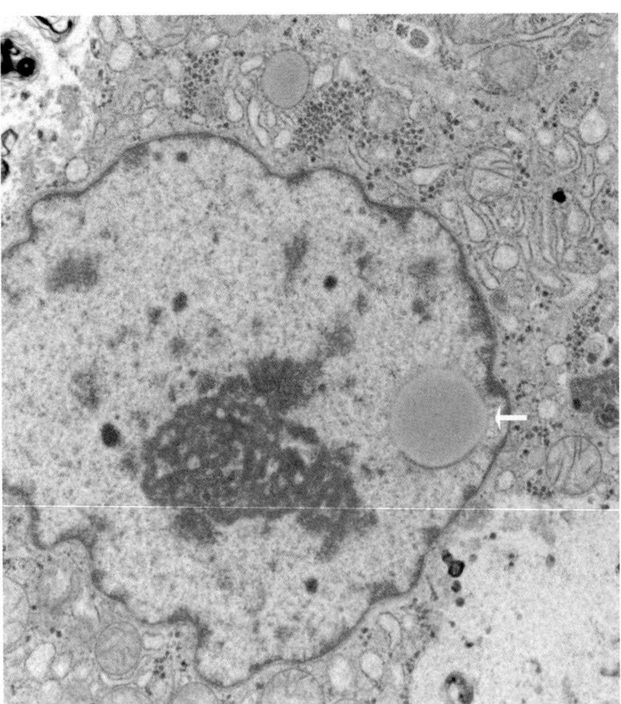

Figure 5.16 The normal hepatocyte: nuclear inclusions. Lipid inclusions (lipid droplet, *arrow*) are often seen in pathologic conditions, but can occasionally be seen in normal hepatocytes.

The cytoskeleton

The hepatocellular cytoskeleton has three components:

Microfilaments. In hepatocytes, microfilaments, whose main function involves motility, are composed mostly of actin filaments. The microfilaments abound in microvilli and are located beneath the cell membrane, especially around the bile canaliculus.[50–52] In the pericanalicular region, microfilaments are visible as an organelle-free ectoplasmic zone, which acts as miniature musculature for the bile canaliculi, facilitating bile flow.[32,53,54]

Intermediate filaments. Intermediate filaments constitute the cytoskeletal framework of hepatocytes and consist mainly of cytokeratin fibrils. Of note, Mallory bodies are pathological alteration of the hepatocellular intermediate filaments (see Alcoholic liver disease).[55–58]

Microtubules. In hepatocytes, microtubules consist predominantly of tubulin.[59] Their function involves intracytoplasmic movement of vesicles, mitosis, and secretory functions (e.g., very low-density lipoprotein secretions).[60]

Zonal differences in hepatocellular ultrastructure

The hepatocytes have different functions depending on their location in the lobules, such as increased bile acid uptake in Zone 1 hepatocytes and drug detoxification in Zone 3 hepatocytes. These specialized functions are also reflected by some ultrastructural differences. The following zonal differences are noteworthy[20]:

1. Increased and more oval-shaped mitochondria in Zone 3 hepatocytes.
2. More abundant rough endoplasmic reticulum in Zone 1 hepatocytes.[37]
3. More abundant smooth endoplasmic reticulum in Zone 3 hepatocytes.
4. Increased peroxisomes in Zone 3 hepatocytes (can outnumber mitochondria) (Fig. 5.17).
5. Larger bile canaliculi with more prominent microvilli in Zone 1 hepatocytes.[37]
6. Increased hemosiderin-filled lysosomes in Zone 1 hepatocytes.

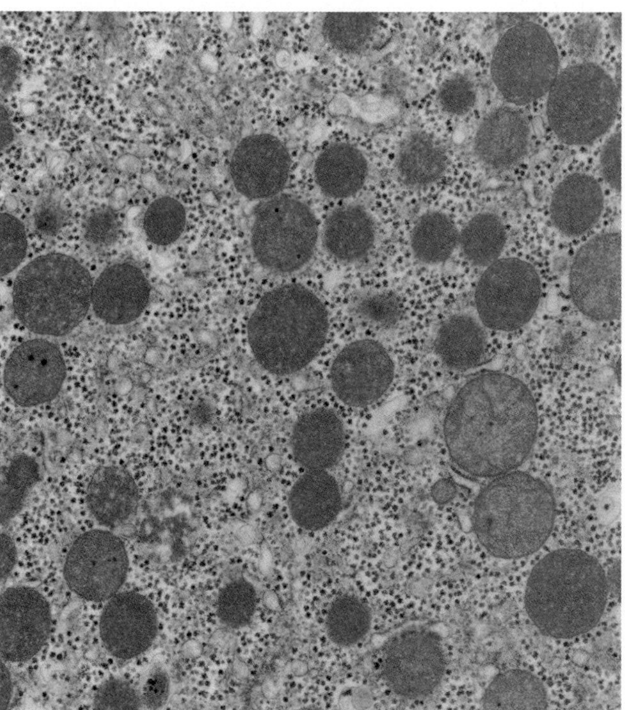

Figure 5.17 The normal hepatocyte: zonal differences. Peroxisomes can be increased in Zone 3 hepatocytes, sometimes outnumbering mitochondria.

The sinusoids

The sinusoidal lining allows direct bathing of hepatocytes with plasma, although protecting them from the mechanical trauma of blood flow.[8,9,61] The following cells constitute the structure of the sinusoids and space of Disse (Figs. 5.18 and 5.19).

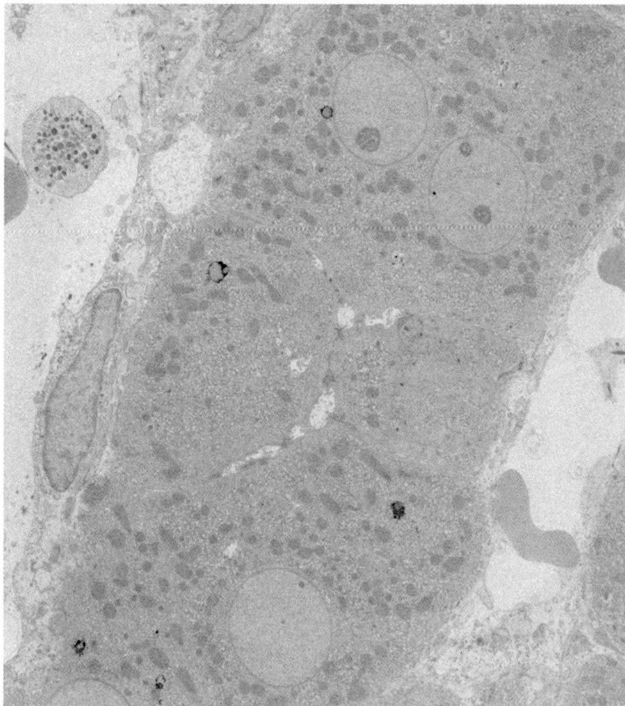

Figure 5.18 Endothelial cells. Endothelial cells line the sinusoidal spaces.

The endothelial cells

Endothelial cells are separated from hepatocytes by the space of Disse. The space of Disse is occupied by hepatocellular microvilli, some collagen fibers, and hepatic stellate cells. Endothelial cells are flattened and elongated and have numerous cytoplasmic projections separated by characteristic fenestrae. The latter allow the endothelium to act as a filtration barrier, permitting contact between the hepatocytes and plasma, although excluding the cellular components of the blood and protecting the hepatocytes from trauma.[20]

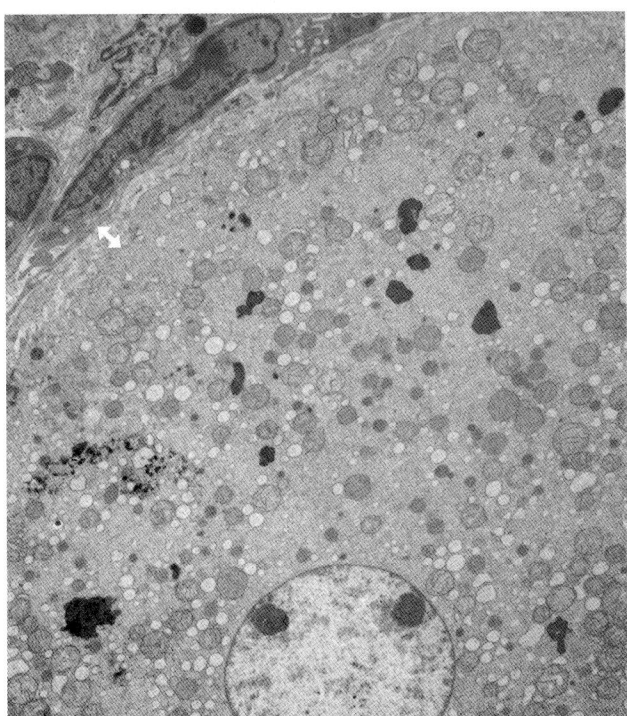

Figure 5.19 Endothelial cells. Endothelial cells are separated from hepatocytes by the space of Disse (*white arrow*).

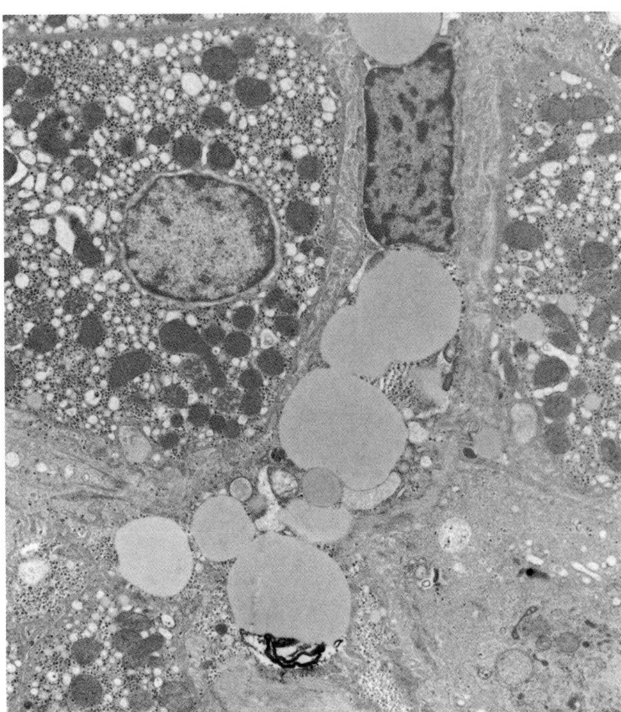

Figure 5.20 Hepatic stellate cells. Hepatic stellate cells have round to oval, eccentrically placed nucleus, and many large lipid droplets occupying most of the cytoplasm.

Another characteristic feature of sinusoidal endothelial cells is the presence of numerous pinocytotic pits and vesicles. Each endothelial cell is loosely attached to its neighboring endothelial cells by junctions.[62] Unlike other endothelia, the sinusoidal endothelium lacks a basement membrane.[9]

The hepatic stellate cells

Although usually indiscernible by routine light microscopy in normal livers, hepatic stellate cells are relatively easy to identify ultrastructurally in the space of Disse (Fig. 5.20), where they tend to occupy perisinusoidal recesses. There is approximately one hepatic stellate cell per 20 hepatocytes, and they tend to be more abundant in Zone 3. The hepatic stellate cell in its inactivated state has a round to oval, eccentrically placed nucleus, and many large lipid droplets occupying the bulk of the cytoplasm.

Kupffer cells

Kupffer cells occupy one-third of the endothelial volume.[20] They have a pyramidal or star shape (Figs. 5.21 and 5.22), with many cytoplasmic pseudopodia and are rich in lysosomes. They are more frequently observed in Zone 1 and their primary function is phagocytosis. Many lysosomal storage disorders manifest mostly in Kupffer cells (see Lysosomal storage disorders).

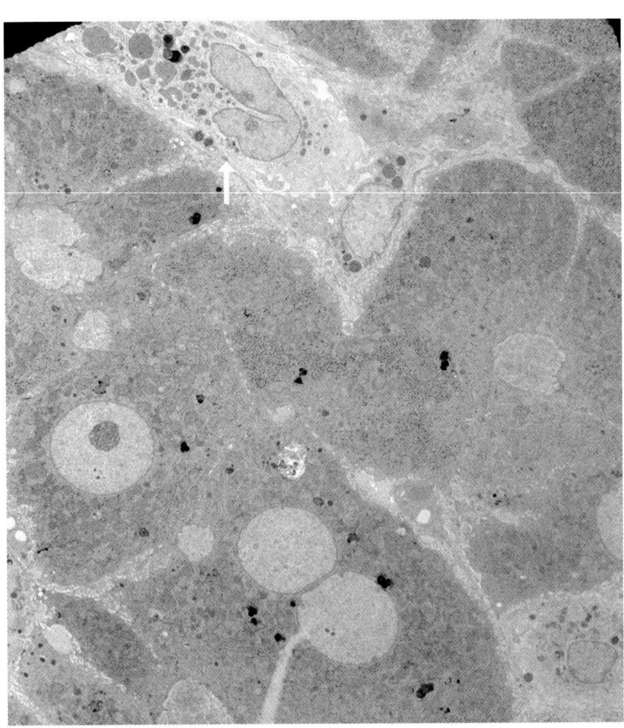

Figure 5.21 Kupffer cells. Kupffer cells (*arrow*) are frequently seen in sinusoidal spaces.

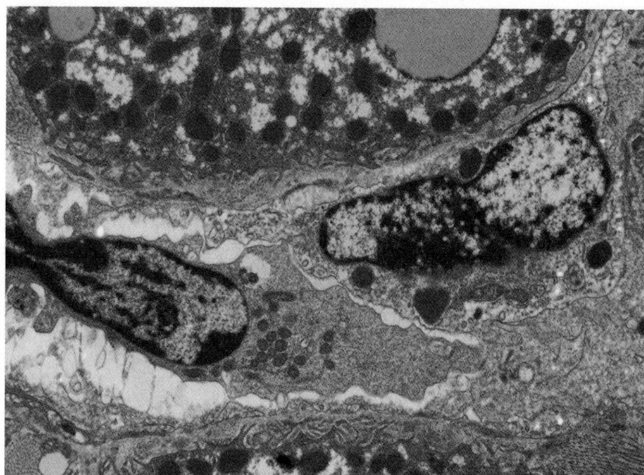

Figure 5.22 Kupffer cells. Kupffer cells have abundant cytoplasm with many cytoplasmic projections.

Biliary epithelial cells

Unlike hepatocytes, biliary epithelial cells (Figs. 5.23 and 5.24) rest on a well-formed basement membrane, which completely surrounds the bile duct. They have basally located nuclei and are smaller and have less cytoplasm than hepatocytes. Their mitochondria are sparse and smaller than those of hepatocytes, and have characteristic cristae, which traverse the entire mitochondrion rather than being shelf-like. Numerous microvilli project into the bile duct lumen and many pinocytic vacuoles underlie the luminal plasma membrane of the biliary epithelial cell. Desmosomes between neighboring cells are clustered near the apical border, and apical tight junctions are present as well. The most relevant ultrastructural abnormalities evaluated in routine practice involve hepatocytes and Kupffer cells; evaluation of biliary epithelial fine structure seldom reveals additional critical ultrastructural findings.

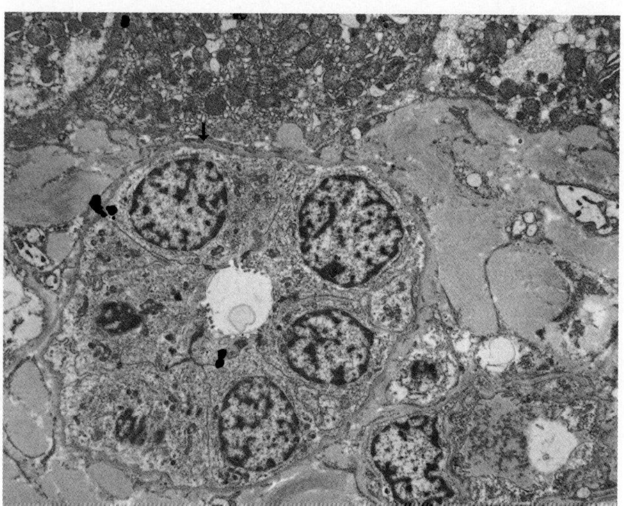

Figure 5.23 Biliary epithelial cells. Biliary epithelial cells rest on a basement membrane (*arrow*). They have basally located nuclei and are smaller and have less cytoplasm than hepatocytes. Notice the abundance of collagen (**right** and **left**), typically seen in portal tracts.

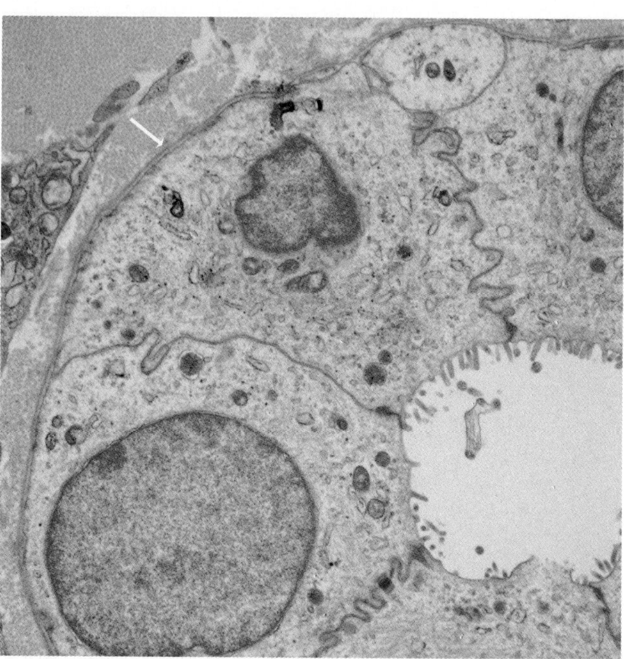

Figure 5.24 Biliary epithelial cells. Biliary epithelial cells, resting on a basement membrane (*arrow*), have sparse and smaller mitochondria than those of hepatocytes. Microvilli project into the bile duct lumen, which is sealed by many desmosomes that are clustered near the apical border of biliary epithelial cells.

5.4 GENERAL FEATURES IN ULTRASTRUCTURAL HEPATOPATHOLOGY

Before discussing specific disease conditions, it is important to identify common abnormalities seen in electron microscopy images and understand their significance.

Hepatocellular injury

In general, ultrastructural features of hepatocellular injury follow this sequence of events: cytoplasmic edema, mitochondrial swelling, cristolysis, flocculated mitochondrial matrix, clumping of nuclear chromatin, nuclear apoptosis (characterized by chromatin margination and fragmentation), rough endoplasmic reticulum degranulation, dense deposits in mitochondria and peroxisomes, and, finally, cell necrosis. In practice, general ultrastructural patterns of hepatocyte injury include the following:

1. Ballooning degeneration (Fig. 5.25) reflects ongoing hepatocyte damage.[63,64] Of note, the term ballooning degeneration, when used in ultrastructural descriptions, refers to extensive dilatation of the endoplasmic reticulum and is a different finding than the ballooning seen on hematoxylin and eosin (H&E) in diseases, such as fatty liver disease. In electron microscopy studies, ballooning is characterized by marked dilatation of the rough endoplasmic reticulum with detachment of the ribosomes, sometimes to a degree that hinders distinction between the rough endoplasmic reticulum and the smooth endoplasmic reticulum. The dilated rough endoplasmic reticulum often displaces other organelles. Although ballooning degeneration is considered a hallmark of viral hepatitis, it can be seen in many other conditions. As this pattern of hepatocellular damage continues, it can be followed by injury of the plasma membrane, which results in flattening of the villi and bleb formation (especially at the vascular pole), and by mitochondrial changes (swelling, low matrical density, fragmentation of cristae, and loss of matrical granules); these latter ultrastructural changes indicated an irreversible damage to the hepatocyte.[63]

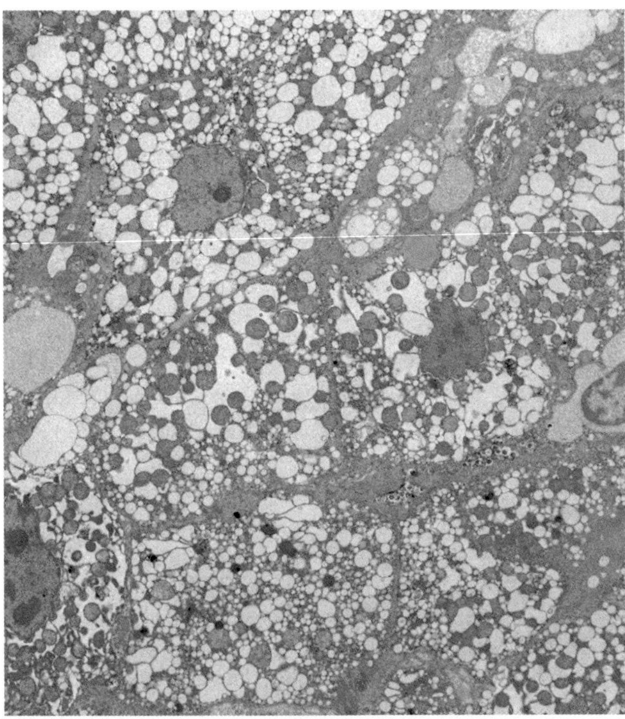

Figure 5.25 Hepatocellular injury: ballooning. Ballooning degeneration is characterized by marked and diffuse dilatation of the endoplasmic reticulum

2. Focal cytoplasmic degeneration (Fig. 5.26) is a pattern of hepatocellular injury that is characterized by necrosis of a portion of the hepatocellular cytoplasm, which is recognized ultrastructurally by the appearance of empty spaces in the cytoplasm, followed by breaking down of organelles and accumulation of amorphous electron-dense and granular material in the affected areas. Foci of focal cytoplasmic degeneration have irregular margins and vary in size; they are initially surrounded only by well-preserved organelles but eventually become bound by a distinct membrane, eventually producing an autophagic vacuole, then a cytolysosome.

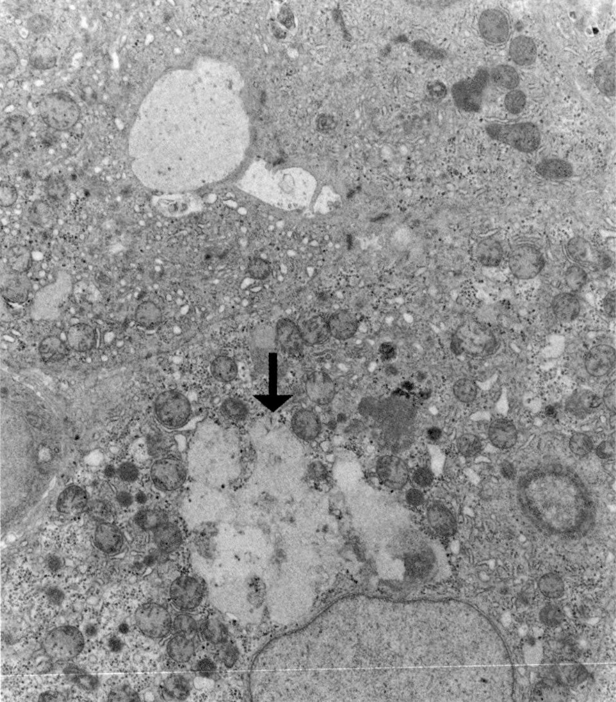

Figure 5.26 Hepatocellular injury: focal cytoplasmic degeneration. Focal cytoplasmic degeneration represents necrosis of a portion of the hepatocellular cytoplasm and features organelle-free, empty-looking spaces in the cytoplasm (*arrow*), containing some amorphous and granular material.

3. Oxyphilic/oncocytic change (Fig. 5.27) is characterized by increased mitochondria, some of which might show minor changes such as reduction of dense granules. It is considered to represent an adaptive change in response to various stimuli, including hypoxia and toxic injury. It is not a specific change because it can be seen in viral hepatitis, drug reactions, and in up to 50% of livers with cirrhosis.[65]

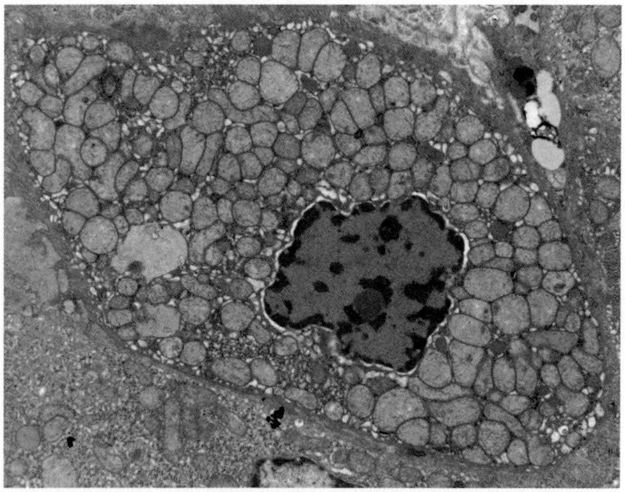

Figure 5.27 Hepatocellular injury: oncocytic change. Hepatocytes with oncocytic change are packed with numerous mitochondria.

4. Acidophil bodies, in contrast to ballooning degeneration, are characterized by cytoplasmic water loss, with cells becoming shrunken because of plasma membrane injury.[63,66] In addition to shrinkage, the cell loses its microvilli and plasma membrane junctions, resulting in detachment from neighboring hepatocytes.[64,67] Acidophil bodies are eventually engulfed by macrophages.

Cholestasis

Given that electron microscopy is frequently performed to evaluate hyperbilirubinemia in infants, cholestasis is commonly encountered in liver samples. Furthermore, electron microscopy is extremely sensitive in detecting cholestasis; signs of hepatocellular bile retention can be seen in the absence of clinical or biochemical evidence of jaundice.[68–71] For instance, focal subcellular cholestasis can be seen in asymptomatic gallstone patients whose livers are otherwise normal clinically, by laboratory testing, and by routine histology.[68,69,71]

The ultrastructural features of cholestasis include[20] the following changes:

1. Retained bile pigment in hepatocellular (Figs. 5.28 and 5.29) and Kupffer cell lysosomes. Occasionally, the biliary pigment in hepatocytes can be associated with cholesterol deposits (e.g., in cases of total parenteral nutrition), mimicking cholesteryl ester storage disease.
2. Canalicular changes with cholestasis include the following findings:
   a. Canalicular dilatation (most prominent in Zone 3) with retention of biliary material (Figs. 5.30 and 5.31), which can have variable appearances (filamentous, granular, lamellar, membranous, amorphous, and vesicular)
   b. Reduced or absent microvilli
   c. Swollen microvilli with or without bleb formation
   d. Thickening of the pericanalicular ectoplasm
   e. Increased pericanalicular lysosomes (with bile pigment)
   f. Prominent Golgi apparatus
   g. Increased pericanalicular vesicles
   h. Dilatation of pericanalicular rough endoplasmic reticulum and proliferation of the smooth endoplasmic reticulum
3. Mitochondrial changes include the following (Fig. 5.32):
   a. Curled or circular cristae
   b. Paracrystalloid mitochondrial inclusions (Figs. 5.33 and 5.34)
4. Focal cytoplasmic degeneration/necrosis (Fig. 5.35)

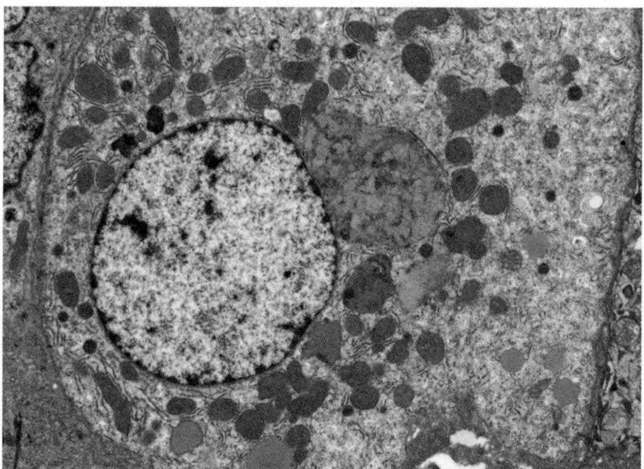

Figure 5.28 Hepatocellular cholestasis. Retained biliary material is identified in hepatocytes.

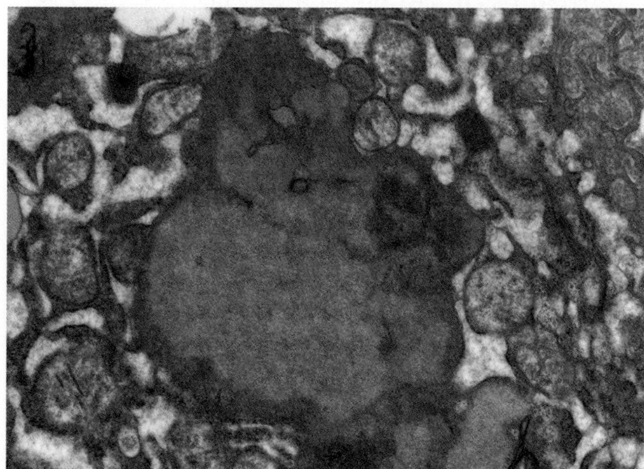

Figure 5.29 Hepatocellular cholestasis. The biliary material is contained in lysosomes and has a moderate to high electron density.

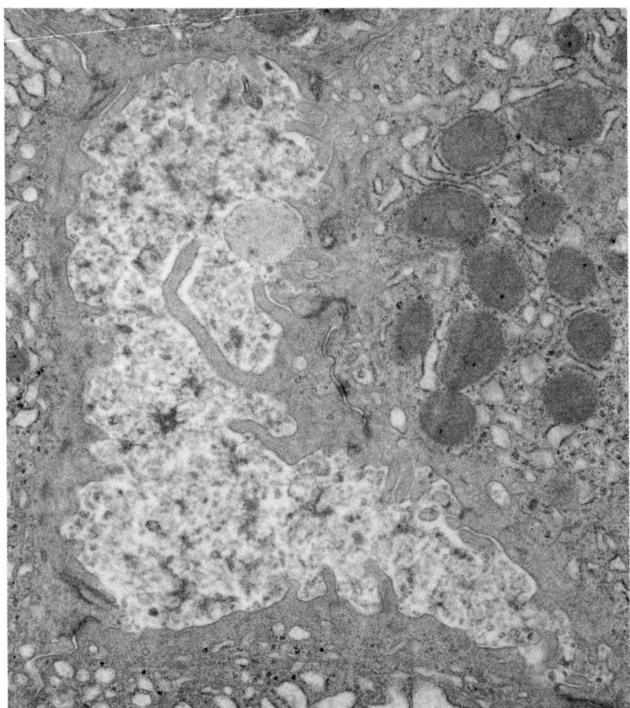

Figure 5.30 Canalicular cholestasis. Canalicular cholestasis is characterized by dilatation of canaliculi with retention of biliary material. The canalicular microvilli are reduced and swollen. Notice the thickening of the pericanalicular ectoplasm.

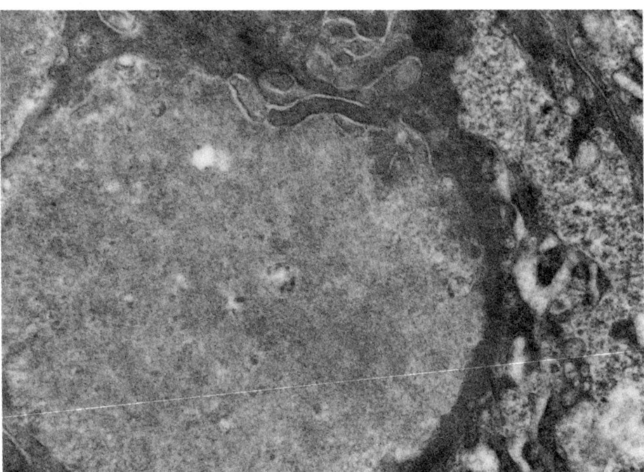

Figure 5.31 Canalicular cholestasis. In this instance, the biliary material retained in the canalicular lumen has a filamentous appearance.

Cholestasis is a nonspecific ultrastructural feature, but the nature of the canalicular material can provide hints to the etiology. Examples include the distinctive canalicular bile plugs seen in Byler bile, which is typical of progressive familial intrahepatic cholestasis or phospholipid-rich canalicular deposits that are characteristic of amiodarone toxicity.

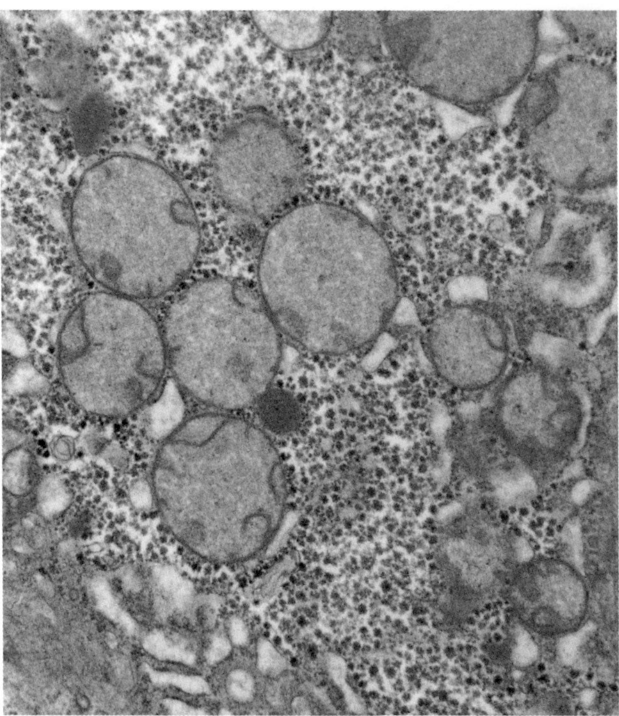

Figure 5.32 Cholestasis: mitochondrial changes. In cholestasis, the mitochondria often show curled or circular cristae.

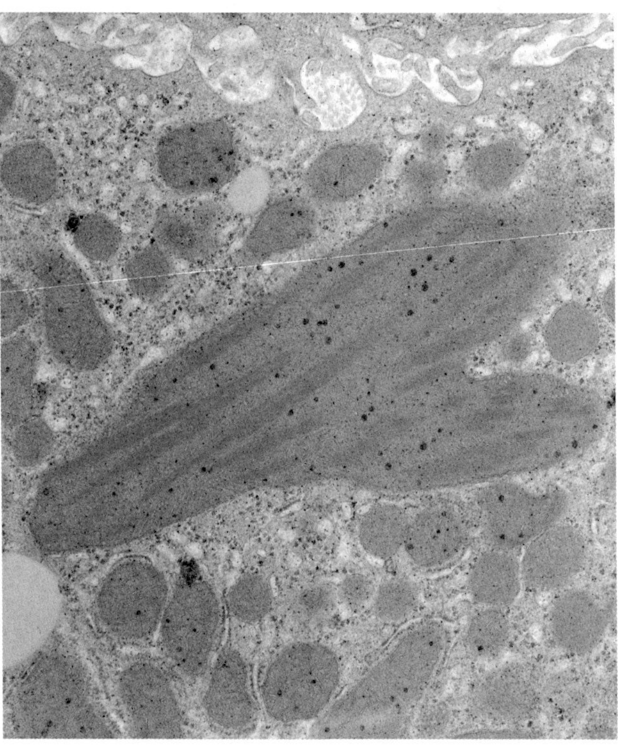

Figure 5.33 Cholestasis: mitochondrial changes. In cholestasis, the mitochondria often show paracrystalline inclusions.

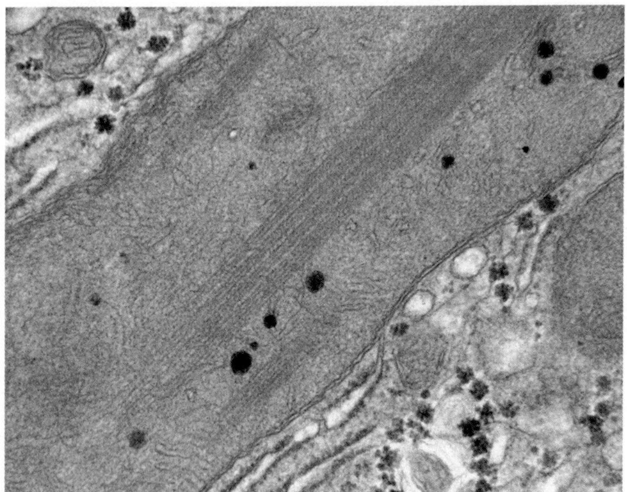

Figure 5.34 Cholestasis: mitochondrial changes. Another example of paracrystalline inclusions.

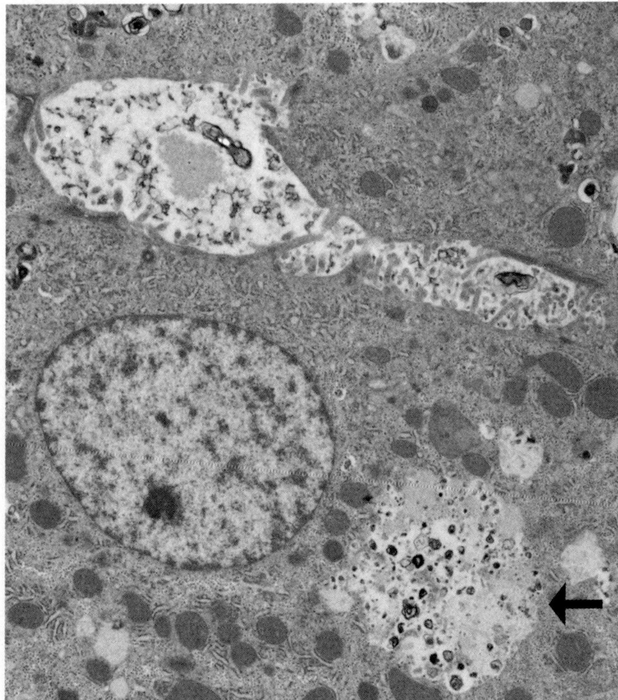

Figure 5.35 Hepatocellular cholestasis. Hepatocytes with marked cholestasis can contain areas of focal cytoplasmic degeneration (*arrow*).

Mitochondrial changes

The following pathologic abnormalities can be seen in mitochondria:

1. Giant mitochondria (Figs. 5.36 and 5.37) occur in drug-induced injury, fatty liver disease, and various metabolic disorders.

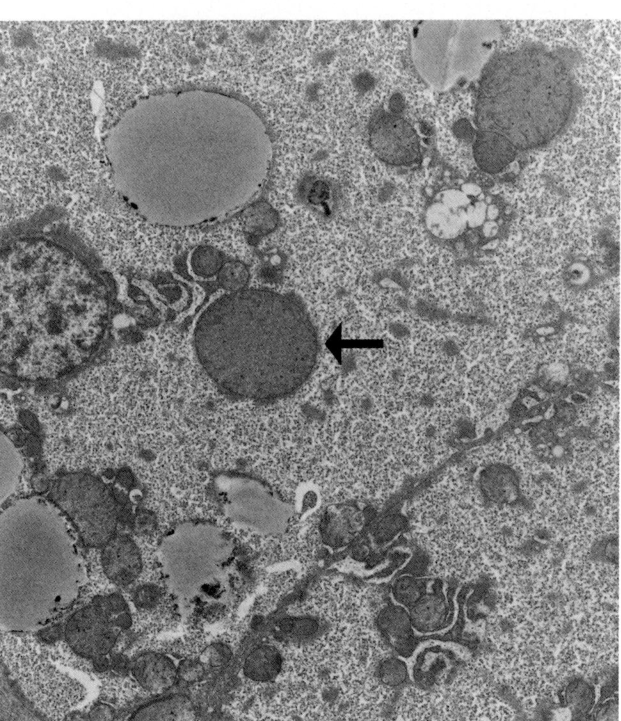

Figure 5.36 Mitochondrial changes: giant mitochondria. Giant mitochondria (*arrow*) are almost of the same size of the hepatocellular nucleus and are seen in a variety of pathologic conditions.

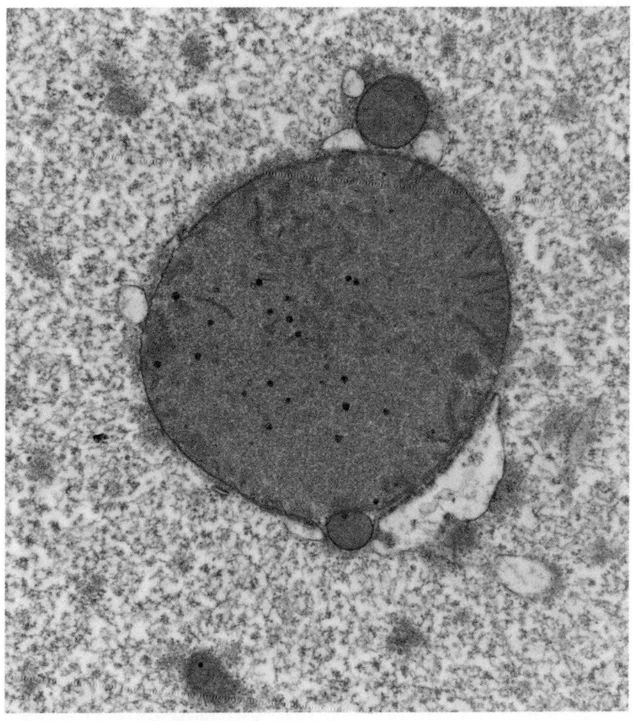

Figure 5.37 Mitochondrial changes: giant mitochondria. Another example.

2. Oxyphilic/oncocytic change (increased mitochondria in hepatocyte) is considered to represent adaptive changes in response to a variety of stimuli, including hypoxia and toxic injury. This finding is generally found in association with mitochondrial DNA deficiencies[72] but can also be frequently seen in various conditions, including viral hepatitis, drug-induced changes, and cirrhosis.[65]
3. Curled or circular cristae are generally associated with cholestasis.[69]
4. Condensed mitochondrial matrix (Fig. 5.38) can be seen in Wilson disease and mitochondrial cytopathies, but can also be mimicked by edge artifact (artifactual condensation seen at the periphery of the thin section). Mistaking this artifact for true pathology can be avoided by assessing mitochondria away from the tissue edge.
5. Cristolysis (Fig. 5.39) is a term referring to the loss of portions of the mitochondrial cristae. This finding usually indicates injury, but is somewhat nonspecific and can be seen in a wide variety of conditions, ranging from fixation artifact to Reye syndrome.[73]

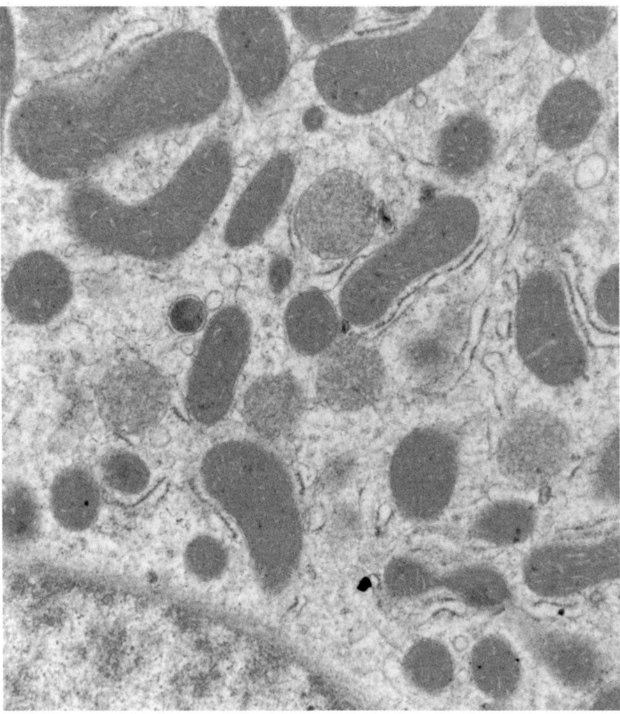

Figure 5.38 Mitochondrial changes: increased matrical density. The mitochondria have an abnormally increased electron density, significantly exceeding that of neighboring peroxisomes. This indicates a mitochondrial abnormality.

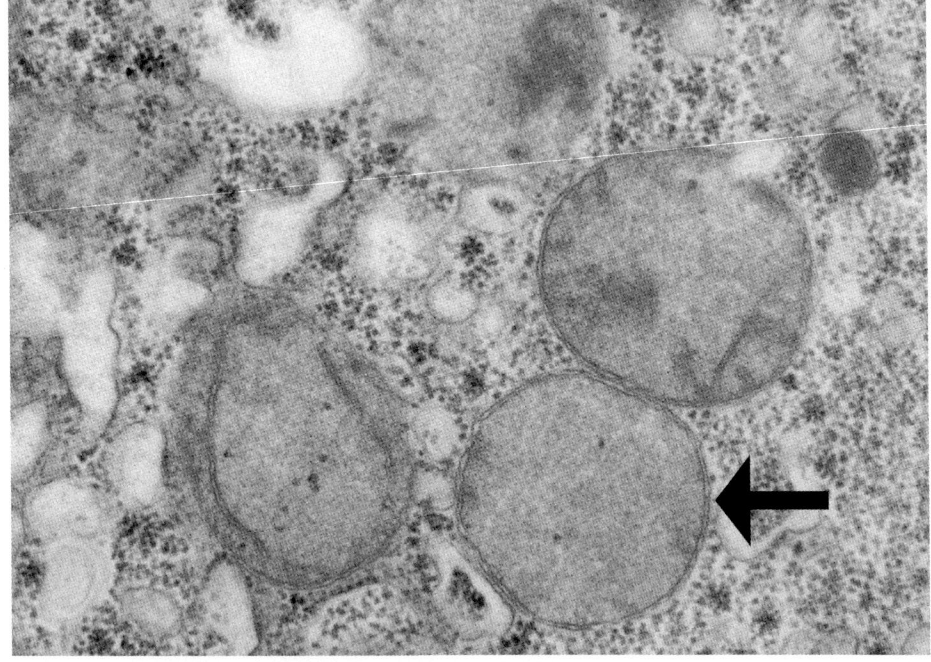

Figure 5.39 Mitochondrial changes: cristolysis. Cristolysis is characterized by loss of portions of the mitochondrial cristae. Notice that one of the mitochondrion (*arrow*) is completely devoid of cristae.

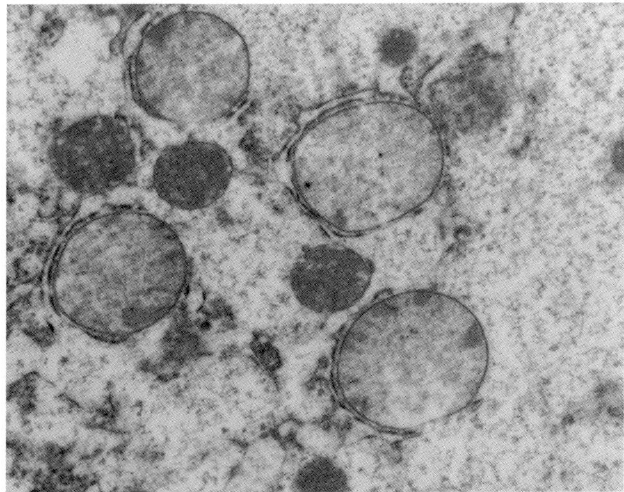

Figure 5.40 Mitochondrial changes: "empty-looking" mitochondria. Delayed fixation or autolysis can lead to "empty-looking" mitochondria, featuring low matrical density and lacking cristae.

6. "Empty-looking" mitochondria (Fig. 5.40) result from delayed fixation that leads to the loss of mitochondrial matrix and cristae, resulting in "empty-looking" mitochondria. This change can also be seen in autolyzed tissue (autopsy material).
7. The absence of matrical dense granules in mitochondria (Fig. 5.41) is considered an abnormality, but is a nonspecific finding that can be a feature of drug-induced injury or metabolic disorders.
8. Various inclusions can be seen in mitochondria, including crystalline/paracrystalline inclusions that can be found in the mitochondria of normal hepatocytes, but can also be seen in various pathologic conditions.[36]

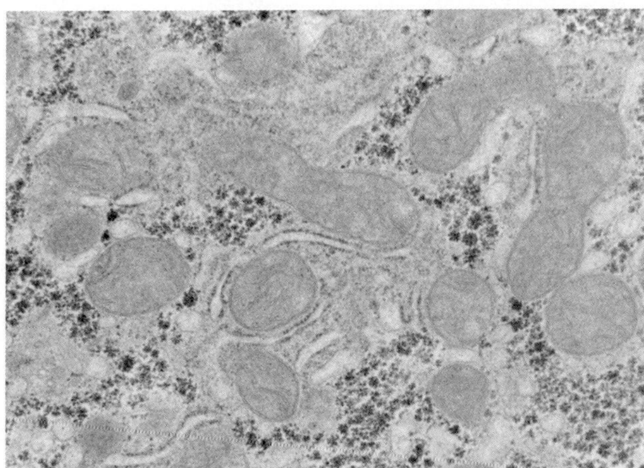

Figure 5.41 Mitochondrial changes: absence of matrical dense granules. The absence of matrical dense granules in mitochondria is a nonspecific finding that can be a feature of drug-induced injury or metabolic disorders.

Steatosis

Cytoplasmic lipid can be seen in normal hepatocytes, but excessive amounts are pathological. Steatosis features nonmembrane-bound cytoplasmic lipid deposits within hepatocytes. In contrast, the presence of a binding membrane, by definition, indicates that the structure is a lipolysosome rather than steatosis (Figs. 5.42 and 5.43). Macrovesicular steatosis (Figs. 5.44 and 5.45) can be seen in a variety of conditions including alcoholic and nonalcoholic liver disease, diabetes mellitus, Wilson disease, total parenteral nutrition, hyperlipidemia, familial lipoprotein deficiency, abetalipoproteinemia, total lipodystrophy, and carnitine palmoyl transferase deficiency.[73] Microvesicular steatosis (Fig. 5.46) can be seen in mitochondriopathies, urea cycle enzyme defects, Reye and Reye-like syndromes, drug-induced toxicities, lysosomal storage disorders, and lipodystrophies.[74]

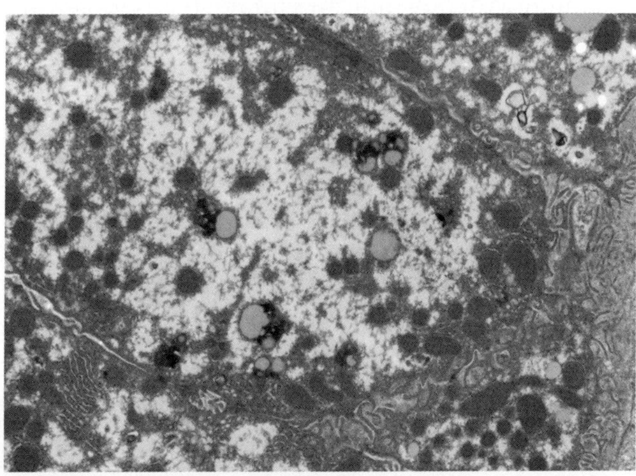

Figure 5.42 Lipolysosomes. Lipolysosomes are clusters of membrane-bound lipid droplets, usually admixed with other electron-dense lysosomal material.

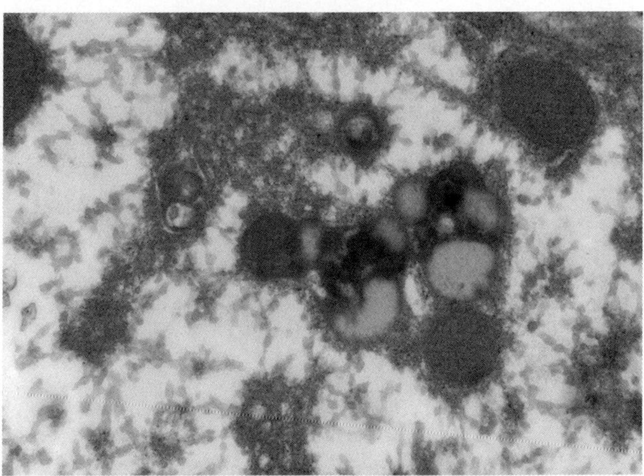

Figure 5.43 Lipolysosomes. Another example.

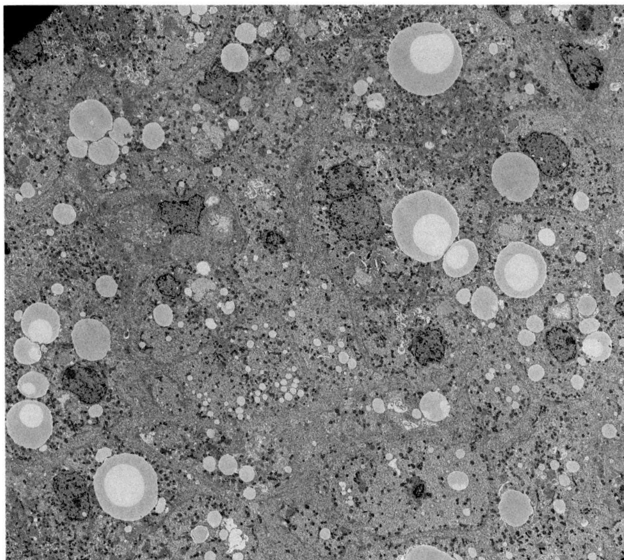

Figure 5.44 Macrovesicular steatosis. Lipid droplets in steatosis, in contrast to lipolysosomes, are nonmembrane-bound cytoplasmic lipid droplets found in hepatocellular cytoplasm.

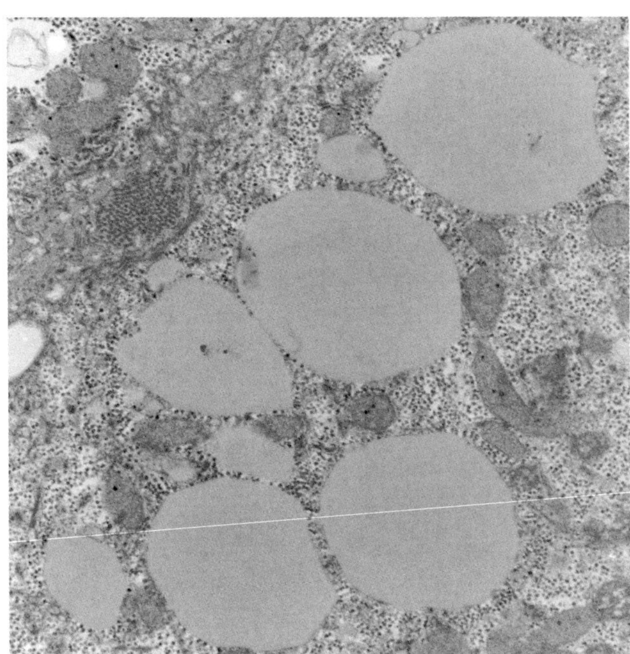

Figure 5.45 Macrovesicular steatosis. Another example.

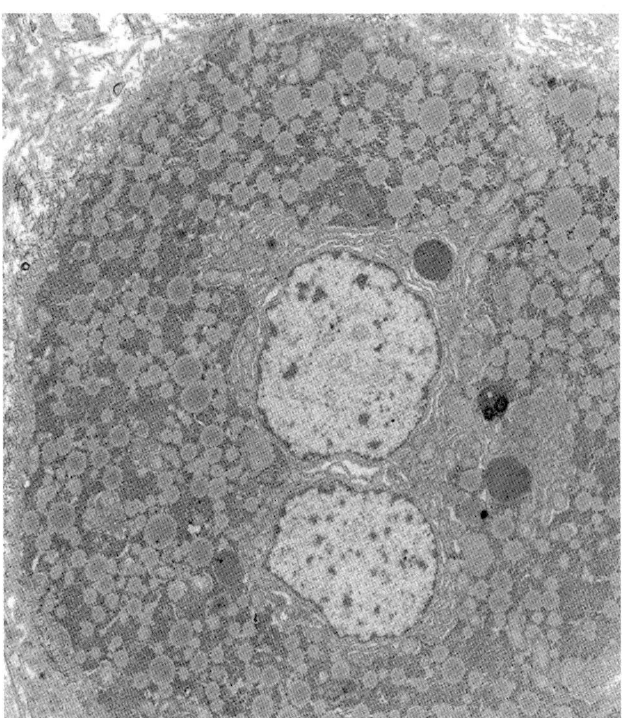

Figure 5.46 Microvesicular steatosis. This binucleated hepatocyte contains numerous small lipid droplets characteristic of microvesicular steatosis.

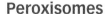

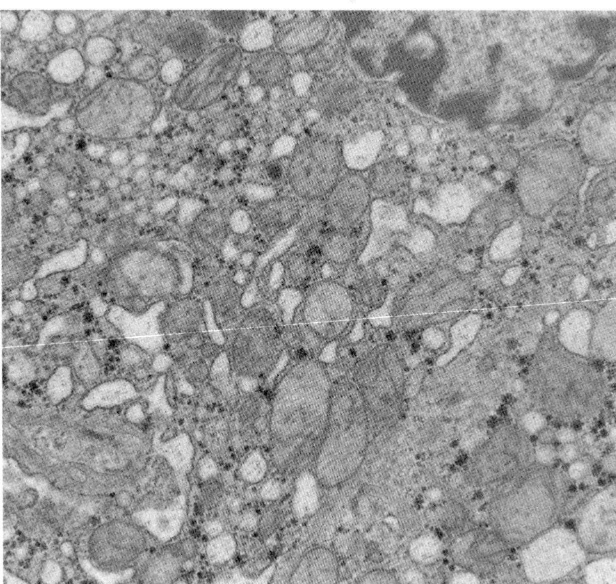

Figure 5.47 Zellweger syndrome. The absence of peroxisomes is pathognomic of Zellweger syndrome.

Peroxisomes

Peroxisomes are absent in Zellweger syndrome (Fig. 5.47), markedly decreased or absent in infantile Refsum disease and neonatal adrenoleukodystrophy, and can be increased in Reye syndrome, alcoholic liver disease, some drug-induced reactions (6-mercaptourine), and in cholestatic jaundice of pregnancy.[33]

5.5 METABOLIC LIVER DISEASE

In current practice, evaluation for the possibility of inherited metabolic diseases has become the main indication for electron microscopy evaluation of liver biopsies. Although electron microscopy information can greatly aid in achieving a diagnosis of a specific metabolic disorder, the definitive diagnosis is only achieved by demonstration of the underlying metabolic defect by molecular or biochemical methods. Electron microscopy findings in a liver biopsy can generally be placed into one of three categories:

1. Electron microscopy findings are very characteristic (virtually diagnostic) of a specific disease (or there is very small number of conditions in the differential). Examples of this category include the following:
   - Glycogen storage disease Types II and IV
   - α-1 antitrypsin deficiency
   - Wilson disease (a combination of electron microscopy findings, not a single feature, is very characteristic)
   - Gaucher disease
   - Farber disease
   - Dubin–Johnson syndrome
   - Zellweger syndrome
   - Fructosemia
   - Metachromatic leukodystrophy
   - Erythropoietic protoporphyria
   - Tay–Sachs disease
2. Electron microscopy findings are suggestive but not diagnostic of a specific disease. Examples include the following:
   - Progressive familial intrahepatic cholestasis
   - Cholesteryl ester storage disease
   - Rotor syndrome
   - Galactosemia

This category also includes cases where the electron microscopy findings provide broad categorization of the ultrastructural pattern, narrowing down the differential diagnosis (e.g., hepatocellular glycogenosis and phospholipidosis), but the ultimate diagnosis can only achieved by molecular and biochemical methods. Although not pathognomic, the electron microscopy findings in this category are still very helpful in achieving diagnosis.

3. Electron microscopy findings are important for their ability to exclude entities in the clinical or histologic differential diagnoses.

Numerous inherited metabolic disorders are known to involve the liver; including all of them is beyond the scope of this chapter. Instead, this chapter discusses those metabolic diseases that are the most common or that have the most characteristic ultrastructural features.

Disorders of carbohydrate metabolism and related disorders

Glycogen storage disease

The ultrastructural features of the following types of glycogen storage diseases have been characterized.[74]

1. Type I (Von Gierke disease): The hepatocytes are expanded and filled by pools of glycogen particles, displacing the hepatocellular organelles into the cytoplasmic periphery (Figs. 5.48, 5.49, and 5.50). Glycogen is not confined to the cytoplasm; nuclear glycogenation is a prominent and consistent finding in glycogen storage disease Type I. The presence of lipid droplets in hepatocellular cytoplasm is also a consistent finding.

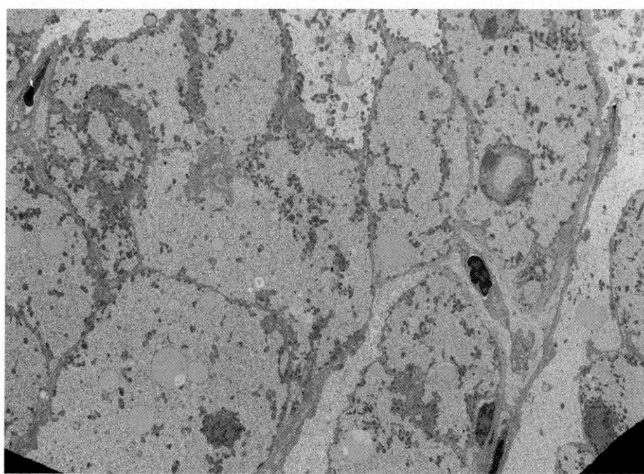

Figure 5.48 Glycogen storage disease, Type I. The hepatocytes are expanded and filled by pools of glycogen particles, displacing hepatocellular organelles into the cytoplasmic periphery.

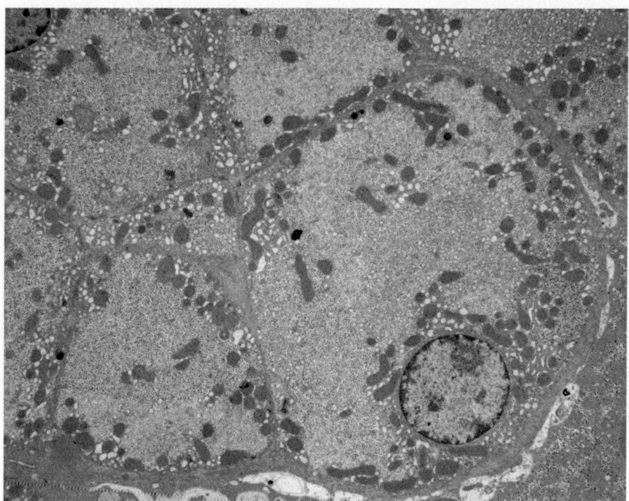

Figure 5.49 Glycogen storage disease, Type I. Another example.

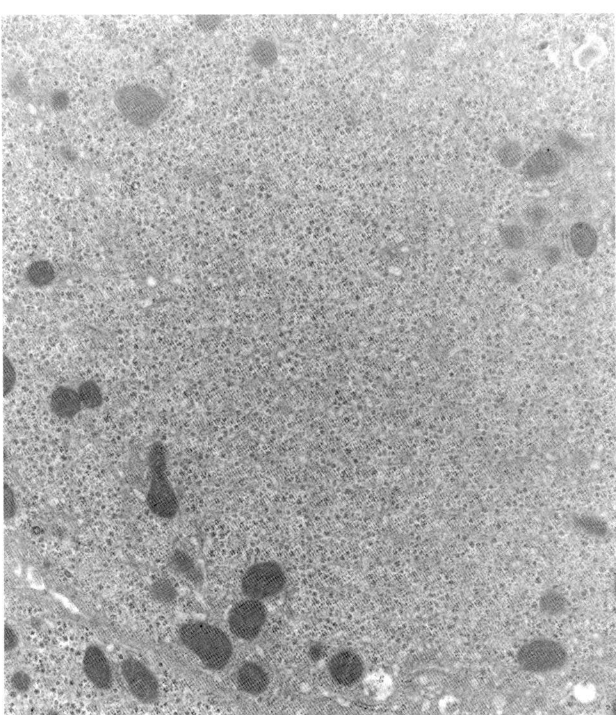

Figure 5.50 Glycogen storage disease, Type I. Another example.

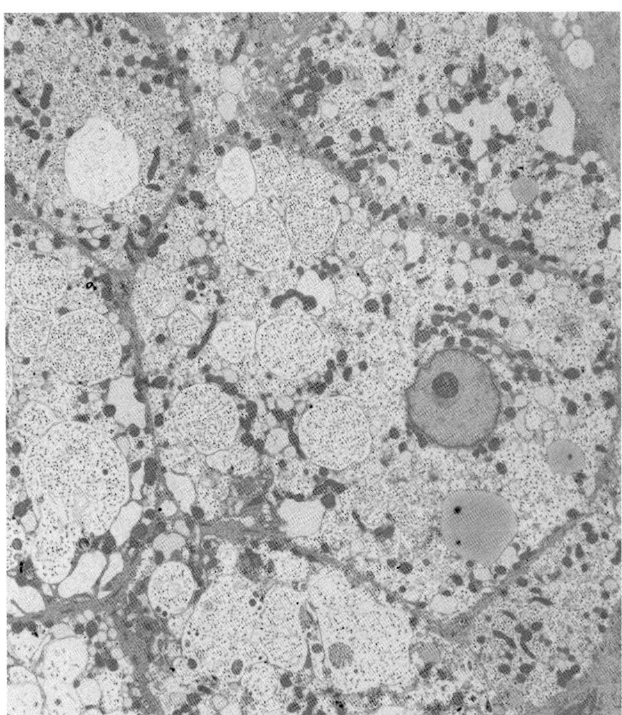

Figure 5.51 Glycogen storage disease, Type II. The ultrastructural features of glycogen storage disease, Type II are very characteristic, featuring excessive glycogen pools located in lysosomes.

2. Type II (Pompe disease): The electron microscopy findings are very distinctive (Fig. 5.51); the excessive glycogen pools are centered more in lysosomes than in the cytoplasm. These "glycogenosomes," typically laden with monoparticulate glycogen, are round to oval and can be large enough to displace other organelles into the cytoplasmic periphery. Although a few glycogenosomes can be seen in other glycogen storage disease types, they are the hallmark of Pompe disease if they are the predominant ultrastructural finding.[74,75] Like glycogen storage disease Type I, lipid droplets are usually present in the cytoplasm.
3. Type III: Glycogen storage disease Type III has a very similar ultrastructural appearance to that of glycogen storage disease Type I.[74,76] The main difference is the prominent collagen deposition seen in glycogen storage disease Type III, which is not usually seen in glycogen storage disease Type I.[74,76,77]
4. Type IV: The ultrastructural features of glycogen storage disease Type IV are essentially pathognomic[74,78–81]; they are characterized by cytoplasmic inclusions that are irregular, large, nonmembrane bound, and sharply demarcated. The inclusions consist of randomly oriented fibrils representing abnormal glycogen (Figs. 5.52 and 5.53). Ill-defined glycogen rosettes are often admixed with the fibrils. Furthermore, very large glycogen rosettes

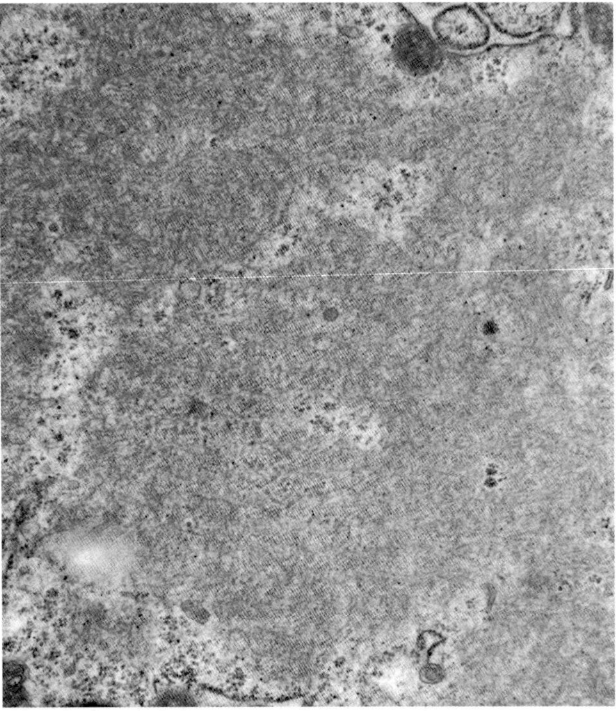

Figure 5.52 Glycogen storage disease, Type IV. The ultrastructural features of glycogen storage disease Type IV are essentially pathognomic, featuring large cytoplasmic inclusions consisting of randomly oriented fibronectin fibrils representing abnormal glycogen.

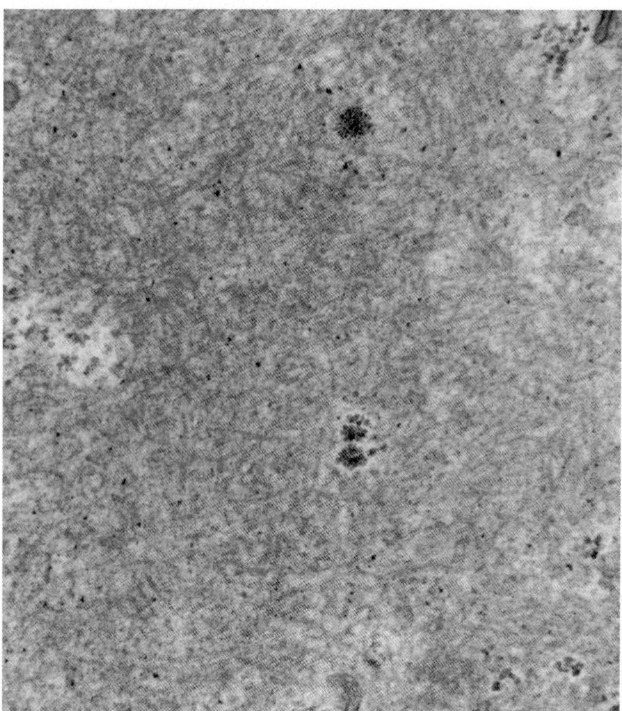

Figure 5.53 Glycogen storage disease, Type IV. Scattered ill-defined glycogen rosettes are often admixed with the fibrils.

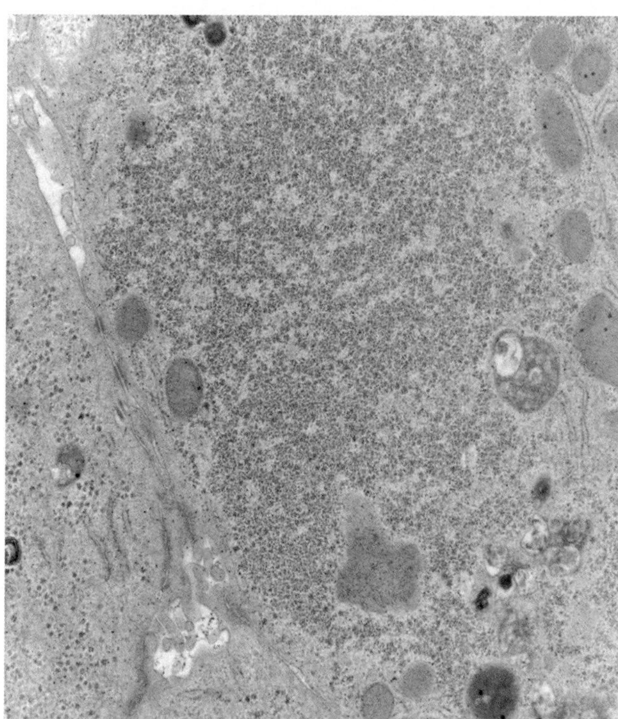

Figure 5.54 Glycogen storage disease, Type VI. The glycogen deposits in glycogen storage disease, Types VI and IX often have a "starry-sky" appearance, resulting from scattered foci of granular material of low electron density scattered within the glycogen pools.

often delineate the fibrillary deposits from the surrounding cytoplasm. In some cases, the fibrillary deposits have a "spider-like" appearance. Lipid droplets are frequently seen in the vicinity of the glycogen inclusions.

5. Type VI: Glycogen storage disease Type VI features pools of glycogen, predominantly monoparticulate, but with scattered interspersed glycogen rosettes, displacing other organelles into the cytoplasmic periphery. The glycogen deposits often have a "starry-sky" appearance (Fig. 5.54), resulting from scattered foci of granular material of low electron density scattered within the glycogen pools.
6. Type IX: Electron microscopy examination shows pools of glycogen occupying most of the cytoplasm, consisting of a mixture of monoparticulate and rosette forms; the presence of scattered foci of granular, organelle-free zones within the glycogen deposits imparts a "starry-sky" appearance that is typical of glycogen storage disease Type IX. Although the "starry-sky" appearance is typical of glycogen storage disease Type IX, it can be seen in other types of glycogen storage disease, such as glycogen storage disease Types III and VI. The presence of cytoplasmic lipid droplets is a consistent finding.
7. Type XI: This glycogen storage disease is characterized by the accumulation of various amounts of glycogen, predominantly in rosette forms, as well as lysosomal glycogen deposits, in the monoparticulate form.

Although the ultrastructural features of glycogen storage disease Types II and IV are characteristic, increased hepatocellular glycogen that closely mimics the other types of glycogen storage diseases can be seen in other conditions, including glycogenic hepatopathy, glycogenosis sometimes seen in Type 2 diabetes mellitus, carnitine deficiency, and long-term corticosteroid use.[74,82,83] The distinction between these conditions is often difficult or even impossible based on electron microscopy findings alone; correlation with the clinical findings and/or molecular/biochemical methods is also required.

Galactosemia

Ultrastructurally, galactosemia shows canalicular and hepatocellular cholestasis, multinucleated giant cell change in hepatocytes, dilatation of the endoplasmic reticulum, and large lipid droplets within hepatocytes. The dilated endoplasmic reticulum can displace other organelles, and sometimes contains flocculent clear material. Glycogen deposits are often diminished. Although none of these findings is specific for galactosemia, their collective presence can suggest this disorder[74] in the appropriate clinical setting.

Hereditary fructose intolerance (fructosemia)

The most characteristic ultrastructural finding in hereditary fructose intolerance is "fructose holes," which are numerous, variably sized, membrane bound, lucent structures scattered in the hepatocellular cytoplasm, either completely devoid of contents or only containing sparse glycogen particles.[84] Occasionally, the fructose holes can be rich in glycogen, resembling the "glycogenosomes" of glycogen storage disease Type II, and the distinction can be made by the presence of typical lucent lesions elsewhere in the cytoplasm. In addition to fructose holes, fructosemia also shows lipid droplets, an abundance of glycogen, myelin figures, and focal cytoplasmic degeneration.[74]

Diabetes mellitus

The ultrastructural findings seen in Type II diabetes are nonspecific but include steatosis (most frequent finding) and nuclear glycogenosis. Large hepatocellular glycogen stores can be observed, similar to glycogen storage disease.

Lafora disease

Lafora bodies are characteristic hepatocellular inclusions composed of aggregates of smooth endoplasmic reticulum membranes associated with irregular glycogen rosettes.[74] They occupy most of the hepatocellular cytoplasm, displacing other organelles, and are not limited by a membrane. They are not seen in all hepatocytes and are most prominent in Zone 1. Entrapped organelles or lipid droplets can sometimes be identified within the inclusion. A minority of hepatocytes can show a diffuse increase in glycogen instead of inclusions.

Lysosomal storage disorders

Various inherited deficiencies in lysosomal enzymes lead to the accumulation of the undigested metabolites of the deficient enzyme within the lysosomes of hepatocytes and/or Kupffer cells.

Gaucher disease

Ultrastructurally, Gaucher cells represent markedly enlarged Kupffer cells with characteristic cytoplasmic inclusions (Figs. 5.55, 5.56, and 5.57).[74] The inclusions

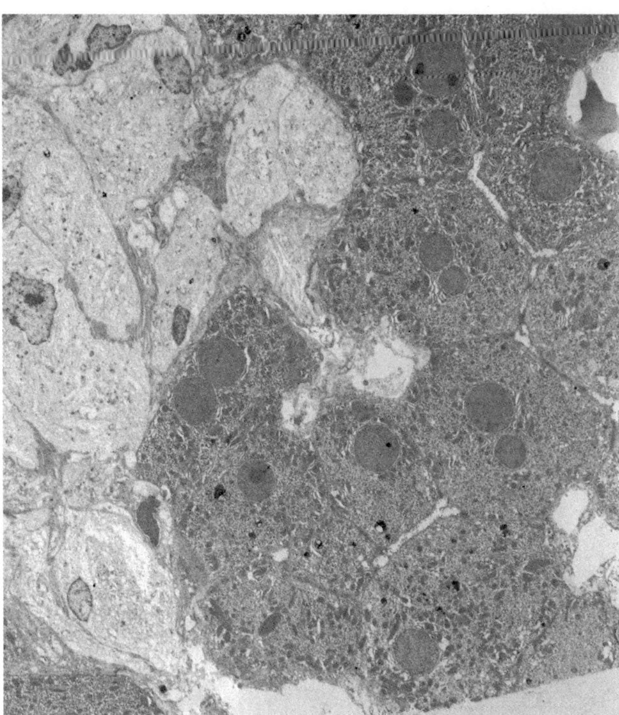

Figure 5.55 Gaucher disease. Gauchers cells are distended Kupffer cells, laden with inclusions (representing accumulation of glucocerbroside, phospholipids, cholesterol, and lipoprotein), often forming aggregates (**left side**). Notice that the hepatocytes are essentially normal (**right side**).

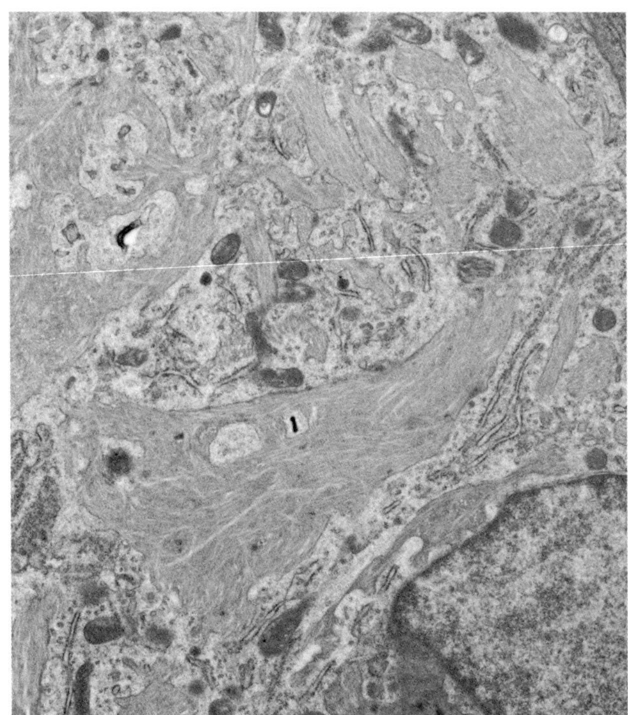

Figure 5.56 Gaucher disease. The inclusions within Gaucher cells are well demarcated but irregularly shaped and consist of numerous long tubules (circular on cross sections) arranged in bundles and bound by a single membrane.

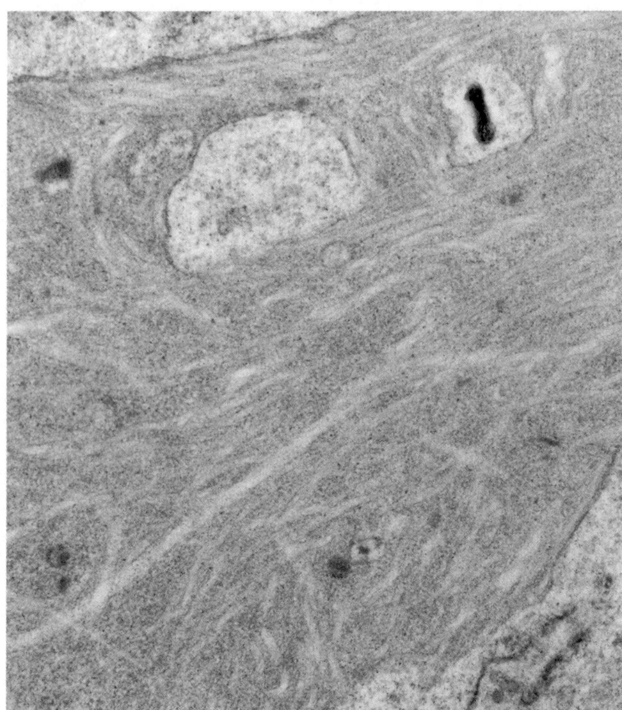

Figure 5.57 Gaucher disease. Another example.

are well demarcated but irregularly shaped and consist of numerous long tubules (circular on cross section) arranged in bundles and bound by a single membrane[73]; they tend to cluster together, forming large aggregates that push the nucleus to the periphery of the cell. The inclusions represent the accumulation of glucocerbroside, phospholipids, cholesterol, and lipoprotein.[85] These inclusions are absent in hepatocytes; instead, the hepatocytes sometimes show "zebra bodies," which are lamellar deposits in the hepatocyte cytoplasm.[85] Although these findings are almost pathognomic, confirmation by mutation analysis or by glucocerebrsidase activity determination in leukocytes or cultured fibroblasts is usually required.

Cholesteryl ester storage disease and Wolman disease

These two conditions are clinically distinct, but are ultrastructurally similar.[74,86–95] They are both characterized by lipid droplets and cholesterol crystals expanding the cytoplasm of hepatocytes and Kupffer cells. Lipolysosomes are also frequent.

Metachromatic leukodystrophy (sulphatidosis)

Metachromatic leukodystrophy has very characteristic lysosomal inclusions,[74] which are found in Kupffer cells and fibroblasts. These inclusions feature closely packed structures alternating between leaflets and a tubular appearance (depending on the orientation), an arrangement that produces a prismatic herringbone appearance.

Niemann–Pick disease

Electron microscopy in Niemann–Pick disease shows characteristic whorled lysosomes (Fig. 5.58) within Kupffer cells, distending their cytoplasm. The whorls consist of pleomorphic membrane-bound, concentric/parallel leaflets that alternate with loosely arranged lipid, representing sphingomyelin deposits.[74,85,96–99] The inclusions are also present in hepatocytes, but are less abundant. When present, they have a pericanalicular location. In hepatocytes, lipid droplets, cholesterol crystals, and focal cytoplasmic degeneration are also seen. The hepatocellular inclusions are essentially indistinguishable from other forms of phospholipidosis, such as can be seen in association with amiodarone use. A definitive diagnosis is achieved by mutation analysis and sphingomyelinase assays and/or assaying cultured fibroblasts for cholesterol esterification.[100] The only advantage of liver electron microscopy over these methods is rapid turnaround time.[101]

Gangliosidosis (GM1 and GM2)

In GM1 gangliosidosis, hepatocytes and Kupffer cells contain lysosomal inclusions, which appear as electron lucent vacuoles containing fine granular material; these inclusions are responsible for the vacuolated appearance seen by light microscopy. Concentric membranous arrays can also be seen. In GM2 gangliosidosis (Tay–Sachs disease and Sandhoff disease), numerous characteristic "zebra bodies" are seen; they consist of membrane-bound inclusions containing parallel arrays of electron-dense material.

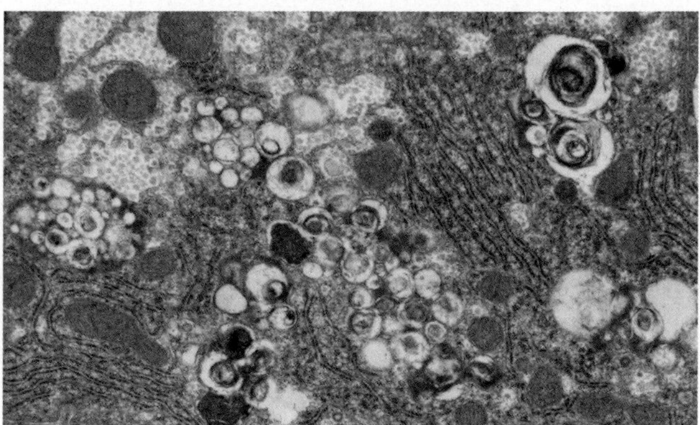

Figure 5.58 Niemann–Pick disease. Niemann–Pick disease is characterized by typical whorled lysosomes within Kupffer cells. These whorls consist of pleomorphic membrane-bound, concentric/parallel leaflets that alternate with loosely arranged lipid, representing sphingomyelin deposits.

Mucopolysaccharidoses

Although various enzymatic defects result in various clinical syndromes (Hurler, Hunter, Scheie, etc.),[74,88,98,102–111] the ultrastructural features of mucopolysaccharidoses are the same. Hepatocytes contain numerous electron lucent, round, membrane-bound vacuoles (lysosomal inclusions) containing flocculent material. Sometimes electron-dense structures are seen within the center of the flocculent material, generating a "bull's eye" appearance. Membranous arrays can also be seen at the margins of the inclusions. Mucopolysaccharidoses can be mimicked by various other disorders that can produce empty-looking lysosomes with occasional electron-sense deposits (e.g., gangliosidosis, sialidosis, and mannosidosis).

Farber disease

In Farber disease, Kupffer cells demonstrate lysosomes packed with comma-shaped structures and short tubules formed by two parallel membranes separated by electron lucent spaces. The hepatocytes, on the other hand, demonstrate ultrastructural findings similar to those of mucopolysaccharidoses.[74,85,112–115]

Mucolipidoses

In mucolipidoses, Kupffer cells, endothelial cells, and to a lesser extent hepatocytes and biliary cells contain membrane-bound vacuoles containing flocculent material.[74]

Oligosaccharidoses

All variants of oligosaccharidoses have the same ultrastructural characteristic. These findings include numerous membrane-bound electron lucent vacuoles containing flocculent material expanding the cytoplasm of hepatocytes, Kupffer cells, endothelial cells, and hepatic stellate cells, and displacing nuclei and organelles. These vacuoles result in a foamy appearance on H&E histology.

Fabry disease

The ultrastructural features of Fabry disease are similar to those of phospholipidosis.[74,116] Hepatocytes, Kupffer cells, and endothelial cells contain markedly pleomorphic, membrane-bound, electron-dense lysosomal inclusions, which consist of concentric and geometrical membranous arrays. In hepatocytes, the inclusions have a pericanalicular distribution. The inclusions can sometimes be angulated or curved. Steatosis is also a frequent finding.

Disorders of lipid and lipoprotein metabolism

Abetalipoproteinemia

Electron microscopy findings in abetalipoproteinemia are characterized by numerous membrane-bound lipid droplets occupying the hepatocellular cytoplasm, hypertrophy of the Golgi apparatus, and dilatation of the rough endoplasmic reticulum. In the prominent Golgi apparatus, a lack of very low-density lipoprotein inclusions constitutes a constant feature of the disease.

Carnitine deficiency

Carnitine deficiency has an ultrastructural picture featuring multiple lipid droplets within hepatocytes. The glycogen stores vary in amount; they can be either reduced or excessive. When excessive, the can form massive pools of glycogen rosettes, mimicking glycogen storage disease. In fact, differentiation between carnitine deficiency and glycogen storage disease can be impossible on ultrastructural analysis. Mitochondrial changes, including enlargement, pleomorphism, and increased numbers of cristae, along with the microvesicular steatosis, can also mimic Rye syndrome. However, the characteristic mitochondria of Rye syndrome (swollen ameboid mitochondria with collapsed membranes) are absent in carnitine deficiency, allowing ultrastructural differentiation.[74]

Tangier disease

Ultrastructural changes can be seen both in Kupffer cells and hepatocytes. Kupffer cells are distended by many lipid droplets, displacing the nucleus and cytoplasmic organelles. Kupffer cells also contain membranous arrays within lysosomes. The hepatocytes, on the other hand, display lipid droplets and occasional cholesterol clefts.

Familial hypercholesterolemia

The main ultrastructural finding in this disease is the presence of lipid droplets and cholesterol crystal clefts.

Fatty acid oxidation defect (acyl CoA dehydrogenase deficiency)

Fatty acid oxidation defects are characterized by a peculiar accumulation of irregularly shaped lipid droplets with electron-dense margins within the hepatocytes, surrounded by crystal clefts. Entrapped mitochondria and glycogen can sometimes be found in the periphery of the lipid inclusions.

Congenital total lipodystrophy

In congenital total lipodystrophy, the hepatocytes demonstrate numerous lipid droplets, lipofuscin laden lysosomes, and lipolysosomes. Peroxisomal changes have also been reported, including dense matrix granules. Mitochondrial pleomorphism is seen, with crystal-like inclusions that likely represent cholesterol.[117] Macrophages laden with lipid droplets and cholesterol crystals can also be found.

Endoplasmic reticulum storage disorders

α-1 antitrypsin deficiency

The hepatocytes of patients with α-1 antitrypsin deficiency demonstrate dilated sacs of rough endoplasmic reticulum containing moderately electron-dense material (sometimes flocculent), representing the abnormally accumulated protein (Figs. 5.59 and 5.60). An electron lucent halo separates the inclusions from the endoplasmic reticulum membrane. Although communication with the rough endoplasmic reticulum persists, large inclusions often lose their membrane associated ribosomes. In infants, cholestasis is also a prominent feature, which may overshadow the inclusions. Classical inclusions can be less conspicuous and therefore very difficult to identify in young infants (<3 months).[74,118–124]

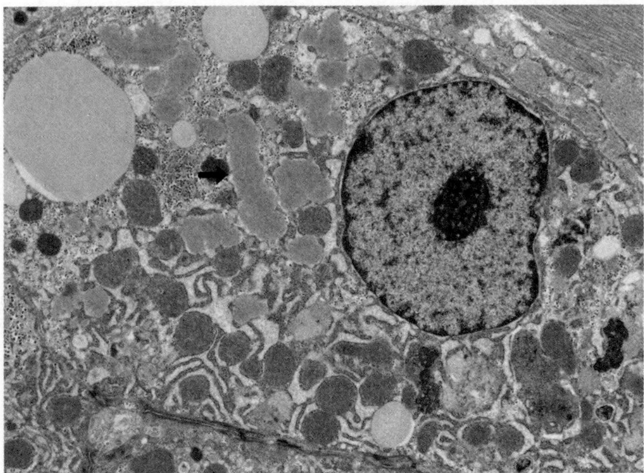

Figure 5.59 α-1 antitrypsin deficiency. The hepatocytes in α-1 antitrypsin deficiency demonstrate dilated sacs of rough endoplasmic reticulum containing moderately electron-dense material, representing the abnormally accumulated protein. An electron lucent halo (arrow) separates the inclusions from the endoplasmic reticulum membrane.

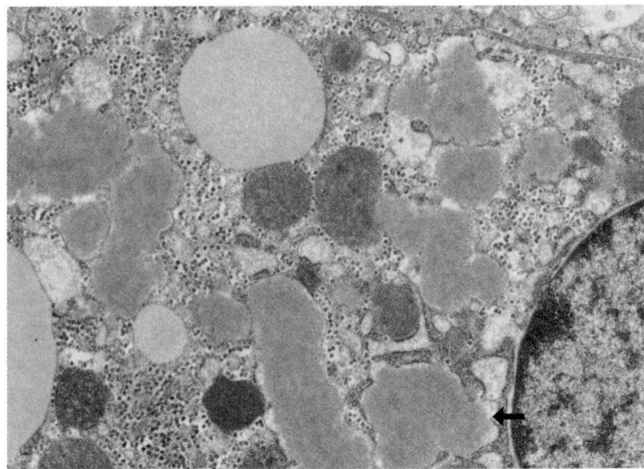

Figure 5.60 α-1 antitrypsin deficiency. Notice the communication between the inclusions and the endoplasmic reticulum (*arrow*).

Disorders of amino acid metabolism

Tyrosinemia

The ultrastructural findings in liver biopsies are nonspecific. The hepatocytes show variable amounts of lipid droplets, which can bulge into dilated rough endoplasmic reticulum, and contain granular material with a lucent background. Mitochondrial pleomorphism and rough endoplasmic reticulum dilatation are frequent findings.

Cystinosis and homocystinuria

In cystinosis, the lysosomes of Kupffer cells contain crystalloid inclusion; these can be recognized as empty rectangular spaces made by the cysteine crystals that are dissolved during processing.[125,126] In homocystinuria, mitochondrial pleomorphism, smooth endoplasmic reticulum proliferation, and increased pericanalicular lysosomes can be observed.[73,125,127]

Urea cycle disorders

The hepatocytes in urea cycle disorders have characteristic elongated, tortuous and branching mitochondria, often containing paracrystalline inclusions, and dilated endoplasmic reticulum.[104]

Disorders of bile acid and bilirubin metabolism

Progressive familial intrahepatic cholestasis

Progressive familial intrahepatic cholestasis Type 1 has two distinctive ultrastructural features.[74] First, Byler bile (Fig. 5.61) consists of coarsely particulate biliary

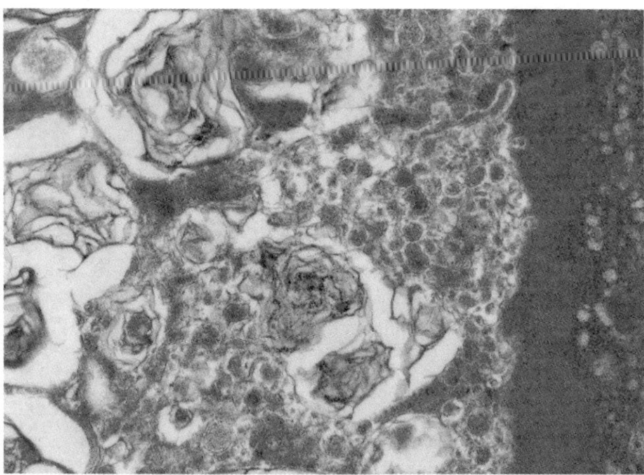

Figure 5.61 Progressive familial intrahepatic cholestasis, Type 1. Progressive familial intrahepatic cholestasis Type 1 features the distinctive Byler bile, which consists of coarsely particulate biliary material distending bile canaliculi. Notice the presence of membranous elements within the biliary material as well. The bile canaliculi containing Byler bile are distended and their microvilli are lost. Notice the marked thickening of the pericanalicular ectoplasm.

material seen in the bile canaliculi, which also includes membranous and vesicular elements.[74,128] The bile canaliculi containing Byler bile are distended, and their microvilli are damaged or lost. Secondly, marked thickening of the pericanalicular ectoplasm is seen.

Byler bile is not entirely specific for progressive familial intrahepatic cholestasis Type 1 and can be seen in other conditions, such as benign recurrent intrahepatic cholestasis. Byler bile is not generally considered to be a feature of progressive familial intrahepatic cholestasis Types 2 and 3, although some have described similar findings in progressive familial intrahepatic cholestasis Type 2.[129–131] Filamentous looking bile has also been described in progressive familial intrahepatic cholestasis Type 2, but this is not distinctive and can be seen in other cholestatic conditions.

Gilbert syndrome

The electron microscopy findings are variable in Gilbert syndrome. A common finding is increased lipofuscin deposits within lysosomes.[74,132,133] Some patients have mitochondrial changes including giant forms and paracrystalline inclusions.[74] Other cases have shown changes in the sinusoidal membrane of hepatocytes, with flattening of the membrane and loss of microvilli.[134] Reduced rough endoplasmic reticulum and proliferated smooth endoplasmic reticulum have also been reported.[73]

Dubin–Johnson syndrome

Characteristic Dubin–Johnson pigment is distinct from lipofuscin. The pigment consists of very dense particles, often associated with lipid droplets, located within lysosomes, in a background of more homogenous moderately dense granular material occupying the rest of the lysosome. Like lipofuschin, Dubin–Johnson pigment is more abundant in Zone 3 hepatocytes.

Rotor syndrome

In Rotor syndrome, the H&E morphology of the liver is usually normal, but the ultrastructural features are variable. The most characteristic findings are seen in the lysosomes, which contain electron-dense material with a "two-tone" appearance, resulting from alternating electron dense and fine granular material. This material can also resemble lipofuscin.[135] The material differs from Dubin–Johnson pigment by the lack of dense lipid droplets. Another common finding is nuclear glycogenosis. Bile canaliculi can either be normal or demonstrate some dilatation and reduction of microvilli. Mitochondrial pleomorphism, giant mitochondria, and paracrystalline inclusions have been reported.

Disorders of metal metabolism

Wilson disease

Although there is not a single pathognomic ultrastructural feature for Wilson disease, the constellation electron microscopy features are virtually diagnostic. Nowadays, however, the diagnosis of Wilson disease is made by evaluation of serum ceruloplasmin, 24 hours urine copper levels, quantitation of hepatic copper levels, and genetic testing. Electron microscopy is seldom required for diagnosis in current practice. Nonetheless, the ultrastructural features remain important.

The hepatocytes in Wilson disease show very characteristic mitochondrial changes (Figs. 5.62, 5.63, and 5.64). These changes include mitochondrial pleomorphism and enlargement, with the presence of giant mitochondria. The cristae are abnormal, with dilatation of the intracristal space and formation of sacs and/or microcysts at the tips of the cristae, which often appear as free-floating vacuoles in the mitochondrial lumen. The mitochondria also have large matrical granules and often contain paracrystalloid inclusions or lipid droplets. Sometimes, electron-dense deposits, likely representing copper, are observed in the mitochondria. In addition to the typical mitochondrial changes, copper deposits are seen in lysosomes

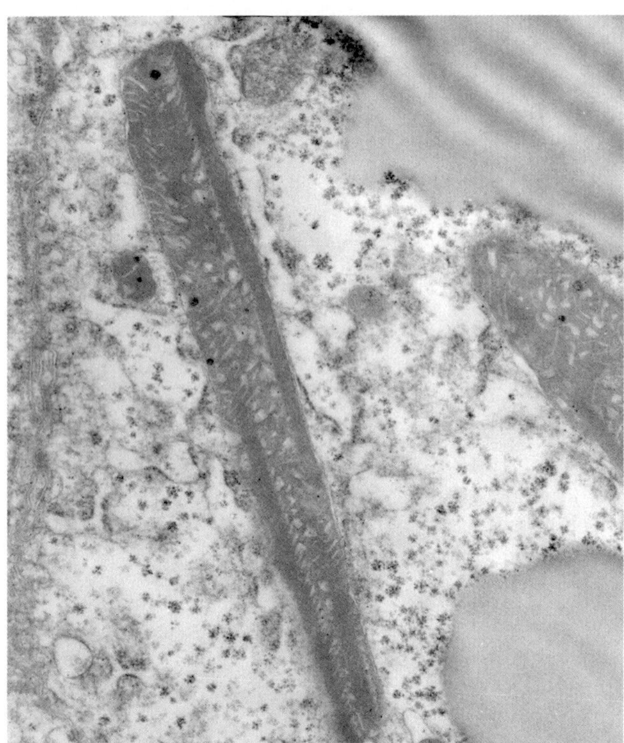

Figure 5.62 Wilson disease, mitochondrial changes. The hepatocytes in Wilson disease show very characteristic mitochondrial changes. These include large, pleomorphic, and bizarre-shaped mitochondria, including giant mitochondria.

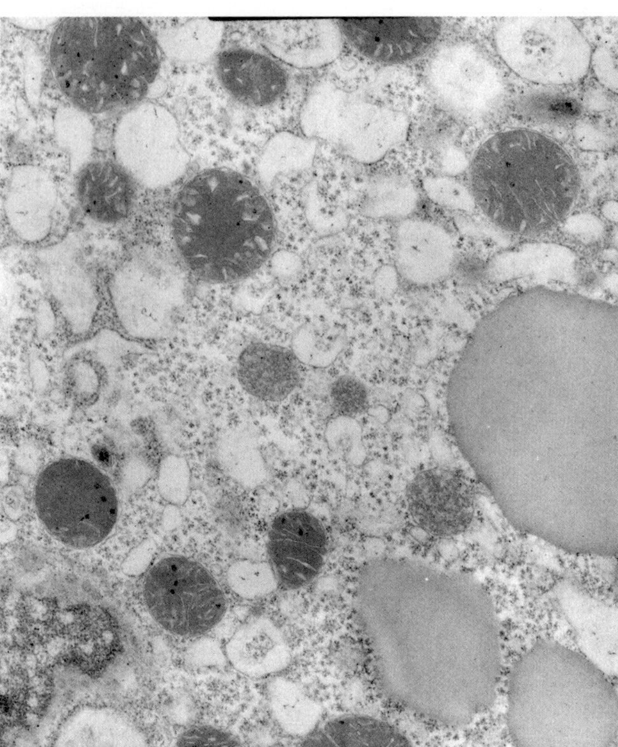

Figure 5.64 Wilson disease, mitochondrial changes. The mitochondrial cristae are abnormal, showing abnormal dilatation and sac formation, which often appear as free-floating vacuoles in the mitochondrial lumen.

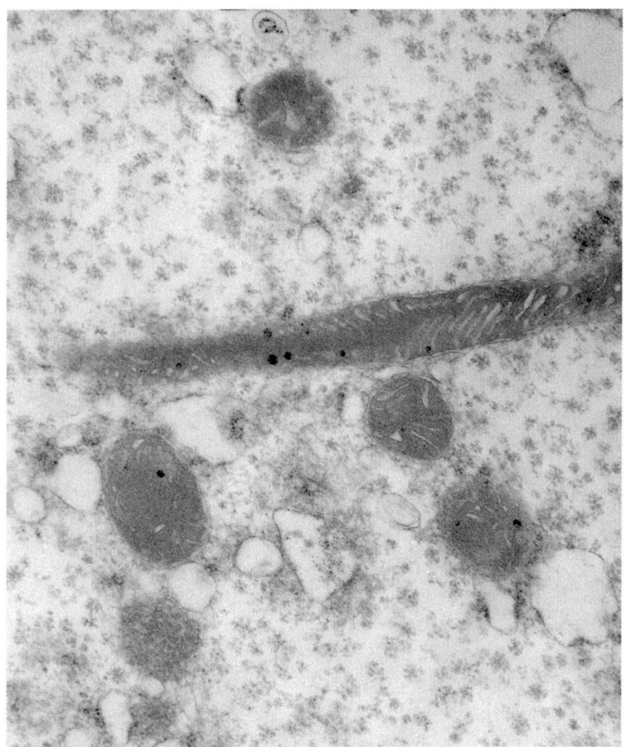

Figure 5.63 Wilson disease, mitochondrial changes. Another example of giant mitochondria.

(coppersomes) (Figs. 5.65 and 5.66), most prominent in Zone 1 hepatocytes. The copper deposits are usually associated with lipofuscin and display marked electron density and pleomorphism.

The hepatocytes in Wilson disease also sometimes feature abnormalities in the bile canaliculi, including elongation and increased numbers of microvilli that fill the canalicular lumen, sometimes producing a "fish-mouth" appearance. Other consistent ultrastructural features include steatosis and glycogenated nuclei. Mallory hyaline (see Alcoholic liver disease) and glycogen bodies (see Drug-induced injury) are sometimes seen.

Hereditary hemochromatosis

In hereditary hemochromatosis, siderosomes are ultrastructurally recognized as membrane-bound pleomorphic deposits representing hemosiderin and ferritin, with a pericanalicular distribution. The deposits have a finely granular matrix containing variable electron-dense masses (Fig. 5.67), and can sometimes be arranged in geometric arrays. In addition to lysosomal hemosiderin, very fine iron particles can be found freely in the hepatocellular cytoplasm. In secondary hemochromatosis, similar lysosomal deposits exist,

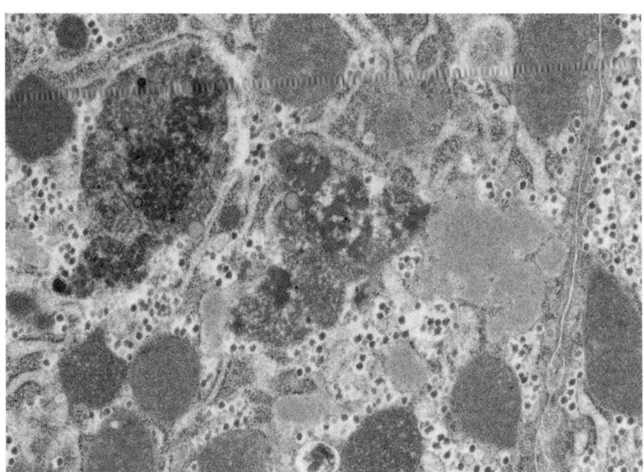

Figure 5.65 Wilson disease, copperosomes. Copperosomes represent excessive lysosomal copper deposits, often admixed with lipofuscin, characterized by marked electron density and pleomorphism.

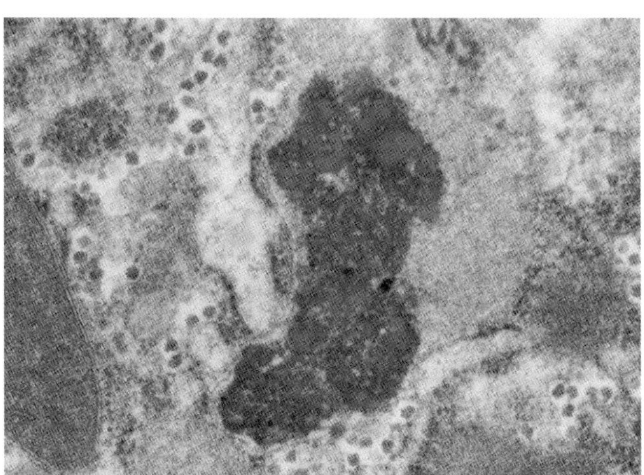

Figure 5.66 Wilson disease, copperosomes. Another example.

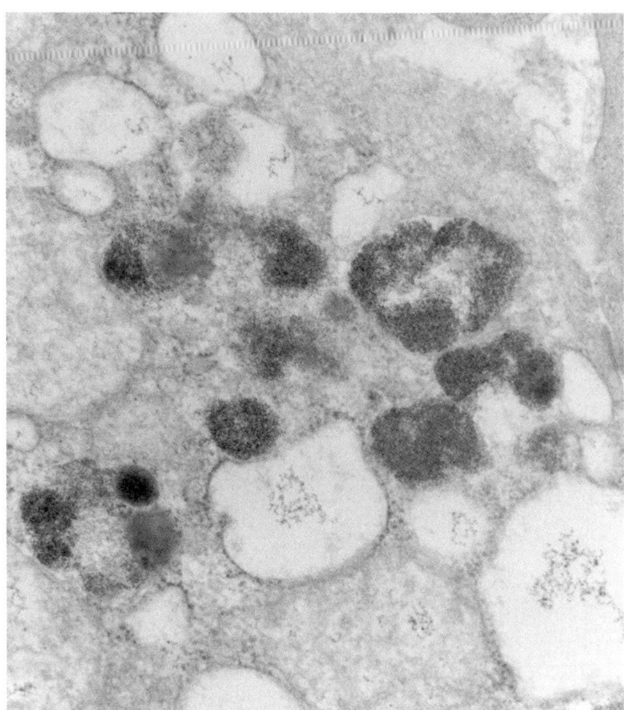

Figure 5.67 Hereditary hemochromatosis. The hepatocytes in hereditary hemochromatosis contain excessive amounts of hemosiderin. Hemosiderin consists of lysosomal aggregates of finely granular electron-dense material.

but they predominate in the Kupffer cells as opposed to the hepatocytes. Hemosiderin deposits are also found both in hepatocytes and Kupffer cells in neonatal hemochromatosis, but are also accompanied by hepatocellular cytoplasmic necrosis.

Peroxisomal disorders

The ultrastructural features of Zellweger syndrome are pathognomonic.[74] The disease is characterized by the complete absence of peroxisomes, sometimes with the presence of ill-formed vesicular forms resembling incompletely developed peroxisomes. Although the electron microscopy findings are characteristic, the diagnosis can be easily missed because the presence or absence of peroxisomes was not evaluated. Therefore, it is essential to examine electron microscopy images methodically, and pathologists examining liver ultrastructure should routinely verify the presence of lysosomes in every case. Infantile Refsum disease can also show total absence of peroxisomes in some hepatocytes, whereas other hepatocytes have underdeveloped peroxisomes, often containing an unusual dense matrix. In both disorders, Kupffer cells have angulated lysosomes containing needle-shaped inclusions that are admixed with lipid droplets.[136] Other peroxisomal disorders include neonatal adrenoleukodystrophy, which demonstrates decreased and diminutive peroxisomes and Kupffer cells that show features similar to those seen in infantile Refsum disease (angulated lysosomes).[73] It is important to note that the presence of peroxisomes does not rule out a peroxisomal disorder (other than Zellweger syndrome) because some of these disorders affect the function rather than the biogenesis of peroxisomes.

Mitochondrial cytopathies

Ultrastructural features of mitochondrial cytopathies include several mitochondrial structural abnormalities including pleomorphism, loss of crista, and matrical changes (granular fluffy matrix).[125,137,138]

Other metabolic disorders

Cystic fibrosis

The eosinophilic plugs that sometimes can be seen by light microscopy in the bile ducts and the proliferating ductules are ultrastructurally characterized by a filamentous or fibrillo-granular appearance. There are also changes in the bile duct basement membrane, including thickening, duplication, and deposition of coarse, granular, electron-dense material (Fig. 5.68). This material can also be seen in intercellular spaces and interstitium. However, this electron-dense material it is not specific for cystic fibrosis because it can be seen in a variety of chronic biliary-type injuries.[74]

Porphyrias

The hepatocytes in porphyria cutanea tarda have typical needle-shaped cytoplasmic inclusions, mitochondrial changes including pleomorphism and paracrystalline inclusions, and lysosomal iron deposition. Mallory hyaline can also be found.[74,139,140] Erythropoietic protoporphyria shows numerous needle-shaped crystals assuming a "starbust" configuration floating freely in the cytoplasm of hepatocytes, as well as many pleomorphic crystal-laden lysosomes in hepatocytes and Kupffer cells. The cytoplasmic crystals are usually surrounded by glycogen. They can sometimes be found in bile canaliculi.

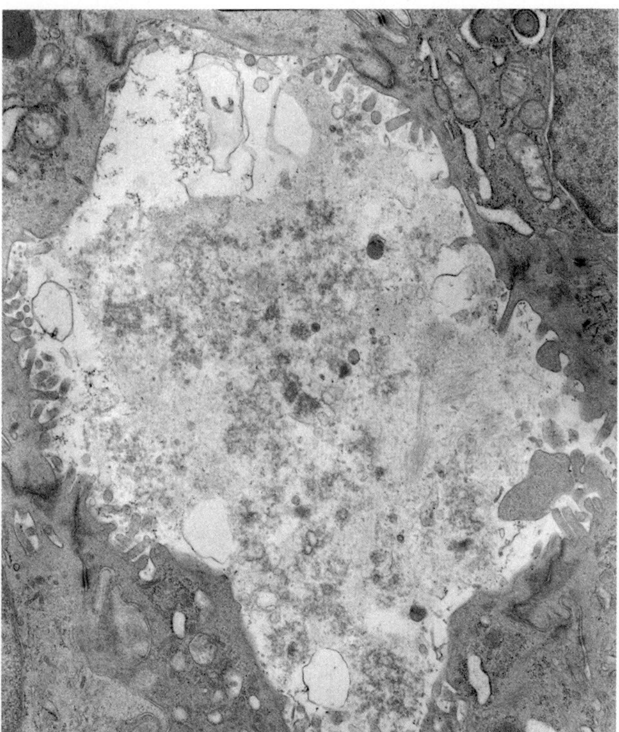

Figure 5.68 Cystic fibrosis. The bile ducts contain coarse granular material corresponding to the inspissated granular eosinophilic material seen in bile ducts by light microscopy.

Congenital disorders of glycosylation

Electron microscopy shows characteristic "grape-like" aggregates of numerous small membrane-bound inclusions in hepatocytes, found in a pericanalicular distribution. These inclusions (aka myelinosome) are either empty-looking or have concentric, multi-lamellar structures (whorls, or an amorphous, electron-dense deposition). Some of these aggregates have lipofuscin in their center.[141]

5.6 DRUG-INDUCED INJURY

Virtually, the entire spectrum of liver pathology can be induced by medications, and a detailed description of all of the ultrastructural features associated with the numerous drugs that produce hepatic injury is beyond the scope of this chapter. However, this chapter describes the general ultrastructural features that suggest drug-induced injury and provides a few examples of characteristic patterns seen on ultrastructural pathology.

In general, the presence of several (two or more) of the following ultrastructural features suggests a drug/toxin-induced injury[74]:

1. Changes involving the endoplasmic reticulum:
   a. Proliferation of the smooth endoplasmic reticulum (adaptive response). Most medications are metabolized by the smooth endoplasmic reticulum, and this is the most common ultrastructural feature seen in drug-induced injury. Importantly, the zonal variation in smooth endoplasmic reticulum prominence (more abundant in Zone 3) should not be misinterpreted as a sign of drug-induced injury. Cyanamide is an example of this phenomenon, wherein the proliferating smooth endoplasmic reticulum is associated with heavy glycogen deposits, producing characteristic inclusions.[142,143]
   b. Concentric membranous arrays (adaptive response). This change also affects the endoplasmic reticulum, which assumes a concentric membranous configuration. When the lamellar membrane formations are associated with heavy glycogen rosette deposit, they are known as "glycogen bodies." This is a common finding in drug-induced injury; tetracycline being a good example.[144,145]
   c. Dilatation, vesiculation, and degranulation (loss of ribosomes) of the rough endoplasmic reticulum. These ultrastructural features are

associated with the H&E finding of hepatocellular ballooning. Carbamazepine produces a classic example of these changes.[146]

2. Mitochondrial changes (adaptive response) are very common in drug-induced injury. These changes include increased numbers of mitochondria, reflected by oncocytic change under light microscopy, for example with valproic acid.[146] Other changes include bizarre mitochondria shapes and giant forms, for example with tetracycline.[144,147] The mitochondria can also have paracrystalline inclusions, for example with methotrexate.[146] Concentric membranous arrays can also be observed, for example with amiodarone.[146,148] Finally, mitochondrial granules can be increased in size or number, for example in methotrexate use.[146] Although the above-described changes are adaptive, more significant changes, such as swelling and membranous breaks, suggest irreversible damage to the hepatocytes.
3. Proliferation of peroxisomes can be seen, for example in oral contraceptives and anabolic steroids.[33,146]
4. Lysosomal changes can be found. The most characteristic lysosomal alteration is lysosomal phospholipidosis (secondary phospholipidosis), featuring myelin figures, exemplified by amiodarone toxicity (Fig. 5.69). These features closely resemble primary phospholipidosis, such as Niemann–Pick disease.[146,149–151]

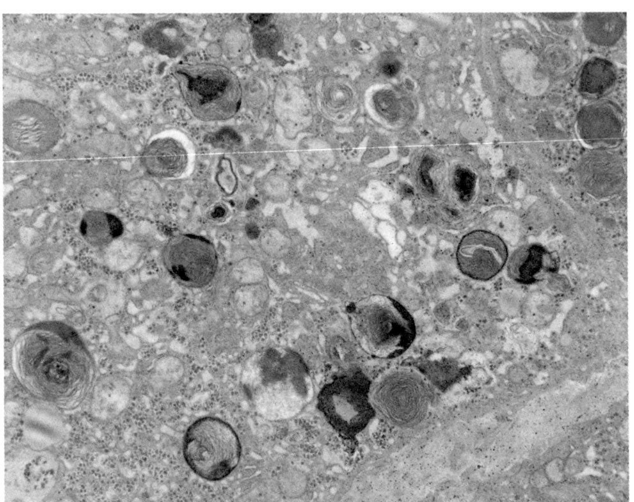

Figure 5.69 Amiodarone toxicity. Amiodarone toxicity is characterized by lysosomal phospholipidosis (secondary phospholipidosis), featuring numerous lysosomal myelin figures. These features closely resemble primary phospholipidosis (i.e., Niemann–Pick disease), but are instead mainly seen in hepatocytes rather than Kupffer cells.

Other nonspecific ultrastructural features frequently occur in drug-induced liver injury. For instance, macrovesicular steatosis is common in drug-induced hepatocellular injury, whereas microvesicular steatosis is less common but can be seen, for example with valproic acid.[146] Another common feature is cholestasis, but this is nonspecific in most cases. As an exception, the presence of phospholipid membranous arrays in bile canaliculi (drug plugs) is characteristic for amiodarone toxicity. Drug-induced Mallory hyaline, for example with amiodarone, is ultrastructurally identical to that seen in alcoholic steatohepatitis (see Alcoholic liver disease).

Certain characteristic ultrastructural features can be seen in association with a few medications. Several examples include the following:

1. Amiodarone toxicity: The electron microscopy picture is typical, featuring lysosomal phospholipidosis (see earlier), Mallory bodies, and ballooning of hepatocytes.[73]
2. Reye syndrome like picture: Electron microscopy changes show microvesicular steatosis, glycogen depletion, and mitochondrial swelling, for example in tetracycline and valproic acid.[146,152,153]
3. Aspirin toxicity: Electron microscopy shows dilated rough endoplasmic reticulum, giant mitochondria, mitochondrial crystalline inclusions, and lipofuscin accumulation.[154]
4. Corticosteroids (long-term use): Electron microscopy is characterized by macrovesicular steatosis and glycogen accumulation,[73] sometimes mimicking glycogen storage disease.

5.7 OTHER DISORDERS

Reye syndrome

The typical ultrastructural features of Reye syndrome include microvesicular steatosis, glycogen depletion, increased peroxisomes, and giant ameboid mitochondria that have cristolysis, flocculent matrix, and paracrystalline inclusions, often lacking matrical granules. Certain medications and several metabolic disorders can produce a similar ultrastructural picture, including defects in fatty acid oxidation, carbohydrate and amino acid metabolism, and disorders of ammonia detoxification.

Viral hepatitis

In the current practice of liver pathology, electron microscopy has limited utility in the diagnosis of viral hepatitis because there are other serologic- and histologic-based detection methods (e.g., immunohistochemistry and in situ hybridization). The hepatocytes in viral hepatitis show nonspecific but reproducible features of hepatocyte injury including ballooning degeneration, focal cytoplasmic degeneration, acidophil bodies, hepatocellular oncocytic change, and cholestasis. These features are found either with or without the identification of the viral organisms. Ultrastructural features of hepatotropic and nonhepatotropic viruses have been well described,[20] but are beyond the scope of this chapter.

In addition to the generic ultrastructural features seen in the hepatocytes with viral infection, certain characteristic features can be seen by electron microscopy. For instance, ground-glass inclusions characteristic of hepatitis B infection correspond ultrastructurally to hepatocytes containing excessive quantities of surface antigen particles, which consist of elongated or spherical structures (depending on the orientation), packed in a proliferating endoplasmic reticulum.[63,155–157] The endoplasmic reticulum plays an important role in the production of hepatitis B surface antigens, and viral proteins can accumulate, leading to the ground-glass inclusions.[158–164] Of note, the inclusions can be ultrastructurally very similar to α-1 antitrypsin inclusions.[63] In contrast to cytoplasmic ground-glass changes, the sanded nucleus sometimes seen by light microscopy in biopsies with hepatitis B correspond to an abundance of core antigen particles within the nucleus; these are tiny (27 nm) ring-shaped structures admixed with or scattered within the chromatin.[63]

Alcoholic liver disease

In acute alcoholic hepatitis, the main findings include steatosis, marked dilatation of the rough endoplasmic reticulum, reduced glycogen, and focal cytoplasmic degeneration. In nonacute alcohol-induced injury, the presence of lipid droplets is almost always present. Lipolysosomes, which represent lipid droplets engulfed by lysosomes, appear as aggregates of vacuoles intermixed with amorphous clumps and granular, electron-dense material. Although these changes are common in alcoholic liver disease, they can also be seen in other conditions, such as hypercholesterolemia. Sometimes, cholesterol clefts can be identified as well. Various mitochondrial changes occur, with giant mitochondria often showing increase in the size and number of dense granules. These changes most often occur in Zone 3 hepatocytes and are found in almost all cases (93%).[165–168] Mallory bodies (Figs. 5.70, 5.71, and 5.72) are frequent in alcoholic liver disease, but can occur in a variety of other types of hepatocellular injury. Three subtypes of Mallory bodies are recognized.[169] In a specific sample, Mallory bodies most often consist of admixtures of all types.

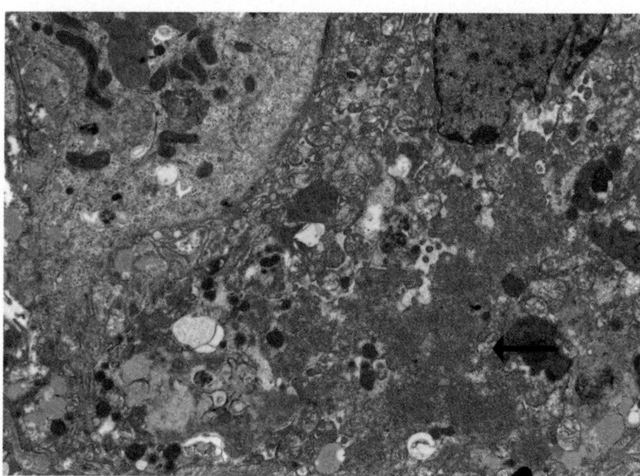

Figure 5.70 Mallory bodies. Mallory bodies (*arrow*) are irregularly shaped cytoplasmic inclusions.

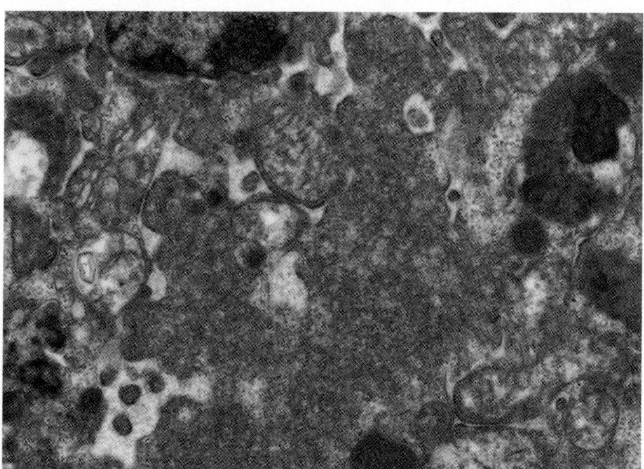

Figure 5.71 Mallory bodies. Another example.

1. Type I: Parallel bundles of filaments, often producing mosaic patterns and concentric arrangements.
2. Type II (most common): Thicker randomly arranged filaments, coated by very fine granules, producing an appearance of periodicity.
3. Type III: Lacks filamentous structures, and rather represents inclusions that consist of markedly electron-dense granular and homogeneous material.

Amyloidosis and light-chain deposition disease

Amyloid and monoclonal light chains can be deposited in various locations in the liver, including the portal tracts and sinusoidal walls. For light-chain deposition disease, sinusoidal localization (space of Disse) is most characteristic. Ultrastructurally, amyloid proteins consist of randomly oriented long fibrils (Fig. 5.73),

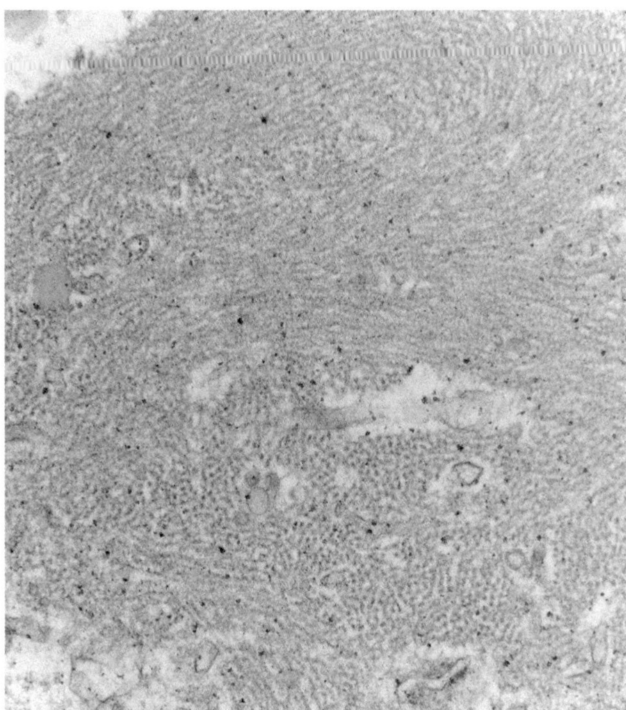

Figure 5.72 Mallory bodies. This example of Type 2 Mallory bodies consists of randomly arranged filaments, with scattered small granules.

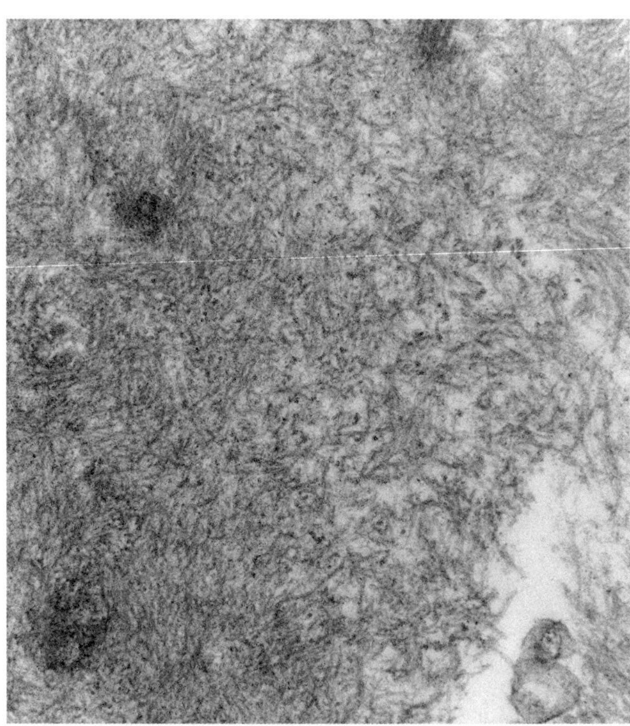

Figure 5.73 Amyloidosis. Amyloid consists of randomly oriented long fibrils, including some with parallel arrangement.

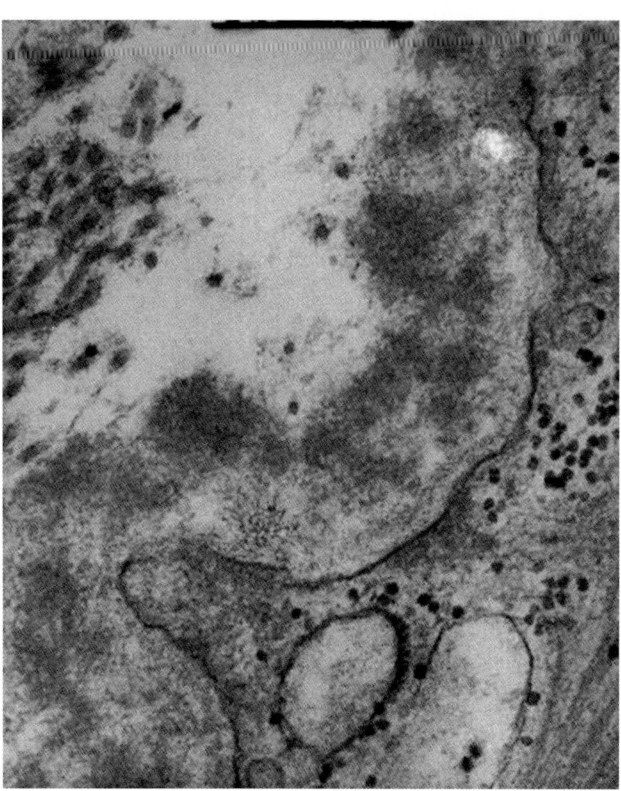

Figure 5.74 Light-chain deposition disease. Monoclonal light chains have a homogenous granular appearance.

including some with parallel arrangement, whereas monoclonal light chains have a homogenous granular appearance (Fig. 5.74).

REFERENCES

1. Geuze HJ. A future for electron microscopy in cell biology? *Trends Cell Biol*. 1999;9(3):92–93.
2. Braet F, Ratinac K. Creating next-generation microscopists: structural and molecular biology at the crossroads. *J Cell Mol Med*. 2007;11(4):759–763.
3. Rockey DC, Caldwell SH, Goodman ZD, et al. Liver biopsy. *Hepatology*. 2009;49(3):1017–1044.
4. Wisse E, Braet F, Duimel H, et al. Fixation methods for electron microscopy of human and other liver. *World J Gastroenterol*. 2010;16(23):2851–2866.
5. Fahimi HD. Perfusion and immersion fixation of rat liver with glutaraldehyde. *Lab Invest*. 1967;16(5):736–750.
6. Wisse E. An electron microscopic study of the fenestrated endothelial lining of rat liver sinusoids. *J Ultrastruct Res*. 1970;31(1):125–150.
7. David H, Uerlings I. Quantitative ultrastructure of the rat liver by immersion and perfusion fixations. *Exp Pathol*. 1983;23(3):131–141.

8. Wisse E, De Zanger RB, Jacobs R, et al. Scanning electron microscope observations on the structure of portal veins, sinusoids and central veins in rat liver. *Scan Electron Microsc.* 1983(Pt 3):1441–1452.
9. Wisse E, De Zanger RB, Charels K, et al. The liver sieve: considerations concerning the structure and function of endothelial fenestrae, the sinusoidal wall and the space of Disse. *Hepatology.* 1985;5(4):683–692.
10. Nation JL. A new method using hexamethyldisilazane for preparation of soft insect tissues for scanning electron microscopy. *Stain Technol.* 1983;58(6):347–351.
11. Braet F, De Zanger R, Wisse E. Drying cells for SEM, AFM and TEM by hexamethyldisilazane: a study on hepatic endothelial cells. *J Microsc.* 1997;186(Pt 1):84–87.
12. DeLeve LD. Hepatic microvasculature in liver injury. *Semin Liver Dis.* 2007;27(4):390–400.
13. Wang NS, Minassian H. The formaldehyde-fixed and paraffin-embedded tissues for diagnostic transmission electron microscopy: a retrospective and prospective study. *Hum Pathol.* 1987;18(7):715–727.
14. Wang NS, Huang SN, Thurlbeck WM. Combined Pneumocystis carinii and cytomegalovirus infection. *Arch Pathol.* 1970;90(6):529–535.
15. Rossi GL, Luginbuhl H, Probst D. A method for ultrastructural study of lesions found in conventional histological sections. *Virchows Arch A Pathol Pathol Anat.* 1970;350(3):216–224.
16. Pinkerton H, Carroll S. Fatal adenovirus pneumonia in infants. Correlation of histologic and electron microscopic observations. *Am J Pathol.* 1971;65(3):543–548.
17. Zeitoun P, Lehy T. Utilization of paraffin-embedded material for electron microscopy. Study of an A2-cell type microadenoma of the endocrine pancreas. *Lab Invest.* 1970;23(1):52–57.
18. Johannessen JV. Use of paraffin material for electron microscopy. *Pathol Annu.* 1977;12(Pt 2):189–224.
19. Miyai K. Ultrastructural basis for toxic liver injury. In: Farber EaFM, ed. *Toxic injury of the liver.* New York, NY: Marcel Dekker; 1979:59–154.
20. Phillips MJ, Poucell S, Patterson J, et al. The normal liver. In: Phillips MJ, Poucell S, Patterson J, et al., ed. *The liver; an atlas and text of ultrastrutctural pathology.* New York, NY: Raven Press; 1987:1–10.
21. Rohr HP, Luthy J, Gudat F, et al. Stereology of liver biopsies from healthy volunteers. *Virchows Arch A Pathol Anat Histol.* 1976;371(3):251–263.
22. Bradley SE, Herz R. Permselectivity of biliary canalicular membrane in rats: clearance probe analysis. *Am J Physiol.* 1978;235(5):E570–576.
23. Lazarow PB, Robbi M, Fujiki Y, et al. Biogenesis of peroxisomal proteins in vivo and in vitro. *Ann N Y Acad Sci.* 1982;386:285–300.
24. Diamond JM. Channels in epithelial cell membranes and junctions. *Fed Proc.* 1978;37(12):2639–2643.
25. Easter DW, Wade JB, Boyer JL. Structural integrity of hepatocyte tight junctions. *J Cell Biol.* 1983;96(3):745–749.
26. Loewenstein WR, Kanno Y, Socolar SJ. The cell-to-cell channel. *Fed Proc.* 1978;37(12):2645–2650.
27. Robenek H, Herwig J, Themann H. The morphologic characteristics of intercellular junctions between normal human liver cells and cells from patients with extrahepatic cholestasis. *Am J Pathol.* 1980;100(1):93–114.
28. Robenek H, Rassat J, Themann H. A quantitative freeze-fracture analysis of gap and tight junctions in the normal and cholestatic human liver. *Virchows Arch B Cell Pathol Incl Mol Pathol.* 1981;38(1):39–56.
29. Dermietzel R, Janssen-Timmen U, Willecke K, et al. Cytoplasmic and cell surface structure of purified liver gap junctions revealed by freeze-drying. *Eur J Cell Biol.* 1984;33(1):84–89.
30. Friend DS, Gilula NB. Variations in tight and gap junctions in mammalian tissues. *J Cell Biol.* 1972;53(3):758–776.
31. Oda M, Phillips MJ. Bile canalicular membrane pathology in cytochalasin B-induced cholestasis. *Lab Invest.* 1977;37(4):350–356.
32. Oshio C, Phillips MJ. Contractility of bile canaliculi: implications for liver function. *Science.* 1981;212(4498):1041–1042.
33. Sternlieb I. Electron microscopy of mitochondria and peroxisomes of human hepatocytes. *Prog Liver Dis.* 1979;6:81–104.
34. Palade G. Intracellular aspects of the process of protein synthesis. *Science.* 1975;189(4206):867.
35. Jezequel AM, Koch M, Orlandi F. A morphometric study of the endoplasmic reticulum in human hepatocytes. Correlation between morphological and biochemical data in subjects under treatment with certain drugs. *Gut.* 1974;15(9):737–747.
36. Ma MH, Goldfisher S, Biempica L. Morphology of the normal liver cell. *Prog Liver Dis.* 1972;4:1–17.
37. Ma MH, Biempica L. The normal human liver cell. Cytochemical and ultrastructural studies. *Am J Pathol.* 1971;62(3):353–390.
38. Amar-Costesec A. Analytical study of microsomes and isolated subcellular membranes from rat liver. VII. Distribution of protein-bound sialic acid. *J Cell Biol.* 1981;89(1):62–69.
39. de Man JC, Blok AP. Relationship between glycogen and agranular endoplasmic reticulum in rat hepatic cells. *J Histochem Cytochem.* 1966;14(2):135–146.
40. Jones AL, Fawcett DW. Hypertrophy of the agranular endoplasmic reticulum in hamster liver induced by phenobarbital (with a review on the functions of this organelle in liver). *J Histochem Cytochem.* 1966;14(3):215–232.

41. Feldman D, Swarm RL, Becker J. Elimination of excess smooth endoplasmic reticulum after phenobarbital administration. *J Histochem Cytochem.* 1980;28(9):997–1006.
42. Rothman JE. The compartmental organization of the Golgi apparatus. *Sci Am.* 1985;253(3):74–89.
43. Novikoff AB. The endoplasmic reticulum: a cytochemist's view (a review). *Proc Natl Acad Sci U S A.* 1976;73(8):2781–2787.
44. Novikoff PM, Yam A. The cytochemical demonstration of GERL in rat hepatocytes during lipoprotein mobilization. *J Histochem Cytochem.* 1978;26(1):1–13.
45. Novikoff AB, Essner E. The liver cell. Some new approaches to its study. *Am J Med.* 1960;29:102–131.
46. Neufeld EF, Lim TW, Shapiro LJ. Inherited disorders of lysosomal metabolism. *Annu Rev Biochem.* 1975;44:357–376.
47. De Duve C, Beaufay H, Jacques P, et al. Intracellular localization of catalase and of some oxidases in rat liver. *Biochim Biophys Acta.* 1960;40:186–187.
48. Sternlieb I, Quintana N. The peroxisomes of human hepatocytes. *Lab Invest.* 1977;36(2):140–149.
49. Watson ML. The nuclear envelope; its structure and relation to cytoplasmic membranes. *J Biophys Biochem Cytol.* 1955;1(3):257–270.
50. Gabbiani G, Montesano R, Tuchweber B, et al. Phalloidin-induced hyperplasia of actin filaments in rat hepatocytes. *Lab Invest.* 1975;33(5):562–569.
51. Oda M, Price VM, Fisher MM, et al. Ultrastructure of bile canaliculi, with special reference to the surface coat and the pericanalicular web. *Lab Invest.* 1974;31(4):314–323.
52. Phillips MJ, Oshio C, Miyairi M, et al. What is actin doing in the liver cell? *Hepatology.* 1983;3(3):433–436.
53. Phillips MJ, Oda M, Mak E, et al. Microfilament dysfunction as a possible cause of intrahepatic cholestasis. *Gastroenterology.* 1975;69(1):48–58.
54. Phillips MJ, Oshio C, Miyairi M, et al. A study of bile canalicular contractions in isolated hepatocytes. *Hepatology.* 1982;2(6):763–768.
55. Denk H, Franke WW. Rearrangement of the hepatocyte cytoskeleton after toxic damage: involution, dispersal and peripheral accumulation of Mallory body material after drug withdrawal. *Eur J Cell Biol.* 1981;23(2):241–249.
56. Denk H, Franke WW, Dragosics B, et al. Pathology of cytoskeleton of liver cells: demonstration of mallory bodies (alcoholic hyalin) in murine and human hepatocytes by immunofluorescence microscopy using antibodies to cytokeratin polypeptides from hepatocytes. *Hepatology.* 1981;1(1):9–20.
57. French SW, Kondo I, Irie T, et al. Morphologic study of intermediate filaments in rat hepatocytes. *Hepatology.* 1982;2(1):29–38.
58. Kimoff RJ, Huang S. Immunocytochemical and immunoelectron microscopic studies on Mallory bodies. *Lab Invest.* 1981;45(6):491–503.
59. Sabesin SM. Microtubules--biological machines at the molecular level. *Gastroenterology.* 1981;81(4):810–813.
60. Reaven EP, Reaven GM. Evidence that microtubules play a permissive role in hepatocyte very low density lipoprotein secretion. *J Cell Biol.* 1980;84(1):28–39.
61. Wisse E, Knook DL. The investigation of sinusoidal cells: a new approach to the study of liver function. *Prog Liver Dis.* 1979;6:153–171.
62. Yee AG, Revel JP. Endothelial cell junctions. *J Cell Biol.* 1975;66(1):200–204.
63. Phillips MJ, Poucell S, Patterson J, et al. Viral hepatitis. In: Phillips MJ, Poucell S, Patterson J, et al., ed. *The liver; an atlas and text of ultrastrutctural pathology.* Raven Press; 1987.
64. Phillips MJ, Poucell S. Modern aspects of the morphology of viral hepatitis. *Hum Pathol.* 1981;12(12):1060–1084.
65. Lefkowitch JH, Arborgh BA, Scheuer PJ. Oxyphilic granular hepatocytes. Mitochondrion-rich liver cells in hepatic disease. *Am J Clin Pathol.* 1980;74(4):432–441.
66. Klion FM, Schaffner F. The ultrastructure of acidophilic "Councilman-like" bodies in the liver. *Am J Pathol.* 1966;48(5):755–767.
67. Biava C, Mukhlova-Montiel M. Electron microscopic observations on councilman-like acidophilic bodies and other forms of acidophilic changes in human liver cells. *Am J Pathol.* 1965;46(5):775–802.
68. Kantrowitz PA, Jones WA, Greenberger NJ, et al. Severe postoperative hyperbilirubinemia simulating obstructive jaundice. *N Engl J Med.* 1967;276(11):590–598.
69. Phillips MJ, Poucell S, Patterson J, et al. Cholestasis. In: Phillips MJ, Poucell S, Patterson J, et al., ed. *The liver; an atlas and text of ultrastrutctural pathology.* Raven Press; 1987.
70. Phillips MJ, Fisher RL, Anderson DW, et al. Ultrastructural evidence of intrahepatic cholestasis before and after chenodeoxycholic acid therapy in patients with cholelithiasis: the national cooperative gallstone study. *Hepatology.* 1983;3(2):209–220.
71. Schaffner F, Popper H, Perez V. Changes in bile canaliculi produced by norethandrolone: electron microscopic study of human and rat liver. *J Lab Clin Med.* 1960;56:623–628.
72. Mandel H, Hartman C, Berkowitz D, et al. The hepatic mitochondrial DNA depletion syndrome: ultrastructural changes in liver biopsies. *Hepatology.* 2001;34(4 Pt 1):776–784.
73. Iancu TC, Manov I. Electron microscopy of liver biopsies. In: Takahashi H, ed. *Liver biopsy.* InTech; 2011:110–132.

74. Phillips MJ, Poucell S, Patterson J, et al. Metabolic liver disease. In: Phillips MJ, Poucell S, Patterson J, et al., ed. *The liver; an atlas and text of ultrastrutctural pathology*. New York, NY: Raven Press; 1987.
75. Murray AK, Brown BI, Brown DH. The molecular heterogeneity of purified human liver lysosomal alpha-glucosidase (acid alpha-glucosidase). *Arch Biochem Biophys*. 1978;185(2):511–524.
76. McAdams AJ, Hug G, Bove KE. Glycogen storage disease, types I to X: criteria for morphologic diagnosis. *Hum Pathol*. 1974;5(4):463–487.
77. Greene HL. Glycogen storage disease. *Semin Liver Dis*. 1982;2(4):291–301.
78. Cantin M, Brochu P, Turgeon-Knaack C, et al. Rectal biopsy in type 4 glycogenosis. An ultrastructural cytochemical study. *Arch Pathol Lab Med*. 1976;100(8):422–426.
79. Kalra V, Arya LS, Nayak NC. Glycogen storage disease (Type IV): a familial cirrhosis diagnosed by electron microscopy (case report). *Indian Pediatr*. 1980;17(7):625–627.
80. Reed GB, Jr, Dixon JF, Neustein JB, et al. Type IV glycogenosis. Patient with absence of a branching enzyme alpha-1,4-glucan:alpha-1,4-glucan 6-glycosyl transferase. *Lab Invest*. 1968;19(5):546–557.
81. Schochet SS, Jr, McCormick WF, Zellweger H. Type IV glycogenosis (amylopectinosis). Light and electron microscopic observations. *Arch Pathol*. 1970;90(4):354–363.
82. Edstrom RD. Low-molecular weight glycogen found in a human with a generalized storage disease. *Arch Biochem Biophys*. 1970;137(1):293–295.
83. Krivit W, Sharp HL, Lee JC, et al. Low molecular weight glycogen as a cause of generalized glycogen storage disease. *Am J Med*. 1973;54(1):88–97.
84. Yu DT, Phillips MJ. Hepatic ultrastructural changes in acute fructose overload. *J Ultrastruct Res*. 1971;36(1):222–236.
85. Hers HG, Van Hoof F. The genetic pathology of lysosomes. *Prog Liver Dis*. 1970;3:185–205.
86. Aubert-Tulkens G, Van Hoof F. Acid lipase deficiency: clinical and biochemical heterogeneity. *Acta Paediatr Belg*. 1979;32(4):239–245.
87. Eto Y, Kitagawa T. Wolman's disease with hypolipoproteinemia and acanthocytosis: clinical and biochemical observations. *J Pediatr*. 1970;77(5):862–867.
88. Ishak KG. Applications of scanning electron microscopy to the study of liver disease. *Prog Liver Dis*. 1986;8:1–32.
89. Lough J, Fawcett J, Wiegensberg B. Wolman's disease. An electron microscopic, histochemical, and biochemical study. *Arch Pathol*. 1970;89(2):103–110.
90. Maehira F, Nakada F, Hokama T. Characteristics of acid esterase in Wolman's disease. *Biochem Med*. 1984;32(3):322–330.
91. Philippart M. Wolman's disease. *J Pediatr*. 1971;79(1):173–174.
92. Byrd JC, 3rd, Powers JM. Wolman's disease: ultrastructural evidence of lipid accumulation in central and peripheral nervous systems. *Acta Neuropathol*. 1979;45(1):37–42.
93. Raafat F, Hashemian MP, Abrishami MA. Wolman's disease: report of two new cases, with a review of the literature. *Am J Clin Pathol*. 1973;59(4): 490–497.
94. Schaub J, Janka GE, Christomanou H, et al. Wolman's disease: clinical, biochemical and ultrastructural studies in an unusual case without striking adrenal calcification. *Eur J Pediatr*. 1980;135(1):45–53.
95. Sloan HR, Fredrickson DS. Enzyme deficiency in cholesteryl ester storage idisease. *J Clin Invest*. 1972;51(7):1923–1926.
96. Ashkenazi A, Yarom R, Gutman A, et al. Niemann-Pick disease and giant cell transformation of the liver. *Acta Paediatr Scand*. 1971;60(3):285–294.
97. Dewhurst N, Besley GT, Finlayson ND, et al. Sea blue histiocytosis in a patient with chronic non-neuropathic Niemann-Pick disease. *J Clin Pathol*. 1979;32(11):1121–1127.
98. Elleder M, Smid F, Hyniova H, et al. Liver findings in Niemann-Pick disease type C. *Histochem J*. 1984;16(11):1147–1170.
99. Takahashi K, Naito M. Lipid storage disease: Part I. Ultrastructure of xanthoma cells in various xanthomatous diseases. *Acta Pathol Jpn*. 1983;33(5):959–977.
100. Meiner V, Shpitzen S, Mandel H, et al. Clinical-biochemical correlation in molecularly characterized patients with Niemann-Pick type C. *Genet Med*. 2001;3(5):343–348.
101. Spiegel R, Raas-Rothschild A, Reish O, et al. The clinical spectrum of fetal Niemann-Pick type C. *Am J Med Genet A*. 2009;149A(3):446–450.
102. Bach G, Eisenberg F, Jr, Cantz M, et al. The defect in the Hunter syndrome: deficiency of sulfoiduronate sulfatase. *Proc Natl Acad Sci U S A*. 1973;70(7):2134–2138.
103. Holzgreve W, Grobe H, von Figura K, et al. Morquio syndrome: clinical findings in 11 patients with MPS IVA and 2 patients with MPS IVB. *Hum Genet*. 1981;57(4):360–365.
104. Loeb H, Tondeur M, Toppet M, et al. Clinical, biochemical and ultrastructural studies of an atypical form of mucopolysaccharidosis. *Acta Paediatr Scand*. 1969;58(3):220–228.
105. Mueller OT, Shows TB, Opitz JM. Apparent allelism of the Hurler, Scheie, and Hurler/Scheie syndromes. *Am J Med Genet*. 1984;18(3):547–556.
106. Petersen EM. Sanfilippo's syndrome type C--the first known case in South Africa. *S Afr Med J*. 1986;69(1):63–68.

107. Rutsaert J, Menu R, Resibois A. Ultrastructure of sulfatide storage in normal and sulfatase-deficient fibroblasts in vitro. *Lab Invest.* 1973;29(5):527–535.
108. Schachern PA, Shea DA, Paparella MM. Mucopolysaccharidosis I-H (Hurler's syndrome) and human temporal bone histopathology. *Ann Otol Rhinol Laryngol.* 1984;93(1 Pt 1):65–69.
109. Sjoberg I, Fransson LA, Matalon R, et al. Hunter's syndrome: a deficiency of L-idurono-sulfate sulfatase. *Biochem Biophys Res Commun.* 1973;54(3):1125–1132.
110. Van Hoof F. Mucopolysaccharidoses and mucolipidoses. *J Clin Pathol Suppl (R Coll Pathol).* 1974;8:64–93.
111. Young ID, Harper PS. The natural history of the severe form of Hunter's syndrome: a study based on 52 cases. *Dev Med Child Neurol.* 1983;25(4):481–489.
112. Rutsaert J, Tondeur M, Vamos-Hurwitz E, et al. The cellular lesions of Farber's disease and their experimental reproduction in tissue culture. *Lab Invest.* 1977;36(5):474–480.
113. Schmoeckel C. Subtle clues to diagnosis of skin diseases by electron microscopy. "Farber bodies" in disseminated lipogranulomatosis (Farber's disease). *Am J Dermatopathol.* 1980;2(2):153–156.
114. Schmoeckel C, Hohlfed M. A specific ultrastructural marker for disseminated lipogranulomatosis (Faber). *Arch Dermatol Res.* 1979;266(2):187–196.
115. Tanaka T, Takahashi K, Hakozaki H, et al. Farber's disease (disseminated lipogranulomatosis)--a pathological, histochemical and ultrastructural study. *Acta Pathol Jpn.* 1979;29(1):135–155.
116. Faraggiana T, Churg J, Grishman E, et al. Light- and electron-microscopic histochemistry of Fabry's disease. *Am J Pathol.* 1981;103(2):247–262.
117. Harbour JR, Rosenthal P, Smuckler EA. Ultrastructural abnormalities of the liver in total lipodystrophy. *Hum Pathol.* 1981;12(9):856–862.
118. Callea F, Fevery J, Desmet VJ. Simultaneous alpha-1-antitrypsin accumulation in liver and pancreas. *Hum Pathol.* 1984;15(3):293–295.
119. Clausen PP, Lindskov J, Gad I, et al. The diagnostic value of alpha 1-antitrypsin globules in liver cells as a morphological marker of alpha 1-antitrypsin deficiency. *Liver.* 1984;4(6):353–359.
120. Hadchouel M, Gautier M. Histopathologic study of the liver in the early cholestatic phase of alpha-1-antitrypsin deficiency. *J Pediatr.* 1976;89(2):211–215.
121. Hirschberger M, Stickler GB. Neonatal hepatitis and alpha-1-antitrypsin deficiency. The prognosis in five patients. *Mayo Clin Proc.* 1977;52(4):241–245.
122. Kidd VJ, Golbus MS, Wallace RB, et al. Prenatal diagnosis of alpha 1-antitrypsin deficiency by direct analysis of the mutation site in the gene. *N Engl J Med.* 1984;310(10):639–642.
123. Nemeth A, Strandvik B. Natural history of children with alpha 1-antitrypsin deficiency and neonatal cholestasis. *Acta Paediatr Scand.* 1982;71(6):993–999.
124. Strobel S, Bender SW, Posselt HG, et al. Alpha-1-antitrypsin deficiency: fulminant course in early infancy. *Helv Paediatr Acta.* 1980;35(1):75–83.
125. Thompson RJ, Portmann BC, Roberts EA. Genetic and metablic liver disease. In: Burt AD, Portmann BC, Ferrell LD, ed. *MacSween's pathology of the liver.* 6th ed. Edinburgh, NY. Churchill Livingstone/ Elsevier; 2012:157–222.
126. Scotto JM, Stralin HG. Ultrastructure of the liver in a case of childhood cystinosis. *Virchows Arch A Pathol Anat Histol.* 1977;377(1):43–48.
127. Gaull G, Sturman JA, Schaffner F. Homocystinuria due to cystathionine synthase deficiency: enzymatic and ultrastructural studies. *J Pediatr.* 1974;84(3):381–390.
128. Linarelli LG, Williams CN, Phillips MJ. Byler's disease: fatal intrahepatic cholestasis. *J Pediatr.* 1972;81(3):484–492.
129. Strautnieks SS, Kagalwalla AF, Tanner MS, et al. Identification of a locus for progressive familial intrahepatic cholestasis PFIC2 on chromosome 2q24. *Am J Hum Genet.* 1997;61(3):630–633.
130. Takahashi A, Hasegawa M, Sumazaki R, et al. Gradual improvement of liver function after administration of ursodeoxycholic acid in an infant with a novel ABCB11 gene mutation with phenotypic continuum between BRIC2 and PFIC2. *Eur J Gastroenterol Hepatol.* 2007;19(11):942–946.
131. Bull LN, Carlton VE, Stricker NL, et al. Genetic and morphological findings in progressive familial intrahepatic cholestasis (Byler disease [PFIC-1] and Byler syndrome): evidence for heterogeneity. *Hepatology.* 1997;26(1):155–164.
132. Barth RF, Grimley PM, Berk PD, et al. Excess lipofuscin accumulation in constitutional hepatic dysfunction (Gilbert's syndrome). Light and electron microscopic observations. *Arch Pathol.* 1971;91(1):41–47.
133. Herman JD, Cooper EB, Takeuchi A, et al. Constitutional hyperbilirubinemia with unconjugated bilirubin in the serum and pigment deposition in the liver. Report of a case. *Am J Dig Dis.* 1964;9:160–169.
134. Tanikawa K, Emura T. Electron microscopic observation of the liver in Gilbert's disease. *Kurume Med J.* 1965;12(1):27–32.
135. Evans J, Lefkowitch J, Lim CK, et al. Fecal porphyrin abnormalities in a patient with features of Rotor's syndrome. *Gastroenterology.* 1981;81(6):1125–1130.
136. Dingemans KP, Mooi WJ, van den Bergh Weerman MA. Angulate lysosomes. *Ultrastruct Pathol.* 1983;5(2–3):113–122.
137. Fayon M, Lamireau T, Bioulac-Sage P, et al. Fatal neonatal liver failure and mitochondrial

cytopathy: an observation with antenatal ascites. *Gastroenterology*. 1992;103(4):1332–1335.
138. Bioulac-Sage P, Parrot-Roulaud F, Mazat JP, et al. Fatal neonatal liver failure and mitochondrial cytopathy (oxidative phosphorylation deficiency): a light and electron microscopic study of the liver. *Hepatology*. 1993;18(4):839–846.
139. Bruguera M, Esquerda JE, Mascaro JM, et al. Erythropoietic protoporphyria. A light, electron, and polarization microscopical study of the liver in three patients. *Arch Pathol Lab Med*. 1976;100(11):587–589.
140. Wolff K. Liver inclusions in erythropoietic protoporphyria. *Eur J Clin Invest*. 1975;5(1):21–26.
141. Iancu TC, Mahajnah M, Manov I, et al. The liver in congenital disorders of glycosylation: ultrastructural features. *Ultrastruct Pathol*. 2007;31(3):189–197.
142. Vazquez JJ, Cervera S. Cyanamide-induced liver injury in alcoholics. *Lancet*. 1980;1(8164):361–362.
143. Vazquez JJ, Guillen FJ, Zozaya J, et al. Cyanamide-induced liver injury. A predictable lesion. *Liver*. 1983;3(4):225–230.
144. Altmann HW. Drug-induced liver reactions: a morphological approach. *Curr Top Pathol*. 1980;69:69–142.
145. Damjanov I, Solter D. Ultrastructure of acute tetracycline induced liver change. *Experientia*. 1971;27(10):1204–1205.
146. Phillips MJ, Poucell S, Patterson J, et al. Drug and toxic effects. In: Phillips MJ, Poucell S, Patterson J, et al., ed. *The liver; an atlas and text of ultrastrutctural pathology*. Raven Press; 1987.
147. Chedid A, Jao W, Port J. Megamitochondria in hepatic and renal disease. *Am J Gastroenterol*. 1980;73(4):319–324.
148. Burns W, Vander Weide G, Chan C. Laminated mitochondrial inclusions in hepatocytes of liver biopsies. *Arch Pathol*. 1972;94(1):75–80.
149. Lullmann H, Lullmann-Rauch R, Wassermann O. Lipidosis induced by amphiphilic cationic drugs. *Biochem Pharmacol*. 1978;27(8):1103–1108.
150. Lullmann H, Lullmann-Rauch R, Wassermann O. Drug-induced phospholipidoses. II. Tissue distribution of the amphiphilic drug chlorphentermine. *CRC Crit Rev Toxicol*. 1975;4(2):185–218.
151. Poucell S, Ireton J, Valencia-Mayoral P, et al. Amiodarone-associated phospholipidosis and fibrosis of the liver. Light, immunohistochemical, and electron microscopic studies. *Gastroenterology*. 1984;86(5 Pt 1):926–936.
152. Zimmerman HJ, Ishak KG. Valproate-induced hepatic injury: analyses of 23 fatal cases. *Hepatology*. 1982;2(5):591–597.
153. Keene DL, Humphreys P, Carpenter B, et al. Valproic acid producing a Reye-like syndrome. *Can J Neurol Sci*. 1982;9(4):435–437.
154. Iancu T, Elian E. Ultrastructural changes in aspirin hepatotoxicity. *Am J Clin Pathol*. 1976;66(3):570–575.
155. Hoofnagle JH, Schafer DF. Serologic markers of hepatitis B virus infection. *Semin Liver Dis*. 1986;6(1):1–10.
156. Huang SN, Millman I, O'Connell A, et al. Virus-like particles in Australia antigen-associated hepatitis. An immunoelectron microscopic study of human liver. *Am J Pathol*. 1972;67(3):453–470.
157. Huang SN, Neurath AR. Immunohistologic demonstration of hepatitis B viral antigens in liver with reference to its significance in liver injury. *Lab Invest*. 1979;40(1):1–17.
158. Alberti A, Tremolada F, Fattovich G, et al. Virus replication and liver disease in chronic hepatitis B virus infection. *Dig Dis Sci*. 1983;28(11):961–966.
159. Bianchi L, Gudat F. Immunopathology of hepatitis B. *Prog Liver Dis*. 1979;6:371–392.
160. Bonino F, Recchia S, Farci P, et al. Hepatitis B virus replication and clinical outcome in carriers of HBsAg. Perspectives of treatment with DNA inhibitors. *Liver*. 1983;3(1):30–35.
161. Rizzetto M, Shih JW, Verme G, et al. A radioimmunoassay for HBcAg in the sera of HBsAg carriers: serum HBcAg, liver HBcAg immunofluorescence as markers of chronic liver disease. *Gastroenterology*. 1981;80(6):1420–1427.
162. Scullard GH, Smith CI, Merigan TC, et al. Effects of immunosuppressive therapy on viral markers in chronic active hepatitis B. *Gastroenterology*. 1981;81(6):987–991.
163. Takahashi K, Akahane Y, Gotanda T, et al. Demonstration of hepatitis B e antigen in the core of Dane particles. *J Immunol*. 1979;122(1):275–279.
164. Thomas HC, Lok AS. The immunopathology of autoimmune and hepatitis B virus-induced chronic hepatitis. *Semin Liver Dis*. 1984;4(1):36–46.
165. Bruguera M, Bertran A, Bombi JA, et al. Giant mitochondria in hepatocytes: a diagnostic hint for alcoholic liver disease. *Gastroenterology*. 1977;73(6):1383–1387.
166. Ma MH. Ultrastructural pathologic findings of the human hepatocyte. I. Alcoholic liver disease. *Arch Pathol*. 1972;94(6):554–571.
167. Stewart RV, Dincsoy HP. The significance of giant mitochondria in liver biopsies as observed by light microscopy. *Am J Clin Pathol*. 1982;78(3):293–298.
168. Uchida T, Kronborg I, Peters RL. Giant mitochondria in the alcoholic liver diseases--their identification, frequency and pathologic significance. *Liver*. 1984;4(1):29–38.
169. Yokoo H, Minick OT, Batti F, et al. Morphologic variants of alcoholic hyalin. *Am J Pathol*. 1972;69(1):25–40.

6

Basic patterns of injury in medical liver pathology

Roger K. Moreira, MD

A pattern of injury represents individual histologic findings that cluster into a meaningful and recognizable histologic pattern. Identification of basic patterns of injury is the first and most fundamental step in the evaluation of medical liver biopsies because most patterns are associated with fairly well-established differential diagnoses and accompanying pitfalls. Whenever possible, we should try to fit all individual findings into one pattern of injury, always keeping in mind that any given feature is part of a spectrum and may vary, within certain limits, from case to case. Occasionally, more than one pattern is present in the same sample, with one pattern usually predominating. In spite of their importance, no universal consensus exists regarding the precise nomenclature, definition, or characterization of many of the basic patterns of injury in the liver presented here. Nonetheless, there is general agreement on the core elements that make up these patterns of injury and in this chapter we discuss the patterns most commonly seen in our practice, along with their significance.

6.1 THE NORMAL/NEAR-NORMAL LIVER

Definition

In this pattern, a liver sample is either completely normal or only shows minimal, nonspecific changes.

Dealing with a normal/nearly normal liver sample can be frustrating, especially when significant clinical abnormalities have been identified. The obvious concern is that the pathologist is missing something meaningful or not recognizing subtle, yet diagnostic features. Therefore, the first and perhaps most important step in this setting is to ascertain that the basic pattern is truly "normal/near-normal," rather than a mild form of another pattern. Four steps should be followed before labeling a liver sample as normal/nearly normal: (1) carefully evaluate the adequacy of the biopsy specimen. A specimen with too few portal tracts, marked crush or other artifacts, or severe fragmentation should be considered inadequate or suboptimal and a diagnosis of "normal" should be rendered with caution; (2) thoroughly review the specimen to ascertain that all expected portal and lobular structures are present, show a normal appearance, and that no abnormal elements are present (also refer to Chapter 1, "Normal liver"); (3)

carefully review the "checklist" (Table 6.1) of the most commonly missed histologic findings in this setting (Figs. 6.1, 6.2, 6.3, 6.4, 6.5, 6.6, and 6.7); and (4) correlate with clinical features, specifically searching for subtle changes related to clinically suspected condition and for features of diseases most commonly associated with a normal/near-normal pattern (Table 6.2). Chapter 7 discusses the "normal/near-normal" differential in more detail.

6.2 HEPATITIS

Definition

Histologically, the term hepatitis is used to describe a combination of various degrees of inflammation (a *sine qua non* feature) and associated liver cell injury, necrosis, and regeneration, with or without fibrosis.

Under the "hepatitis" umbrella, several basic patterns of injury are recognized.

Nonspecific inflammation (also referred to as "reactive hepatitis")

This pattern is characterized by a mild, predominantly lymphocytic infiltrate involving portal tracts, hepatic lobules, or both, usually not accompanied by any other abnormalities. As the name implies, this pattern is typically not associated with any primary liver disease, but rather with systemic inflammatory processes (infections, connective tissue disorders, celiac disease,[1,2] primary immunodeficiencies,[3] etc.). When features of other patterns concomitantly occur (fatty liver, for example), the latter should be regarded as the primary pattern for differential diagnosis purposes.

Acute hepatitis

Acute liver injury can occur either *de novo* or as a flare of various chronic liver diseases. The term "acute hepatitis" is largely a clinical term, defined by the length of time for liver enzyme elevations. The histological correlates of acute hepatitis include various degrees of lobular inflammation, injury, necrosis, and regeneration, in the absence of features of chronic hepatitis (e.g., well-formed portal lymphoid aggregates, fibrosis). In typical cases of acute hepatitis, therefore, the process is primarily inflammatory and primarily involves the hepatic lobules (Fig. 6.8). Although a fairly long list of etiologies is associated with this histologic appearance (Table 6.3), the etiology of the acute injury is often clinically known or strongly suspected (e.g., acute viral hepatitides, drug reaction) and a liver biopsy may not be indicated. In practice, most biopsied cases showing this pattern will represent either drug-induced liver injury or an unsuspected viral hepatitis, usually by a nonhepatotropic virus, which may not have been included in the prebiopsy clinical evaluation. Other entities in the differential include autoimmune hepatitis and Wilson disease. The features of an acute hepatitis may overlap with those of "chronic hepatitis," "panlobular hepatitis," and "cholestatic hepatitis" patterns (see later).

Table 6.1 Most common "easy-to-miss" findings in otherwise normal/nearly normal liver samples

Feature	Associated clinical scenario	Comment
Ductopenia	Cholestasis, drug reaction, Allagille syndrome, PSC, BMT/GVHD, liver transplant	Identification of hepatic arteries without associated bile ducts is helpful
Bile duct injury in graft versus host disease	BMT	GVHD may present with minimal bile duct damage and little or no inflammation
Hepatoportal sclerosis	Clinical, laboratory, and imaging findings related to portal hypertension with no cirrhosis	Findings may be rather subtle and may require a high index of suspicion; look for atrophic or absent portal veins; dilated portal veins with herniation into the lobules, NRH
Focal viral inclusions	Immunosuppression, immunodeficiencies, known viral infection	CMV inclusions may be very focal and not apparent on all levels; search should focus on inflammatory foci or microabscesses, if present. Adenovirus inclusions can be very inconspicuous (small samples may not include areas of necrosis)
Amyloid	Plasma cell dyscrasias, paraproteinemia, chronic infections, chronic inflammatory processes	Small amounts of amyloid are notoriously difficult to recognize on H&E; examine arterioles carefully
α-1 antitrypsin globules	Abnormal α-1 antitrypsin levels or phenotype	Small globules, particularly in the neonatal period, are very difficult to recognize; search periportal hepatocytes carefully; immunostain may also be helpful
Focal hepatocanalicular cholestasis	Elevated bilirubin, usually >2	Search should focus on centrilobular areas; look for small canalicular plugs
Other pigments	Dubin–Johnson, PCT, EPP	Dubin–Johnson syndrome shows abundant, coarse, brown pigment similar to lipofuscin; PCT can show needle-shaped crystals within hepatocytes, best seen using unstained paraffin sections under polarized light; EPP pigment may resemble other pigments but shows a typical red-birefringence and a "Maltese cross" configuration under polarized light
Ito/stellate cell hyperplasia	Vitamin A or multivitamin supplements	Ito/stellate cells are small and inconspicuous and can be missed even when present in large numbers. Multivacuolated cytoplasm with nuclear indentation represent the key cytologic features
Hairy cell leukemia	Hematologic abnormalities, known HCL	HCL cells are typically very bland and may mimic Kupffer cells. A high index of suspicion is required
Nodular regenerative hyperplasia	Portal hypertension, certain medications such as azathioprine, collagen-vascular diseases, vascular malformations and hepatic hemangiomas	NRH can be very subtle on H&E stain. Reticulin stain is very helpful
Hepatitis B	Chronic hepatitis B infection	Ground-glass inclusions may be absent or be difficult to recognize in chronic hepatitis B, and the diagnosis may be missed if no clinical history is available; HBV surface antigen immunohistochemistry typically shows strong and diffuse cytoplasmic positivity in spite of the normal/near-normal appearance on H&E

(continued)

Table 6.1 Most common "easy-to-miss" findings in otherwise normal/nearly normal liver samples (*Continued*)

Feature	Associated clinical scenario	Comment
Kupffer cell clusters (resolving hepatitis)	Evidence of significant improvement of liver enzymes previous to biopsy procedure (spontaneous or treatment-related), most commonly in the setting of proven or suspected drug reaction or systemic infections	PAS-D stain is very helpful in highlighting Kupffer cell and portal macrophage clusters in an otherwise relatively unremarkable liver, indicative of recent, resolving injury (resolving hepatitis pattern)
Sickled red blood cells	Sickle cell disease or trait	Sickled red blood cells often form small clusters within sinusoids but sinusoidal dilatation and iron pigment may be absent
Microvesicular steatosis	Mitochondrial injury or dysfunction, drug toxicity (e.g., tetracycline, valproic acid), Reye syndrome, acute fatty liver of pregnancy	"True" microvesicular steatosis presents exclusively as very small fat droplets in the cytoplasm and can be very difficult to recognize. Fat stains such as Sudan and oil-red-O are useful
Vascular thrombi	Hypercoagulability, suspected ischemia	Thrombi can be easily overlooked in the liver, often dismissed as nonspecific fibrinous debris or hyalinized/fibrous areas; endothelial makers and elastic stains (e.g., Verhoeff–Van Gieson) can be useful

Abbreviations: PSC, primary sclerosing cholangitis; BMT, bone marrow transplant; GVHD, graft versus host disease; NRH, nodular regenerative hyperplasia; PCT, porphyria cutanea tarda; EPP, erythropoietic protoporphyria; HCL, hairy cell leukemia.

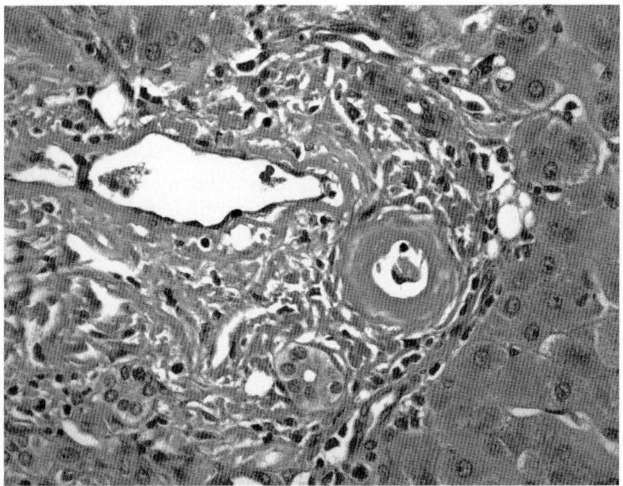

Figure 6.1 Focal amyloid. Amyloid material focally involving the wall of a hepatic artery branch.

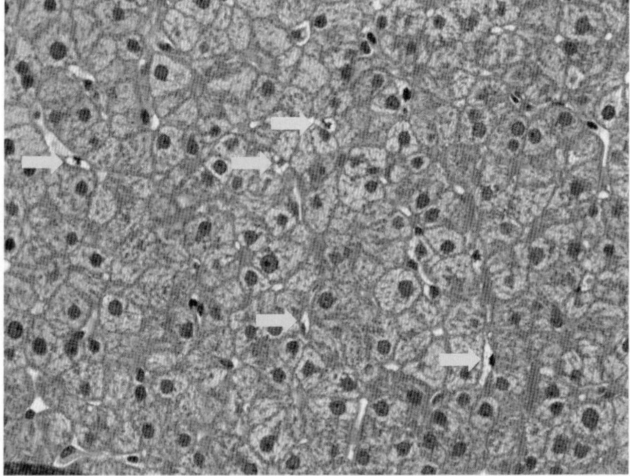

Figure 6.2 Ito (stellate) cell hyperplasia. Several Ito cells, characterized by multiple small clear cytoplasmic vacuoles indenting the nuclei, are present within spaces of Disse.

Chronic hepatitis, NOS

This is one of the most common patterns of injury seen in practice and its hallmark is the presence of dense chronic inflammatory infiltrates in the portal tracts, often associated with lymphoid aggregates (occasionally with germinal centers) and with varying degrees of interface activity (Fig. 6.9). Although the associated lobular activity is highly variable, it is typically less pronounced relative to the portal infiltrate. This stands in contrast to the acute hepatitis pattern, where lobular inflammation is the predominant pattern of injury, with relative less portal inflammation and interface activity. The prototype etiology associated with this pattern is chronic viral hepatitis (B and C). Many different etiologies, however, can potentially show a "chronic hepatitis" histology, including drug-induced liver injury, Wilson disease, α-1 antitrypsin deficiency, autoimmune hepatitis, and primary biliary diseases

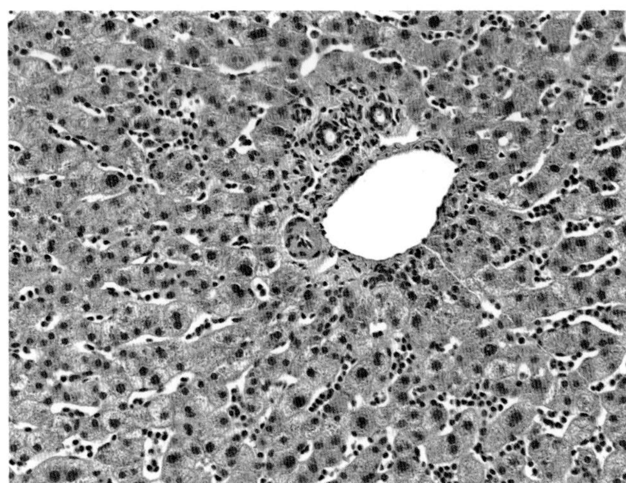

Figure 6.3 Hairy cell leukemia. A sinusoidal infiltrate by bland cells, mimicking Kupffer cell hyperplasia, is seen in this example of hairy cell leukemia.

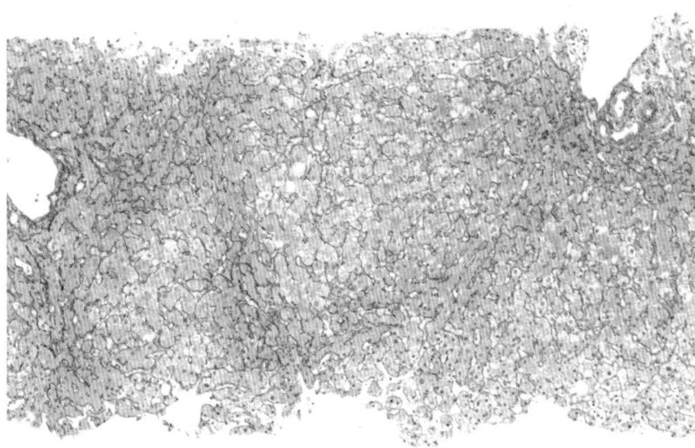

Figure 6.4 Nodular regenerative hyperplasia (NRH). Subtle areas of hepatocyte regeneration alternating with slightly compressed/atrophic areas in this example of mild NRH.

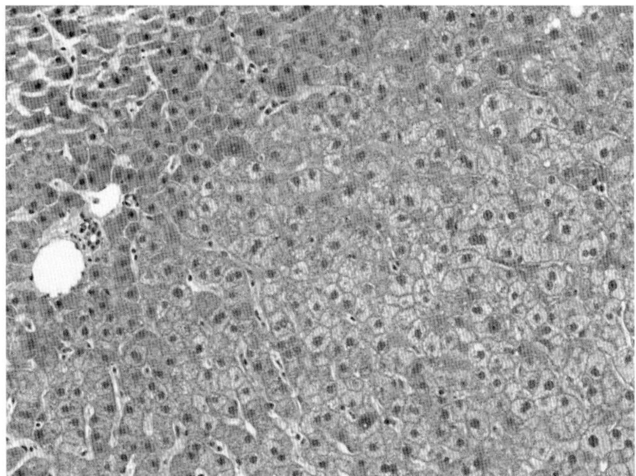

Figure 6.5 Hepatitis B. An essentially normal H&E appearance of the liver in this patient with congenital hepatitis B.

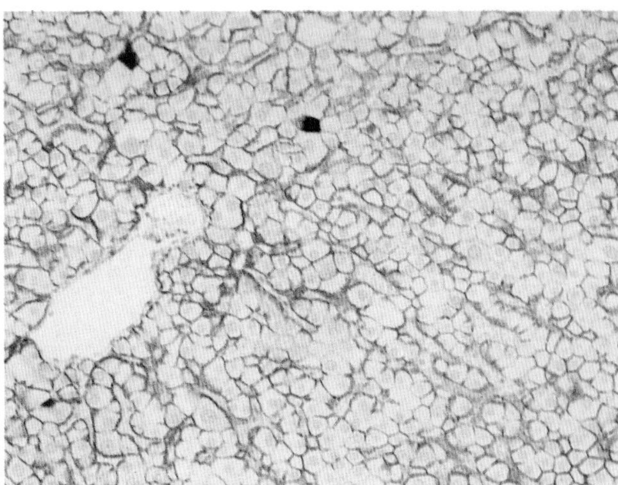

Figure 6.6 Hepatitis B. A hepatitis B surface antigen immunostain in a diffuse membranous and focal cytoplasmic pattern in the same case of congenital hepatitis B illustrated in this igure.

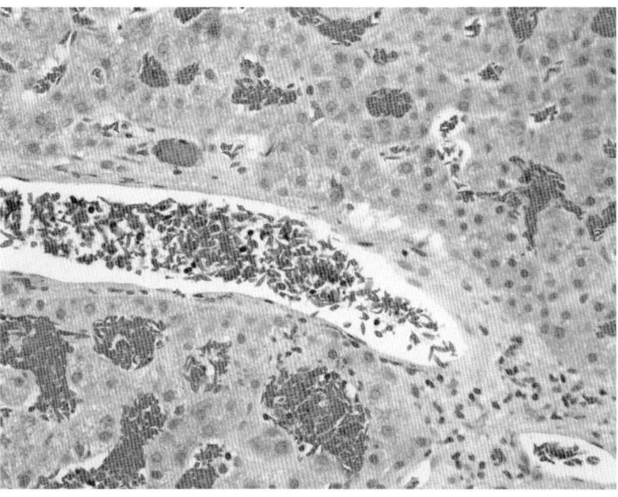

Figure 6.7 Sickle cell disease. Focal areas in this biopsy showed dilated sinusoids with clusters of sickled red blood cells, which are also present within the blood vessel in the center of the image.

(especially primary biliary cirrhosis) (Table 6.4). Fatty liver disease, especially in the setting of advanced fibrosis, can also show relatively dense portal infiltrate as a nonspecific finding, mimicking a superimposed chronic hepatitis. Cases with a pronounced plasma cell component are best classified as "plasma cell rich/ autoimmune" pattern.

Plasma cell rich/autoimmune pattern

This pattern is characterized by dense portal infiltrates, with increased plasma cells (which should

Table 6.2 Diseases and conditions associated with clinical liver dysfunction and normal/nearly normal histology

Disease/condition	Histology
Drug reaction	Normal/near-normal histology is common in spite of significant laboratory abnormalities; subtle histologic changes include nonspecific portal/lobular inflammation, mild cytoplasmic eosinophilia (endoplasmic reticulum "induction"), pseudoground glass change, megamitochondria, minimal cholestasis
Celiac disease	Mild nonspecific portal/lobular inflammation
Crohn disease	Mild nonspecific portal/lobular inflammation
Intestinal bacterial overgrowth	Mild nonspecific portal/lobular inflammation
Wilson disease	May be normal; mild steatosis, inflammatory changes and glycogenated nuclei are common
Sepsis	Mild nonspecific inflammatory changes and/or minimal cholestasis
Early biliary tract disease	PBC, PSC, cystic fibrosis, and TPN-associated liver disease, in their early phases, can be very patchy, and findings may be absent in a biopsy sample
Hyperviscosity syndromes	Caused by multiple myeloma, Waldenstrom macroglobulinemia, polycythemia vera, and various autoimmune disorders; may present histologically as normal liver, minimal nonspecific inflammatory changes, minimal sinusoidal dilatation, or lobular disarray
Various genetic/metabolic conditions	Storage diseases, cystinosis, urea cycle defects, hereditary intrahepatic cholestasis syndromes, phenylketonuria, aminoacidopathies, etc.

Abbreviations: PBC, primary biliary cirrhosis; PSC, primary sclerosing cholangitis; TPN, total parenteral nutrition.

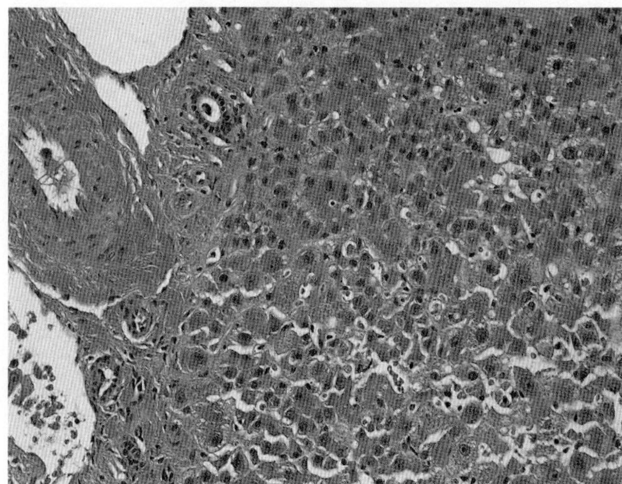

Figure 6.8 Acute hepatitis pattern. Lobular injury and disarray with apoptotic hepatitis (acidophilic bodies) but no significant lobular inflammation in this example of hepatitis A.

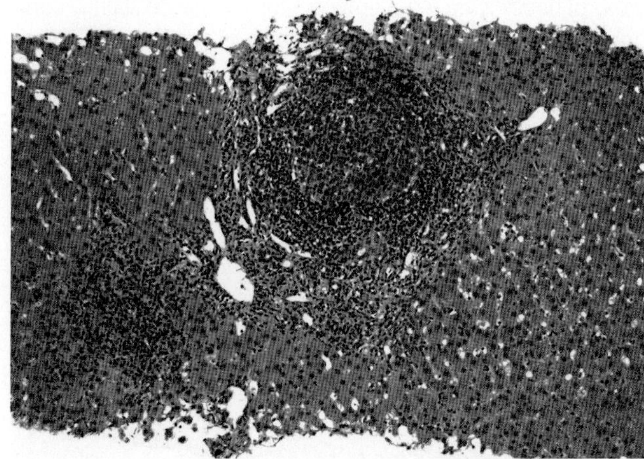

Figure 6.9 Chronic hepatitis pattern. Marked portal inflammation with a lymphoid aggregate and germinal center as well as mild interface activity in this example of chronic viral hepatitis.

Table 6.3 Etiologies associated with the "acute hepatitis" pattern

Etiology	Related findings/comments
Acute infections by hepatotropic viruses (HAV, HBV with or without HDV, less commonly HCV and HEV)	Ground-glass inclusions typically absent in acute HBV infection but may be present in acute flair of chronic HBV infection; "sanded nuclei" in HDV
Nonhepatotropic viruses (CMV, EBV, adenovirus, HSV, VZV, HHV-6, yellow fever, dengue, hemorrhagic fever-associated viruses)	Lobular microabscesses and/or microgranulomas in CMV; prominent (mononucleosis-like or "beaded") sinusoidal infiltrate in EBV; localized, "punched-out" necrosisin HSV and adenovirus; hemophagocytosis in HHV-6; Zone 2-predominant necrosis in yellow fever; hemorrhagic zonal necrosis in dengue and yellow fever; prominent hemorrhage in hemorrhagic fevers
Other infections (leptospirosis, tick-borne diseases, malaria, visceral leishmaniasis, Q fever)	Travel history to endemic areas; brown-black pigment in Kupffer cells and portal macrophages in malaria; small round 2–3 μm organisms within histiocytes in leishmaniasis; fibrin ring granulomas in Q fever
Drug reaction	Should be suspected when either prominent eosinophils or a mixed pattern (bile duct inflammation/injury, granulomas, and cholestasis) are present
Miscellaneous: hemophagocytic lymphohistiocytosis/macrophage activation syndrome	Hemophagocytosis

Abbreviations: HAV, hepatitis a virus; HBV, hepatitis B virus; HCV, hepatitis C virus; HDV, hepatitis D virus; HEV, hepatitis E virus; CMV, cytomegalovirus; EBV, Epstein–Barr virus; HSV, herpes simplex virus; VZV, varicella-zoster virus; HHV-6, human herpesvirus 6.

Table 6.4 Diseases associated with the "chronic hepatitis" pattern

Etiology	Related findings/comments
Viral hepatitis (HBV±HDV, HCV, HEV)	Ground-glass hepatocytes in HBV; sanded nuclei in HDV; HEV has only been associated with chronic hepatitis in immunosuppressed patients
Autoimmune hepatitis	Plasma cells can be focal or absent in histologically "atypical" autoimmune hepatitis
Drug reaction	As in acute hepatitis, drug reaction should be suspected when prominent eosinophils or other associated findings such as bile duct inflammation/injury, granulomas, and cholestasis are seen
Chronic biliary tract disease (PBC and less commonly PSC)	Early PBC may lack florid bile duct lesions, granulomas, or features of "biliary tract disease" but portal inflammation may still be prominent. This is less common but also occurs in PSC
Wilson disease	Glycogenated nuclei are common (but nonspecific); chronic hepatitis pattern may become more prominent as disease progresses
α-1 antitrypsin deficiency	A minority of cases shows a chronic hepatitis pattern; α-1 antitrypsin globules may be focal and difficult to visualize on H&E
Late-onset acute cellular rejection	Typical acute rejection-related findings may be minimal or absent
Sarcoidosis	A minority of cases will show a chronic hepatitis pattern in the background; granulomas may be focal and are not always sampled

Abbreviations: HAV, hepatitis a virus; HBV, hepatitis B virus; HCV, hepatitis C virus; HDV, hepatitis D virus; HEV, hepatitis E virus; PBC, primary biliary cirrhosis; PSC, primary sclerosing cholangitis.

be easily recognizable), often forming clusters, typically associated with brisk interface and lobular activity (Fig. 6.10). Cases showing typical histology most commonly represent autoimmune hepatitis, although clinical correlation is required to establish this diagnosis. Occasionally, this pattern in seen in viral hepatitis B and C (rarely in other infections), as well as in drug-induced liver injury (most notably nitrofurantoin, minocycline, halothane, statins, hydralazine, and methyldopa).[4]

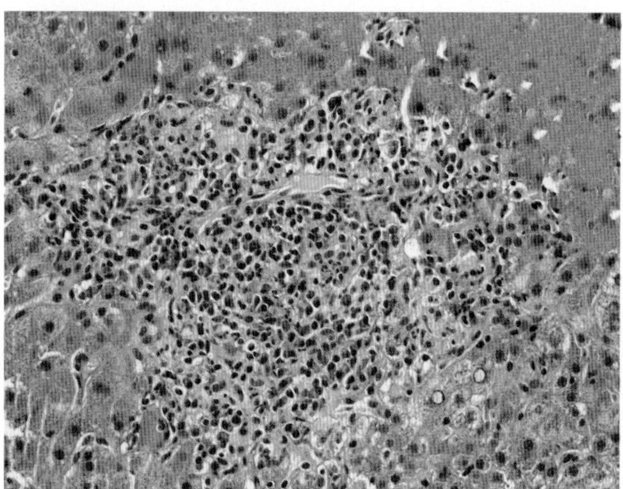

Figure 6.10 Plasma cell rich/autoimmune pattern. Chronic portal inflammation with numerous plasma cells in this case of autoimmune hepatitis.

Panacinar hepatitis

The term "panacinar hepatitis" (or "panlobular hepatitis") refers to a lymphocytic or lymphoplasmacytic inflammatory process, usually of at least moderate degree, involving both portal tracts and hepatic lobules in a relatively diffuse and uniform manner (Fig. 6.11). This pattern is typically seen in the setting of significant transaminase elevation and may represent either an acute process or an acute flare of a chronic disease. The main entities that should be considered in the differential diagnosis of panacinar hepatitis include acute viral hepatitis (including non-hepatotropic viruses), chronic viral hepatitis with an acute flare (primarily hepatitis B), drug-induced liver injury, Wilson disease, and autoimmune hepatitis. This pattern may overlap with acute hepatitis (with more prominent portal inflammation), chronic hepatitis (with significant activity), and cholestatic hepatitis (if cholestatic changes are pronounced).

Giant cell hepatitis

This pattern is defined by the presence of large, multinucleated hepatocytes (Fig. 6.12). Focal giant cell

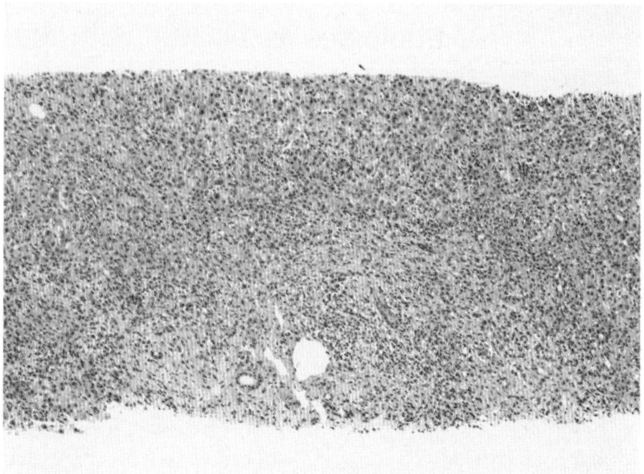

Figure 6.11 Panacinar/panlobular hepatitis pattern. A moderate or severe hepatitis involving both portal tracts and hepatic lobules in a somewhat diffuse manner, as in this case of drug-induced liver injury.

transformation may be seen in various settings, and the term "giant cell hepatitis" is generally reserved for cases in which this finding is either pronounced or predominant. Giant cell transformation is most commonly seen in the setting of neonatal cholestasis, either as a dominant finding in cases of "neonatal/giant cell hepatitis" or as a secondary/nonspecific finding in biliary atresia and other forms of cholestatic liver disease (see Chapter 13). When seen in adults, this pattern is usually referred to as postinfantile (or adult)-type giant cell hepatitis and can be associated with various autoimmune conditions, including primary liver diseases such as autoimmune hepatitis and primary biliary cirrhosis, and extrahepatic/systemic

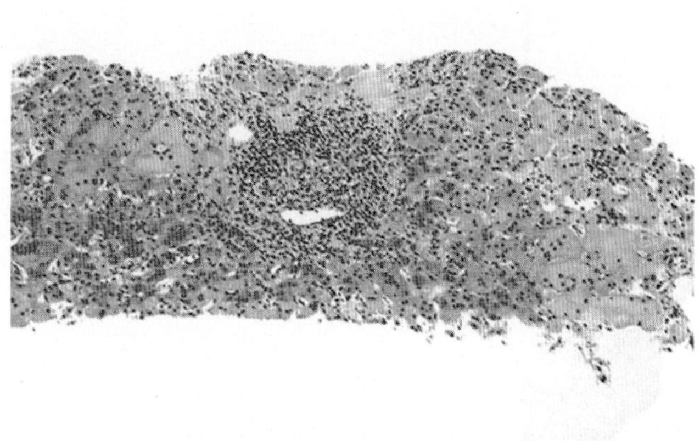

Figure 6.12 Giant cell hepatitis pattern. Multiple multinucleated hepatocytes throughout the hepatic lobules are seen in this case of neonatal giant cell hepatitis.

diseases such as lupus erythematosus, immune thrombocytopenic purpura, autoimmune hemolytic anemia, and various infections (CMV, HHV-6, HCV, HEV, EBV, and HIV).[5–8]

Isolated central perivenulitis

This is a somewhat uncommon pattern in which there is inflammation and hepatocyte injury essentially restricted to the areas around the central veins (Fig. 6.13). Outside of the liver transplant setting, this pattern is usually associated with either autoimmune hepatitis (thought to represent an early feature of this disease, occurring before a "chronic hepatitis" histology develops) or drug-induced liver injury. In liver allografts, central perivenulitis is a common acute cellular rejection-related feature, but one usually seen in combination with portal-based findings. Isolated central perivenulitis becomes more common in the late posttransplantation period, as one of the "atypical" histologic presentations of rejection[9] (see Chapter 19 for further discussion). Auto/alloimmune phenomena and drug reactions are also in the differential for isolated central perivenulitis in the posttransplant setting, but the presence of associated central vein endotheliitis strongly favors rejection.

Resolving hepatitis

This term refers to a pattern showing clusters of Kupffer cells and portal macrophages, with or without mild nonspecific inflammatory findings and hepatocyte regeneration, indicating recent (but resolving) injury (Fig. 6.14). This pattern is typically seen in patients with prominent elevation of liver enzymes on initial clinical evaluation, which subsequently improve, but do not completely normalize, and whose workup (viral hepatitis, autoimmune markers, etc.) is often negative. The underlying etiology in these cases is often never found but is most commonly attributed to either a drug reaction or a systemic viral infection.

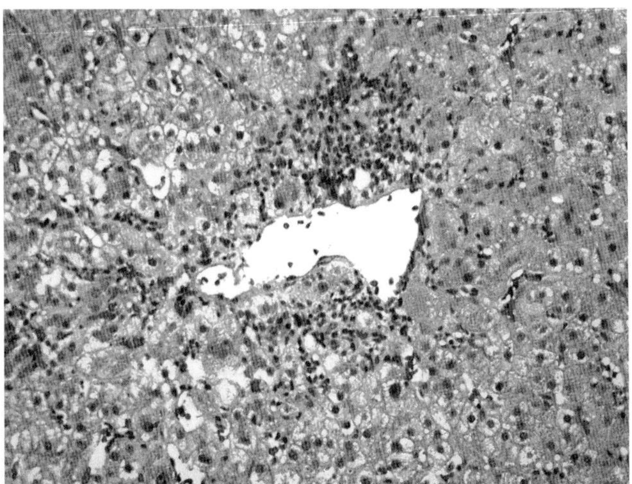

Figure 6.13 Isolated central perivenulitis pattern. Inflammation and hepatocyte injury around central veins. The portal tracts (not shown) are essentially uninvolved.

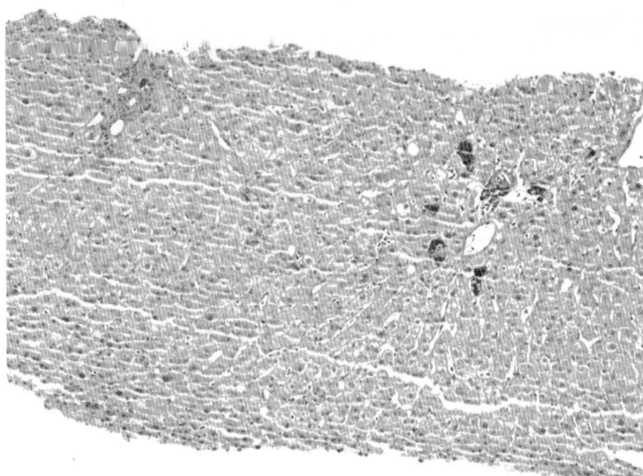

Figure 6.14 Resolving hepatitis. Clusters of ceroid-laden Kupffer cells in centrilobular areas, indicating recent/resolving injury.

6.3 FATTY LIVER DISEASE

Definition

Fatty liver disease results from the accumulation of fat droplets in the cytoplasm of hepatocytes, with or without associated inflammation, hepatocyte injury, or fibrosis.

Although classically subdivided into "simple steatosis" and "steatohepatitis," fatty liver disease actually represents a spectrum of histologic changes with increasing degrees of inflammation, hepatocellular injury, and associated fibrosis. The histologic appearance of alcoholic and nonalcoholic fatty liver disease is histologically very similar (a few differences exist, refer to Chapter 15 for details) and the distinction between these two entities ultimately relies on clinical correlation (i.e., history of alcohol abuse and features of metabolic syndrome) in most cases.

Simple steatosis

This is a common pattern seen by liver pathologist in western countries and is characterized by the presence of variable degrees of fat accumulation

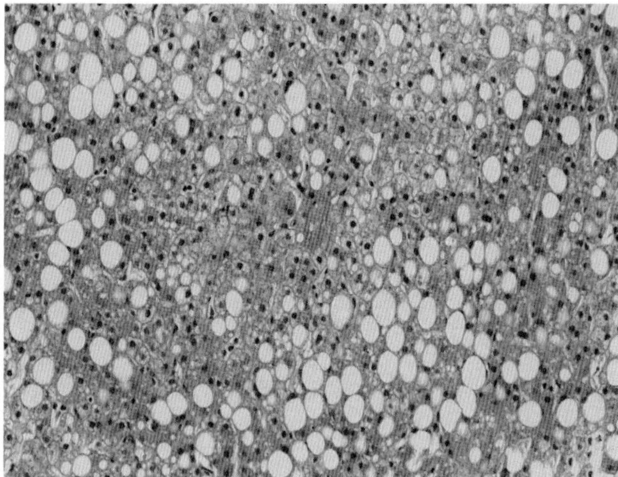

Figure 6.15 Simple steatosis pattern. Steatosis without hepatocyte ballooning or Mallory hyaline.

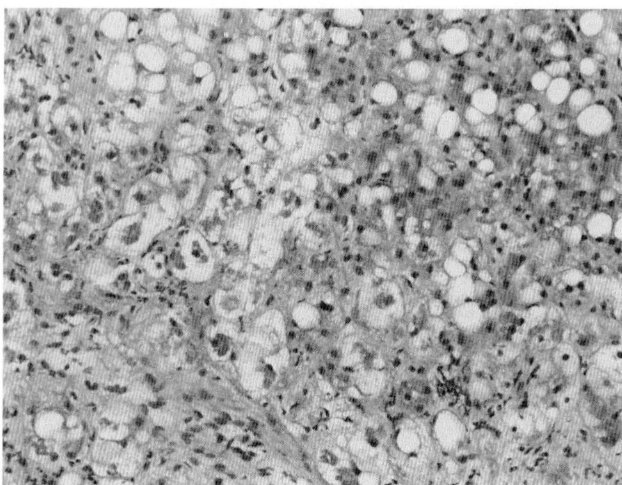

Figure 6.16 Steatohepatitis pattern. Steatosis with associated hepatocyte ballooning, Mallory hyaline, and inflammation in this example of alcoholic steatohepatitis.

within hepatocytes, without identifiable features of steatohepatitis (hepatocyte ballooning, Mallory hyaline, lobular inflammation, and/or sinusoidal fibrosis) (Fig. 6.15). Steatosis is traditionally subdivided into micro and macrovesicular patterns. Most liver pathologists now reserve the term microvesicular steatosis for cases showing very small fat droplets (often difficult to identify on H&E stain, but that are readily seen on oil-red-O or other fat stains done on frozen tissue), typically occurring in specific (and uncommon) settings such as acute fatty liver of pregnancy, HELLP syndrome, Rye syndrome, toxicity by certain medications (tetracycline, valproic acid), and mitochondrial toxicity/dysfunction. Therefore, the steatosis seen in typical cases of fatty liver disease is best described as "large droplet" and "small droplet" (both of which are part of the spectrum of macrovesicular steatosis). Although most commonly due to metabolic syndrome and/or alcohol, steatosis can result from a long list of etiologies (see Chapter 15).

Steatohepatitis

This pattern represents the histologically more severe end of the fatty liver disease spectrum, in which steatosis occurs in association with various combinations of hepatocyte ballooning, Mallory hyaline, inflammation,[10] and fibrosis (Fig. 6.16). A significant proportion of cases of steatohepatitis, but not simple steatosis, is thought to progress to advanced fibrosis/cirrhosis, hence the importance of the histologic distinction between these two patterns. Although no universally accepted definition exists for the minimal criteria necessary to distinguish steatohepatitis from simple steatosis, most experts would agree that unequivocal hepatocyte ballooning, with or without Mallory hyaline, indicates steatohepatitis.[11,12] Pericellular fibrosis, likewise, most often represents a steatohepatitis-related finding in this setting, whether or not ballooning or Mallory hyaline is present in a given sample. The interpretation of steatosis plus "more than minimal" inflammatory changes and acidophil bodies, in the absence of ballooning and Mallory, is more variable, even among specialists, and whether inflammation or acidophil bodies[13] by themselves (combined with steatosis) can characterize steatohepatitis is still unsettled.

Steatohepatitis is associated with a relatively limited differential diagnosis. In older patients, it is usually due to either alcohol abuse or metabolic syndrome (i.e., NASH). Some forms of drug injury, such as Amiodarone toxicity, can also show a steatohepatitis-like pattern[14] and represent an important consideration, particularly in cases showing prominent and easily identifiable Mallory hyaline and significant neutrophilic inflammation (including neutrophilic "satellitosis" around dying hepatocytes), often with little or no steatosis. Other medications such as steroids and estrogen therapy are also occasionally implicated. Severe steatohepatitis with numerous ballooned hepatocytes and Mallory hyaline, sometimes accompanied by cholestasis (which is not part of the spectrum of NASH in a noncirrhotic liver), are more typical of alcoholic liver disease. In young individuals (age 40 to 45 years or younger), especially in those without a clinically identifiable reason to have steatohepatitis, Wilson disease must be excluded because steatohepatitis is one of the several histologic presentations of this disease.[15]

6.4 CHOLESTATIC PATTERNS

Definition

This injury pattern can show hepatocanalicular cholestasis, obstructive-type changes, or features of chronic cholestasis as the main or only finding.

The hallmark of cholestatic patterns is the presence of hepatocanalicular cholestasis and/or changes of chronic cholestasis (also referred to as cholate stasis), characterized by periportal hepatocyte swelling/feathery degeneration (often containing Mallory hyaline) and copper/copper-binding protein.[16] The presence or absence of inflammation and biliary obstructive-type changes will allow further characterization of the pattern of cholestasis in most cases (refer to Table 6.5 for a list of etiologies associated with each pattern).

"Bland" cholestasis

In this pattern, hepatocanalicular cholestasis is seen as an isolated finding (i.e., without significant inflammation, hepatocyte injury, obstructive changes, or features of chronic cholestasis) (Fig. 6.17). Bile pigment characteristically involves centrilobular (Zone 3) hepatocytes, with variable, but less prominent, involvement of other regions of the lobule. Canalicular bile plugs (often small) represent the most reliable finding to identify cholestasis and should be present in most or all cases, usually associated with intracytoplasmic bile (i.e., hepatocanalicular cholestasis). Although bile may conceivably be exclusively intracytoplasmic, it is very difficult in practice to reliably distinguish this from various other pigments, especially lipofuscin, which also has a centrilobular-predominant distribution (in contrast to iron and copper deposits, which are mainly periportal). The differential diagnosis for this pattern is relatively broad, but cholestatic drug reactions and systemic infections/sepsis account for most cases seen in practice.

Cholestatic hepatitis

The association of hepatocanalicular cholestatis with inflammation and hepatocyte injury characterizes the "cholestatic hepatitis" pattern (Fig. 6.18). The main diagnostic considerations in this pattern are cholestatic drug reactions, acute viral hepatitis (especially hepatitis A, B, and E), and other systemic infections. Most forms of severe inflammatory liver injury, especially those with significant necrosis (as could be seen in autoimmune hepatitis or Wilson disease) often show cholestasis as a secondary finding.

Table 6.5 Conditions associated with various "cholestatic" patterns

Pattern
Bland cholestasis
Drug reaction (estrogen therapy, androgenic steroids)
Sepsis/systemic infections
Benign recurrent intrahepatic cholestasis
Thyroid dysfunction (hyper or hypothyroidism)
Cholestasis of pregnancy
Paraneoplastic syndromes (especially lymphomas)
Cholestatic hepatitis
Drug reaction (amoxicillin, penicillins, cephalosporins, rifampin, sulfonylureas)
Viral infections (including HAV, HBV, HEV, and nonhepatotropic viruses)
Biliary obstruction
Choledocholithiasis
Biliary stricture(s)
Tumors (primarily or secondarily involving bile ducts)
Primary sclerosing cholangitis
Pancreatic tumors, tumor-like lesions, and chronic pancreatitis
Biliary atresia
Chronic biliary tract disease, NOS
Primary biliary cirrhosis
Primary sclerosing cholangitis
Chronic biliary obstruction of any etiology
Ductopenia
Primary biliary cirrhosis
Primary sclerosing cholangitis
Chronic rejection
Drug reaction (same drugs as in "cholestatic hepatitis")
Syndromic (Alagille) and nonsyndromic paucity of bile ducts
Graft versus host disease
Ischemic cholangiopathy
Late-stage biliary obstruction or biliary atresia
Paraneoplastic syndromes (Hodgkin, T-cell lymphomas)
Neonatal infections

Abbreviations: HAV, hepatitis A virus; HBV, hepatitis B virus; HEV, hepatitis E virus.

Biliary obstruction

This pattern is essentially characterized by portal findings, which are often, but not always, associated with hepatocanalicular cholestasis. In acute biliary obstruction, the first changes to occur are portal edema and mild mixed inflammation, with ductular reaction appearing shortly thereafter (Fig. 6.19). These

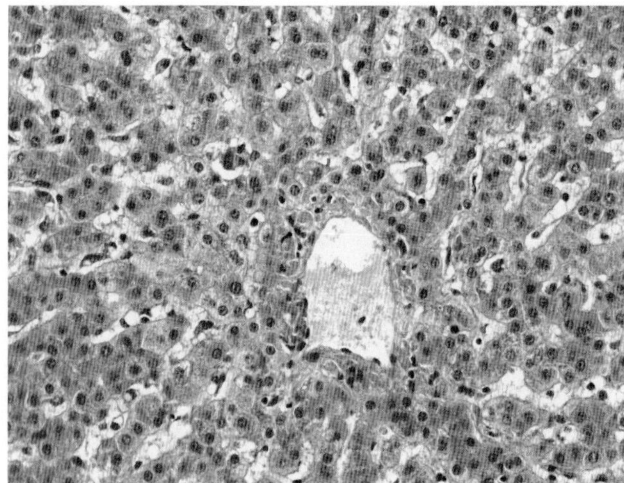

Figure 6.17 Bland cholestasis pattern. Prominent cholestasis, including numerous canalicular bile plugs, is seen in this case of cholestatic drug reaction.

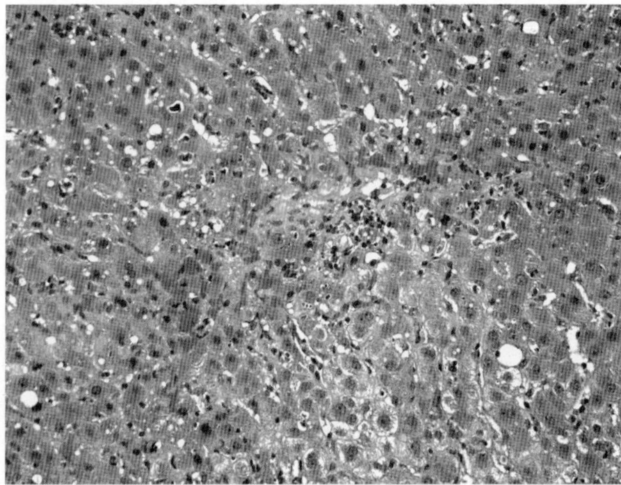

Figure 6.18 Cholestatic hepatitis pattern. In addition to cholestasis, there is inflammation and hepatocyte injury in cholestatic hepatitis.

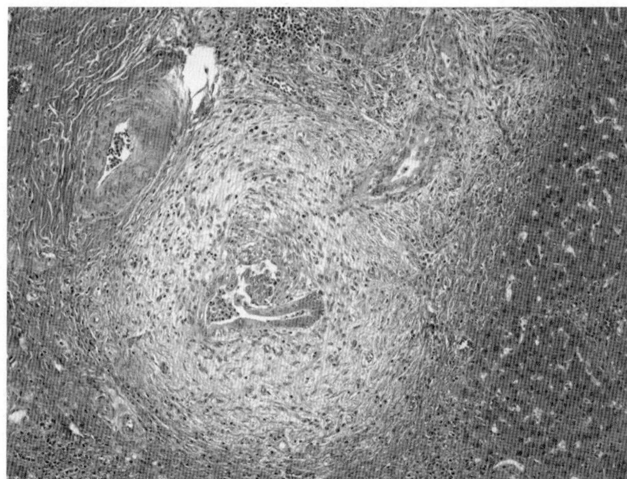

Figure 6.19 Biliary obstruction pattern. Mixed portal inflammation and prominent portal edema in this example of acute biliary obstruction. Cholestasis was also present in Zone 3 in this case (not shown). Acute cholangitis is also occasionally present in these cases.

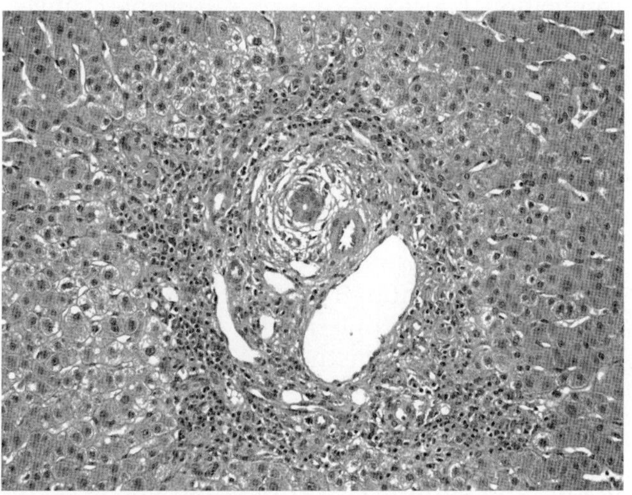

Figure 6.20 Chronic biliary obstruction pattern. Significant ductular reaction and mild mixed inflammation, characteristic of chronic biliary obstruction.

changes are usually associated with variable degrees of hepatocanalicular cholestasis. As cholestasis becomes chronic, there is an increasingly prominent ductular reaction (with or without portal edema or fibrosis) and features of cholate stasis (discussed later) develop. Any cause of biliary obstruction (stones, strictures, tumors, or extrinsic compression) can lead to a biliary obstructive pattern.

Chronic biliary tract disease, NOS

Many forms of chronic disease of the biliary tract lead to a common histologic appearance characterized by a ductular reaction (Fig. 6.20) and changes involving periportal hepatocytes, including swelling/feathery degeneration (often with Mallory hyaline) (Fig. 6.21), and accumulation of copper/copper-binding protein (best seen with special stains such as rhodanine, orcein, and Victoria Blue) (Fig. 6.22). This pattern may be seen in obstructive processes of various etiologies, primary ductopenic processes (vanishing bile duct syndrome, chronic rejection) as well as in primary sclerosing cholangitis and primary biliary cirrhosis.

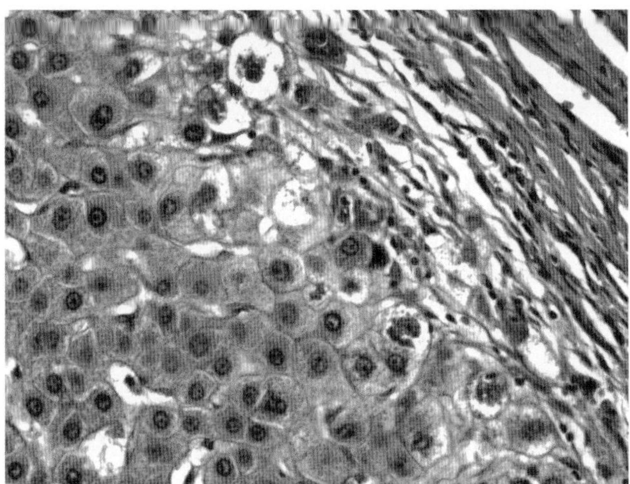

Figure 6.21 Chronic biliary obstruction pattern. Chronic cholestatic changes can also present in the form of periportal or periseptal hepatocyte swelling (feathery degeneration) and Mallory hyaline, referred to as "cholate stasis."

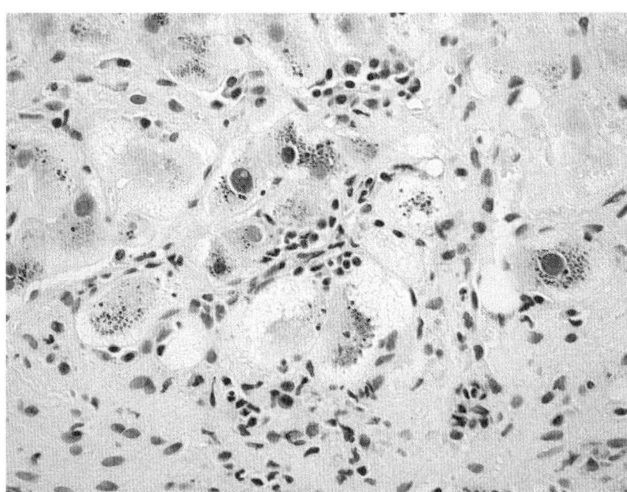

Figure 6.22 Chronic biliary obstruction pattern. Copper accumulation in hepatocytes, highlighted here with a rhodanine stain, is also part of cholate stasis (chronic cholestasis).

Ductopenia

The loss of interlobular bile ducts represents the hallmark of this pattern (Fig. 6.23). Although historically defined as "absence of bile ducts in >50% of portal tracts", the recognition of the normal relationship between bile ducts and hepatic artery branches within portal tracts is important in this setting because the vast majority of arterial profiles should be accompanied by a nearby bile duct of similar size.[17] When several portal tracts within a sample show "unpaired" arteries, ductopenia is likely present[18] (see further discussion in Chapter 12). Ductopenia is typically accompanied

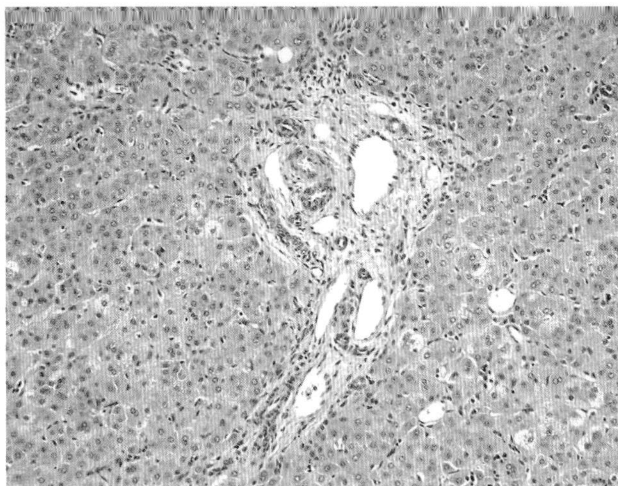

Figure 6.23 Ductopenia pattern. A portal tract is shown here with several hepatic artery branches without an accompanying bile duct in this example of Alagille syndrome. Most portal tracts in this case showed similar findings.

by cholestasis, cholate stasis, and various features related to its primary cause. Ductular reaction, however, may be minimal or absent depending on the etiology. In the setting of liver transplantation, ductopenia usually represents chronic ductopenic rejection. In the nontransplant setting, the differential includes syndromic (Alagille) and nonsyndromic ductopenia, primary biliary cirrhosis, primary sclerosing cholangitis, and various infections (particularly in the neonatal period).

6.5 VENOUS OUTFLOW IMPAIRMENT

Definition

Venous outflow impairment represents a pattern of injury showing sinusoidal dilatation/congestion, with or without fibrosis, as its primary feature.

The hallmark of the venous outflow impairment pattern is the presence of sinusoidal dilatation and congestion centered around Zone 3 (Fig. 6.24). Hepatic plate atrophy and sinusoidal fibrosis can also be seen within congested areas, depending on the degree and duration of the process. The portal tracts are often unremarkable in this setting, although ductular reaction is not uncommon. Prominent ductular reaction, mimicking biliary obstruction,[19] can also occur. However, biopsies in this setting typically lack other "biliary" features, such as portal edema and cholestasis. Aberrant CK-7 expression[20] and the presence of PAS+, diastase resistant hyaline globules[21] in centrilobular hepatocytes are also within the spectrum of changes seen in this pattern. Although subtle differences are described among the different etiologies of venous outflow impairment (refer to Chapter 20 for further

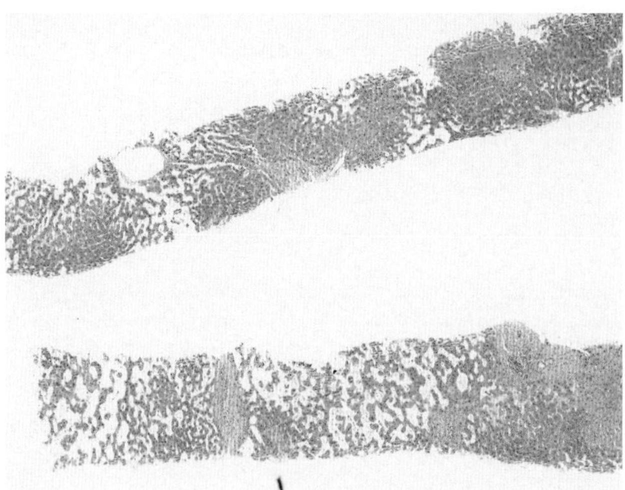

Figure 6.24 Venous outflow impairment pattern. Prominent sinusoidal dilatation, primarily involvings Zone 3.

discussion), recognition of the general pattern represents the main step.

One of the main difficulties in this setting is the interpretation of mild sinusoidal dilatation/congestion. In our experience, this is most commonly nonspecific in nature because the majority of patients have no clinical evidence of any conditions related to venous outflow impairment. Hepatocyte atrophy in the areas of sinusoidal dilatation/congestion suggests the finding most likely represents true venous outflow impairment. Another helpful hint that the sinusoidal congestion/dilatation is pathologic (i.e., caused by increased sinusoidal pressure) is the presence of associated sinusoidal fibrosis, however mild it may be (a technically optimal trichrome stain, without under or overstaining, is necessary for this evaluation) (Fig. 6.25). The differential diagnosis of venous outflow impairment includes: (1) cardiovascular disease with right sided or congestive heart failure (leading to "passive" venous congestion) or restrictive cardiac physiology (constrictive pericarditis, diastolic dysfunction, tamponade, etc.); (2) thrombotic/obstructive processes involving the vena cava and/or hepatic veins (Budd–Chiari syndrome, tumors, etc.); and (3) obstructive/thrombotic process involving the hepatic sinusoids (veno-occlusive disease/sinusoidal obstruction syndrome, and less commonly neoplastic proliferations with widespread sinusoidal infiltration).

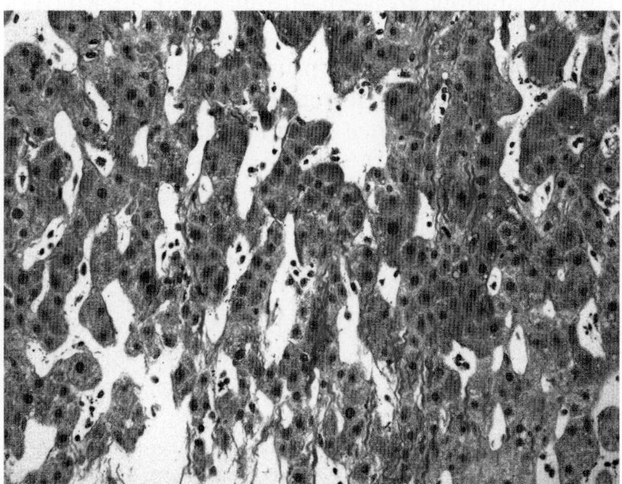

Figure 6.25 Venous outflow impairment. A trichrome stain highlights unequivocal sinusoidal fibrosis in a case of venous outflow impairment otherwise showing only mild sinusoidal dilatation and congestion.

6.6 BLAND (NONINFLAMMATORY) NECROSIS

Definition

A pattern of injury characterized primarily by the presence of hepatocellular necrosis, with minimal or no inflammation.

Severe injury with large areas of necrosis can occur in aggressive forms of many types of primarily inflammatory liver diseases; these cases are best classified as one of the hepatitis patterns. In cases in which necrosis represents the dominant (or only) finding, with little to no associated inflammation, the differential diagnosis largely depends on the pattern of necrosis itself. These are discussed here under the pattern "bland necrosis" (Table 6.6).

Zonal necrosis

Bland necrosis with a zonal distribution is seen in a variety of types of insults, as listed on Table 6.6. In practice, Zone 3 (or Zones 2 to 3) necrosis is the most common form and can result from ischemia, cocaine abuse (largely representing ischemic injury

Table 6.6 Primarily necrotic patterns and their differential diagnosis

Bland (noninflammatory/pauci-inflammatory) necrosis
- Zonal necrosis:
  - Zone 1: ferrous sulfate, phosphorus, and bacterial endotoxin (e.g., Proteus vulgaris)
  - Zone 2: yellow fever
  - Zone 3: ischemia, acetaminophen
- Massive/submassive necrosis: medications, severe ischemia
- Geographic necrosis: HSV, adenovirus, occasionally CMV
- Hemorrhagic necrosis: yellow fever, dengue fever, other hemorrhagic fever viruses

Abbreviations: HSV, herpes simplex virus; CMV, cytomegalovirus.

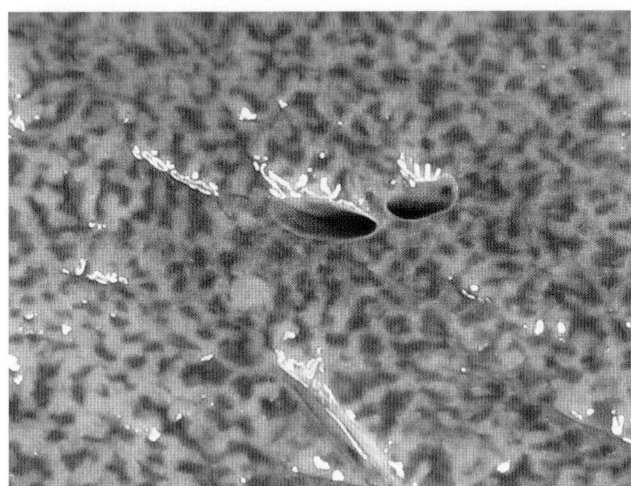

Figure 6.26 Zonal necrosis. A gross specimen (liver explant) showing zonal necrosis in the setting of acetaminophen toxicity.

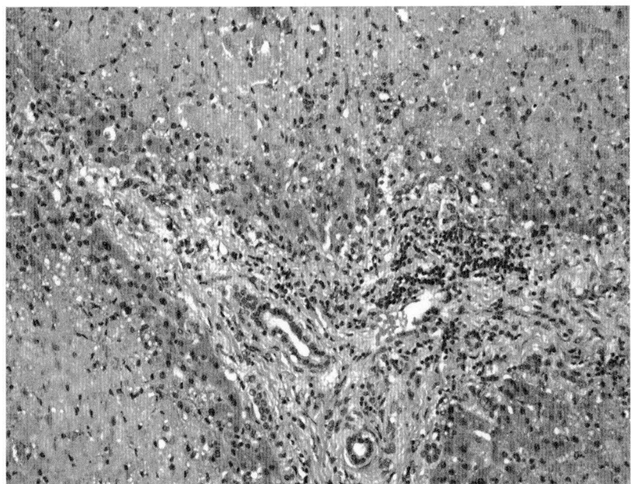

Figure 6.27 Bland necrosis pattern. Centrilobular (Zones 2 to 3) zonal necrosis in the same case of acetaminophen toxicity shown in Figure 6.26.

related to cocaine-induced vasoconstriction), and acetaminophen toxicity (Figs. 6.26 and 6.27). Necrosis with a predominantly Zone 1 or 2 distribution is significantly less common. Zone 1 necrosis is most often related to ferrous sulfate, phosphorus, and some bacterial endotoxin (e.g., Proteus vulgaris), whereas Zone 2 necrosis—recognized by the sparing of a periportal and perivenular ring of hepatocytes—can be seen in yellow fever.

Geographic necrosis

Bland necrosis with a "geographic" distribution is characterized by well-delineated areas of confluent necrosis with an irregular, nonzonal, map-like pattern. Adenovirus and herpes simplex virus infection should be carefully excluded in these cases.

Massive/submassive necrosis

This pattern is characterized by extensive necrosis and parenchymal collapse, involving the majority of the lobular areas (without a recognizable zonal distribution) (Fig. 6.28). The portal tracts are located closer to one another than normal (due to collapse of the intervening lobules), show varying degree of inflammation, and often have a pronounced ductular reaction. Islands of regenerating hepatocytes are also variably present and commonly show prominent rosetting and cholestasis (Fig. 6.29). In some cases, the regenerating hepatocytes can form large nodules, resembling a tumor on imaging studies. Patients almost invariably show signs of acute/subacute or fulminant liver failure. In fact, if the patient is not in liver failure, these findings most commonly represent localized areas of liver injury, as can be seen in intrahepatic or segmental arterial thrombosis.

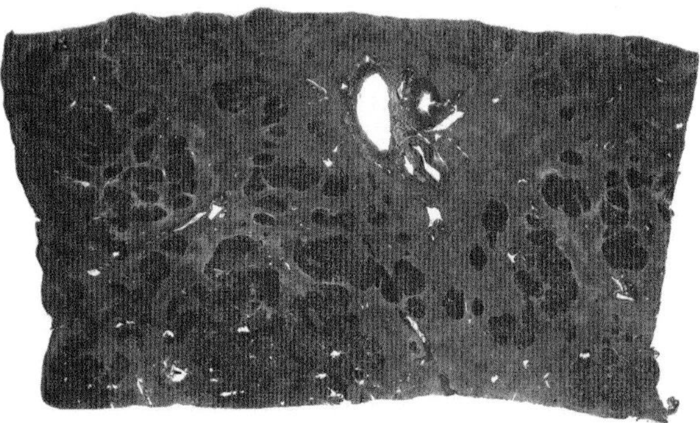

Figure 6.28 Massive necrosis. A low power image of a trichrome stain in a case of isoniazid-associated massive necrosis. Approximately 50% of the parenchyma in this example is necrotic/collapsed, appearing as pale blue areas, in contrast to the dark blue native portal tracts and red areas of nonnecrotic parenchyma.

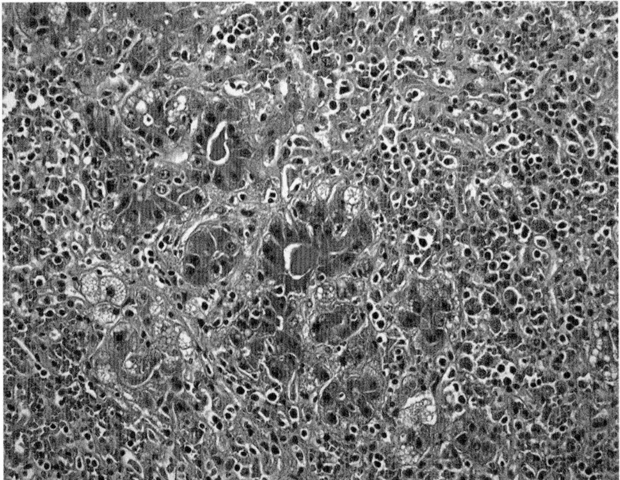

Figure 6.29 Massive necrosis. Residual hepatocyte islands forming rosettes and containing canalicular bile plugs. Marked ductular reaction is also common in these cases (not shown).

Bona fide massive/submassive necrosis can be due to a variety of etiologies, but pathologists should specifically search for features of autoimmune hepatitis (especially plasma cells, which can be present only focally), viral inclusions (CMV, herpesvirus), and ground-glass inclusions (hepatitis B), with the appropriate stains/immunostains, as applicable. Ground-glass inclusions are not seen in acute hepatitis B, but can be seen if there is a superimposed injury on top of chronic hepatitis B. Increased eosinophils suggest the possibility of a severe drug reaction or parasites. In young patients, Wilson disease should also be excluded because acute liver failure is one of several possible presentations.

6.7 GRANULOMATOUS PATTERN

Definition

In this pattern of injury, granulomas (necrotizing or nonnecrotizing) represent either the primary or the only finding in the specimen.

The first step with this pattern is the appropriate characterization of the granulomas (Table 6.7). Granulomas are defined by the presence of an organized cluster of histiocytes forming a nodular, somewhat cohesive structure, in contrast to nonspecific histiocyte clusters lacking the organization of a *bona fide* granuloma, often seen in fatty liver disease, mineral oil ingestion (i.e., lipogranulomas), or in any process associated with necroinflammation (i.e., microgranulomas). True granulomatous processes should be further subclassified into necrotizing and nonnecrotizing categories. Necrotizing granulomas are usually related to infections (bacterial, mycobacterial, or fungal) regardless of their location (Fig. 6.30). Occasional cases of sarcoidosis with large granulomas will also show areas of central hyalinization and fibrinous debris, superficially resembling a necrotizing granulomatous process. Nonnecrotizing granulomas can be found in the portal tracts, lobules, or both. Although the differential diagnosis for nonnecrotizing granulomatous inflammation in the liver is broad, the four most commonly encountered entities are primary biliary cirrhosis (Fig. 6.31), sarcoidosis (Fig. 6.32), granulomatous drug reactions, and infections. The granulomas in primary biliary cirrhosis are found primarily within portal tracts, with small granulomas occasionally present within lobular areas. They are often relatively poorly formed and typically seen adjacent to or around a bile

Table 6.7 Etiologies associated with granulomatous hepatitis
Nonnecrotizing granulomas PBC Sarcoidosis Drug reaction Paraneoplastic (e.g., Hodgkin disease) Idiopathic (approximately one-third of cases) Infections (brucellosis, listeriosis, salmonella, tick-borne diseases [Lyme, ehrlichiosis, tularemia], fungal infections, occasional cases of tuberculosis, schistosomiasis, and some viral infections [EBV, CMV, acute hepatitis A, hepatitis E])
Necrotizing granulomas Mycobacterium tuberculosis Fungal infections (histoplasmosis, cryptococcosis, occasionally others) *Bartonella henselae* (cat scratch disease) Sarcoid (very rare cases show fibrinoid, necrotizing-type changes)
Fibrin ring granulomas Bacteria: *Coxiella burnetti* (Q fever), Rickettsia conorii (Boutonneuse fever) Viruses: EBV, CMV, hepatitis A, hepatitis C Parasites: toxoplasmosis, leishmaniasis Drugs: allopurinol Miscellaneous: giant cell arteritis, Hodgkin disease
Miscellaneous granulomatous processes Lipogranuloma (nonspecific finding in fatty liver disease, mineral oil ingestion) Microgranuloma (nonspecific finding in necroinflammatory processes) Foreign body granulomas (talc granulomas in IV drug users, prior abdominal surgery, tumor embolization)

Abbreviations: PBC, primary biliary cirrhosis; EBV, Epstein–Barr virus; CMV, cytomegalovirus.

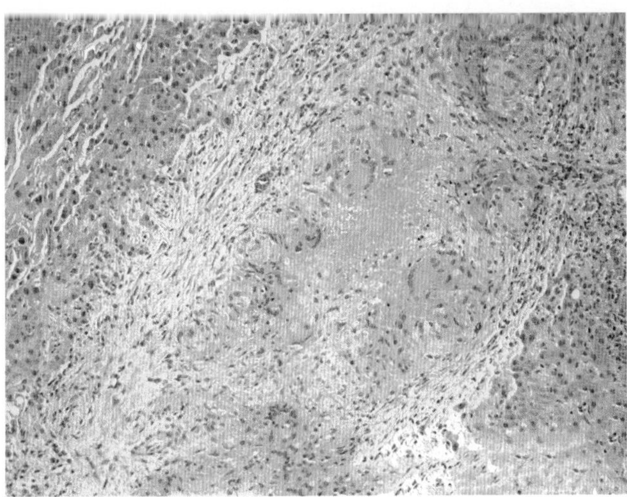

Figure 6.30 Granulomatous pattern. A necrotizing granuloma with a rim of histiocytes/giant cells and a necrotic center is shown here.

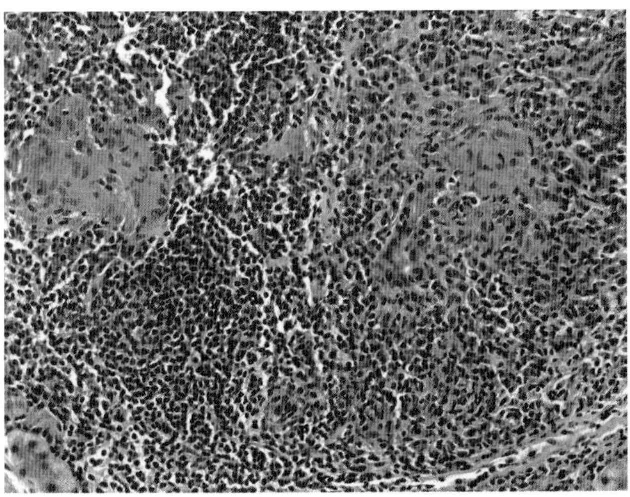

Figure 6.31 Granulomatous pattern. Nonnecrotizing granulomas are shown here within a densely inflamed portal tract, associated with an injured bile duct (at the center of the image to the **right**), in this case of primary biliary cirrhosis.

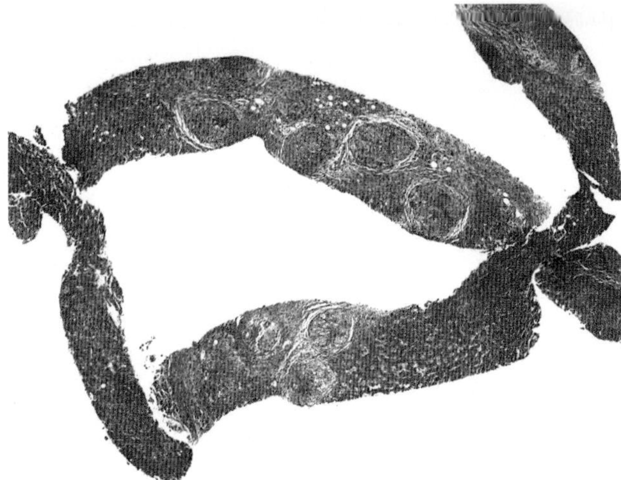

Figure 6.32 Granulomatous pattern. A case of hepatic sarcoidosis showing numerous well-formed granulomas involving both portal tracts and hepatic lobules, surrounded by a thin rim of fibrosis.

duct branch (multiple H&E levels and/or cytokeratin immunostains often help identify the injured duct). In contrast, the granulomas in sarcoidosis tend to be better formed, larger, located either in portal tracts or lobules, and are often associated with fibrosis. Granulomas in drug reactions can have essentially any appearance and distribution, but usually occur in combination with other findings (inflammatory infiltrates, lobular injury, cholestasis, etc.), as part of a mixed pattern. Fibrin ring granulomas represent a granuloma variant with distinct morphology, characterized by a central fatty droplet surrounded by a thin rim of eosinophilic/fibrinous material and an outer layer of histiocytes. Fibrin ring granulomas are most commonly seen in the setting of infections such as *Coxiella burnetti* (Q fever), EBV, CMV, toxoplasmosis, leishmaniasis, and rarely in hepatitis A and hepatitis C. Other etiologies include allopurinol toxicity, giant cell arteritis, and Hodgkin disease. Finally, although typically necrotizing, the granulomas associated with fungal infections and mycobacteria can be nonnecrotizing, and these organisms should also be excluded in the histologic workup.

6.8 ABNORMAL DEPOSITION

Definition

In this pattern of injury, there are abnormal substances/inclusions within various cell types in the liver and/or within the extracellular compartment.

The differential diagnosis for this pattern is rather broad, but mostly related to genetic/metabolic diseases and less commonly to infections or drug effects. Although the final diagnosis will usually require enzymatic and/or genetic testing, narrowing of the differential diagnosis is usually possible by careful characterization of the appearance of the abnormal substance and assessment of its location (i.e., cell type involved). Please refer to Chapters 4, 17, and 18 for further discussion.

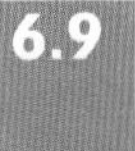

6.9 HEPATOPORTAL SCLEROSIS/ NONCIRRHOTIC PORTAL HYPERTENSION

This pattern is characterized by a combination of features (often very subtle) that include: (1) portal vein

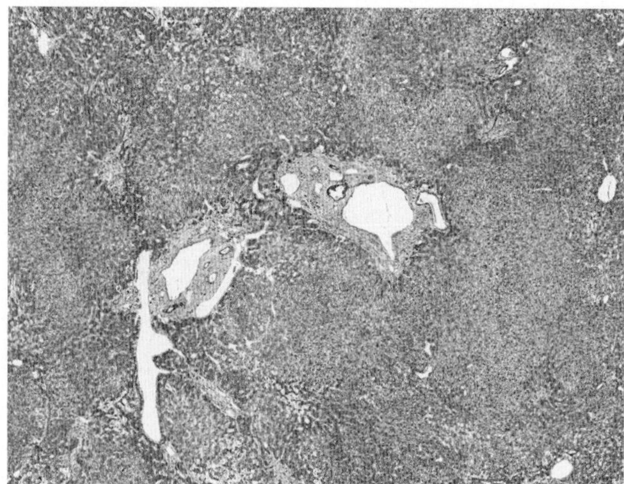

Figure 6.33 Hepatoportal sclerosis. Two portal tracts in close proximity at the center of the image show dilated portal veins with herniation into the hepatic lobules, whereas some of the smaller portal tracts around them show no recognizable portal veins.

abnormalities (absent or atrophic/obliterated portal veins and/or dilated portal veins with "herniation" into the lobular area) (Fig. 6.33) and (2) vague parenchymal nodularity in the form of either nodular regenerative hyperplasia or subtle macronodules surrounded by a rim of very thin fibrous septa. Although some of these may occasionally be seen as incidental, nonspecific findings, it is important to carefully search for these features in cases of unexplained portal hypertension in noncirrhotic liver.

6.10 MIXED PATTERNS

Basic patterns in liver pathology sometimes coexist, but establishing the presence of a mixed pattern requires careful consideration of whether all features may be part of a single pattern. For example, cases showing a "fatty liver disease" pattern may also show portal inflammation resembling a chronic hepatitis and cases with a "venous outflow impairment" pattern may be associated with a prominent ductular reaction, mimicking biliary tract disease. These changes, however, are still within the spectrum of their respective categories and do not usually represent a mixed pattern. True mixed patterns, however, do exist (representing one or more underlying conditions), and examples include "chronic biliary tract disease" and "hepatitis" (e.g., primary biliary cirrhosis/autoimmune hepatitis overlap), "cholestatic hepatitis" and "granulomatous" (e.g., drug-induced injury), and "steatohepatitis" and "abnormal deposition" (NASH with α-1 antitrypsin deficiency).

6.11 PATTERNS OF FIBROSIS AND CIRRHOSIS

Although fibrosis represents a common final pathway for most forms of chronic liver disease, distinct patterns of fibrosis can often be recognized in association with certain diseases or disease groups (Table 6.8).

Portal-based fibrosis

This is the typical pattern of fibrosis seen in many forms of liver disease, including chronic viral hepatitides, chronic biliary tract diseases, autoimmune hepatitis, Wilson disease, hemochromatosis, etc. (Fig. 6.34). Initially, there is fibrous expansion of portal tracts with associated periportal fibrosis—a process driven by ductular reaction and activation of stellate cells in periportal areas. This is followed by the formation of bridging fibrosis (portal–portal or portal–central).

Table 6.8 Patterns of fibrosis

Portal-based: chronic viral hepatitis, AIH, chronic biliary tract diseases, Wilson disease, hemochromatosis
Sinusoidal fibrosis:
Centrilobular: steatohepatitis, venous outflow impairment, post-ACR
Periportal: diabetic hepatosclerosis, fibrosing cholestatic hepatitis
Biliary-type: PBC, PSC, biliary obstruction, TPN, cystic fibrosis

Abbreviations: AIH, autoimmune hepatitis; ACR, acute cellular rejection; PBC, primary biliary cirrhosis; PSC, primary sclerosing cholangitis; TPN, total parenteral nutrition.

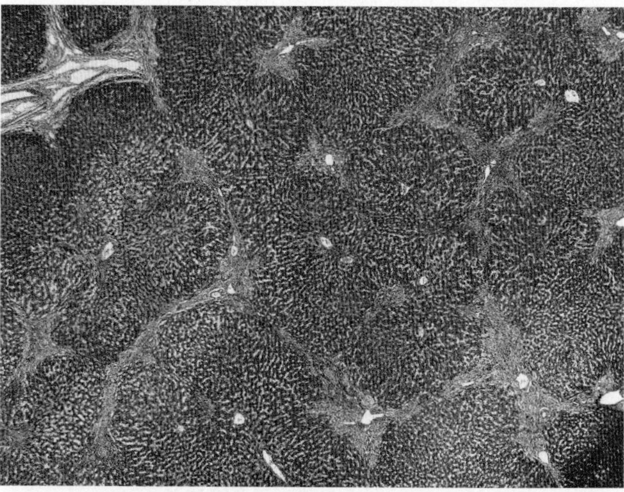

Figure 6.34 Portal-based fibrosis. The fibrosis in this case of chronic biliary obstruction primarily involves portal tracts, with multiple areas of portal–portal fibrous bridges.

Finally, the intervening hepatic lobules become increasingly disorganized and nodular, characterizing cirrhosis. The various staging systems essentially use slight variations of the same features (i.e., portal/periportal fibrosis, fibrous bridges, and parenchymal nodularity) to ascribe a specific score (i.e., stage). Please refer to Chapter 7 for further details.

Sinusoidal and centrilobular fibrosis

This pattern of fibrosis is characterized by the presence of generally very thin, linear deposits of collagen fibers along the hepatic sinusoids, thought to be triggered by the activation of stellate cells within the spaces of Disse by various insults. Sinusoidal fibrosis is easily recognizable on a good-quality collagen stain because no Type I collagen (which stains blue on Masson trichrome and red on Sirius red stain) is normally present along hepatic sinusoids. Collagen stains, however, are frequently "overstained" and can show artifactual bluish discoloration along sinusoidal spaces, which can be mistaken for fibrosis. Type I collagen can also be identified on reticulin stains as brown fibers along the sinusoids, in contrast to black (silver)-staining normal sinusoidal reticulin fibers. This pattern of fibrosis is seen in a more limited number of conditions. Most commonly, it occurs in the setting of steatohepatitis or venous outflow impairment—prototypes of centrilobular processes (Fig. 6.35). Other rare conditions associated with sinusoidal fibrosis include diabetic hepatosclerosis and long standing vitamin A toxicity.

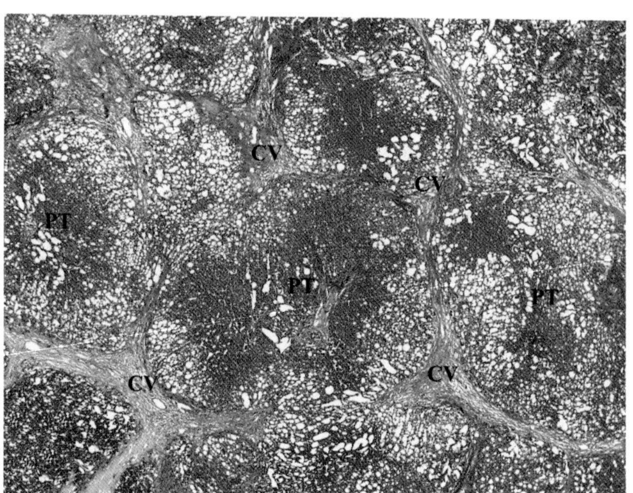

Figure 6.35 Centrilobular fibrosis. There is extensive bridging fibrosis in this case of nonalcoholic steatohepatitis, primarily involving central areas (central–central fibrosis).

Congenital hepatic fibrosis

Congenital hepatic fibrosis represents a distinctive pattern that is characterized by prominent portal fibrosis with thick portal–portal bridges in a cirrhosis-like pattern. Unlike typical cirrhosis, the lobular areas do not typically appear regenerative/nodular and expansile, in spite of the prominent fibrosis. The main feature in this pattern, however, is the presence of well-formed irregularly shaped ductal structures at the periportal/periseptal areas, as well as foci analogous to Von-Meyenburg complexes (bile duct hamartomas), characteristic of duct plate malformations (Fig. 6.36). Although present congenitally, the manifestations of this disease may not appear until well into adulthood, and this diagnosis/pattern needs to be kept in mind in the differential diagnosis of cirrhosis.

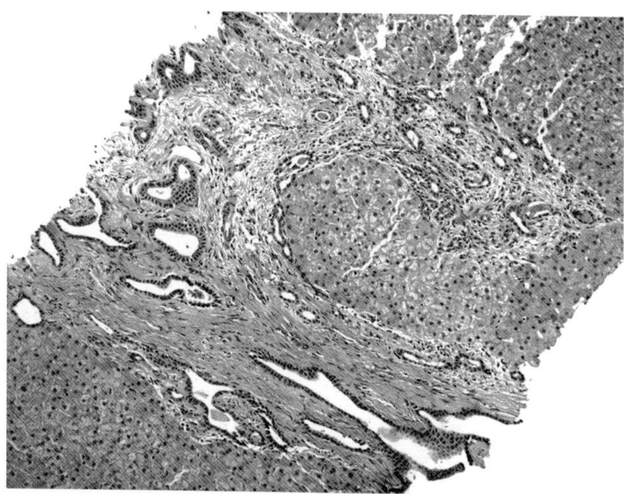

Figure 6.36 Congenital hepatic fibrosis. Numerous abnormal, relatively well-formed ductal structures are present within portal tracts and along the portal–lobular interface, characteristic of a duct plate malformation. This change was present throughout the sample in this case, associated with thick fibrous bridges, typical of congenital hepatic fibrosis.

6.12 CIRRHOSIS

Definition

Cirrhosis is a chronic process whereby continuous or recurrent injury leads to fibrous tissue deposition, fibrous bridging between portal tracts and central veins, distorted microanatomy, and regenerative nodule formation.

A few patterns of cirrhosis are worth recognizing in practice. Historically, cases of cirrhosis were classified into micronodular (nodule size <0.3 cm) (Fig. 6.37), macronodular (nodule size >0.3 cm) (Fig. 6.38), and mixed patterns. Alcoholic cirrhosis, NASH, and α-1 antitrypsin deficiency have traditionally been considered the prototype of micronodular cirrhosis, whereas various forms of "post-hepatitic" cases of cirrhosis (viral hepatitis, autoimmune hepatitis) typically

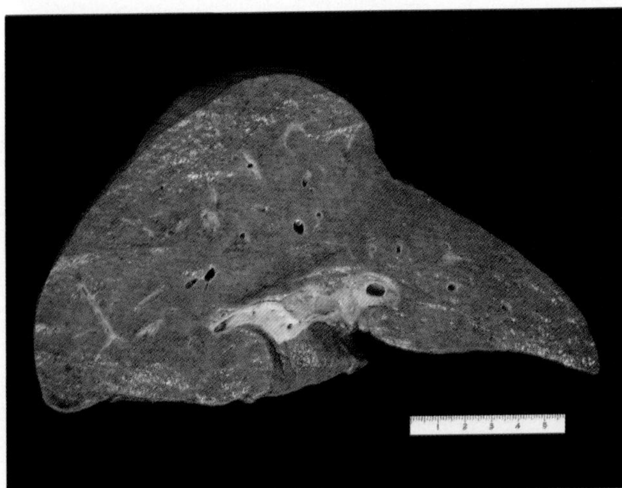

Figure 6.37 Micronodular cirrhosis. Gross appearance of a liver with alcoholic hepatitis-related (Laenec) cirrhosis. Very small nodules (average 1 to 2 mm) are present throughout.

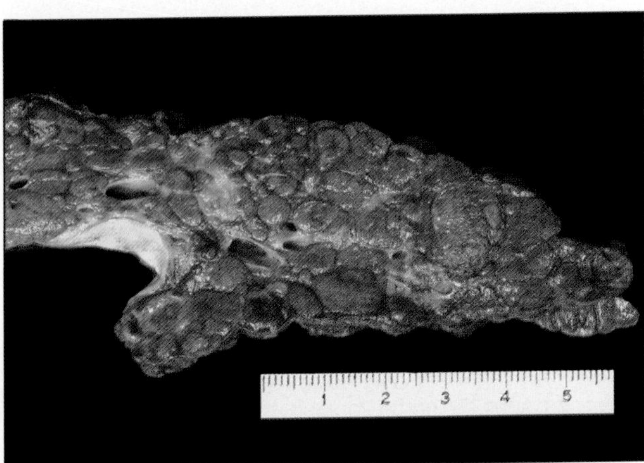

Figure 6.38 Macronodular cirrhosis. A gross image of a case of hepatitis B-related cirrhosis with mostly large nodules. The largest nodule on the right side of the image is a hepatocellular carcinoma.

showed a macronodular pattern. Although reflecting aspects of the pathogenesis of these conditions, this classification has now largely become obsolete with the availability of accurate methods of diagnosing the specific etiology of underlying chronic liver diseases. What remains relevant is the recognition of the fact that micronodular cirrhosis is generally easy to sample properly and to recognize as such on small biopsy samples, whereas macronodular cirrhosis can potentially pose challenges related to staging (along with cases of "incomplete septal cirrhosis"[22] and "partial nodular transformation,"[23] as well as cases of "remodeling" or "resolving" cirrhosis, with nodules measuring up to several centimeters in diameter).

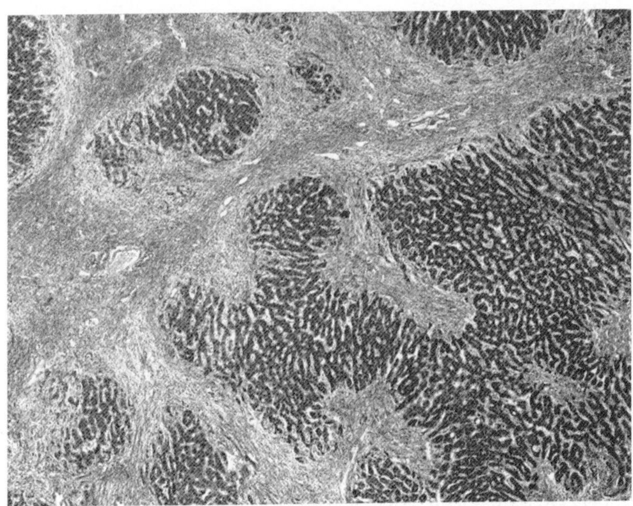

Figure 6.39 Biliary-type fibrosis. Prominent bridging fibrosis with irregular regenerative nodules resembling a jigsaw puzzle pattern.

The "biliary-type" fibrosis (or cirrhosis) is a somewhat distinctive pattern associated with chronic biliary tract diseases of various etiologies (primary biliary cirrhosis, primary sclerosing cholangitis, biliary obstruction, biliary atresia, etc.), in which there is a geographic, or jigsaw puzzle parenchymal configuration to the cirrhotic nodules, rather than distinct, round nodules (Fig. 6.39). The presence of edema, prominent bile ductular reaction, and cholate stasis with feathery degeneration of periportal hepatocytes often imparts a characteristic clear "halo" at the periphery of regenerating nodules—a helpful feature on low power magnification in the recognition of biliary-type cirrhosis.

Finally, certain biliary tract diseases—most commonly cystic fibrosis—can show cirrhosis in a highly heterogeneous pattern, with areas of well-established cirrhosis alternating with regions of mild or no fibrosis (i.e., "focal biliary cirrhosis"). A similar phenomenon can be seen in cases of primary sclerosing cholangitis, particularly those with one or more dominant strictures, whereby the affected segments are significantly more fibrotic.

REFERENCES

1. Rubio-Tapia A, Murray JA. The liver in celiac disease. *Hepatology*. 2007;46(5):1650–1658. doi:10.1002/hep.21949.
2. Mounajjed T, Oxentenko A, Shmidt E, et al. The liver in celiac disease: clinical manifestations, histologic features, and response to gluten-free diet in 30 patients. *Am J Clin Pathol*. 2011; 136(1):128–137. doi:10.1309/AJCPDOMY5RI5TPMN.

3. Daniels JA, Torbenson M, Vivekanandan P, et al. Hepatitis in common variable immunodeficiency. *Hum Pathol.* 2009;40(4):484–488. doi:10.1016/j.humpath.2008.09.008.
4. Stine JG, Northup PG. Autoimmune-like drug-induced liver injury: a review and update for the clinician. *Expert Opin Drug Metab Toxicol.* 2016;12(11):1–11. doi:10.1080/17425255.2016.1211110.
5. Potenza L, Luppi M, Barozzi P, et al. HHV-6A in syncytial giant-cell hepatitis. *N Engl J Med.* 2008;359(6):593–602. doi:10.1056/NEJMoa074479.
6. Welte S, Gagesch M, Weber A, et al. Fulminant liver failure in Wilson's disease with histologic features of postinfantile giant cell hepatitis; cytomegalovirus as the trigger for both? *Eur J Gastroenterol Hepatol.* 2012;24(3):328–331. doi:10.1097/MEG.0b013e3283506843.
7. Harmanci O, Onal IK, Ersoy O, et al. Postinfantile giant cell hepatitis due to hepatitis E virus along with the presence of autoantibodies. *Dig Dis Sci.* 2007;52(12):3521–3523. doi:10.1007/s10620-006-9698-8.
8. Lau JY, Koukoulis G, Mieli-Vergani G, et al. Syncytial giant-cell hepatitis--a specific disease entity? *J Hepatol.* 1992;15(1–2):216–219. http://www.ncbi.nlm.nih.gov/pubmed/1506641. Accessed July 23, 2016.
9. Krasinskas AM, Demetris AJ, Poterucha JJ, et al. The prevalence and natural history of untreated isolated central perivenulitis in adult allograft livers. *Liver Transpl.* 2008;14(5):625–632. doi:10.1002/lt.21404.
10. Neuschwander-Tetri B, Caldwell SH. Nonalcoholic steatohepatitis: summary of an AASLD Single Topic Conference. *Hepatology.* 2003;37(5):1202–1219. doi:10.1053/jhep.2003.50193.
11. Matteoni C, Younossi Z, Gramlich T, et al. Nonalcoholic fatty liver disease: a spectrum of clinical and pathological severity. *Gastroenterology.* 1999;116(6):1413–1419. doi:10.1016/S0016-5085(99)70506-8.
12. Gramlich T, Kleiner DE, McCullough AJ, et al. Pathologic features associated with fibrosis in nonalcoholic fatty liver disease. *Hum Pathol.* 2004;35(2):196–199. doi:10.1016/j.humpath.2003.09.018.
13. Yeh MM, Belt P, Brunt EM, et al. Acidophil bodies in nonalcoholic steatohepatitis. *Hum Pathol.* 2016;52:28–37. doi:10.1016/j.humpath.2016.01.001.
14. Raja K, Thung SN, Fiel MI, et al. Drug-induced steatohepatitis leading to cirrhosis: long-term toxicity of amiodarone use. *Semin Liver Dis.* 2009;29(4):423–428. doi:10.1055/s-0029-1240011.
15. Ala A, Walker AP, Ashkan K, et al. Wilson's disease. *Lancet.* 2007;369(9559):397–408. doi:10.1016/S0140-6736(07)60196-2.
16. Li MK, Crawford JM. The pathology of cholestasis. *Semin Liver Dis.* 2004;24(1):21–42. doi:10.1055/s-2004-823099.
17. Crawford AR, Lin X-ZZ, Crawford JM. The normal adult human liver biopsy: a quantitative reference standard. *Hepatology.* 1998;28(2):323–331. doi:10.1002/hep.510280206.
18. Moreira RK, Chopp W, Washington MK. The concept of hepatic artery-bile duct parallelism in the diagnosis of ductopenia in liver biopsy samples. *Am J Surg Pathol.* 2011;35(3):392–403. doi:10.1097/PAS.0b013e3182082ef6.
19. Kakar S, Batts KP, Poterucha JJ, et al. Histologic changes mimicking biliary disease in liver biopsies with venous outflow impairment. *Mod Pathol.* 2004;17(7):874–878. doi:10.1038/modpathol.3800073.
20. Pai RK, Hart JA. Aberrant expression of cytokeratin 7 in perivenular hepatocytes correlates with a cholestatic chemistry profile in patients with heart failure. *Mod Pathol.* 2010;23(12):1650–1656. doi:10.1038/modpathol.2010.175.
21. Klatt EC, Koss MN, Young TS, et al. Hepatic hyaline globules associated with passive congestion. *Arch Pathol Lab Med.* 1988;112(5):510–513. http://www.ncbi.nlm.nih.gov/pubmed/2451899. Accessed July 31, 2016.
22. Sciot R, Staessen D, Van Damme B, et al. Incomplete septal cirrhosis: histopathological aspects. *Histopathology.* 1988;13(6):593–603. http://www.ncbi.nlm.nih.gov/pubmed/2466750. Accessed July 18, 2016.
23. Wanless IR, Lentz JS, Roberts EA. Partial nodular transformation of liver in an adult with persistent ductus venosus. Review with hypothesis on pathogenesis. *Arch Pathol Lab Med.* 1985;109(5):427–432. http://www.ncbi.nlm.nih.gov/pubmed/3838656. Accessed July 18, 2016.

7 The almost normal liver biopsy

Michael S. Torbenson, MD

7.1 OVERVIEW

Liver biopsies can sometimes be almost normal on histological examination, even when performed for clinical indication. The clinical indication is typically abnormal liver enzyme elevations, but can be other laboratory abnormalities, such as elevated ammonia levels. Unexplained clinical findings or abnormal hepatic imaging can also prompt biopsy, such as ascites, hepatomegaly, or fevers of unknown origin. Generating a diagnosis and a differential can be very challenging when these biopsies appear almost normal on hematoxylin and eosin stain (H&E), or have minimal nonspecific changes. When minimal inflammation is the only finding, the differential is so long that it is essentially meaningless. However, these cases sometimes have subtle changes that can lead to a more specific diagnosis.

A specific diagnosis is most likely to be identified when using a disciplined, systematic approach. One approach is shown in Table 7.1, where the biopsy is systematically analyzed for subtle changes. Because the changes can be subtle, many cases benefit from being set aside and reexamined for clues a second time later that day or the next day. Additional H&E recuts can also help.

A broad differential for the almost normal liver biopsy is shown in Table 7.2. These entities are discussed in more detail in the relevant sections of this book, but this table provides a useful compilation of possible diagnoses when the biopsy looks almost normal. These entities are also briefly discussed in the next section. Following that, the differential for cryptogenic cirrhosis is briefly considered. Finally, the differential is discussed for the almost normal, nonfibrotic liver when all of the other potential causes discussed in this chapter have been carefully excluded.

In cases where no specific diagnosis is evident, the histological findings can still be valuable when they help clinicians to rule out specific clinical concerns; for example, autoimmune hepatitis in the setting of positive autoimmune markers or ruling out cirrhosis as the cause of portal hypertension.

7.2 CLINICAL HISTORY

Achieving a meaningful diagnosis in an almost normal liver biopsy depends heavily on integrating the clinical findings, laboratory

Table 7.1 Approach to the almost normal liver biopsy

Questions	Comments
What clinical finding prompted the biopsy?	The clinical findings can provide critical clues that can help guide histology evaluation. This information is often not provided to the pathologists; it can be well worth the extra effort and phone calls to get it
What are the imaging findings?	Hepatomegaly? Vascular flow changes? Steatosis? Different imaging findings can help when evaluating liver biopsies
What are the lab tests?	What do the predominant enzyme patterns suggest?
Are the bile ducts normal?	Rule out ductopenia, subtle duct proliferation
Are the portal veins normal?	Rule out portal vein atrophy, loss, muscularization
Are the hepatic arteries normal?	Rule out amyloid
Are the hepatocytes normal?	Rule out inclusions, apoptosis, endoplasmic reticulum proliferation
Are the sinusoids normal?	Rule out amyloid, light chain deposition disease, diabetic sclerosis, stellate cell hyperplasia, Kupffer cell hyperplasia, abnormal cell infiltrates
Are the central veins normal?	Rule out veno-occlusive disease

Table 7.2 The differential for an almost normal liver biopsy includes these conditions

Diagnoses	Major findings
α-1-antitrypsin deficiency	Zone 1 hepatocytes with cytoplasmic globules—in infants and children, the globules may not be evident
Amyloid	Acellular deposits in sinusoids or vessels
Celiac disease	Mild nonspecific inflammatory changes
Crohn's disease of the small bowel	Mild nonspecific inflammatory changes
Cystic fibrosis	Patchy areas of bile ductular proliferation and fibrosis. May also see nodular regenerative hyperplasia
Drug effect	Some can show minimal nonspecific inflammatory and reactive changes
Ferroportin disease	Moderate iron deposits, Kupffer cells >> hepatocytes, in a person with elevated ferritin but low transferrin saturation levels
Glycogenic hepatopathy	Big pale hepatocytes cells in a person with poorly controlled diabetes
Glycogen psuedoground glass inclusions	Large amphophilic hepatocyte inclusions in immunosuppressed patients on many medications
Hemochromatosis	Hepatocellular iron accumulation
Hepatoportal sclerosis	Loss or atrophy of portal veins, often accompanied by nodular regenerative hyperplasia
Hypervitaminosis A	Stellate cell hyperplasia
Ischemia, low grade	Scattered apoptotic cells in the lobules
Light chain deposition disease	Sinusoids lined by irregularly thickened deposits that can mimic pericellular fibrosis

(continued)

Table 7.2 The differential for an almost normal liver biopsy includes these conditions (*continued*)

Diagnoses	Major findings
Mitochondrial injury	Microvesicular steatosis
Nodular regenerative hyperplasia	Distinct nodularity to the liver parenchyma but without fibrosis; best seen on low-power magnification
Sickle cell hepatopathy	Dilated sinusoids, sickled red blood cells, Kupffer cell iron
Small bowel bacterial overgrowth	Mild nonspecific inflammatory changes
Thyroid disease	Mild cholestasis with hyperthyroidism Fatty change (may be minimal) with hypothyroidism
Urea cycle defects	Affects all ages; can range from essentially normal to mild changes including fat and glycogenosis
Wilson's disease	Mild fatty change with glycogenated nuclei

findings, and histology findings. Important clinical information includes the use of medications, vitamins, and other herbal supplements. Histories of systemic illnesses are also very important, as many can involve the liver (discussed in more detail in Chapter 19). Family histories of unexplained liver disease in siblings or parents can be important clues. Some of the key aspects of integrating the liver enzyme patterns into the histology evaluation are discussed below. In addition, imaging studies of the liver are often performed prior to the biopsy and can help solidify the diagnosis in some cases. Vascular flow changes can be particularly subtle to diagnosis on histology, and the imaging can provide helpful corroboration.

In some difficult cases, the diagnosis is only evident after an iterative process. First, the histology findings are discussed with the hepatologist/clinician and with the radiologist. Next, each of these three groups of experts then take the information obtained from the discussions and go back and reexamine the patient, the histology, and the radiology. A subsequent joint discussion can then often bring the proper diagnosis into focus or suggest further lines of investigation. This process is the most effective method for making the best diagnosis in the most difficult cases. Unfortunately, time pressures and other complexities in the practice of modern medicine make this very challenging to do on a routine basis. That being said, there is no substitute as effective as this iterative process in resolving the most challenging cases.

7.3 CLUES IN THE LIVER ENZYMES

Alkaline phosphatase

A predominately alkaline phosphatase elevation (compared to aspartate transaminase (AST) and alanine transaminase (ALT)) is most commonly seen in the setting of biliary tract disease. In this situation, AST and ALT levels are also commonly above normal, but typically less than 5× the upper limit of normal. Examine the biopsy carefully for evidence of bile duct injury, including bile ductular proliferation and ductopenia. The differential for a predominant elevation in the alkaline phosphatase levels also includes granulomatous disease, nodular regenerative hyperplasia, chronic venous outflow impairment, and sinusoidal infiltrative processes. A subset of patients with nonalcoholic fatty liver disease can also present with isolated alkaline phosphatase elevations, particularly older aged women.[1] The histology findings in these cases can range from minimal steatosis to active steatohepatitis with cirrhosis.

Don't forget that there are nonhepatic causes for alkaline phosphatase elevations (Table 7.3); these possibilities should be considered more strongly if the liver is negative after full histological evaluation. Serum γ-glutamyltransferase levels can also be helpful, as they are elevated with liver disease but not in the conditions listed in Table 7.3.

Low levels of alkaline phosphatase are only rarely encountered, but the differential includes Wilson disease, generalized malnutrition, and hypothyroidism.[2]

Table 7.3 Nonhepatic causes of persistent elevations in serum alkaline phosphatase levels

Causes
Bone disease
Renal failure
Heart failure
Malignancy (e.g., lymphoma)
Parathyroid disease
Thyroid disease
Pregnancy

AST and ALT

Predominate elevations in the AST and ALT (compared to alkaline phosphatase) usually indicate a hepatitis injury pattern or a direct toxin exposure. In many cases of inflammatory hepatitis, such as viral hepatitis, the AST is less elevated than the ALT. In contrast, as we all learned in medical school, the AST is often 2× or greater than the ALT in alcohol-related liver disease. However, this observation is most useful as an exam question for medical students, as the clinical reality is much more complicated, with many exceptions,[3] including alcoholic hepatitis that does not show this AST:ALT relationship, as well as non–alcohol-related diseases that do.

Isolated hyperammonemia

Isolated elevations in serum ammonia are seen primarily with urea cycle defects[4] or with drug effects, in particular valproate.[5] The biopsies can look normal or have mild and nonspecific changes (Fig. 7.1). In the transplant setting, isolated hyperammonemia can result from anastomotic strictures of the portal or hepatic veins or with a patent portosystemic shunt.[6] Many of the transplant patients in this setting also have ascites from the anastomotic strictures.

7.4 PORTAL TRACT CHANGES

Bile duct changes

The biopsy should be examined for bile duct changes, including ductopenia, cholangitis, periductal fibrosis, duct duplication, or ductular proliferation. In all of these settings, the alkaline phosphatase should be elevated. The most commonly used definition for

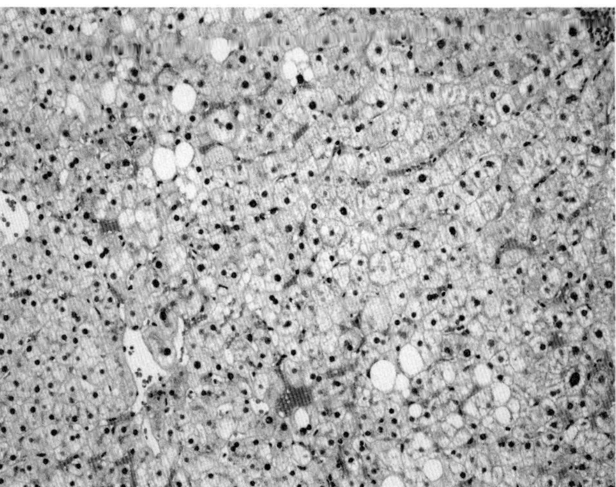

Figure 7.1 Almost normal biopsy, isolated hyperammoniemia. This biopsy is from a patient taking valproic acid. There was very focal fatty change and rare foci of lobular inflammation, but the biopsy was otherwise normal.

ductopenia is loss of 50% or more of the bile ducts. Immunostains such as CK7 or CK19 can highlight both bile duct loss and/or subtle bile ductular proliferation. Copper stains may also be useful if a biliary disease is in consideration.

Portal vein changes

Portal vein changes can be subtle, but can include portal vein muscularization (Fig. 7.2), thrombosis (Fig. 7.2), portal vein herniation (Fig. 7.3), and portal vein atrophy or loss. There is no well-established cutoff for determining portal vein loss, but the changes should be convincing and reasonably diffuse to be diagnostically useful. Portal vein atrophy is even more

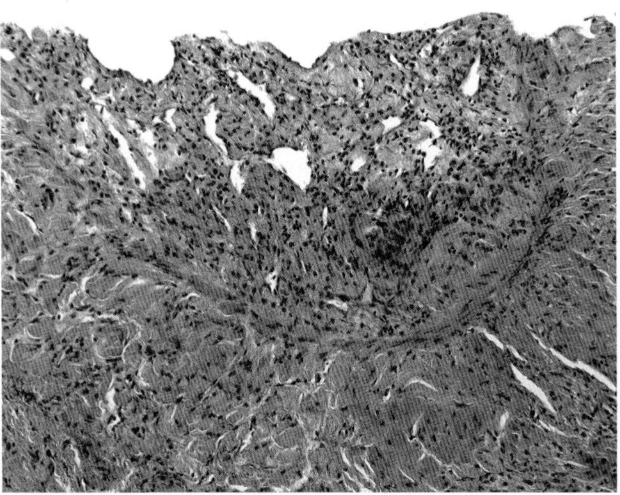

Figure 7.2 Portal vein thrombosis. The portal vein is thrombosed. In response, the portal vein wall had developed striking muscularization.

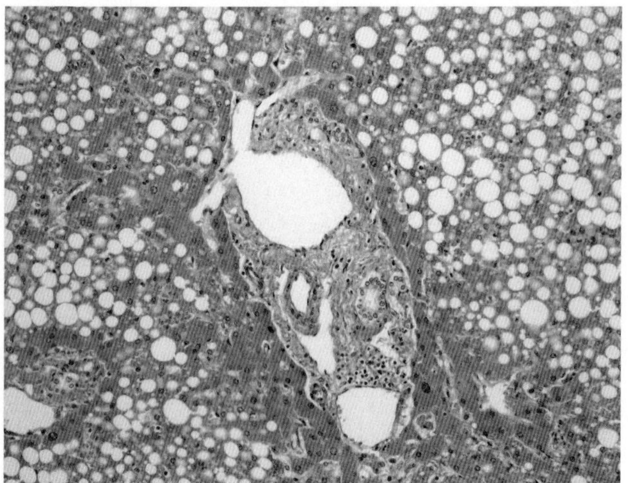

Figure 7.3 Portal vein herniation. In this case of portal vein thrombosis, the portal vein appears to herniate out of the portal tract into the adjacent parenchyma.

challenging to confidently diagnose in the early stages. When most of the portal veins are clearly smaller than normal, this diagnosis should be considered. In many cases with portal vein abnormalities, the lobules will show nodular regenerative hyperplasia-like changes.

Hepatic artery changes

Hepatic artery changes in the nontransplant setting can be very subtle. Look carefully for amyloid, as some types of familial amyloid can have a predominately arterial pattern of amyloid deposition (Fig. 7.4). Hepatic artery arteriolosclerosis can be seen in the setting of hypertension and/or diabetes,[7] particularly in the elderly, but usually this is an incidental finding (Fig. 7.5).

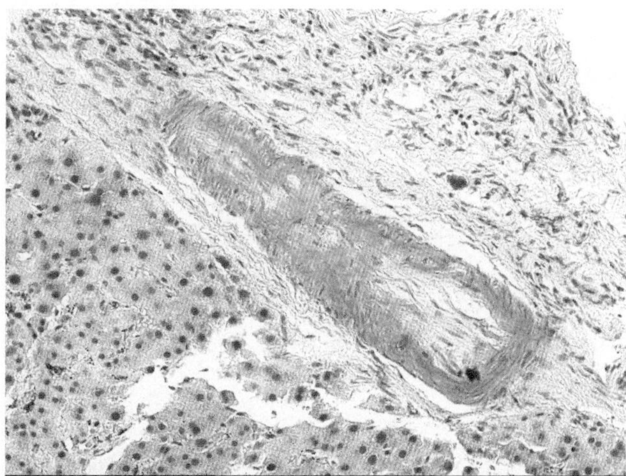

Figure 7.4 Familial amyloidosis, Congo red stain. The biopsy was essentially normal on H&E, but a Congo red stain showed amyloid deposition limited to the hepatic arteries.

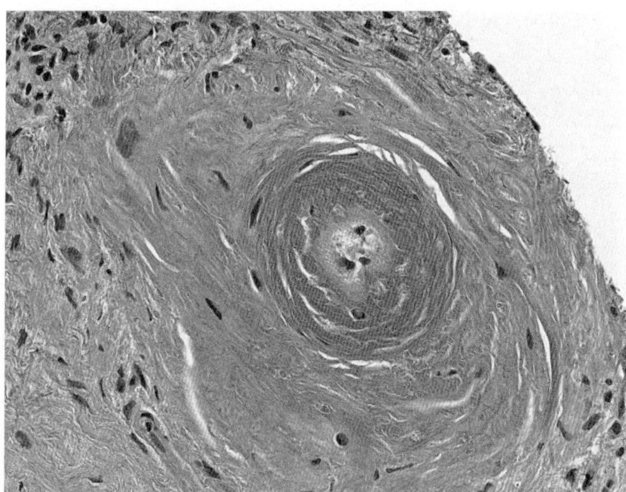

Figure 7.5 Hepatic artery, hypertensive changes. The walls are thickened and hyalinized.

7.5 HEPATOCYTE CHANGES

The hepatocytes should be examined carefully in the almost normal liver biopsy for any changes, even if the changes are mild and patchy. Hepatocyte changes generally fall into the category of either subtly increased apoptosis or abnormal cytoplasmic changes. A subtle increase in apoptosis, without significant inflammation or cholestasis, usually results from a mild drug effect, early acute viral hepatitis, or low-grade or transient ischemia.

Increased hepatocyte apoptosis is almost invariably accompanied by increased hepatocyte proliferation, which can be highlighted by a Ki-67 immunostain. In this regard, a Ki-67 stain can show active regeneration even if apoptotic bodies are sparse or subtle, serving as an excellent screen for a recent or ongoing liver injury that has led to active hepatocyte regeneration. The opposite is also true: a Ki-67 immunostain can help identify impaired liver regeneration, when there is active hepatocyte injury, but little or no regeneration.

Abnormal cytoplasmic changes include the presence of globules, such as those seen with α-1-antitrypsin deficiency, megamitochondria, ground glass changes, pseudground glass changes, glycogenosis, microvesicular steatosis, cholestasis, or other pigment accumulation.

Eosinophilic globules

The globules of α-1-antitrypsin deficiency are typically in zone 1 hepatocytes. Not all hepatocytes will have globules, but those that do will have multiple globules. The globules can be highlighted by a PASD stain or by an immunostain.

Prominent megamitochondria are most commonly seen in the setting of fatty liver disease or with cholestatic liver disease, in which case they are considered to be part of the ordinary disease pattern and are ignored. However, in rare biopsies the only significant finding is that of prominent hepatocyte megamitochondria. In adults, this findings can be associated with drug effects, though usually the biopsy will also have other findings to point to a possible drug reaction, such as mild inflammatory changes.[8] In children, prominent megamitochondria can be seen as one of the earliest changes in several different metabolic diseases, including inherited mitochondrial defects, various urea cycle defects, or with other inherited metabolic defects, such as lysinergic protein intolerance (Fig. 7.6) or hypermethioninemia.[9]

Ground glass and related changes

Ground glass changes refer to large amphophilic inclusions found in the hepatocyte cytoplasm (Fig. 7.7). The most common causes by far are chronic hepatitis B and drug effects, but there is a longer differential that includes rare genetic conditions, such as glycogen storage disease type IV. The differential for ground glass change is discussed in more detail in the drug effect and other relevant chapters. Globular amyloid (Fig. 7.8) can also show somewhat similar changes, with subtle inclusions in the hepatocyte cytoplasm. The inclusions are positive on Congo red stains and on LECT2 immunostains.[10]

Some drugs lead to proliferation of the smooth endoplasmic reticulin, resulting in a distinctive amphophilic change to the hepatocyte cytoplasm, called induced hepatocytes (Fig. 7.9). In contrast to glycogen pseudoground inclusions, induced hepatocytes do not have well-defined inclusions. The cytoplasmic

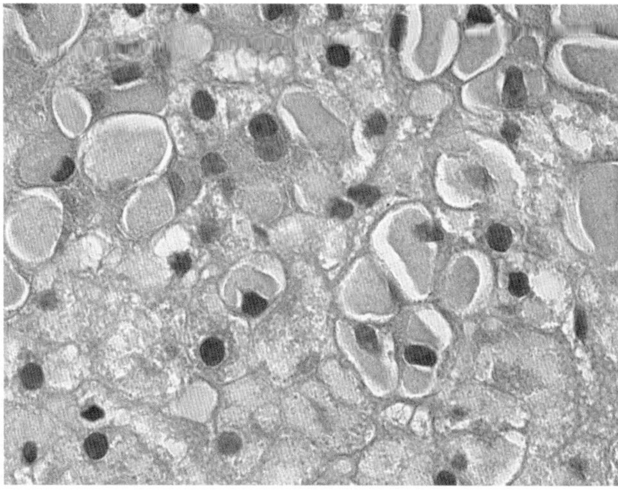

Figure 7.7 Pseudoground glass change. The hepatocytes have distinct round amphophilic inclusions. HBV testing was negative, and these changes represent a drug effect.

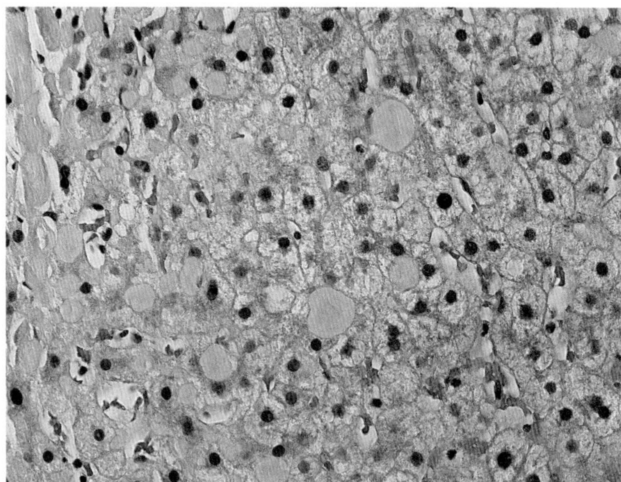

Figure 7.8 Globular amyloid. Subtle hepatocyte inclusions are seen.

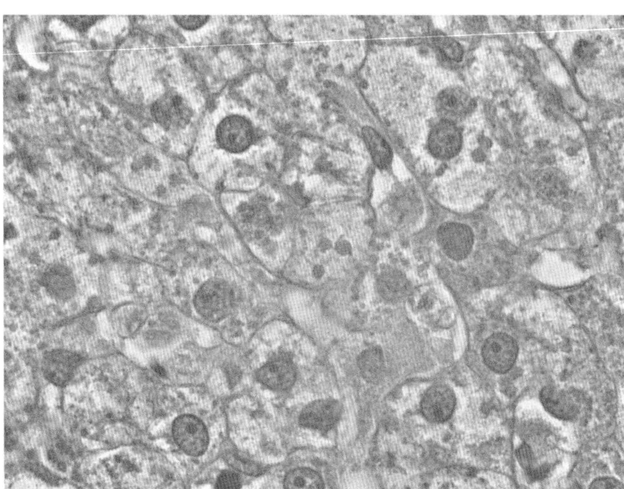

Figure 7.6 Megamitochondria, lysinergic protein intolerance. This biopsy showed mild lobular disarray and prominent megamitochondria.

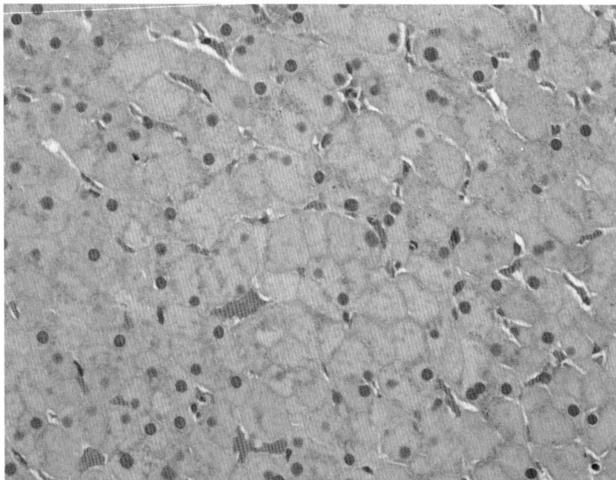

Figure 7.9 Smooth ER proliferation. The patient was on phenobarbital and the hepatocytes show a distinctive cytoplasmic change that represents smooth endoplasmic reticulum proliferation.

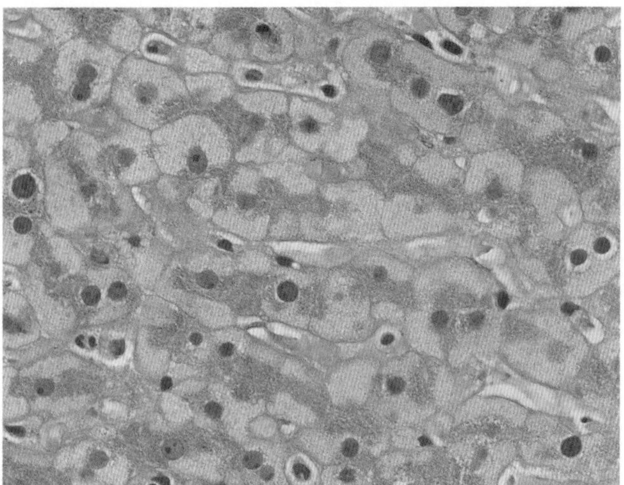

Figure 7.10 Two-tone hepatocytes. In this case, the induced hepatocytes have a distinctive "two-tone appearance."

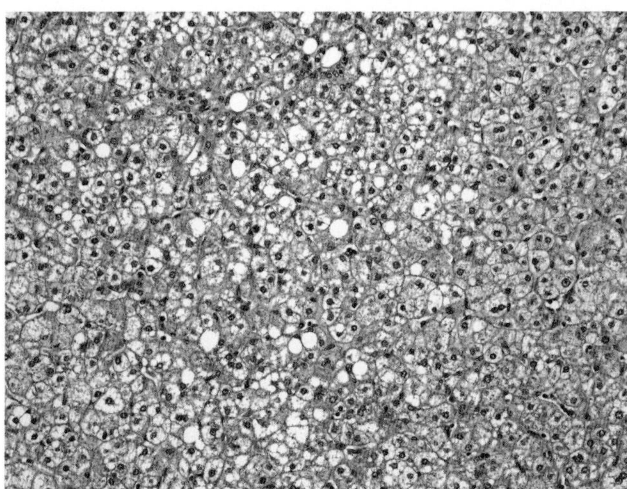

Figure 7.12 Urea cycle defect, ornithine transcarbamylase deficiency. The biopsy showed subtle hepatocyte glycogen accumulation and very mild fatty change.

change can be diffuse or affect only a portion of the cytoplasm, giving the hepatocytes a distinctive "two-toned" appearance (Fig. 7.10).

Glycogen accumulation

Glycogenic hepatopathy is often quite striking, as the hepatocytes throughout the biopsy are swollen and clear, filled with glycogen (Fig. 7.11). However, in some cases the findings can be more subtle, only being identified after thinking to look for it. The most common cause of glycogenic hepatopathy is poorly controlled blood sugar levels, usually in the setting of type I diabetes mellitus. Glycogenic hepatopathy is discussed in more detail in the chapters on drug reactions and systemic diseases involving the liver. Subtle glycogen accumulation in the hepatocytes can also be seen in various urea cycle defects, where liver biopsies can look essentially normal, other than for the subtle glycogen accumulation and often minimal steatosis (Fig. 7.12). Prednisone can also lead to glycogen accumulation, especially after pulse steroids.

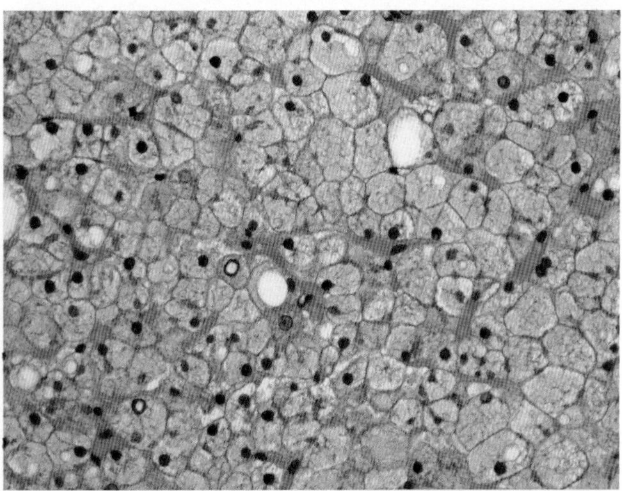

Figure 7.11 Glycogenic hepatopathy. The hepatocytes are diffusely enlarged, filled with glycogen.

Microvesicular steatosis

Microvesicular steatosis can be subtle, with the biopsy looking almost normal at low and medium power. Microvesicular steatosis results from mitochondrial injuries of various sorts, ranging from drug effects to inherited diseases, to a rare complication of pregnancy. The cytoplasm is filled with tiny vacuoles, often just at the resolution of light microscopy. Also commonly present are rare scattered fat droplets of intermediate or larger size.

Cholestasis

Some almost normal liver biopsies can show minimal lobular cholestasis with no inflammation and no evidence for obstructive biliary tract disease. This subtle pattern of injury is most commonly seen with drug reactions, but there is a longer differential (Table 7.4). In some cases, the changes can be sufficiently mild to leave you uncertain as to whether the pigment is bile or lipofuscin, or mostly lipofuschin with a bit of bile. Checking the serum bilirubin levels is very helpful in this situation. A Hall's bile stain is not very helpful, but if needed the lipofuschin can be stained with glypican 3 or with a Fontana Masson. Copper and CK7 stains can also be helpful, looking for periportal copper deposition in hepatocytes and intermediate hepatocytes, respectively.

Table 7.4 Causes of minimal bland lobular cholestasis without ductopenia, obstructive changes, or significant hepatitis

Causes
Benign recurring intrahepatic cholestasis
Drug effect
Hypothyroid disease
Hyperthyroid disease
Intrahepatic cholestasis of pregnancy
Paraneoplastic syndrome
Sepsis

7.6 LOBULAR INJURY PATTERNS

The resolving hepatitis pattern

In this pattern, the biopsy shows little or no inflammation, but there are scattered clusters of macrophages (Fig. 7.13), which are often pigmented, located in the lobules and portal tracts. The scattered clusters of pigmented macrophages represent foci of prior hepatocyte injury and death. A Ki-67 often shows a mild increase in proliferation (normal quiescent liver <1%). This pattern of injury is most commonly seen with an idiosyncratic drug reaction, when the offending agent is stopped some days to weeks before the liver biopsy is performed. The differential also includes acute self-limited viral hepatitis.

Lobular disarray

Lobular disarray refers to the loss of the normal, largely parallel organization of hepatocytes. Instead of lining up in thin parallel trabecula, the hepatocytes have more irregular nuclear spacing, and the trabeculae are more variable in width. There can also be mild nuclear pleomorphism in the hepatocytes. Lobular disarray results from injury and regeneration and is present in all sorts of liver injuries. However, sometimes the biopsy shows only isolated lobular disarray, with no other clear pattern of injury, including no significant inflammation, no fatty change, no cholestatic injury, and no vascular flow changes. In some cases, mild lobular disarray can co-occur with the resolving hepatitis pattern, and overall tends to have the same differential of resolving drug effect or acute self-limited viral infection.

The broader differential for isolated lobular disarray also includes low-grade chronic ischemia. In clinical practice, low-grade chronic ischemia is very rare but can be seen with significant vascular compromise. Finally, the hyperviscosity syndromes can also show lobular disarray as the main pattern of injury (Fig. 7.14). This syndrome rarely prompts a liver biopsy, as the patient's systemic disease is typically known, but the hyperviscosity syndrome can be seen with multiple myeloma, Waldentrom's macroglobulinemia, and polycythemia vera. In additional to hematopathology abnormalities, the hyperviscosity syndrome can be seen with various autoimmune diseases, including Sjögren's syndrome, systemic lupus erythematosus, and rheumatoid arthritis.

Figure 7.13 Resolving hepatitis pattern. The lobules shows rare small clusters of macrophages and lymphocytes.

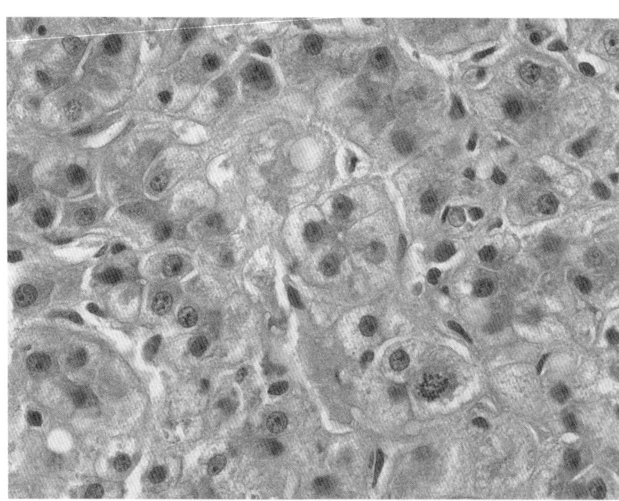

Figure 7.14 Hyperviscosity syndrome. The hepatocytes show lobular disarray with no inflammation, fatty change, or cholestasis.

7.7 SINUSOIDAL CHANGES

Sinusoidal dilation and congestion is an important clue to vascular outflow abnormalities, but is usually easy to see and the biopsy is usually not "almost normal" However, in other cases the sinusoidal dilatation is subtle and downright equivocal, especially when you show it your colleague, the one who seems enjoy disagreeing with you. Two findings can increase the likelihood that the changes are real: any zone 3 pericellular fibrosis, or convincing zone 3 hepatocyte atrophy. Of these, finding convincing hepatocyte atrophy is most often helpful. Of course, when the changes are equivocal, it is best to indicate that in the pathology report too.

Vascular outflow disease is the most common cause of sinusoidal dilation, but the differential is actually much longer and includes systemic inflammatory diseases, infectious granulomatous diseases, autoimmune diseases, and paraneoplastic effects from carcinomas in other organs.[11,12] Two of the more common autoimmune conditions associated with mild sinusoidal dilatation are the antiphospholipid syndrome[13] and rheumatoid arthritis.[14] Also of note, rapid blood volume expansion can lead to sinusoidal dilatation.

Nodular regenerative hyperplasia is most commonly seen with vascular flow abnormalities. In some cases, there is obvious parenchymal nodularity without fibrosis (Fig. 7.15), but in other cases this injury pattern is best appreciated with the help of a reticulin stain (Fig. 7.16). Other subtle changes in the sinusoids include Kupffer cell hyperplasia, sometimes with hemophagocytosis. This reactive finding is usually related to drug reactions or to viral infection, in particular cytomegalovirus (CMV) or Epstein–Barr virus (EBV), and can involve the liver even if the infection does not. Stellate cell hyperplasia (Ito cell hyperplasia) is very subtle and should also be searched for carefully (Fig. 7.17). Most cases result from herbal or vitamin supplements. Finally, amyloid deposition and light chain deposition disease can also be subtle and easily overlooked on H&E stains, but tend to be more evident on trichrome stains and confirmed on Congo red stains.

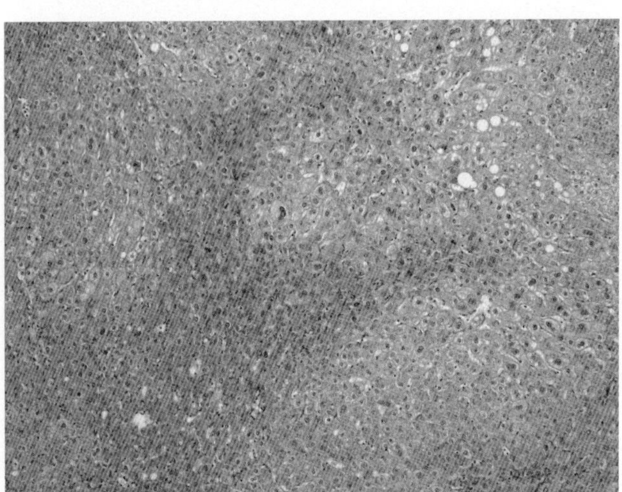

Figure 7.15 Nodular regenerative hyperplasia. In this case, the changes of nodular regenerative hyperplasia are not very subtle.

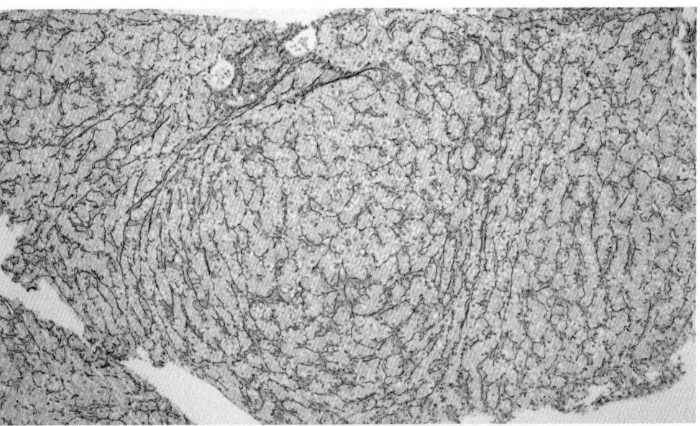

Figure 7.16 Nodular regenerative hyperplasia, reticulin stain. In this case, the H&E findings were essentially normal, but the reticulin stain brought out subtle changes of nodular regenerative hyperplasia.

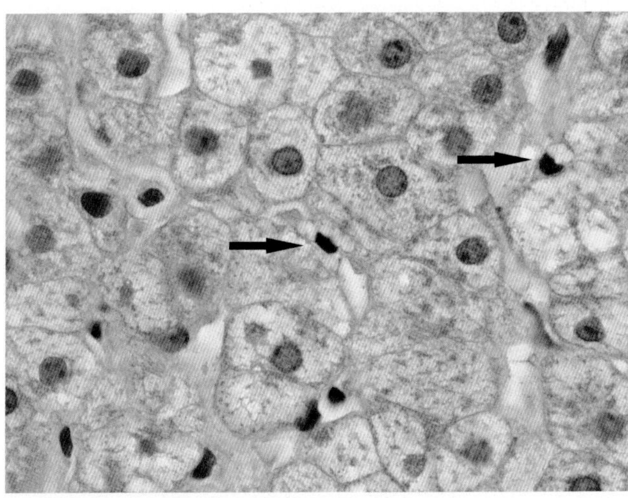

Figure 7.17 Stellate cell (Ito cell) hyperplasia. The sinusoids show small cells with numerous cytoplasmic vacuoles, some indenting the stellate cell nuclei (*arrows*).

7.8 CRYPTOGENIC FIBROSIS/ CIRRHOSIS

In some cases, liver biopsies are obtained because of unexplained chronic elevations in liver enzymes, but the only significant finding is advanced fibrosis or cirrhosis. For most of these biopsies, you won't be diagnosing a specific etiology no matter what approach you use, but in this section we will consider a reasonable approach that optimizes your chance of being useful and, in some cases, brilliant.

First, get the best history and all of the laboratory test results reasonably available. This step is really important. The patient's age can also provide some broad guidance. Advanced fibrosis in infants or toddlers suggests a genetic disorder. Overall, biliary atresia is one of the most common causes of cirrhosis in this age group, but there are many other causes (Table 7.5). Older children and teenagers can also have cirrhosis from chronic inflammatory conditions of the liver, such as autoimmune hepatitis, fatty liver disease, and chronic viral hepatitis. For example, in one study 20% of pediatric age individuals with autoimmune hepatitis had cirrhosis at presentation.[15] Cirrhosis in adults can result from genetic or acquired conditions, but most commonly result from acquired conditions.

If serological testing to rule out viral hepatitis or autoimmune hepatitis has not been performed, then testing can be suggested in the pathology report. If hepatitis C virus (HCV) antibodies or HBcAb antibodies are positive, but there are no viral nucleic acids in the blood and no HBsAg (for hepatitis B virus, HBV), then the differential includes resolved chronic hepatitis C or hepatitis B. Overall, the vast majority of cases of resolved chronic viral hepatitis are never biopsied because the infection was known and clinically treated. However, spontaneous viral clearance can occur. In either case, the liver enzymes can remain mildly elevated for several years after viral clearance. If the individual comes to medical attention during this time, the chronic enzyme elevations can prompt biopsy. The biopsies in this setting typically show minimal to mild nonspecific inflammatory changes. Also of note, a subset of individuals with clinically resolved hepatitis B can have very low levels of persistent viral DNA in their liver, despite the lack of viral DNA in the blood, a finding called occult hepatitis B.[16] Immunosuppression can reactivate the infection and the patient can present with a sudden flare of liver enzymes.

Many individuals with cryptogenic cirrhosis also have risk factors for the metabolic syndrome, such truncal obesity, insulin resistance, and hypertension. Or there may be a remote history of heavy alcohol use. However, finding mild fat or a rare ballooned hepatocyte in a cirrhotic liver is insufficient to establish an etiology of cirrhosis from either the metabolic syndrome or alcohol use. Instead, a presumptive diagnosis of cirrhosis caused by fatty liver disease should be considered if there is a history of the metabolic syndrome, or remote but heavy alcohol use, and no other clinical or histological findings that suggest a more likely cause.

Table 7.5 Causes of pediatric cirrhosis

Etiology	Comment/reference
Genetic disorders, known genes	
α-1-antitrypsin deficiency	
Cystic fibrosis	
Gaucher's disease	Typical Gaucher cells will be seen
Glycogen storage diseases	Mostly types III, IV, VI, and IX
GLIS3 mutations	Present with neonatal diabetes; can also have thyroid, renal, and liver disease, including cirrhosis [18]
Lysosomal acid lipase deficiency	[19]
Tyrosinemia	
North American Indian childhood cirrhosis	Children of Ojibway-Cree descent. Mutations in the UTP4 gene in some individuals
Peroxismal disorders	[20]
PFIC	Mostly types 2 and 3 [21]
Wilson's disease	
Unknown etiology	
Alagille syndrome	
Biliary atresia	Typically not cryptogenic clinically or histologically
Indian childhood cirrhosis	Marked copper deposition in the liver
Neonatal hemochromatosis	[22]
Other causes	
Autoimmune hepatitis	Usually type 1, can be type 2 [15]
Fatty liver disease	
Chronic viral hepatitis	
Status post-Fontan procedure	
TPN	

A somewhat analogous situation can be seen when a biopsy shows advanced fibrosis with minimal chronic inflammation in the setting of a positive antinuclear antibody (ANA) and/or antismooth muscle antibody

(ASMA) serology and elevated serum immunoglobulin G (IgG) levels. Autoimmune hepatitis can lose the typical inflammatory changes over time, including the plasma cells, leaving behind only scarred liver parenchyma with minimal or mild nonspecific inflammatory changes. This pattern is not specific, but once all other likely causes have been excluded, then a presumptive diagnosis of autoimmune hepatitis can be considered.

Family histories of liver diseases can be helpful when dealing with a biopsy that shows advanced fibrosis alone. In particular, histories of siblings with unexplained advanced fibrosis or histories of parents with unexplained advanced fibrosis suggest an inherited cause. Many of these cases occur in children, but there is a growing recognition that adults can present with diseases historically associated with pediatric presentations (Table 7.6). Some examples include urea cycle defects and mutations in the bile salt transporters, such as PFIC3. The diagnosis of the telomere shortening syndrome should be considered in individuals with both unexplained pulmonary fibrosis and cryptogenic liver cirrhosis.[17] The cirrhosis in these cases is nondescript with little to no inflammation. The cirrhosis also can be incomplete, with some degree of patchiness and with rather thin bands of fibrosis (Fig. 7.18).

Table 7.6 Possible etiologies for adult cryptogenic cirrhosis

Etiology	Comment/reference
"Burned out" chronic liver disease	
Previous steatohepatitis	Can be either alcoholic or nonalcoholic [23]
"Burned out" autoimmune hepatitis	[24, 25]
Resolved chronic viral hepatitis	[26]
Chronic biliary tract disease	[24]
Portal venopathy	[24]
Genetic mutations	
Short telomere syndromes	[27]
Keratin 18 mutations	[28, 29]
ABCB4 mutations	Biliary pattern of cryptogenic cirrhosis [30]
Familial Mediterranean fever	[31]
Apolipoprotein B mutations	[32]

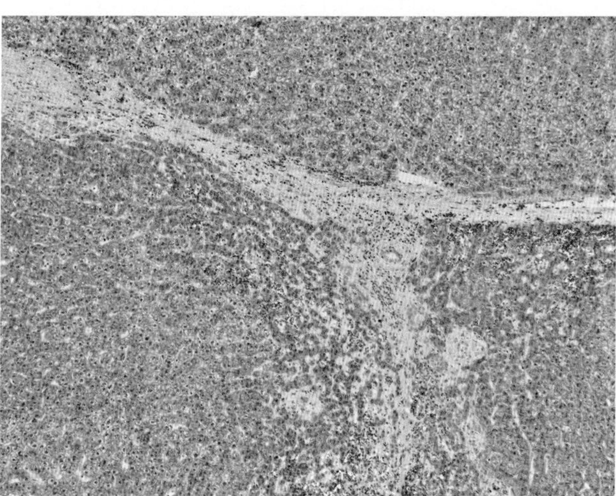

Figure 7.18 Telomere shortening syndrome. This patient presented with idiopathic pulmonary fibrosis and cryptogenic cirrhosis.

Finally, be systematic in your approach to the histology. For example, start in the portal tracts and make sure there is no ductopenia or periductal fibrosis. Make sure the hepatic arteries and the portal veins appear normal. Examine the hepatocytes for cytoplasmic changes or inclusions. Examine the sinusoids for subtle changes, such as can be seen with diabetic sclerosis. On a PASD stain, examine the lobules for the globules of α-1-antitrypsin deficiency. Examine an iron stain for iron accumulation. Mild iron accumulation in the setting of advanced fibrosis is most often a secondary result of impaired hepcidin and does not suggest any specific etiology. Wilson's disease should also be considered in younger individuals with unexplained advanced fibrosis or cirrhosis.

7.9 THE DIFFERENTIAL FOR THE ALMOST NORMAL LIVER BIOPSY

In this final section, the differential is considered for biopsies that are essentially normal after all of the subtle entities discussed above have been excluded. Overall, approximately 5% of biopsies performed for unexplained liver enzyme elevations (excluding protocol biopsies and posttransplant biopsies) have an "almost normal" appearance and fall into this category of having no probable or definite diagnosis, despite a systematic, analytical approach (Table 7.1), including careful correlation with current laboratory and clinical findings.

Although data on this topic is quite limited, approximately 80% of these cases will have been biopsied for mild elevations in liver enzymes and the remaining 20% for unexplained ascites. Almost all of these cases will fall into one of the six categories discussed below.

Category 1. In 15% of cases, the patients will have known systemic autoimmune conditions, such as systemic lupus erythematosus or rheumatoid arthritis. The biopsies can be essentially normal or show trivial inflammatory changes. As such, the minimal inflammation does not support a diagnosis of autoimmune hepatitis, even though the autoimmune serologies can be very striking. Instead, the changes reflect the systemic disease, and more significant liver disease does not develop. In some older pathology text books, the term "nonspecific reactive hepatitis" was used in this setting.

Category 2. In another 10% of cases, a more typical autoimmune hepatitis, primary biliary cirrhosis, or sarcoidosis will develop clinically over the months to years following the liver biopsy. Even when you go back and retrospectively reexamine these cases, there typically are no biopsy findings that could have foretold the subsequent clinical course.

Category 3. Despite the lack of fat in the biopsy, another 10% of cases with no diagnosis are associated with the metabolic syndrome. In fact, imaging studies can also suggest mild fatty liver disease in these cases. Presumably the fatty change was not sampled on the biopsy. However, the imaging studies are not specific, so in the end these cases should be given a prioritized differential and should not be called fatty liver disease if the fatty liver disease is not histologically present. On the other hand, some individuals with the metabolic syndrome truly appear to have no histological fat (as seen in wedge biopsies or autopsies), but do have mild enzyme elevations and show minimal to mild portal and lobular inflammation.

Category 4. Another 5% of "almost normal biopsies" are seen in the setting of chronic inflammatory conditions of the gut, usually the small intestine. In some cases, the inflammatory disease of the gut is not diagnosed for some time after the liver biopsy. Examples of these intestinal conditions include celiac disease, Crohn's disease, and common variable immunodeficiency.

Category 5. Approximately 1% of the almost normal liver biopsies are seen in the setting of low-grade hepatic ischemia, where the degree of ischemia is insufficient to cause the typical ischemic injury patterns in the liver, and instead causes only mild nonspecific changes on biopsy. In these cases, the eventual diagnosis is made on imaging of the hepatic vasculature.

Category 6. The remaining 50% of essentially normal liver biopsies do not fall into any of the above categories and the enzyme elevations remain unexplained. In these cases where no cause is identified at the time of biopsy or in the subsequent clinical course, the hepatic enzymes self-normalize in about half of cases and remain persistently but mildly elevated in the remaining half of cases.

REFERENCES

1. Pantsari MW, Harrison SA. Nonalcoholic fatty liver disease presenting with an isolated elevated alkaline phosphatase. *J Clin Gastroenterol.* 2006;40(7):633–635.
2. Siddique A, Kowdley KV. Approach to a patient with elevated serum alkaline phosphatase. *Clin Liver Dis.* 2012;16(2):199–229.
3. Botros M, Sikaris KA. The de ritis ratio: the test of time. *Clin Biochem Rev.* 2013;34(3):117–130.
4. Açikalin A, Disel NR. A rare cause of postpartum coma: isolated hyperammonemia due to urea cycle disorder. *Am J Emerg Med.* 2016;34(9):1894.
5. Wadzinski J, Franks R, Roane D, et al. Valproate-associated hyperammonemic encephalopathy. *J Am Board Fam Med.* 2007;20(5):499–502.
6. Belenky A, Igov I, Konstantino Y, et al. Endovascular diagnosis and intervention in patients with isolated hyperammonemia, with or without ascites, after liver transplantation. *J Vasc Interv Radiol.* 2009;20(2):259–263.
7. Balakrishnan M, Garcia-Tsao G, Deng Y, et al. Hepatic arteriolosclerosis: a small vessel complication of diabetes and hypertension. *Am J Surg Pathol.* 2015;39(7):1000
8. Itoh S, Yamaba Y, Matsuo S, et al. Sodium valproate-induced liver injury. *Am J Gastroenterol.* 1982;77(11):875–879.
9. Gaull GE, Bender AN, Vulovic D, et al. Methioninemia and myopathy: a new disorder. *Ann Neurol.* 1981;9(5):423–432.
10. Chandan VS, Shah SS, Lam-Himlin DM, et al. Globular hepatic amyloid is highly sensitive and specific for LECT2 amyloidosis. *Am J Surg Pathol.* 2015;39(4):558–564.
11. Kakar S, Kamath PS, Burgart LJ. Sinusoidal dilatation and congestion in liver biopsy: is it always due to venous outflow impairment? *Arch Pathol Lab Med.* 2004;128(8):901–904.
12. Bruguera M, Aranguibel F, Ros E, et al. Incidence and clinical significance of sinusoidal dilatation in liver biopsies. *Gastroenterology.* 1978;75(3):474–478.
13. Saadoun D, Cazals-Hatem D, Denninger MH, et al. Association of idiopathic hepatic sinusoidal dilatation with the immunological features of the antiphospholipid syndrome. *Gut.* 2004;53(10):1516–1519.

14. Laffon A, Moreno A, Gutierrez-Bucero A, et al. Hepatic sinusoidal dilatation in rheumatoid arthritis. *J Clin Gastroenterol.* 1989;11(6):653–657.
15. Jiménez-Rivera C, Ling SC, Ahmed N, et al. Incidence and characteristics of autoimmune hepatitis. *Pediatrics.* 2015;136(5):e1237–e1248.
16. Torbenson M, Thomas DL. Occult hepatitis B. *Lancet Infect Dis.* 2002;2(8):479–486.
17. Alder JK, Chen JJ, Lancaster L, et al. Short telomeres are a risk factor for idiopathic pulmonary fibrosis. *Proc Natl Acad Sci.* 2008;105(35):13051–13056.
18. Dimitri P, Habeb AM, Garbuz F, et al. Expanding the clinical spectrum associated with GLIS3 mutations. *J Clin Endocrinol Metab.* 2015;100(10):E1362–E1369.
19. Tylki-Szymańska AN, Rujner J, Lugowska A, et al. Clinical, biochemical and histological analysis of seven patients with cholesteryl ester storage disease. *Pediatr Int.* 1997;39(6):643–646.
20. Roels F, Espeel M, De Craemer D. Liver pathology and immunocytochemistry in congenital peroxisomal diseases: a review. *J Inherit Metab Dis.* 1991;14(6):853–875.
21. Englert C, Grabhorn E, Richter A, et al. Liver transplantation in children with progressive familial intrahepatic cholestasis. *Transplantation.* 2007;84(10):1361–1363.
22. Collardeau-Frachon S, Heissat S, Bouvier R, et al. French retrospective multicentric study of neonatal hemochromatosis: importance of autopsy and autoimmune maternal manifestations. *Pediatr Dev Pathol.* 2012;15(6):450–470.
23. Maheshwari A, Thuluvath PJ. Cryptogenic cirrhosis and NAFLD: are they related? *Am J Gastroenterol.* 2006;101(3):664.
24. Ayata G, Gordon FD, Lewis WD, et al. Cryptogenic cirrhosis: clinicopathologic findings at and after liver transplantation. *Human Pathol.* 2002;33(11):1098–1104.
25. Berg T, Neuhaus R, Klein R, et al. Distinct enzyme profiles in patients with cryptogenic cirrhosis reflect heterogeneous causes with different outcomes after liver transplantation (OLT): a long-term documentation before and after OLT. *Transplantation.* 2002;74(6):792–798.
26. Chan HL, Tsang SW, Leung NW, et al. Occult HBV infection in cryptogenic liver cirrhosis in an area with high prevalence of HBV infection. *Am J Gastroenterol.* 2002;97(5):1211–1215.
27. Carulli L, Dei Cas A, Nascimbeni F. Synchronous cryptogenic liver cirrhosis and idiopathic pulmonary fibrosis: a clue to telomere involvement. *Hepatology.* 2012;56(5):2001–2003.
28. Schöniger-Hekele M, Petermann D, Müller C. Mutation of keratin 8 in patients with liver disease. *J Gastroenterol Hepatol.* 2006;21(9): 1466–1469.
29. Ku NO, Darling JM, Krams SM, et al. Keratin 8 and 18 mutations are risk factors for developing liver disease of multiple etiologies. *Proc Natl Acad Sci.* 2003;100(10):6063–6068.
30. Wendum D, Barbu V, Rosmorduc O, et al. Aspects of liver pathology in adult patients with MDR3/ABCB4 gene mutations. *Virchows Arch.* 2012;460(3):291–298.
31. Tweezer-Zaks N, Doron-Libner A, Weiss P, et al. Familial Mediterranean fever and cryptogenic cirrhosis. *Medicine.* 2007;86(6):355–362.
32. Bonnefont-Rousselot D, Condat B, Sassolas A, et al. Cryptogenic cirrhosis in a patient with familial hypocholesterolemia due to a new truncated form of apolipoprotein B. *Eur J Gastroenterol Hepatol.* 2009;21(1):104–108.

8

Viral hepatitis

Roger K. Moreira, MD and Douglas A. Simonetto, MD

8.1 GRADING AND STAGING OVERVIEW

In a fashion somewhat analogous to tumor pathology—where grade refers to features that reflect disease aggressiveness and stage refers to how advanced the disease is—grading and staging of various forms of liver diseases are a widely adopted practice around the world. Other disease categories, such as fatty liver disease, which show biologically distinct forms of fibrosis progression, have their own specific grading and staging systems.

Regardless of the specific method that is used, grading and staging systems provide prognostic value and are important tools when evaluating the effectiveness of new therapeutic modalities for chronic hepatitis. In clinical practice, most pathologists provide a descriptive term for grading (no activity, mild, moderate, or severe activity) and for staging (no fibrosis, portal/periportal fibrosis, bridging fibrosis, or cirrhosis). In our practice, we generally use a four-tiered staging system (Batts–Ludwig) for biopsies of chronic viral hepatitis (Figs. 8.1, 8.2, 8.3, 8.4, and 8.5).

Adequacy criteria

Although most forms of chronic viral hepatitis represent diffuse, relatively homogeneous processes, in some cases there can be challenges with regard to grading and staging. First, subcapsular samples should be interpreted with caution when they are superficial. The subcapsular area commonly shows nonspecific fibrous septa extending from the liver capsule into the hepatic parenchyma. This is usually restricted to tissue a few millimeters deep to the capsule but can mimic true advanced fibrosis with biopsies that are both superficial and tangential to the capsule. The subcapsular area may also show nonspecific inflammation that does not reflect the status of the remainder of the liver.

When needle core biopsies—the preferred type of sample for grading and staging—are performed, specimen adequacy evaluation should focus on two parameters: fragmentation and number of portal tracts. Even though no universally accepted consensus exists regarding the specific characteristics of an adequate sample, the overall literature seems conclusive about larger samples being better for grading and staging.[1] One study[2] suggested a minimum of 11 complete portal tracts, preferably

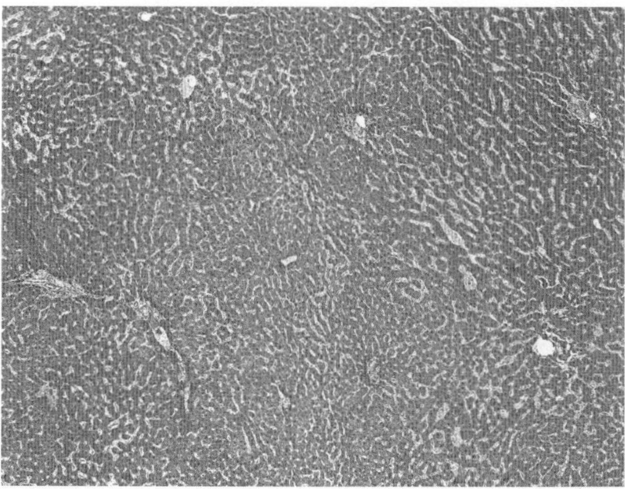

Figure 8.1 Stage 0 of 4. Small, normal portal tracts with no fibrosis.

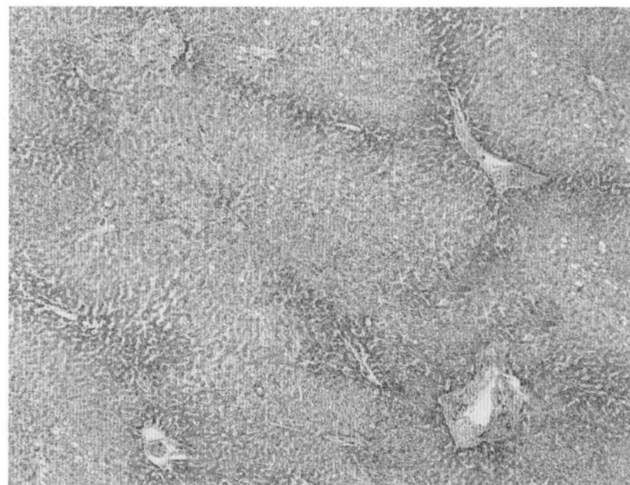

Figure 8.2 Stage 1 of 4. Mild fibrous expansion of portal tracts.

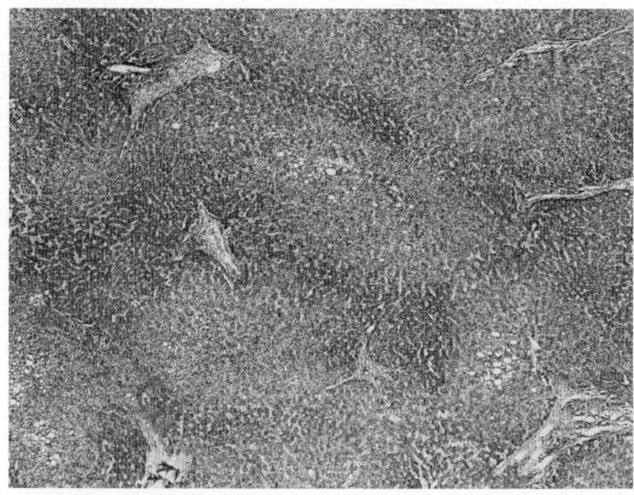

Figure 8.3 Stage 2 of 4. Enlarged, irregular portal tracts with focal periportal septa.

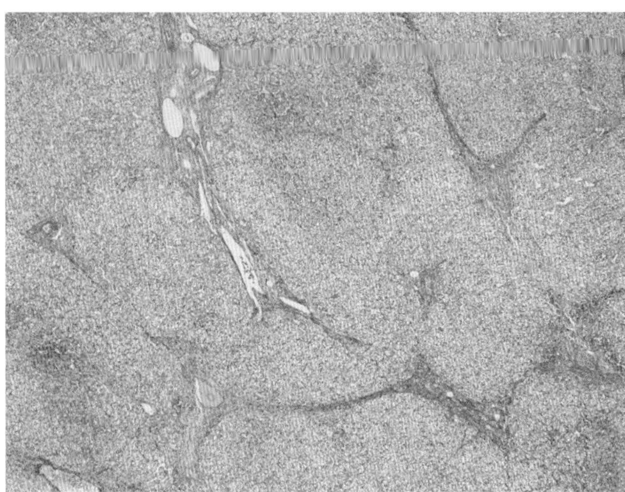

Figure 8.4 Stage 3 of 4. Bridging fibrosis without parenchymal nodularity.

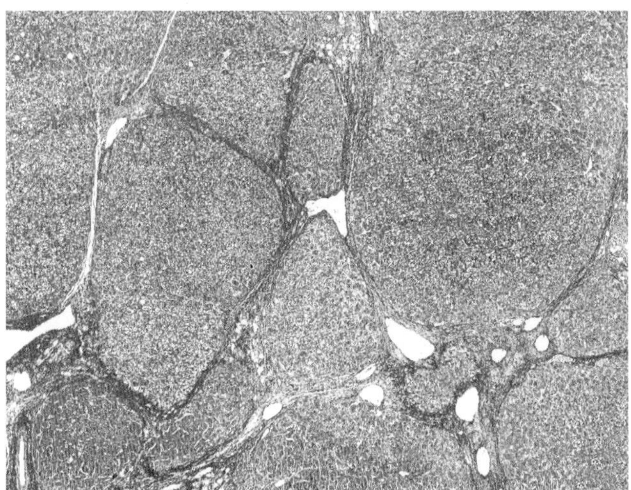

Figure 8.5 Stage 4 of 4. Extensive bridging fibrosis with parenchymal nodularity, i.e., cirrhosis.

Table 8.1 Potential pitfalls in grading and staging liver biopsy samples

Cause	Pitfall
Disease heterogeneity	Biliary tract disease (especially PSC and CF) and venous outflow impairment (especially congestive heart failure) can show heterogeneous fibrosis/cirrhosis, leading to both under- and over-staging
Sample size	Under-grading and under-staging in small samples
Biopsy location	Presence of nonspecific subcapsular fibrous septa and inflammation leading to overestimation of grade and stage
Bridging necrosis	Cases of severe parenchymal injury with bridging necrosis are often difficult to reliably differentiate from advanced fibrosis or cirrhosis
Macronodular cirrhosis	Fibrous septa can be very inconspicuous or absent in these cases; subtle parenchymal nodularity with surrounding thin fibrous rims should be carefully searched

PSC, primary sclerosing cholangitis; CF, cystic fibrosis.

in a specimen containing two linear centimeters of tissue and cores being at least 1.4 mm (corresponding to a 16G needle) in thickness, is optimal to avoid underestimating both grading and staging. Fine needles (21G or less), although appropriate for the evaluation of focal lesions (i.e., tumors), have been found to systematically underscore grading and staging histologic variables.[3] Ultimately, these data represent general and useful guidelines, but the final assessment of adequacy is rendered on a case-by-case basis, because even very small samples can sometimes provide all the information that is clinically needed for management purposes. A summary of potential pitfalls in grading/staging liver biopsy samples is presented in Table 8.1.

The first scoring system to be devised was the "histologic activity index" (HAI), by Knodell and colleagues in 1981.[4] This pioneering system, however, incorporated features that are now known to represent both grading and staging parameters into a single score. Nonetheless, the individual histologic features, namely, portal inflammation, "piecemeal" necrosis (interface hepatitis), focal (spotty) lobular necrosis, and confluent necrosis, along with staging parameters, have formed the basis for all major systems that were subsequently developed: Ishak [modified HAI] system, Scheuer system, Batts–Ludwig system, and the METAVIR system (see Tables 8.2, 8.3, 8.4, and 8.5).

All current staging systems are generally comparable, with relatively minor individual strengths and weaknesses. All have acceptable reproducibility. The choice among the different systems will largely depend on local preferences and purposes—with systems using fewer fibrosis stages being more reproducible and hence generally utilized for routine clinical diagnosis. Systems based on higher numbers of fibrosis stages provide more detailed information and are commonly used in research studies and clinical trials. Our group generally uses the Batts and Ludwig system in our daily practice.

Table 8.2 Scheuer system (1991)

Grade	Portal/periportal inflammation	Lobular inflammation
0	None or minimal	None
1	Portal inflammation	Inflammation without necrosis
2	Mild interface activity	Focal necrosis or acidophilic bodies
3	Moderate interface activity	Severe focal cell damage
4	Severe interface activity	Bridging necrosis
Stage	**Degree of fibrosis**	
0	None	
1	Enlarged, fibrotic portal tracts	
2	Periportal or portal–portal septa but intact architecture	
3	Fibrosis with architectural distortion but no obvious cirrhosis	
4	Probable or definite cirrhosis	

From Scheuer PJ. Classification of chronic viral hepatitis: a need for reassessment. *J Hepatol*. 1991;13(3):372–374, with permission from Elsevier.

Table 8.3 Batts–Ludwig system (1995)

Grade	Lymphocytic piecemeal necrosis (interface activity)	Lobular inflammation and necrosis
0	None	None
1	Minimal, patchy	Minimal: occasional spotty necrosis
2	Mild, involving some or all portal tracts	Mild: little hepatocellular damage
3	Moderate involving all portal tracts	Moderate: noticeable hepatocellular damage
4	Severe, may have bridging necrosis	Severe: prominent diffuse hepatocellular damage
Stage	**Degree of fibrosis**	
0	Normal connective tissue (no fibrosis)	
1	Fibrous portal expansion (portal fibrosis)	
2	Periportal fibrosis or rare portal–portal septa	
3	Fibrous septa with architectural distortion; no obvious cirrhosis	
4	Cirrhosis	

From Batts KP, Ludwig J. Chronic hepatitis: an update on terminology and reporting. *Am J Surg Pathol*. 1995;19(12):1409–1417. http://journals.lww.com/ajsp/pages/default.aspx

Table 8.4 METAVIR system (1996) grading

Piecemeal necrosis, PN (0–3)	Lobular necrosis, LN (0–2)	Activity score, A (0–3)
0	0	0
0	1	1
0	2	2
1	0–1	1
1	2	2
2	0–1	2
2	2	3
3	0–3	3
The overall activity score (A) is reported as: no activity (A0), mild activity (A1), moderate activity (A2), and severe activity (A3).Staging		
Stage	**Degree of fibrosis**	
F0	No fibrosis	
F1	Portal fibrosis without septa	
F2	Portal fibrosis with rare septa	
F3	Numerous septa without cirrhosis	
F4	Cirrhosis	

From Bedossa P, Poynard T. An algorithm for the grading of activity in chronic hepatitis C. The METAVIR Cooperative Study Group. *Hepatology*. 1996;24(2):289–293. doi:10.1002/hep.510240201

Table 8.5 Ishak system grading

A. Periportal or periseptal interface hepatitis (piecemeal necrosis)	Score
Absent	0
Mild (focal, few portal tracts)	1
Mild/moderate (focal, most portal tracts)	2
Moderate (continuous around <50% of tracts or septa)	3
Severe (continuous around >50% of tracts or septa)	4
B. Confluent necrosis	
Absent	0

Table 8.5 Ishak system grading (*continued*)

B. Confluent necrosis	
Focal confluent necrosis	1
Zone 3 necrosis in some areas	2
Zone 3 necrosis in most areas	3
Zone 3 necrosis plus occasional portal-central bridging necrosis	4
Zone 3 necrosis plus multiple portal-central bridging necrosis	5
Panacinar or multiacinar necrosis	6
C. Focal (spotty) lytic necrosis, apoptosis, and focal inflammation	
Absent	0
One focus or less per ×10 objective	1
Two to four foci per ×10 objective	2
Five to ten foci per ×10 objective	3
More than ten foci per ×10 objective	4
D. Portal inflammation	
Absent	0
Mild, some or all portal tracts	1
Moderate, some or all portal tracts	2
Moderate/marked, all portal tracts	3
Marked, all portal tracts	4

The overall grade is reported as a sum of individual scores (total score range: 0–18).
From Callea F, De Grootes J, Gudat F, et al. Histological grading and staging of chronic hepatitis. *J Hepatol*. 1995;22(6):696–699, with permission from Elsevier.

Table 8.5 Ishak system grading (*continued*)

Staging	
Stage	**Degree of fibrosis**
0	No fibrosis
1	Fibrous expansion of some portal tracts, with or without short septa
2	Fibrous expansion of most portal tracts, with or without short septa
3	Fibrous expansion of most portal tracts with occasional portal–portal bridging
4	Fibrous expansion of portal tracts with marked portal–portal as well as portal-central bridging
5	Marked bridging with occasional nodules (incomplete cirrhosis)
6	Cirrhosis, probable or definite

8.2 HEPATITIS A

Etiology and pathogenesis

Hepatitis A is caused by a small, nonenveloped RNA virus belonging to the Picornaviridae family, which is spread almost exclusively by fecal-oral transmission, either directly or through contaminated food or water. Upon entry into the hepatocyte, the viral RNA is uncoated, viral proteins are synthetized, and the assembled viral particles are shed into the biliary system and excreted in the feces. Viral infection of hepatocytes is thought to have little or no direct cytotoxic effect, with liver injury stemming predominantly from immune-mediated attack.

Clinical manifestations

Hepatitis A virus (HAV) infection has three main clinical phases: incubation, symptomatic, and convalescence. The incubation period of acute hepatitis A varies from 14 to 50 days. The clinical manifestations also vary and are age dependent. Only 30% of children (age 6 or less) will develop symptoms, whereas more than 70% of adults develop jaundice with markedly elevated transaminases. Additional symptoms include fatigue, anorexia, nausea, vomiting, diarrhea, fever, headaches, and arthralgia.[5] The symptomatic phase typically lasts 1 to 8 weeks and coincides with the presence of IgM anti-HAV antibodies. Positive IgM antibodies are used to confirm the diagnosis of HAV infection and may persist for up to 6 months. Total anti-HAV IgG antibody levels rise in parallel with a decrease in IgM titers and reflect long-term immunity against hepatitis A.[6] A small subset of patients with hepatitis A will develop severe forms of infection, including cholestatic hepatitis, relapsing hepatitis, and rarely, fulminant hepatitis.[7,8]

Histologic features and differential diagnosis

The histopathology of hepatitis A will largely depend on the severity of the clinical presentation. A large proportion of cases is either asymptomatic or associated with very mild signs/symptoms and hence is not biopsied. Sampled cases most commonly show prototypical features of an acute, lobular-predominant hepatitis (Fig. 8.6), with variable inflammation (mostly CD8+ T cells), numerous acidophilic bodies, lobular disarray, hepatocyte swelling, Kupffer cell hyperplasia, sometimes with hepatocanalicular cholestasis. Acute HAV infection can also show relatively dense portal inflammation with interface activity, sometimes with increased plasma cells,[9] mimicking autoimmune hepatitis. This pattern can also be seen in cases with a clinically protracted or relapsing course. In a small minority of cases, fulminant hepatitis occurs, and the histologic picture is that of a massive/submassive necrosis (Fig. 8.7), with prominent regenerative changes and cholestasis of the residual hepatocytes, sometimes with striking ductular reaction.[10]

Prognosis and treatment

Hepatitis A infection will spontaneously resolve in over 99% of cases. The treatment is mainly supportive, including adequate hydration and avoidance of hepatotoxic drugs. Liver transplantation may be required in as many as 30% of patients with fulminant hepatitis A.[11] Hepatitis A is a vaccine-preventable disease, and the fundamental management of hepatitis A remains active immunization.

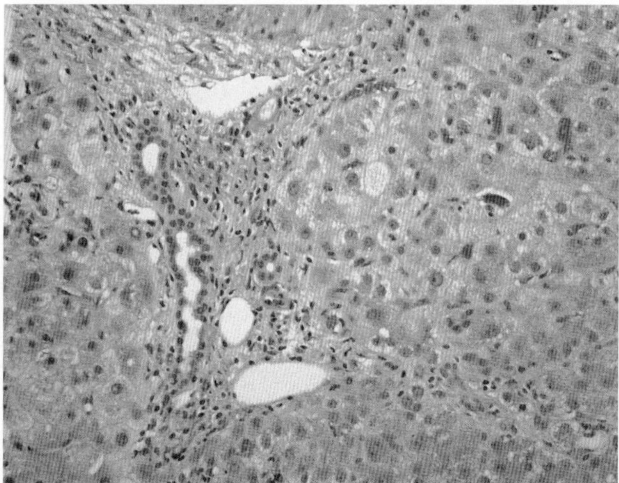

Figure 8.6 Hepatitis A. Acute hepatitis pattern, featuring a predominantly lobular process, with mild necroinflammation, disarray, and acidophilic bodies.

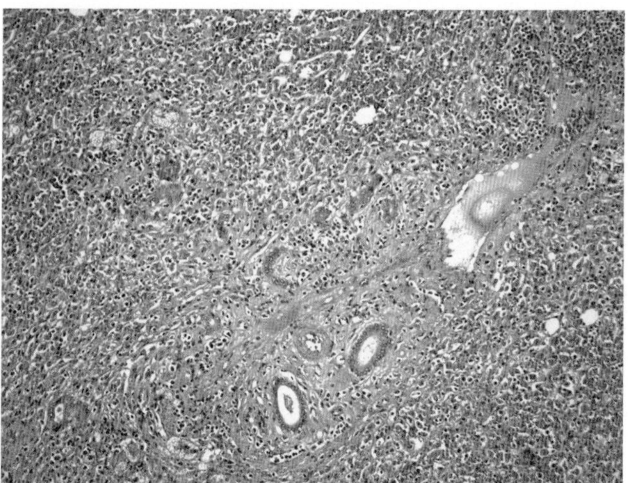

Figure 8.7 Hepatitis A. A case of fulminant hepatitis with massive parenchymal necrosis.

8.3 HEPATITIS B AND DELTA VIRUS

Etiology and pathogenesis

Although hepatitis B has a relatively low prevalence in the United States, an estimated 250 million people (approximately 3.6% of the world's population) are HBsAg positive worldwide, representing one of the main causes of chronic liver disease. The prevalence of hepatitis B virus (HBV) infection is highly variable, being highest in sub-Saharan Africa and certain countries in the Middle-East, Asia, and Western Pacific region.[12] HBV is an enveloped DNA virus, a member of the Hepadnaviridae family. Transmission occurs through blood and body fluid exchange, taking place predominantly during the perinatal period (vertical transmission) or during childhood in high-prevalence areas. In low-prevalence areas, such as the United States and Western Europe, infections are acquired mostly during young adulthood through sexual contact or injection drug abuse (horizontal transmission). The natural history of the disease is also deeply influenced by the timing of initial infection. The infection becomes chronic in approximately 90% of cases in perinatal transmission, whereas the opposite is seen in infections acquired in adulthood, where over 90% of infections have spontaneous resolution.

Patients with chronic infection, especially those acquired during the perinatal period or early childhood years, as well as those with high levels of HBV replication (high HBeAg and HBV DNA levels), have the highest risk for developing hepatocellular carcinoma.[13] Several HBV genotypes have been described (eight in total, A–H), showing distinct geographic and ethnic distributions around the world, as well as different risk levels for the development of cirrhosis and hepatocellular carcinoma.[14–17] Finally, HBV viral replication occurs through reverse transcription but without an effective proof reading mechanism, leading to a high rate of viral mutations. Precore and basal core mutations[18,19] have been linked to diminished or loss of HBeAg production, and YMDD mutants are associated with drug resistance.[20]

Following acute infection, the disease goes through several phases, with different serological, histologic, and immunophenotypic characteristics (Table 8.6). In the initial phase—immune tolerance—there is a low level of immunologic response to the virus, variable but generally mild necroinflammatory activity, and high levels of viral replication, with corresponding serology that is HBeAg positive and anti-HBe negative. In the immune clearance phase, there is heightened immune response to the virus, and the histologic activity tends to be correspondingly high. This is followed by a low-replicative phase in which both viral replication and histologic activity are low. This sequence of events, however, is complex and variable from case to case. Disease activity can also flare above baseline for several reasons, including emergence of viral mutants, coinfection with delta virus, and treatment-related factors.

The hepatitis D virus (HDV, also called delta virus) is known as a "defective virus," because it requires hepatocytes being also infected with HBV in order to replicate. HDV can be transmitted either as a coinfection with HBV or as a superinfection in patients with chronic hepatitis B. In cases of coinfection, HDV confers an increased risk of fulminant hepatitis,[21] while superinfection has been associated with increased inflammatory activity (mimicking hepatitis B flares or other superimposed acute injuries). Higher rates of chronicity, increased liver-related mortality, and higher risk of hepatocellular carcinoma have also been reported with hepatitis D.[22]

Clinical manifestations

Acute hepatitis B symptoms are nonspecific and mainly constitutional, including low-grade fever, fatigue, nausea, myalgia, and arthralgia. Approximately 70% of patients will present with subclinical or anicteric hepatitis. Jaundice, present in only 30% of acute HBV infections, typically begins within 10 days after the onset of symptoms. Marked transaminase elevations

Table 8.6 Clinical features of different phases of chronic hepatitis B

Phases of chronic hepatitis B	Serologic markers	Findings
Immune tolerant phase	HBeAg positive	• High-serum HBV DNA levels • Normal aminotransferases • Mild or no hepatic necroinflammation • Mild or no fibrosis progression
Immune active or immune clearance phase	HBeAg positive	• Low-serum HBV DNA levels • Elevated aminotransferases • Moderate–severe liver necroinflammation • Fibrosis progression
Inactive HBV carrier state	HBeAg negative HBeAb positive	• Low-serum HBV DNA levels • Normal aminotransferases • No hepatic necroinflammation • No fibrosis progression
Reactivation phase	HBeAg negative HBeAb positive	• Fluctuating levels of serum HBV DNA • Elevated aminotransferases • Mild–moderate liver necroinflammation • Fibrosis progression
HBsAg-negative phase or occult HBV infection	HBeAg negative HBeAb positive HBsAg negative HBsAb negative	• Undetectable serum HBV DNA • Detectable HBV DNA in the liver • At risk for reactivation with immunosuppressive therapy

HBV, hepatitis B virus; HBeAg, hepatitis B e antigen; HBeAb, hepatitis B e antibody; HBsAb, hepatitis B s antibody; HBsAg, hepatitis B s antigen.

are often seen, with levels over 1,000 to 2,000 IU/L, followed by hyperbilirubinemia. These symptoms usually resolve spontaneously within 1 to 3 months.

The vast majority of patients with chronic hepatitis B are asymptomatic, but acute exacerbations can manifest as fatigue, anorexia, nausea, and jaundice. The transaminase levels are often normal or only mildly elevated in chronic hepatitis B. Extrahepatic manifestations of chronic hepatitis B occur in 10% to 20% of patients and have been attributed to circulating immune complexes containing HBsAg. Extrahepatic manifestations include polyarteritis nodosa, membranous and membranoproliferative glomerulonephritis, and papular acrodermatitis.[23]

The diagnosis of hepatitis B is based on serologic markers and confirmed by the presence of HBsAg and/or HBV DNA in the serum (Table 8.7).[24] The presence of HBsAg for longer than 6 months in the blood defines a hepatitis B infection as chronic. HDV exposure can be detected by the presence of IgG anti-HDV antibodies. The diagnosis of active HDV infection is confirmed by detection of serum HDV RNA by polymerase chain reaction (PCR).

Histologic features

Acute hepatitis B

Acute hepatitis B is rarely an indication for liver biopsies, but biopsies do occur when acute hepatitis B is not clinically suspected. The histologic findings in acute hepatitis B are similar to other causes of acute hepatitis, including a lobular-predominant process characterized by various degrees of necroinflammation. Ground-glass inclusions are absent in acute infection, and HBV-related immunohistochemical markers (see discussion later) are usually negative.

Table 8.7 Serologic markers in hepatitis B

Serologic marker	Interpretation
Hepatitis B surface antigen (HBsAg)	Current hepatitis B infection
Hepatitis B surface antibody (HBsAb)	Resolved hepatitis B infection or immunization
Hepatitis B e antigen (HBeAg)	Indicates high level of viral replication and infectivity
Hepatitis B e antibody (HBeAb)	Indicates HBeAg seroconversion and usually marks the transition to inactive carrier state
IgM hepatitis B core antibody (IgM anti-HBc)	Indicates acute hepatitis B or reactivation. The only positive marker during the window period (between disappearance of HBsAg and appearance of HBsAb)
IgG hepatitis B core antibody (IgG anti-HBc)	Indicates past or current HBV infection

Chronic hepatitis B

In chronic infection, the findings are broadly similar to those seen in other forms of chronic viral hepatitis (e.g., chronic hepatitis C), with the presence of variably dense portal inflammatory infiltrates containing lymphoid aggregates, rarely with germinal centers, and variable interface activity and lobular activity. In contrast to hepatitis C, however, in which a chronic hepatitis with low-grade inflammation is virtually the rule, chronic hepatitis B can show a spectrum of injury that ranges from essentially no inflammation (mimicking a normal liver, often seen in congenital cases) to prominent inflammation with extensive necrosis in severe hepatitis B flares. In practice, the main unique feature of chronic HBV infection is ground-glass inclusions in hepatocytes, which consist of eosinophilic, glassy, minimally granular-appearing cytoplasmic inclusions that often (but not always) show a peripheral clear halo of displaced hepatocyte cytoplasm (Fig. 8.8). Ground-glass hepatocytes may be seen scattered throughout a sample but commonly cluster in a heterogeneous manner. Biologically, ground-glass hepatocytes result from markedly distended endoplasmic reticulum filled with viral HBsAg. Ground-glass hepatocytes are seen in only a subset of cases of chronic hepatitis, unusually with

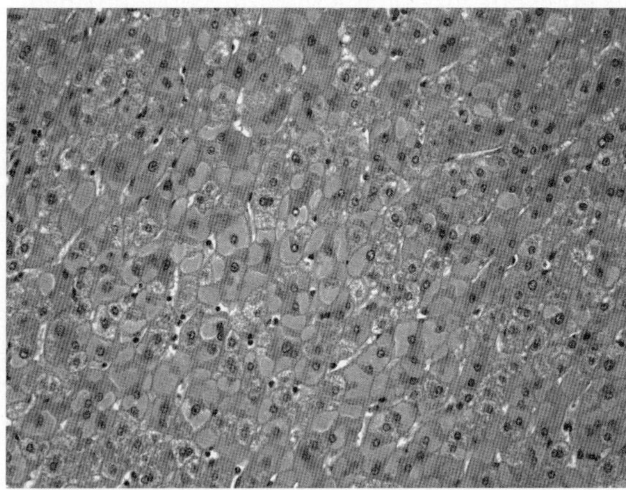

Figure 8.8 Chronic hepatitis B. Numerous ground-glass hepatocyte inclusions are shown here, characterized by eosinophilic, finely granular material distending the cytoplasm, sometimes with a thin peripheral rim of displaced normal cytoplasm.

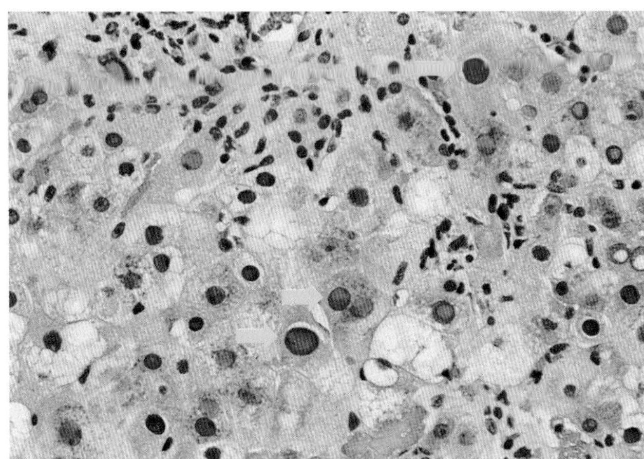

Figure 8.9 Hepatitis B, sanded nuclei. Occasionally, hepatocyte nuclei in the setting of hepatitis B show a smudgy appearance due to accumulation of core antigen.

long standing infection. Even less commonly seen, hepatocyte nuclei can show pale, slightly eosinophilic, finely granular inclusions, referred to as "sanded nuclei," which represent nuclear accumulation of core antigen (HBcAg) in the presence of high viral replication (Fig. 8.9).[25]

Fibrosing cholestatic hepatitis B represents a severe, rapidly progressive form of the disease, which is caused by unchecked viral replication in the setting of immunosuppression. Initially described in liver transplant patients,[26–28] it has since been described in other forms of immunosuppression. Histologically, it is characterized by a relative paucity of inflammation, marked ductular reaction, sinusoidal fibrosis, marked hepatocyte swelling, and hepatocanalicular cholestasis. With the advent of effective antiviral therapy, fibrosing cholestatic hepatitis B has become vanishingly rare.

Special stains and immunostains

HBsAg is expressed in essentially all chronic cases, including those that lack ground-glass inclusions hepatocytes. Therefore, if HBV infection is suspected (or has not been excluded clinically), HBsAg immunostain is a valuable tool. HBcAg immunostain may occasionally be positive before HBsAg early in the course of the infection and may be useful in this context. Both stains, however, are usually negative in the acute phase. HBsAg typically shows cytoplasmic expression but may also be membranous in cases with higher levels of active viral replication (Fig. 8.10). The degree of HBcAg expression (Fig. 8.11) generally parallels HBV DNA and HBeAg levels in the serum. Abundant nuclear HBcAg expression usually indicates unchecked viral replication in the setting of tolerance or immunosuppression, while cytoplasmic expression

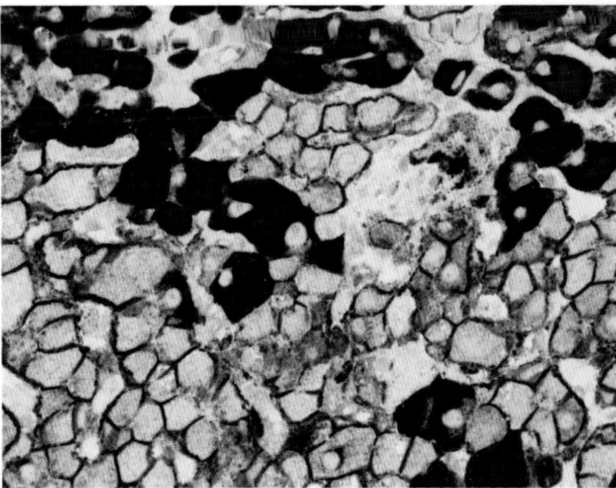

Figure 8.10 Hepatitis B, surface antigen. HBs immunohistochemistry, highlighting intracytoplasmic and membranous surface antigen.

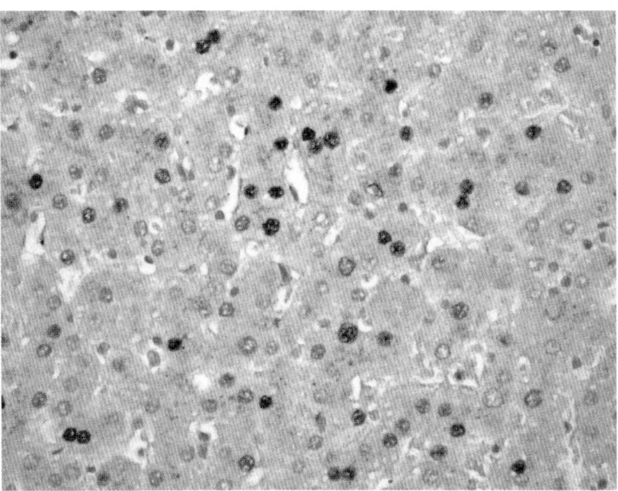

Figure 8.11 Hepatitis B, core antigen. HBc immunohistochemistry showing scattered positive nuclei.

correlates mainly with high necroinflammatory activity.[29–33] Special stains such as Orcein and Victoria blue (Fig. 8.12) also stain ground-glass inclusions and may be used if immunostains are not available.

Differential diagnosis

Various forms of liver disease are in the histologic differential diagnosis of hepatitis B. In acute hepatitis B, the findings are generally nonspecific and are similar to those seen in other forms of acute hepatitis; therefore, clinical and serological correlation is essential. It must be kept in mind, however, that acute HBV can vary from a very mild hepatitis to a fulminant hepatitis with massive necrosis. In some cases, plasma cells may be rather conspicuous,[34] potentially mimicking autoimmune hepatitis. In its chronic phase, hepatitis B

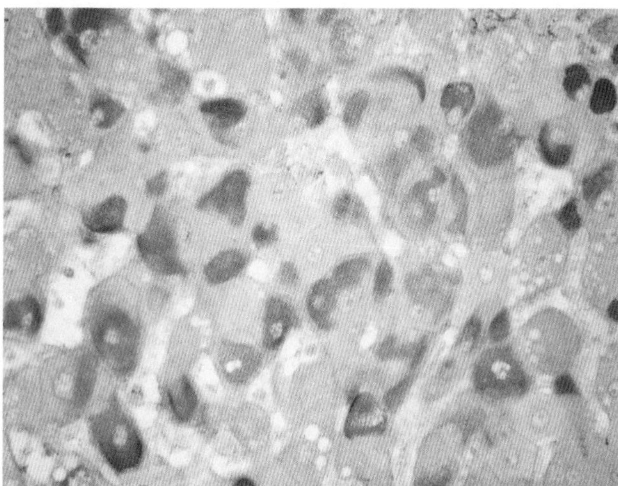

Figure 8.12 Hepatitis B, surface antigen. Victoria blue stain represents an alternative method to detect surface antigen.

can range from essentially no inflammation to severe activity in acute flares. Although the general pattern of a chronic hepatitis is overall nonspecific (largely overlapping with chronic hepatitis C and other forms of chronic hepatitis), most cases will show immunohistochemical evidence of HBsAg or HBcAg, which are diagnostic. Occasionally, there will be clinical suspicion for superimposed diseases such as alcoholic or nonalcoholic steatohepatitis, biliary tract disease, or autoimmune hepatitis. Features of steatohepatitis are not part of the spectrum of typical HBV infection. Likewise, features of biliary tract disease are not seen in typical cases of hepatitis B, except for cholestasis (which can be seen in fibrosing cholestatic hepatitis B and acute flares) and prominent ductular reaction (seen in fibrosing cholestatic hepatitis B). Copper and CK-7 immunostains could also assist in this differential in a manner analogous to hepatitis C-related fibrosing cholestatic hepatitis (see Chapter 20 for further discussion). On the other hand, excluding a component of autoimmune hepatitis in the context of HBV infection can be more difficult histologically because a significant number of plasma cells can be seen in hepatitis B alone, and the disease activity is equally variable in both diseases. Finally, hepatitis D should be suspected histologically in hepatitis B flares or fulminant disease because such cases can be associated with superinfection and coinfection, respectively. Histologically, the only distinctive feature that has been described in hepatitis D is the presence of sanded nuclei (owing to the nuclear accumulation of HDVAg[35]), with identical appearance to what is seen in HBV infection with nuclear HBcAg deposition, but they are not always present. HDVAg immunostain, although not widely available, can accurately diagnose HDV infection.

Prognosis and treatment

The majority of acute HBV infections will resolve spontaneously in adults and do not require antiviral treatment. Less than 1% of adult patients will develop fulminant liver failure and fewer than 5% will go on to develop chronic infection. In the pediatric population, however, the disease becomes chronic in a much higher percentage of patients (inversely proportional to the child's age), with approximately 90% of infants and 6% to 50% of older children developing chronic infection.[36]

Treatment for chronic hepatitis B is based mainly on three criteria: serum HBV DNA levels, serum alanine aminotransferase (ALT) levels, and severity of liver disease. Patients with active hepatitis, defined as ALT above two times the upper limit of normal and/or serum HBV DNA greater than 20,000 IU/mL, and those with advanced liver fibrosis and detectable HBV DNA, should be considered for antiviral treatment.[37]

Current treatments for chronic hepatitis B include interferon, pegilated-interferon, nucleoside analogues (lamivudine, telbivudine, and entecavir), and nucleotide analogues (adefovir and tenofovir). Tenofovir and entecavir carry the lowest rates of viral resistance and are currently considered first-line therapy. Long-term nucleoside/nucleotide analogues are the most commonly utilized therapy, with the goal to maintain serum HBV DNA at the undetectable level.[38]

Acute HBV/HDV coinfections typically result in spontaneous recovery, with less than 2% of patients progressing to chronic HDV infection. On the other hand, HDV superinfection usually progress to chronic hepatitis D. The treatment of chronic hepatitis D is primarily PEG-interferon, which results in only 20% to 40% sustained viral clearance.[39] Approximately 20% of patients with chronic HBV infection will progress to cirrhosis, of which 10% to 25% will decompensate or develop hepatocellular carcinoma within 5 years.[40,41]

8.4 HEPATITIS C

Etiology and pathogenesis

Hepatitis C virus (HCV) is a single-stranded RNA virus belonging to the Flaviviridae family. HCV currently infects an estimated 2.7 to 3.9 million people (approximately 0.8% to 1.2% of the population) in the United States according to the Center of Disease Control (2014 data). Worldwide, 130 to 170 million people (2% to 3% of the world population) are estimated to be infected, with Eastern Europe, Southeast Asia, the Middle-East, and Northern Africa having the highest disease prevalence.[42,43] The disease is most often transmitted parenterally, although transmission through sexual contact (especially in immunosuppressed individuals) and maternal transmission also occurs.[44–47] After acute infection, a minority of patients (15% to 25%) clear the virus spontaneously—a phenomenon that has been associated with several genetic factors, including IL28B and DQB1*0301 major histocompatibility complex class II.[48] The remaining patients (75% to 85%) go on to develop chronic HCV infection. Once infection occurs, the virus establishes itself in the liver and mainly replicates within hepatocytes, but other potential replication sites also exist, such as peripheral mononuclear cells[49] and dendritic cells.[50] Owing to its inherently high mutational rate, genetic heterogeneity can rapidly develop within an infected patient—referred to as quasispecies—which in part enables the virus to successfully evade the host's immune response.[51] This genetic variability has given rise to the seven currently recognized genotypes (1 to 7), and over 60 subtypes,[52] with markedly different distribution across geographic locations and specific populations, as well as important implications with regard to treatment response.

Clinical manifestations

Acute hepatitis C is mild and essentially asymptomatic in the vast majority of cases. In symptomatic individuals, the presentation is similar to an acute hepatitis due to other etiologies, including hepatotrophic and nonhepatotropic viruses. Transaminases can be markedly elevated (>1,000 IU/L), and bilirubin can be normal to markedly elevated. Signs and symptoms include jaundice, abdominal pain, decreased appetite, fatigue, and rash.[53] Chronic HCV infection has also been associated with several extrahepatic manifestations, including mixed cryoglobulinemia vasculitis, lymphoproliferative malignancies, sicca syndrome, rheumatoid-arthritis-like polyarthritis, autoantibody production, depression, and insulin resistance. Mixed cryoglobulinemia is the most common extrahepatic manifestation of chronic HCV infection, identified in as many as 50% of patients with HCV infection. Manifestations of HCV-associated cryoglobulinemia include palpable purpura (18% to 33%), fatigue (35% to 54%), arthralgia-myalgia (35% to 54%), sicca syndrome (10% to 25%), neuropathy (11% to 30%), and renal complications including membranoglomerulonephritis (27%).[54]

Histologic features

Acute hepatitis C

Little is known about the histopathology of typical/asymptomatic cases of acute hepatitis C, because these are rarely biopsied. In well-characterized symptomatic cases of acute HCV infection,[53] there is a predominantly lobular hepatitis with variable necroinflammatory activity, cholestasis, and ductular reaction (which may mimic biliary tract disease) early in the course of the infection. Subsequently (weeks to a few months), the activity and cholestasis are less pronounced. Portal infiltrates become more prominent within several months, because the hepatitis transits histologically into its chronic form. Bile duct injury and lymphocytic cholangitis (or "Poulsen-Christoffersen" lesion) are also a reported feature.[55] In HIV-infected patients, acute hepatitis C has also been associated with denser portal inflammatory infiltrates, interface activity, and periportal fibrosis, mimicking the appearance of a chronic hepatitis.

Chronic hepatitis C

Portal findings The portal findings in chronic hepatitis C are fairly predictable and present in the vast majority of cases (Fig. 8.13). Although relatively patchy in nature and variable from biopsy to biopsy, most portal tracts show mildly to moderately dense chronic inflammation, composed predominantly of mature-appearing lymphocytes. Loose lymphoid aggregates are frequently present.[56] Clearly recognizable germinal centers are also found in a minority of cases. The lymphoid aggregates are usually located away from the interlobular bile ducts and vasculature, or at least not centered around these structures. Although eosinophils are usually not prominent, they are at least focally present in most cases. Likewise, scattered plasma cells are a fairly common finding. Both mild lymphocytic cholangitis (Poulsen-Christoffersen lesions, more common with genotype 3a[57]) and focal portal vein endotheliitis are also part of the spectrum of chronic hepatitis C.[58]

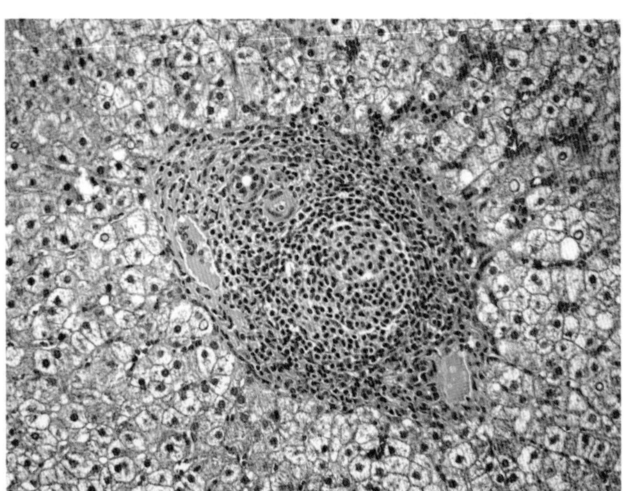

Figure 8.13 Hepatitis C, portal findings. A typical case of chronic hepatitis C showing chronic portal inflammation with the presence of lymphoid aggregate (and a small germinal center), with minimal interface activity.

Interface hepatitis The chronic inflammation in hepatitis C commonly shows at least focal interface activity—a process also referred to as interface hepatitis (formerly known as "piecemeal necrosis") (Fig. 8.14).[59] A mild amount of ductular reaction with associated mixed inflammatory infiltrate may also be present, further contributing to the effacement of the interface area. The ductular reactions are usually inconspicuous on H&E but are highlighted by keratin immunostains.

Lobular findings As with other forms of chronic hepatitis, there is variable lobular necroinflammatory activity in chronic hepatitis C. In typical cases, there are scattered clusters of lymphocytes and Kupffer cells, often surrounding a necrotic/apoptotic hepatocyte (collectively referred to as "necroinflammatory foci" or "spotty necrosis"), as well as isolated apoptotic hepatocytes (Fig. 8.15). The lobules commonly show concomitant features of regeneration, such as hepatocyte binucleation, slightly thickened and irregular hepatocyte plates, occasional mitotic figures, and anisonucleosis, referred to as lobular "disarray." In addition to injury, steatosis is also a common feature in chronic hepatitis C and can develop either as a result of direct viral cytopathic effect in genotype 3 infection (Fig. 8.16), whereby HCV directly elicits intrahepatocytic metabolic derangement leading to steatosis, or indirectly thorough increased insulin resistance.[60,61] Many of these patients also have the metabolic syndrome. Hepatocyte multinucleation (giant cell transformation) is relatively uncommon and may be seen in the setting of HCV infection alone or in HCV/HIV coinfection (Fig. 8.17).[62] Finally, mildly increased hepatic iron is relatively common in HCV

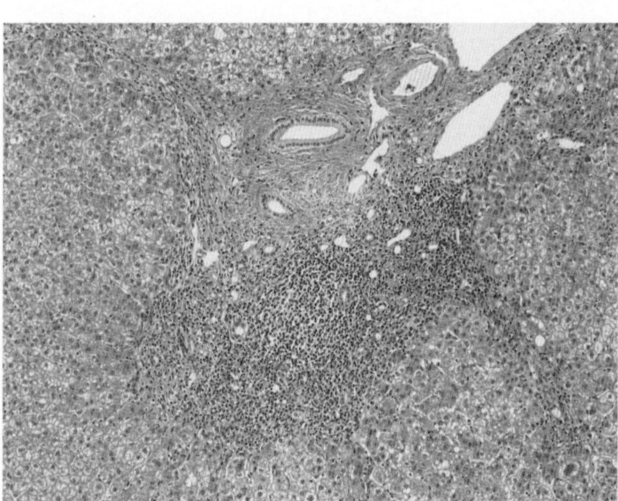

Figure 8.14 Hepatitis C, portal findings. Interface hepatitis (along the inferior edge of this portal tract) is shown, characterized by lymphocytic infiltrate invading the lobular area adjacent to the portal tract.

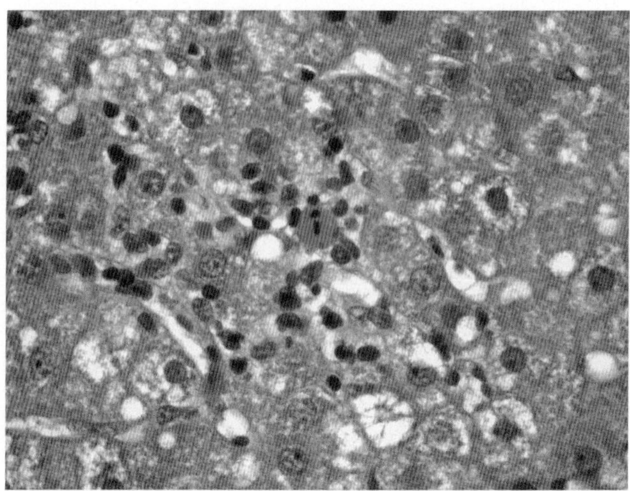

Figure 8.15 Hepatitis C, lobular findings. A typical necroinflammatory focus in hepatitis C, with a cluster of lymphocytes and histiocytes around an apoptotic hepatocyte (acidophilic body, at the center of the image).

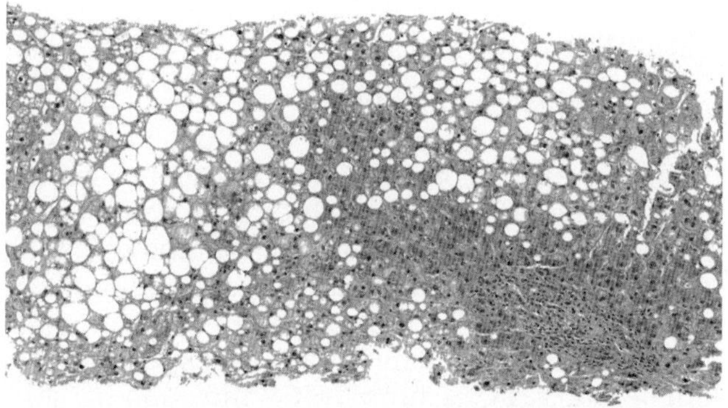

Figure 8.16 Hepatitis C, lobular findings. Prominent steatosis in this case of HCV genotype 3 infection.

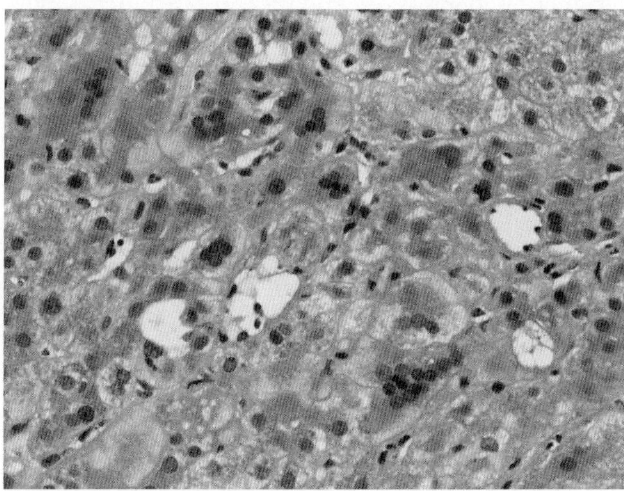

Figure 8.17 Hepatitis C, lobular findings. Giant cell transformation. Multiple nuclei are seen in several of the hepatocytes in this image.

infection, currently thought to be at in part related to HCV-mediated decreased hepcidin transcription activity, leading to iron accumulation.[63]

Special stains and immunostains

No commercially available special stains or immunostains are widely utilized diagnostically to detect HCV. Special stains such as trichome, reticulin, PAS with diastase, and iron are useful for grading and staging as well as for exclusion of other disease processes.

Differential diagnosis

The differential diagnosis of chronic hepatitis C will depend on the phase of the disease. Acute hepatitis C can resemble a drug reaction or biliary tract disease. The histopathology of chronic HCV infection is the prototype of a "chronic hepatitis" pattern but has no unique or diagnostic features. Chronic hepatitis B is certainly in the differential diagnosis. However, serologic testing is virtually always performed before a biopsy is obtained, and this differential is usually not a clinical problem, except for cases of HCV/HBV coinfection. HBsAg and HBcAg immunohistochemistry can be useful. Autoimmune hepatitis is a more challenging problem, both clinically and histologically, particularly in patients with high autoantibody titers. As a general rule, the necroinflammatory activity in chronic hepatitis C is mild or mild-to-moderate, and, while plasma cells are present, they should be few and generally restricted to the portal tracts. Larger numbers of plasma cells, plasma cell clusters, and readily identifiable lobular plasma cells, prominent central perivenulitis, and hepatocyte cholestatic rosetting are not part of the typical histologic spectrum of chronic hepatitis C and suggest autoimmune hepatitis in this setting. Higher grade of necroinflammation in a known hepatitis C patient should also raise the possibility of a superimposed drug reaction. Although a few eosinophils are common in hepatitis C, large numbers are unusual. Central perivenulitis, prominent bile duct injury, granulomas, and cholestasis are also features that are commonly seen in drug reaction but not in chronic hepatitis.

Prognosis and treatment

An estimated 5% to 20% of infected patients eventually develop cirrhosis over a period of 20 to 30 years, and 1% to 5% ultimately die from end-stage liver disease and/or hepatocellular carcinoma. The natural history of chronic hepatitis C in individual patients, however, is very heterogeneous, with studies showing that the fibrosis progression may be faster in individuals acquiring the infection at an older age and in the presence of comorbidities, including other liver diseases (NASH,[64] alcohol,[65] α-1 antitrypsin deficiency, and hepatitis B), and unrelated conditions such as HIV.[66] In spite of the sharp decline in the incidence of HCV infection since the 1990s, largely related to successful blood screening and other public health measures, the incidence of HCV-related complications is predicted to keep increasing in the coming decades.[42] The treatment of hepatitis C has dramatically changed in the last few years with the introduction of highly effective direct-acting oral agents, and numerous additional new drugs are being evaluated in clinical trials. Treatment is currently recommended for most patients with chronic hepatitis C with the goal of virologic cure. Cure of HCV infection reduces the progression of liver fibrosis and lowers the risk of both hepatocellular carcinoma[67] and liver-related mortality.[68] The antiviral regimen of choice varies according to the HCV genotype, history of prior treatment, and stage of liver disease (AASLD-IDSA updated recommendations for testing, managing, and treating hepatitis C can be found at www.hcvguidelines.org).

8.5 HEPATITIS E VIRUS

Etiology, pathogenesis, and clinical manifestations

Hepatitis E is caused by a single-stranded RNA virus belonging to the Hepeviridae family, which is mainly transmitted enterically (fecal-oral route). The virus has a worldwide distribution but occurs most commonly in Asia, where numerous water-borne epidemics have been reported. The clinical manifestations and severity of the disease are highly variable, with the vast majority of cases being either asymptomatic or mild and self-limited. Cholestatic and fulminant hepatitis, however, do occur, and pregnant women are particular vulnerable.[69] A chronic form of hepatitis E virus (HEV) infection was identified in 2008 as a cause of potentially progressive chronic hepatitis in liver transplantation patients in many European countries,[70] and HEV infection was subsequently identified in North American transplant recipients, although the prevalence of chronic infection/chronic hepatitis in this population is unclear.[71]

Histologic features

The histologic appearance of HEV infection is very similar to that seen in hepatitis A, including the range of severity. Milder forms show typical features of a mildly to moderately active acute hepatitis, with more severe cases showing increasing cholestasis and variable amounts of confluent necrosis. Chronic HEV infection is uncommon and primarily described in

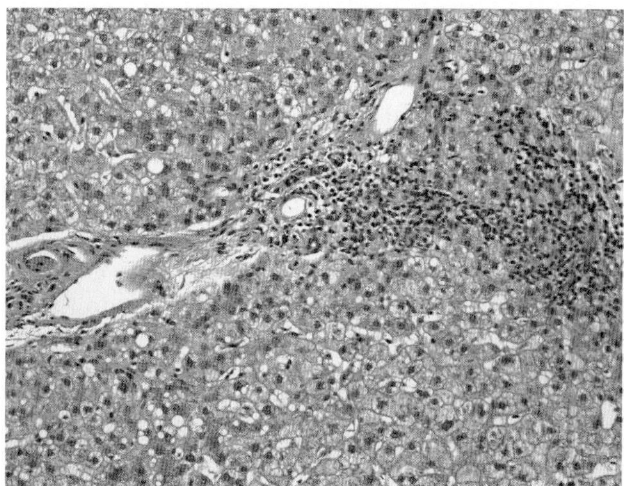

Figure 8.18 Hepatitis E. A mildly active hepatitis (nonspecific pattern) is seen in this liver transplant patient with chronic hepatitis E.

transplanted patients (also see Chapter 20). In this setting, the histological findings are typically nonspecific, showing primarily a mildly active chronic hepatitis (Fig. 8.18).

Special stains and immunostains

No immunostains or special stains are currently available commercially, but several medical centers are actively working on the development of clinically useful immunostains or in situ hybridization (Fig. 8.19).

Prognosis and treatment

Acute hepatitis E has a self-limited course in immunocompetent patients, and the treatment is mainly supportive. Ribavirin monotherapy is the treatment of choice for chronic hepatitis E in immunosuppressed patients, with a sustained viral response rate of 85%.[72]

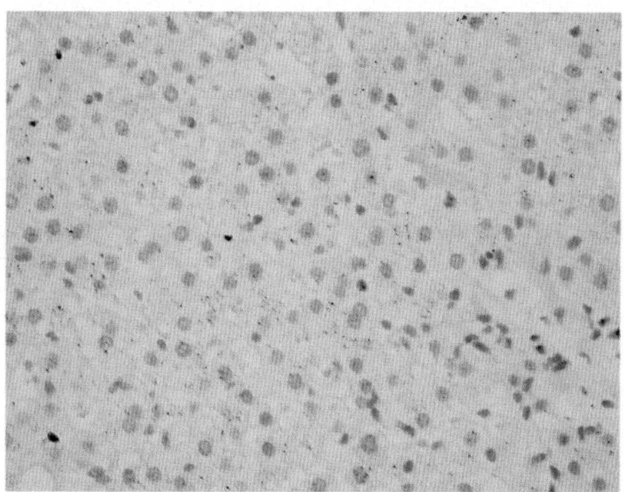

Figure 8.19 Hepatitis E. In situ hybridization for hepatitis E shows multifocal areas of cytoplasmic positivity within hepatocytes (***brown dots***).

8.6 CYTOMEGALOVIRUS

Clinical manifestations

Cytomegalovirus (CMV) is one of the most common viral infections in the world. Nowadays, it is most commonly seen by pathologists in the context of liver transplantation. Outside of the liver transplant setting, CMV hepatitis is also seen in other immunosuppressed individuals, rarely in immunocompetent individuals, and rarely in the neonatal period.

Neonatal CMV infection

CMV is one of the most common congenital infections, although only a minority of infected neonates is symptomatic. When present, clinical manifestations include hepatosplenomegaly, chorioretinitis, low birth weight, microcephaly, central nerve system calcifications, seizures, and rash.

Immunocompetent hosts

In teenagers and immunocompetent adults, CMV infection is often asymptomatic. Symptomatic cases typically present as an "infectious mononucleosis-like" illness, with fever, lymphocytosis, hepatosplenomegaly, lymphadenopathy, and rash. A minority of cases also presents with jaundice, and occasional cases of fulminant hepatitis have been reported.[73]

Immunosuppressed hosts

In this population, the presentation of CMV infection/hepatitis is highly variable and overall similar to that seen in the liver transplant population (refer to Chapter 20).

Histologic features and differential diagnosis

CMV inclusions represent the only specific histologic finding. The histological/cytological features (described in detail in Chapter 20) are similar regardless of the clinical context. In the neonatal population, CMV may present histologically as a nonspecific acute hepatitis or show a giant cell hepatitis pattern (Fig. 8.20). Typical CMV inclusions on H&E, however, are usually absent. In immunocompetent teenagers and adults, the most common histologic picture is similar to what is seen in Epstein–Barr virus (EBV)-related hepatitis, with predominantly lobular (sinusoidal)

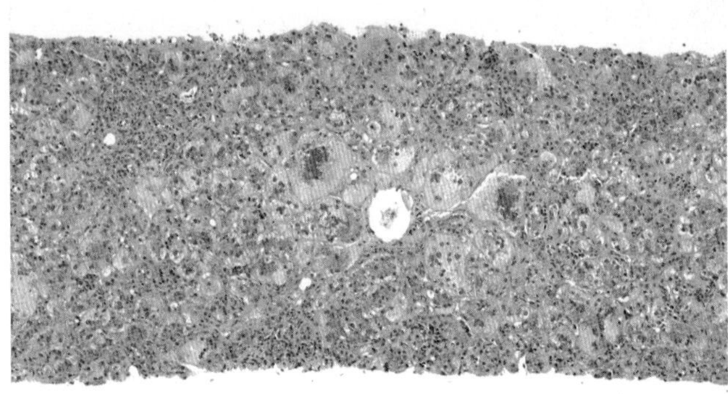

Figure 8.20 Cytomegalovirus, giant cell hepatitis. This case of congenital cytomegalovirus infection showed prominent and diffuse giant cell transformation of hepatocytes with associated cholestasis and pronounced lobular disarray.

infiltrates by lymphocytes, generally mild lobular necroinflammation, Kupffer cell hyperplasia, and typically mild portal inflammation (i.e. mononucleosis-like histologic pattern). Occasional lobular microabscesses can be seen in some cases (Fig. 8.21). In nonliver transplant immunosuppressed hosts (i.e., HIV, primary immunodeficiency, immunosuppressive medications, or chemotherapy), the histologic features of CMV infection and its differential are largely analogous to those seen in the transplant setting.

Prognosis and treatment

The majority of primary CMV infections in immunocompetent individuals are self-limited and do not require antiviral therapy. Severe cases of CMV cholestatic hepatitis may be treated with ganciclovir[74] or valganciclovir.[75]

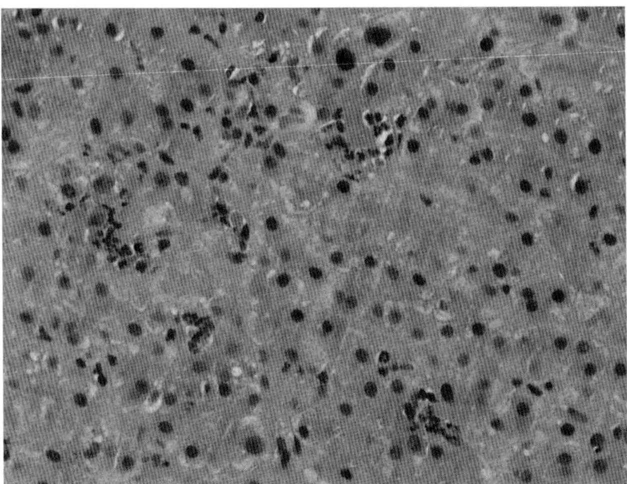

Figure 8.21 Cytomegalovirus microabscesses. Several clusters of neutrophils around apoptotic hepatocytes (microabscesses) are seen in this field. This finding is often associated with CMV infection.

8.7 EPSTEIN–BARR VIRUS

Etiology and pathogenesis

EBV is a double-stranded DNA enveloped virus transmitted predominantly through an oral–oral route and can cause disease in immunocompetent or immunosuppressed hosts by primary infection, reactivation, or reinfection. Immediately after infection, EBV replicates within epithelial cells in the upper respiratory tract, subsequently infecting B lymphocytes and reaching other organs thorough the systemic circulation. EBV then elicits a CD8+ T cell response, linked to its systemic manifestations and organ damage.

Histologic features

EBV hepatitis is histologically highly variable. Most cases present with a nonspecific "acute hepatitis" pattern. A "mononucleosis pattern" can also be seen, characterized by prominent sinusoidal lymphocytic infiltrates, which is often referred as a "beaded pattern," with generally mild nonspecific portal inflammation and mild hepatocyte injury. There can be a prominent Kupffer cell hyperplasia as well as small epithelioid granulomas. Fibrin ring granulomas can rarely be seen. EBV infection in immunosuppressed patients can also lead to lymphoma (see Chapter 20).

8.8 HERPES SIMPLEX VIRUS

Etiology, pathogenesis, and clinical findings

Herpes Simplex virus (HSV) hepatitis can be caused by either HSV Type I or HSV Type II and can represent reactivation, reinfection, or primary infection. Liver involvement (i.e., HSV hepatitis), although fairly uncommon, is often associated with massive/fulminant liver failure, leading to death in the majority of cases. Many patients are immunosuppressed, and approximately one-third of cases occur in the setting of solid organ or bone marrow transplantation. In the setting of solid organ transplantation, HSV tends to occur in the early posttransplant period (days 5 to 46).[77]

Liver enzymes typically show a hepatitic pattern, with marked transaminase elevations, commonly associated with signs of acute/fulminant liver failure, including coagulopathy and encephalopathy.

Mucocutaneous herpetic rashes can be important clinical clues, but are seen in less than half of cases, where they can be either localized or disseminated. The majority of cases reported in the literature were clinically unsuspected before tissue confirmation (either on autopsy or biopsy).[76,77] The diagnosis of HSV hepatitis can be established by PCR assays from tissue sampling or blood, which has replaced tissue culture and direct fluorescent antibody as the preferred diagnostic test.[78] Serology testing is not useful for diagnosis.

Histologic findings

The typical histologic pattern of HSV hepatitis is characterized by relatively well-demarcated ("punched out") areas of necrosis that vary from small necrotic foci involving a few hepatocytes, often surrounded by macrophages and neutrophils, to massive areas of geographic necrosis. HSV cytopathic effect generally involves hepatocytes adjacent to necrotic areas and is characterized by either a distinct nuclear inclusion surrounded by a halo (Cowdry type A) or, most commonly, by a diffuse glassy nuclear appearance, with margination of the chromatin toward the edge of the nucleus (Cowdry type B). Syncytial giant cell transformation and multinucleation of affected hepatocytes is also common, and molding of juxtaposed infected nuclei may be present in some cases. The "3 M's" of HSV cytopathic effect is a useful mnemonic and stands for margination, multinucleation, and molding (see Chapter 20). The inclusions can be subtle and should be confirmed by immunostains.

Special stains and immunostains

Specific antibodies directed to HSV 1 and HSV 2 (and combined HSV1/2) by immunohistochemistry are very helpful and should be used to confirm the H&E findings.

Differential diagnosis

Typical cases generally pose little diagnostic difficulty. In many cases, however, areas of cytopathic effect may be sparse and obscured by the necrotic debris. In addition, hepatocytes undergoing necrosis or apoptosis will commonly show some degree of nuclear "smudging" which is a common diagnostic pitfall. CMV nuclear inclusions can mimic HSV cytopathic effect but are often associated with cytoplasmic inclusions, which are not seen in HSV infection. Adenovirus is also in the differential because it may cause geographic areas of liver parenchymal necrosis and similar nuclear inclusions. Neither CMV nor adenovirus, however, shows hepatocyte multinucleation, which suggests HSV infection when present. Varicella-Zoster Virus (VZV) is very rare but shares most of the histologic changes with HSV and cannot be reliably distinguished from the latter without the aid of immunohistochemistry.

Prognosis and treatment

Although sampling may represent a problem given the patchy/geographic nature of the diseases, the degree of liver involvement on biopsies has prognostic implications. In one study, all patients with "diffuse disease" (presumably necrosis) died, while nearly half of the patients with "focal disease" survived.[77] Disseminated, visceral or extensive cutaneous, or mucosal HSV infection is treated with intravenous acyclovir.[79] Foscarnet can be used for acyclovir-resistance HSV infection.[80]

8.9 ADENOVIRUS

Adenovirus—a double-stranded DNA virus—is a common cause of upper respiratory tract infection in children. Like EBV, adenovirus remains latent within lymphoid cells and can occasionally cause hepatitis when reactivated due to immunodeficiency or therapeutic immunosuppression.

Histologic features and differential diagnosis

Adenovirus-related liver disease typically presents clinically and histologically as a moderate to severe hepatitis with numerous, randomly distributed "punched out" areas of parenchymal necrosis. The diagnosis can be suggested by adenovirus-type nuclear inclusions, typically found along the edges of necrotic

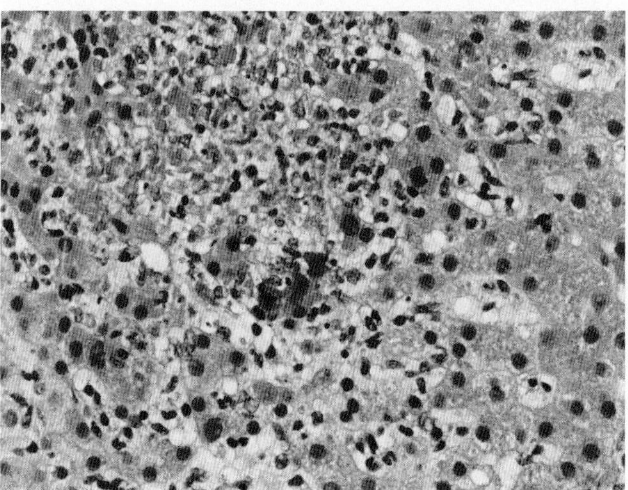

Figure 8.22 Adenovirus. "Punched out" areas of necrosis are typical for adenovirus hepatitis, often with the presence of subtle nuclear smudging of hepatocytes immediately around necrotic areas.

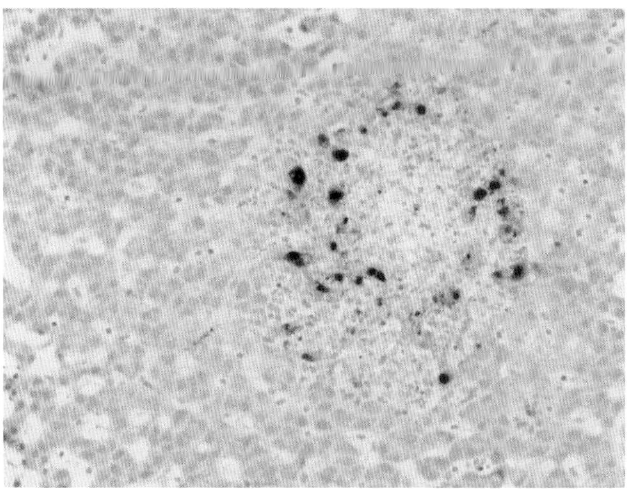

Figure 8.23 Adenovirus. In situ hybridization highlighting adenovirus-infected cells (nuclei) around a small necrotic area.

areas, characterized by slightly basophilic, glassy material that replaces most of the nucleus and leads to a "smudgy" appearance (somewhat similar to HSV inclusions, but without multinucleation) (Fig. 8.22). These nuclear changes are sometimes associated with basophilic cytoplasmic aggregates, thought to represent viral material. Variable nonspecific portal and lobular inflammation (typically mild) may also be seen. When inclusions are present, the main differential diagnosis is with HSV infection, which can also cause well-delineated areas of necrosis, similar to the pattern seen in adenovirus. Although the nuclear inclusions are also rather similar, prominent multinucleation is common in HSV infection but not in adenovirus infection. Although very rare, cases of VZV hepatitis may also show overlapping histologic features and should be considered in the differential. Ischemic necrosis and acetaminophen toxicity are also associated with well-defined areas of necrosis, but these are zonal in nature (centrilobular), in contrast to the nonzonal pattern seen in adenovirus infection. Nuclear inclusions are absent in these cases.

Immunohistochemistry

Immunostains and in situ hybridization studies (Fig. 8.23) for adenovirus are available and can be very helpful in confirming the diagnosis, especially in cases with suspicious but nondiagnostic nuclear inclusions (Fig. 8.23).

8.10 VARICELLA-ZOSTER VIRUS

VZV hepatitis is rare and typically occurs in the setting of disseminated VZV infection, almost exclusively in immunocompromised patients. The histologic findings and the viral cytopathic effect seen in VZV infection overlap significantly with adenovirus and HSV. Specific immunohistochemical antibodies are available and are very useful. We have seen some cross-reactivity with HSV antibodies (typically week), which could represent a diagnostic pitfall.

8.11 MISCELLANEOUS VIRUSES

Several other viruses have been associated with hepatitis of various degrees of severity. HHV-6 and parvovirus, both predominantly seen in childhood in the form of systemic viral illnesses (exanthema subitum and erythema infectiosum, respectively), have been associated with cases of acute hepatitis, including occasional fulminant cases. In tropical and subtropical regions of the world, mosquito-borne diseases such as yellow fever and dengue are rather common, often occurring in epidemics. In cases of yellow fever, there can be hemorrhagic hepatocyte necrosis with a predominantly zone 2 distribution (panacinar in more severe cases). The recognition of rims of preserved hepatocytes around portal structures and central veins represents a useful histologic hint for the zone 2-predominant nature of this infection. Numerous acidophil (Councilman) bodies in the lobules are also typical. Specific immunohistochemical antibodies are available in some centers within endemic areas. Otherwise, correlation with travel history and clinical/laboratory diagnosis of the disease is essential.

In dengue fever, liver involvement is typically seen in severe (hemorrhagic) forms of the disease and is thought to be largely due to endothelial cell injury related to the infection. Like yellow fever, there may be a predominantly zone 2 pattern of necrosis (typically with sparse inflammation). But contrary to yellow fever, periportal and centrilobular necrosis are also common.

REFERENCES

1. Scheuer PJ. Liver biopsy size matters in chronic hepatitis: bigger is better. *Hepatology*. 2003;38(6):1356–1358. doi:10.1016/j.hep.2003.10.010.
2. Colloredo G, Guido M, Sonzogni A, et al. Impact of liver biopsy size on histological evaluation of chronic viral hepatitis: the smaller the sample, the milder the disease. *J Hepatol*. 2003;39(2):239–244. http://www.ncbi.nlm.nih.gov/pubmed/12873821. Accessed August 26, 2016.
3. Brunetti E, Silini E, Pistorio A, et al. Coarse vs. fine needle aspiration biopsy for the assessment of diffuse liver disease from hepatitis C virus-related

chronic hepatitis. *J Hepatol*. 2004;40(3):501–506. doi:10.1016/j.jhep.2003.11.008.

4. Knodell RG, Ishak KG, Black WC, et al. Formulation and application of a numerical scoring system for assessing histological activity in asymptomatic chronic active hepatitis. *Hepatology*. 1981;1(5):431–435. http://www.ncbi.nlm.nih.gov/pubmed/7308988. Accessed August 26, 2016.
5. Tong MJ, el-Farra NS, Grew MI. Clinical manifestations of hepatitis A: recent experience in a community teaching hospital. *J Infect Dis*. 1995;171(1):S15–S18. http://www.ncbi.nlm.nih.gov/pubmed/7876641. Accessed November 13, 2016.
6. Liaw YF, Yang CY, Chu CM, et al. Appearance and persistence of hepatitis A IgM antibody in acute clinical hepatitis A observed in an outbreak. *Infection*. 1986;14(4):156–158. http://www.ncbi.nlm.nih.gov/pubmed/3759243. Accessed November 13, 2016.
7. Ciocca M. Clinical course and consequences of hepatitis A infection. *Vaccine*. 2000;18 suppl 1:S71–S74. http://www.ncbi.nlm.nih.gov/pubmed/10683554. Accessed November 13, 2016.
8. Jeong S-H, Lee H-S. Hepatitis A: clinical manifestations and management. *Intervirology*. 2010;53(1):15–19. doi:10.1159/000252779.
9. Abe H, Beninger PR, Ikejiri N, et al. Light microscopic findings of liver biopsy specimens from patients with hepatitis type A and comparison with type B. *Gastroenterology*. 1982;82(5 Pt 1):938–947. http://www.ncbi.nlm.nih.gov/pubmed/6174391. Accessed August 26, 2016.
10. Masada CT, Shaw BW, Zetterman RK, et al. Fulminant hepatic failure with massive necrosis as a result of hepatitis A infection. *J Clin Gastroenterol*. 1993;17(2):158–162. http://www.ncbi.nlm.nih.gov/pubmed/8409320. Accessed August 26, 2016.
11. Taylor RM, Davern T, Munoz S, et al. Fulminant hepatitis A virus infection in the United States: incidence, prognosis, and outcomes. *Hepatology*. 2006;44(6):1589–1597. doi:10.1002/hep.21439.
12. Schweitzer A, Horn J, Mikolajczyk RT, et al. Estimations of worldwide prevalence of chronic hepatitis B virus infection: a systematic review of data published between 1965 and 2013. *Lancet*. 2015;386(10003):1546–1555. doi:10.1016/S0140-6736(15)61412-X.
13. El-Serag HB. Epidemiology of viral hepatitis and hepatocellular carcinoma. *Gastroenterology*. 2012;142(6):1264-1273.e1. doi:10.1053/j.gastro.2011.12.061.
14. Kao J-H, Chen P-J, Lai M-Y, et al. Basal core promoter mutations of hepatitis B virus increase the risk of hepatocellular carcinoma in hepatitis B carriers. *Gastroenterology*. 2003;124(2):327-334. doi:10.1053/gast.2003.50053.
15. Ni Y-H, Chang M-H, Wang K-J, et al. Clinical relevance of hepatitis B virus genotype in children with chronic infection and hepatocellular carcinoma. *Gastroenterology*. 2004;127(6):1733-1738. http://www.ncbi.nlm.nih.gov/pubmed/15578511. Accessed August 27, 2016.
16. Liu C-J, Chen B-F, Chen P-J, et al. Role of hepatitis B viral load and basal core promoter mutation in hepatocellular carcinoma in hepatitis B carriers. *J Infect Dis*. 2006;193(9):1258-1265. doi:10.1086/502978.
17. Yang H-I, Yeh S-H, Chen P-J, et al. Associations between hepatitis B virus genotype and mutants and the risk of hepatocellular carcinoma. *J Natl Cancer Inst*. 2008;100(16):1134-1143. doi:10.1093/jnci/djn243.
18. Hadziyannis SJ, Vassilopoulos D. Hepatitis B e antigen-negative chronic hepatitis B. *Hepatology*. 2001;34(4 Pt 1):617–624. doi:10.1053/jhep.2001.27834.
19. Locarnini S, McMillan J, Bartholomeusz A. The hepatitis B virus and common mutants. *Semin Liver Dis*. 2003;23(1):5–20. doi:10.1055/s-2003-37587.
20. Lai C-L, Dienstag J, Schiff E, et al. Prevalence and clinical correlates of YMDD variants during lamivudine therapy for patients with chronic hepatitis B. *Clin Infect Dis*. 2003;36(6):687–696. doi:10.1086/368083.
21. Caredda F, Rossi E, d'Arminio Monforte A, et al. Hepatitis B virus-associated coinfection and superinfection with delta agent: indistinguishable disease with different outcome. *J Infect Dis*. 1985;151(5):925–928. http://www.ncbi.nlm.nih.gov/pubmed/3989325. Accessed August 28, 2016.
22. Abiad H, Ramani R, Currie JB, et al. The natural history of hepatitis D virus infection in Illinois state facilities for the developmentally disabled. *Am J Gastroenterol*. 2001;96(2):534–540. doi:10.1111/j.1572-0241.2001.03555.x.
23. Han S-HB. Extrahepatic manifestations of chronic hepatitis B. *Clin Liver Dis*. 2004;8(2):403–418. http://www.ncbi.nlm.nih.gov/pubmed/15481347. Accessed November 13, 2016.
24. Hatzakis A, Magiorkinis E, Haida C. HBV virological assessment. *J Hepatol*. 2006;44(1 suppl):S71–S76. doi:10.1016/j.jhep.2005.11.017.
25. Bianchi L, Gudat F. Sanded nuclei in hepatitis B: eosinophilic inclusions in liver cell nuclei due to excess in hepatitis B core antigen formation. *Lab Invest*. 1976;35(1):1–5. http://www.ncbi.nlm.nih.gov/pubmed/781402. Accessed August 28, 2016.
26. O'Grady JG, Smith HM, Davies SE, et al. Hepatitis B virus reinfection after orthotopic liver transplantation. Serological and clinical implications. *J Hepatol*. 1992;14(1):104–111. http://www.ncbi.nlm.nih.gov/pubmed/1737910. Accessed November 15, 2016.
27. Davies SE, Portmann BC, O'Grady JG, et al. Hepatic histological findings after transplantation for

chronic hepatitis B virus infection, including a unique pattern of fibrosing cholestatic hepatitis. *Hepatology*. 1991;13(1):150–157. http://www.ncbi.nlm.nih.gov/pubmed/1988336.

28. Xiao S-Y, Lu L, Wang HL. Fibrosing cholestatic hepatitis: clinicopathologic spectrum, diagnosis and pathogenesis. *Int J Clin Exp Pathol*. 2008;1(5):396–402. http://www.pubmedcentral.nih.gov/articlerender.fcgi?artid=2480579&tool=pmcentrez&rendertype=abstract.
29. Chu CM, Liaw YF. Immunohistological study of intrahepatic expression of hepatitis B core and E antigens in chronic type B hepatitis. *J Clin Pathol*. 1992;45(9):791–795. http://www.ncbi.nlm.nih.gov/pubmed/1401209. Accessed August 28, 2016.
30. Trevisan A, Gudat F, Busachi C, et al. An improved method for HBcAg demonstration in paraffin-embedded liver tissue. *Liver*. 1982;2(4):331–339. http://www.ncbi.nlm.nih.gov/pubmed/6762478. Accessed August 28, 2016.
31. Chu CM, Yeh CT, Chien RN, et al. The degrees of hepatocyte nuclear but not cytoplasmic expression of hepatitis B core antigen reflect the level of viral replication in chronic hepatitis B virus infection. *J Clin Microbiol*. 1997;35(1):102–105. http://www.ncbi.nlm.nih.gov/pubmed/8968888. Accessed August 28, 2016.
32. Ballaré M, Lavarini C, Brunetto MR, et al. Relationship between the intrahepatic expression of "e" and "c" epitopes of the nucleocapsid protein of hepatitis B virus and viraemia. *Clin Exp Immunol*. 1989;75(1):64–69. http://www.ncbi.nlm.nih.gov/pubmed/2467769. Accessed August 28, 2016.
33. Serinoz E, Varli M, Erden E, et al. Nuclear localization of hepatitis B core antigen and its relations to liver injury, hepatocyte proliferation, and viral load. *J Clin Gastroenterol*. 2003;36(3):269–272. http://www.ncbi.nlm.nih.gov/pubmed/12590241. Accessed August 28, 2016.
34. Farci P, Diaz G, Chen Z, et al. B cell gene signature with massive intrahepatic production of antibodies to hepatitis B core antigen in hepatitis B virus-associated acute liver failure. *Proc Natl Acad Sci U S A*. 2010;107(19):8766–8771. doi:10.1073/pnas.1003854107.
35. Bean P. Latest discoveries on the infection and coinfection with hepatitis D virus. *Am Clin Lab*. 2002;21(5):25–27. http://www.ncbi.nlm.nih.gov/pubmed/12122781. Accessed August 28, 2016.
36. Shepard CW, Simard EP, Finelli L, et al. Hepatitis B virus infection: epidemiology and vaccination. *Epidemiol Rev*. 2006;28(1):112–125. doi:10.1093/epirev/mxj009.
37. European Association For The Study Of The Liver. EASL clinical practice guidelines: management of chronic hepatitis B virus infection. *J Hepatol*. 2012;57(1):167–185. doi:10.1016/j.jhep.2012.02.010.
38. Martin P, Lau DT-Y, Nguyen MH, et al. A treatment algorithm for the management of chronic hepatitis B virus infection in the United States: 2015 update. *Clin Gastroenterol Hepatol*. 2015;13(12):2071–87.e16. doi:10.1016/j.cgh.2015.07.007.
39. Wedemeyer H, Yurdaydìn C, Dalekos GN, et al. Peginterferon plus adefovir versus either drug alone for hepatitis delta. *N Engl J Med*. 2011;364(4):322–331. doi:10.1056/NEJMoa0912696.
40. Chen C-J, Yang H-I. Natural history of chronic hepatitis B REVEALed. *J Gastroenterol Hepatol*. 2011;26(4):628–638. doi:10.1111/j.1440-1746.2011.06695.x.
41. Poh Z, Goh B-BG, Chang P-EJ, et al. Rates of cirrhosis and hepatocellular carcinoma in chronic hepatitis B and the role of surveillance. *Eur J Gastroenterol Hepatol*. 2015;27(6):638–643. doi:10.1097/MEG.0000000000000341.
42. Mohd Hanafiah K, Groeger J, Flaxman AD, et al. Global epidemiology of hepatitis C virus infection: new estimates of age-specific antibody to HCV seroprevalence. *Hepatology*. 2013;57(4):1333–1342. doi:10.1002/hep.26141.
43. Averhoff FM, Glass N, Holtzman D. Global burden of hepatitis C: considerations for healthcare providers in the United States. *Clin Infect Dis*. 2012;55(suppl 1):S10–S15. doi:10.1093/cid/cis361.
44. Terrault NA. Sexual activity as a risk factor for hepatitis C. *Hepatology*. 2002;36(5 suppl 1):S99–S105. doi:10.1053/jhep.2002.36797.
45. Thomas DL, Seeff LB. Natural history of hepatitis C. *Clin Liver Dis*. 2005;9(3):383–398, vi. doi:10.1016/j.cld.2005.05.003.
46. Eyster ME, Alter HJ, Aledort LM, et al. Heterosexual co-transmission of hepatitis C virus (HCV) and human immunodeficiency virus (HIV). *Ann Intern Med*. 1991;115(10):764–768. http://www.ncbi.nlm.nih.gov/pubmed/1656825. Accessed August 14, 2016.
47. Roberts EA, Yeung L. Maternal-infant transmission of hepatitis C virus infection. *Hepatology*. 2002;36(5 suppl 1):S106–S113. doi:10.1053/jhep.2002.36792.
48. Westbrook RH, Dusheiko G. Natural history of hepatitis C. *J Hepatol*. 2014;61(1 suppl):S58–S68. doi:10.1016/j.jhep.2014.07.012.
49. Lerat H, Hollinger FB. Hepatitis C virus (HCV) occult infection or occult HCV RNA detection? *J Infect Dis*. 2004;189(1):3–6. doi:10.1086/380203.
50. Goutagny N, Fatmi A, Ledinghen VD, et al. Evidence of viral replication in circulating dendritic cells during hepatitis C virus infection. *J Infect Dis*. 2003;187(12):1951–1958. doi:10.1086/375350.
51. Di Lello FA, Culasso ACA, Campos RH. Inter and intrapatient evolution of hepatitis C virus. *Ann Hepatol*. 2015;14(4):442–449. http://www.ncbi.nlm.nih.gov/pubmed/26019029. Accessed August 14, 2016.

52. Echeverría N, Moratorio G, Cristina J, et al. Hepatitis C virus genetic variability and evolution. *World J Hepatol*. 2015;7(6):831–845. doi:10.4254/wjh.v7.i6.831.
53. Johnson K, Kotiesh A, Boitnott JK, et al. Histology of symptomatic acute hepatitis C infection in immunocompetent adults. *Am J Surg Pathol*. 2007;31(11):1754–1758. doi:10.1097/PAS.0b013e318093f90e.
54. Jacobson IM, Cacoub P, Dal Maso L, et al. Manifestations of chronic hepatitis C virus infection beyond the liver. *Clin Gastroenterol Hepatol*. 2010;8(12):1017–1029. doi:10.1016/j.cgh.2010.08.026.
55. Tsuang W, Subramanian R, Liu Q, et al. The need for liver biopsy in a patient with acute HCV infection. *Nat Clin Pract Gastroenterol Hepatol*. 2008;5(1):54–57. doi:10.1038/ncpgasthep1030.
56. Luo JC, Hwang SJ, Lai CR, et al. Clinical significance of portal lymphoid aggregates/follicles in Chinese patients with chronic hepatitis C. *Am J Gastroenterol*. 1999;94(4):1006–1011. doi:10.1111/j.1572-0241.1999.01004.x.
57. Mihm S, Fayyazi A, Hartmann H, et al. Analysis of histopathological manifestations of chronic hepatitis C virus infection with respect to virus genotype. *Hepatology*. 1997;25(3):735–739. doi:10.1002/hep.510250340.
58. Souza P, Prihoda TJ, Hoyumpa AM, et al. Morphologic features resembling transplant rejection in core biopsies of native livers from patients with Hepatitis C. *Hum Pathol*. 2009;40(1):92–97. doi:10.1016/j.humpath.2008.06.020.
59. French SW, Enbom ET. Piecemeal necrosis of the liver revisited a review. *Exp Mol Pathol*. 2014;96(3):307–309. doi:10.1016/j.yexmp.2014.03.009.
60. González-Reimers E, Quintero-Platt G, Rodríguez-Gaspar M, et al. Liver steatosis in hepatitis C patients. *World J Hepatol*. 2015;7(10):1337–1346. doi:10.4254/wjh.v7.i10.1337.
61. Kralj D, Virović Jukić L, Stojsavljević S, et al. Hepatitis C virus, insulin resistance, and steatosis. *J Clin Transl Hepatol*. 2016;4(1):66–75. doi:10.14218/JCTH.2015.00051.
62. Micchelli STL, Thomas D, Boitnott JK, et al. Hepatic giant cells in hepatitis C virus (HCV) mono-infection and HCV/HIV co-infection. *J Clin Pathol*. 2008;61(9):1058–1061. doi:10.1136/jcp.2008.058560.
63. Foka P, Dimitriadis A, Karamichali E, et al. Alterations in the iron homeostasis network: a driving force for macrophage-mediated hepatitis C virus persistency. *Virulence*. 2016;7(6):679–690. doi:10.1080/21505594.2016.1175700.
64. Adinolfi LE, Rinaldi L, Guerrera B, et al. NAFLD and NASH in HCV infection: prevalence and significance in hepatic and extrahepatic manifestations. *Int J Mol Sci*. 2016;17(6):pii: E803. doi:10.3390/ijms17060803.
65. Federico A, Ormando VM, Dallio M, et al. Alcoholic liver disease and hepatitis C chronic infection. *Rev Recent Clin Trials*. 2016;11(3):201–207. http://www.ncbi.nlm.nih.gov/pubmed/27457351. Accessed August 15, 2016.
66. Zhang Y-H, Zhao Y, Rajapaksa US, et al. A comprehensive analysis of the impact of HIV on HCV immune responses and its association with liver disease progression in a unique plasma donor cohort. *PLoS One*. 2016;11(7):e0158037. doi:10.1371/journal.pone.0158037.
67. Morgan RL, Baack B, Smith BD, et al. Eradication of hepatitis C virus infection and the development of hepatocellular carcinoma. *Ann Intern Med*. 2013;158(5 Pt 1):329. doi:10.7326/0003-4819-158-5-201303050-00005.
68. van der Meer AJ, Veldt BJ, Feld JJ, et al. Association between sustained virological response and all-cause mortality among patients with chronic hepatitis c and advanced hepatic fibrosis. *JAMA*. 2012;308(24):2584. doi:10.1001/jama.2012.144878.
69. Lhomme S, Marion O, Abravanel F, et al. Hepatitis E pathogenesis. *Viruses*. 2016;8(8):E212. doi:10.3390/v8080212.
70. Unzueta A, Rakela J. Hepatitis E infection in liver transplant recipients. *Liver Transpl*. 2014;20(1):15–24. doi:10.1002/lt.23764.
71. Sue PK, Pisanic N, Heaney CD, et al. Hepatitis E virus infection among solid organ transplant recipients at a north american transplant center. *Open forum Infect Dis*. 2016;3(1):ofw006. doi:10.1093/ofid/ofw006.
72. Dalton HR, Kamar N. Treatment of hepatitis E virus. *Curr Opin Infect Dis*. 2016;29(6):639–644. doi:10.1097/QCO.0000000000000316.
73. Yu Y-D, Park G-C, Park P-J, et al. Cytomegalovirus infection-associated fulminant hepatitis in an immunocompetent adult requiring emergency living-donor liver transplantation: report of a case. *Surg Today*. 2013;43(4):424–428. doi:10.1007/s00595-012-0209-6.
74. Serna-Higuera C, González-García M, Milicua JM, et al. Acute cholestatic hepatitis by cytomegalovirus in an immunocompetent patient resolved with ganciclovir. *J Clin Gastroenterol*. 1999;29(3):276–277. http://www.ncbi.nlm.nih.gov/pubmed/10509956. Accessed November 13, 2016.
75. Fernández-Ruiz M, Muñoz-Codoceo C, López-Medrano F, et al. Cytomegalovirus myopericarditis and hepatitis in an immunocompetent adult: successful treatment with oral valganciclovir. *Intern Med*.

2008;47(22):1963–1966. http://www.ncbi.nlm.nih.gov/pubmed/19015608. Accessed November 13, 2016.

76. Norvell JP, Blei AT, Jovanovic BD, et al. Herpes simplex virus hepatitis: an analysis of the published literature and institutional cases. *Liver Transpl.* 2007;13(10):1428–1434. doi:10.1002/lt.21250.

77. Kusne S, Schwartz M, Breinig MK, et al. Herpes simplex virus hepatitis after solid organ transplantation in adults. *J Infect Dis.* 1991;163(5):1001–1007. http://www.ncbi.nlm.nih.gov/pubmed/1850439. Accessed June 25, 2016.

78. Wald A, Huang M-L, Carrell D, et al. Polymerase chain reaction for detection of herpes simplex virus (HSV) DNA on mucosal surfaces: comparison with HSV isolation in cell culture. *J Infect Dis.* 2003;188(9):1345–1351. doi:10.1086/379043.

79. Basse G, Mengelle C, Kamar N, et al. Disseminated herpes simplex type-2 (HSV-2) infection after solid-organ transplantation. *Infection.* 2008;36(1):62–64. doi:10.1007/s15010-007-6366-7.

80. Safrin S, Crumpacker C, Chatis P, et al. A controlled trial comparing foscarnet with vidarabine for acyclovir-resistant mucocutaneous herpes simplex in the acquired immunodeficiency syndrome. The AIDS Clinical Trials Group. *N Engl J Med.* 1991;325(8):551–555. doi:10.1056/NEJM199108223250805.

81. Scheuer PJ. Classification of chronic viral hepatitis: a need for reassessment. *J Hepatol.* 1991;13(3):372–374. http://www.ncbi.nlm.nih.gov/pubmed/1808228. Accessed October 22, 2016.

82. Batts KP, Ludwig J. Chronic hepatitis. An update on terminology and reporting. *Am J Surg Pathol.* 1995;19(12):1409–1417. http://www.ncbi.nlm.nih.gov/pubmed/7503362. Accessed October 22, 2016.

83. Bedossa P, Poynard T. An algorithm for the grading of activity in chronic hepatitis C. The METAVIR Cooperative Study Group. *Hepatology.* 1996;24(2):289–293. doi:10.1002/hep.510240201.

84. Callea F, Grootes J De, Gudat F, et al. Histological grading and staging of chronic hepatitis. 1995;22(6):696–699.

9 Parasites in the liver

Bobbi S. Pritt, MD, MSc

9.1 INTRODUCTION

Parasites are an important cause of infections in the liver and biliary tract and are responsible for significant morbidity and mortality in many parts of the world.[1,2] The spectrum of parasites includes single-celled protozoa, as well as multicellular roundworms (nematodes), tapeworms (cestodes), flukes (trematodes), and rarely, arthropods (Tables 9.1, 9.2, 9.3, 9.4, and 9.5). Several parasitic infections are classified by the World Health Organization (WHO) as neglected tropical diseases on the basis of their impact on billions of individuals living in developing countries.[1] The Centers for Disease Control and Prevention (CDC) has also identified five neglected parasitic infections in the United States as priorities for public health action, of which four can involve the liver.[3] This chapter will focus on the most important members of these groups that are likely to be encountered by the anatomic pathologist. It is important to note that the prevalence of these parasites varies widely with the travel history and immune status of the host. It is therefore essential to obtain a good clinical history when evaluating a specimen for parasites.

9.2 PROTOZOA

Entamoeba histolytica (amebiasis, amebic liver abscess)

Definition, etiology, and pathogenesis

The term *amebiasis* refers to infection with the parasitic ameba, *Entamoeba histolytica*. This protozoan causes primary intestinal infection and is a rare but important cause of liver disease.[4,5] Transmission is through the fecal–oral route, in which individuals become infected primarily through ingestion of cysts in fecally contaminated food and water.[6] It is, therefore, unsurprising that infection is most common in resource-limited settings where poor sanitary conditions exist. In developed countries, infection is usually limited to travelers and immigrants from endemic areas.[4] It is estimated that 1% of the world's population (74,000,000 individuals) is infected with *E. histolytica* and that there are approximately 50 million symptomatic cases and 100,000 deaths each year.[7]

Following ingestion of the infectious cyst form, the parasite excysts and releases a trophozoite, which colonizes the large intestine and replicates by binary fission.[6US] Some trophozoites eventually form

Table 9.1 Protozoan infections of the human liver

Parasite (infection)	Pathology	Epidemiology
Cryptosporidium spp. (cryptosporidiosis)[a]	Cholangitis; intracellular parasites in bile duct epithelium below the brush border; extension from intestinal disease	Worldwide, usually profoundly immunocompromised hosts
Cyclospora cayetanensis (cyclosporiasis)	Cholangitis; intracellular parasites in the cytoplasm of bile duct epithelial cells; extension from intestinal disease	Regions of the tropics and subtropics with poor sanitation; outbreaks in nonendemic countries due to imported produce
Cystoisospora (*Isospora*) *belli* (cyclosporiasis)	Cholangitis; intracellular parasites in the cytoplasm of bile duct epithelial cells; extension from intestinal disease	Regions of the tropics and subtropics with poor sanitation
Entamoeba histolytica[a,b] (amebiasis)	Acute nonsuppurative hepatitis and hepatic abscess (i.e., pseudoabscess); can involve an entire lobe. Extracellular trophozoites primarily at periphery of lesion; concurrent intestinal disease may be absent.	Regions of the tropics and subtropics with poor sanitation
Leishmania spp.[a] (visceral leishmaniasis, kala-azar)	Hepatomegaly (may be massive) due to parasite infiltration, fibrosis; amastigotes within Kupffer cells; Usually concurrent lymph node, spleen, and bone marrow involvement	Tropics and subtropics
Plasmodium falciparum[a] (malaria)	Hepatomegaly, gray-black decolorization due to hemozoin pigment in macrophages and infected erythrocytes; component of systemic disease	Tropics and subtropics
Toxoplasma gondii[a] (toxoplasmosis)	Hepatomegaly, hepatocellular necrosis; intracellular and extracellular tachyzoites in necrotic regions. Liver involvement is rare and a component of systemic disseminated disease.	Worldwide; usually neonates and profoundly immunocompromised hosts

[a]Most common parasites causing human disease.
[b]The term *amebiasis* is most commonly used to describe infection with *Entamoeba histolytica* but may also be used to describe infection with the free-living amebae.

Table 9.2 Nematode (roundworm) infections of the human liver

Parasite (infection)	Pathology	Epidemiology
Ascaris lumbricoides[a] (ascariasis)	Cholangitis, biliary obstruction due to ectopic migration of adult worm; pyogenic abscess and eggs in liver; concurrent intestinal infection	Regions of the tropics and subtropics worldwide with poor sanitation
Baylisascaris procyonis (baylisascariasis, visceral larva migrans)	Hepatomegaly, sinuous tracts formed by migrating larvae, necrosis, and eosinophilic abscesses; larvae rarely seen in histologic sections	North America and other locations where raccoons are found
Capillaria hepatica (hepatic capillariasis)	Hepatomegaly, remnants of adults and eggs within hepatic granulomas	Worldwide; rare cases reported
Filarial worms: *Wuchereria bancrofti, Brugia malayi, B. timori* (filariasis)	Pericaval filariasis with obliterative hepatocavopathy and Budd–Chiari syndrome due to obstruction by the adult worm	Asia (India, Nepal), rare cases of liver involvement reported
Gnathostoma spinigerum (gnathostomiasis)	Visceral larva migrans-like: hepatomegaly, sinuous tracts formed by migrating larvae, necrosis, and eosinophilic abscesses	Primarily regions of Southeast Asia and Mexico where undercooked frog, fish, or snake is ingested
Strongyloides stercoralis[a] (strongyloidiasis, *Strongyloides* hyperinfection syndrome)	Liver involvement with hyperinfection syndrome; abdominal pain, peritoneal signs, hepatomegaly, mild jaundice; usually seen with respiratory and intestinal symptoms; larvae may be seen in histologic sections. Concurrent intestinal infection	Regions of the tropics and subtropics with poor sanitation, including part of the rural southeastern United States (e.g., Appalachia). Hyperinfection in immunocompromised hosts
Toxocara canis and *Toxocara cati*[a] (toxocariasis, visceral larva migrans)	Hepatomegaly, sinuous tracts formed by migrating larvae, necrosis, and eosinophilic abscesses; larvae rarely seen in histologic sections	Worldwide

[a]Most common parasites causing human disease.

Table 9.3 Cestode (tapeworm) infections of the human liver

Parasite (infection)	Pathology	Epidemiology
Echinococcus granulosus[a] (cystic echinococcosis), *E. multilocularis* (alveolar echinococcosis), *E. vogeli* and *E. oligarthrus* (polycystic echinococcosis)	*E. granulosus* causes a slowly growing cyst; may be massive, compress adjacent structures; may contain daughter cysts. Protoscoleces commonly seen. *E. multilocularis* cysts grow in an infiltrative destructive manner, invading extrahepatic structures. Protoscoleces rarely formed. *E. vogeli* and *E. oligarthrus* cause a slowly growing cystic mass, with secondary cysts forming off the initial cyst. Protoscoleces may be present.	*E. granulosus*—Worldwide, rural sheep-rearing regions where dogs ingest viscera of infected animals; most common form; *E. multilocularis*—Rural regions of the northern hemisphere *E. vogeli* and *E. oligarthrus*—Central and South America (rare cases reported)
Spirometra spp. (sparganosis)	Mass ± abscess due to presence of larval form (sparganum)	Worldwide where undercooked frog or snake flesh is ingested or used it as a wound poultice
Taenia solium (cysticercosis)	Hepatomegaly, cysts (cysticerci) formed throughout liver parenchyma. Liver involvement rare; component of systemic infection	Worldwide; found where undercooked pork is ingested (prerequisite for acquiring the intestinal tapeworm and shedding eggs in stool; cysticercosis is acquired via ingestion of eggs)

[a]Most common parasites causing human disease.

cysts, and both cysts and trophozoites are shed in the stool. If the cysts enter the environment and contaminate food or water, then the infection can be passed to other individuals. Infection can also be passed directly through oral–anal intercourse.

The trophozoites are normally commensal organisms that feed on intestinal bacteria and do not cause disease. However, they are also capable of invading the bowel wall and causing amebic colitis. In rare cases, the trophozoites will enter the portal blood supply and disseminate to other organs. Importantly, dissemination can occur months to years after initial infection. The liver is the most common site of extraintestinal spread, with the right lobe being four times more likely to be involved than the left lobe because it receives the majority of venous drainage

Table 9.4 Trematode (fluke) infections of the human liver

Parasite (infection)	Pathology	Epidemiology
Clonorchis sinensis[a] (clonorchiasis)	Cholangitis, choledocholithiasis, cholangiocarcinoma; adult flukes in the bile ducts	Primarily regions of Asia where undercooked fish is ingested
Dicrocoelium dendriticum	Hepatomegaly, liver abscess; adult flukes in the bile ducts	Regions of the Americas, Europe, Asia, and Africa where raw ants are ingested
Fasciola hepatica[a] (fascioliasis)	Hepatomegaly, parenchymal necrosis and fibrosis, cholangitis, biliary obstruction; adult flukes in bile ducts or parenchyma	Worldwide; sheep and cattle-rearing regions where raw watercress is ingested
Metorchis spp. (metorchiasis)	Cholangitis; adult flukes in bile ducts	Regions of North America, Europe, and Asia where undercooked fish is ingested
Opisthorchis spp.[a] (opisthorchiasis)	Cholangitis, choledocholithiasis, cholangiocarcinoma; adult flukes in bile ducts	Regions of Europe, Asia, and Southeast Asia where undercooked fish is ingested
Schistosoma species[a] (schistosomiasis)	Hepatomegaly, portal fibrosis ("pipestem fibrosis") due to egg deposition and granuloma formation	Regions of Asia, Africa, and South America

[a]Most common parasites causing human disease.

Table 9.5 Miscellaneous parasites/parasite-like organisms of the human liver

Parasite (infection)	Liver manifestations	Epidemiology
Pentastomids[a]		
Armillifer spp., *Linguatula serrata* (pentastomiasis)	Motile nodule (larval parasite) in the liver parenchyma or peritoneal tissue around the liver	Worldwide; highest prevalence in the Middle East where individuals have close contact to infected dogs and in Africa and Asia where undercooked snake flesh is ingested
Fungi-like organisms (previously considered parasites)		
Microsporidia species (microsporidiosis)	Cholangitis, hepatic necrosis; liver involvement is a component of systemic disease	Worldwide; profoundly immunocompromised hosts

[a]Pentastomids (a.k.a. "tongue worms") are genetically related to arthropods, although their exact taxonomic placement is unclear.

from the right colon.[8] Extraintestinal spread can also occur because of direct intraperitoneal spread.[8] In the liver, invasive trophozoites release chemical mediators, which result in hepatocyte death and necrosis. The lesions are devoid of neutrophils unless there is secondary bacterial infection, and therefore the term *abscess* is a misnomer.[8] Some have advocated the use of "pseudoabscess" as an alternate description for *E. histolytica* liver involvement.

Clinical features

Greater than 80% of patients with *E. histolytica* intestinal infection do not have invasive disease and are asymptomatic.[4,9] The symptoms of invasive disease range from self-limited watery diarrhea to fulminant necrotizing colitis. Amebic liver abscess occurs in less than 1% of infected individuals and presents as right-upper-quadrant pain and tender hepatomegaly.[8] Fever is reported in greater than 90% of cases of amebic liver abscess and is commonly accompanied by profuse perspiration, chills, and weakness.[8] Concomitant diarrhea is only reported in <30% of cases of amebic liver abscess, whereas jaundice is seen in approximately 5%.[8] For reasons that are not well understood, amebic liver abscess is up to 20 times more common in males than in females and is rare in children.[8] The presentation is usually acute, but occasionally is chronic and associated with significant anorexia and weight loss.[9]

Complications of amebic liver abscess include bacterial superinfection, spread of the lesion across the diaphragm, and rupture into the peritoneal, pleural, or pericardial cavities. Rupture is one of the most commonly reported complications, occurring in up to 20% of cases, and is associated with significant morbidity and mortality.[8]

Recognition of amebic liver abscess requires a high index of suspicion, particularly in nonendemic settings where this disease is rarely encountered. Laboratory findings include mild anemia, mild to moderate leukocytosis, and normal liver function tests.[8] Less commonly, patients may have significant leukocytosis and elevated alkaline phosphatase and transaminases, particularly in the setting of multiple or large abscesses or with secondary bacterial infection. Material aspirated from liver lesions is usually sterile and rarely contains recognizable trophozoites. Furthermore, concurrent intestinal infection is seldom detected in patients with amebic liver abscess using stool microscopy or stool antigen testing. When organisms are identified by microscopy in stool specimens, they must be differentiated by the morphologically identical *Entamoeba* species, *E. dispar, E. moshkovskii,* and *E. bangladeshi.*[4,10] Given these limitations, *E. histolytica* serology is the test of choice for confirmation of invasive disease and has a high sensitivity (>94%) and specificity (>95%) for detection of amebic liver abscess.[9] Highly sensitive nucleic acid amplification tests have also been described for use on liver specimens and stool, but their use is limited to specialized reference centers.[9]

Imaging

Plain film radiographs demonstrate nonspecific findings such as hepatomegaly and right hemidiaphragm elevation (with right lobe involvement), whereas ultrasonography (US) and computed tomography (CT) are useful for defining the nature and extent of the lesions.[8,11] Amebic liver abscesses appear as round to oval, hypoechoic lesions with well-defined margins on US and low-density lesions with internal fluid on CT.[8]

Gross findings

Liver lesions are usually solitary and located in the right lobe near the liver capsule.[8] Multiple lesions may also occur. They can vary greatly in size, with extreme cases occupying 80% or more of the lobe.[8,12] Lesions contain yellow-gray-red liquid material, which is commonly described as having an "anchovy paste" appearance (Fig. 9.1), whereas the wall has a fibrinous and shaggy appearance.[12]

Microscopic findings

As mentioned above, the liver lesion does not contain neutrophils unless there is bacterial superinfection. The center of the lesion consists of amorphous necrotic material, and there is generally little inflammation in the surrounding liver (Fig. 9.2).[12] Trophozoites may be rare and are usually located in the fibrin at the periphery of the lesion near viable liver tissue. They range in size from 10 to 60 μm in greatest dimension in stool specimens, but rarely exceed 35 μm in biopsy or autopsy specimens.[12] Trophozoites have a vacuolated cytoplasm that may contain engulfed erythrocytes and a small, round nucleus with peripheral rim of condensed chromatin and small central karyosome (Fig. 9.3). Cysts are not seen in invasive disease. Since the other *Entamoeba* spp. do not cause disseminated disease, identification of morphologically compatible trophozoites in liver in the appropriate histologic and clinical setting is diagnostic of amebic liver abscess.

Special stains and immunohistochemistry

Routine hematoxylin and eosin (H&E) is generally sufficient for identification. Periodic Acid Schiff staining may aid in locating amebae by staining their abundant cytoplasmic glycogen, although the deep staining of the trophozoites may obscure the nuclear details needed for confirmation. The rarely used Gridley ameba stain may also be useful for phagocytosed erythrocytes in the trophozoite cytoplasm, but is not commonly available.[12]

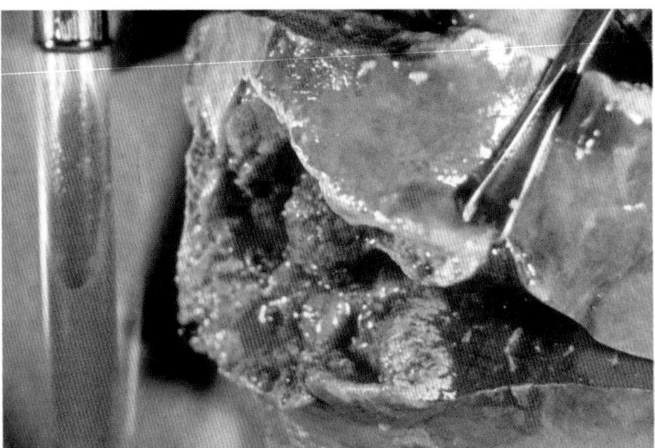

Figure 9.1 Amebic liver abscess demonstrating necrotic parenchyma. The material removed from the abscess within the vial on the left has a characteristic "anchovy paste" appearance. Image courtesy of Dr. Mae Melvin, Dr. E. West, and the CDC Public Health Image Library.

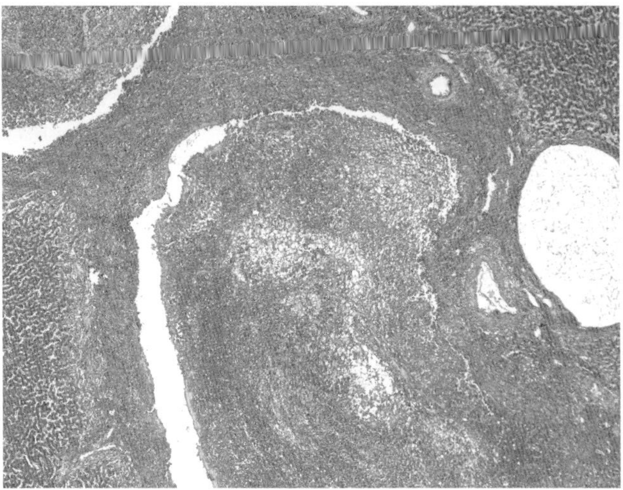

Figure 9.2 Low-power magnification of an amebic liver abscesses consisting of paucicellular necrotic material (H&E, 40×). Despite the name, this entity does not generally contain neutrophils.

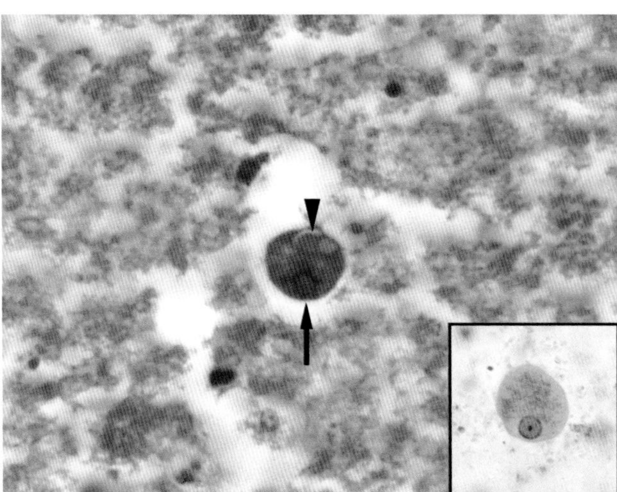

Figure 9.3 Trophozoite of *Entamoeba histolytica* in an amebic liver abscess demonstrating a characteristic nucleus with a peripheral condensed rim of chromatin and small central karyosome (*arrow*; H&E, 1,000×). Ingested red blood cells are also seen within the cytoplasm (*arrow head*). The cellular features are less clear than those generally seen in trichrome-stained stool preparations (inset, 1,000×), but are still recognizable.

Differential diagnosis

The clinical and radiologic differential for amebic liver abscess is broad and includes bacterial abscess, tuberculosis, echinococcal cyst, and metastatic malignancy; these

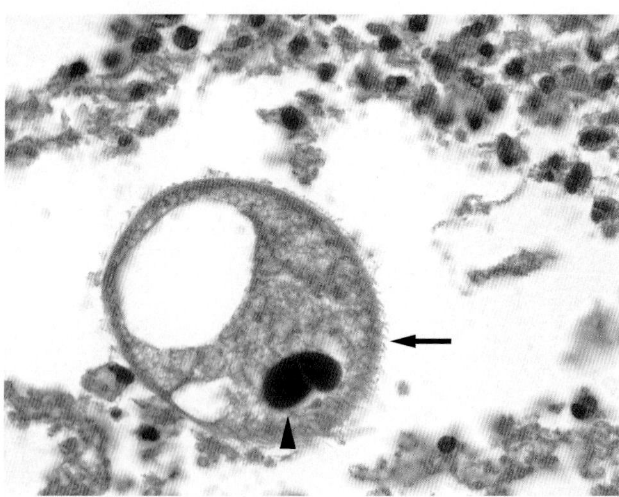

Figure 9.4 Trophozoite of *Balantidium coli* with circumferential cilia (*arrow*) and large "kidney-bean" shaped macronucleus (*arrow head*, H&E, 1,000×).

entities can be excluded during histologic examination by the lack of neutrophils, granulomas, protoscoleces, and malignant cells, respectively. Rarely, trophozoites of the intestinal protozoal parasite, *Balantidium coli*, can disseminate to the liver and cause similar-appearing necrotic lesions. *B. coli* trophozoites can be differentiated from *E. histolytica* trophozoites by their larger size (40 to 100 μm in greatest dimension), large deeply basophilic kidney-bean-shaped macronucleus, and circumferential cilia (Fig. 9.4).[13]

Prognosis and treatment

Amebic liver abscess results in progressive and invariably fatal disease if untreated.[8] Fortunately, rapid recognition and management has decreased mortality rates to 1% to 3%.[9] Treatment of invasive intestinal disease and extraintestinal disease is with metronidazole or tinidazole, followed by paromomycin or iodoquinol to possibly eradicate intestinal carriage.[14] Percutaneous drainage is only indicated for large liver abscesses in which there is a concern for rupture or when bacterial superinfection is suspected.[8]

Leishmania species (visceral leishmaniasis)

Definition, etiology and pathogenesis

Leishmaniasis is an infection of the reticuloendothelial system caused by protozoan hemoflagellate parasites in the genus *Leishmania*. There are both visceral and cutaneous forms of infection, and the type and severity depends on the infecting species and host immune response.[6] Visceral leishmaniasis, also known as kala-azar, is a potentially fatal form of infection caused by parasites in the *Leishmania donovani* complex (e.g., *L. donovani donovani, L. donovani infantum, L. donovani chagasi*).[1] The WHO classifies leishmaniasis as a neglected tropical disease, with an estimated 300,000 cases and over 20,000 deaths caused by visceral leishmaniasis each year.[1] Visceral infection is found in 82 countries worldwide, with the predominance of cases reported from Brazil, East Africa, and India.[1] Factors contributing to ongoing infection include poverty, crowding, and poor access to health care.

Transmission is through the bite of an infected female phlebotomine sandfly.[6] Sandflies inject the infective form of the parasite (the flagellated promastigote) into the skin while taking a blood meal, and these forms enter host phagocytic cells through receptor-mediated phagocytosis. The parasite then converts to the non-motile amastigote stage and replicates inside the host cell. In visceral leishmaniasis, the infected macrophages spread to the local lymph nodes and then disseminate hematogenously to the bone marrow, liver, and spleen, as well as other organs. Infected cells rupture because of ongoing parasite replication, releasing the amastigotes into the tissue to infect new phagocytic cells.[6] Humans and canines are important reservoir hosts and serve as ongoing sources of infection.[15]

Clinical features

Clinical disease usually manifests 2 to 6 months after initial infection, but the organism may remain dormant for many years.[15] Patients without preexisting immunity usually present with acute onset of high fever, chills, and malaise. In comparison, patients in *Leishmania*-endemic regions have some degree of immunity and commonly present with subacute or chronic disease, manifested by an insidious onset of fever, weight loss, weakness, and failure to thrive.[6,15] Hepatosplenomegaly is present and may be massive in both acute and subacute/chronic disease.[15] Secondary bacterial infections including pneumonia and tuberculosis are important contributions to overall mortality with visceral leishmaniasis. Cirrhosis is uncommon.[15] Patients with HIV or those receiving immunosuppressive medications are at increased risk of severe disease and disease relapse.[1,15] Visceral leishmaniasis is now recognized as an important opportunistic infection of late-stage HIV, with high coinfection rates reported from Ethiopia, India, and Brazil.[1]

Recognition of visceral leishmaniasis requires a high index of suspicion, particularly since latent infection may only become clinically apparent years after initial infection, or when patient immunity is compromised. Common laboratory findings in visceral leishmaniasis are normocytic anemia, leukopenia, thrombocytopenia, polyclonal hypergammaglobulinemia, and elevated erythrocyte sedimentation rate. Liver transaminases are often mildly elevated, but serum bilirubin is usually within normal limits.[15] Definitive diagnosis is made through visualization of amastigotes in tissue aspirates or biopsies and by culture or molecular testing of involved tissues.[6,16] Testing for antiparasitic antibodies or parasite antigens can also be performed. Microscopic examination of bone marrow smears has an estimated 60% to 80% sensitivity for diagnosis of visceral leishmaniasis, whereas the sensitivity of examining a splenic aspirate exceeds 95%. Splenic aspirate is rarely performed in nonendemic settings because of the risk of fatal hemorrhage but is a widely used and relatively safe procedure when performed by experienced practitioners.[17] Parasites are less commonly seen in the liver, lymph nodes, and buffy coat of peripheral blood.[16]

In the United States, bone marrow examination is commonly paired with culture, serology, and molecular analysis at the CDC. It is important to contact the CDC before obtaining a biopsy so that they can provide a collection instructions and a kit for specimen transport to their laboratories; further information is available at http://www.cdc.gov/parasites/leishmaniasis/health_professionals/.

Imaging

Ultrasonography and CT usually reveal an enlarged liver and spleen. While the spleen enlarges at a relatively constant rate (approximately 1 inch/month) until it fills the abdomen, the liver undergoes less predictable enlargement and may even be normal in size.[11]

Gross findings

The liver is generally enlarged and has a smooth capsule.[18] The cut surface may be firm with a nodular appearance in cases with significant fibrosis.

Microscopic findings

The predominant microscopic finding is *Leishmania* amastigotes within macrophages (Fig. 9.5). Amastigotes are 2 to 5 μm in diameter and have a small nucleus and rod-shaped kinetoplast. These important morphologic features are difficult to appreciate in formalin-fixed tissues, but are often more apparent on air-dried aspirates and smears (Fig. 9.6). Other histologic findings include sinusoidal enlargement, lymphoplasmacytic inflammation in the lobules and portal tracts, nonnecrotizing granulomatous inflammation, ballooning degeneration of hepatocytes, and focal cellular necrosis. Diffuse fibrosis (so-called "Roger cirrhosis") has also been described, particularly from cases of visceral leishmaniasis in India.[15,18,19]

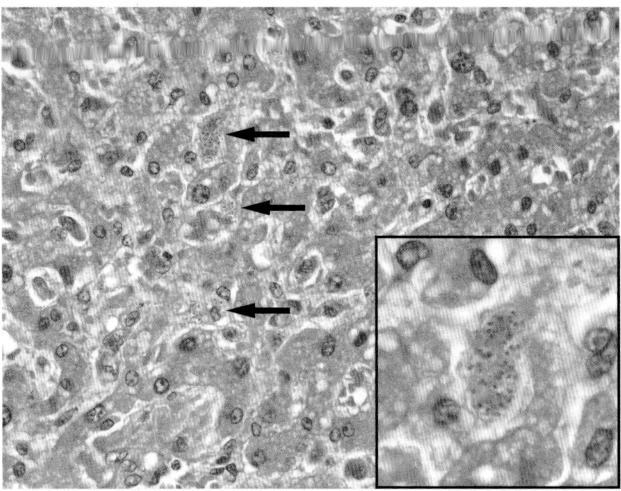

Figure 9.5 Visceral Leishmaniasis of the liver, in which small intracellular objects are seen within Kupffer cells (*arrows*, H&E, 400×; inset 1,000×). It is challenging to make out the characteristic features in formalin-fixed paraffin-embedded sections.

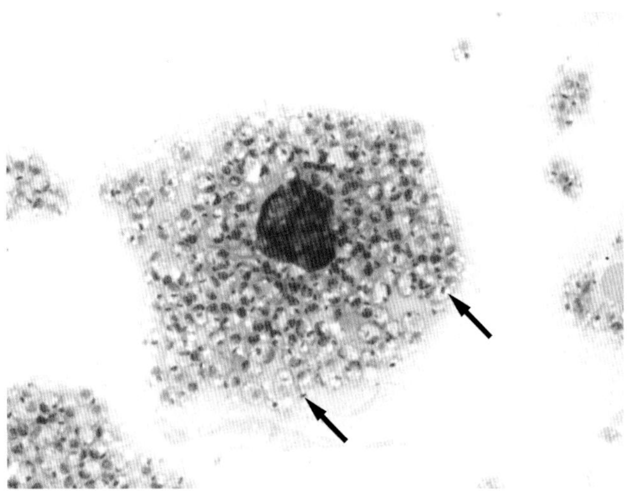

Figure 9.6 Giemsa-stained air-dried preparation of a liver aspirate showing a macrophage containing numerous *Leishmania* sp. amastigotes (1,000×). Each amastigote contains a small oval-to-round nucleus and a rod-shaped kinetoplast (*arrows*).

Special stains and immunohistochemistry

Although amastigotes are readily apparent using H&E, the characteristic nucleus and kinetoplast may be difficult to identify, thus raising the possibility of other small intracellular organisms such as yeasts. Gomori methenamine-silver (GMS) is useful for differentiating amastigotes from yeasts since they are GMS negative, whereas the Brown and Hopps tissue Gram stain and combined H&E/Jones silver stain are useful for highlighting the kinetoplast. Other stains such as periodic acid–Schiff (PAS), Giemsa, and Wilder reticulum stain offer no additional diagnostic advantage.

Molecular findings

Molecular amplification and sequencing methods are commonly used at specialized reference centers such as the CDC for detection and species identification. These methods are best performed on fresh tissue and culture isolates, but may also be performed on formalin-fixed paraffin-embedded tissues.

Differential diagnosis

The primary clinical differential diagnosis for patients with fever and recent travel to a *Leishmania*-endemic setting includes malaria, typhoid, and tuberculosis.[17] On microscopic examination, the differential diagnosis includes other small intracellular objects such as *Histoplasma capsulatum* (also found inside of histiocytes), *Toxoplasma gondii,* and *Trypanosoma cruzi.* As mentioned earlier, yeasts are GMS positive whereas amastigotes are GMS negative. *Toxoplasma gondii* can infect any nucleated cell and appears as tissue cysts and tachyzoites. The tachyzoites are 2 to 5 µm in size and may have a similar appearance to *Leishmania* amastigotes (Fig. 9.7), but can be differentiated by their arc shape (not always seen in tissue sections) and lack of a kinetoplast. Commercially available *T. gondii* immunohistochemistry may also be helpful. *Leishmania* spp. amastigotes are indistinguishable from amastigotes of *Trypanosoma cruzi,* but the latter are rarely seen in the liver and generally form larger collections of amastigotes. Clinical correlation is useful for differentiating infection with the two parasites.

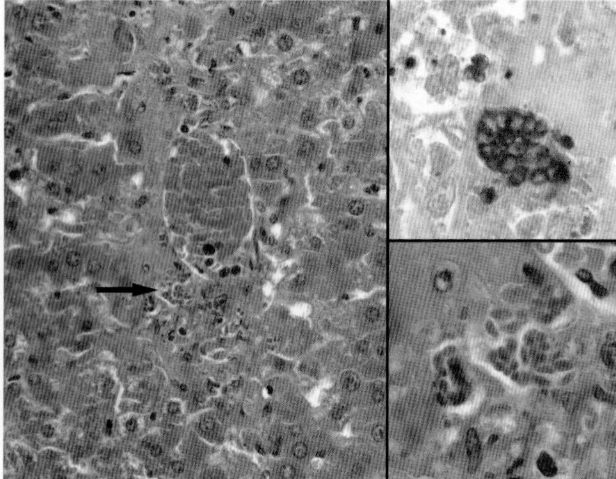

Figure 9.7 Toxoplasmosis in a liver biopsy demonstrating collections of intracellular and extracellular tachyzoites within the liver parenchyma (*arrow*, H&E, 400×). On higher magnification (inset, **bottom right**, 1,000×), the oval-to-arc shape of the tachzyoites can be appreciated. Because of their small size, the organisms are best highlighted using *T. gondii* immunohistochemistry (inset, above right, 1,000×).

Prognosis and treatment

Visceral leishmaniasis is a potentially fatal disease that should be treated promptly. Treatment options are potentially toxic and availability may be limited; therefore treatment should be provided by an infectious disease physician or other specialist. The conventional therapy is a pentavalent antimonial compound (e.g., Pentostam), which is available through the CDC to U.S. physicians.[14] Parental liposomal amphotericin B and miltefosine are additional options. Antiretroviral therapy should be considered for HIV coinfected patients since it improves survival and decreases the risk of relapse.[6]

Plasmodium falciparum (malaria)

Definition, etiology, and pathogenesis

Malaria is caused primarily by four species in the genus *Plasmodium: P. falciparum, P. vivax, P. ovale,* and *P. malariae.*[20] Of these, *Plasmodium falciparum* is the deadliest species to cause human malaria and is found in the tropics and subtropics worldwide. The WHO estimates that 3.2 billion individuals are at risk of infection worldwide.[21] In 2015, there were approximately 214 million cases and over 400,000 deaths.[21] The highest morbidity and mortality is in nonimmune individuals (e.g., travelers) and children under the age of 5 years who live in endemic areas (primarily Sub-Saharan Africa).

Transmission to humans occurs primarily through the bite of an infected female *Anopheles* mosquito. Less commonly, the organism is transmitted through congenital infection and blood transfusion.[6,20] Mosquitoes inject the infective form of the parasite (the sporozoite) into the blood while feeding, and this form travels to the liver to undergo a short-term asexual reproductive phase in hepatocytes.[6] Within 7 to 10 days, parasites are then released into the blood stream to infect and replicate within erythrocytes. With *P. ovale* and *P. vivax* infection, some parasites also remain behind in the liver in a dormant phase called a hypnozoite, which can reactivate months to years later.[6] Within erythrocytes, parasites feed on the host's hemoglobin and form hemozoin as a waste product. After 48 to 72 hours of replication, the infected erythrocyte bursts and newly formed parasites are released into the blood to infect new erythrocytes.[6US] Some parasites also form gametocytes, which are the infective stage for the mosquito; the parasite life cycle continues when gametocytes are taken up by a female *Anopheles* during a blood meal.[6]

There are several reasons why *Plasmodium falciparum* is responsible for the greatest burden of human morbidity and mortality. Unlike the other species, it is capable of infecting all stages of erythrocytes and can therefore reach very high levels of parasitemia. Furthermore, *P. falciparum*–infected erythrocytes will adhere to other erythrocytes (i.e., cytoadherence) and sequester in the microcirculation, resulting in blood-flow sludging and hypoxia. Cytoadherence and sequestration does not occur with other *Plasmodium* species.

Clinical features

Clinical symptoms typically appear 2 to 3 days after parasites are released from the liver into the peripheral blood (total time: 9 to 13 days after infection). The clinical manifestations may mimic many other infections and therefore malaria must be considered in the differential in patients with recent exposure to malaria-endemic areas. The classical feature is the fever paroxysm, characterized by abrupt onset of chills, followed by fever, and then sweats.[6,20] Each species is associated with a characteristic fever cycle (e.g., every 48 hours or less with *P. falciparum* infection) that peaks with erythrocyte rupture and release of pyrogens into the blood, although this is not reliably seen. Other symptoms include myalgia, headache, anorexia, nausea, vomiting, diarrhea, and shortness of breath.[20] Falciparum malaria commonly presents with gastrointestinal symptoms and progresses to high fever, hepatic tenderness, hepatomegaly, jaundice, and splenic tenderness with ongoing erythrocyte rupture and sequestration of infected cells in visceral capillaries.[22] Complications of falciparum malaria include hypotension, pulmonary edema, hypoglycemia, disseminated intravascular coagulopathy, glomerulonephritis, mental status alterations, seizures, and death. Adverse fetal outcomes are also seen in pregnancy.[22] Laboratory testing commonly reveals anemia and elevated bilirubin and transaminases.

Definitive diagnosis is usually made by detecting intact parasites, or their DNA in peripheral blood. Microscopic examination of Giemsa-stained thin and thick blood films is considered the gold standard diagnostic test and allows for calculation of percent parasitemia.[20] Commercially available rapid diagnostic tests are also commonly used for detection of *Plasmodium* antigens in peripheral blood, but are less sensitive than blood film examination, particularly for non-*falciparum* species and low levels of parasitemia. Finally, nucleic acid amplification tests such as polymerase chain reaction (PCR) generally offer increased sensitivity over blood films and are useful for detecting low-level parasitemia and mixed infections. However, they are not widely available and limited to specialized research facilities and reference labs. Serologic testing is used primarily for blood donor screening and has no role for diagnosis of acute infection.[20]

Gross findings

The spleen is commonly enlarged, particularly in patients with repeated or long-standing infections, and perisplenic fibrosis and adhesions may be present.[11] There is variable liver enlargement, and the parenchyma may have a diffuse slate-gray discoloration because of hemozoin pigment accumulation in Kupffer cells.[22] Patients with chronic falciparum malaria may have a lobular pattern of pigmentation because of hemozoin deposition in portal tracts.

Microscopic findings

The most common microscopic findings in the liver and other organs are vascular congestion and malaria pigment (hemozoin)–laden erythrocytes and phagocytes within capillaries (Fig. 9.8). Hemozoin appears as granular clumps of variably sized brown-black pigment that is birefringent using polarized light.[22,23] Intraerythrocytic parasites may also be seen; on H&E, they appear as faintly staining, blue-gray, spherical masses measuring 2 to 4 µm, with one or more associated pigment clumps.[22] The infected erythrocytes are often nearly depleted of hemoglobin and are very pale. A study of autopsy-diagnosed malaria deaths detected involvement of the liver in 78% of cases, whereas involvement of the brain, spleen, lungs, and myocardium were seen in 100%, 67%, 56%, and 43% of cases, respectively.[24]

Differential diagnosis

The clinical differential diagnosis of malaria is broad and includes other febrile illnesses such as bacteremia,

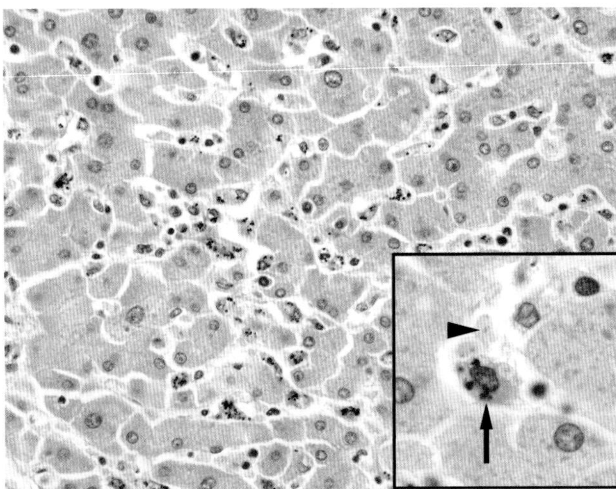

Figure 9.8 Liver biopsy in a fatal case of malaria due to *Plasmodium falciparum* (H&E, 400×). Evidence of the parasites is seen primarily as hemozoin pigment (inset, 1,000×) within erythrocytes and Kupffer cells (*arrow*). Faintly staining blue-gray intraerythrocytic parasites may also be seen (*arrow head*).

dengue, African trypanosomiasis, and cholera. In histologic sections, the primary differential is formalin pigment, which has a similar appearance to hemozoin pigment. Formalin pigment may deposit in congested tissues, especially when phosphate-buffered neutral formalin is not used. Like hemozoin, it appears as granular brown-black clumps and is birefringent with polarized light. However, it is usually extracellular and commonly rod-shaped, whereas hemozoin is intracellular, associated with intraerythrocytic parasites, and spherical.

Prognosis and treatment

Malaria is a potentially life-threatening disease, and treatment should be begun promptly.[20] When diagnosed early, the prognosis is very good, but untreated *P. falciparum* is associated with high mortality. Treatment varies by the infecting species, the region where infection was acquired, percent parasitemia, clinical status (including comorbidities and pregnacy), and drug allergies.[6,20] Most *P. falciparum* worldwide is resistant to chloroquine, and therefore other drugs such as atovaqunone-proguanil (Malarone), artemether-lumefantrine (Coartem), quinine, and mefloquine must be used.[14] Although uncomplicated *P. falciparum* disease can be treated with oral agents, severe malaria is usually treated with parenteral quinine, quinidine, or artimisinin agents.[14] Exchange transfusion may be considered for patients with percent parasitemia of 10% or higher although it is no longer recommended by the CDC.[20] Primaquine is added to treatment regiments for *P. ovale* and *P. vivax* malaria to eradicate the dormant hypnozoite stage in the liver.[14]

Cryptosporidium species (cryptosporidiosis)

Definition, etiology, and pathogenesis

Cryptosporidium are small intracellular apicomplexan parasites that infect the intestinal and biliary epithelium of humans and a wide array of other animals.[6] They were previously classified as coccidia along with *Cyclospora cayetanensis* and *Cystoisospora* (*Isospora*) *belli*, but are now known to be more closely related to the gregarines, which are parasites of invertebrates.[25] Nearly 20 *Cryptosporidium* species have been reported to infect humans. The two most common species are *C. hominis* (a human/anthroponotic parasite) and *C. parvum* (a zoonotic parasite).[25]

Cryptosporidium is found worldwide and causes human disease in both tropical and temperate climates. There are an estimated 750,000 cases of cryptosporidiosis each year in the United States alone, with the vast majority thought to be undiagnosed or unreported.[25] Transmission is through the fecal–oral route. Humans become infected through ingestion (and possibly inhalation) of infective oocysts in contaminated food or drinking and recreational water sources, as well as through direct contact with infected humans or animals.[25] Many outbreaks in the United States have been associated with swimming pools, waterparks, day care centers, petting zoos, and faulty municipal water supplies.[25] Patients with AIDS and other immunocompromised states are at increased risk for acquiring infection and developing prolonged or severe disease.

After ingestion, the oocysts excyst and release sporozoites, which infect the epithelial cells of the gastrointestinal tract. The parasites then go through a complicated life cycle in the epithelial cells consisting of both asexual and sexual stages.[25] The parasites are localized in the brush border, just below the cell membrane (intracellular, extracytoplasmic) and may interfere with host absorption and digestion.[25] Ultimately, larger numbers of oocysts are produced and shed in the stool. These oocysts are infective upon excretion, which contributes to the ease of transmission to others.[25]

Clinical features

The primary clinical features of cryptosporidiosis are profuse watery diarrhea, nausea, vomiting, abdominal cramps, and low-grade fever.[25] Symptoms may last for 2 to 3 weeks but usually resolve spontaneously in the immunocompetent host. In contrast, patients with AIDS and other causes of profound immune compromise may have chronic, life-threatening diarrhea and dehydration. This population is also more likely to have extraintestinal involvement, including infection of the stomach, esophagus, and hepatobiliary, pancreatic, and respiratory tracts.[26] In particular, cryptosporidiosis is a well-recognized cause of AIDS cholangiopathy, with up to 15% of AIDS patients having hepatobiliary tract infection.[26,27] Symptoms include right-upper-quadrant pain, epigastric pain, diarrhea, and, less commonly, fever and jaundice. Although immunocompetent individuals may also have involvement of the biliary tract, symptomatic infection is primarily in patients with AIDS. Complications of hepatobiliary disease include papillary sclerosis, extrahepatic and intrahepatic sclerosing cholangitis, and acalculous cholecystitis.[25]

Diagnosis is usually made by identification of parasite forms, or parasite antigens or DNA in stool specimens.[27] Direct sampling of the biliary tree via endoscopic retrograde cholangiopancreatography (ERCP) may increase the diagnostic yield, particularly for patients with papillary stenosis.[28] In stool, The oocysts are small spherical structures, measuring 4 to

6 µm in diameter and stain deep red with modified acid-fast and safranin stains. Stool immunoassays offer increased sensitivity over stool microscopic examination and come in numerous formats such as direct fluorescence and enzyme immunoassays.[25] More recently, multiplex nucleic acid amplification tests for multiple stool pathogens including *Cryptosporidium* spp. have become commercially available and have been increasingly implemented in the clinical microbiology laboratory for testing stool specimens.[25]

Imaging

Cryptosporidiosis of the biliary tract is seen by US and CT as duct wall thickening and dilation, thickening of the gallbladder wall, and the presence of pericholecystic fluid.[29] Cholangiograms may show papillary stenosis, dilation of the common bile duct, and attenuation of the intrahepatic ducts.[29]

Microscopic findings

Cryptosporidium parasites may be found in epithelial cells throughout the intestinal and hepatobiliary tract, but are most commonly found in the jejunum and ileum in immunocompetent individuals.[27] On H&E-stained sections, these intracellular parasites appear as small basophilic spherical structures bulging from the brush border and may appear to be extracellular (Fig. 9.9). On high power, different asexual and sexual forms can be appreciated.[27] Structural changes include mild villous blunting and crypt elongation.[27] In immunocompromised hosts, infection may result in more pronounced architectural changes including severe villous atrophy, dense inflammatory infiltrates, and larger numbers of parasites.[27]

Biliary tract involvement is more focal than diffuse and may occasionally be associated with mixed periductal inflammation and edema.[27] Infected intrahepatic ducts may be dilated and contain intraluminal debris and parasites, whereas the epithelium may be focally flattened and eroded.[27]

Special stains

Cryptosporidium parasites are usually identified easily using H&E and do not require the use of additional stains. In cases where the diagnosis is not clear, use of select histochemical stains may be helpful. *Cryptosporidium* are red to purple on tissue Gram stain, focally GMS and Warthin–Starry positive (depending on the life-cycle stage), and dark blue by Giemsa.[27] Of these, Giemsa is the most helpful for highlighting the parasites along the brush border. The parasites are mucicarmine negative which aids in their differentiation from extruded mucin. It is important to note that modified acid-fast stains do not reliably highlight the parasites like they do in stool specimens.

Differential diagnosis

The clinical differential of hepatobiliary cryptosporidiosis includes several infectious and noninfectious cholangiopathies. In patients with AIDS, important causes of cholangiopathy include cytomegalovirus infection, microsporidiosis, cyclosporiasis, and cystoisosporiasis.[26] The latter three parasites appear as intracytoplasmic parasites (Figs. 9.10 and 9.11) and therefore can be easily differentiated from the apical

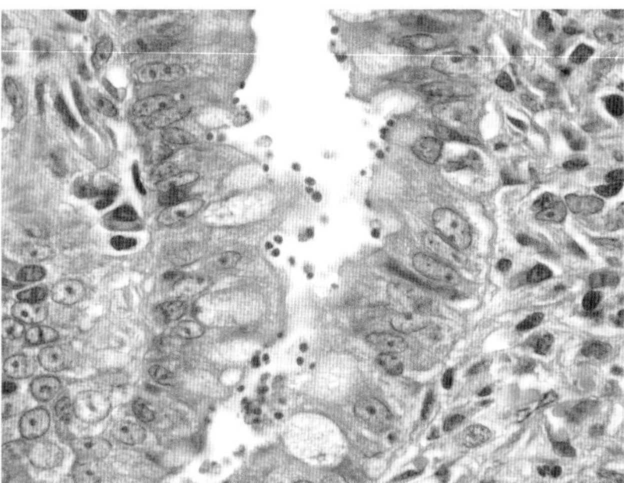

Figure 9.9 Intestinal biopsy demonstrating multiple *Cryptosporidium* forms at the enterocyte brush border (H&E, 1,000×). The objects are intracellular, lying just below the apical portion of the cell membrane. This appearance is also seen in cryptosporidiosis involving the biliary epithelium.

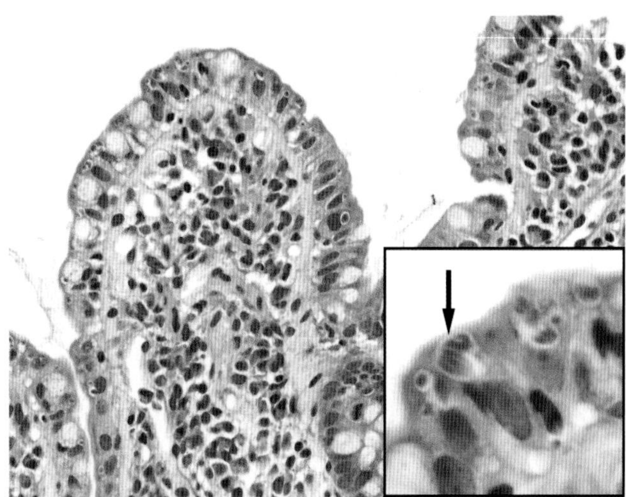

Figure 9.10 Intestinal biopsy in a patient with cyclosporiasis in which multiple parasite forms (*arrow*) are seen within the enterocyte cytoplasm (H&E, 400×; inset 1,000×).

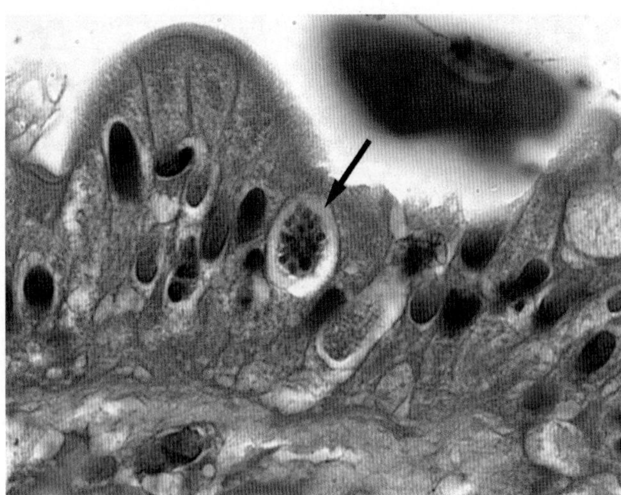

Figure 9.11 Parasite form (schizont) of *Cystoisospora belli* in an intestinal biopsy (*arrow*, H&E, 1,500×). Image courtesy of the CDC Division of Parasitic Diseases and Malaria.

parasites of *Cryptosporidium* spp.[27] Finally, nonparasitic structures such as extruded mucin can occasionally be mistaken for *Cryptosporidium* parasites. In this instance, careful morphologic examination with use of high-power magnification (e.g., oil immersion) is helpful for differentiating these structures.

Prognosis and treatment

Infection is usually self-limited in immunocompetent individuals and may require only fluid and electrolyte replacement. Nitazoxinide can be used to shorten the course of disease.[14] Unfortunately, immunocompromised patients usually experience chronic and relapsing intestinal disease and have limited response to nitazoxinide. Restoration of immunity is essential for achieving disease resolution in this population. Treatment of some infection-related cholangiographic abnormalities may be accomplished through endoscopic interventions including sphincterotomy for papillary stenosis and stenting of isolated common bile duct strictures, but these techniques are not helpful for extrahepatic or intrahepatic sclerosing cholangitis.[26] Some patients with AIDS-associated cholangiopathy may also respond to treatment with ursodeoxycholic acid (UDCA).[30]

9.3 NEMATODES (ROUND WORMS)

Toxocara spp. (toxocariasis, visceral larva migrans)

Definition, etiology, and pathogenesis

Toxocara canis, also known as the dog round worm, is the most common cause of visceral larva migrans in humans.[6,31] Visceral larva migrans is a syndrome in which larvae migrate through the liver, lungs, eye (ocular larva migrans), brain (neural larva migrans), and other viscera and cause eosinophilic granulomatous inflammation, abscess formation, and tissue destruction.[32] Infection with *Toxocara* spp. is also called *toxocariasis*.

Other important, but less common, causes of visceral larva migrans or similar syndromes are *Toxocara cati* (the cat roundworm), *Baylisascaris procyonis* (the raccoon roundworm), *Gnathostoma* spp., and *Capillaria hepatica*.[6]

Dogs harbor the adult *T. canis* worms in their intestines and release immature eggs in their stool.[6] If the stool is allowed to contaminate the environment, the eggs will embryonate and become infective to humans and other mammals within weeks of being deposited.[31] Humans become infected primarily through ingestion of embryonated *Toxocara* eggs in contaminated soil, but can also become infected through ingestion of larvae in the undercooked flesh of other infected mammals (e.g., rabbits, cows).[6,33] Following ingestion of eggs, larvae are released and penetrate the intestinal wall to disseminate hematogenously to other organs. The larvae cannot mature in humans and will continue to migrate until they ultimately die in the host tissues.[6]

Toxocariasis is one of the most common zoonotic diseases in the United States.[3] Data from the CDC National Health and Nutrition Examination Survey (1988 to 1994) detected antibodies to *Toxocara* in nearly 14% of the U.S. population, indicating that millions of Americans have been exposed to infection.[3] Young children (<5 years) are most likely to develop visceral larva migrans, whereas ocular larva migrans is usually seen in older children and young adults.[6] Toxocariasis is classified by the CDC as a neglected parasitic infection owing to the number of individuals infected, the potential severity of illness, and the preventable nature of infection.[3] Risk factors for infection include young age (≤20 years), close contact with infected dogs, history of geophagia, and living in warm humid environments that favor egg survival in the soil.[3,6] Children from socioeconomically disadvantaged populations are disproportionately affected.[3]

Clinical features

The clinical presentation depends on the ingested egg burden and localization of the migrating larvae. Many light infections are asymptomatic and are discovered incidentally during investigation of eosinophilia.[33,34] When present, symptoms include high fever, abdominal pain, hepatosplenomegaly, cough, wheezing, and rash. Hypereosinophilia (up to 90%) and hypergammaglobulinemia (primarily IgE) are characteristic.[35] Ocular involvement can result in blindness, whereas neurologic involvement is associated with seizures and mental status changes.[35]

The presence of eosinophilia in a pediatric patient with an unexplained febrile illness should prompt an investigation for visceral larva migrans.[31] Diagnosis is usually made by detection of antibodies to *Toxocara* species in conjunction with supportive clinical and radiographic features.[6,31] Several commercial immunoassays are available and have sensitivities of 78% to 90% depending on the interpretative criteria used.[6,31] The specificity is >90%, but cross-reactivity may be seen with other helminth infections.[6] Since the larvae do not mature in humans, a parasite exam will not detect *Toxocara* eggs in stool specimens.[6] Definitive diagnosis is by histopathologic identification of larvae in biopsies or autopsy specimens.[35]

Imaging

The imaging features of visceral larva migrans are nonspecific and reflect the larval migration and resultant tissue inflammation. The liver is commonly involved. Lesions are hypoechoic on US and appear as ill-defined low-attenuating nodules on CT.[32] They are commonly small (1 to 1.5 cm in diameter), round, oval, or asymmetrical, but can coalesce and involve an entire segment or lobe in extensive disease.[32]

Gross findings

The liver is enlarged, soft, and commonly contains multiple small (0.5 to 1 cm) white nodules on the surface and throughout the parenchyma.[35]

Microscopic findings

Compared with other organs, the liver commonly has the highest burden of larvae. Characteristic features include eosinophilic granulomas, abscesses, and evidence of previous migration tracts in the parenchyma (Fig. 9.12).[35] Portal tracts are commonly expanded by an inflammatory infiltrate consisting of lymphocytes, plasma cells, and eosinophils.[35] The larvae may be rare and not seen in random biopsies, so examination of serial sections is recommended to increase the likelihood of detection.[35] *Toxocara* larvae are most commonly identified within granulomas, but may less commonly be found in the walls of arteries and veins associated with a focal granulomatous vasculitis. They measure 290 to 350 μm in length by 12 to 20 μm in diameter, have a single pair of small lateral alae (external ridges on either side of the worm when seen on cross-section), and contain simple internal cellular structures (Fig. 9-12).[13,35] Only a single intestinal cell is seen in cross-section, with no apparent intestinal lumen.[13]

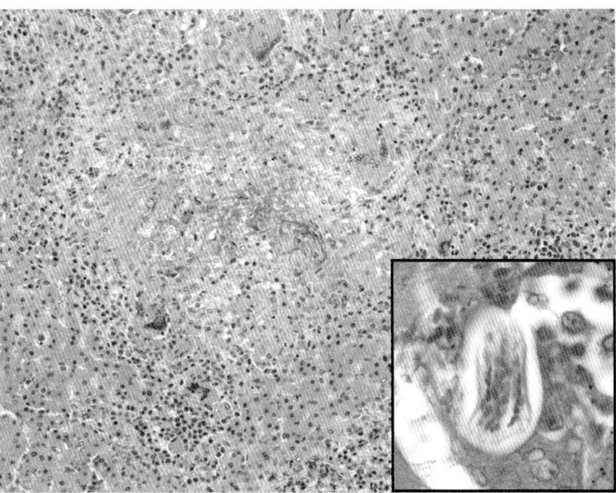

Figure 9.12 Liver biopsy from a patient with visceral larva migrans diagnosed by *Toxocara* serology (H&E, 200×). Multiple eosinophilic granulomas were present throughout the liver, but no larvae were seen. The inset shows a portion of a *Toxocara* larva from a different case (PAS, 1,000×). Note the simple internal cellular structures.

Differential diagnosis

The clinical differential for fever and hypereosinophilia includes multiple infectious and noninfectious entities. Other parasites that can cause similar clinical findings with hypereosinophilia include baylisascariasis, gnathostomiasis, fascioliasis, echinococcosis, paragonimiasis, strongyloidiasis, and trichinellosis.[6] The differential of roundworm larvae found in the liver is more limited and includes *B. procyonis, Gnathostoma* spp., and *Strongyloides stercoralis*, all of which can be seen in conjunction with granulomatous inflammation. Careful correlation with the clinical presentation and other laboratory findings is helpful for differentiating these entities. The raccoon roundworm, *B. procyonis*, causes a severe form of visceral larva migrans that is most commonly diagnosed on autopsy.[36] Like toxocariasis, children are the usual host. A history of geophagia or exposure to raccoon feces is helpful in supporting the diagnosis. When seen in tissue, *Baylisascaris* larvae can be differentiated from *Toxocara* larvae by their larger size (60 to 70 μm in diameter), presence of large paired lateral alae, and centrally located patent intestine. Gnathostomiasis is rare in the United States and most commonly reported in adults in Mexico and Asia.[6] Patients are infected with *Gnathostoma* spp. through ingestion of undercooked infected intermediate hosts (fish, frogs) or by drinking water containing infected copepods.[6] Like *B. procyonis,* the migrating larvae of *Gnathostoma* spp. are larger than those of *Toxocara* (200 to 300 μm in diameter) and have recognizable internal organs, including a patent intestine. They also have prominent cuticular spines. The larvae of

S. stercoralis bear the closest resemblance to *Toxocara* spp. larvae in terms of size (15 to 16 μm in diameter) and their simple internal structures without patent intestine. They have a small pair of double lateral alae unlike the single pair of lateral alae of *Toxocara* larvae, but these can be difficult to appreciate in tissue sections. The primary means for differentiating these two nematodes is through consideration of the clinical picture and results of microbiology testing. *Strongyloides stercoralis* larvae are only found in the liver during hyperinfection syndrome and therefore the host is generally immunocompromised and larvae are also found in the stool and sputum.

Prognosis and treatment

Infection is usually self-limited in humans, but is associated with severe sequelae, particularly with ocular and neurologic involvement.[31] Treatment is with albendazole or mebendazole, as well as systemic corticosteroids if indicated to control the associated inflammation.[6]

9.4 CESTODES (TAPEWORMS)

Echinococcus spp. (echinococcosis, hydatid disease)

Definition, etiology, and pathogenesis

Echinococcosis, also known as hydatid disease, is caused by tapeworm larvae in the genus *Echinococcus*.[6US] *Echinococcus granulosus* is the common species to infect humans and causes cystic echinococcosis, whereas *E. multilocularis* less commonly infects humans and causes alveolar echinococcosis. Rarely, humans can be infected by *E. vogeli* and *E. oligarthrus*, resulting in polycystic echinococcosis.[6US,37] Recently, molecular analyses have identified several other species of *Echinococcus* that can cause cystic echinococcosis in humans; these are described in further detail elsewhere.[38]

Echinococcosis is a neglected tropical disease that infects more than 1 million people worldwide.[1] *Echinococcus granulosus* is most common in sheep-rearing regions throughout the world, including parts of the United States.[6US] In comparison, *E. multilocularis* is found in the northern hemisphere, and *E. vogeli* and *E. oligarthrus* occur in South and Central America.[6,37]

The natural life cycle of all species involves a carnivore definitive host (e.g., canid, hyenid, felid) and an intermediate host. The typical intermediate hosts of *Echinococcus granulosus* are herbivores such as sheep, goats, cattle, swine, horses, deer, and camels, whereas rodents are the intermediate hosts of the other *Echinococcus* species.[6US] The definitive host is infected with the adult tapeworm in its intestine and sheds microscopic eggs in its feces, which then go on to contaminate the environment. Humans and other animals become infected through ingestion of eggs on contaminated hands, or in food, or water.[6US] Following ingestion, the egg hatches to release an oncosphere that penetrates the intestinal wall and disseminates hematogenously to other organs.[6US,38]

In cystic echinococcosis, the oncosphere forms a fluid-filled cyst (hydatid cyst) that slowly enlarges over a period of several years. The outside of the cyst (the pericyst) is formed by compressed host tissue, while the inside of the cyst (the endocyst) is derived from the larval parasite.[38] The endocyst comprises a mitotically active inner germinal layer, from which immature tapeworms (protoscoleces) arise, and an outer acellular laminated layer. Protoscoleces are commonly contained within a thin-walled brood capsule within the cyst. Over time, daughter cysts may form within the larger cyst, and each daughter cyst may also form protoscoleces and brood capsules. Depending on the location, infection may go unnoticed for years until the cyst ruptures or impinges upon neighboring structures.[38] The vast majority (70%) of cystic echinococcosis cases are found in the liver, whereas 20% are found in the lung and the remaining 10% are found in other organs.[38]

In comparison with cystic echinococcosis, other forms of echinococcosis are more aggressive and infiltrative in nature. Nearly all arise in the liver. In alveolar echinococcosis, small cysts infiltrate host tissue like a malignancy, forming an ill-defined fibrous mass. In polycystic echinococcosis, variably sized cysts develop both internally and externally, forming a large vesicular mass.[37] Both can involve the bulk of the liver and extend into surrounding organs.

If infected viscera containing cysts with viable protoscoleces are ingested by a definitive host, then the life cycle continues. Each protoscolex becomes an adult tapeworm, which attaches to the intestinal mucosa and produces thousands of eggs each day. Humans are considered dead-end hosts because they are unlikely to perpetuate the disease cycle.[38]

Clinical features

The clinical presentation varies with the location of the cyst and the infecting species.[38] Liver involvement due to *E. granulosus* may remain asymptomatic for many years.[39] When present, signs and symptoms include abdominal mass, anorexia, and abdominal pain.[6,39,40] The most common complication of cystic echinococcosis of the liver is cysto-biliary fistula formation (seen in 13% to 37% of liver cysts).[38] Cysts can become secondarily infected because of communication with the biliary tree, resulting in bacterial abscess.[39] Other important complications include jaundice due to biliary tree compression, portal hypertension due to compression of the portal or hepatic veins, and cyst rupture.[37,40] Liver cysts may rupture into the peritoneum, or across the diaphragm into the pleural or pericardial cavities, resulting in formation of new cysts in the adjoining spaces. Rupture or leakage of antigenic cyst contents can also cause allergic reactions ranging from hives and angioedema to life-threatening anaphylaxis.[39] Laboratory testing may reveal a mild leukocytosis, but peripheral eosinophilia is usually absent unless there is cyst rupture. Other laboratory abnormalities include moderate elevations of alkaline phosphatase and transaminases. Bilirubin is rarely elevated.

The infiltrative nature of the other *Echinococcus* species may result in involvement of adjacent organs.[39] Cysts can also disseminate hematogenously to distant organs.[6,39] The nature of the symptoms is dependent on the organs involved.

Diagnosis is usually made by serologic testing in conjunction with supportive clinical and radiologic findings and a compatible exposure history.[39] Immunodiagnostic tests for IgG, IgM, IgA, and IgE against *E. granulosus* antigens are commercially available in EIA, immunoblot, indirect hemagglutination assay (IHA), and indirect fluorescent antibody formats. The sensitivity of serology ranges from 60% to 90% for detection of cystic echinococcosis depending on the size, number, viability, and integrity of the cysts and prior treatment.[39] Small intact cysts are less likely to elicit an immune response, whereas ruptured cysts produce a rapid increase in antibody production.[6US] Generally, an EIA or IHA is used for screening for *E. granulosus*, whereas confirmation of positive reactions is performed using an immunoblot assay.[41] False-positive results may be seen in up to 25% of patients with cysticercosis, but these diseases can usually be distinguished on clinical and radiologic grounds.[6US]

Patients with other causes of echinococcosis will usually have detectable antibodies using commercially available *E. granulosus* tests.[6US] Specific *E. multilocularis* serologic tests are not commercially available in the United States, but are available through specialized laboratories in Europe.[6US]

When serologic tests are negative and echinococcosis is still suspected on the basis of clinical and radiologic grounds, identification of protoscoleces or free hooklets from aspirated or excised cyst material allows for definitive diagnosis. Care must be taken when puncturing an echinococcal cyst to avoid rupture and anaphylactic reactions.[6US]

Imaging

Imaging plays an important role in diagnosis.[38] Findings vary with the stage of the cyst and the infecting species. Ultrasound is commonly used for cystic echinococcosis screening, particularly in resource-limited settings, and has a diagnostic accuracy approaching 90%.[39] Both simple and multivesicular cysts can be appreciated, whereas repositioning the patient may reveal punctate echogenic foci within the cyst, representing free-floating protoscoleces.[39] When the inner endocyst layer detaches from the outer pericyst, the membrane appears to "float" within the cystic cavity; this is the so-called "water lily" sign. The widely used WHO Informal Working Group on Echinococcosis classification divides the cysts of *E. granulosus* into five categories on the basis of their composition (simple cyst vs. multiple septations/daughter cysts) and degree of viability (active, transitional, or inactive).[11,38,39] This classification is used to guide treatment decisions on the basis of the suitability for therapeutic aspiration or surgical removal. CT and magnetic resonance imaging (MRI) offer increased sensitivity (94%) over US for detection of cystic echinococcosis and are important methods for detecting vascular and biliary involvement.[39] CT is also commonly used to guide needle aspiration and monitor for perisurgical complications.[39]

Alveolar and polycystic echinococcosis have a much more heterogeneous appearance on imaging, with irregular infiltrative lesions that may be mistaken for a malignancy. Postobstructive dilation of the biliary ducts and narrowing of hepatic and portal veins is commonly seen.[11]

Gross findings

An active lesion of cyst of *E. granulosus* may be a simple fluid-filled cyst or contain multiple thin-walled daughter cysts (Fig. 9.13). Forty percent to 80% of patients have a single cyst.[38] Brood capsules are sometimes seen as small, 1-to-2-mm granular nodules on

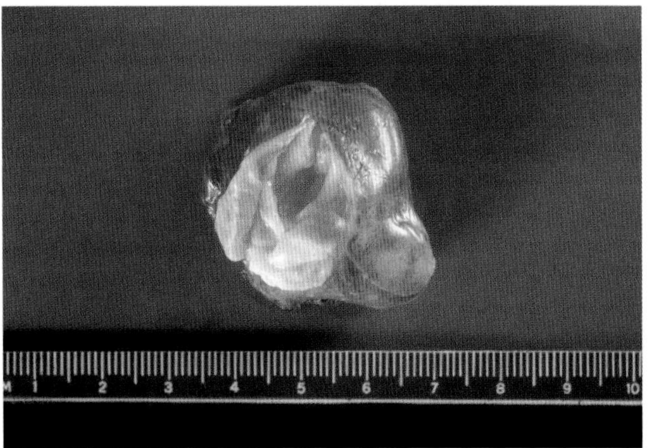

Figure 9.13 Hydatid cyst of *Echinococcus granulosus*. The outer cyst wall has been incised to reveal the numerous internal daughter cysts. Image courtesy of Dr. I. Kagan and the CDC public health image library.

the inner surface of the cyst wall. Over time, cysts of *E. granulosus* can reach massive proportions (35 cm or more) and contain innumerable variably sized daughter cysts.[40] Degenerating or inactive cysts may be partially fibrosed or contain yellow-green pasty material.[40]

In contrast to cystic echinococcosis, the lesion of alveolar echinococcosis appears as firm, relatively solid mass composed of minute cysts and intervening fibrous tissue. The lesion is not contained within a parent cyst and has an infiltrative border (Fig. 9.14). As with its radiologic appearance, its gross appearance is suggestive of malignancy.

The lesions of polycystic echinococcosis are sponge-like and composed of multiple, variably sized macroscopic cysts measuring up to several centimeters in diameter. The cystic mass may replace large portions of the liver and extend into adjacent structures.

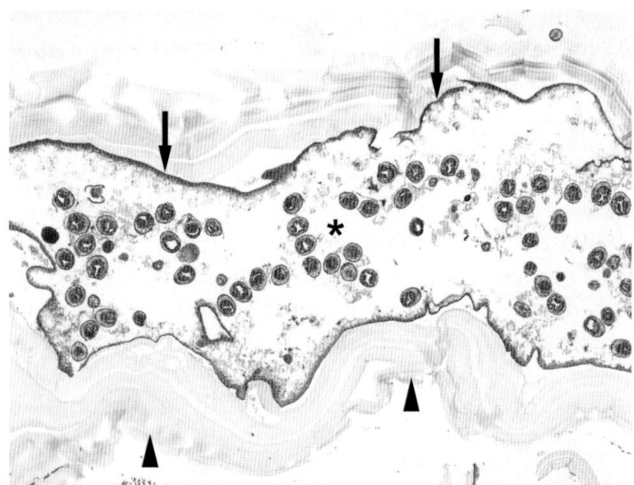

Figure 9.15 Section of an intact *E. granulosus* daughter cyst demonstrating an eosinophilic germinal layer (*arrows*) and surrounding acellular laminated layer (*arrow heads*) (H&E, 40×). Inside the cyst (*asterisk*) are multiple protoscoleces.

Microscopic findings

Both the parent cyst and daughter cysts of *E. granulosus* have an outer acellular laminated layer and thin inner nucleated germinal layer (Fig. 9.15). Over time, the parent cyst becomes surrounded by a thick host–derived fibrous wall (the pericyst) and surrounding compressed liver tissue.[40] Multiple protoscoleces may be seen within each daughter cyst (Figs. 9.15 and 9.16), either free-floating or contained within thin-walled brood capsules.[40] Protoscoleces contain an inverted ring of refractile hooklets (Fig. 9-16) and commonly have stromal calcified bodied (calcareous corpuscles), which are characteristic of all cestodes.[13] Occasionally, everted protoscoleces are seen. The term *hydatid sand* is used to describe the combination of degenerated protoscoleces and free hooklets.[6US,13] This material is commonly encountered in cytology and microbiology preparations of aspirated cyst fluid. Collapsed, degenerating, and ruptured cysts may occasionally pose a diagnostic dilemma when viable protoscoleces are not seen. The presence of a thick, laminated eosinophilic layer on H&E-stained sections is strongly suggestive of cystic echinococcosis, and a careful search may reveal degenerated protoscoleces and/or free hooklets (Fig. 9.17).

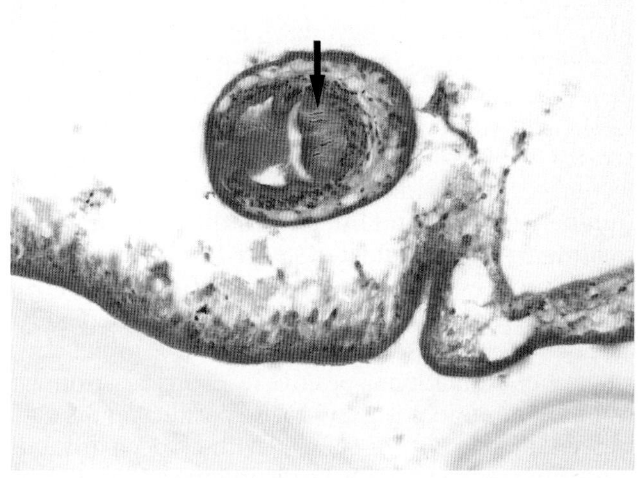

Figure 9.16 Higher magnification of the case shown in Figure 9-14 demonstrating a protoscolex (inverted tapeworm head) with refractile hooklets (*arrow*; H&E, 400×).

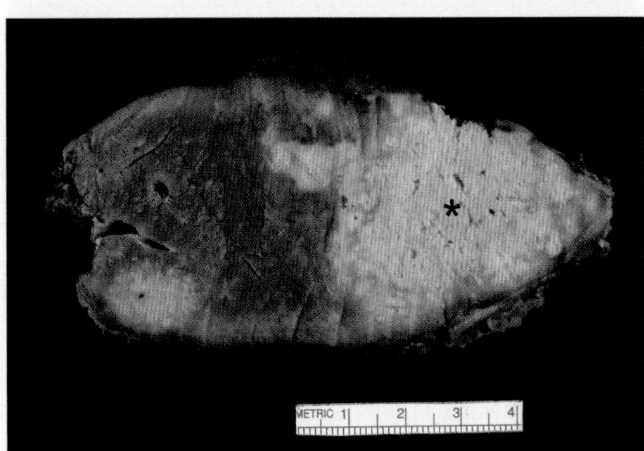

Figure 9.14 Portion of resected liver showing infiltrating lesions of *Echinococcus multilocularis* (asterisks). Image courtesy of Dr. Michael Keeney, MD. © Copyright Mayo Clinic.

Unlike *E. granulosus, E. multilocularis* usually presents as sterile, variably sized, and irregularly shaped cysts infiltrating into adjacent host tissue (Fig. 9.18). The cysts may be thin-walled or lined with an attenuated laminated layer (Fig. 9.19) and are surrounded by a granulomatous, necrotic, or fibrotic host reaction.[40] Protoscoleces are not commonly produced in humans.

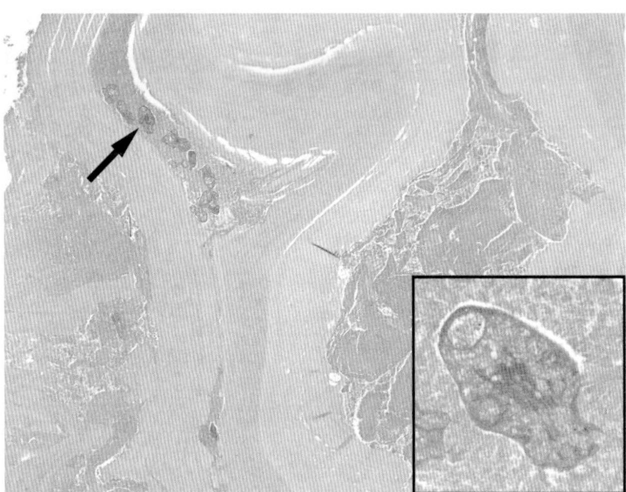

Figure 9.17 Old echinococcal cyst of *E. granulosus* in which only the laminated layer and mummified protoscoleces (*arrow*, inset) are seen (H&E, 40×; inset 400×). A careful search revealed rare free hooklets.

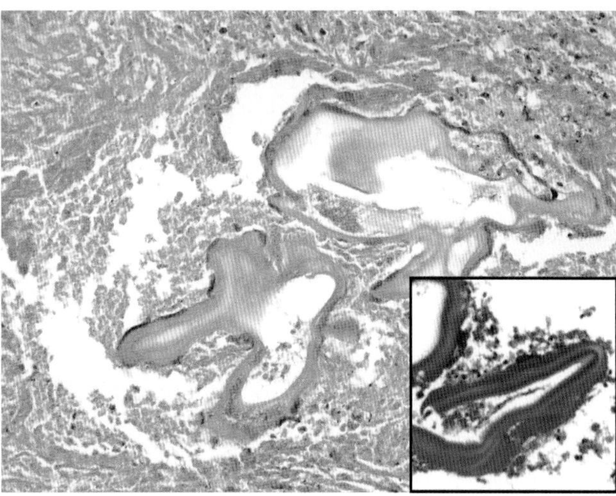

Figure 9.19 Cysts of *E. multilocularis* from the case shown in Figures 9-14 and 9-18. As is common with human infection, the cysts do not contain protoscoleces and only have thin outer laminated layers (H&E 400×; inset Masson Trichrome, 400×).

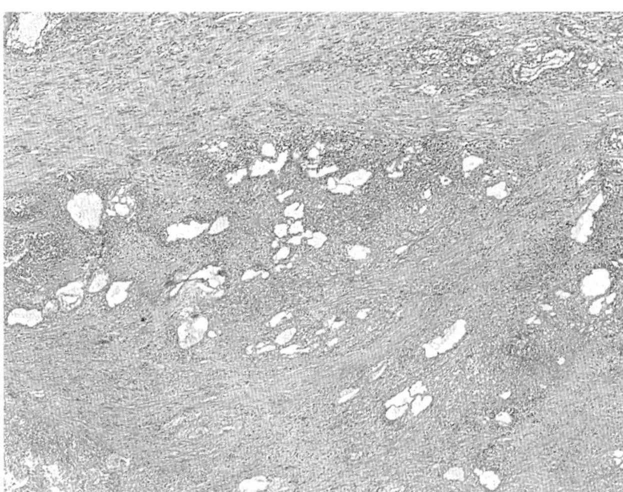

Figure 9.18 Low-power view of invasive *E. multilocularis* cysts in a portion of resected liver (H&E, 40×). Note that the individual cysts are seen invading through host tissue and are not confined by an outer cyst wall as they are in *E. granulosus* infection.

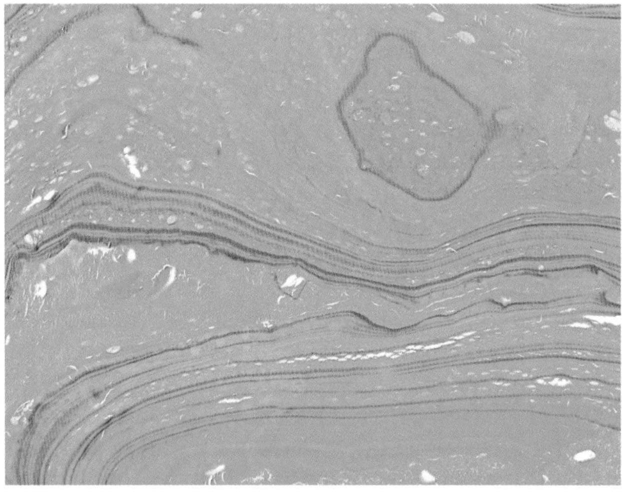

Figure 9.20 GMS highlights the laminated layers of hydatid cysts and is a useful method for differentiating the parasite-derived material from similar-appearing host material such as layered fibrin deposits (40×).

Polycystic echinococcosis appears as distinct infiltrative cysts containing protoscoleces.

Special stains

Cystic echinococcosis can usually be diagnosed using H&E alone. However, GMS (Fig. 9.20), PAS, and Masson trichome may be useful for highlighting the laminated membranes of the endocyst and differentiating them from similar-appearing nonparasitic structures such as laminated deposits of fibrin and lipid pseudomembranes.[13] These stains are also useful for highlighting the attenuated laminated layer of *E. multilocularis* cysts (Fig. 9.19).

Differential diagnosis

Cystic and polycystic echinococcosis have a characteristic histologic appearance, particularly when protoscoleces are seen, and are not usually confused with other cyst-forming tapeworm infections such as cysticercosis and coenurosis.[13] In comparison, alveolar echinococcosis can be very challenging to diagnose owing to its diffuse infiltrative nature and general lack of protoscoleces. In these cases, the differential diagnosis includes benign cystic lesions.[40] The diagnosis can usually be made through careful examination of the cysts and *Echinococcus* serologic testing.

Prognosis and treatment

Cystic echinococcosis does not cause symptoms unless it ruptures, impinges on neighboring structures, or communicates with the biliary tree. Over time, cysts may resolve spontaneously, and therefore a "watch and wait" approach can be taken with degenerating or inactive cysts. Active cysts, on the other hand, should be treated to decrease the risk of rupture, anaphylaxis, and secondary bacterial infection.[40] The type of treatment depends on the size and complexity of the cyst; well-described algorithms are described elsewhere.[39] Medical therapy alone (albendazole or mebendazole) may be used for simple cysts, less than 5 cm in diameter, whereas larger active lesions are generally surgically excised or treated using the PAIR (percutaneous aspiration, injection, and reaspiration) procedure, in conjunction with medical therapy.[39] With the latter procedure, approximately 30% of the cyst contents are percutaneously aspirated, the cyst is injected with a scolicidal agent (e.g., hypertonic saline, 95% alcohol), and then the contents are reaspirated.[39] This serves to sterilize the inner germinal layer of the endocyst so that new protoscoleces cannot be formed. PAIR is often the method of choice for handling single cysts with no or few daughter cysts, but is contraindicated for large cysts with multiple daughter cysts and in cases with cyst communication with the biliary tree.[39]

The aggressive nature of infection by alveolar and polycystic echinococcosis is associated with a worse outcome compared with cystic echinococcosis. Complete excision of the infiltrative mass should be performed whenever possible, in conjunction with medical treatment. When complete excision is not possible, life-long suppression with albendazole or mebendazole may be required. Unchecked growth of the parasite may be fatal.[6US,37]

9.5 TREMATODES (FLUKES)

Schistosoma spp. (schistosomiasis, bilharzia)

Definition, etiology, and pathogenesis

Schistosomiasis, also known as *bilharzia*, is a potentially chronic and debilitating infection caused by blood flukes in the genus *Schistosoma*. The main species that infect humans are *S. mansoni, S. japonicum,* and *S. haematobium*.[6] *S. mekongi* and *S. intercalatum* also cause human disease in geographically localized areas.[6] *S. haematobium* primarily causes urogenital disease, whereas the others primarily cause intestinal and hepatosplenic disease; the latter will be the focus of this section.[6,42]

Schistosomiasis is a major public health problem in the tropics and subtropics worldwide. It is classified by the WHO as a neglected tropical disease and is estimated to affect nearly 240 million people, most of whom live in Africa.[1] *Schistosoma mansoni* is found in parts of Africa, the Middle East, South America, and the Caribbean, whereas *S. haematobium* is found in Africa and the Middle East and *S. japonicum* is found in Asia and Southeast Asia. *S. intercalatum* and *S. mekongi* are only found in regions of central West Africa and Southeast Asia, respectively.[6]

Individuals become infected when they come into contact with microscopic, free-swimming parasite forms (cercariae) in fresh water.[6] The cercariae are capable of penetrating intact skin, after which they travel in the blood stream to the lungs and then the liver. Schistosomes mature into male and female worms in the liver and then travel as a pair to the venous plexus (*S. haematobium*) or mesenteric plexus (all other species) where they remain for their lifespan.[6] The schistosomes are unique from other human-pathogenic flukes in that they have separate sexes rather than being hermaphrodites. The slender female resides in the anterior groove (gynecophoric canal) of the larger male and only leaves periodically to deposit eggs in the terminal venules. Some of these eggs will lodge in the adjacent tissues (bladder or intestine) and are extruded into urine or stool. If human waste containing schistosome eggs is deposited into fresh water, then the eggs will hatch and the parasite can infect its intermediate snail host.[6] The snail infection eventually results in production of more cercariae. Unfortunately, most eggs are retained in the adjacent tissues or are swept away to the liver where they induce a granulomatous host response.[6] The resultant pathology is dependent on the number of deposited eggs, the site of egg deposition, and the extent of the host reaction to the egg antigens.[41] In the liver, eggs are deposited primarily in the presinusoidal portal areas. Although early disease is reversible, ongoing fibrosis results in irreversible organ damage.[42]

Clinical features

Schistosomiasis may manifest in different ways depending on the stage of infection and the organs involved. In some individuals, the first evidence of infection is the production of a pruritic papular rash at the site of cercarial penetration.[41] The rash is short lived and will resolve spontaneously. Four to 6 weeks later, the female schistosome begins to release eggs into the blood stream, which may stimulate a host immune response to the circulating egg antigens.[42] This stage of disease, known as acute schistosomiasis or Katayama fever, is characterized by fever, urticaria, arthralgias, myalgias, cough, wheezing, abdominal pain, cachexia, diarrhea, tender hepatosplenomegaly, lymphadenopathy, eosinophilia, and IgE hypergammaglobulinemia.[41,42] The chronic manifestations of infection occur with ongoing deposition of eggs in surrounding tissues. Genitourinary involvement is characterized by hematuria, dysuria, hydronephrosis, bladder or urethral obstruction, and squamous cell carcinoma of the bladder, whereas intestinal involvement is characterized by bloody diarrhea, polyp formation, and obstruction. The liver is also commonly involved in cases of intestinal disease. The early (compensated) stage of hepatosplenic schistosomiasis is characterized by mild hemolytic anemia, leukopenia, thrombocytopenia, mildly elevated alkaline phosphatase, normal transaminases, and palpable hepatomegaly.[42] Later during decompensated disease, patients present with a small shrunken liver, hepatic encephalopathy, hypoalbuminemia, massive ascites, splenomegaly, esophageal varices, and muscle wasting.[42] Interestingly, cirrhosis does not occur unless there is coinfection with HIV or hepatitis viruses.[42] *Schistosoma japonicum* infection has been identified as a potential risk factor for hepatocellular carcinoma, but other risk factors for cancer development (e.g., alcohol abuse, hepatitis B virus infection) are also commonly present, thus making this association less clear.[42]

Diagnosis is most commonly made by identification of characteristic eggs in urine or stool (Fig. 9.21).[6] The eggs of *S. mansoni* are among the largest parasite eggs found in stool (114 to 180 µm long by 45 to 70 µm wide) and have a large lateral spine. In comparison, the eggs of *S. japonicum* are smaller, measuring 70 to 100 µm long by 55 to 64 µm wide. They have only a small rudimentary spine, which is not commonly appreciated in tissue sections. The eggs of *S. mekongi* have a similar appearance to *S. japonicum*, but are slightly smaller. Finally, the eggs of *S. intercalatum* are elongated, 140 to 240 µm in length, and have a small pinched-off terminal spine. They have a similar appearance to the eggs of *S. haematobium* seen in urine, but are slightly larger. Examination of at least three stool specimens, collected on different days and examined using concentration techniques, is recommended for optimal sensitivity.[41] Less commonly, rectal biopsy is performed for egg detection.

In suspected cases where eggs are not detected, serologic testing can be used for presumptive diagnosis. The assays performed at the CDC have estimated sensitivities of 99%, 95%, and <50% for detection of *S. mansoni, S. haematobium,* and *S. japonicum,* respectively.[6]

Imaging

In chronic hepatosplenic schistosomiasis with periportal fibrosis, the thickened walls of the portal vein and its branches are seen as echogenic bands on US and low-density homogeneous bands on CT.[11,43] Splenomegaly and evidence of portal hypertension may also be seen.[43]

Gross findings

The external surface of the liver may be smooth, bosselated, or nodular, and the cut surface usually shows marked periportal fibrosis with intervening

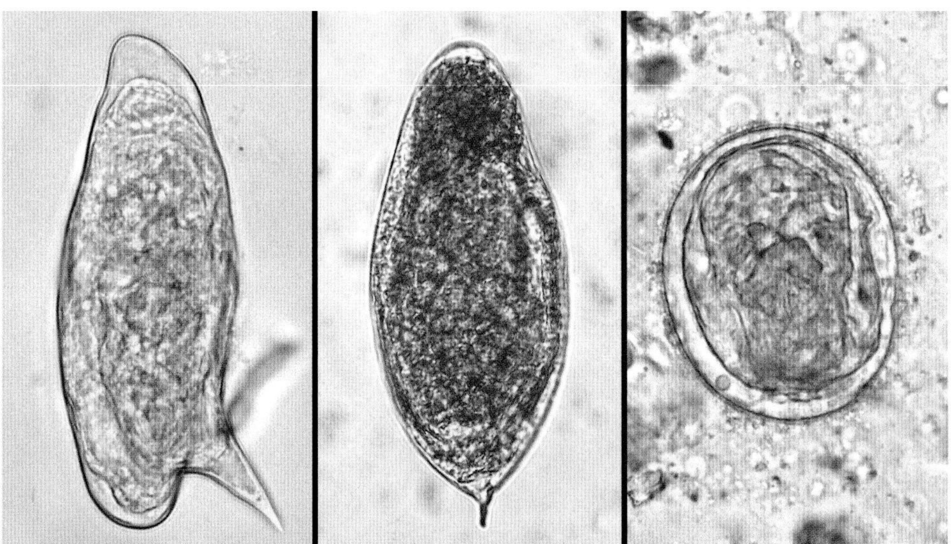

Figure 9.21 ***Schistosoma* eggs.** From left to right are *Schistosoma mansoni, Schistosoma haematobium,* and *Schistosoma japonicum*, showing lateral, terminal, and rudimentary (*arrow*) spines, respectively. Images reproduced from Pritt BS. *Parasitology Benchtop Reference Guide: An Illustrated Guide for Commonly Encountered Parasites*. Northfield, IL: College of American Pathologists; 2014, with permission.

normal-appearing parenchyma.[11,44] This characteristic pattern of fibrosis is also referred to as *Symmers' pipe stem fibrosis*, in reference to the individual who described this pathology and the gross resemblance of the thick fibrotic lesions to the stem of a pipe.[43]

Microscopic findings

The characteristic finding in the liver is periportal fibrosis with pylephlebitis/peripylephlebitis associated with deposited schistosome eggs and granulomatous inflammation (Figs. 9.22 and 9.23).[43] Fibrotic portal areas containing a bile ductule and arteriole without a venule are common.[44] The fibrosis is distinctive in that it is not associated with bridging fibrosis, cirrhosis, hepatocellular injury, or nodule formation.[43] Eggs are seen as round, oval, or elongated structures in cross-section and commonly contain multiple, small basophilic nuclei (Fig. 9.23). The outer contour often becomes irregular and infolded during histologic processing, and care must be taken not to interpret these irregularities as spines. Figure 9.24 shows a rare example of a true lateral spine of *S. mansoni*. The eggs of *S. mansoni* commonly elicit a granulomatous host response, which occasionally includes eosinophils (Fig. 9.24). The Splendore-Hoeppli phenomenon may be observed around eggs within eosinophilic granulomas. *Schistosoma japonicum* eggs are less likely to be associated with a robust immune response. Over time, retained eggs will die and calcify (Fig. 9.25).

The adult flukes are only rarely seen in tissue sections (Fig. 9-22). The female measures up to 26 mm long by 0.5 mm wide and is most commonly found in the anterior groove of larger male. There is typically no associated immune response around the adult worms.[41]

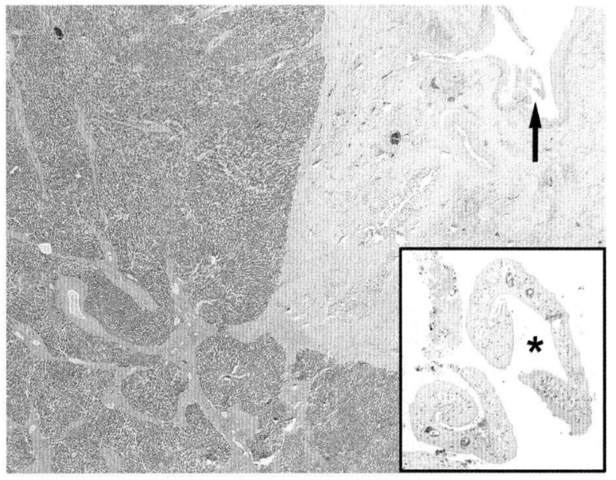

Figure 9.22 Hepatic schistosomiasis due to *S. japonicum*. Numerous eggs are present in the surrounding tissue, and there is increased portal fibrosis in the neighboring liver parenchyma. Two adult schistosome males can be seen in cross-section within a large vessel (H&E, 20×, *arrow*; inset 200×). The female is not seen in this section but would normally be resting in the gynecophoric canal of the male (*asterisk*).

Differential diagnosis

The clinical differential for hepatobiliary schistosomiasis includes visceral leishmaniasis and other causes of portal hypertension. The primary histopathologic differential is other entities that produce eggs in the liver. This includes *Capillaria hepatica,*[45,46] *Ascaris lumbricoides,*[47] and the liver flukes, *Clonorchis sinensis, Opisthorchis* spp., and *Fasciola hepatica.*[2] *Capillaria hepatica* is a roundworm that only rarely

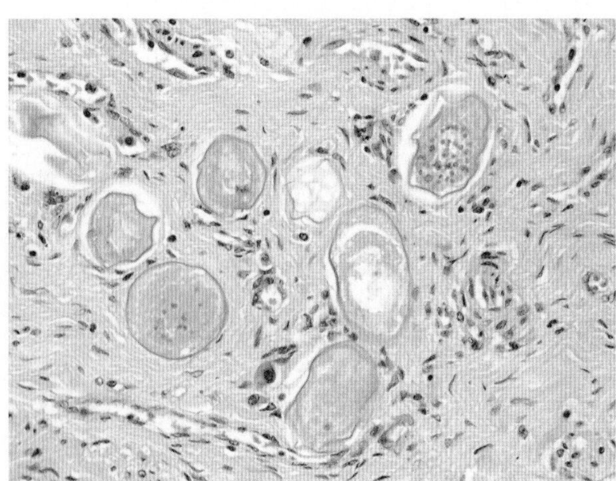

Figure 9.23 Multiple eggs of *S. japonicum* from the case shown in Figure 9-22 in regions of periportal fibrosis (H&E, 400×). Histologic processing results in irregularities of the outer shells of the eggs, and these should not be mistaken for spines. Note the small nuclei within some of the eggs.

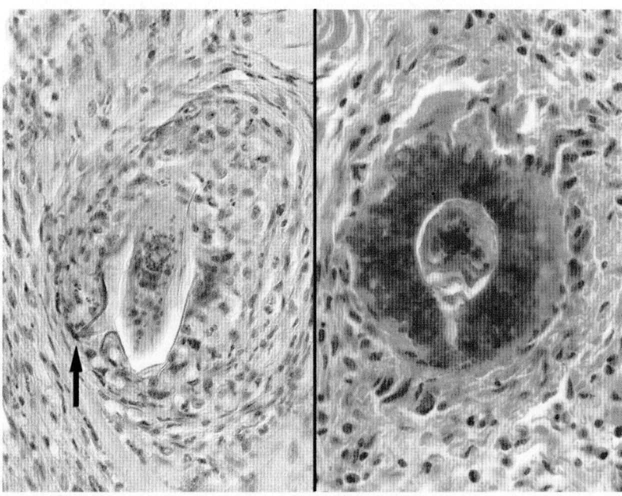

Figure 9.24 *Schistosoma mansoni* eggs from two separate cases (H&E, 400×). The image on the left shows a rarely seen lateral spine (*arrow*), whereas the image on the right shows an egg within an eosinophilic granuloma with surrounding proteinaceous club-like material (Splendore-Hoeppli phenomenon).

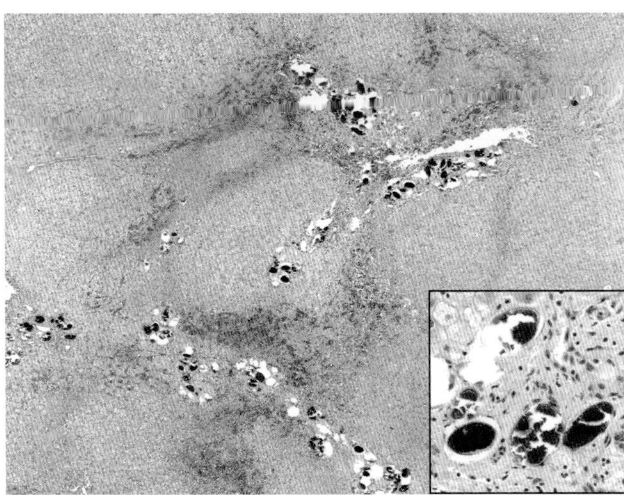

Figure 9.25 Hepatic schistosomiasis due to *Schistosoma japonicum* (H&E, 40×). Note the deposition of calcified eggs in a mostly periportal distribution. Many of the eggs are calcified, indicating a long-standing or previously treated infection (inset, 400×).

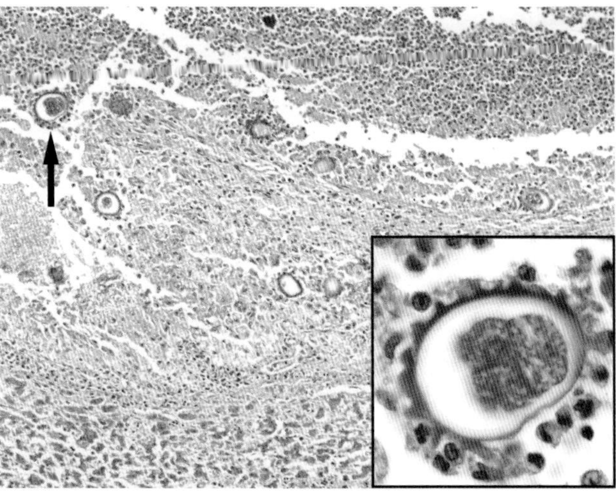

Figure 9.27 Hepatic ascariasis demonstrating several deeply eosinophilic thick-walled eggs with a characteristic outer bumpy layer (mammillations) within an abscess (*arrow*; H&E, 100×; inset 1,000×).

infects humans.[6] *Capillaria hepatica* produces eggs that resemble those of the whipworm, *Trichuris trichiura,* but have distinct striated walls that allow their differentiation (Fig. 9.26). Eggs of the roundworms *Ascaris lumbricoides* (Fig. 9.27) and *Enterobius vermicularis* (Fig. 9.28) may be found in the liver when the adult worms aberrantly migrate up the biliary tree from the intestine. They are usually seen within a hepatic abscess that is formed in response to the dying worm and deposited eggs. Again, characteristics of the eggs can be used to differentiate these organisms. Finally, the eggs of the liver flukes may be found in the liver, usually within the biliary tree associated with adult worms. The liver flukes are discussed later in further detail.

Prognosis and treatment

The prognosis of chronic hepatosplenic schistosomiasis is relatively good, considering that hepatic function is preserved until late in the disease.[42] Praziquantel is the drug of choice and will kill the adult worms, thus stopping egg production.[6] Unfortunately, much of the long-term damage is irreversible. Surgical therapy may be required for alleviation of portal hypertension.[42]

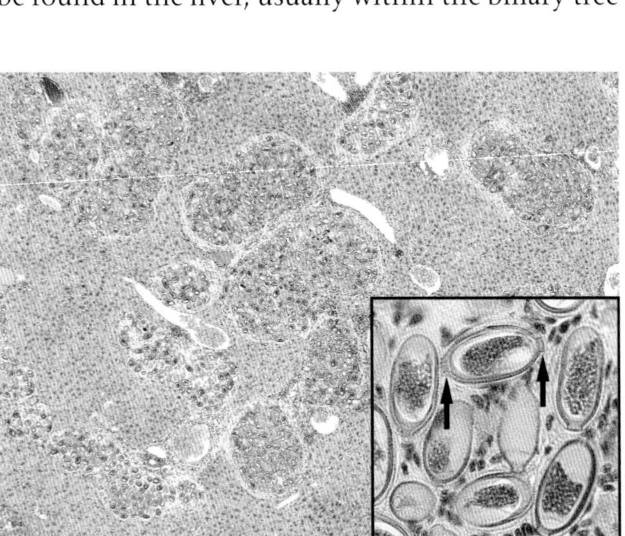

Figure 9.26 Hepatic capillariasis in which large collections of eggs are present in the parenchyma (H&E, 40×). Higher magnification (inset, 400×) shows the characteristic nature of the eggs with striated walls (accentuated by narrowing the condenser on the microscope) and bipolar plugs (*arrows*).

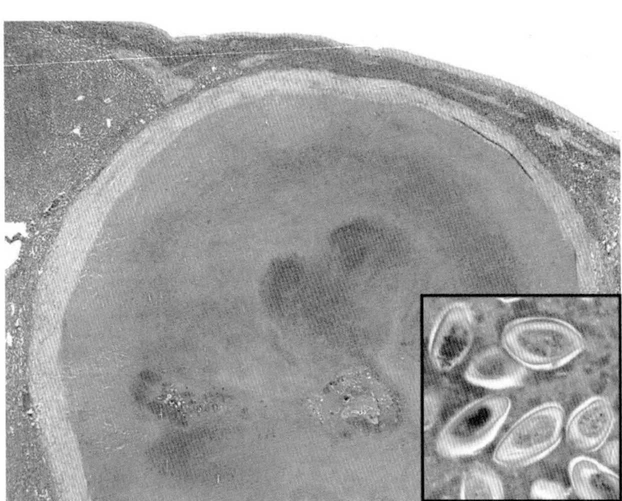

Figure 9.28 Hepatic abscess due to *Enterobius vermicularis.* Numerous characteristic eggs are seen within the abscess (H&E, 20×; inset 400×). The eggs are ovoid, measure approximately 60 μm in length and are slightly flattened on one side.

Clonorchis sinensis/Opisthorchis spp. (clonorchiasis/opisthorchiasis)

Definition, etiology, and pathogenesis

Clonorchis and *Opisthorchis* are closely related small trematodes that preferentially infect the biliary tree.[2,6] *Clonorchis sinensis*, also known as the Chinese liver fluke, is found in parts of Asia, including China, Korea, Vietnam, and Taiwan; *Opisthorchis viverrini* (the Southeast Asian liver fluke) is found in northeast Thailand, Kampuchea, and Laos; and *Opisthorchis felis* (the cat liver fluke) is found in parts of Europe and Asia, including Russia.[6,48]

These flukes are acquired through ingestion of undercooked fish and are therefore considered to be a foodborne trematodiases.[1] The WHO classifies the foodborne trematodiases as neglected tropical diseases and estimates at least 12.5 million individuals are infected with *Clonorchis sinensis* in China alone.[1]

Clonorchis and *Opisthorchis* require three different hosts for completion of their life cycle. When the definitive host (humans, dogs, cats, and other fish-eating mammals) ingests the encysted parasite (the metacercariae) in undercooked fish, the parasite excysts in the duodenum and migrates through the ampulla of Vater into the biliary tree. Within 3 to 4 weeks of infection, the flukes reach maturity and reside within the intrahepatic bile ducts where they feed on ductular epithelial cells.[49] These flukes are hermaphrodites, containing both male and female reproductive organs, and therefore a single worm is capable of producing infective eggs. The eggs are released into the bile, which then enters the feces. When feces containing eggs is allowed to enter fresh water, the eggs may be ingested by the first intermediate host (a snail). Further maturation in the snail results in the production of cercariae, which leave the snail and encyst within the flesh of the second intermediate host (freshwater fish). When undercooked or raw fish is eaten by humans or other definitive hosts, the parasite's life cycle continues.

The pathogenesis of clonorchiasis and opisthorchiasis encompasses several factors, including mechanical obstruction of the bile ducts by the adult flukes, epithelial injury caused by flukes' feeding activities, and toxic effects caused by the flukes' excretory-secretory products.[48] The worms may also act as a nidus for biliary stone formation or secondary bacterial infection, resulting in cholangitis, ductal wall fibrosis, and subsequent dilatations and strictures of the biliary tree. Cholangiocarcinoma is an uncommon but important complication of long-term infection.[6,48]

Clinical features

The clinical presentation is dependent on the worm burden and degree of associated bile duct inflammation. Patients with a low parasite burden are often asymptomatic.[50] When present, symptoms may change over the course of infection. During the acute stage, patients commonly present with nausea, diarrhea, headache, and abdominal pain, usually in the right upper quadrant, and tender hepatomegaly.[48] Eosinophilia, leukocytosis, and elevated bilirubin levels are commonly seen. Chronic infection is associated with cholangitis, intrahepatic lithiasis, hepatic abscess, and cholangiocarcinoma.[48,50] Patients with clonorchiasis and opisthorchiasis have a 15-fold higher risk of developing cholangiocarcinoma than do noninfected individuals.

Diagnosis is usually accomplished by microscopic identification of characteristic eggs in stool or duodenal aspirates.[6,48] Adult flukes may also be recovered during ERCP or surgery. Serologic testing is an ancillary method for supporting the diagnosis, but is not widely available in nonendemic settings.[6]

Imaging

The most significant findings are seen with heavy infection. The common bile duct may be dilated (2.5 cm or more in diameter) and stones, adult worms and debris may be seen within the ducts.[11] Adult flukes are 1 to 2 cm in length and appear as small, curved filling defects on ERCP and hyperdense material on CT.[11] Diffuse dilation of intrahepatic ducts, especially in the liver periphery, with less extrahepatic duct dilation is characteristic of clonorchiasis. Evidence of fibrosis and thickening of bile duct walls may be seen as echogenic areas on US. MRI shows similar findings as CT, but provides increased sensitivity for detection of early cholangiocarcinoma.[11]

Gross findings

The liver is commonly enlarged and demonstrates pale cystic areas on the external surface corresponding with dilated bile ducts.[51] On cut surfaces, dilated bile ducts with thickened walls are often visible. The parenchyma has a normal appearance unless malignancy or coinfecting viruses are present.[51] Adult flukes may be grossly visible in the medium-to-large bile ducts, particularly in the left lobe. Biliary stones or sludge may also be noted within the bile ducts.

Microscopic findings

The primary pathology is seen in the bile ducts. The ducts are dilated and there is usually periductal inflammation and fibrosis. The ductal epithelium may exhibit desquamation, adenomatous hyperplasia, goblet cell metaplasia, and occasionally, dysplasia.[50] When dysplasia is seen, this should prompt a careful search for early cholangiocarcinoma. The hepatocytes appear relatively normal unless there is secondary bacterial cholangiohepatitis and abscess.[51]

Flattened, leaf-like flukes may be seen within the ducts and allow for definitive diagnosis (Fig. 9.29). *Clonorchis sinensis* adults measures 10 to 25 mm in length by 3 to 5 mm in width, whereas *Opisthorchis* adults are approximately half this size.[52] On cross-section, these flukes have a thin body wall, measuring 25 to 30 μm in thickness. The external cuticle is smooth without spines (in contrast to the spines of *Fasciola hepatica*), and portions of the oral and ventral suckers may be seen. Eggs are commonly seen in the uterus and aid in making the diagnosis. The eggs of *Clonorchis* and *Opisthorchis* species are small, measuring approximately 30 μm long by 15 μm wide, and have an operculum (lid-like opening) at one end (Fig. 9.30). On either side of the operculum is an external bump; thus, the operculum is said to be "shouldered." An important feature for differentiating *C. sinensis* and *Opisthorchis* spp. adults from *Fasciola* spp. is the presence of only two gut branches when seen in cross-section (Fig. 9-30). As discussed in the section below, *Fasciola* species are larger flukes with multiple gut branches, which aids in identification.

Differential diagnosis

The clinical differential includes fascioliasis, schistosomiasis, *Strongyloides stercoralis* hyperinfection, ectopic ascariasis with biliary involvement, choledocholithiasis, and primary sclerosing cholangitis.[53] When flukes are seen within the biliary tree, the differential diagnosis includes the liver fluke, *Fasciola hepatica* (discussed below), as well as some lesser-known flukes such as *Metorchis bilis, Metorchis conjunctus, M. orientalis, Dicrocoelium dendriticum, Dicrocoelium hospes,* and *Pseudamphistomum truncatum.*[53] *Metorchis bilis,* in particular, has recently been identified as a main agent of liver fluke infection in Russia, along with *O. felineus.*[53] It is not possible to reliably differentiate *Clonorchis, Opisthorchis,* and *Metorchis* from their eggs alone or from the fluke morphology in tissue sections.[53] However, anatomic differences of intact adult flukes can be used for differentiation; examination is best performed by an experienced parasitologist. Molecular methods may also be used.[53] It is not clinically important to differentiate *C. sinensis* from *Opisthorchis* spp., but it may be useful to accurately identify *Metorchis* spp. because they have not been definitively associated with cholangiocarcinoma.[53]

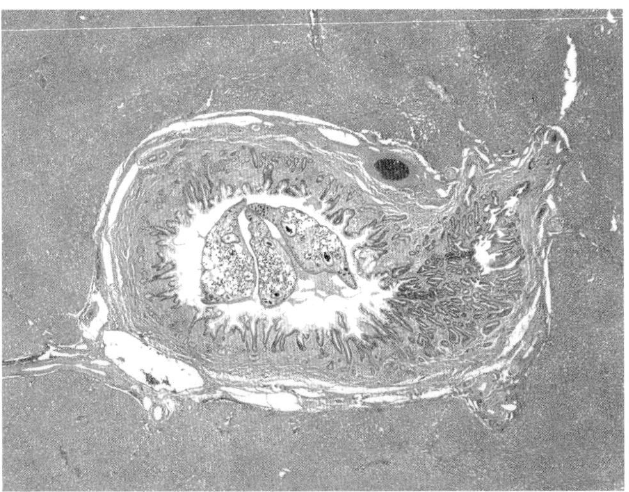

Figure 9.29 Three *Clonorchis sinensis* adult flukes in a bile duct (H&E, 20×). The surrounding liver appears relatively normal.

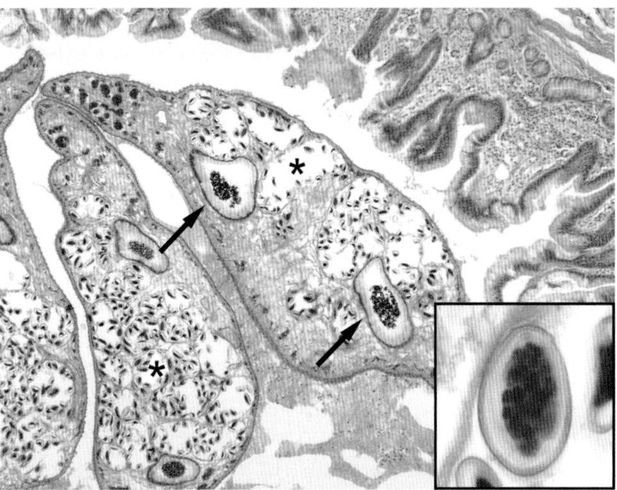

Figure 9.30 Higher magnification of the flukes in Figure 9-29 demonstrates the characteristic morphologic features including two gut branches (*arrows*) and uterus with numerous eggs (*asterisks*) (H&E, 100×). The intrauterine eggs measure approximately 30 microns in length and have a shouldered operculum, which is characteristic of *Clonorchis* and *Opisthorchis* species (1,000×).

Prognosis and treatment

Prognosis is generally good in early disease, but cases with severe hepatobiliary damage or cholangiocarcinoma have a significantly worse prognosis. Treatment is with praziquantel.[6] Ductal abnormalities may persist following successful treatment.[11]

Fasciola hepatica (fascioliasis)

Definition, etiology, and pathogenesis

Fascioliasis is caused primarily by *Fasciola hepatica,* and less commonly by *Fasciola gigantica.*[6] Like clonorchiasis and opisthorchiasis, fascioliasis is a foodborne trematodiasis and is classified as a neglected tropical disease by the WHO.[1] Fascioliasis is a disease with a global distribution, affecting an estimated 2.4 million individuals in 70 countries.[1] High-transmission regions include East and Southeast Asia, the Caspian Sea basin, the Nile river valley, and the highlands of South America.[1] Fascioliasis is primarily a zoonosis (disease of animals), and therefore its biggest economic impact is on livestock. However, humans are also capable of being definitive, albeit dead-end, hosts and may experience severe associated morbidity.[6]

The life cycle is complex and involves three hosts.[6] Humans and various herbivores become infected through ingestion of parasitic forms (metacercariae) on uncooked water plants such as watercress and water mint.[1,6] The metacercariae excyst in the duodenum, but rather than entering the bile duct through the ampulla of Vater like *Clonorchis* and *Opisthorchis*, they penetrate the bowel wall and migrate through the peritoneal cavity into the liver.[6] They then migrate through the liver parenchyma until they reach a large bile duct where they mature and reside. *Fasciola* spp. are hermaphrodites, and thus a single worm is capable of producing viable eggs. Eggs are released into the bile and are then shed in the feces. If feces containing eggs enters fresh water, then the eggs hatch and the parasite invades the first intermediate snail host.[6] After further maturation steps in snail, the parasite emerges as free-swimming cercariae, which encyst onto the second intermediate host (an aquatic plant) and form metacercariae.[6]

Fasciola spp. are large flukes that cause considerable damage when migrating through the liver parenchyma.[6] They later cause significant inflammation and obstruction when inhabiting the bile ducts. Despite their location in the bile ducts, *Fasciola* do not cause cholangiocarcinoma like *Clonorchis* and *Opisthorchis*.[6]

Clinical features

Acute fascioliasis occurs with the migration of the immature flukes from the duodenum into the liver. Associated symptoms include fever, nausea, diarrhea, anorexia, and mild to severe abdominal pain.[51] Urticaria with dermatographism is also frequently seen, as well as asthma. Hepatomegaly, ascites, anemia, and jaundice are common.[51]

Following the acute phase is a latent period that can last for months to years.[51] This phase is characterized by ongoing gastrointestinal symptoms and eosinophilia. The chronic obstructive phase then follows when the large adult flukes are located in the bile ducts. Ongoing mechanical obstruction and cholangitis manifests as epigastric pain, jaundice, pruritus, right-upper-quadrant pain, hepatosplenomegaly, ascites, and hemobilia.[51] Eosinophilia is common in all phases and may exceed 80% of the circulating leukocytes.[51] Leukocytosis, anemia, elevated erythrocyte sedimentation rate, and bilirubinemia are also seen. Less commonly, immature flukes may migrate outside of the liver. This usually results in production of painful migratory subcutaneous swellings.[51]

Definitive diagnosis is made by identification of characteristic eggs in feces or duodenal aspirates. False-positive results can occur when the patient has recently ingested liver of an infected animal and passes *Fasciola* eggs from the liver in the stool.[6] In this setting, it is important to inquire about the patient's diet and repeat the exam if liver was recently consumed. The eggs of the large intestinal fluke, *Fasciolopsis buski,* are indistinguishable from those of *F. hepatica,* and therefore egg identification must be carefully correlated with the clinical presentation.[6] Serology may be used to support the diagnosis, but availability is limited in nonendemic areas.[6]

Imaging

CT commonly reveals hypodense nodules throughout the parenchyma corresponding with microabscesses caused by the migrating fluke.[11] These nodules are characteristic but not diagnostic of fascioliasis because they cannot be differentiated from other causes of abscess and necrotic neoplasms. More diagnostic is the identification of tortuous channels representing migration tracks; these are present in 55% to 75% of cases.[11] Identification of adult flukes within dilated bile ducts is best appreciated using US.[11]

Gross findings

The liver is commonly enlarged, may have an irregular bosselated surface, and often has a thickened capsule with white to yellow striae.[51] Soft yellow to gray-white subcapsular nodules, 0.2 to 3 cm in diameter, may also be seen, which correspond histologically to eosinophilic abscesses.[51] Cut surfaces demonstrate extensive hemorrhage, with visible necrotic migration tracks. In the chronic obstructive phase of the disease, the bile ducts are dilated with thickened walls and may contain adult flukes.[51]

Microscopic findings

Fluke migration tracts are filled with necrotic cellular debris and commonly surrounded by eosinophilic infiltrates.[51] Adult flukes may be seen within the liver parenchyma (Fig. 9.31) or in bile ducts. When the ducts are involved, the epithelium usually shows extensive hyperplasia and dilation.[51] *Fasciola hepatica* adults are 2 to 5 cm long by 0.6 to 1.3 cm wide and

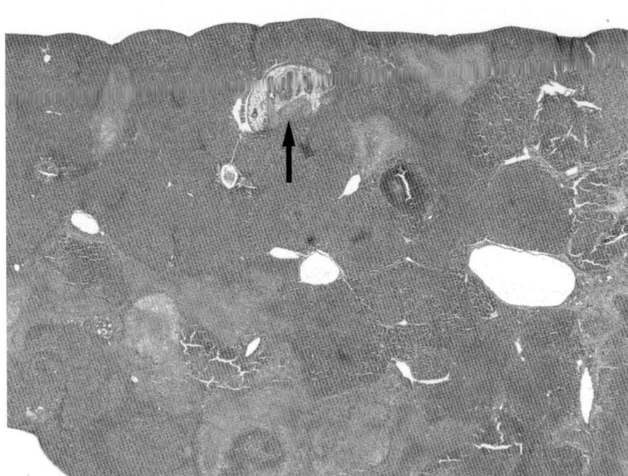

Figure 9.31 ***Fasciola hepatica*** **in a liver biopsy (*arrow*, H&E, 20×).** Note the extensive inflammation and disruption of the lobular architecture caused by the fluke's migration.

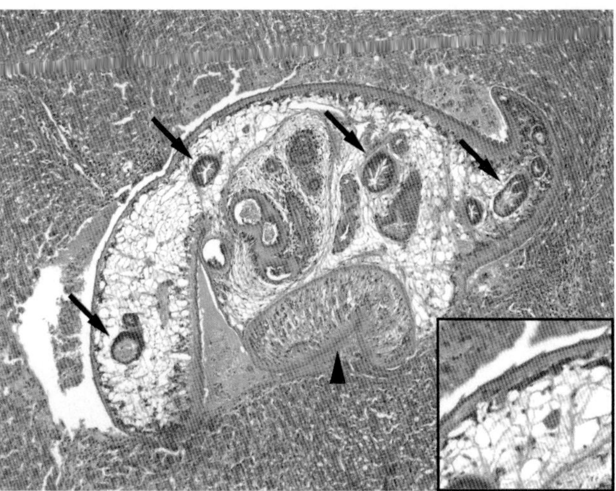

Figure 9.32 Higher magnification of Figure 9-31 demonstrates the characteristic morphologic features of *F. hepatica*, including multiple gut branches (*arrows*), sucker (*arrowhead*), and outer cuticular spines (inset); (H&E, 100×; inset 1,000×).

measure approximately 30 to 50 μm thick in tissue sections.[51] *Fasciola gigantica* is considerably larger than *F. hepatica,* measuring up to 7.5 cm long by 1.3 cm wide. Its body wall is approximately 50 μm thick.[51] Both *Fasciola* species have a thick spiny cuticle, and portions of the oral or ventral suckers are commonly seen (Fig. 9.32). Both also have multiple gut branches in cross-section, which is helpful for differentiating *Fasciola* spp. from *Clonorchis* and *Opisthorchis*.[13] The presence of characteristic eggs also aids in the diagnosis. The eggs of *F. hepatica* are large, 70 to 100 μm long by 63 to 90 μm wide, thin walled, and have a small indistinct operculum.[13] The eggs of *F. gigantica* have a similar appearance but can be up to twice as large.[6] Eggs may be seen within the uterus or bile ducts, or associated with granulomas in the biliary epithelium.[51]

Differential diagnosis

The clinical differential depends on the stage of infection. During the acute phase of infection, the differential includes other causes of fever, right-upper-quadrant pain, and eosinophilia, such as visceral larva migrans and acute schistosomiasis.[51] Identification of multiple liver lesions on imaging raises the possibility of malignancy or pyogenic abscesses. In the chronic obstructive phase, the differential includes other causes of cholangitis and biliary obstruction, such as choledocholithiasis, ectopic ascariasis, clonorchiasis, opisthorchiasis, and cholangiocarcinoma.[51]

When seen, adult flukes of *Fasciola* spp. must be differentiated from the other liver flukes such as *Clonorchis sinensis* and *Opisthorchis* spp. See the previous section for further information on identifying features.

Prognosis and treatment

The treatment of choice is triclabendazole, which is active against all stages of the fluke.[6] The prognosis is generally good, although some degree of fibrosis may remain after treatment.

REFERENCES

1. Neglected Tropical Diseases. World Health Organization, 2015. http://www.who.int/neglected_diseases/diseases/en/. Accessed July 31, 2016.
2. Rana SS, Bhasin DK, Nanda M, et al. Parasitic infestations of the biliary tract. *Curr Gastroenterol Rep*. 2007;9:156–164.
3. Neglected Parasitic Infections (NPIs) in the United States. 2014. http://www.cdc.gov/parasites/npi/. Accessed April 15, 2016.
4. Pritt BS, Clark CG. Amebiasis. *Mayo Clinic Proc*. 2008;83:1154–1159; quiz 9–60.
5. Stanley SL, Jr. Amoebiasis. *Lancet*. 2003;361:1025–1034.
6. DPDx—Laboratory Identification of Parasitic Diseases of Public Health Concern. Centers for Disease Control and Prevention, 2016. http://www.cdc.gov/dpdx/. Accessed November 8, 2016.
7. Walsh JA. Problems in recognition and diagnosis of amebiasis: estimation of the global magnitude of morbidity and mortality. *Rev Infect Dis*. 1986;8:228–238.
8. Salles JM, Moraes LA, Salles MC. Hepatic amebiasis. *Braz J Infect Dis*. 2003;7:96–110.

9. Fotedar R, Stark D, Beebe N, et al. Laboratory diagnostic techniques for Entamoeba species. *Clin Microbiol Rev*. 2007;20:511–532, table of contents.
10. Royer TL, Gilchrist C, Kabir M, et al. Entamoeba bangladeshi nov. sp., Bangladesh. *Emerg Infect Dis*. 2012;18:1543–1545.
11. Palmer PES, Reeder MM. *The Imaging of Tropical Diseases*. 2nd ed. Berlin: Springer; 2000.
12. Klassen-Fischer MK, Wear DJ, Neafie RC. Amebiasis. In: Meyers WM, Firpo A, Wear DJ, eds. *Topics on the Pathology of Protozoan and Invasive Arthropod Diseases*. Washington, DC: Armed Forces Institute of Pathology; 2011:1–15.
13. Orihel TC, Ash LR. *Parasites in Human Tissues*. Chicago, IL: ASCP Press; 1995.
14. Letter TM. *Drugs for Parasitic Infections*. 3rd ed. New Rochelle, NY: The Medical Letter, Inc.; 2013.
15. Magill AJ, Meyers WM, Klassen-Fischer MK, et al. Visceral leishmaniasis. In: Meyers WM, Firpo A, Wear DJ, eds. *Topics on the Pathology of Protozoan and Invasive Arthropod Diseases*. Washington, DC: Armed Forces Institue of Pathology; 2011:1–15.
16. Sundar S, Rai M. Laboratory diagnosis of visceral leishmaniasis. *Clin Diagn Lab Immunol*. 2002;9:951–958.
17. Sundar S, Maurya R, Singh RK, et al. Rapid, noninvasive diagnosis of visceral leishmaniasis in India: comparison of two immunochromatographic strip tests for detection of anti-K39 antibody. *J Clin Microbiol*. 2006;44:251–253.
18. el Hag IA, Hashim FA, el Toum IA, et al. Liver morphology and function in visceral leishmaniasis (Kala-azar). *J Clin Pathol*. 1994;47:547–551.
19. Duarte MI, Corbett CE. Histopathological patterns of the liver involvement in visceral leishmaniasis. *Rev Inst Med Trop Sao Paulo*. 1987;29:131–136.
20. Pritt BS. *Plasmodium* and *Babesia*. In: Jorgensen JH, Pfaller MA, Carroll KC, et al., eds. *Manual of Clinical Microbiology*. Washington, DC: ASM Press; 2015.
21. World Health Organization. *World Malaria Report 2015*. Geneva: World Health Organisation; 2015.
22. Klassen-Fischer MK, Neafie RC, Meyer AC. Malaria. In: Meyers WM, Firpo A, Wear DJ, eds. *Topics on the Pathology of Protozoan and Invasive Arthropod Diseases*. Washington, DC: Armed Forces Institue of Pathology; 2011.
23. Pritt BS. Protozoal infections. In: Procop GW, Pritt BS, eds. *Pathology of Infectious Diseases: A Volume in the Series Foundations in Diagnostic Pathology*. Philadelphia, PA: Elsevier; 2015:610–643.
24. Menezes RG, Pant S, Kharoshah MA, et al. Autopsy discoveries of death from malaria. *Leg Med (Tokyo)*. 2012;14:111–115.
25. Xiao L, Cama V. Cryptosporidium. In: Jorgensen JH, Pfaller MA, Carroll KC, et al., eds. *Manual of Clinical Microbiology*. Washington, DC: ASM Press; 2015:2435–2447.
26. Cello JP. Acquired immunodeficiency syndrome cholangiopathy: spectrum of disease. *Am J Med*. 1989;86:539–546.
27. Klassen-Fischer MK, Neafie RC, Wear DJ, et al. Cryptosporidiosis, isosporiasis, cyclosporiasis & sarcocystosis. In: Meyers WM, Firpo A, Wear DJ, eds. *Topics on the Pathology of Protozoan and Invasive Arthropod Diseases*. Washington, DC: Armed Forces Institue of Pathology; 2011.
28. Bouche H, Housset C, Dumont JL, et al. AIDS-related cholangitis: diagnostic features and course in 15 patients. *J Hepatol*. 1993;17:34–39.
29. Teixidor HS, Godwin TA, Ramirez EA. Cryptosporidiosis of the biliary tract in AIDS. *Radiology*. 1991;180:51–56.
30. Castiella A, Iribarren JA, Lopez P, et al. Ursodeoxycholic acid in the treatment of AIDS-associated cholangiopathy. *Am J Med*. 1997;103:170–171.
31. Despommier D. Toxocariasis: clinical aspects, epidemiology, medical ecology, and molecular aspects. *Clin Microbiol Rev*. 2003;16:265–272.
32. Lim JH. Toxocariasis of the liver: visceral larva migrans. *Abdom Imaging*. 2008;33:151–156.
33. Kwon NH, Oh MJ, Lee SP, et al. The prevalence and diagnostic value of toxocariasis in unknown eosinophilia. *Ann Hematol*. 2006;85:233–238.
34. DPDx: Amebiasis [*Entamoeba histolytica*]. Centers for Disease Control and Prevention, 2014. http://www.cdc.gov/dpdx/amebiasis/index.html. Accessed August 9, 2015.
35. Marty AM. Toxocariasis. In: Meyers WM, Neafie RC, Marty AM, et al., eds. *Pathology of Infectious Diseases*. Washington, DC: Armed Forces Institue of Pathology; 2000:411–422.
36. Graeff-Teixeira C, Morassutti AL, Kazacos KR. Update on baylisascariasis, a highly pathogenic zoonotic infection. *Clin Microbiol Rev*. 2016;29:375–399.
37. D'Alessandro A. Polycystic echinococcosis in tropical America: Echinococcus vogeli and E. oligarthrus. *Acta Trop*. 1997;67:43–65.
38. Agudelo Higuita NI, Brunetti E, McCloskey C. Cystic echinococcosis. *J Clin Microbiol*. 2016;54:518–523.
39. Pakala T, Molina M, Wu GY. Hepatic echinococcal cysts: a review. *J Clin Transl Hepatol*. 2016;4:39–46.
40. Marty AM, Johnson LK, Neafie RC. Hydatidosis (echinococcosis). In: Meyers WM, Neafie RC, Marty AM, et al., eds. *Pathology of Infectious Diseases*. Washington, DC: Armed Forces Institue of Pathology; 2000:145–164.
41. Fritsche TR, Pritt BS. Medical parasitology. In: McPherson, RA, Pincus, MR, et al. *Henry's Clinical Diagnosis and Management by Laboratory Methods*. 23rd ed. Philadelphia: Elsevier; 2016.

42. Shaker Y, Samy N, Ashour E. Hepatobiliary schistosomiasis. *J Clin Transl Hepatol.* 2014;2:212–216.
43. Lambertucci JR. Revisiting the concept of hepatosplenic schistosomiasis and its challenges using traditional and new tools. *Rev Soc Bras Med Trop.* 2014;47:130–136.
44. Cheever AW, Neafie RC. Schistosomiasis. In: Meyers WM, Neafie RC, Marty AM, et al., eds. *Pathology of Infectious Diseases.* Washington, DC: Armed Forces Institue of Pathology; 2000:23–48.
45. Wang Z, Lin X, Wang Y, et al. The emerging but neglected hepatic capillariasis in China. *Asian Pac J Trop Biomed.* 2013;3:146–147.
46. Klenzak J, Mattia A, Valenti A, et al. Hepatic capillariasis in Maine presenting as a hepatic mass. *Am J Trop Med Hygiene.* 2005;72:651–653.
47. Khuroo MS. Hepatobiliary and pancreatic ascariasis. *Indian J Gastroenterol.* 2001;20 suppl 1:C28–32.
48. Qian MB, Utzinger J, Keiser J, et al. Clonorchiasis. *Lancet.* 2016;387:800–810.
49. Sripa B, Brindley PJ, Mulvenna J, et al. The tumorigenic liver fluke Opisthorchis viverrini--multiple pathways to cancer. *Trends Parasitol.* 2012;28:395–407.
50. Hong ST, Fang Y. Clonorchis sinensis and clonorchiasis, an update. *Parasitol Int.* 2012;61:17–24.
51. Mas-Coma S, Castello MDB, Marty AM, et al. Hepatic trematodiases. In: Meyers WM, Neafie RC, Marty AM, et al., eds. *Pathology of Infectious Diseases.* Washington, DC: Armed Forces Institue of Pathology; 2000:69–92.
52. Ash LR, Orihel TC. *Ash & Orihel's Atlas of Human Parasitology.* 5th ed. Chicago, IL: ASCP Press; 2007.
53. Mordvinov VA, Yurlova NI, Ogorodova LM, et al. Opisthorchis felineus and Metorchis bilis are the main agents of liver fluke infection of humans in Russia. *Parasitol Int.* 2012;61:25–31.
54. Pritt BS. *Parasitology Benchtop Reference Guide: An Illustrated Guide for Commonly Encountered Parasites.* Northfield, IL: College of American Pathologists; 2014.

10 Other infections of the liver

Michael S. Torbenson, MD

10.1 INTRODUCTION

This chapter discusses nonviral and nonparasitic infections of the liver, though infections that are primarily granulomatous are discussed with other granulomatous diseases in Chapter 11, including fungal infections, *Mycobacterium tuberculosis*, *Mycobacterium leprae*, Brucellosis, and Q fever. Of course, not all organisms that can possibly infect the liver can be covered in this chapter, because the list of specific organisms is vast and ever growing. Instead, this chapter will focus on the most common infections.

The histologic findings vary considerably with these infections. Many cases have only nonspecific findings such as mild portal and lobular chronic inflammation with Kupffer cell hyperplasia. In contrast, some biopsies will have findings that more strongly suggest infection (Table 10.1). Special stains are key tools in identifying organisms (Table 10.2). When infection is strongly considered clinically before the biopsy, an additional core of tissue for culture can be very helpful in establishing a diagnosis.

10.2 MALARIAL INFECTION

Malaria is caused by the protozoan parasite Plasmodium, of which there are four species: falciparum, vivax, malariae, and ovale. The organism is transmitted by the anopheline mosquito. The World Health Organization (WHO, http://www.who.int/malaria/en/) estimates that there are more than 200 million malarial infections per year worldwide, leading to approximately 438,000 deaths per year, 90% occurring in Africa. Almost all of the infections are in the tropical areas of the world. Malaria is very uncommon outside of the tropics but can be encountered because of the increasingly global nature of medicine, with patients traveling widely for health care. The large increase in vacations to endemic areas also increases exposure. Finally, the infection can be encountered as populations emigrate from endemic areas to nonendemic areas.

The classic clinical presentation for malaria is cyclic fevers that occur every 48 to 72 hours, often preceded by shaking chills. That being said, in many cases the presentation is not classic, consisting of milder and less-specific complaints. Jaundice is reported in about 5% of infected individuals but can be as high as 60% during epidemic

Table 10.1 Overview of histologic findings of infections in liver

Association with infection	Histologic findings
Common but nonspecific	• Mild to moderate portal and mild lobular chronic inflammation • Kupffer cell hyperplasia • Cholestasis
Strongly suspicious for infection	• Numerous small clusters of sinusoidal histiocytes (consider listeriosis, typhoid) • Small abscesses (consider listeriosis, tularemia) • Abscesses • Necrotizing granulomas • Irregular geographic areas of necrosis (viral infection and malignancy should also be excluded) • Malakoplakia • Inflammatory pseudotumor
Strongly suspicious for a specific organisms	• Malarial pigment (malaria) • Sulfur granules (*Actinomyces*)
Other findings	• Peliosis • Steatosis

Table 10.2 Special stains used to identify organisms

Stain	Comment
For fungi	
Gomori Methenamine-Silver (GMS)	Fungi *Pneumocystis carini* Also stains some bacteria: *Actinomyces* and related species, Nocardia, some encapsulated bacteria
PAS	Fungi Foamy macrophages in Whipple's disease
Alcian Blue	Mucoid capsule of *Cryptococcus neoformans*
Mucicarmine	Mucoid capsule of *Cryptococcus neoformans*
For bacteria	
Gram-Weigert	Gram-positive organisms, blue. Fibrin also stains blue. Bacteria that are negative on the stain are assumed to be gram-negative. Some acid-fast bacteria can stain red.
Brown–Hopps	Gram-positive organisms, blue. Gram-negative organisms, red. Rickettsia are also positive.
Giemsa	Rickettsia lack cell walls so don't stain with gram stains. Same for other organisms such as Leishmania, Plasmodium.
For acid-fast bacteria	
Kinyoun/Ziehl Neelsen	Stains all mycobacteria red/purple. Non–acid-fast bacteria will be blue.
Fite	Nocardia, *Mycobacterium leprae*
For spirochetes	
Warthin–Starry	Stain is dirty and hard to read, but can stain spirochetes including Bartonella, *Treponema pallidum*. Legionella also can stain. In fact, many different bacteria stain, so morphology of the organism is also important.
Dieterle	Similar to Warthin–Starry
Steiner Stains	Similar to Warthin–Starry
Immunostains	
Treponema pallidum	Spirochetes
Tropheryma whipplei	

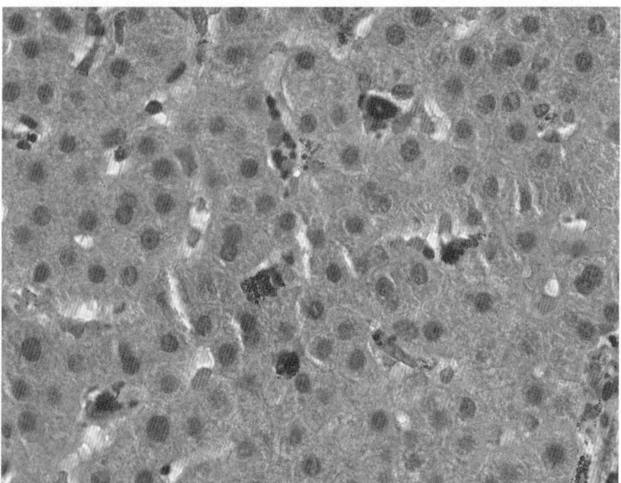

Figure 10.1 Hemozoin or malarial pigment. This biopsy was prompted by unexplained liver enzyme elevations and showed malarial pigment.

outbreaks.[1] Children are more likely than adults to be jaundiced.[2]

The histologic findings in liver vary in severity and can be mild and subtle, even with fatal cases.[3,4] The actual malarial organisms are generally not seen.[3] The major pattern is that of variable degrees of Kupffer cell hyperplasia, sinusoidal congestion, and generally minimal to mild portal chronic inflammation.[5] However, moderate to marked portal chronic inflammation has been reported in more severe cases.[5] The Kupffer cells can show prominent hemophagocytosis. In some cases, the Kupffer cells or the portal macrophages will have distinctive brown-black malarial pigment, also called hemozoin (Fig. 10.1). Other lobular changes include cholestasis and, rarely, fatty change in more severe cases.[6] In fatal cases, hemorrhagic necrosis of the zone 3 hepatocytes can be seen.[3] Additional findings will be seen in those individuals with comorbid conditions, such as a more significant hepatitis in the setting of chronic viral hepatitis, or iron deposits in the setting of glucose-6-phosphate dehydrogenase deficiency.

10.3 TICK-BORNE DISEASES

Ticks can transmit a variety of infectious agents, including protozoa, bacteria, and viruses. Most tick-borne infections do not present with hepatitis as their primary clinical manifestation, but the liver is commonly involved, as evidenced by elevated liver enzymes. Of the tick-borne infections, the bacterial infections are particularly likely to involve the liver. Three of the tick-borne diseases that most commonly cause liver dysfunction are discussed later, but all known tick-borne diseases can lead to liver biochemical and histologic abnormalities.[7]

Clinical findings are quite variable and often quite confusing, but gastrointestinal manifestations are common, including nausea, vomiting, abdominal pain, diarrhea, and hepatomegaly. Unfortunately, the histologic findings remain incompletely defined because of the relative rarity of these diseases and the challenges of making a definite diagnosis. Nonetheless, our current state of knowledge is that the histologic changes range from mild nonspecific inflammatory changes to predominately cholestatic changes to small abscesses. Granulomas are not particularly common in any of the tick-borne diseases but can be seen in many of them, especially Lyme disease, ehrlichiosis, and tularemia. When granulomas are present, most are poorly formed and lack the circumscription and epithelioid morphology of fungal infection-associated granulomas. Q fever (*Coxiella burnetii*) is not transmitted directly by ticks, but ticks serve as a major reservoir, infecting domesticated sheep, goats, and cattle, with subsequent spread to human through unpasteurized milk, cheese, or undercooked meats. Q fever is discussed in more detail in Chapter 11.

Ehrlichiosis

Ehrlichiosis is a bacterial disease caused by *Ehrlichia* and *Anaplasma* organisms and transmitted by the lone star tick. The bacteria are obligate intracellular organisms that infect white blood cells. Mild and transitory elevations in liver enzymes are found in greater than 80% of infections.[7] In about 3% of cases, the infection can be fatal.[8,9] Liver biopsies are only rarely performed, so the full histologic spectrum of changes is unknown, but biopsy specimens can show lobular cholestasis and diffuse Kupffer cell hyperplasia. The cholestasis can be severe. The biopsies can also show mild lobular hepatitis, including scattered discrete foci of lymphocytes and macrophages (often 50 to 100 cells in size) associated with hepatocyte necrosis and drop out.[8,10] The organisms are present in the liver and can be identified by immunostains,[10] but can't really be seen on the hematoxylin and eosin (H&E). They are best identified on peripheral blood smears, where cytoplasmic morulae are found in monocytes or granulocytes, with the infection burden ranging from 0.2% to 10% of cells.[11]

Lyme disease

Lyme disease results from infection with the spirochete, *Borrelia burgdorferi*. At presentation, patients can have fevers, chills, headaches, arthralgias, and fatigue. The typical bull's eye skin rash and a history of a tick bite are very helpful in suggesting a diagnosis, but are not evident in most cases. Gastrointestinal findings are also common at presentation but are not very specific, including anorexia, nausea, and vomiting. About 1/3 of individuals with localized disease will have a mild hepatitis, whereas 2/3 of individuals with disseminated disease have a mild hepatitis, primarily with elevated aspartate aminotransferase (AST) and alanine aminotransferase (ALT) levels in both cases.[12–15] The enzyme elevations resolve within a few weeks following appropriate antibiotic therapy.[7,14]

The histologic findings have been described only in a few cases, but show a mild lobular predominant hepatitis with Kupffer cell hyperplasia.[7,16] The lobular infiltrates are predominately lymphocytic but can also have admixed neutrophils. Granulomatous hepatitis has been reported in several cases,[17–19] including one with large necrotizing granulomas, palisading histiocytes and multinucleated giant cells.[18] In one case report with chronic infection, the biopsy showed portal-based inflammation that was initially interpreted as suggestive of primary biliary cirrhosis.[19] In this same case, the authors identified mulberry shaped granules within the Kupffer cells on periodic acid–Schiff diastase (PASD) stain. In some reports, spirochetes have been identified on Dieterle silver stains and/or immunostains.[16,19,20]

Rocky Mountain spotted fever

Rickettsia rickettsia is a gram-negative intracellular bacteria that is transmitted by the wood tick and the dog tick, causing Rocky Mountain spotted fever, a serious and sometimes life threatening illness. Risk factors for severe disease include older age, male gender, and glucose-6-phosphate dehydrogenase deficiency,[21] which most commonly affects African Americans. In the first 2 to 3 days of illness, the clinical findings are largely gastrointestinal tract related, including anorexia, nausea, vomiting, and diarrhea. The classic constellation of findings takes longer to develop, but consists of fever, headache, and a rash following a tick bite. The liver is commonly involved in symptomatic individuals, as evidenced by hepatomegaly and abnormal liver enzymes.

The organism infects endothelial cells throughout the body. The resulting vasculitis can involve the stomach, pancreas, small bowel, and colon, leading to significant clinical disease. Within the liver, the histologic findings are often mild and not very specific. The histologic findings are primarily portal-based, showing mild to moderate inflammation with mixed lymphocytes and neutrophils.[22,23] In some cases, the portal tract inflammation shows a prominent neutrophilia. Portal vein vasculitis and fibrin thrombi can occasionally be seen, with the inflammation composed of both lymphocytes and neutrophils. Cholestasis is not uncommon and can be striking.[24] Kupffer cell hyperplasia and erythrophagocytosis can be prominent.

Tularemia

Tularemia is caused by *Francisella tularensis*, a gram-negative coccobacillus. *Francisella tularensis* was first isolated in 1912 by GW McCoy of the US Public Health Services and named after Tulare County, California. However, the disease was well known anciently, though by different names of course, names that often included the term plague. As one example, tularemia infection has been proposed as the etiologic agent for the "Hittite plague."[25]

In the USA, the majority of tularemia cases are found in the southeast and southwest. Tularemia is not transmitted from humans to humans. However, the infection is highly contagious, transmitted to humans from rodents, rabbits, and deerfly or tick bites (*Amblyomma americanum, Dermacentor andersoni,* and *Dermacentor variabilis*). The organism can also live for many weeks in the soil, causing rare infections through aerosolization of organisms in the soil by gardeners, farmers, and construction workers. There is a bimodal epidemiologic distribution over the course of a year, reflecting these two primary sources for infection, with one peak in the summer driven by tick bites and a peak in the winter due largely to rabbit/rodent exposure. For the latter, there are a number of ways for disease transmission to occur, including skinning rabbits/rodents and recent contact with domestic cats that have eaten infected rodents.

The incubation period is usually short, averaging 3 to 5 days, but can extend out to 14 days. Tuleremia infection is broadly classified into a localized ulceroglandular pattern or a disseminated typhoidal pattern. The typhoidal pattern often has pneumonia as one of its manifestations, contributing to its overall worse prognosis.[26]

Histologic descriptions are sparse, but there is hepatic involvement in more than 75% of cases.[7] The liver shows small abscesses, 1 to 2 mm in size, with central necrosis surrounded by a thin rim of mixed neutrophils, lymphocytes, and macrophages.[27–30] Organisms are only rarely found on gram stain.[7] Scattered granulomas can also be seen.[30] Outside of these abscesses/granulomatous areas, the lobules show mild nonspecific inflammatory changes and varying degrees of cholestasis.

10.4 HEPATIC ABSCESSES

An abscess is a localized collection of inflammatory exudate, often admixed with necrotic debris, which is surrounded by a rim of inflamed fibrous tissue. Liver abscesses can result from amebic, fungal, or bacterial infections. Mixed bacterial and fungal abscesses are also frequent but bacterial (or pyogenic) abscess are the most common. The two major risk factors for hepatic abscesses are immunosuppression and chronic biliary tract disease. As an example, bacterial abscesses can result from biliary obstruction due to cancer involving the biliary tree or pancreas.[31] Colon cancer is also associated with an increased risk for hepatic abscesses, even if there is no metastatic disease.[32] The most common organisms in bacterial abscesses occurring in adults are streptococcal or *Pseudomonas* species, whereas in children, most hepatic abscesses are due to *Staphylococcus aureus*.[33]

In many cases, hepatic abscesses are not biopsied because the clinical history and imaging studies can make the diagnosis. However, a number of abscesses remain challenging to diagnose by imaging findings and so undergo biopsy. On histology, an abscess is composed of a rim of inflamed fibrous tissue (Fig. 10.2), often with scattered reactive bile ducts (Fig. 10.3), and an inner layer of necrotic debris and inflammatory exudate (Fig. 10.4). The adjacent hepatic parenchyma also shows nonspecific inflammatory changes, edema, fibrosis, and sometimes cholestasis. This histologic pattern is very typical of a hepatic abscess and a diagnosis is usually straightforward. Gram and GMS stains are helpful to identify organisms (Fig. 10.5) and Table 10.2.

In time, the inner layer of the abscess can become increasingly fibrotic, losing the necrotic debris and exudate, leaving an inflamed nodule of fibrous tissue. The inflammation at this stage is composed mostly of lymphocytes and pigmented macrophages, but there can be numerous plasma cells and admixed eosinophils and neutrophils. Eventually, the fibrotic tissue can become less inflamed and more densely

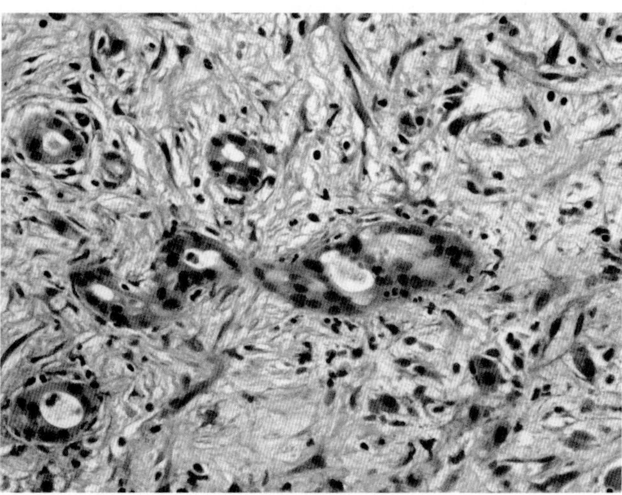

Figure 10.3 Abscess wall. The abscess wall often contains inflamed and reactive bile ducts.

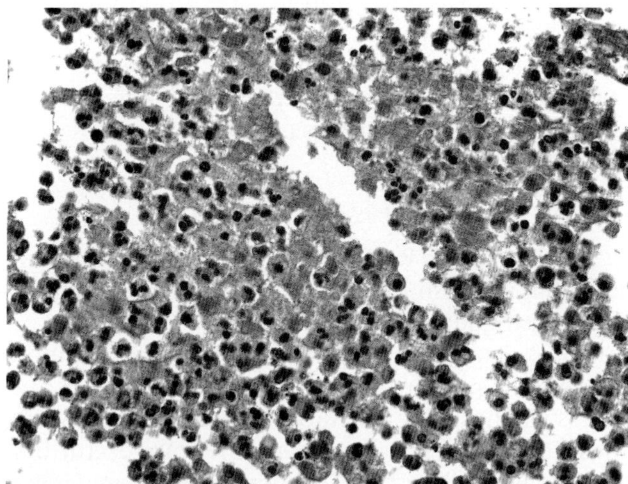

Figure 10.4 Abscess center. The center of this abscess shows necrotic debris and inflammatory exudate.

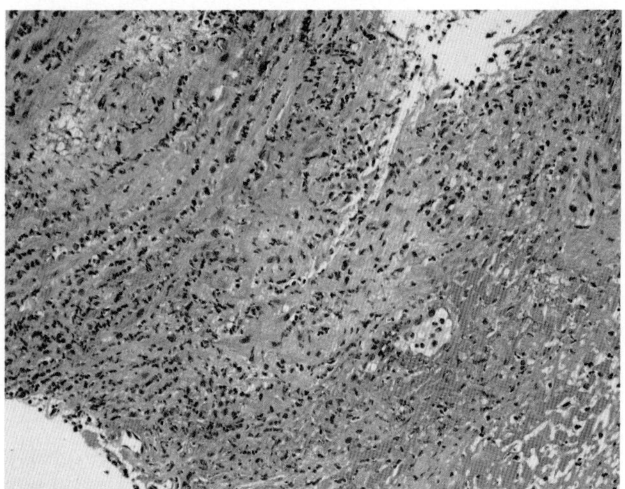

Figure 10.2 Abscess wall. This biopsy is from the edge of an abscess and shows inflamed fibrous tissue in the upper left and the abscess center in the lower right. Cultures were positive for *Klebsiella pneumoniae*.

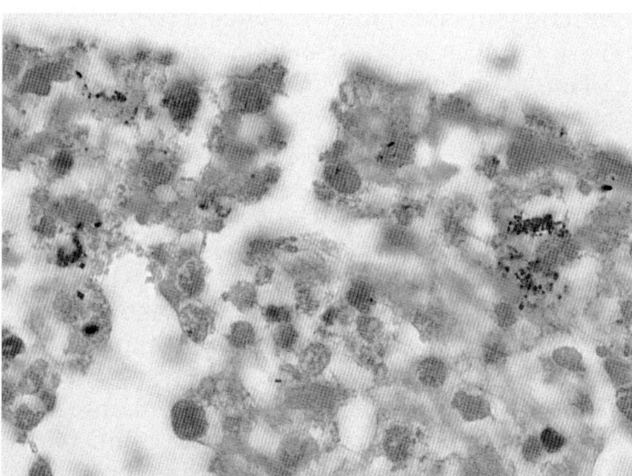

Figure 10.5 Gram-Weigert stain. Clusters of gram-positive cocci are seen (same case as preceding image).

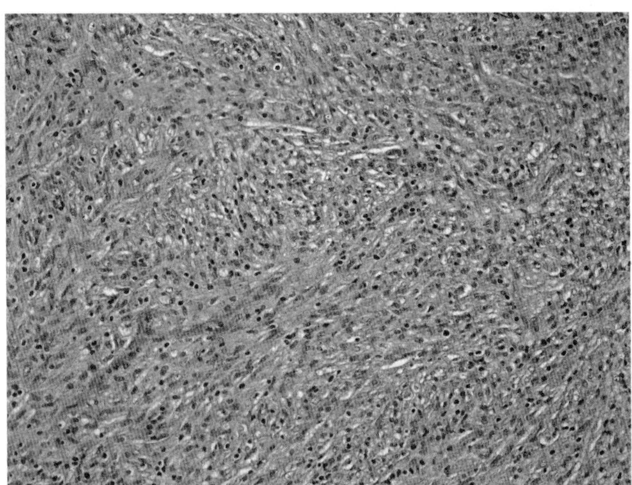

Figure 10.6 Inflammatory pseudotumor. Cultures were positive for *Bacteroides fragilis and Dialister pneumosintes* (formerly named *Bacteroides pneumosintes*).

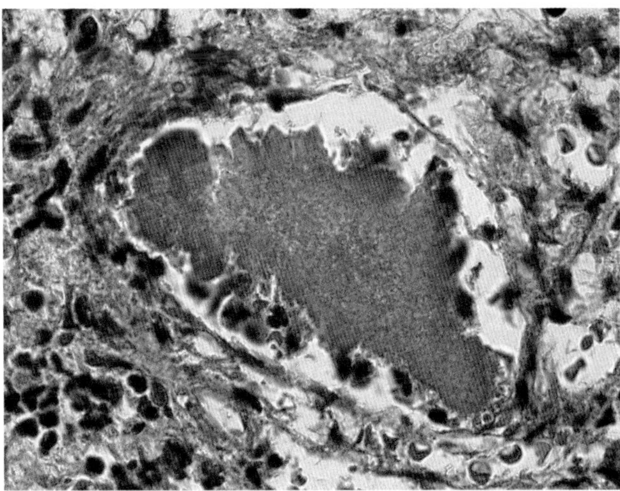

Figure 10.7 Hepatic *Actinomyces*. A large colony or "sulfur granule" is seen, composed of filamentous bacteria.

hyalinized. At this point, the histologic findings are that of an inflammatory pseudotumor (Fig. 10.6). However, inflammatory pseudotumors do have a larger differential, including IgG4-related disease and syphilis. Immunostains can be helpful in this differential, but in most cases are negative.

Actinomycosis

Actinomyces is part of the normal flora of the gastrointestinal tract and the female genital tract. Infections of the liver are rare and most individuals present with very mild and nonspecific clinical findings because the organism is of relatively low pathogenicity. Despite the low pathogenicity, most individuals are immunocompetent. There also is a modest male predominance of about 2:1.[34] *Actinomyces* infection of the liver is usually seen in the setting of multiorgan disease, but can be primary to the liver, in which cases the diagnosis can be challenging to make on imaging and clinical findings, often prompting biopsies. To illustrate, the average time between presentation and diagnosis was 3 months in one review of the literature.[35]

Actinomyces infection commonly forms mass like lesions in the liver, which can mimic hepatic tumors.[34] The mass lesions can be single (2/3 of cases) or multiple (1/3 of cases)[35] and can be very large, up to 11 cm.[35] In fact, many cases are first diagnosed on liver biopsy performed to evaluate a radiographic mass lesion. The histologic findings are overall similar to those seen in any biopsy of an abscess. There is a rind of inflamed fibrotic tissue and the center can show areas of necrosis or may show loose, inflamed myofibroblastic proliferation. In some cases, the findings can closely resemble an inflammatory pseudotumor.

Actinomyces is a filamentous bacteria that can mimic fungal infection because of hyphal like structures. *Actinomyces* can also grow in large colonies surrounding sulfur granules. These foci tend to appear purple in color on H&E stain (Fig. 10.7). These sulfur granules are found in about 2/3 of biopsy specimens[35] and have also been reported in cytology smears.[36] Also of note, 20% to 30% of *Actinomyces* infections are polymicrobial,[35] so other organisms may also be present on bacterial stains. Cultures are negative in about 50% of cases,[35] highlighting the importance of adequate sectioning and careful histologic examination.

Actinomyces is always GMS-positive (Fig. 10.8) and usually gram-positive, but the gram staining qualities are more variable in formalin fixed tissue specimens. Nocardia is also GMS-positive and can have similar filamentous morphology, but the organisms do not

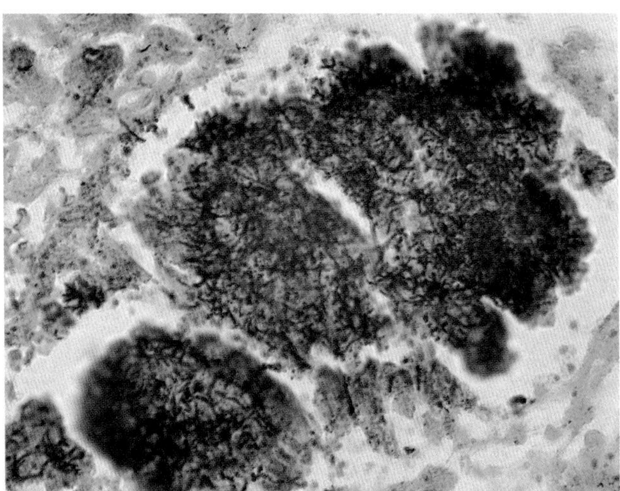

Figure 10.8 Hepatic *Actinomyces*, GMS stain. The filamentous bacteria are highlighted by the GMS stain.

clump like *Actinomyces* and are Fite-positive, whereas *Actinomyces* is Fite-negative. The best place to hunt for organisms is in the fibrinoinflammatory exudate or areas of central necrosis, especially in those areas that are macrophage rich.

10.5 OTHER BACTERIAL INFECTIONS

Listeria monocytogenes

Listeriosis is relatively rare, with about 25,000 infections per year throughout the world,[37] but the frequency is increasing slowly.[38] Infections can be sporadic or occur as part of outbreaks. The infection usually results from ingestion of contaminated foods.[38] The organism is fairly ubiquitous in the environment and very stable, with the ability to replicate at 0°C.[39] These attributes allow transmission in a variety of food products, such as unpasteurized milk, cheeses—particularly soft cheeses, raw fruits and vegetables, undercooked meats and seafood. As examples, a large outbreak in 2011 in the USA was associated with cantaloupes.[40] Another large outbreak in 2006 to 2007 in Germany was associated with cheese, even though it was made from pasteurized milk.[41]

Most infections occur in individuals who are immunosuppressed, are very young, are very old, are pregnant, or have cancer or lymphoma/leukemia.[42] Overall, infections in pregnant women make up 30% of all cases. In the solid organ transplant population, mortality can be very high. One study found a 30 day mortality rate of 27% in the liver transplant population.[43]

The primary site of infection is the small intestine, in particular the Peyer's patches, but the infection can spread from there to the liver.[44] The histologic findings in the liver vary, but most biopsies show scattered small abscesses of 1 to 2 mm in size or small clusters of sinusoidal histiocytes.[45,46] Rarely, larger epithelioid granulomas can be found.[47] Hepatic abscesses have also been reported[48–51] and can be single or multiple. Almost all individuals with single abscess recover following antibiotic therapy, but most individuals with multiple abscesses die from disease even with antibiotic therapy.[51,52] The organism is a short pleomorphic gram-positive rod, but organisms are typically sparse and hard to find on special stains. Rarely, the gallbladder and biliary tree can also be infected.[53]

Leptospirosis

Leptospirosis is caused by leptospira, a spirochete bacteria. The infection is a major health concern worldwide, with 1 million infections per year, leading to 60,000 deaths.[54] Most infections result from exposure to rodent urine. The disease is endemic in the tropics, with peaks during the rainy season. Increased global travel and tourism have dramatically changed the epidemiology of leptospirosis.[55] Infections in the nontropical parts of the world are most commonly identified in travelers who have visited tropical areas. Bathing in fresh water or participation in fresh water sports are major risk factors.[56] Most infections are asymptomatic.

When symptoms develop, infections are classically biphasic, with an early acute phase of 5 to 10 days manifesting as high fevers, headaches, chills, and rigors, which is followed by a brief clinical recovery and then by a subsequent phase of 5 to 30 days, called the immune phase, with the recurrence of high fevers, along with increased liver damage, renal failure, and hemorrhagic complications.[1,57] At the end of the early phase, about 30% of individuals develop conjunctival suffusion, with redness of the conjunctiva without inflammatory exudates.

About 90% of symptomatic infections are self-limited.[1] However, the development of jaundice indicates more severe disease that can require medical intervention. If jaundice develops (about 10%), then the term Weil's disease is used, named after Adolf Weil, a German physician, who described the constellation of an infectious disease with jaundice, splenomegaly, and nephritis in 1886.[58] The mortality rate with anicteric disease is close to 0% but climbs to 20% with jaundice.[59] Age >60 years or the development of the pulmonary hemorrhagic syndrome are also important risk factors for mortality.[59,60]

The liver is affected in essentially all symptomatic cases, as measured by elevated liver enzymes.[56] However, the histologic findings vary and can be very mild. The most common findings are varying degrees of cholestasis and generally mild portal and lobular chronic inflammation (Fig. 10.9).[61] Kupffer cell hyperplasia is common, even if there is no cholestasis. Scattered small clusters of sinusoidal histiocytes can also be found (Fig. 10.10). Fulminant hepatic failure can rarely occur and the liver shows extensive zone 3 hemorrhagic necrosis.[62] In another case report, leptospirosis appeared to induce the subsequent development of autoimmune hepatitis in a child.[63]

Several studies have noted that the hepatocytes, especially in zone 1, appear discohesive.[57,61] E-cadherin staining also appears to be diminished.[61] However, it is not clear if this finding is associated with leptospirosis, versus a nonspecific finding of hepatic injury.

Salmonella (typhoid fever)

Salmonella hepatitis is caused by either *Salmonella typhi* or *Salmonella paratyphi*, gram-negative bacilli. Contaminated food and water are the most common sources of infection. Humans are the only known

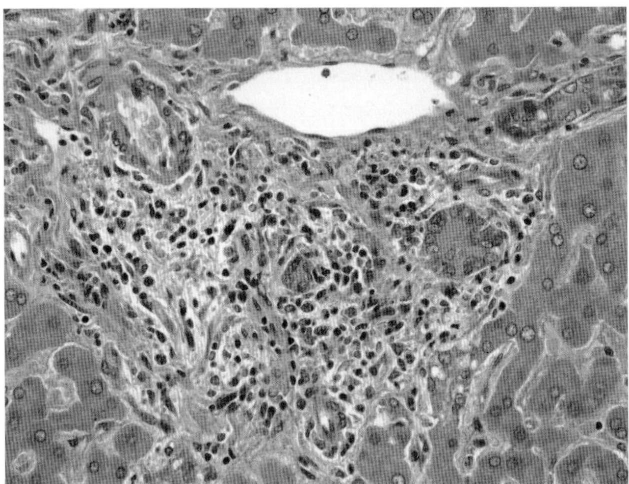

Figure 10.9 Leptosirosis. The biopsy shows mild nonspecific mixed portal inflammation.

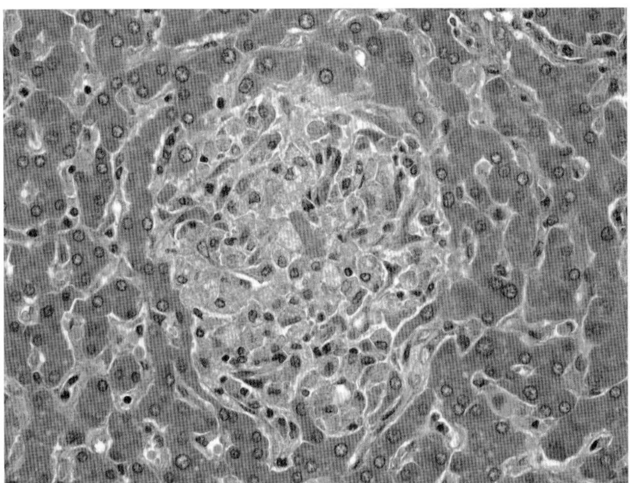

Figure 10.10 Leptosirosis. In the lobules, clusters of histiocytes were found.

natural reservoir, so infections are transmitted either by actively infected individuals with typhoid fever, or more commonly by chronic carriers. Chronic carriers are commonly asymptomatic older women with colonization of the biliary tree. Mary Mallon (Typhoid Mary) is the archetype, a cook in New York who is thought to have infected >50 individuals. She evaded detection for many years by rapidly switching jobs whenever household members or staff developed enteric fever, which happened in almost all of the homes where she worked. Health officials finally traced an outbreak back to her in 1907 and she was eventually quarantined after refusing to stop working as cook, dying therein 26 years later.

Salmonella is primarily a gastrointestinal infection, but almost all individuals have some elevations in liver enzymes and 10% to 20% develop clinical liver disease. A travel history is not uncommon, being identified in about 40% of individuals.[64] About 40% of individuals will be febrile.[64] The organism replicates in macrophages of the Peyer's patches, spleen, and lymph nodes. Liver involvement is associated with delayed treatment and or poor overall health of the patient. The liver disease manifests primarily as jaundice, which develops about 2 weeks after initial infection.[65] Fulminant hepatitis can rarely develop.[66] The diagnosis is primarily made by culture of blood or stool samples or by polymerase chain reaction (PCR) from tissue specimens such as the blood or bone marrow.

The liver is commonly enlarged and enzyme elevations can range from very mild to moderate.[65,67] The liver is only rarely biopsied. The main histologic finding in *Salmonella* hepatitis is a generalized lobular Kupffer cell hyperplasia. The lobules can also show a mild to moderate lymphocytosis, resembling Epstein-Barr virus (EBV) infection. In more severe and long standing cases, the Kupffer cells can focally aggregate into "typhoid nodules", granuloma-like nodules in the lobules. These nodules can show a zone 3 predominance, but when marked will show a panlobular distribution.[65] Other common findings in the lobules include mild lymphocytic inflammation, occasional acidophil bodies, and cholestasis. The portal tracts mostly show mild nonspecific inflammation, but increased numbers of macrophages may be seen.

Syphilis

Syphilis can involve the liver in any of its stages. The frequency of liver disease with congenital syphilis is high, whereas in acquired syphilis it is typically less than 50%. For example, in the HIV-positive population, 20% to 30% of individuals with syphilis will have elevated liver enzymes.[68,69]

In congenital syphilis, the findings are variable but the classic pattern is diffuse sinusoidal fibrosis and mild sinusoidal lymphocytosis. In untreated individuals, organisms are easily found on Warthin–Starry stains. Another pattern found with congenital syphilis is neonatal giant cell hepatitis,[70] with some cases also showing paucity of intrahepatic bile ducts.[71] In some cases, macrophage rich infiltrates are found around the vessels.[72]

Several broad patterns of infection have been described in acquired syphilis. In most cases, the biopsies show an essentially normal liver.[73,74] In the remaining cases, the liver shows mild nonspecific inflammatory changes (Fig. 10.11), often with Kupffer cell hyperplasia as the most prominent finding.[74,75] However, a small number of cases show moderate portal chronic inflammation, occasionally with prominent plasma cells.[76] Epithelioid granulomas are occasionally

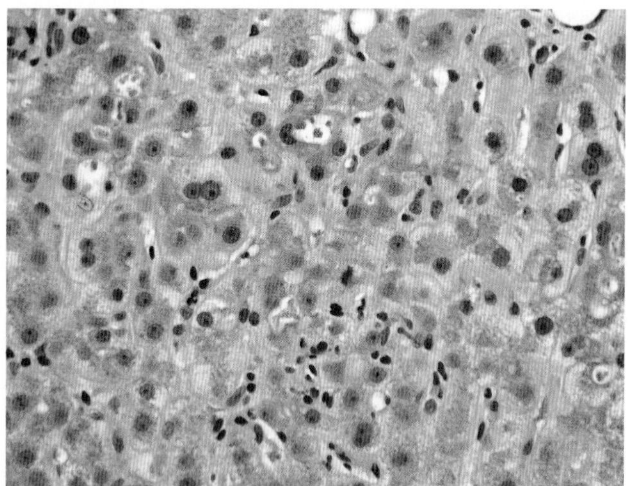

Figure 10.11 Syphilis. The biopsy shows cholestasis and mild nonspecific lobular inflammation

present. Spirochetes can be identified even when the histologic findings are minimal, though the number of organisms may be few. Immunostains are much more sensitive than silver stains (Fig. 10.12), but can stain other spirochetes, so correlation with serologic findings is still very important.

In late syphilis, the gumma can be found. This lesion is rarely encountered today but looks pretty similar to an abscess, with central necrosis surrounded by a rim of inflamed fibrous tissue. However, the area of central necrosis is more hyalinized than a typical bacterial abscess and can contain recognizable, though necrotic, normal liver tissue. The inflammation in the inflamed fibrous rim is predominately lymphocytic but is also enriched for plasma cells and may have scattered multinucleated giant cells and small granulomas. In some cases, an adjacent vessel will show active inflammation and fibrosis. In time, some

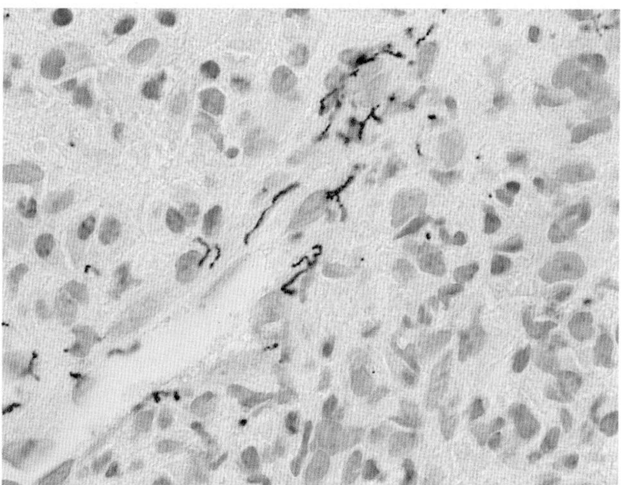

Figure 10.12 Syphilis, T. pallidum immunostain. Organisms cluster around a vein.

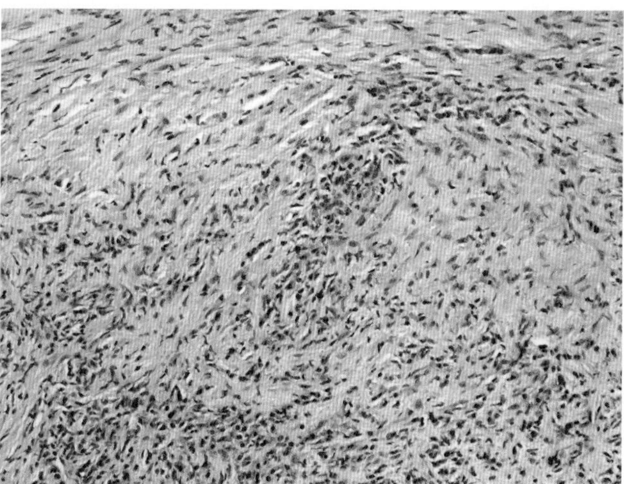

Figure 10.13 Syphilis. This biopsy was directed against a mass lesion and showed an inflammatory pseudotumor. Serology and immunostains on the inflammatory pseudotumor were both positive for syphilis.

of these lesions can transform to an inflammatory pseudotumor (Fig. 10.13).[77] Both gummas and inflammatory psuedotumors can present as mass lesion that mimic neoplasms.

Whipple's disease

Whipple's disease was first recognized in an autopsy of a young medical missionary in 1907.[78] although the organism itself was not identified until 1992.[79] The infection is caused by *Tropheryma whipplei*, a gram-positive organism. Whipple's disease can be very difficult to diagnosis, sometimes taking many years before a firm diagnosis is established.[80] The clinical presentation is nonspecific but typically includes variable degrees of arthralgia, weight loss, diarrhea (often prominent), and abdominal pain. The liver can be secondarily involved when there is systemic disease, but isolated infections of the liver haven't been reported. Immunosuppression therapy for other autoimmune conditions can exacerbate the infection, bringing it clinical attention.[81] On the other hand, successful treatment of Whipple's disease with antibiotics can lead to the immune reconstitution syndrome, with new onset fevers and arthralgias.[82]

The histologic findings in the liver are similar to those seen in other organs, with numerous PAS-positive foamy macrophages. The macrophage infiltrates can involve the lobules and/or the portal tracts, usually forming small and discrete clusters. In some cases, the macrophages will be relative few in number. Epithelioid granulomas can also form, although these will be PAS-negative.[83,84] The granulomas can be mistaken for involvement by sarcoidosis.[85] In addition to the macrophage infiltrate, the liver shows mild nonspecific lymphocytic inflammation in the portal tracts and lobules. In many cases, the lobules also show Kupffer cell hyperplasia.[86,87] If the biopsy samples the larger branches of the hepatic artery, PAS-positive macrophages can also be found within the arterial walls.[88]

REFERENCES

1. Talwani R, Gilliam BL, Howell C. Infectious diseases and the liver. *Clin Liver Dis*. 2011;15(1):111–130.
2. Khan W, Zakai HA, Umm EA. Clinico-pathological studies of *Plasmodium falciparum* and *Plasmodium vivax*—malaria in India and Saudi Arabia. *Acta Parasitol*. 2014;59(2):206–212.
3. Rupani AB, Amarapurkar AD. Hepatic changes in fatal malaria: an emerging problem. *Ann Trop Med Parasitol*. 2009;103(2):119–127.
4. Whitten R, Milner DA Jr, Yeh MM, et al. Liver pathology in Malawian children with fatal encephalopathy. *Hum Pathol*. 2011;42(9):1230–1239.
5. Viriyavejakul P, Khachonsaksumet V, Punsawad C. Liver changes in severe *Plasmodium falciparum* malaria: histopathology, apoptosis and nuclear factor kappa B expression. *Malar J*. 2014;13:106.
6. Srivastava A, Khanduri A, Lakhtakia S, et al. Falciparum malaria with acute liver failure. *Trop Gastroenterol*. 1996;17(3):172–174.
7. Zaidi SA, Singer C. Gastrointestinal and hepatic manifestations of tickborne diseases in the United States. *Clin Infect Dis*. 2002;34(9):1206–1212.
8. Sosa-Gutierrez CG, Solorzano-Santos F, Walker DH, et al. Fatal monocytic ehrlichiosis in woman, Mexico, 2013. *Emerg Infect Dis*. 2016;22(5):871–874.
9. Pavelites JJ, Prahlow JA. Fatal human monocytic ehrlichiosis: a case study. *Forensic Sci Med Pathol*. 2011;7(3):287–293.
10. Sehdev AE, Dumler JS. Hepatic pathology in human monocytic ehrlichiosis. *Ehrlichia chaffeensis* infection. *Am J Clin Pathol*. 2003;119(6):859–865.
11. Hamilton KS, Standaert SM, Kinney MC. Characteristic peripheral blood findings in human ehrlichiosis. *Mod Pathol*. 2004;17(5):512–517.
12. Fathi R, Huang WW, Brown K. Disseminated Lyme borreliosis preceded by hepatitis in an African American male. *Dermatol Online J*. 2012;18(10):4.
13. Benedix F, Weide B, Broekaert S, et al. Early disseminated borreliosis with multiple erythema migrans and elevated liver enzymes: case report and literature review. *Acta Derm Venereol*. 2007;87(5):418–421.
14. Horowitz HW, Dworkin B, Forseter G, et al. Liver function in early Lyme disease. *Hepatology*. 1996;23(6):1412–1417.
15. Kazakoff MA, Sinusas K, Macchia C. Liver function test abnormalities in early Lyme disease. *Arch Fam Med*. 1993;2(4):409–413.
16. Goellner MH, Agger WA, Burgess JH, et al. Hepatitis due to recurrent Lyme disease. *Ann Intern Med*. 1988;108(5):707–708.
17. Chavanet P, Pillon D, Lancon JP, et al. Granulomatous hepatitis associated with Lyme disease. *Lancet*. 1987;2(8559):623–624.
18. Zanchi AC, Gingold AR, Theise ND, et al. Necrotizing granulomatous hepatitis as an unusual manifestation of Lyme disease. *Dig Dis Sci*. 2007;52(10):2629–2632.
19. Middelveen MJ, McClain SA, Bandoski C, et al. Granulomatous hepatitis associated with chronic *Borrelia burgdorferi* infection: a case report. *Biol Environ Sci Faculty Publications*. 2014; Paper 33. doi:10.13070/rs.en.1.875.
20. Duray PH, Steere AC. Clinical pathologic correlations of Lyme disease by stage. *Ann N Y Acad Sci*. 1988;539:65–79.
21. Walker DH, Hawkins HK, Hudson P. Fulminant Rocky Mountain spotted fever. Its pathologic characteristics associated with glucose-6-phosphate dehydrogenase deficiency. *Arch Pathol Lab Med*. 1983;107(3):121–125.
22. Adams JS, Walker DH. The liver in Rocky Mountain spotted fever. *Am J Clin Pathol*. 1981;75(2):156–161.
23. Jackson MD, Kirkman C, Bradford WD, et al. Rocky mountain spotted fever: hepatic lesions in childhood cases. *Pediatr Pathol*. 1986;5(3–4):379–388.
24. Ramphal R, Kluge R, Cohen V, et al. Rocky Mountain spotted fever and jaundice. Two consecutive cases acquired in Florida and a review of the literature on this complication. *Arch Intern Med*. 1978;138(2):260–263.
25. Trevisanato SI. The "Hittite plague", an epidemic of tularemia and the first record of biological warfare. *Med Hypotheses*. 2007;69(6):1371–1374.
26. Evans ME, Gregory DW, Schaffner W, et al. Tularemia: a 30-year experience with 88 cases. *Medicine (Baltimore)*. 1985;64(4):251–269.
27. Case records of the Massachusetts General Hospital. Weekly clinicopathological exercises. Case 22-2001. A 25-year-old woman with fever and abnormal liver function. *N Engl J Med*. 2001;345(3):201–205.
28. Gourdeau M, Lamothe F, Ishak M, et al. Hepatic abscess complicating ulceroglandular tularemia. *Can Med Assoc J*. 1983;129(12):1286–1288.
29. Ortego TJ, Hutchins LF, Rice J, et al. Tularemic hepatitis presenting as obstructive jaundice. *Gastroenterology*. 1986;91(2):461–463.
30. Lamps LW, Havens JM, Sjostedt A, et al. Histologic and molecular diagnosis of tularemia: a potential bioterrorism agent endemic to North America. *Mod Pathol*. 2004;17(5):489–495.

31. Huang CJ, Pitt HA, Lipsett PA, et al. Pyogenic hepatic abscess. Changing trends over 42 years. *Ann Surg*. 1996;223(5):600–607; discussion 607–609.
32. Qu K, Liu C, Wang ZX, et al. Pyogenic liver abscesses associated with nonmetastatic colorectal cancers: an increasing problem in Eastern Asia. *World J Gastroenterol*. 2012;18(23):2948–2955.
33. Mishra K, Basu S, Roychoudhury S, et al. Liver abscess in children: an overview. *World J Pediatr*. 2010;6(3):210–216.
34. Kanellopoulou T, Alexopoulou A, Tanouli MI, et al. Primary hepatic actinomycosis. *Am J Med Sci*. 2010;339(4):362–365.
35. Yang XX, Lin J-M, Xu K-J, et al. Hepatic actinomycosis: report of one case and analysis of 32 previously reported cases. *World J Gastroenterol*. 2014;20(43):16372–16376.
36. Xing J, Rodriguez EF, Monaco SE, et al. Cytopathology of hepatobiliary-related actinomycosis. *Acta Cytol*. 2016;60(2):179–184.
37. de Noordhout CM, Devleesschauwer B, Angulo FJ, et al. The global burden of listeriosis: a systematic review and meta-analysis. *Lancet Infect Dis*. 2014;14(11):1073–1082.
38. Hernandez-Milian A, Payeras-Cifre A. What is new in listeriosis? *Biomed Res Int*. 2014;2014:358051.
39. Rocourt J, Jacquet C, Reilly A. Epidemiology of human listeriosis and seafoods. *Int J Food Microbiol*. 2000;62(3):197–209.
40. McCollum JT, Cronquist AB, Silk BJ, et al. Multistate outbreak of listeriosis associated with cantaloupe. *N Engl J Med*. 2013;369(10):944–953.
41. Koch J, Dworak R, Prager R, et al. Large listeriosis outbreak linked to cheese made from pasteurized milk, Germany, 2006-2007. *Foodborne Pathog Dis*. 2010;7(12):1581–1584.
42. Goulet V, Hebert M, Hedberg C, et al. Incidence of listeriosis and related mortality among groups at risk of acquiring listeriosis. *Clin Infect Dis*. 2012;54(5):652–660.
43. Fernandez-Sabe N, Cervera C, López-Medrano F, et al. Risk factors, clinical features, and outcomes of listeriosis in solid-organ transplant recipients: a matched case-control study. *Clin Infect Dis*. 2009;49(8):1153–1159.
44. Rouquette C, Berche P. The pathogenesis of infection by Listeria monocytogenes. *Microbiologia*. 1996;12(2):245–258.
45. Gebauer K, Hall JC, Donlon JB, et al. Hepatic involvement in listeriosis. *Aust N Z J Med*. 1989;19(5):486–487.
46. Vargas V, Alemán C, de Torres I, et al. Listeria monocytogenes-associated acute hepatitis in a liver transplant recipient. *Liver*. 1998;18(3):213–215.
47. De Vega T, Echevarria S, Crespo J, et al. Acute hepatitis by Listeria monocytogenes in an HIV patient with chronic HBV hepatitis. *J Clin Gastroenterol*. 1992;15(3):251–255.
48. Marino P, Maggioni M, Preatoni A, et al. Liver abscesses due to Listeria monocytogenes. *Liver*. 1996;16(1):67–69.
49. Lopez-Prieto MD, Aller Garciía AI, Alcaraz Garciía S, et al. Liver abscess due to Listeria monocytogenes. *Clin Microbiol Infect*. 2000;6(4):226–227.
50. Bronnimann S, Baer HU, Malinverni R, et al. Listeria monocytogenes causing solitary liver abscess. Case report and review of the literature. *Dig Surg*. 1998;15(4):364–368.
51. Braun TI, Travis D, Dee RR, et al. Liver abscess due to Listeria monocytogenes: case report and review. *Clin Infect Dis*. 1993;17(2):267–269.
52. Scholing M, Schneeberger PM, van den Dries P, et al. Clinical features of liver involvement in adult patients with listeriosis. Review of the literature. *Infection*. 2007;35(4):212–218.
53. Charlier C, Fevre C, Travier L, et al. Listeria monocytogenes-associated biliary tract infections: a study of 12 consecutive cases and review. *Medicine (Baltimore)*. 2014;93(18):e105.
54. Costa F, Hagan JE, Calcagno J, et al. Global morbidity and mortality of leptospirosis: a systematic review. *PLoS Negl Trop Dis*. 2015;9(9):e0003898.
55. Bandara M, Ananda M, Wickramage K, et al. Globalization of leptospirosis through travel and migration. *Global Health*. 2014;10:61.
56. van de Werve C, Perignon A, Jauréguiberry S, et al. Travel-related leptospirosis: a series of 15 imported cases. *J Travel Med*. 2013;20(4):228–231.
57. Haake DA, Levett PN. Leptospirosis in humans. *Curr Top Microbiol Immunol*. 2015;387:65–97.
58. Adler B. History of leptospirosis and leptospira. *Curr Top Microbiol Immunol*. 2015;387:1–9.
59. Taylor AJ, Paris DH, Newton PN. A systematic review of the mortality from untreated leptospirosis. *PLoS Negl Trop Dis*. 2015;9(6):e0003866.
60. McBride AJ, Athanazio DA, Reis MG, et al. Leptospirosis. *Curr Opin Infect Dis*. 2005;18(5):376–386.
61. De Brito T, Menezes LF, Lima DM, et al. Immunohistochemical and in situ hybridization studies of the liver and kidney in human leptospirosis. *Virchows Arch*. 2006;448(5):576–583.
62. Shintaku M, Itoh H, Tsutsumi Y. Weil's disease (leptospirosis) manifesting as fulminant hepatic failure: report of an autopsy case. *Pathol Res Pract*. 2014;210(12):1134–1137.
63. Urganci N, Kalyoncu D, Cayonu N, et al. Acute liver failure, autoimmune hepatitis, and leptospirosis: a case report. *Pediatr Emerg Care*. 2011;27(10):963–965.
64. El-Newihi HM, Alamy ME, Reynolds TB. Salmonella hepatitis: analysis of 27 cases and

comparison with acute viral hepatitis. *Hepatology*. 1996;24(3):516–519.
65. Pramoolsinsap C, Viranuvatti V. Salmonella hepatitis. *J Gastroenterol Hepatol*. 1998;13(7):745–750.
66. Khan FY, Kamha AA, Alomary IY. Fulminant hepatic failure caused by Salmonella paratyphi A infection. *World J Gastroenterol*. 2006;12(32):5253–5255.
67. Ahmed A, Ahmed B. Jaundice in typhoid patients: differentiation from other common causes of fever and jaundice in the tropics. *Ann Afr Med*. 2010;9(3):135–140.
68. Jung N, Kümmerle T, Brengelmann SD, et al. Liver involvement in HIV-infected patients diagnosed with syphilis. *Infection*. 2012;40(5):543–547.
69. Palacios R, Navarro F, Narankiewicz D, et al. Liver involvement in HIV-infected patients with early syphilis. *Int J STD AIDS*. 2013;24(1):31–33.
70. Shet TM, Kandalkar BM, Vora IM. Neonatal hepatitis—an autopsy study of 14 cases. *Indian J Pathol Microbiol*. 1998;41(1):77–84.
71. Sugiura H, Hayashi M, Koshida R, et al. Nonsyndromatic paucity of intrahepatic bile ducts in congenital syphilis. A case report. *Acta Pathol Jpn*. 1988;38(8):1061–1068.
72. Guarner J, Greer PW, Bartlett J, et al. Congenital syphilis in a newborn: an immunopathologic study. *Mod Pathol*. 1999;12(1):82–87.
73. Wright DJ, Berry CL. Letter: liver involvement in congenital syphilis. *Br J Vener Dis*. 1974;50(3):241.
74. Terry SI, Hanchard B, Brooks SE, et al. Prevalence of liver abnormality in early syphilis. *Br J Vener Dis*. 1984;60(2):83–86.
75. Pareek SS. Liver involvement in secondary syphilis. *Dig Dis Sci*. 1979;24(1):41–43.
76. Khambaty M, Singal AG, Gopal P. Spirochetes as an almost forgotten cause of hepatitis. *Clin Gastroenterol Hepatol*. 2015;13(2):A21–A22.
77. Hagen CE, Kamionek M, McKinsey DS, et al. Syphilis presenting as inflammatory tumors of the liver in HIV-positive homosexual men. *Am J Surg Pathol*. 2014;38(12):1636–1643.
78. Whipple G. A hitherto undescribed disease characterized anatomically by deposits of fat and fatty acids in the intestinal and mesenteric lymphatic tissues. 190. *Bull Johns Hopkins Hospital*. 1907;18:382–393.
79. Relman DA, Schmidt TM, MacDermott RP, et al. Identification of the uncultured bacillus of Whipple's disease. *N Engl J Med*. 1992;327(5):293–301.
80. Arnold CA, Moreira RK, Lam-Himlin D, et al. Whipple disease a century after the initial description: increased recognition of unusual presentations, autoimmune comorbidities, and therapy effects. *Am J Surg Pathol*. 2012;36(7):1066–1073.
81. Kneitz C, Suerbaum S, Beer M, et al. Exacerbation of Whipple's disease associated with infliximab treatment. *Scand J Rheumatol*. 2005;34(2):148–151.
82. Biagi F, Moos V, Schinnerling K, et al. Previous immunosuppressive therapy is a risk factor for immune reconstitution inflammatory syndrome in Whipple's disease. *Dig Liver Dis*. 2012;44(10):880–882.
83. Torzillo PJ, Bignold L, Khan GA. Absence of PAS-positive macrophages in hepatic and lymph node granulomata in Whipple's disease. *Aust N Z J Med*. 1982;12(1):73–75.
84. Saint-Marc Girardin MF, Zafrani ES, Chaumette MT, et al. Hepatic granulomas in Whipple's disease. *Gastroenterology*. 1984;86(4):753–756.
85. Dutly F, Altwegg M. Whipple's disease and "Tropheryma whippelii". *Clin Microbiol Rev*. 2001;14(3):561–583.
86. Cho C, Linscheer WG, Hirschkorn MA, et al. Sarcoidlike granulomas as an early manifestation of Whipple's disease. *Gastroenterology*. 1984;87(4):941–947.
87. Viteri AL, Stinson JC, Barnes MC, et al. Rod-shaped organism in the liver of a patient with Whipple's disease. *Dig Dis Sci*. 1979;24(7):560–564.
88. James TN. The protean nature of Whipple's disease includes multiorgan arteriopathy. *Trans Am Clin Climatol Assoc*. 2001;112:196–214.

11 Granulomatous liver disease

Vishal S. Chandan, MD and Tsung-Teh Wu, MD, PhD

11.1 INTRODUCTION

Granulomas are localized collections of macrophages and other inflammatory cells, such as lymphocytes, that usually develop in response to chronic antigen exposure. Granulomas also may contain multinucleated giant cells due to fusion of the macrophages. The prevalence of granulomas within liver biopsies ranges from 2% to 15% and up to a third of cases may not have a known etiology, even after full clinical workup.[1–6] Granulomas within the liver may be related to primary hepatic disease (PBC), or may be due to systemic diseases involving the liver and other organ systems, or may even be just an incidental finding. Table 11.1 summarizes the causes of hepatic granulomas. Sarcoidosis, primary biliary cirrhosis, drug-induced liver injury, and infection are the most common identifiable causes of hepatic granulomas in the United States.[1,7] In developing countries such as India, tuberculosis infection is the most common cause of hepatic granulomas. Careful assessment of the morphology and location of the granulomas can provide helpful clues regarding the etiology and a prioritized differential, information that can be very helpful to our clinical colleagues. In contrast, simply listing the generic differential for hepatic granulomas in the surgical pathology report is not of much help to most physicians. The term granulomatous hepatitis is used when the granulomas are poorly formed and are associated with significant inflammation within the liver parenchyma.

11.2 MORPHOLOGY OF GRANULOMAS AND THEIR DISEASE CORRELATES

Hepatic granulomas can be broadly divided in the following morphologic types.

Epithelioid granulomas

Epithelioid granulomas are composed of distinct collections of histiocytes, often with admixed lymphocytes. They often have well-defined edges separating them from the adjacent tissue (Fig. 11.1). Epithelioid granulomas are one of the most frequently seen types of granuloma within the liver and are associated with both primary and secondary

Table 11.1 Causes of hepatic granulomas

Infections	Sarcoidosis
Bacterial *Mycobacterium tuberculosis* *Mycobacterium avium-intracellulare* *Mycobacterium leprae* Bartonella *henselae* (cat scratch disease) Brucella Rickettsia (Q fever)	*Intrinsic liver disease* Primary biliary cirrhosis Primary sclerosing cholangitis Acute cellular rejection
Fungal Histoplasmosis Cryptococcus	*Drugs* Allopurinol Sulfonamides Isoniazid Phenytoin Hydralazine Quinidine
Parasitic Schistosomiasis Visceral leishmaniasis (kala-azar)	*Neoplasms* Hodgkin lymphoma Leukemia Hepatic adenoma Hepatocellular carcinoma Metastatic carcinoma
Viral Hepatitis C virus Cytomegalovirus Epstein-Barr virus Hepatitis A virus Hepatitis B virus	*Other diseases* Crohn's disease Chronic ulcerative colitis Common variable immunodeficiency Chronic granulomatous disease Collagen vascular diseases

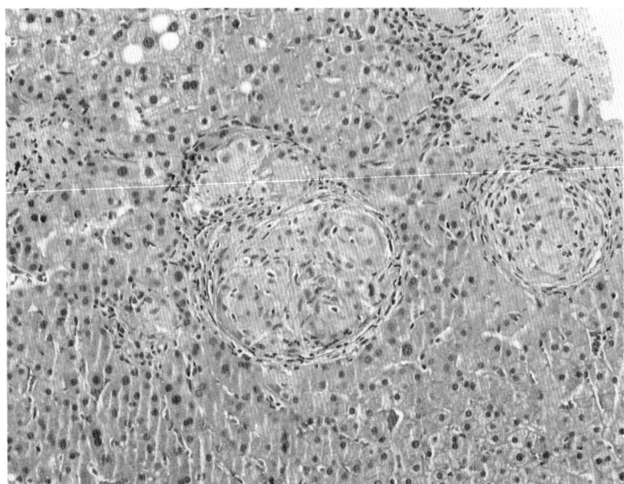

Figure 11.1 Epithelioid granuloma. A well-defined collection of histiocytes is seen.

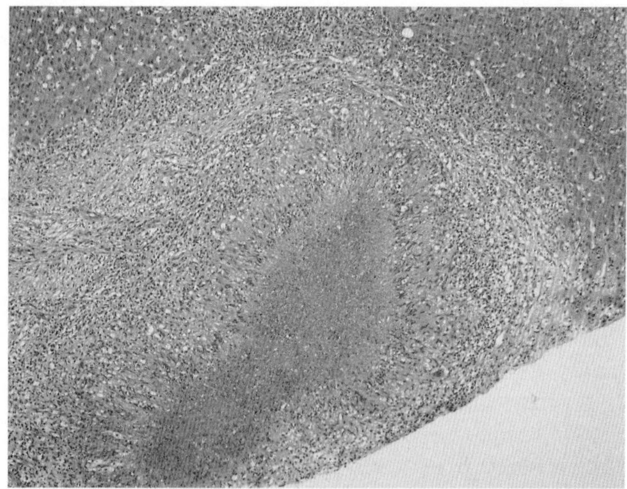

Figure 11.2 Necrotizing granuloma. A central area of necrosis is surrounded by histiocytes and lymphocytes.

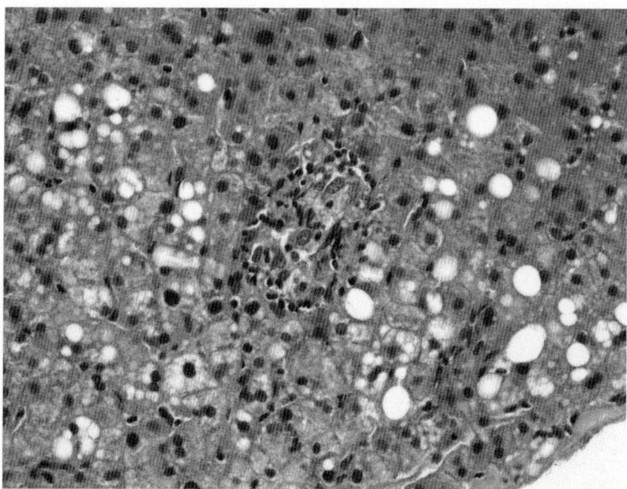

Figure 11.3 Micrograto granuloma. A small collection of a few histiocytes and lymphocytes is seen.

liver diseases. Special stains for microorganisms should be performed, as epithelioid granulomas can be associated with infectious organisms.

Necrotizing/caseating granulomas

These granulomas show central "dirty" necrosis composed of nuclear debris and are almost always infectious in origin, although no organisms are found in many cases (Fig. 11.2). The mononuclear cells tend to be palisading at the periphery. These granulomas often destroy the adjacent liver parenchyma and do not respect the hepatic architecture.

Microgranulomas

These are small collections (about 3 to 7) of Kupffer cells in the hepatic lobules and can be admixed with other inflammatory cells or apoptotic hepatocytes (Fig. 11.3). Microgranulomas usually represent a reparative response to an episode of acute lobular injury and are nonspecific in nature. The macrophage cytoplasm may contain light pigment and they are usually highlighted on the periodic acid–Schiff (PAS) stain. Although this pattern is important to recognize within the liver, the term microgranuloma is probably best avoided in the pathology report as the clinical colleagues may misunderstand this term.

Granulomatous inflammation

Sometimes the granulomas are so indistinct that it is better to use the term *granulomatous inflammation*. These are poorly formed, ill-defined histiocytic aggregates that often are admixed with other inflammatory cells (Fig. 11.4). This pattern can be seen with a wide variety of conditions. Portal-based granulomatous inflammation is more likely to be associated with drug effect or biliary tract disease, whereas lobular granulomatous inflammation is more likely to be infectious or drug-induced.

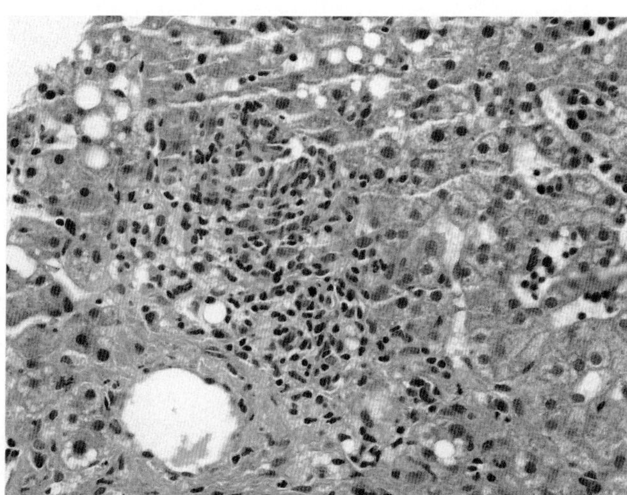

Figure 11.4 Granulomatous inflammation. An ill-defined aggregate of histiocytes and other inflammatory cells is seen.

Florid duct lesions and granulomatous inflammation

A florid duct lesion is characterized by lymphocytes and plasma cells cuffing a medium-sized bile duct. The bile duct epithelium is damaged/injured by infiltrating lymphocytes and is associated with granulomatous inflammation (Fig. 11.5). Sometimes the florid duct lesion can be associated with epithelioid granulomas. Florid duct lesions are typically associated with primary biliary cirrhosis or less commonly with drug effects.

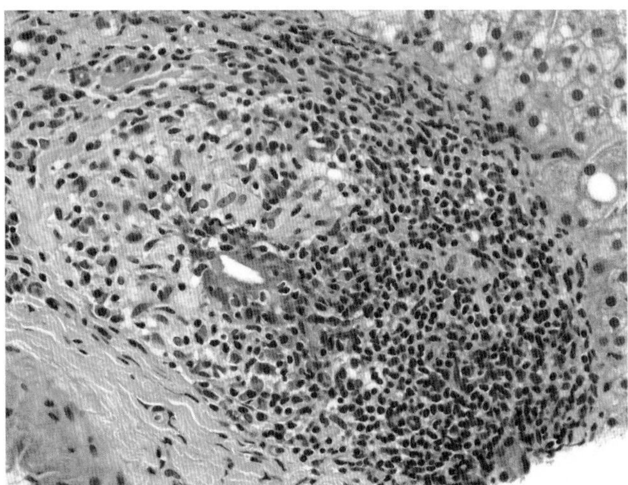

Figure 11.5 Florid duct lesion and granulomatous inflammation. In this portal tract, granulomatous inflammation is associated with bile duct injury.

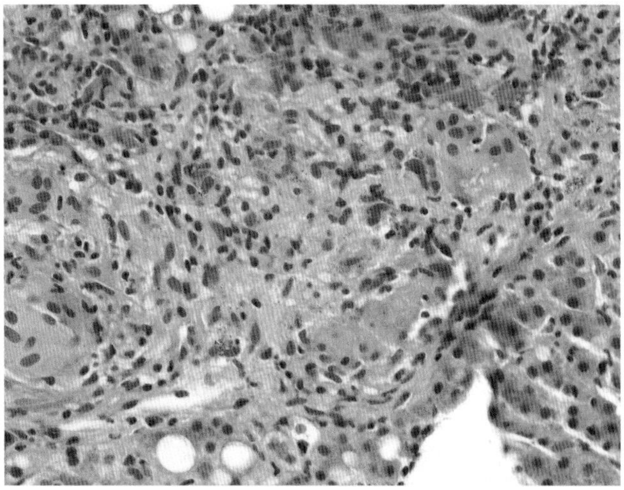

Fibrin-ring granulomas

Fibrin-ring granulomas are epithelioid granulomas with a central lipid droplet surrounded by an eosinophilic fibrin ring that stains positively with Masson trichrome stain and phosphotungstic acid hematoxylin (PTAH) stain (Fig. 11.6).[8,9] They were first described in association with Q fever, but are now considered quite nonspecific, as they can be seen in a number of conditions such as hepatitis A, chronic hepatitis C, Epstein–Barr virus (EBV) infection, cytomegalovirus (CMV) infection, toxoplasmosis, leishmaniasis, Rickettsia typhus, Hodgkin disease, allopurinol reaction.[1,5,8,10,11] Nonetheless, fibrin-ring granulomas are most commonly associated with infections or drug effects.

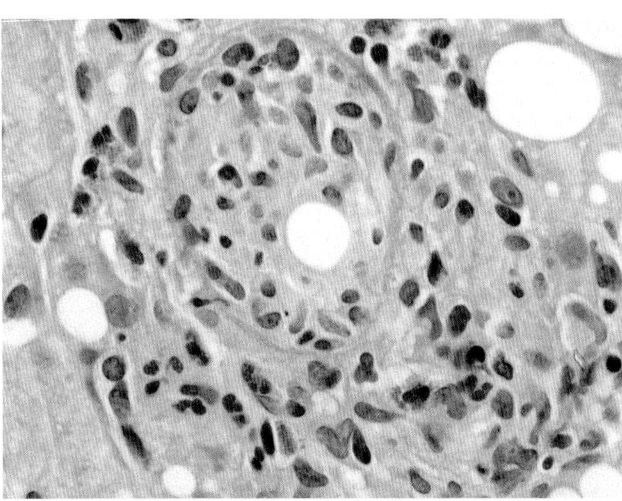

Figure 11.6 Fibrin-ring granuloma. Epithelioid granulomas with a central lipid droplet surrounded by an eosinophilic fibrin ring.

Figure 11.7 Foreign body granuloma. This biopsy in patient with IV drug use showed aggregates of histiocytes and giant cells containing the foreign brownish titanium pigment.

Foreign body granulomas

Foreign body granulomas contain particulate material within cytoplasmic vacuoles. The foreign material may be seen on hematoxylin and eosin (H&E) stain or on polarization of the granuloma (Figs. 11.7 and 11.8). Foreign body granulomas in the liver can be caused by silicone, starch, or talc from injection drug use. They also may be related to prior abdominal surgery or therapeutic tumor embolization.

Lipogranulomas

Lipogranulomas are composed of small aggregates of histiocytes surrounding vacuoles of lipid/mineral

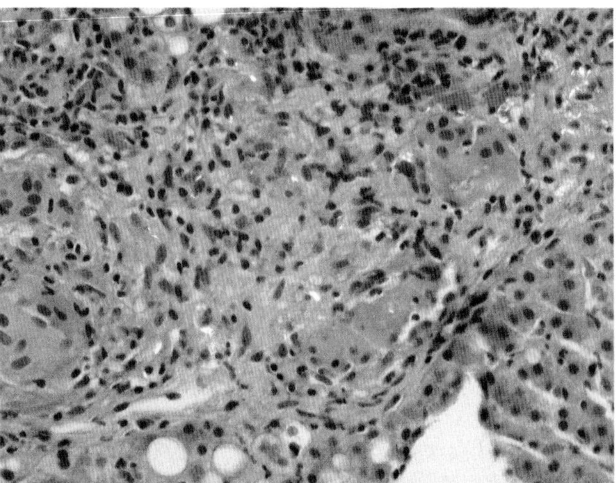

Figure 11.8 Foreign body granuloma, polarized light. Same case as in Figure 11.6, highlighting the titanium granules under polarized light.

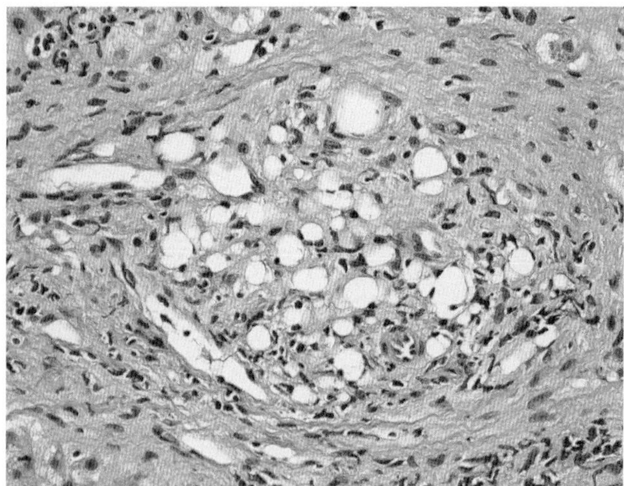

Figure 11.9 Lipogranuloma. A collection of histiocytes surrounds vacuoles of fat in a portal tract.

oil and may be stained with Oil red O on frozen sections (Fig. 11.9). Lipogranulomas often have a bit of associated fibrosis, but overall do not contribute to liver fibrosis. They are commonly associated with fatty liver disease or chronic hepatitis C but can also be incidental findings. They are usually found within the portal areas or next to the central veins.

11.3 GRANULOMAS ASSOCIATED WITH BACTERIAL INFECTIONS

Mycobacterium tuberculosis

Almost all cases of miliary tuberculosis have liver disease characterized by granulomas, which typically involving the portal areas.[12] Hepatic involvement is also commonly seen in cases of pulmonary tuberculosis and cases of localized extrapulmonary tuberculosis.[10,13,14] Tuberculous hepatic granulomas are especially prevalent in HIV-positive populations. Sometimes on radiography, the confluent granulomas are concerning for a neoplastic process because the liver has a mass lesion and there can be periportal lymphadenopathy.

Mycobacterium tuberculosis granulomas are usually small to medium-sized epithelioid granulomas with caseating necrosis, often surrounded by a ring of lymphocytes and histiocytes. These granulomas may coalesce by central liquefactive necrosis to form larger nodules. Older granulomas may also be calcified or fibrotic. The *Mycobacterium tuberculosis* organisms are small and often sparse and hence may be difficult to identify on the acid-fast bacillus (AFB) stain. A repeat AFB stain on the deeper sections may be useful. Polymerase chain reaction (PCR) and cultures are also important tools for detecting this infection.

Mycobacterium avium-intracellulare

This infection is frequently seen in HIV-positive or other severely immunosuppressed individuals. Liver involvement can be seen in more than 50% of patients with disseminated *Mycobacterium avium-intracellulare* (MAI) infection.[15,16] In immunosuppressed patients, MAI infections within the liver usually show aggregates of foamy histiocytes in the hepatic parenchyma and portal tracts (Fig. 11.10). Immunocompetent patients may have well-defined epithelioid granulomas with other inflammatory cells, such as lymphocytes and neutrophils. Large numbers of organisms are identified on the AFB stain in immunosuppressed patients, whereas organisms are usually rare in immunocompetent individuals (Fig. 11.11). In such cases performing culture and PCR studies may be useful. Infections such

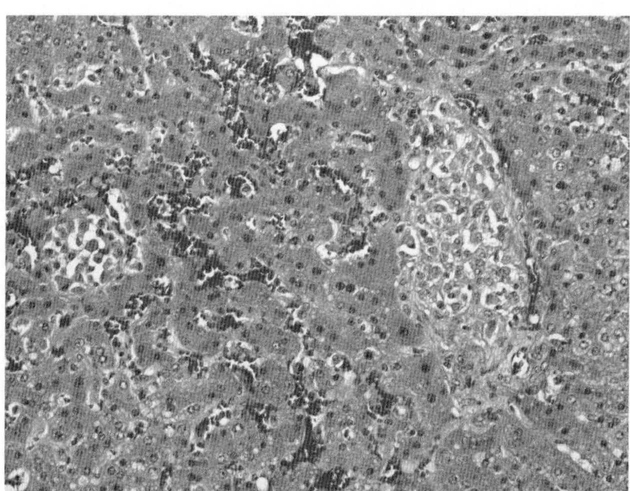

Figure 11.10 *Mycobacterium avium-intracellulare*. Aggregates of foamy histiocytes are found within the lobule.

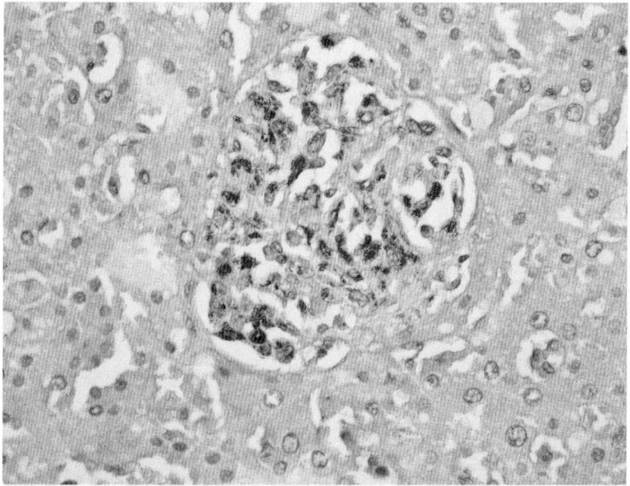

Figure 11.11 *Mycobacterium avium-intracellulare*, Fite stain. A Fite stain highlights numerous acid-fast microorganisms within the histiocytes.

as Whipple's disease and *Rhodococcus equi* may also cause foamy histiocytic aggregates within the liver.

Mycobacterium leprae

Studies have shown liver involvement in greater than 50% of patients with lepromatous leprosy and in up to 20% of patients with tuberculoid leprosy.[17–19] In lepromatous leprosy, scattered aggregates of foamy histiocytes containing multiple acid-fast bacilli are usually seen within the hepatic lobules and the portal areas, with minimal accompanying inflammation. Epithelioid granulomas with giant cells are usually seen in tuberculoid leprosy, but the organisms are difficult to identify on the AFB stains.

Bartonella species

Bartonella henselae causes cat scratch disease. When the liver is involved, there can be multiple lesions and associated abdominal lymphadenopathy, which radiologically can resemble a neoplastic process. Typical histologic lesions show geographic foci of neutrophilic inflammation or stellate microabscesses surrounded by three zones: an inner layer of palisading histiocytes, an intermediate lymphocytic rim, and an outermost layer of fibrous tissue.[20,21] Silver stains such as Warthin–Starry can be useful in highlighting the organisms on tissue sections, but these stains are negative in many cases. The silver stains can also be difficult to read, as they tend to have a lot of background staining. For this reason, it can be very helpful to have a positive control on the slide to compare the morphology of definite organisms to what you are seeing while reading the stain. A clinical history of cat exposure can be useful, but is often not available to the pathologist. The diagnosis can also be made on serologic studies. Immunohistochemistry and molecular assays are available at some institutions.

Brucella

Infection with Brucella is uncommon in the general population but can be seen in people working with farm and barnyard animals. Hepatomegaly and lymphadenopathy is commonly seen with Brucella infection. Hepatic involvement can be seen in up to 50% of patients with brucellosis. The liver typically shows nonnecrotizing granulomatous inflammation.[22–24] The granulomas may be small and ill defined or they may be epithelioid and well formed. The Brucella organisms are usually not seen on the special stains and they are also difficult to culture. The diagnosis can be suggested by an animal exposure history and made on appropriate serology studies.

Rickettsia and similar species

Coxiella burnetii, the causative organism for Q fever, causes fibrin-ring granulomas.[9,25] However, as mentioned earlier, fibrin-ring granulomas within the liver can also be seen in a number of other conditions.

11.4 GRANULOMAS ASSOCIATED WITH FUNGAL INFECTIONS

Histoplasmosis

Histoplasmosis is caused by Histoplasma capsulatum and is one of the most frequent fungal causes of hepatic granulomatous inflammation. This infection is most common in the lower Mississippi and Ohio River valleys. Lymphohistiocytic inflammation and sinusoidal Kupffer cell hyperplasia are the most common morphologic findings (Fig. 11.12).[26,27] Well-formed granulomas are infrequently seen, but when present they can be both portal and lobular. Occasionally, the organisms may also be visible on the H&E stain, especially when numerous. Gomori methenamine-silver (GMS) stains can highlight these organisms (Fig. 11.13).

Cryptococcus

Infection by cryptococcus neoformans is typically seen in immunosuppressed individuals. Liver involvement usually shows ill-defined granulomas and small aggregates of foamy histiocytes within the hepatic lobules.[28,29] Well-formed granulomas are rare. Cryptococcus can also involve the biliary tract. Periodic acid–Schiff (PAS) and mucicarmine stains can highlight the thick capsule of the yeast. Some

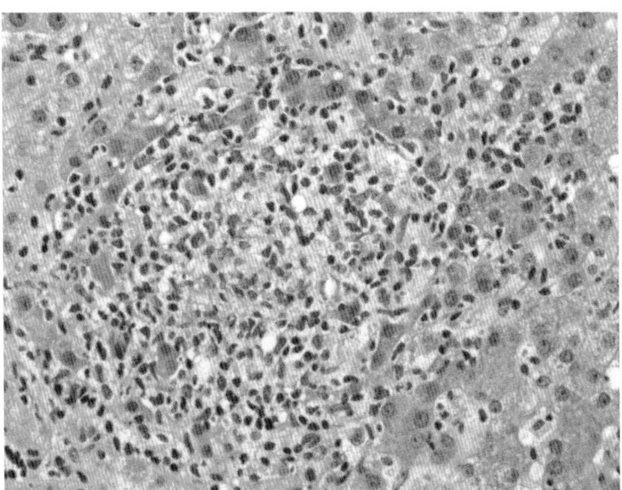

Figure 11.12 Histoplasmosis. The biopsy showed lymphohistiocytic aggregates within the hepatic lobules.

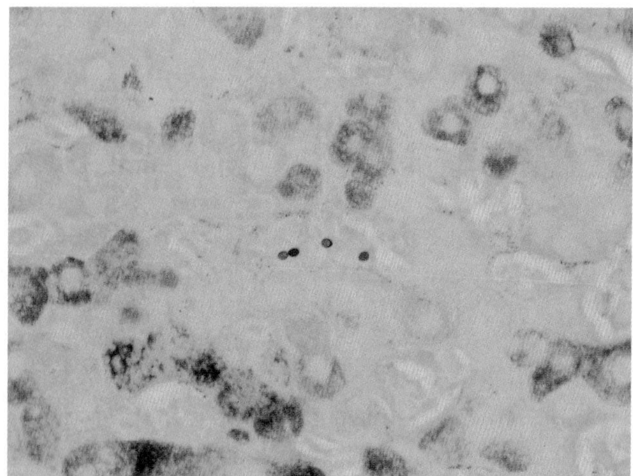

Figure 11.13 Histoplasmosis, GMS stain. A GMS stain highlights a few narrow-based budding yeasts.

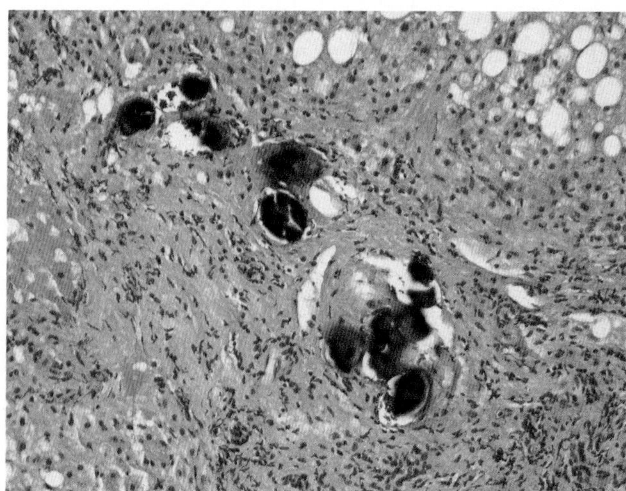

Figure 11.14 Schistosomiasis. Calcified schistosomal eggs with portal fibrosis are present.

strains of cryptococcus may be capsule deficient and hence may be negative or only focally positive on mucicarmine stain. In such cases, a Fontana–Masson stain may be helpful.

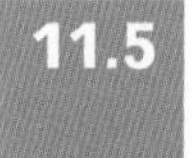

11.5 PARASITIC INFECTIONS FEATURING GRANULOMATOUS LIVER DISEASE

Schistosomiasis

Parasitic hepatobiliary disease is mostly caused by Schistosoma mansoni, Schistosoma japonicum, or Schistosoma mekongi. These are waterborne parasites in which the freshwater snails are the intermediary host (see Chapter 9 for more details). The disease is transmitted via drinking or swimming in parasite-contaminated water. Infections are found in Southeast Asia, the Caribbean, the Middle East, and tropical Africa, where waterborne parasitic diseases remain a source of significant illness.[30,31] Schistosomiasis can also be seen in United States due to global travel and immigration, and nearly half a million people with schistosomiasis are estimated to live in the United States.[32]

Adult worms produce eggs within the portal and mesenteric veins. These eggs become trapped in the portal veins and hepatic parenchyma. The body's reaction to the eggs is the underlying cause of disease and the resultant inflammation leads to fibrosis and obstructive hepatobiliary disease.

The liver is grossly enlarged and nodular. The cut surface may show a pipestem or Symmers pattern of fibrosis. Microscopic features vary depending on the duration of disease. The eggs may get trapped in the hepatic parenchyma or portal tracts and elicit a granulomatous inflammatory response. Prominent eosinophils may be seen within the granulomatous response. Adult worms are usually not seen. Later on, the portal tracts become densely sclerotic and fibrosis develops. The eggs often get calcified (Fig. 11.14). As the fibrosis progresses, the eggs become increasingly difficult to identify. Ultimately, the portal veins become sclerotic and destroyed, with a subsequent proliferation of the hepatic arterial branches.

Visceral leishmaniasis (kala-azar)

This disease is most often seen in patients with AIDS. The liver usually shows organisms within hyperplastic Kupffer cells. Sometimes, ill-defined granulomas, epithelioid granulomas, or fibrin-ring granulomas can be seen.[33,34]

11.6 GRANULOMAS IN VIRAL INFECTIONS

Hepatitis C

The reported prevalence of hepatic granulomas in hepatitis C varies from 1% to 10%.[35,36] These granulomas are usually small and epithelioid (Fig. 11.15). They can be found within the lobules and the portal tracts. In most cases they are idiopathic. Studies have suggested granulomas in some cases are related to hepatitis C treatment.[36] For unclear reasons, other studies have linked granulomatous disease in hepatitis C infection to a higher mortality rate,[37] but this is not a widely replicated finding.

Other viral infections

Viral infections typically do not present primarily with hepatic granulomas as their pattern of injury.

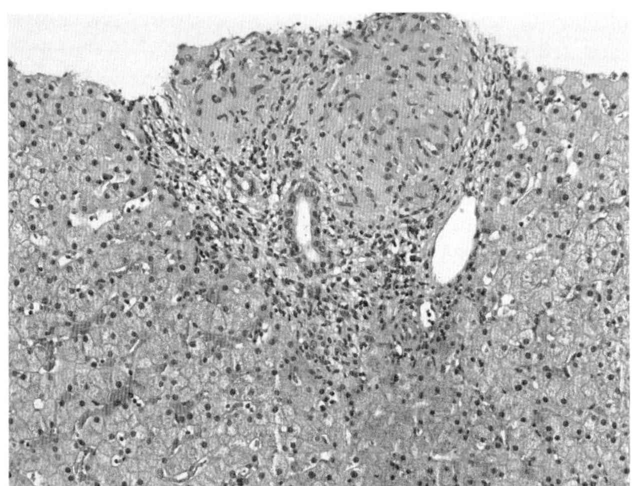

Figure 11.15 Hepatitis C granuloma. This biopsy in a case of chronic hepatitis C also showed an epithelioid granuloma within the portal area.

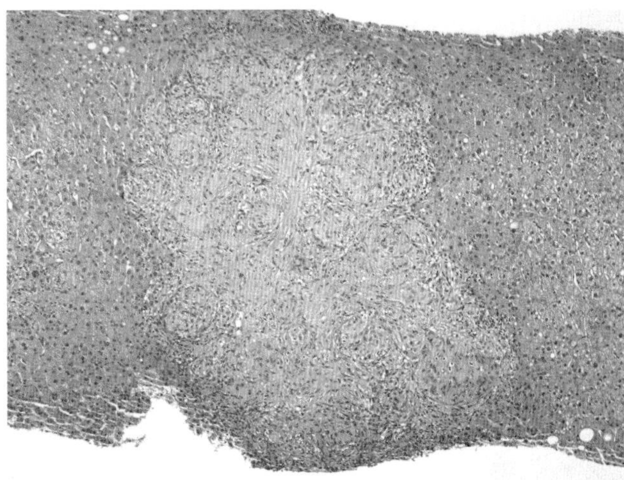

Figure 11.16 Sarcoidosis. In this case of sarcoidosis, a large confluent well-defined epithelioid granuloma is present within the hepatic lobule.

However, granulomas can accompany a hepatitic pattern of injury in a number of acute viral infections, including hepatitis B, EBV hepatitis, CMV hepatitis, hepatitis E, and hepatitis A.[38]

11.7 SARCOIDOSIS

Sarcoidosis is a multisystem granulomatous disease of unknown etiology. The disease primarily involves the lungs and lymph nodes, but the incidence of hepatic granulomas in sarcoidosis is high, ranging from 50% to 90%.[10] However, liver disease is clinically evident in only 15% to 20% of cases and is generally mild. Sarcoidosis is one of the more common causes of hepatic granulomas in the United States.[6,39]

Sarcoid granulomas are typically well-defined, noncaseating epithelioid granulomas with variable giant cell change (Fig. 11.16). A bland, hyalinized or fibrinoid pattern of central necrosis can rarely be seen in sarcoid granulomas, but these granulomas tend to be very large and are usually not sampled on a liver biopsy. In these cases, the necrosis lacks the "dirty" nuclear and cellular debris seen in typical infectious necrotizing granulomas. Small- or medium-sized granulomas in sarcoidosis do not show caseating necrosis. In many cases, the granulomas in sarcoidosis have asteroid bodies and/or Schaumann bodies, but this finding is not specific for sarcoidosis.

Histologically there are four main patterns of liver involvement by sarcoidosis. The first and the most common is that of well-defined noncaseating granulomas within the portal areas (primarily) and the hepatic lobules. The granulomas typically show varying degrees of fibrosis. Those granulomas that are fibrotic show fibrosis extending into and through the granulomas. The second pattern is less common and shows portal-based granulomas along with changes of chronic obstructive biliary tract disease, characterized by varying degree of bile ductular proliferation and even ductopenia. These changes are related to the obstructive effect of the hilar lymphadenopathy on the extrahepatic biliary system. A third pattern in sarcoidosis shows portal granulomatous venulitis and loss of portal veins, clinically presenting as portal hypertension. In these cases, the lobules can also show nodular regenerative hyperplasia. The fourth pattern, which is very rare, presents as a mass lesion that is caused by confluent fibrotic granulomas.

11.8 PRIMARY BILIARY CIRRHOSIS

Granulomas are a well-known morphologic component of primary biliary cirrhosis and have been reported in 20% to 60% of cases.[40–42] They can be portal or lobular and are often associated with inflammatory bile duct lesions (florid duct lesions) (Fig. 11.5). Primary biliary cirrhosis is discussed in more detail in Chapter 13.

11.9 OTHER DISEASES WITH GRANULOMAS

Primary sclerosing cholangitis

Hepatic granulomas have also been reported in a minority of cases with primary sclerosing cholangitis.[10,43,44] Granulomas in primary sclerosing cholangitis are almost always related to bile extravasation. These granulomas are usually small, discrete, epithelioid and noncaseating.

Crohn's disease

Liver granulomas can be seen in patients with Crohn's disease. The granulomas can be part of Crohn's disease itself, but infection and drug effect need to be clinically excluded.

Common variable immunodeficiency

Small epithelioid granulomas in the hepatic lobules and portal areas can be seen in some patients with common variable immunodeficiency.[45] In some cases, the granulomatous disease also involves multiple organs and hence cannot be distinguished from sarcoidosis, both clinically and pathologically. Some authors believe that granulomatous common variable immunodeficiency is a manifestation of sarcoidosis in common variable immunodeficiency patients.

Chronic granulomatous disease

Patients with chronic granulomatous disease can have hepatic granulomas, varying from small poorly formed histiocytic aggregates to large multiloculated granulomatous abscesses.[46–48] Please see Chapter 19 for additional discussion.

Acute cellular rejection

Granulomatous inflammation has been reported in few cases of acute cellular rejection.[49,50] In one report, the granulomatous inflammation was seen with other typical histologic features of acute cell rejection and disappeared after response to antirejection therapy.[3] However, granulomas are not part of the typical pattern of rejection and a full work is needed, with exclusion of infection, drug effect, and recurrent disease.

Vasculitis/collagen vascular diseases

Hepatic granulomas involving the hepatic vasculature have been also reported in rare cases of lupus, giant cell arteritis, polyarteritis nodosa, and Churg–Strauss disease.[10,11,43]

Rheumatoid nodule

Rare cases of hepatic rheumatoid nodules have also been reported.[51,52] These can appear as discrete fibrotic nodules within the liver, often with a central area of hyalinization when they are large. The edges can show histiocytic aggregates and chronic inflammation.

Idiopathic

Up to one third of cases with hepatic granulomas may not have an identifiable cause despite a full clinical and pathologic workup.[1,10,29,53,54]

11.10 ADVERSE DRUG REACTION AND GRANULOMAS

Numerous drugs have been associated with hepatic granulomas and this list is continually growing. A complete discussion of drugs and medications causing hepatic granulomas is beyond the scope of this chapter. It is better to consult an online source with an actively managed database to check if there is any association between the patient's medications and hepatic granulomas. However it may be useful to remember a few drugs that are most commonly associated with hepatic granulomas such as allopurinol, sulfonamides, isoniazid, phenytoin, hydralazine, and quinidine.[55,56]

Drug-induced granulomas are usually noncaseating and can be found within the hepatic lobules and/or the portal areas. When present in the portal areas, there can rarely be associated bile duct injury, mimicking primary biliary cirrhosis. Granulomatous liver disease with moderate to severe lobular hepatitis is usually due to a drug effect or infection. Bacillus Calmette–Guérin (BCG) vaccination and intravesical therapy for urinary bladder carcinoma can also cause hepatic granulomas.[57]

11.11 GRANULOMAS AND NEOPLASMS

Benign and malignant hepatic neoplasms, including metastatic tumors, have been associated with hepatic granulomas. The best known association is with Hodgkin disease (Figs. 11.17 and 11.18). In one study, 6% of liver biopsies with granulomas

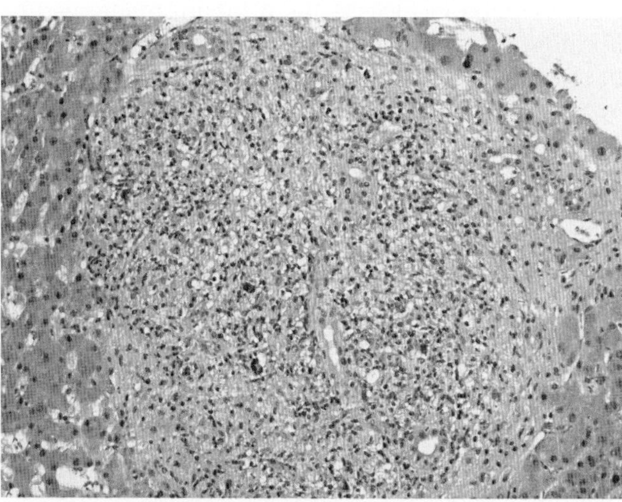

Figure 11.17 Hodgkin lymphoma. In this biopsy from a patient with Hodgkin lymphoma, granulomas were found in the portal areas.

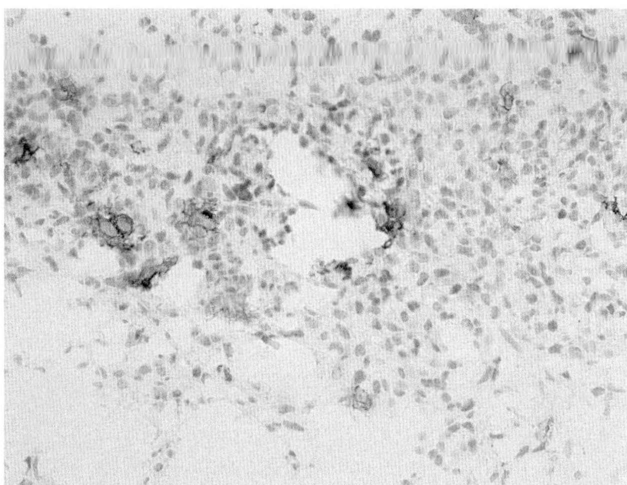

Figure 11.18 Hodgkin lymphoma, CD30 immunostain. Same case as in Figure 11.16, the CD30 immunostain highlights the Reed-Sternberg cells within the granuloma.

were associated with Hodgkin disease.[1] Other neoplasms have also been linked to neoplasms, including non-Hodgkin lymphoma, leukemia, hepatic adenomas, hepatocellular carcinoma, cholangiocarcinoma, and metastatic gastrointestinal adenocarcinomas.[1,39,58,59]

11.12 SUMMARY

Identifying granulomas within the liver can have varied clinical implications, ranging from none in the case of lipogranulomas, to being the most important finding, for example in cases of granulomatous infections or drug reactions. The most common conditions should be considered first, including infection, sarcoidosis, drug effect, and primary biliary cirrhosis. In most cases, an exact etiology will not be evident on histology alone, but will require clinical and serologic correlation. Special stains for microorganisms (fungal and acid-fast stains) should be routinely performed and epithelioid granulomas should be polarized. Granulomatous disease that is primarily portal based and is associated with bile duct injury is most likely to be primary biliary cirrhosis, drug effect, or sarcoidosis. Granulomatous liver disease presenting as acute onset hepatitis with fever is most likely to be an infection or drug reaction. Caseating granulomas are most likely infectious, even if organisms are not identified on special stains. Molecular testing for infections is available and may be useful. The presence of rare small granulomas in a liver biopsy is most often an incidental finding and up to a third of cases with hepatic granulomas do not have an identifiable cause despite complete work up.

REFERENCES

1. Gaya DR, Thorburn D, Oien KA, et al. Hepatic granulomas: a 10 year single centre experience. *J Clin Pathol*. 2003;56(11):850–853.
2. Bhardwaj SS, Saxena R, Kwo PY. Granulomatous liver disease. *Curr Gastroenterol Rep*. 2009;11(1):42–49.
3. Lagana SM, Moreira RK, Lefkowitch JH. Hepatic granulomas: pathogenesis and differential diagnosis. *Clin Liver Dis*. 2010;14(4):605–617.
4. Lamps LW. Hepatic granulomas, with an emphasis on infectious causes. *Adv Anat Pathol*. 2008;15(6):309.
5. Lamps LW. Hepatic granulomas: a review with emphasis on infectious causes. *Arch Pathol Lab Med*. 2015;139(7):867–875.
6. Zakim D, Boyer TD. Hepatology, a textbook of liver diseases. 3rd ed. Philadelphia, PA: WB Saunders 1996:1472.
7. Matheus T, Munoz S. Granulomatous liver disease and cholestasis. *Clin Liver Dis*. 2004;8(1):229–246, ix.
8. Marazuela M, Moreno A, Yebra M, et al. Hepatic fibrin-ring granulomas: a clinicopathologic study of 23 patients. *Hum Pathol*. 1991;22(6):607–613.
9. Srigley JR, Vellend H, Palmer N, et al. Q-fever. The liver and bone marrow pathology. *Am J Surg Pathol*. 1985;9(10):752–758.
10. Ishak KG. Granulomas of the liver. In: Joachim HL ed. *Pathology of Granulomas*. New York, NY: Raven Publishers; 1983:307–369.
11. Restrepo MI, Vasquez EM, Echeverri C, et al. Fibrin ring granulomas in Rickettsia typhi infection. *Diagn Microbiol Infect Dis*. 2010;66(3):322–325.
12. Flamm S. Hepatic granulomas. In: Chopra S, ed. UpToDate: Hepatology, Waltham, MA: UpToDate; 2008.
13. Essop AR, Posen JA, Hodkinson JH, et al. Tuberculosis hepatitis: a clinical review of 96 cases. *Q J Med*. 1984;53(212):465–477.
14. Oliva A, Duarte B, Jonasson O, et al. The nodular form of local hepatic tuberculosis: a review. *J Clin Gastroenterol*. 1990;12(2):166–173.
15. Farhi DC, Mason UG III, Horsburgh CR Jr. Pathologic findings in disseminated Mycobacterium avium-intracellulare infection. A report of 11 cases. *Am J Clin Pathol*. 1986;85(1):67–72.
16. Klatt EC, Jensen DF, Meyer PR. Pathology of Mycobacterium aviumintracellulare infection in acquired immunodeficiency syndrome. *Hum Pathol*. 1987;18(7):709–714.
17. Karat ABA. Liver in leprosy: histological and biochemical findings. *Br Med J*. 1971;1(5744):307–310.
18. Chen TSN, Drutz DJ, Whelan GE. Hepatic granulomas in leprosy. Their relation to bacteremia. *Arch Pathol Lab Med*. 1976;100(4):182–185.

19. Sehgal VN, Tyagi SP, Kumar S, et al. Microscopic pathology of the liver in leprosy patients. *Int J Dermatol*. 1972;11(3):168–172.
20. Lamps LW, Gray GF, Scott MA. The histologic spectrum of hepatic cat scratch disease: a series of six cases with confirmed *Bartonella henselae* infection. *Am J Surg Pathol*. 1996;20(10):1253–1259.
21. Murano I, Yoshii H, Kurashige H, et al. Giant hepatic granuloma caused by *Bartonella henselae*. *Pediatr Infect Dis J*. 2001;20(3):319–320.
22. Akritidis N, Tzivras M, Delladetsima I, et al. The liver in brucellosis. *Clin Gastroenterol Hepatol*. 2007;5(9):1109–1112.
23. Williams RK, Crossley K. Acute and chronic hepatic involvement of brucellosis. *Gastroenterology*. 1982;83(2):455–458.
24. Cervantes F, Bruguera M, Carbonell J, et al. Liver disease in brucellosis. A clinical and pathological study of 40 cases. *Postgrad Med J*. 1982;58(680):346–350.
25. Pellegrin M, Delsol G, Auvergnat JC, et al. Granulomatous hepatitis in Q fever. *Hum Pathol*. 1980;11(1):51–57.
26. Lamps LW, Molina CP, West AB, et al. The pathologic spectrum of gastrointestinal and hepatic histoplasmosis. *Am J Clin Pathol*. 2000;113(1): 64–72.
27. Heninger E, Hogan LH, Karman J, et al. Characterization of the histoplasma capsulatum-induced granuloma. *J Immunol*. 2006;23:161–169.
28. Bonacini M, Nussbaum J, Ahluwalia C. Gastrointestinal, hepatic, and pancreatic involvement with cryptococcus neoformans in AID. *J Clin Gastroenterol*. 1990;12(3):295–297.
29. Washington K, Gottfried MR, Wilson ML. Gastrointestinal cryptococcosis. *Mod Pathol*. 1991;4(6):707–711.
30. Wainwright H. Hepatic granulomas. *Eur J Gastroenterol Hepatol*. 2007;19(2):93.
31. Wilson MS, Mentink-Kane MM, Pesce JT, et al. Immunopathology of schistosomiasis. *Immunol Cell Biol*. 2007;85(2):148–154.
32. Sharma S. Granulomatous diseases of the liver. In Zakim D, Boyer T, eds.: *Hepatology – A Textbook of Liver Disease*. 4th ed. Philadelphia, PA: Saunders Elsevier Science; 2003:1317–1330.
33. Daneshbod K. Visceral leishmaniasis (kala-azar) in Iran: a pathologic and electron microscopic study. *Am J Clin Pathol*. 1972;57(2):156–166.
34. Moreno A, Marazuela M, Yebra M, et al. Hepatic fibrin-ring granulomas in visceral leishmaniasis. *Gastroenterology*. 1988;95(4):1123–1126.
35. Desai N, Thakur N, Amrapurkar N, et al. Hepatic granuloma in chronic hepatitis C. *Trop Gastroenterol*. 2004;25(4):174–175.
36. Mert A, Tahan V, Mert A, et al. Hepatic granulomas in chornic hepatitis C. *J Clin Gastroenterol*. 2001;33(4):342–343.
37. Ozaras R, Tahan V, Mert A, et al. The prevalence of hepatic granulomas in chronic hepatitis C. *J Clin Gastroenterol*. 2004;38(5):449–452.
38. Tahan V, Ozaras R, Lacevic N, et al. Prevalence of hepatic granulomas in chronic hepatitis B. *Dig Dis Sci*. 2004;49(10):1575–1577.
39. Drebber U, Kasper HU, Ratering J, et al. Hepatic granulomas: histological and molecular pathological approach to differential diagnosis-a study of 442 cases. *Liver Int*. 2008;28(6):828–834.
40. Sherlock S, Scheuer PJ. The presentation and diagnosis of 100 patients with primary biliary cirrhosis. *N Engl J Med*. 1973;289(13):674–678.
41. Lee RG, Epstein O, Jauregui H, et al. Granulomas in primary biliary cirrhosis: a prognostic feature. *Gastroenterology*. 1981;81(6):983–986.
42. Fagan EA, Moore-Gillon JC, Turner-Warwick M. Multiorgan granulomas and mitochondrial antibodies. *N Engl J Med*. 1983;308(10):572–575.
43. Kleiner DE. Granulomas in the liver. *Semin Diagn Pathol*. 2006;23(3–4):161–169.
44. Ludwig J, Colina F, Poterucha JJ. Granulomas in primary sclerosing cholangitis. *Liver*. 1995;15(6):307–312.
45. Daniels JA, Torbenson M, Vivekanandan P, et al. Hepatitis in common variable immunodeficiency. *Hum Pathol*. 2009;40(4):484–488.
46. Garcia-Eulate R, Hussain N, Heller T, et al. CT and MRI of hepatic abscess in patients with chronic granulomatous disease. *Am J Roentgenol*. 2006;187(2):482–490.
47. Levine S, Smith VV, Malone M, et al. Histopathological features of chronic granulomatous disease (CGD) in childhood. *Histopathology*. 2005;47(5):508–516.
48. Lublin M, Bartlett DL, Danforth DN, et al. Hepatic abscess in patients with chronic granulomatous disease. *Ann Surg*. 2002;235(3):383–391.
49. Alenezi B, Lamoureux E, Alpert L, et al. Effect of ursodeoxycholic acid on granulomatous liver disease due to sarcoidosis. *Dig Dis Sci*. 2005;50(1):196–200.
50. Ferrell LD, Lee R, Brixko C, et al. Hepatic granulomas following liver transplantation: clinicopathologic features in 42 patients. *Transplantation*. 1995;60(9):926–933.
51. Smits JG, Kooijman CD. Rheumatoid nodules in liver. *Histopathology*. 1986;10(11):1211–1213.
52. Saeed SA, Kelly DR, Hardin WD Jr. Pseudorheumatoid nodule in the liver of an adolescent male. *J Pediatr Surg*. 2006;41(8):1479–1482.

53. Holla RG, Gupta A, Dubey AK. Idiopathic granulomatous hepatitis. *Indian Pediatr.* 2004;41(6):610–613.
54. Dourakis SP, Saramadou R, Alexopoulou A, et al. Hepatic granulomas: a 6-year experience in a single center in Greece. *Eur J Gastroenterol Hepatol.* 2007;19(2):101–104.
55. Vial T, Descotes J. Drug-induced granulomatous hepatitis. *Gastroenterol Clin Biol.* 1993;17(5 Pt 2):H44–48.
56. Zhang X, Ouyang J, Thung SN. Histopathologic manifestations of drug-induced hepatotoxicity. *Clin Liver Dis.* 2013;17(4):547–564.
57. Villamil-Cajoto I, Iove MI, Serrano M, et al. Granulomatous hepatitis due to Mycobacterium complex following Bacillus Calmette-Guerin intravesical instillation. *Enferm Infecc Microbiol Clin.* 2010;28(10):759–761; author reply 761–762.
58. McCluggage WG, Sloan JM. Hepatic granulomas in Northern Ireland: a thirteen year review. *Histopathology.* 1994;25(3):219–228.
59. Bieze M, Bioulac-Sage P, Verheij J, et al. Hepatocellular adenomas associated with hepatic granulomas: experience in five cases. *Case Rep Gastroenterol.* 2012;6(3):677–683.

12 Autoimmune hepatitis

Rish K. Pai, MD, PhD

12.1 INTRODUCTION

Autoimmune hepatitis is defined as an unresolving hepatitis characterized by an aberrant immune response against self-liver antigens. This aberrant immune response occurs in genetically susceptible individuals and is associated with characteristic clinical, pathologic, and serologic features, although no one feature is specific for autoimmune hepatitis. The diagnosis of autoimmune hepatitis relies heavily on the liver biopsy, which can support the diagnosis and rule out other entities including primary biliary cirrhosis, primary sclerosing cholangitis, and steatohepatitis, among others. The liver biopsy also plays an important role in assessing response to therapy.

12.2 CLINICAL FEATURES

Demographics and etiology

The incidence of autoimmune hepatitis is somewhat unclear given that many early studies did not exclude the possibility of viral hepatitis C in patients with idiopathic chronic active hepatitis. Furthermore, standard diagnostic criteria for autoimmune hepatitis have only been recently developed. The likely incidence of autoimmune hepatitis ranges from 0.7 to 2.0/100,000; however, the prevalence and incidence of autoimmune hepatitis varies widely among different populations.[1] In particular, autoimmune hepatitis is more common in Caucasian and North American populations, compared with those from Asia. In the United States, the highest prevalence is seen in Alaska Natives (42.9/100,000).[2] The incidence of autoimmune hepatitis is roughly similar to primary biliary cirrhosis, but is twice as common as primary sclerosing cholangitis.

The current hypothesis is that hepatocyte injury due to a variety of factors (viral hepatitis, toxin, medication injury, etc.) triggers an aberrant and dysregulated immune response resulting in an autoimmune hepatitis.[3] The factors that increase the risk of autoimmune hepatitis have not been fully characterized. The strongest associations are with major histocompatibility complex class I and II alleles.

As with other autoimmune diseases, autoimmune hepatitis is more common in women than in men, with a ratio of roughly 4:1. Autoimmune hepatitis can affect any age, but may be somewhat more aggressive in younger-age populations. Although more common in younger individuals, one-fifth of autoimmune hepatitis patients are diagnosed after the age of 60 years. Older individuals are more likely to have concomitant autoimmune thyroid or collagen-vascular disease.

Clinical presentation

The clinical presentation of autoimmune hepatitis is quite varied, ranging from mild elevations in serum liver enzymes to liver failure. The majority of patients present with fatigue, lethargy, anorexia, and abdominal pain. Concurrent autoimmune diseases are common, including type 1 diabetes, celiac disease, autoimmune thyroiditis, and rheumatoid arthritis. The serum liver enzymes may fluctuate quite dramatically because of the waxing and waning nature of autoimmune hepatitis (Fig. 12.1). Up to 33% of patients, mainly those with advanced age, present with sequelae of cirrhosis including ascites, splenomegaly, and esophageal varices. Furthermore, many patients will have some degree of fibrosis on liver biopsy at first presentation, indicating that autoimmune hepatitis has a prolonged subclinical course in many patients.[4]

Up to 20% of patients may be entirely asymptomatic and only have elevations in liver enzymes that are detected during routine medical examination. Autoimmune hepatitis can uncommonly present clinically as an acute hepatitis with scleral icterus. Autoimmune hepatitis is thought to only rarely present as acute liver failure; however, many patients in this setting do not undergo a liver biopsy because of the risk of hemorrhage and it is likely that some patients with unexplained acute liver failure have an autoimmune etiology.

Serologic studies

Often the trigger for gastroenterologists and hepatologists to consider a diagnosis of autoimmune hepatitis is the presence of increased serum transaminases and autoantibodies. Serum transaminase levels vary widely in patients with autoimmune hepatitis and do not accurately reflect disease severity. Bilirubin is often elevated, but alkaline phosphatase levels are usually normal or only mildly elevated in most patients.

Autoantibodies commonly seen in autoimmune hepatitis include antinuclear antibody (ANA), anti-smooth muscle antibodies (anti-SMAs), and anti-liver/kidney microsomal (anti-LKM) antibodies (Table 12.1).[5] Anti-SMAs are the most common antibodies seen in autoimmune hepatitis and have been shown to be directed against filamentous-actin (F-actin). Measurement of F-actin antibodies may be more sensitive than measurement of anti-SMA.[6] Anti-LKM antibodies are uncommon, but occur more frequently in children. Other rare autoantibodies include antibodies against soluble liver antigen/liver-pancreas antigen, liver cytosol Type 1, and asialoglycoprotein receptor, among others. Serum immunoglobulins are often elevated, usually 1.1 to 1.3 times normal levels.

Autoimmune hepatitis has been classified into two different types based on clinical and serologic features (Table 12.1).[1,3,5,7] Type 1 autoimmune hepatitis is characterized by elevations in ANA and/or anti-SMA, often with marked elevations in serum IgG levels. Type 1 autoimmune hepatitis can occur at any age and is by far the most common subtype. Type 2 autoimmune hepatitis is characterized by elevations in anti-LKM antibody and/or anti-liver cytosol antibodies

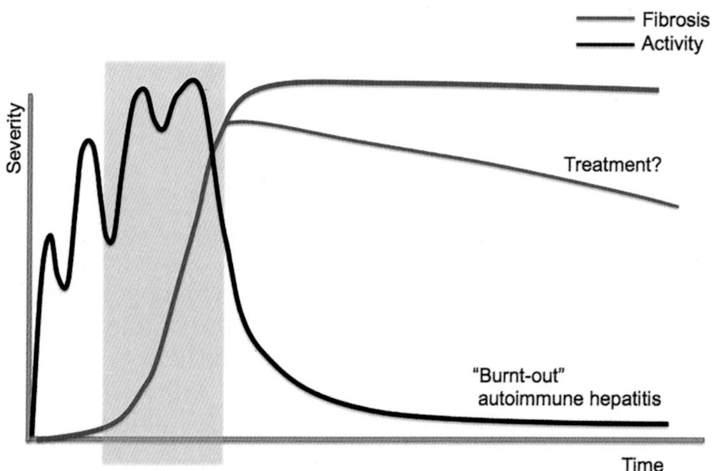

Figure 12.1 Natural history of autoimmune hepatitis. Autoimmune hepatitis is characterized by variations in liver enzymes although they are often ≥5-fold the upper limit of normal. Over time, fibrosis develops. At advanced fibrosis, the degree of inflammatory activity decreases. Treatment may cause regression of fibrosis. The gray box is the window when most patients present clinically and undergo a liver biopsy.

Table 12.1 Clinical and serologic features of autoimmune hepatitis

Feature	Type 1	Type 2
Approximate frequency	95%	5%
Auto-antibodies[9]	ANA Anti-SMA F-actin antibodies Atypical perinuclear antineutrophil antibody	Anti-liver/kidney microsomal antibody (LKM type 1) Anti-liver cytosol (LC1)
Elevated serum IgG levels	+++	+
Most common affected age group	Any age	Childhood and young adulthood
Gender prediction	~75% female	95% female
Clinical severity	Broad range	Generally severe
Histologic findings	Hepatitis with prominent plasma cells, varying fibrosis	Hepatitis with prominent plasma cells, often advanced fibrosis
Relapse after withdrawal of immune suppression	Variable	Common, often long-term maintenance is needed

with only mild elevations in serum IgG. This subtype is more common in the pediatric population and may progress to cirrhosis more often than type 1 autoimmune hepatitis. Histologically, there are no differences between these subtypes. A third type of autoimmune hepatitis has been proposed based on elevations in soluble liver antigen/liver-pancreas antibodies; however, this type has not been proven to be a distinct subtype.[8]

Autoantibodies are useful in the diagnosis of autoimmune hepatitis, but the presence of autoantibodies in the setting of elevated liver enzyme levels does not necessarily indicate autoimmune hepatitis. Autoantibodies, particular ANA, can be elevated in a variety of diseases of the liver and in patients with other autoimmune diseases.[9] Importantly, autoantibody negative autoimmune hepatitis also occurs and accounts for 5% to 10% of cases.[10–12] Although the majority of autoantibody negative patients will have elevations in serum immunoglobulins, IgG levels may also be normal. Patients with autoantibody negative autoimmune hepatitis may have a more aggressive course. Although these patients respond to immunosuppressive therapy, they are less likely to achieve remission.[10]

Clinical scoring systems

Given the importance of making the diagnosis of autoimmune hepatitis, clinical scoring systems have been developed. The International Autoimmune Hepatitis Group in 1999 modified a scoring system

Table 12.2 Simplified criteria for the diagnosis of autoimmune hepatitis

Variable	Cut-off	Points
ANA or anti-SMA	≥1:40	1
ANA or anti-SMA	≥1:80	2[a]
or anti-LKM	≥1:40	2[a]
or anti-SLA	Positive	2[a]
IgG	>Upper normal limit	1
	>1.10 times upper normal limit	2
Liver histology (evidence of hepatitis is necessary)	Compatible with AIH	1
	Typical of AIH	2
Absence of viral hepatitis	Yes	2
Interpretation	≥7: definite AIH	
	≥6: probable AIH	

[a] The maximum total point for all autoantibodies is 2 points, even if the patient scores more than 2.

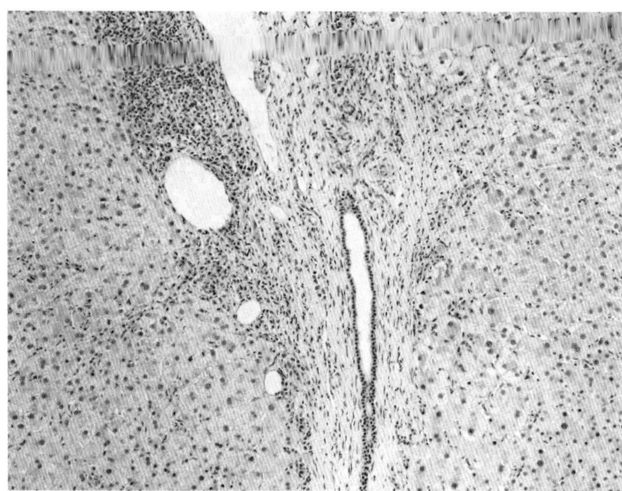

Figure 12.2 Portal inflammation. Prominent lymphoplasmacytic portal inflammation with interface activity.

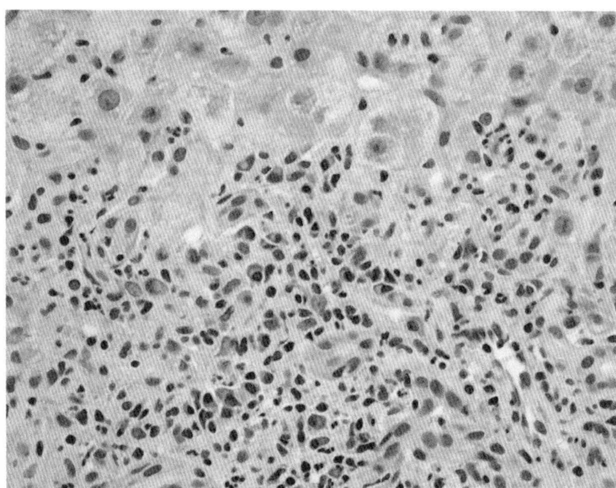

Figure 12.3 Portal inflammations. Clusters of plasma cells are readily identified.

that evaluates clinical, serologic, and histologic data.[13] More recently a simplified autoimmune hepatitis scoring system has been developed that again relies predominantly on serologic and histologic features (Table 12.2).[14] Both have similar sensitivity and specificity for the diagnosis of autoimmune hepatitis.[15] In both of these scoring systems, a high-titer ANA or anti-SMA receives additional points; however, many laboratories in the United States do not report titer levels, which decreases the utility of these scores. Moreover, the titers may not reflect the severity of the liver disease.[16]

12.3 PATHOLOGIC FEATURES

Classic findings

The liver biopsy plays an important role when clinicians are considering a diagnosis of autoimmune hepatitis. Classically, autoimmune hepatitis is characterized by dense lymphoplasmacytic portal inflammation with brisk interface activity, wherein portal inflammatory cells extend from the portal tract into the adjacent hepatic parenchyma, resulting in hepatocyte injury (Fig. 12.2).[17,18] The hepatic parenchyma also demonstrates marked lobular inflammation with clusters of lymphocytes, macrophages, and plasma cells (Fig. 12.3). The hepatocytes are often swollen and occasional multinucleated hepatocytes are seen. The hepatic plate architecture is disrupted by the inflammatory infiltrates and hepatocyte injury (Figs. 12.4 and 12.5). Often the necroinflammatory activity is more severe than seen in chronic viral hepatitis, particularly viral hepatitis C; however, in some cases, autoimmune hepatitis may be quite mild with only minimal to

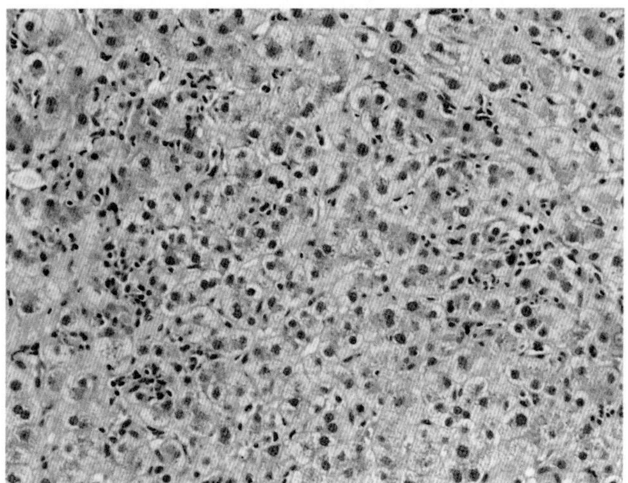

Figure 12.4 Lobular inflammation. Autoimmune hepatitis often demonstrates lobular disarray with numerous inflammatory cells and disruption of the hepatic plate architecture.

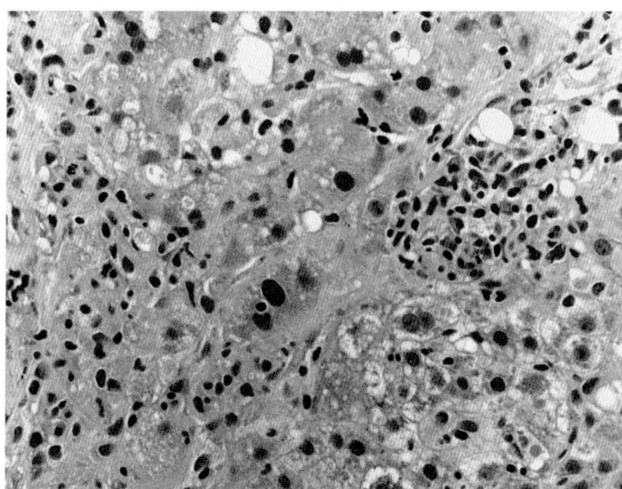

Figure 12.6 Emperipolesis in autoimmune hepatitis. The presence of mononuclear cells within hepatocytes (emperipolesis) can suggest the diagnosis of autoimmune hepatitis.

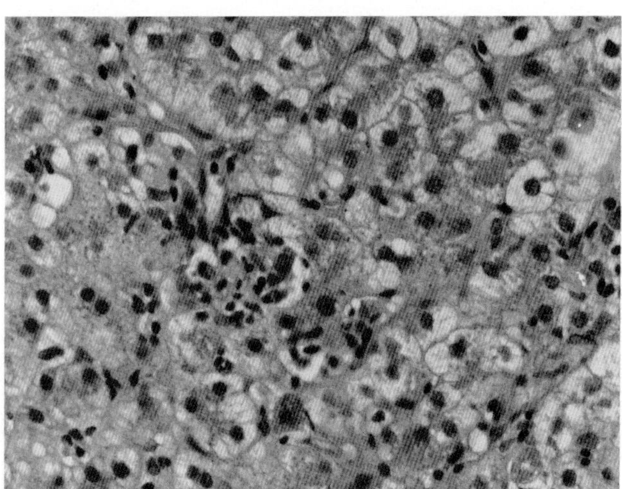

Figure 12.5 Lobular inflammation. Acidophil bodies are readily identified.

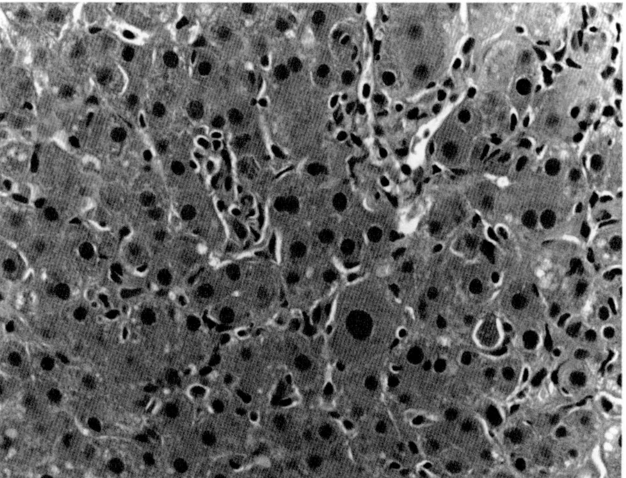

Figure 12.7 Rosettes in autoimmune hepatitis. Hepatic rosette formation (center of image) is commonly seen in autoimmune hepatitis; however, this feature is not specific to autoimmune hepatitis.

mild interface and lobular activity. These cases can be quite difficult to arrive at the correct diagnosis.

There have been numerous studies looking at histologic features that are helpful in differentiating autoimmune hepatitis from other forms of hepatitis, including viral hepatitis as well as drug-induced liver injury. Compared with chronic viral hepatitis, autoimmune hepatitis on average demonstrates more interface hepatitis, heavier plasma cell infiltrates, rosettes, and emperipolesis (lymphocytes within hepatocytes).[19] Emperipolesis (Fig. 12.6) and rosette formation (Fig. 12.7) were found to be superior to plasma cell infiltration and marked interface hepatitis in some studies.[19–21] Indeed, these features were also identified as features characteristic of autoimmune hepatitis in the simplified autoimmune hepatitis scoring system published in 2008.[14] However, while emperipolesis and rosettes appear useful in studies, at the practical level emperipolesis is not reliably identified and the rosettes are a nonspecific finding, so most liver pathologists still rely on dense lymphoplasmacytic portal inflammation with brisk interface and lobular activity in the proper clinical setting to arrive at the correct diagnosis.

More recently, the presence of Kupffer cells with prominent, glassy, intracytoplasmic inclusions has been described in patients with autoimmune hepatitis, both adults and children.[22] Immunohistochemically, this material is shown to be immunoglobulin. Although this feature may be seen more commonly in patients with autoimmune hepatitis, it is unlikely to be used as a major criterion for diagnosis.

Immunohistochemical stains for various T cell and B cell markers have limited utility in the diagnosis of autoimmune hepatitis; however, the lymphocytes within autoimmune hepatitis tend to be CD4+ T cells. The IgG:IgM ratio is distinct in autoimmune hepatitis compared with primary biliary cirrhosis (IgM positive plasma cells predominate in primary biliary cirrhosis; IgG in autoimmune hepatitis), and immunostains can be helpful when the differential is autoimmune hepatitis versus primary biliary cirrhosis. However, IgG-positive plasma cells also predominate in other conditions such as infections and drug effects, so are not specific for autoimmune hepatitis. Finally, IgG4-positive plasma cells are scattered and rare in liver biopsies with autoimmune hepatitis. Marked IgG4-positive plasma cells should raise the possibility of IgG4-mediated disease.[23]

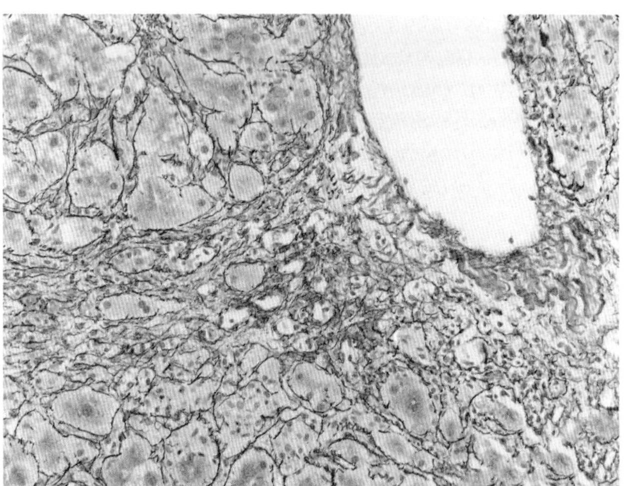

Figure 12.9 Assessment of fibrosis in autoimmune hepatitis. A reticulin stain confirms collapse of the reticulin fibers (same case as 12.8).

Fibrosis in autoimmune hepatitis

Fibrosis in a liver biopsy indicates chronic injury and, as autoimmune hepatitis is a chronic liver disease, liver biopsies in this setting often demonstrate some degree of fibrosis.[24,25] Determining the degree of fibrosis, however, can be quite challenging when there is marked necroinflammatory activity. In cases of confluent or bridging necrosis, one should carefully evaluate the trichrome and reticulin stains to not overestimate the degree of fibrosis. Bridging necrosis should appear more pale blue on a trichrome stain and demonstrate a collapse of reticulin fibers (Figs. 12.8 and 12.9). If there is any uncertainty regarding the degree of fibrosis, this should be clearly stated in the pathology report because bridging necrosis can heal without marked collagen deposition. Given that elastic fibers are deposited only in areas of long-standing fibrosis, evaluation for the presence of elastic fibers using an orcein stain may be helpful to separate reticulin collapse from true fibrosis (Fig. 12.10). Often in the setting of marked inflammatory activity and necrosis, it may be adequate just to indicate that there is or is not advanced fibrosis (bridging or cirrhosis). If the clinicians are concerned about advanced fibrosis, treatment with immune suppression followed by a

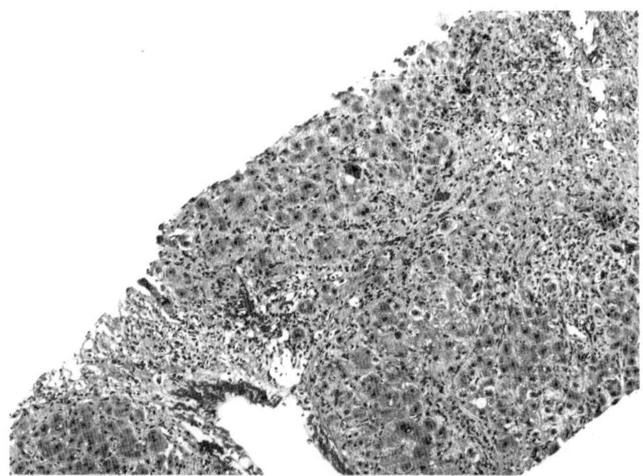

Figure 12.8 Assessment of fibrosis in autoimmune hepatitis. Trichrome stain demonstrating central–portal bridging necrosis. Reticulin fibers stain paler than dense collagen fibers on a trichrome stain. Care must be made to not overestimate the degree of fibrosis.

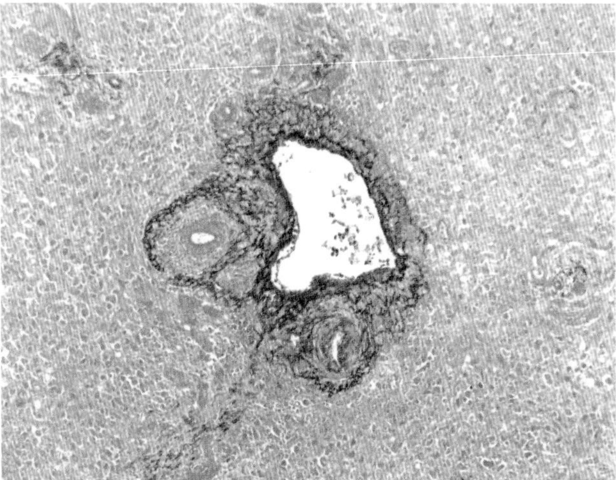

Figure 12.10 Orcein stain. An orcein stain for elastic fibers may be useful in cases where it is uncertain if there is necrosis or fibrosis. Elastic fibers are only deposited in mature fibrous tissue and are limited to the portal tract in this case. The absence of elastic fibers on an orcein stain favors necrosis.

repeat biopsy may be the best way to document the stage of disease. In addition, acute autoimmune hepatitis without evidence of fibrosis does occur.[24] This finding should be recognized so as not to automatically assume the presence of fibrosis when considering a diagnosis of autoimmune hepatitis.

Grading autoimmune hepatitis

After making a diagnosis of autoimmune hepatitis, it is important to provide an estimate of the degree of hepatocyte injury. There are numerous scoring systems available, including the Batts–Ludwig, Scheuer, and Metavir systems. More complicated grading systems are also available, including the Modified Hepatic Activity Index, but these are used predominantly in the research setting. The Batts–Ludwig system has been shown to be reproducible and is the one used at our institution.[26] In this system, untreated autoimmune hepatitis is often grade 3 (moderate interface and lobular activity with interface activity present completely around most portal areas) and grade 4 (confluent and/or bridging necrosis). However, as autoimmune hepatitis progresses to advanced fibrosis, the inflammatory activity often decreases and may resemble a mild chronic hepatitis, similar to that typically seen in chronic viral hepatitis C (Fig. 12.11). These cases of "burned out" autoimmune hepatitis can be somewhat difficult to diagnose. Indeed, some cases of cryptogenic cirrhosis may be a result of end-stage autoimmune hepatitis that is unrecognized/undiagnosed.

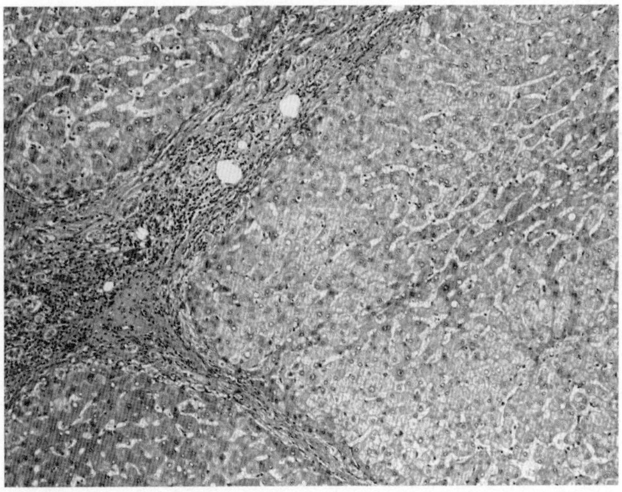

Figure 12.11 "Burnt out" autoimmune hepatitis. In this explant from a patient with known autoimmune hepatitis, there is only minimal septal inflammation without significant interface and lobular activity.

Variants of autoimmune hepatitis

There are a few patterns of autoimmune hepatitis that deserve mention. The earliest injury in autoimmune hepatitis occurs around central veins in Zone 3.[27,28] In this Zone 3 pattern, the inflammatory activity is exclusively or largely in Zone 3, resulting in confluent necrosis around central veins (Fig. 12.12). The inflammatory infiltrate often consists of lymphocytes and clusters of plasma cells. In this pattern, portal tracts are often spared, and these cases often have no fibrosis.

Fulminant autoimmune hepatitis with panacinar necrosis can be life-threatening and require immediate liver transplantation (Figs. 12.13, 12.14, and 12.15). The degree of necrosis, however, can be quite heterogeneous

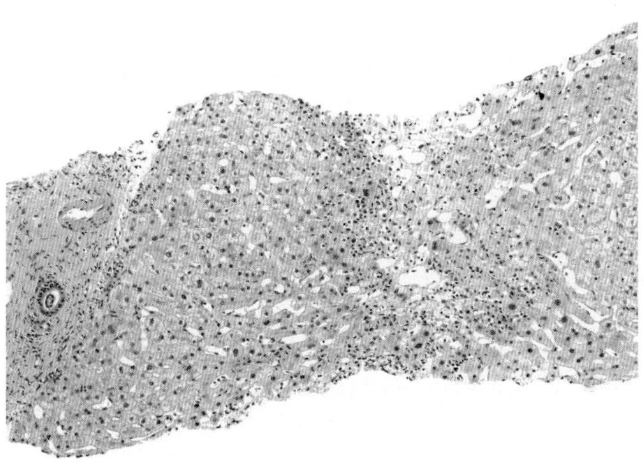

Figure 12.12 Centrilobular variant of autoimmune hepatitis. In this variant, there is prominent inflammation around central veins with relative sparing of the portal tracts.

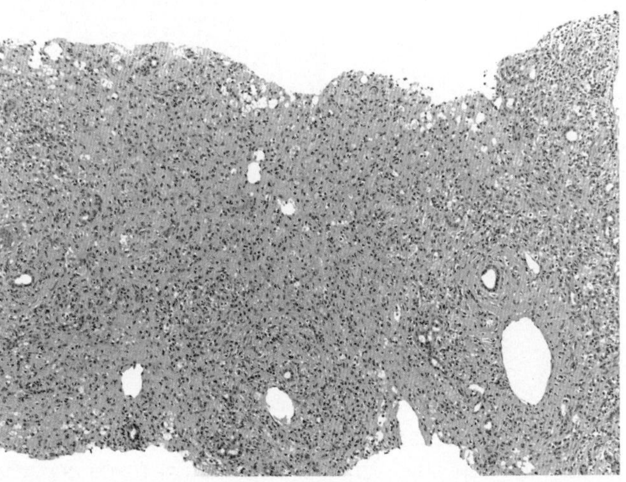

Figure 12.13 Severe autoimmune hepatitis with panacinar necrosis. The portal tracts are in close approximation due to panacinar necrosis.

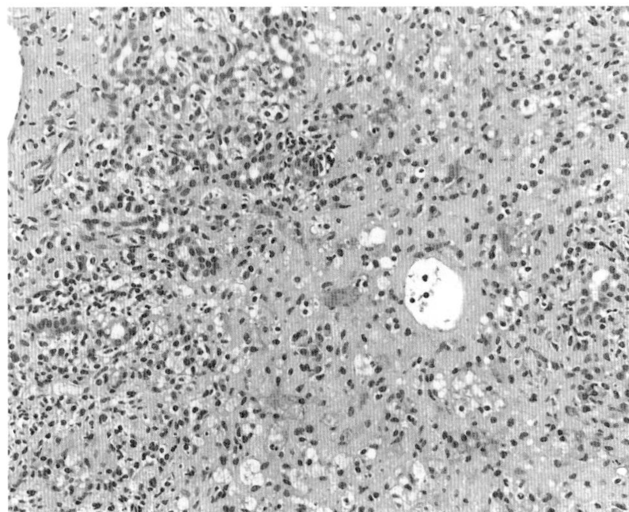

Figure 12.14 Severe autoimmune hepatitis with panacinar necrosis. The inflammation is rich in plasma cells. A bile duct proliferation is also identified as a response to hepatocyte injury. Same case as above.

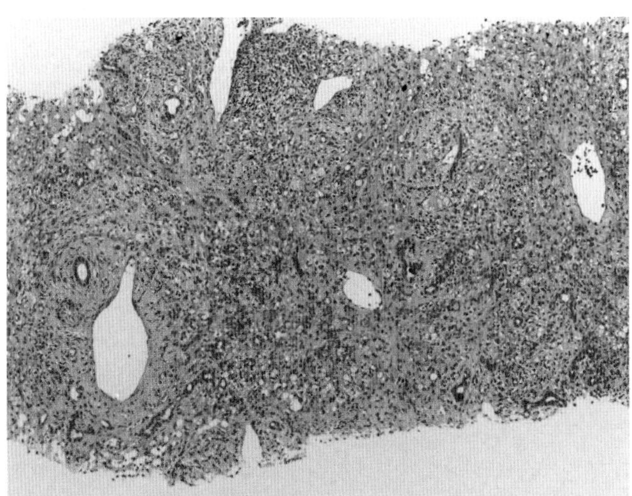

Figure 12.15 Severe autoimmune hepatitis with panacinar necrosis. A trichrome stain demonstrates no evidence of fibrosis. Same case as above.

within the liver and explant specimens often show irregular areas of panacinar necrosis with sparing of other parts of the liver. Thus, using a liver biopsy to determine the need for liver transplantation may be problematic. Rather, in cases of fulminant autoimmune hepatitis, correlation with liver function may be more useful.

Syncytial giant cell hepatitis is an uncommon pattern of liver injury defined by giant cell transformation of hepatocytes.[18] Occasional giant cells in autoimmune hepatitis can be seen in adults (Fig. 12.16), but tends to be more common in children. If prominent, other etiologies should be excluded, particularly viral hepatitis, including hepatitis E and paramyxovirus. Medications can also result in this particular pattern of injury.

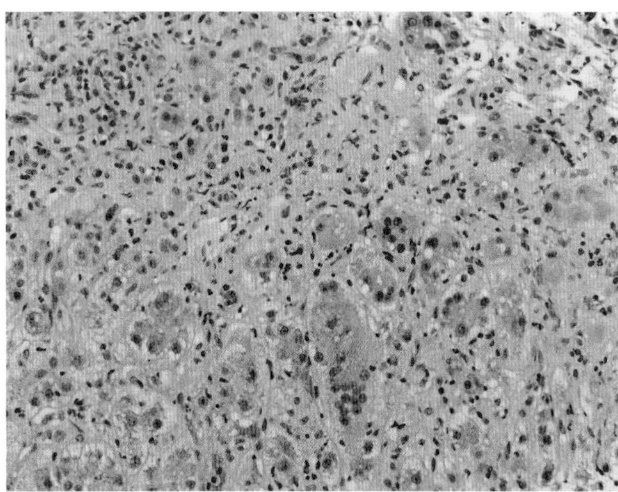

Figure 12.16 Giant cells in autoimmune hepatitis. Multinucleated hepatocytes are occasionally encountered in autoimmune hepatitis.

12.4 DRUG-INDUCED AUTOIMMUNE HEPATITIS

Drug-induced liver injury is becoming increasingly common given the polypharmacy in today's patient population. Drug-induced liver injury can result in bile duct injury, fatty liver disease, acute hepatitis, cholestatic hepatitis, and chronic hepatitis. Two patterns of drug-induced chronic hepatitis have been described, one of which resembles chronic viral hepatitis, whereas others resemble an autoimmune hepatitis. The autoimmune hepatitis pattern of drug injury accounts for 10% to 15% of all autoimmune hepatitis cases.[29,30] Classically, drugs such as minocycline (Fig. 12.17) and nitrofurantoin result in an autoimmune hepatitis pattern of injury and are likely responsible for ~90% of all drug-induced cases that mimic autoimmune hepatitis.[30] Determining if a medication has resulted in autoimmune hepatitis can be quite challenging, and no specific histologic features are useful to point to drug-induced autoimmune hepatitis.[20,31] In order to determine that drug exposure is the cause of the liver injury, a strong temporal association between the medication and liver enzyme elevations is useful. Patients with drug-induced autoimmune hepatitis often respond to drug withdrawal and, when needed, conventional autoimmune hepatitis treatment.

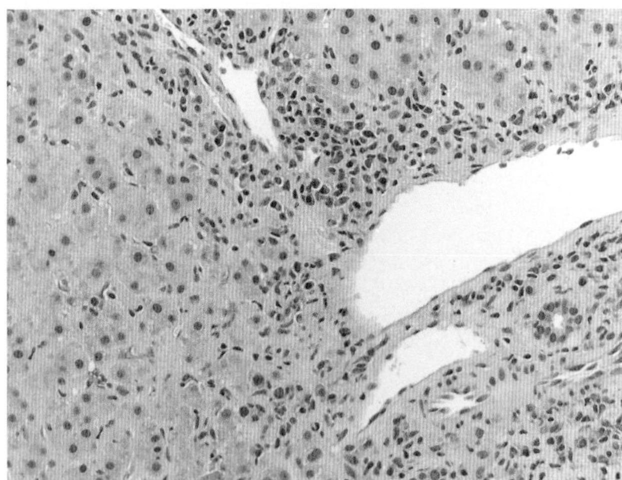

Figure 12.17 Drug-induced autoimmune hepatitis. This 17-year-old female developed autoimmune hepatitis due to minocycline. There is dense lymphoplasmacytic portal inflammation with interface and lobular activity.

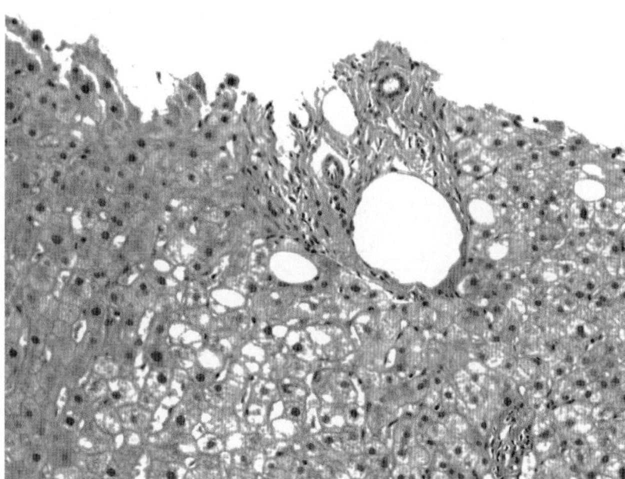

Figure 12.18 Autoimmune hepatitis on therapy. The goal of medical therapy is to induce clinical, biochemical, and histologic remission. This biopsy demonstrates complete histologic remission with no portal inflammation, interface activity, and lobular inflammation.

12.5 AUTOIMMUNE HEPATITIS BIOPSIES IN PATIENTS ON MEDICAL THERAPY

Although the survival of autoimmune hepatitis patients is quite good, there is a decline in long-term survival (beyond the first decade) after the diagnosis. Many clinicians use serum transaminases as a method to determine efficacy of treatment. Currently, complete normalization of aspartate aminotransferase and alanine aminotransferase (ALT) is widely accepted as a measure of effective therapy. More recently, normalization of serum immunoglobulins has also been recommended as a target. Until recently, the role of histologic remission was uncertain, and biopsies to assess the degree of activity were not that frequent. In an early trial from the Mayo Clinic that included follow-up liver biopsies, histologic remission lagged significantly behind biochemical remission by months and was only achieved in 60% of patients after 2 years of immunosuppressive therapy.[32] More recent studies have indicated that histologic remission (Fig. 12.18) is a necessary target.[33,34] In a recent study from the United Kingdom, 120 patients with autoimmune hepatitis who received therapy underwent a follow-up liver biopsy. Despite normalization of serum transaminases, 46% of patients had persistent histologic activity. These patients with persistent histologic activity had less frequent regression of fibrosis and increased liver-specific disease mortality. Multivariate analysis demonstrated that persistent histologic activity was independently associated with death and transplantation.[33] Thus, persistent histologic activity may be useful to guide additional therapy (Fig. 12.19). In keeping with this, a liver biopsy is recommended by the American Association for the Study of Liver Diseases before considering cessation of immune suppression.

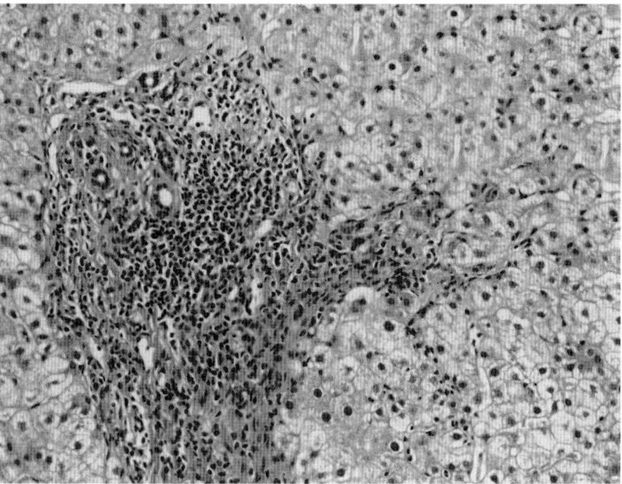

Figure 12.19 Autoimmune hepatitis on therapy. In this example, there is persistent portal inflammation, mostly lymphocytic, with focal areas of interface activity. This patient would likely not be considered for withdrawal of immune suppression.

12.6 DIFFERENTIAL DIAGNOSIS

Given that autoimmune hepatitis often has dense portal inflammation, other chronic hepatitides enter the differential diagnosis; however, these are usually easy to separate based on serologic studies. In cases of severe necrosis, it may be difficult to arrive at the diagnosis of autoimmune hepatitis, and other causes of fulminant hepatic necrosis, such as drug/toxin injury, must be excluded. The hepatocyte swelling in autoimmune hepatitis may be quite severe, raising the possibility that these changes represent ballooned hepatocytes seen in steatohepatitis. However, steatosis is uncommon in autoimmune hepatitis, and the inflammation in fatty liver disease is typically less prominent than what is seen in autoimmune hepatitis. Some cases with brisk periportal inflammation may have a prominent ductular reaction. The proliferation of ductules is an attempt by the liver to regenerate lost hepatocytes because the stem cell compartment lies in the canals of Hering. When marked, the ductular reaction in this setting can be confused with the ductular reaction seen in biliary tract disease. However, biliary tract disease lacks the prominent lobular hepatitis seen in autoimmune hepatitis.

Differentiating drug injury from autoimmune hepatitis often is quite challenging clinically and can be difficult histologically. In the end, this distinction is not made by histology alone, but instead is made by the combination of clinical findings, serologic findings, drug history including the types of medications and when they were started, and the histologic findings. Features that favor autoimmune hepatitis over typical idiosyncratic drug injury include plasma cell-rich portal inflammation and emperipolesis, if you can find it.[20] Of note, eosinophils are not helpful in most cases because they are not a prominent feature of most drug reactions. In fact, one study found that eosinophils were more frequently seen in autoimmune hepatitis cases than in idiosyncratic drug-induced liver injury.[20]

Wilson disease should always be considered in the differential diagnosis of acute liver failure or a chronic hepatitis in young patients. In fact, the histologic findings in Wilson disease can sometimes by indistinguishable from autoimmune hepatitis, including features such as dense portal inflammation with interface activity. Although copper tissue stains often reveal increased copper within the hepatocytes in Wilson disease, stains can be negative and quantitative copper analysis is the preferred method for detecting the increased liver copper seen in Wilson disease.

12.7 CHOLESTATIC VARIANT PATTERNS

Primary biliary cirrhosis and autoimmune hepatitis overlap syndrome

Pathologists are often asked to rule out the possibility of overlap syndrome. The published frequency depends heavily on the strictness of the definition. Using more generous criteria, primary biliary cirrhosis/autoimmune hepatitis overlap occurs in up to ~10% of patients.[35,36] More rigorous criteria provide estimates closer to 1% to 5%. There are two main scenarios when one considers the diagnosis of primary biliary cirrhosis/autoimmune hepatitis overlap: (1) when classic features of primary biliary cirrhosis are present, but the lobular inflammation is more than what is usually seen and (2) when classic features of autoimmune hepatitis are identified, but there is prominent duct lymphocytosis and injury (Figs. 12.20 and 12.21; Table 12.3).

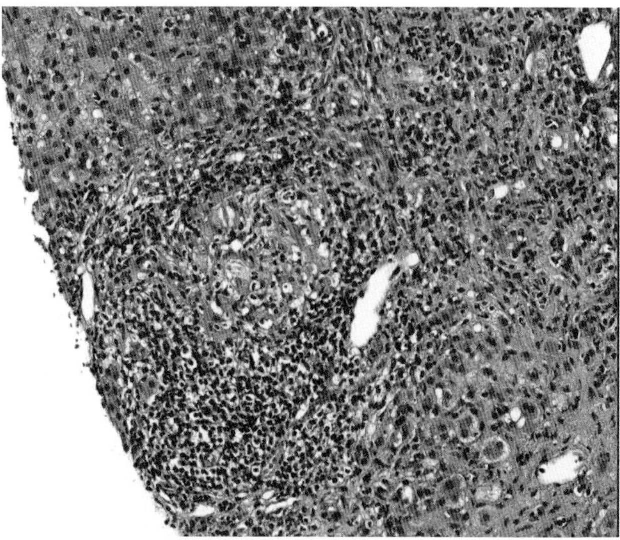

Figure 12.20 Primary biliary cirrhosis/autoimmune hepatitis overlap syndrome. This patient had marked elevations in serum transaminases, elevated ANA, elevated AMA. Histologically, there is interface hepatitis along with a florid duct lesion.

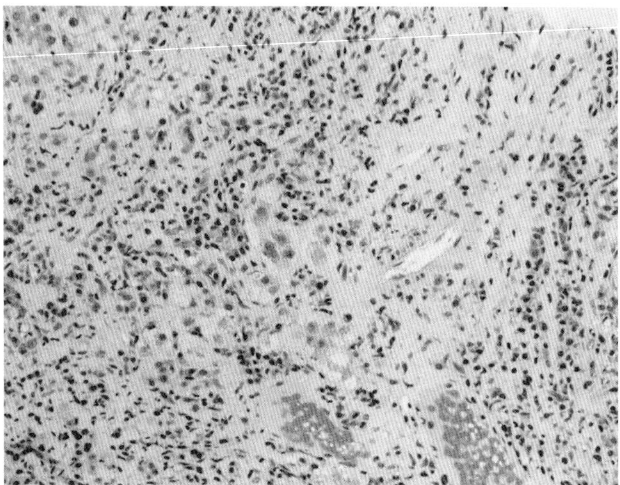

Figure 12.21 Primary biliary cirrhosis/autoimmune hepatitis overlap syndrome. In other areas, there is dense portal inflammation with interface activity and evidence of bile duct loss as demonstrated by an unpaired artery. Same case as above.

Table 12.3 Overlap syndromes (cholestatic variant syndromes)

Overlap syndrome	Laboratory and radiologic features	Histologic	Treatment
Autoimmune hepatitis/ primary biliary cirrhosis	Autoimmune hepatitis features: • *Usually ALT ≥ 5-fold upper limit of normal* • *IgG ≥ 2-fold upper limit of normal or anti-SMA or ANA* • Primary biliary cirrhosis features: • *Alkaline phosphatase ≥2-fold upper limit of normal or γ-glutamyl transferase ≥ 5-fold upper limit of normal* • *Positive antimitochondrial antibodies*	Interface and lobular activity along with florid duct lesions	Immune suppression and ursodeoxycholic acid May consider just immune suppression of the primary biliary cirrhosis component is minimal
Autoimmune hepatitis/primary sclerosing cholangitis	Autoimmune hepatitis features: • *Usually ALT ≥ 5-fold upper limit of normal* • *Usually IgG ≥ 2-fold upper limit of normal or anti-SMA or ANA* Primary sclerosing cholangitis features: • *Characteristic imaging appearance of the biliary tree* • *Lack of antimitochondrial antibodies*	Interface and lobular activity along with features of chronic large duct obstruction (fibro-obliterative lesions are rare on biopsy)	Immune suppression and ursodeoxycholic acid
Autoimmune hepatitis/ indeterminate cholestatic syndrome	Autoimmune hepatitis features: • *Usually ALT ≥ 5-fold upper limit of normal* • *Usually IgG ≥ 2-fold upper limit of normal or anti-SMA or ANA* Chronic cholestatic features: • *Alkaline phosphatase ≥2-fold upper limit of normal or γ-glutamyl transferase ≥5-fold upper limit of normal* • *Lack of antimitochondrial antibodies* • *Normal imaging of the biliary tree*	Interface and lobular activity along with chronic cholestatic features such as bile duct loss and cholate stasis	Unclear, may be dictated by predominant component

It is important to remember that in primary biliary cirrhosis, mild patchy lobular inflammation is quite common, and portal-based plasma cells are usually numerous. Given these features, there is a tendency to over diagnose an overlap with autoimmune hepatitis. One should be cautious of over diagnosing primary biliary cirrhosis/autoimmune hepatitis overlap given the significant morbidity associated with chronic immunosuppressive therapy. In particular, bone loss in primary biliary cirrhosis is accelerated by corticosteroid use.

Chazouillères et al. in 1998 proposed criteria (Paris criteria) to diagnose autoimmune hepatitis/ primary biliary cirrhosis overlap syndrome.[37] These Paris criteria include a combination of laboratory and histologic findings. The Paris criteria were modified slightly by the European Associated for the Study of the Liver in 2011.[38] Of note, interface hepatitis is required for the diagnosis of autoimmune hepatitis/ primary biliary cirrhosis overlap. However, at least focal interface activity is found in the majority of primary biliary cirrhosis biopsies without overlap syndrome. Thus, to have any specificity, the interface hepatitis should be a prominent feature on the biopsy and not simply a small focus of inflammation extending beyond the limiting plate. Although the Paris criteria have a relatively high sensitivity and specificity, some patients with autoimmune hepatitis/ primary biliary cirrhosis overlap may not meet these criteria. Particularly, the ALT and alkaline phosphatase elevations may not be ≥5 times and ≥2 times the upper limit of normal, respectively. Given the wide variations in ALT encountered in patients with autoimmune hepatitis and similar wide variations in alkaline phosphatase in patients with primary biliary cirrhosis, it is not surprising that some patients with overlap would not quality based on the stringent Paris criteria. Such patients may still be classified as having autoimmune hepatitis/primary biliary cirrhosis overlap if other clinical and pathologic features fit well with the diagnosis.

In the setting of definitive autoimmune hepatitis, one may occasionally see prominent duct injury, raising the possibility of primary biliary cirrhosis. One must keep in mind that in autoimmune hepatitis, lymphocytic cholangitis can be seen in up to 30% of biopsies, correlating overall with the degree of portal inflammation, and this feature by itself should not result in a diagnosis of overlap syndrome.[18,19] Rather one should consider superimposed primary biliary cirrhosis in the setting of definite autoimmune hepatitis only if there is a florid duct lesion, disproportionately heavy duct lymphocytosis and injury for the degree of portal inflammation, elevations in antimitochondrial antibody, and disproportionate elevations in alkaline phosphatase. Given that the treatment of primary biliary cirrhosis, ursodeoxycholic acid, is fairly innocuous, the consequence of over diagnosing primary biliary cirrhosis in the setting of *definite* autoimmune hepatitis is less of a problem than in the scenario when considering a diagnosis of autoimmune hepatitis in the setting of *definite* primary biliary cirrhosis. Nonetheless, this observation should not tempt one in to overcalling primary biliary cirrhosis in the setting of *definite* autoimmune hepatitis.

Finally, some patients with autoimmune hepatitis have elevations in antimitochondrial antibodies without any clinical, laboratory, or pathologic findings to suggest a cholestatic disorder. Although some patients may develop overlap with primary biliary cirrhosis in the future, many will not.[39] These patients are often treated with standard immunosuppressive therapy for autoimmune hepatitis without the addition of ursodeoxycholic acid.

Primary sclerosing cholangitis and autoimmune hepatitis overlap syndrome

Primary sclerosing cholangitis and autoimmune hepatitis overlap syndrome has been termed autoimmune sclerosing cholangitis by some experts and occurs in 6% to 11% of young patients with autoimmune hepatitis (Figs. 12.22, 12.23, and 12.24), but is very rare in middle-aged and older individuals.[35,36] Autoimmune sclerosing cholangitis should not be confused with autoimmune cholangitis, another term used to describe antimitochondrial antibody-negative primary biliary cirrhosis.

Autoimmune sclerosing cholangitis patients are younger than patients with primary sclerosing cholangitis. Patients with autoimmune sclerosing cholangitis have typical serologic features of autoimmune hepatitis, namely elevations in autoantibodies (particularly ANA and/or anti-SMA) along with elevated serum IgG. Radiologically, these patients have typical findings of primary sclerosing cholangitis including multifocal stricturing of the extrahepatic biliary tree (Table 12.3). Given the strong link between inflammatory bowel disease and primary sclerosing cholangitis, the presence of autoimmune hepatitis in a patient with inflammatory bowel disease should prompt imaging of the biliary tree to exclude autoimmune sclerosing cholangitis.

Complicating the diagnosis of autoimmune sclerosing cholangitis is the finding that autoimmune hepatitis may precede or follow the diagnosis of

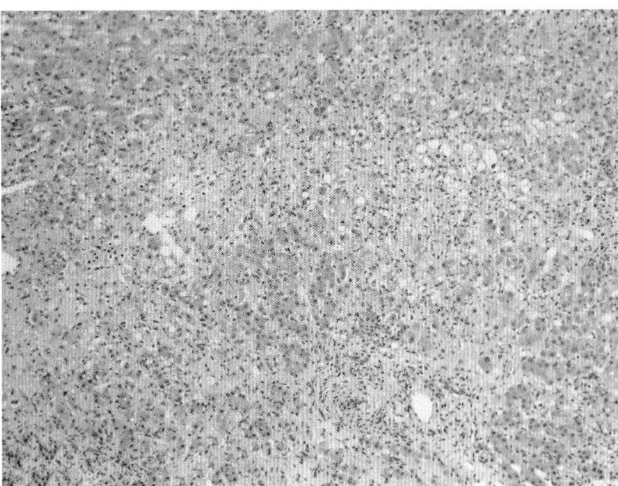

Figure 12.22 Primary sclerosing cholangitis/autoimmune hepatitis overlap syndrome. This patient with known ulcerative colitis developed a marked flare in serum transaminases. There is portal and lobular inflammation with areas of bridging necrosis.

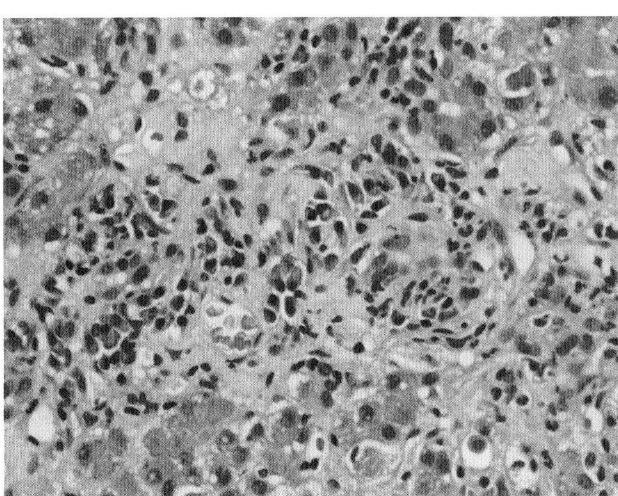

Figure 12.23 Primary sclerosing cholangitis/autoimmune hepatitis overlap syndrome. Numerous plasma cell clusters are identified within portal areas. Same case as above.

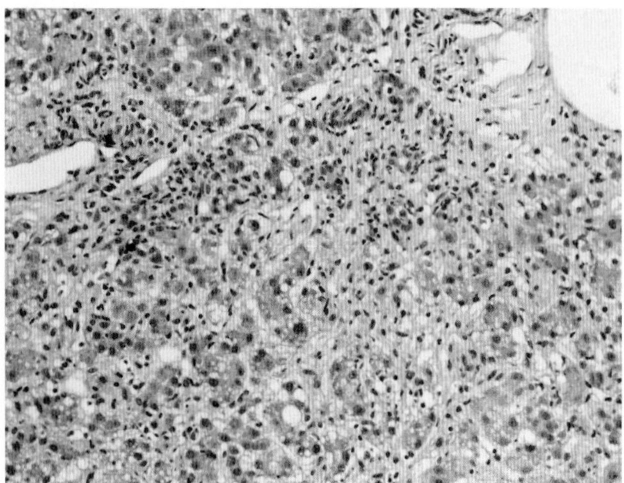

Figure 12.24 Primary sclerosing cholangitis/autoimmune hepatitis overlap syndrome. Some portal areas demonstrate a prominent ductular reaction with associated neutrophilic inflammation. Imaging studies demonstrated segmental biliary strictures consistent with primary sclerosing cholangitis overlap. Same case as above.

primary sclerosing cholangitis. In particular, a subset of pediatric patients with autoimmune hepatitis has been shown to develop biliary strictures in long-term follow-up studies.[40–42] At initial presentation, these patients often lack a cholestatic chemistry profile, and the diagnosis is made based on subsequent elevations in alkaline phosphatase along with imaging studies. Given that a mild ductular reaction can be seen in autoimmune hepatitis, the diagnosis of autoimmune sclerosing cholangitis can be challenging in some cases. The presence of duct loss, ductular reaction out of proportion to the degree of hepatocyte injury, and cholate stasis are helpful findings to suggest a superimposed chronic obstructive biliary process and prompt imaging of the biliary tree. Similar to primary sclerosing cholangitis, the finding of "onion-skinning" fibrosis on a needle biopsy is rare.

Autoimmune hepatitis and indeterminate cholestatic syndrome

Some patients may have features of autoimmune hepatitis and a cholestatic phenotype that does not quite fit with either primary biliary cirrhosis or primary sclerosing cholangitis.[35,36] These patients have clinical, laboratory, and pathologic findings of autoimmune hepatitis in combination with bile duct injury/loss with concomitant elevations in alkaline phosphatase or γ-glutamyl transferase. By definition, they lack antimitochondrial antibodies and have normal imaging studies of the biliary tree. The cholestatic syndrome may represent antimitochondrial antibody-negative primary biliary cirrhosis, small duct primary sclerosing cholangitis, or some other undefined cholestatic syndrome (possibly drug/toxin induced).

12.8 AUTOIMMUNE HEPATITIS AND CHRONIC HEPATITIS C

Autoimmune disease and autoantibodies, often low titer, are quite common in chronic hepatitis C (20% to 40% of patients with hepatitis C have low-titer autoantibodies).[43] Patients with chronic hepatitis C with low-titer autoantibodies without pathologic or other clinical features of autoimmune hepatitis are not a distinct subgroup and behave similarly to hepatitis C patients without autoantibodies. However, a subset of hepatitis C patients have features concerning for true overlap with autoimmune hepatitis, including young age, female gender, high-titer autoantibodies, hypergammaglobulinemia, and a history of extrahepatic autoimmune disorders.[44,45] Hepatitis C with autoimmune features may also be more common in African Americans.[46] It is important to confirm hepatitis C infection with polymerase chain reaction-based studies because autoimmune hepatitis patients may have spurious elevations in antihepatitis C antibodies.

The degree of portal inflammation, plasma cells, interface activity, and lobular activity are increased in these patients compared to liver biopsies from patients with typical chronic hepatitis C. They often have advanced fibrosis at presentation.[46] Although immunosuppression has been used in some patients and results in decreased serum enzymes, patients can also be successfully treated with antiviral therapy.[45] It is likely that patients with chronic hepatitis C with autoimmune features represent a more aggressive variant of hepatitis C with autoimmune features that will resolve with antiviral therapy, rather than true overlap with autoimmune hepatitis.

12.9 AUTOIMMUNE HEPATITIS AND FATTY LIVER DISEASE

Autoantibodies are fairly common in fatty liver disease, occurring in ~20% to 30% of patients. For this reason, patients with risk factors for fatty liver disease and elevations in autoantibodies often undergo a liver biopsy to determine the etiology of the liver dysfunction. Often, the patient is found to have steatosis or steatohepatitis on liver biopsy rather than autoimmune hepatitis. The presence of autoantibodies does not affect the course of fatty liver disease. Concurrent autoimmune hepatitis and steatohepatitis is uncommon, occurring in <1% of patients with steatohepatitis.[47] Portal inflammation can be quite prominent in steatohepatitis, particularly at advanced stages of fibrosis, and does not usually indicate a concomitant chronic hepatitis such as autoimmune hepatitis.[48] Thus, a diagnosis of autoimmune hepatitis and steatohepatitis overlap syndrome should be made with caution.

12.10 TREATMENT AND PROGNOSIS

The American association of the study of Liver Diseases provides absolute, relative, and contraindications to therapy in patients with autoimmune hepatitis.[5] Of note, bridging or multiacinar necrosis on liver biopsy is an absolute indication for therapy, and the pathology report should mention these findings when present. Treatment of autoimmune hepatitis consists predominantly of immunosuppression and has changed very little over the past decades. Immune suppression with corticosteroids is used to induce remission in autoimmune hepatitis patients, followed by maintenance therapy. In some cases, steroids plus azathioprine is used to induce remission, depending on other clinical features. More recently, budesonide, which is a GI-specific steroid, has been shown to be effective in inducing remission with fewer side effects.[49] This is likely due to the high absorption of budesonide by the gut and metabolism in the liver. If remission is not achieved using standard therapy, other immunosuppressive agents can be added, such as mycophenolate mofetil, tacrolimus, and cyclosporin A.

The goal of therapy is to induce complete remission, which is defined by the disappearance of symptoms, normal serum transaminases, bilirubin, γ globulin levels, and no portal or lobular inflammation on liver biopsy.[5] Complete normalization of serum transaminases and liver histology usually requires >12 months of therapy. For those patients with normalization of serum transaminases for at least 2 years, a liver biopsy should be performed before discontinuation of therapy. As mentioned, histologic complete remission is the best predictor of long-term outcomes in autoimmune hepatitis.

Protracted therapy that induces improved clinical, laboratory, and histologic findings, but has not induced remission, is classified as an incomplete response. This occurs in ~10% to 15% of patients who are treated for at least 3 years. Continued prednisone in addition to long-term azathioprine is used to stabilize serum transaminases in these patients.

A small but significant subset of patients fail treatment and experience worsening of clinical, laboratory, and histologic findings. Treatment failure can usually be determined within 3 to 6 weeks of initial immunosuppressive therapy. Institution of high-dose prednisone can be used to rescue these patients; however, even with aggressive therapy, only 20% will achieve histologic remission. Liver transplantation may be considered in these patients if there is development of hepatic decompensation or variceal bleeding.

REFERENCES

1. Wang Q, Yang F, Miao Q, et al. The clinical phenotypes of autoimmune hepatitis: a comprehensive review. *J Autoimmun*. 2016;66:98–107.
2. Hurlburt KJ, McMahon BJ, Deubner H, et al. Prevalence of autoimmune liver disease in Alaska Natives. *Am J Gastroenterol*. 2002;97(9):2402–2407.
3. Liberal R, Vergani D, Mieli-Vergani G. Update on autoimmune hepatitis. *J Clin Transl Hepatol*. 2015;3(1):42–52.
4. Manns MP, Czaja AJ, Gorham JD, et al. Diagnosis and management of autoimmune hepatitis. *Hepatology*. 2010;51(6):2193–2213.
5. Frenzel C, Herkel J, Lüth S, et al. Evaluation of F-actin ELISA for the diagnosis of autoimmune hepatitis. *Am J Gastroenterol*. 2006;101(12):2731–2736.
6. Czaja AJ, Manns MP. The validity and importance of subtypes in autoimmune hepatitis: a point of view. *Am J Gastroenterol*. 1995;90(8):1206–1211.
7. Kanzler S, Weidemann C, Gerken G, et al. Clinical significance of autoantibodies to soluble liver antigen in autoimmune hepatitis. *J Hepatol*. 1999;31(4):635–640.
8. Czaja AJ. Autoantibodies in autoimmune liver disease. *Adv Clin Chem*. 2005;40:127–164.
9. Gassert DJ, Garcia H, Tanaka K, et al. Corticosteroid-responsive cryptogenic chronic hepatitis: evidence for seronegative autoimmune hepatitis. *Dig Dis Sci*. 2007;52(9):2433–2437.
10. Krawitt EL. Autoimmune hepatitis. *N Engl J Med*. 2006;354(1):54–66.
11. Czaja AJ. Autoantibody-negative autoimmune hepatitis. *Dig Dis Sci*. 2012;57(3):610–624.
12. Alvarez F, Berg PA, Bianchi FB, et al. International Autoimmune Hepatitis Group Report: review of criteria for diagnosis of autoimmune hepatitis. *J Hepatol*. 1999;31(5):929–938.
13. Hennes EM, Zeniya M, Czaja AJ, et al. Simplified criteria for the diagnosis of autoimmune hepatitis. *Hepatology*. 2008;48(1):169–176.
14. Czaja AJ. Performance parameters of the diagnostic scoring systems for autoimmune hepatitis. *Hepatology*. 2008;48(5):1540–1548.
15. Czaja AJ. Behavior and significance of autoantibodies in type 1 autoimmune hepatitis. *J Hepatol*. 1999;30(3):394–401.

16. Czaja AJ, Carpenter HA. Sensitivity, specificity, and predictability of biopsy interpretations in chronic hepatitis. *Gastroenterology*. 1993;105(6):1824–1832.
17. Tiniakos DG, Brain JG, Bury YA. Role of histopathology in autoimmune hepatitis. *Dig Dis*. 2015;33(suppl 2):53–64.
18. de Boer YS, van Nieuwkerk CMJ, Witte BI, et al. Assessment of the histopathological key features in autoimmune hepatitis. *Histopathology*. 2015;66(3):351–362.
19. Suzuki A, Brunt EM, Kleiner DE, et al. The use of liver biopsy evaluation in discrimination of idiopathic autoimmune hepatitis versus drug-induced liver injury. *Hepatology*. 2011;54(3):931–939.
20. Miao Q, Bian Z, Tang R, et al. Emperipolesis mediated by CD8 T cells is a characteristic histopathologic feature of autoimmune hepatitis. *Clin Rev Allergy Immunol*. 2015;48(2–3):226–235.
21. Tucker SM, Jonas MM, Perez-Atayde AR. Hyaline droplets in Kupffer cells: a novel diagnostic clue for autoimmune hepatitis. *Am J Surg Pathol*. 2015;39(6):772–778.
22. Moreira RK, Revetta F, Koehler E, et al. Diagnostic utility of IgG and IgM immunohistochemistry in autoimmune liver disease. *World J Gastroenterol*. 2010;16(4):453–457.
23. Zen Y, Nakanuma Y, Portmann B. Immunoglobulin G4-related sclerosing cholangitis: pathologic features and histologic mimics. *Semin Diagn Pathol*. 2012;29(4):205–211.
24. Burgart LJ, Batts KP, Ludwig J, et al. Recent-onset autoimmune hepatitis. Biopsy findings and clinical correlations. *Am J Surg Pathol*. 1995;19(6):699–708.
25. Nikias GA, Batts KP, Czaja AJ. The nature and prognostic implications of autoimmune hepatitis with an acute presentation. *J Hepatol*. 1994;21(5):866–871.
26. Batts KP, Ludwig J. Chronic hepatitis. An update on terminology and reporting. *Am J Surg Pathol*. 1995;19(12):1409–1417.
27. Misdraji J, Thiim M, Graeme-Cook FM. Autoimmune hepatitis with centrilobular necrosis. *Am J Surg Pathol*. 2004;28(4):471–478.
28. Te HS, Koukoulis G, Ganger DR. Autoimmune hepatitis: a histological variant associated with prominent centrilobular necrosis. *Gut*. 1997;41(2):269–271.
29. Yeong TT, Lim KHJ, Goubet S, et al. Natural history and outcomes in drug-induced autoimmune hepatitis. *Hepatol Res*. 2016;46(3):E79–88.
30. Czaja AJ. Drug-induced autoimmune-like hepatitis. *Dig Dis Sci*. 2011;56(4):958–976.
31. de Boer YS, Kosinski AS, Urban TJ, et al. Features of autoimmune hepatitis in patients with drug-induced liver injury. *Clin Gastroenterol Hepatol*. 2017;15(1):103–112.e2.
32. Czaja AJ, Wolf AM, Baggenstoss AH. Laboratory assessment of severe chronic active liver disease during and after corticosteroid therapy: correlation of serum transaminase and gamma globulin levels with histologic features. *Gastroenterology*. 1981;80(4):687–692.
33. Dhaliwal HK, Hoeroldt BS, Dube AK, et al. Long-term prognostic significance of persisting histological activity despite biochemical remission in autoimmune hepatitis. *Am J Gastroenterol*. 2015;110(7):993–999.
34. Verma S, Gunuwan B, Mendler M, et al. Factors predicting relapse and poor outcome in type I autoimmune hepatitis: role of cirrhosis development, patterns of transaminases during remission and plasma cell activity in the liver biopsy. *Am J Gastroenterol*. 2004;99(8):1510–1516.
35. Vierling JM. Autoimmune hepatitis and overlap syndromes: diagnosis and management. *Clin Gastroenterol Hepatol*. 2015;13(12):2088–2108.
36. Czaja AJ. Cholestatic phenotypes of autoimmune hepatitis. *Clin Gastroenterol Hepatol*. 2014;12(9):1430–1438.
37. Chazouillères O, Wendum D, Serfaty L, et al. Primary biliary cirrhosis-autoimmune hepatitis overlap syndrome: clinical features and response to therapy. *Hepatology*. 1998;28(2):296–301.
38. Boberg KM, Chapman RW, Hirschfield GM, et al. Overlap syndromes: the International Autoimmune Hepatitis Group (IAIHG) position statement on a controversial issue. *J Hepatol*. 2011;54(2):374–385.
39. O'Brien C, Joshi S, Feld JJ, et al. Long-term follow-up of antimitochondrial antibody-positive autoimmune hepatitis. *Hepatology*. 2008;48(2):550–556.
40. Rodrigues AT, Liu PMF, Fagundes EDT, et al. Clinical characteristics and prognosis in children and adolescents with autoimmune hepatitis and overlap syndrome. *J Pediatr Gastroenterol Nutr*. 2016;63(1):76–81.
41. Abdo AA, Bain VG, Kichian K, et al. Evolution of autoimmune hepatitis to primary sclerosing cholangitis: a sequential syndrome. *Hepatology*. 2002;36(6):1393–1399.
42. Gregorio GV, Portmann B, Karani J, et al. Autoimmune hepatitis/sclerosing cholangitis overlap syndrome in childhood: a 16-year prospective study. *Hepatology*. 2001;33(3):544–553.
43. Bortolotti F, Vajro P, Balli F, et al. Non-organ specific autoantibodies in children with chronic hepatitis C. *J Hepatol*. 1996;25(5):614–620.
44. Czaja AJ, Carpenter HA. Histological findings in chronic hepatitis C with autoimmune features. *Hepatology*. 1997;26(2):459–466.
45. Cassani F, Cataleta M, Valentini P, et al. Serum autoantibodies in chronic hepatitis C: comparison

with autoimmune hepatitis and impact on the disease profile. *Hepatology*. 1997;26(3):561–566.

46. Jenkins E, Tai R, Hart J, et al. Autoimmune hepatitis (AIH) features in patients with chronic hepatitis C (CHC) is associated with more advanced fibrosis. *Hepatology*. 2009;50(S4):1054A.

47. Yatsuji S, Hashimoto E, Kaneda H, et al. Diagnosing autoimmune hepatitis in nonalcoholic fatty liver disease: is the International Autoimmune Hepatitis Group scoring system useful? *J Gastroenterol*. 2005;40(12):1130–1138.

48. Brunt EM, Kleiner DE, Wilson LA, et al. Portal chronic inflammation in nonalcoholic fatty liver disease (NAFLD): a histologic marker of advanced NAFLD-Clinicopathologic correlations from the nonalcoholic steatohepatitis clinical research network. *Hepatology*. 2009;49(3):809–820.

49. Manns MP, Woynarowski M, Kreisel W, et al. Budesonide induces remission more effectively than prednisone in a controlled trial of patients with autoimmune hepatitis. *Gastroenterology*. 2010;139(4):1198–1206.

13 Cholestatic liver disease and biliary tract disease

Jason Lewis, MD

13.1 INTRODUCTION

Cholestasis is defined as impaired bile flow. It may be secondary to either hepatocyte abnormalities or compromise of the biliary tree.[1] From an etiologic perspective, compromise of the biliary tree can be primary or secondary, and from an anatomic standpoint either intra- and/or extrahepatic. Biliary tract compromise typically leads to a characteristic constellation of portal-based changes (see below).[1]

Clinically, cholestasis is characterized by hyperbilirubinemia and an elevated alkaline phosphatase and γ-glutamyltransferase (GGT). Because GGT can be elevated in other conditions, alkaline phosphatase is the more specific indicator. Importantly, clinical and histologic cholestasis may not occur simultaneously. It is not uncommon for there to be an elevated alkaline phosphatase with no histologic features of cholestasis.

There are five elements to assess when considering a diagnosis of cholestatic or chronic biliary disease. The combination of these features will vary with the type and stage of disease.

1. **Cholestasis:** Bile can be identified in hepatocytes, Kupffer cells, canaliculi, proliferative bile ductules, or bile ducts (Fig. 13.1). *Cholate stasis* is the term given to the cytologic changes which occur in

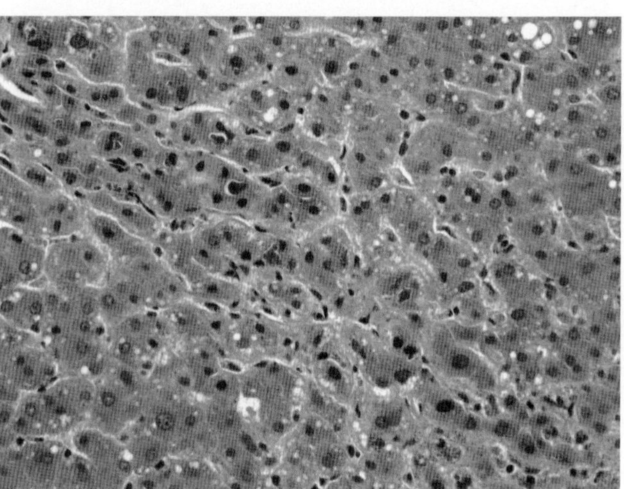

Figure 13.1 Cholestasis. Canaliculi are not visible under normal circumstances but can be seen in cholestasis when they become dilated with inspissated bile plugs.

hepatocytes secondary to the toxic effects of retained bile: cytoplasmic swelling with protein condensation (feathery degeneration) and Mallory–Denk bodies (Figs. 13.2 and 13.3).[1] In severe cases, foci of hepatocyte necrosis with extravasated bile can be seen, which is referred as bile infarcts. In chronic biliary disease, cholestasis is typically not seen until late in the course of the disease.

2. **Ductular reaction:** A reactive process that consists of a mixture of ductular proliferation, inflammation, and stromal cells along the limiting plate.[2] Ductular reactions can occur in many types of disease, and the morphology does not always indicate the precise cause.[2] It may be seen as a secondary pattern in cases of fulminant necrosis or chronic hepatitis in which it is accompanied by other significant portal and lobular changes.[2] Conversely, a primary injury pattern of ductular reaction is one of the earliest and most sensitive indicators of bile flow impairment. With obstruction,

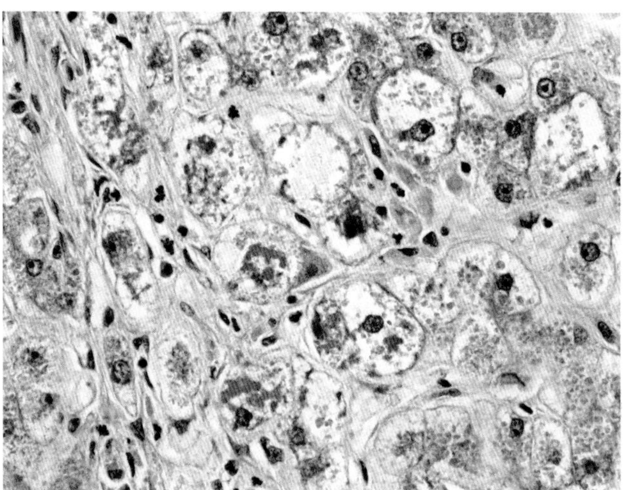

Figure 13.2 Cholestasis. Bile pigment can be identified as golden granular material within hepatocytes or as phagocytosed debris within Kupffer cells. Cholate stasis is characterized by feathery degeneration (cytoplasmic swelling with protein condensation) of hepatocytes. Mallory–Denk bodies are often present.

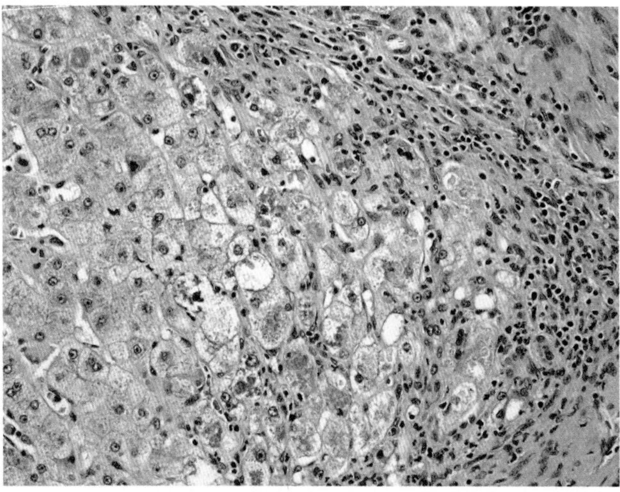

Figure 13.3 Cholestasis. Cholate stasis preferentially affects periportal and periseptal hepatocytes.

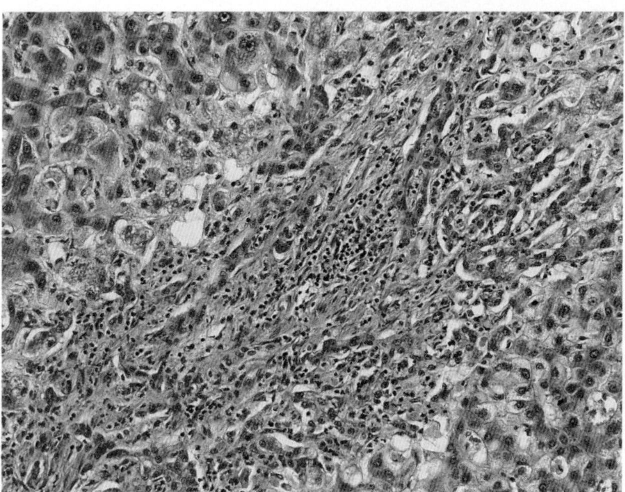

Figure 13.4 Ductular reaction. Marked ductular reaction characterized by an irregular mass of ductules along the limiting plate and focally extending into the periportal lobule. No well-formed lumina are seen in this field. Neutrophilic pericholangitis is present. Note the cholate stasis within the periportal hepatocytes to the left.

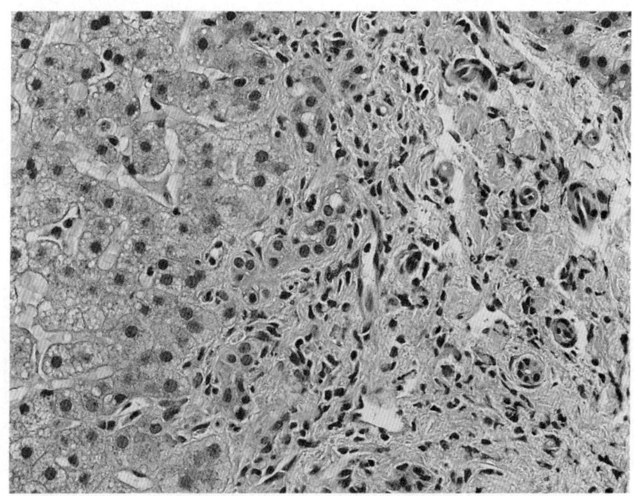

Figure 13.5 Ductular reaction. Ductular reaction is not always pronounced. In the center of the field, there is a subtle ductular reaction extending vertically along the interface of the lobule and the portal tract. There is a poorly formed lumen present within one of the ductule profiles.

there is a visible proliferation of ductules along the perimeter of the portal tracts (Figs. 13.4 and 13.5). The lumina of the ductules are typically not visualized unless they are expanded by bile plugs. Bile plugs within ductules (ductular or cholangiolar cholestasis) is termed *cholangitis lenta*. Although this pattern may be seen in late stage chronic biliary disease, it is also present in other conditions such as sepsis, shock, or uremia (Figs. 13.6 and 13.7).[2] When the obstruction is acute onset and involves a large duct, ductular reaction is typically accompanied by portal edema. With chronicity, the edema subsides and is replaced by fibrosis.[2] Inflammatory cells,

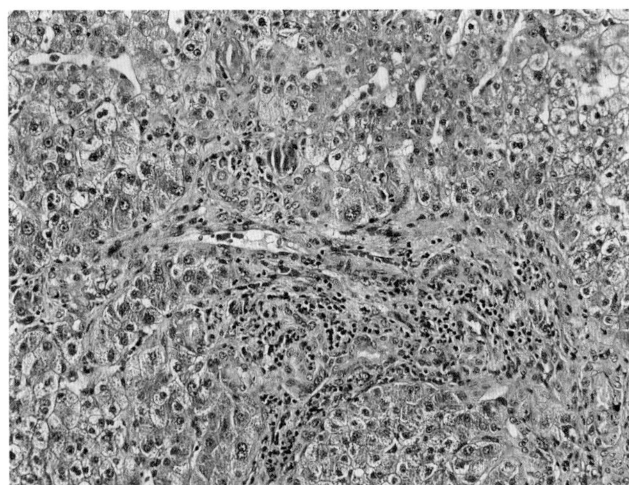

Figure 13.6 Cholangitis lenta. Cholangitis lenta in a case of sepsis. Proliferating ductules along the perimeter of the portal tract are dilated and contain inspissated bile plugs (ductular or cholangiolar cholestasis). There is no significant fibrosis. This finding is often idiopathic but can also be seen in shock, uremia, or any debilitating illness.

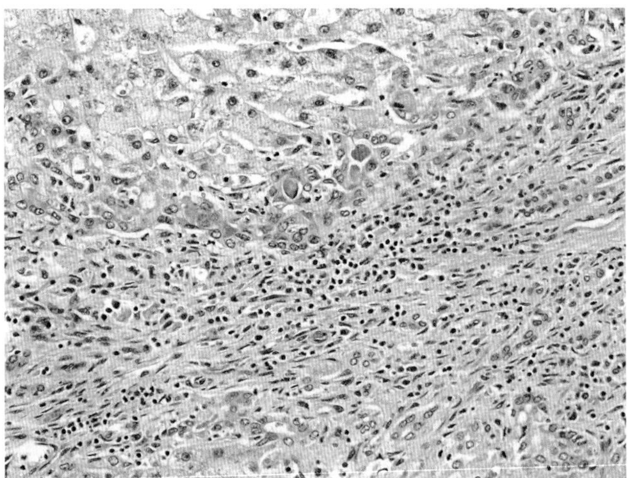

Figure 13.7 Ductular cholestasis. Ductular cholestasis is seen in this case of primary biliary cirrhosis. With prolonged cholestasis of any etiology, bile plugs can be seen within the proliferating ductules. This finding is most commonly seen in the setting of end-stage disease and clinical decompensation.

including lymphocytes, plasma cells, and neutrophils, are an integral component of ductular reaction. The presence of neutrophils along the limiting plate can serve as a valuable clue to the presence of ductular reaction.

3. **Ductopenia:** *Ductopenia* is defined as the absence of a bile duct branch in at least 50% of portal tracts.[3] The number of portal tracts needed for an adequate specimen varies by institution. From a practical standpoint, 8 to 10 portal tracts are usually sufficient to determine if there is significant ductopenia. Because the bile duct branch travels with the hepatic artery, the presence of an artery without a bile duct is a helpful indicator of bile duct loss within that portal tract[3] (Fig. 13.8). Normally, 70% to 80% of arteries have an associated bile duct.[3] At times, portal inflammation may be so dense that it is difficult to identify normal structures. Cytokeratin 7 (CK7) immunostains can aid by highlighting ducts in this situation. Though not typically utilized for this purpose, periodic acid–Schiff diastase (PASD) highlights the basement membranes of bile ducts and can be used to assess for ductopenia. Table 13.1 contains a list of disease processes which can result in ductopenia.

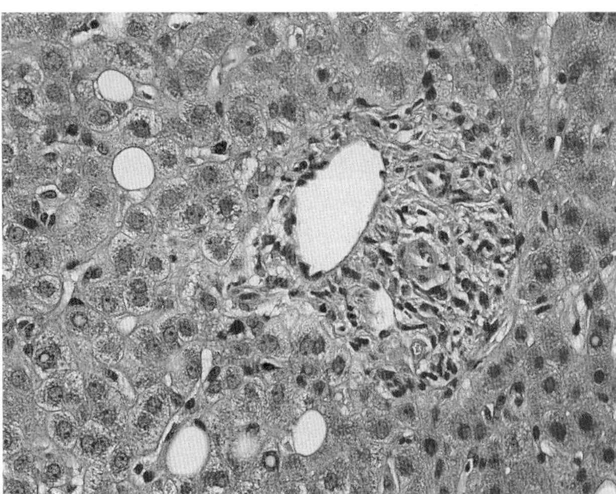

Figure 13.8 Ductopenia. The portal tract contains a portal vein and hepatic artery branch but no bile duct.

4. **Copper accumulation:** In early stage disease, the presence of periportal copper is highly suggestive of a chronic biliary disease. Though rare in chronic hepatitis and steatohepatitis, copper accumulation can be found in a small percent of these cases when there is advanced fibrosis (<10%).[4] In chronic biliary disease, the amount of copper increases with the stage of the disease, such that the absence of copper in the cirrhotic liver is unusual for chronic biliary disease (Figs. 13.9 and 13.10).[4] At Mayo Clinic, rhodanine stain is performed on 10-um thick sections. The orcein stain for copper-associated protein is another commonly utilized stain at other medical centers.
5. **Fibrosis:** Chronic biliary disease has a characteristic pattern of scarring, termed *jigsaw puzzle-like*, in which there is an irregular shape to the cirrhotic nodules (Fig. 13.11). In addition, fibrosis is often unevenly distributed within the liver in early stage disease. When present, fibrosis of any degree

Table 13.1 Common causes of ductopenia in adults
Primary biliary cirrhosis
Primary sclerosing cholangitis
Secondary sclerosing cholangitis
Toxin/drug injury
Sarcoidosis
Graft versus host disease
Liver allograft rejection
Idiopathic adulthood ductopenia

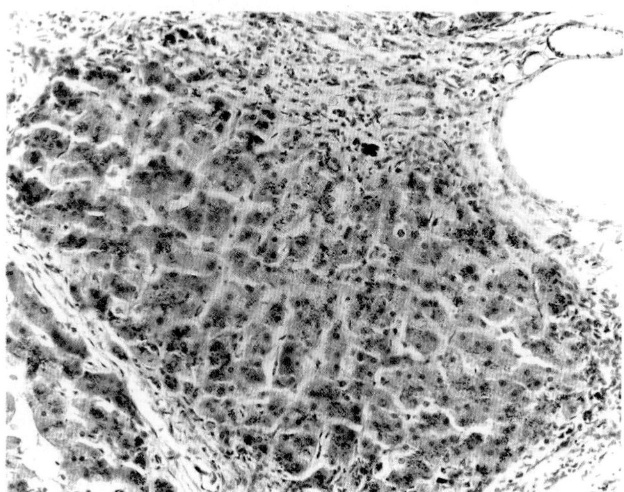

Figure 13.9 Rhodanine stain. In this case of primary biliary cirrhosis, the copper appears as rust-colored granules within hepatocytes. The amount of copper generally increases with the stage of disease and the severity of cholestasis.

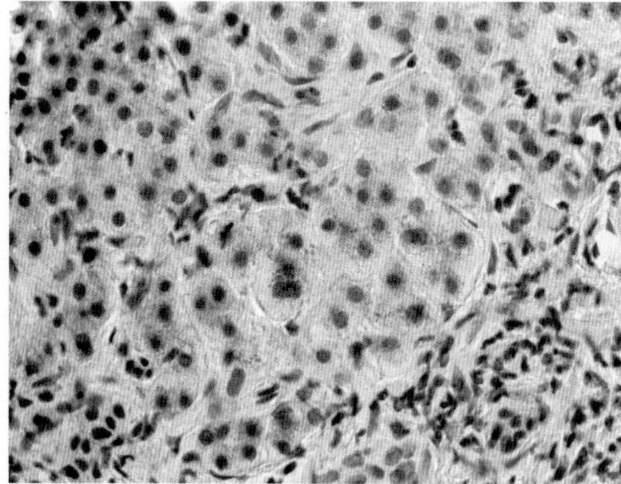

Figure 13.10 Rhodanine stain. In early cholestatic liver disease, copper deposits can be very focal, identified in only rare periportal hepatocytes, requiring careful high-power examination.

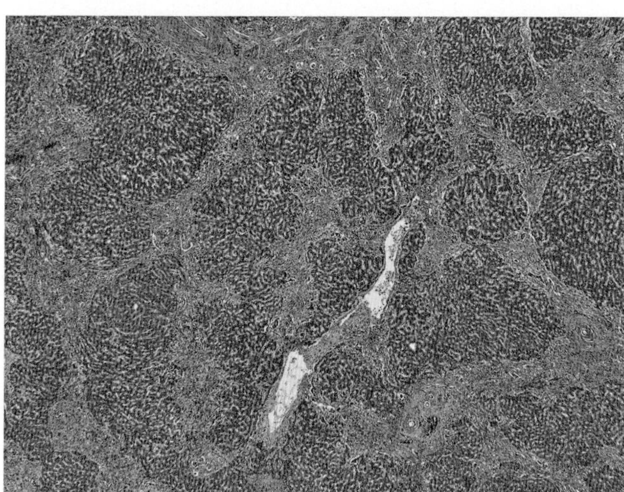

Figure 13.11 Biliary pattern of cirrhosis. In this case of end-stage primary sclerosing cholangitis, there is an irregular pattern of scarring such that the lobular parenchyma appears to fit together like pieces of a puzzle, hence the term *jigsaw puzzle-like*. This pattern is not universally present, and some cases may demonstrate more classic regenerative nodules.

indicates a chronic disorder and argues against an acute process, such as a cholestatic drug reaction or acute large duct obstruction.

Older scoring systems for chronic biliary disease did not give a separate grade and stage for the disease. Instead, inflammation and fibrosis were combined into an overall staging system. For example, the one used historically at the Mayo Clinic was created by Ludwig et al.[5]:

Stage 1: Portal stage—all disease activity is confined to the portal tract; limiting plate intact.

Stage 2: Periportal stage—limiting plate disrupted by lymphocytic interface activity and/or ductular reaction; portal tracts have irregular shape.

Stage 3: Septal stage—fibrous septa (portal–portal bridging fibrosis).

Stage 4: Cirrhotic stage—fibrous septa and parenchymal distortion.

These staging systems are not widely used anymore, but can be encountered in older pathology reports on prior specimens. Currently, at the Mayo Clinic and at most medical centers, fibrosis in biliary tract disease is staged using a standard system such as the Batts–Ludwig, Ishak, or Metavir.

The majority of this chapter will focus on the three main causes of primary chronic biliary tract disease: primary biliary cirrhosis, primary sclerosing cholangitis, and Immunoglobulin G4 (IgG4)–related disease (Table 13.2), followed by brief discussions of secondary causes.

Table 13.2 Clinicopathologic features of the three major autoimmune cholangiopathies

	Primary Biliary Cirrhosis	Primary Sclerosing Cholangitis	IgG4-related Sclerosing Cholangitis
Gender	Females (90%)	Males (70%)	Males (85%)
Peak incidence (age)	50	40	>60
Key diagnostic test	AMA	Cholangiogram	Histology
Serology	AMA	None	Serum IgG4
Hallmark histology	Florid duct lesion	Large duct obstructive disease; fibro-obliterative duct lesions (not always present)	Dense lymphoplasmacytic infiltrate, storiform fibrosis, obliterative phlebitis, increased IgG4+ plasma cell//hpf
Variant(s)	AMA (–) PBC-AIH overlap	Small duct PSC-AIH overlap	None
Associated Condition(s)	Sjogren syndrome, scleroderma, hemolytic anemia, celiac disease, and hypothyroidism	Inflammatory bowel disease	Autoimmune pancreatitis Dacryoadenitis Sialadenitis Retroperitoneal fibrosis
Cancer risk	Hepatocellular carcinoma	Cholangiocarcinoma Colorectal carcinoma Gallbladder carcinoma	Unclear
Therapy	UDCA	Transplantation	Prednisone Rituximab

13.2 PRIMARY BILIARY CIRRHOSIS

Definition

Primary biliary cirrhosis is an autoimmune disease targeting the small, intrahepatic bile ducts.

Clinical features

Primary biliary cirrhosis preferentially affects middle age women (90% of patients are female; median age at diagnosis 50 years).[6–9] It is not diagnosed in children.[10] More than half of patients are asymptomatic at the time of diagnosis and are identified on screening or workup of other conditions.[7,11,12] When present, fatigue and pruritus are the most common symptoms.[7] Fatigue can occur in up to 78% of patients, and pruritus in 20% to 70%, over the course of the disease.[7] It is often associated with other autoimmune conditions, including Sjogren syndrome, scleroderma, celiac disease, and hypothyroidism.[7]

Primary biliary cirrhosis should be ruled out in any patient with a chronic, unexplained elevation in alkaline phosphatase, particularly in middle-age women. Diagnostic criteria include two of the following three findings: (1) chronic elevation of alkaline phosphatase; (2) positive antimitochondrial antibody (AMA); and (3) characteristic histologic features.[13] A liver biopsy is not required in the majority of cases. It is typically performed to diagnose AMA-negative primary biliary cirrhosis (see below), rule out an overlap syndrome or superimposed process, and for staging purposes.

Laboratory findings

Primary biliary cirrhosis is characterized biochemically by elevated alkaline phosphatase levels. Mild elevations in alanine aminotransferase (ALT) and aspartate aminotransferase (AST) are also usually present, but the alkaline phosphatase levels are disproportionately elevated.[13] The AMA is the serologic hallmark of primary biliary cirrhosis, present in 90% to 95% of patients and in less than 1% of the general population.[7,13] AMA may be identified years before the disease manifests clinically.[7] The M2 subtype is the most sensitive and specific.[14] At Mayo Clinic, an enzyme immunoassay is used to detect AMA-M2 autoantibodies. Roughly half of patients will be antinuclear antibody (ANA) and antismooth muscle antibody (ASMA) positive.[7,15]

Imaging

Imaging studies are used to exclude obstructive processes within the biliary tree.

Gross findings

Liver explants show end-stage cirrhosis with a biliary pattern. The liver can be enlarged or mildly atrophic and shows a dark green color because of cholestasis. The cirrhosis usually shows a mixed micro and macronodular pattern.

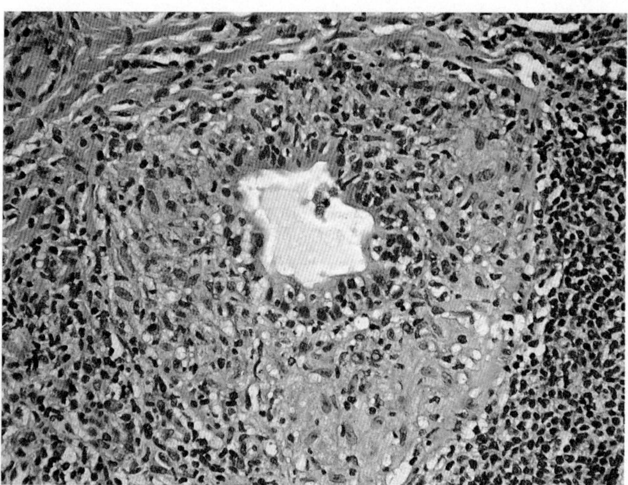

Figure 13.12 Primary biliary cirrhosis. The bile duct in the center of the field is encircled by granulomatous inflammation. A relatively dense aggregate of lymphocytes is visible along the right edge. Note how lymphocytes invade through the basement membrane and infiltrate into the bile duct epithelium (lymphocytic cholangitis). The lymphocytes are surrounded by a clear halo and are more hyperchromatic than the biliary nuclei. There is cytoplasmic swelling of some epithelial cells indicative of injury.

Microscopic findings

General features

In 1965, the term *chronic nonsuppurative destructive cholangitis* was suggested as an alternative to primary biliary cirrhosis because it "accurately describes the basic lesion and has the further merit of avoiding the term cirrhosis."[16,17] Two years later this "basic lesion" was termed the *florid duct lesion,* which is the histologic hallmark of primary biliary cirrhosis.[17] For unknown reasons, the inflammatory injury preferentially affects intrahepatic bile ducts measuring less than 80 to 100 microns in diameter.[16 22]

The florid duct lesion is the histologic manifestation of inflammatory duct destruction (Figs. 13.12, 13.13, and 13.14). It is defined by the presence of both granulomatous inflammation and bile duct damage.[14,16,17,23–25] The inflammatory component comprises lymphocytes, plasma cells, and histiocytes. Lymphocytes may be quite dense, forming aggregates around the bile ducts.[16,17,23] They characteristically infiltrate into the biliary epithelium (lymphocytic cholangitis). The granulomatous component is directed toward the bile duct or is in close proximity, not merely present in the portal tract. It may be well-formed or consist of loose aggregates of macrophages.[16,23,25,26] Bile duct damage manifests as cytologic injury to the biliary epithelial cells and/or disruption of the bile duct basement membrane.[11,16,23,25]

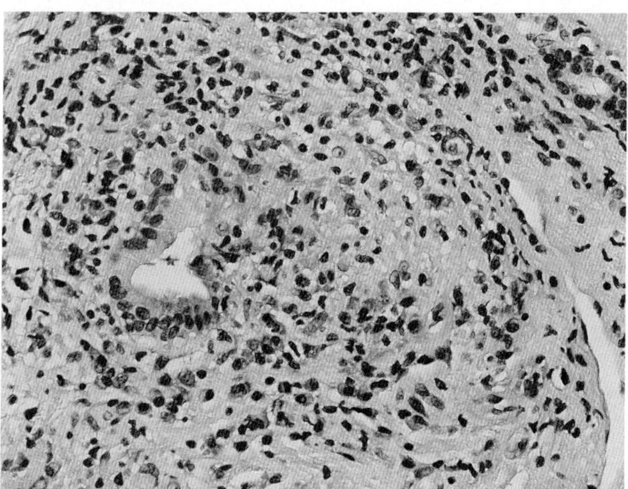

Figure 13.13 Primary biliary cirrhosis. An example of primary biliary cirrhosis in which the granulomatous inflammation is poorly-formed. Lymphocytic cholangitis with destruction of the duct is well-developed. There is rupture of the basement membrane and the biliary nuclei have a disorganized, jumbled appearance along with mild pleomorphism.

Needle biopsy findings

Florid duct lesions are patchy in the liver parenchyma and may not be sampled in needle biopsies. In addition, they decrease in frequency with progression of disease.[5,18] For example, Ludwig et al. identified florid duct lesions in 38% to 45% of early stage (1 or 2) biopsies but only 15% to 19% of late stage (3 or 4) biopsies.[5]

In the appropriate clinical setting (positive AMA and elevated alkaline phosphatase), the presence of patchy, portal-based lymphoplasmacytic inflammation is sufficient to render the diagnosis of "consistent" or

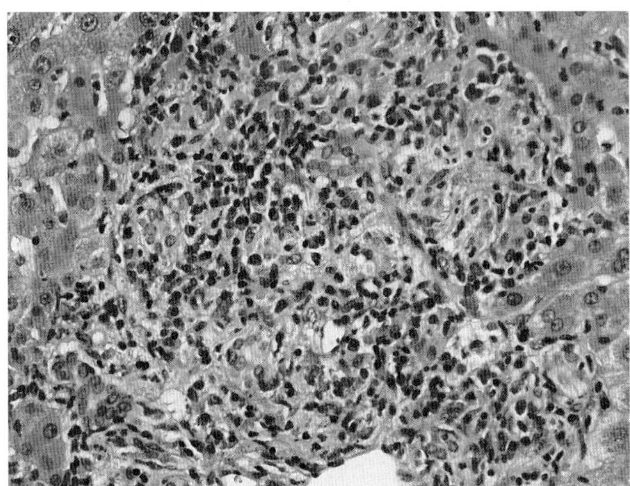

Figure 13.14 Primary biliary cirrhosis. Plasma cells can be conspicuous. This finding does not necessitate a diagnosis of primary biliary cirrhosis–autoimmune hepatitis overlap.

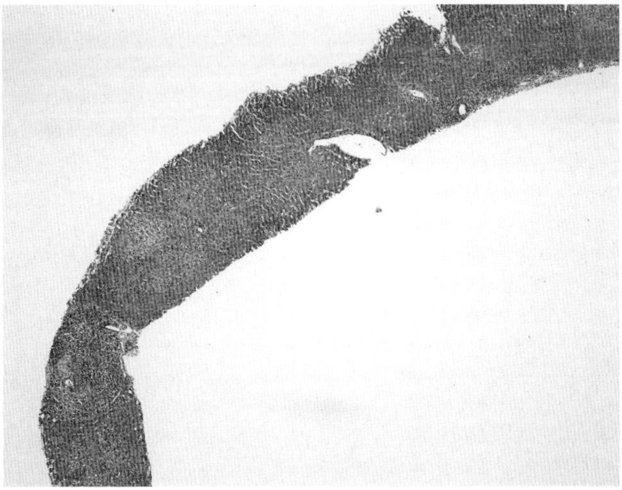

Figure 13.15 Primary biliary cirrhosis. Low-power example of stage 1 primary biliary cirrhosis. Note how there is a dense, portal-based lymphoid aggregate visible at scanning magnification. Even at this power, the process appears confined to the portal tract and the lobule appears quiescent.

"compatible with" the clinical diagnosis of primary biliary cirrhosis, after drug effect has been excluded. After making a diagnosis of primary biliary cirrhosis, attention should next be focused on excluding other disease processes (e.g., steatohepatitis) and accurate staging.

Pertinent findings by disease stage

While disease stages do not correlate exactly with fibrosis stages, they nicely organize the various findings in primary biliary cirrhosis and can be useful for illustrating disease progression

Stage 1: Nascent primary biliary cirrhosis is portal-based, and this can be appreciated at low-power scanning magnification in which a subset of portal tracts contain dense, lymphocytic infiltrates with occasional plasma cells and lymphoid aggregates (Fig. 13.15). Granulomatous cholangitis (florid duct lesion) is common but may be focal, with some normal-appearing portal tracts and some demonstrating only lymphocytic cholangitis. Ductopenia is not seen in this stage. Cholestasis is absent. Lobular inflammation is usually absent or mild, but small granulomas may occasionally be present. A fraction of cases may show focal periportal copper.

Stage 2: Portal tracts show a ductular reaction, often with interface activity (Fig. 13.16). Florid duct lesions may be identified. Some portal tracts may lack intact bile ducts. Cholestasis is rarely seen. Periportal copper accumulation is present in the majority of cases and is moderate in a small percent.

Stage 3: Trichrome stain shows portal–portal bridging fibrosis. Inflammation diminishes and florid duct lesions are less common. Ductular reactions persist and hepatocanalicular cholestasis increases. Ductopenia may be present. There is moderate copper accumulation in the majority of cases.

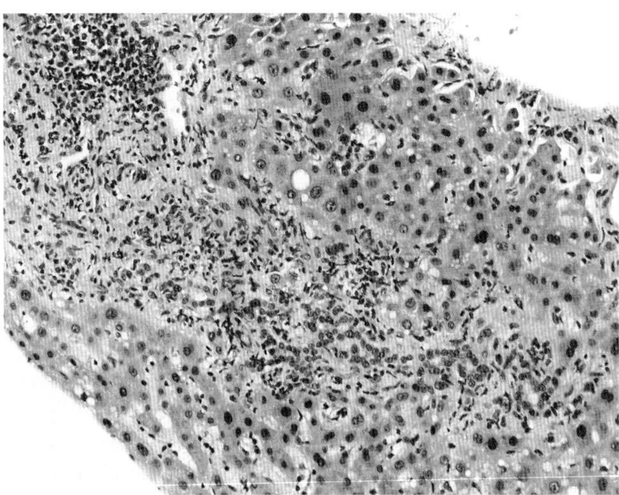

Figure 13.16 Primary biliary cirrhosis. In stage 2 primary biliary cirrhosis, there is eventually disruption of the limiting plate by ductular reaction. Some degree of inflammation may be present, including rare apoptotic hepatocytes.

Stage 4: The Trichrome stain shows a biliary type of cirrhosis. Ductular reactions may be prominent and there can be marked cholestasis and cholate stasis within periportal hepatocytes (Fig. 13.17). Ductopenia is well-developed and copper deposition is present in essentially all cases, being extensive in approximately half.

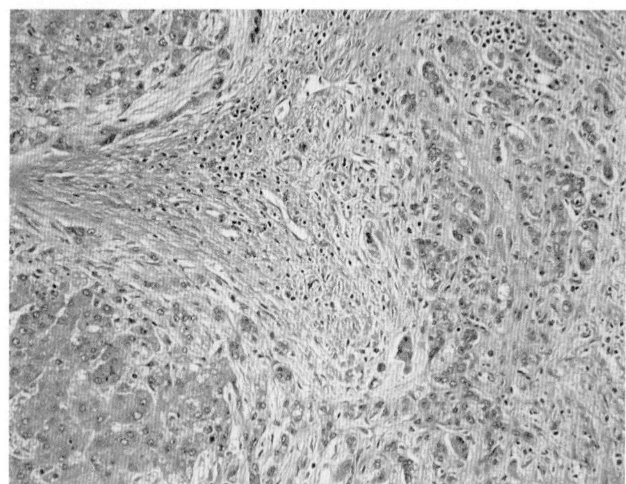

Figure 13.17 Primary biliary cirrhosis. End-stage primary biliary cirrhosis is characterized by exuberant ductular reaction and hepatocanalicular cholestasis. However, the findings are not specific at this stage. There is abundant bile pigment within hepatocytes and Kupffer cells.

Primary biliary cirrhosis variants

AMA-Negative primary biliary cirrhosis

About 5% to 10% of patients will have typical clinical and pathologic features of primary biliary cirrhosis, except for a negative AMA.[13] These individuals are more likely to have positive ANA/ASMA and lower immunoglobulin M (IgM) levels than AMA-positive patients.[13] The natural history of their disease and response to ursodeoxycholic acid (UDCA) are similar to AMA-positive patients.[13,27–29]

Given the absence of AMA, a liver biopsy is required for the diagnosis.[13] Histologic findings, including florid duct lesions and periportal copper accumulation, are similar to AMA-positive cases.[28] Granulomatous cholangitis provides the strongest histologic corroboration of primary biliary cirrhosis.[13]

Primary biliary cirrhosis–autoimmune hepatitis overlap

Rendering the diagnosis of primary biliary cirrhosis–autoimmune hepatitis overlap is challenging because of the variability in diagnostic criteria and the clinical, biochemical, and histologic overlap.[10,13] In one practical approach that combines laboratory and histologic findings, overlap is suggested if 2 of the following 3 features are identified in a patient with primary biliary cirrhosis: (1), ALT > 5 times upper limit of normal; (2), immunoglobulin G (IgG) > 2 times upper limit of normal and/or a positive ASMA; and (3), moderate or severe interface activity.[13,30] This approach is most commonly used by clinicians. An overlap syndrome can be suggested by pathology findings when there is more lobular hepatitis than is typically seen in primary biliary cirrhosis, in particular at the moderate or marked levels. Primary biliary cirrhosis and autoimmune hepatitis can be diagnosed concurrently or sequentially.[10,30,31] Because of the lack of uniform diagnostic criteria, the prevalence of overlap varies by study, ranging from 1% to 9%.[10,30]

It has been this author's anecdotal experience that the typical scenario is one in which a patient has a known history of primary biliary cirrhosis (+AMA) and is then found to have prominent elevations in transaminase levels. Because >30% of primary biliary cirrhosis patients may have a positive ANA, this test is not discriminatory.[7,10] Therefore, a biopsy is undertaken to determine if any histologic features of autoimmune hepatitis are present: specifically to determine the severity of interface and lobular necroinflammatory activities.

As noted above, plasma cells are present in typical cases of primary biliary cirrhosis and are not, in and of themselves, sufficient to suggest an overlap syndrome. Considering that interface activity is also commonly seen in primary biliary cirrhosis, it becomes clear that it would be extremely difficult to diagnose a superimposed minimally or mildly active autoimmune hepatitis (grade 1 or grade 2). For cases of primary biliary cirrhosis that have morphologic features suggestive of, but not diagnostic for, autoimmune hepatitis, the pathology reports can mention that the possibility of an overlap syndrome cannot be ruled out but it is not the predominant component of the liver disease. The clinicians will decide to start corticosteroid therapy or not based on the overall clinical findings.

In typical cases of overlap syndrome, the ALT levels are moderately to severely elevated.[13] Correspondingly, the biopsy shows moderate to severe levels of interface and lobular necroinflammatory activity (grades 3 or 4) or confluent lobular necrosis (grade 4) (Figs. 13.18 and 13.19).[13,28,30] If the patient has been on disease modifying treatment (e.g., corticosteroids), then the diagnostic features of an overlap syndrome may be less evident, a point that can be conveyed in the pathology report.

Immunohistochemistry and special stains

CK7 immunostains can be used to identify interlobular bile ducts and evaluate for ductopenia in cases with marked portal inflammation. They will also highlight

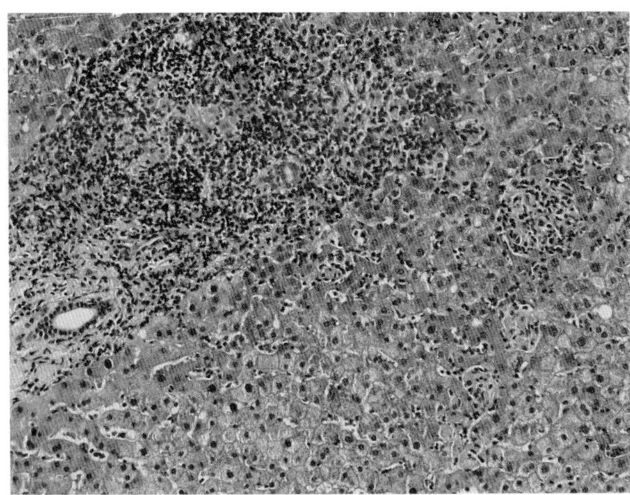

Figure 13.18 Primary biliary cirrhosis–autoimmune hepatitis overlap. Transaminase levels in this well-established case of PBC flared to >10× upper limit of normal. Note the well-developed plasmacytic interface activity within the upper central aspect of the field.

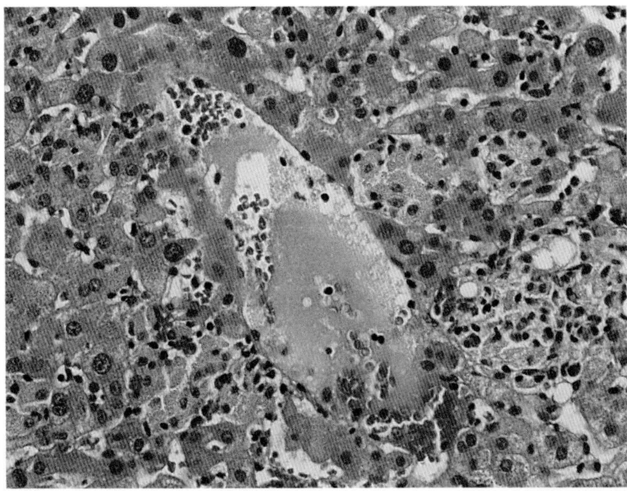

Figure 13.19 Primary biliary cirrhosis–autoimmune hepatitis overlap. Elsewhere within the biopsy were numerous foci of lobular inflammation, like these pericentral aggregates of plasma cells. Marked cholestasis, manifested by collections of macrophages containing phagocytosed bile pigment, was also present.

intermediate hepatocytes when there is chronic cholestatic injury. The rhodanine stain for copper is also a useful ancillary test to support the impression of a chronic biliary disease, as it will show patchy deposition of copper in the periportal hepatocytes.

Immunostains for IgG and IgM can be helpful in difficult cases to distinguish primary biliary cirrhosis from autoimmune hepatitis. The plasma cells in primary biliary cirrhosis are predominantly positive for IgM (equal or greater in number than IgG-positive plasma cells), whereas autoimmune hepatitis is characterized by predominant IgG-positive plasma cells.[32–34] The same portal tracts should be compared when using these stains. Immunostains for Langerhans cells, such as CD1a or Langrin, can also be helpful in diagnosing primary biliary cirrhosis, showing an increased number of intraepithelial Langerhans cells in the bile ducts.[35]

Differential diagnosis

Chronic hepatitis

Chronic hepatitis of viral or autoimmune etiology is characterized by portal-based inflammatory infiltrates which may be very dense and look similar to early stage primary biliary cirrhosis on low power. Although not characteristic, roughly one-fourth of liver biopsies from patients with autoimmune hepatitis can demonstrate biliary changes, including lymphocytic cholangitis or ductopenia.[8] Similarly, bile duct damage has been described in approximately one-third of chronic hepatitis C cases.[36] On the other hand, lymphocytic interface activity also occurs in primary biliary cirrhosis. These challenges can be sorted out by careful attention to clinical, laboratory, and histologic findings. Serologic studies are diagnostic in most viral hepatitis cases, though in acute viral infections nucleic acid testing may be needed. Histologically, the major pattern of injury can help clarify the diagnosis. For example, the presence of well-developed florid duct lesions with only a mild degree of interface and lobular inflammation would support the diagnosis of primary biliary cirrhosis. In contrast, prominent lymphoplasmacytic inflammation with moderate interface and lobular activity, but only focal bile duct injury, suggests autoimmune hepatitis. Confluent lobular necrosis, seen with more severe lobular activity, is also not typical of primary biliary cirrhosis and suggests chronic hepatitis of viral or autoimmune etiology.

Sarcoidosis

Though patients are typically clinically asymptomatic for liver disease, sarcoidosis commonly involves the liver, with granulomas identifiable in 50% to 70% of specimens.[37,38] When a biopsy is performed for biochemically evident liver disease, granulomas are almost universally present.[39] The granulomatous inflammation can be associated with a cholestatic, hepatitic, or vascular pattern of injury.[39] Some features may overlap with primary biliary cirrhosis, including granulomatous cholangitis, hepatocanalicular cholestasis, ductopenia, and copper accumulation.[39] Fibrosis may be present and extensive in some cases.[39]

Sarcoidosis usually affects younger patients than primary biliary cirrhosis and lacks the strong female predilection.[37] Negative serology for AMA, normal IgM serum levels, and the presence of extrahepatic granulomas support the diagnosis of sarcoidosis.[38]

Sarcoid granulomas are typically more numerous than the granulomas in primary biliary cirrhosis. In addition, they are usually well-formed, often contain multinucleated giant cells, and may have associated fibrosis (Figs. 13.20, 13.21, and 13.22). While they are characteristically found in the portal tracts, they are often identified in the lobular parenchyma as well. In some cases, the granulomas coalesce to form tumefactive nodules apparent at low power. In contrast, the granulomas in primary biliary cirrhosis can be either poorly- or well-formed, tend to be smaller, and lack fibrosis.

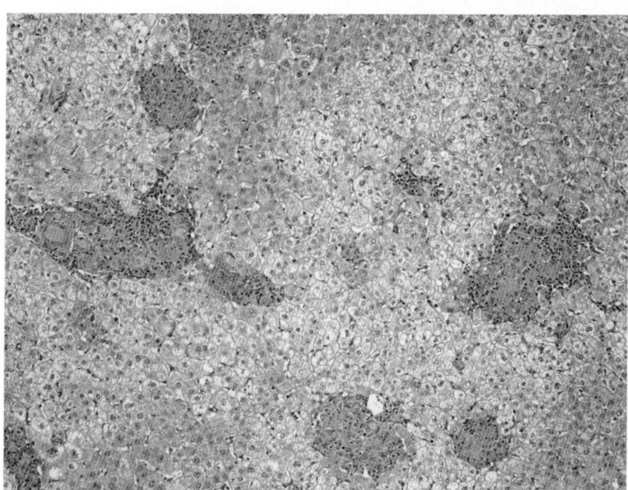

Figure 13.22 Sarcoidosis. Granulomas are often present throughout the lobule, not just within the portal tracts.

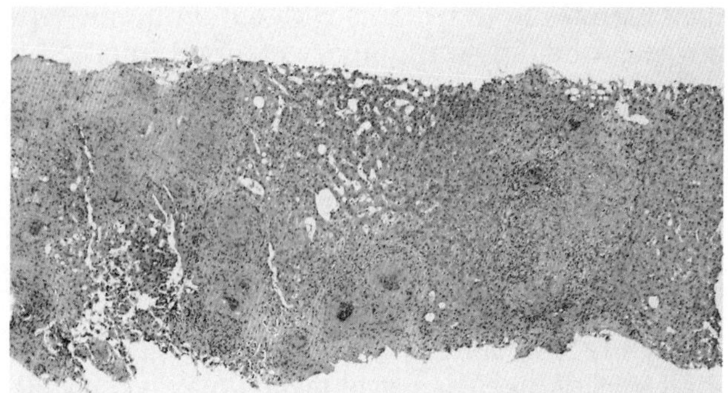

Figure 13.20 Sarcoidosis. Granulomas of sarcoidosis are often tumefactive and readily apparent on low-power inspection. Unlike in primary biliary cirrhosis, giant cells are typically numerous.

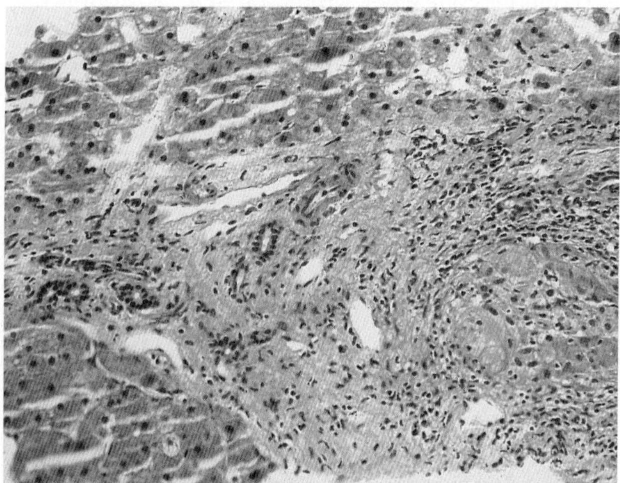

Figure 13.21 Sarcoidosis. Note how the granulomatous component in the right aspect of the field is not centered on the bile duct, as in primary biliary cirrhosis.

Primary sclerosing cholangitis

Primary biliary cirrhosis and primary sclerosing cholangitis can be distinguished in many cases by serology and imaging studies. The primary situation that can cause diagnostic difficulty from a clinical standpoint is differentiating AMA-negative primary biliary cirrhosis (5% to 10% of cases) from small duct primary sclerosing cholangitis (5% of cases). In early stage disease, primary biliary cirrhosis demonstrates more prominent portal inflammation, often with dense lymphoid aggregates.[40] Florid duct lesions support the diagnosis of primary biliary cirrhosis. Although granulomas can rarely be seen in primary sclerosing cholangitis, they are related to bile infarcts extravasated bile in most cases and do not play an active role in duct destruction. The primary pattern of injury seen in primary sclerosing cholangitis is that of large duct obstruction, with bile ductular proliferation and overall mild portal inflammation. Onion skin periductal fibrosis and fibrous scars (fibro-obliterative duct lesions - see below) also indicate a diagnosis of primary sclerosing cholangitis.[40] Liver biopsies in the setting of end-stage cirrhotic livers are more problematic, as both entities can show nonspecific features of chronic biliary disease, including ductopenia, cholate stasis, and copper accumulation.[40]

Prognosis and treatment

Prior to ursodeoxycholic acid, primary biliary cirrhosis was progressive in many patients. The 10 year survival in asymptomatic patients varied from 50% to 70%, but dropped to 5 to 8 years once symptoms appeared.[13] Ursodeoxycholic acid is an effective treatment and slows fibrosis and improves survival in the majority of patients.[13] However, ursodeoxycholic acid is not curative, and patients must remain on treatment indefinitely.

13.3 PRIMARY SCLEROSING CHOLANGITIS

Definition

Primary sclerosing cholangitis is a fibroinflammatory disease which targets the large and/or small bile ducts, resulting in destruction and stricture formation within the biliary tree.

Clinical features

There is geographic variability in the prevalence and incidence of primary sclerosing cholangitis, with higher rates in North America and Northern Europe and lower rates in Southern Europe and Asia.[41–44] North American and European incidence rates are estimated to be 1 per 100,000 persons.[45] Primary sclerosing cholangitis preferentially affects men (M:F = 2:1), with a median age at diagnosis of approximately 40.[45–48]

Approximately half of patients are asymptomatic at the time of diagnosis and are identified on routine workup or for an evaluation related to inflammatory bowel disease.[25,42,44,49] Symptoms are typically vague and include fatigue or abdominal pain.[42,47,50] Jaundice and fever are less common and suggest formation of a dominant stricture.[44,51] Cholelithiasis is common, present in roughly one-fourth of gallbladders.[52,53]

Primary sclerosing cholangitis should be ruled out in any patient with a chronic, unexplained elevation in alkaline phosphatase, particularly in individuals with histories of inflammatory bowel disease.

The diagnostic criteria for primary sclerosing cholangitis include: (1) characteristic cholangiographic findings; (2) cholestatic biochemical profile; and (3) exclusion of secondary causes of sclerosing cholangitis.[42,51] The main roles for liver biopsy are to evaluate for small duct primary sclerosing cholangitis (see below), rule out an overlap syndrome or superimposed process, and for fibrosis staging. A biopsy is not required to diagnose large duct primary sclerosing cholangitis.[51,54]

In the appropriate clinical setting, cholangiography is diagnostic in 95% of patients.[42] The distribution of strictures varies somewhat by study, but involvement of both the intra- and extrahepatic biliary tree is most common, followed by isolated intrahepatic and isolated extrahepatic disease.[47,51] One study demonstrated the following distribution of strictures in over 100 primary sclerosing cholangitis patients: intra- and extrahepatic ducts in 87%, isolated intrahepatic ducts in 11%, and isolated extrahepatic ducts in 2%.[49]

Laboratory findings

Though nonspecific, an elevated alkaline phosphatase level is present in the majority of patients.[46,47,51,55] This and GGT elevations may be the only serum markers that are abnormal, and levels can fluctuate throughout the course of the disease.[44] Transaminase levels are often normal, but may be elevated at 2 to 3× the upper limit of normal.[44,51] As with primary biliary cirrhosis, if AST/ALT levels are greater than 5× upper limit, this raises the possibility of an autoimmune hepatitis overlap syndrome or other superimposed processes.[51]

At presentation, bilirubin levels are normal in the majority of patients and only become elevated in late stage disease, or in the setting of a dominant stricture.[44,51]

Unlike primary biliary cirrhosis, there is no diagnostic serologic test for primary sclerosing cholangitis. Patients may have a variety of nonspecific autoantibodies, with prevalence rates depending upon the population and study. According to one review of 19 studies, the median prevalence of perinuclear antineutrophil cytoplasmic antibodies (p-ANCA) was 68%, with a range of 26% to 94%.[56] ASMA and ANA are also variable, with median prevalence of 17% and 30%, respectively.[56] Hypergammaglobulinemia is present in roughly 60% of patients.[51] Elevated IgM levels are seen in 40% to 50% of cases.[49] AMA is usually negative.[24]

Imaging

Cholangiography is the diagnostic test for large duct primary sclerosing cholangitis. Typical findings include a beaded pattern characterized by short, annular strictures which alternate with normal-to-dilated segments.[49,51,57] Because endoscopic retrograde cholangiography is an invasive test with a complication rate of 10% (e.g., cholangitis and perforation), it has been supplanted by magnetic resonance cholangiography as the initial imaging modality.[51,57] The latter is noninvasive and there is no radiation exposure.[51] It has a sensitivity of >80% and specificity of >87%, providing accurate diagnoses in the majority of patients.[51]

Gross findings

The liver explant in primary sclerosing cholangitis is typically bile stained with well-developed cirrhosis. The hilar area is often densely fibrotic, especially in cases complicated by cholangiocarcinoma. Extensive sections may be necessary to identify dysplasia or carcinoma.

Microscopic findings

General features

The pathologic hallmark of primary sclerosing cholangitis is the fibro-obliterative duct lesion, which begins as concentric rings of periductal "onion-skinning" fibrosis that over time distort and compress the bile duct, resulting in obliteration of the lumen (Figs. 13.23, 13.24, and 13.25). A round scar is often the only clue that a bile duct was present. However, fibro-obliterative lesions are not pathognomonic for primary sclerosing cholangitis and may be seen in other forms of secondary sclerosing cholangitis.[23,58] The most common histologic finding is nonspecific bile ductular proliferation (see below).

In large intra- and extrahepatic bile ducts, there can be mucosal ulceration with mixed inflammation, sometimes including a granulomatous component (Fig. 13.26).[59] The granulomatous inflammation is a response to bile leakage and can be seen in up to 7% of primary sclerosing cholangitis cases.[60]

Needle biopsy findings

Needle biopsy specimens typically demonstrate features of chronic biliary disease, which are a sequelae of strictures in more distal, larger bile ducts. These features vary with the stage of disease, but the main finding in most biopsies is that of bile ductular proliferation and mild, mixed portal inflammation. In general, as disease progresses the biopsies show diminished inflammation and gradually increasing amounts of ductular reaction, cholestatic changes, fibrosis, and ductopenia (Fig. 13.27). The presence of a ductular reaction associated with fibrosis and periportal copper accumulation is sufficient to render a diagnosis of chronic biliary disease, thus alerting the clinicians of the need to perform imaging of the biliary tree.

Primary sclerosing cholangitis tends to progress through a series of histologic patterns that usefully

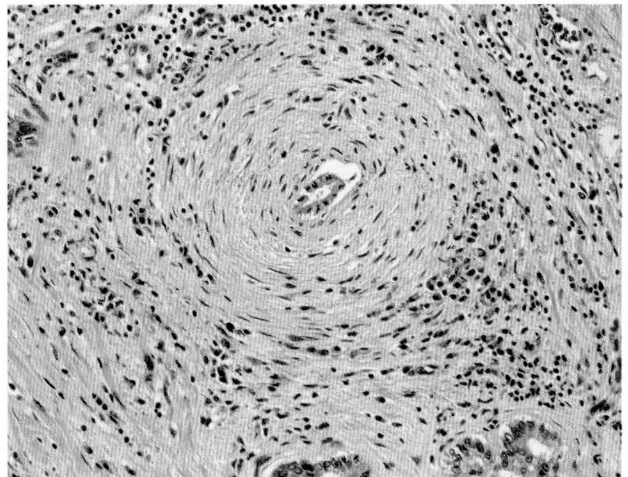

Figure 13.23 Fibro-obliterative lesion. Onion skin fibrosis surrounds the duct in the center of the field. Note the concentric rings of collagen and fibroblasts. Occasional plasma cells are present.

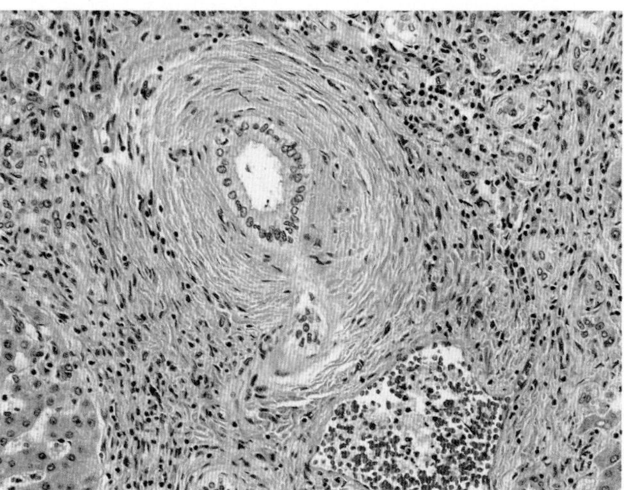

Figure 13.24 Fibro-obliterative lesion. With time, the fibrosis compresses and distorts the lumen leading to complete occlusion of the duct.

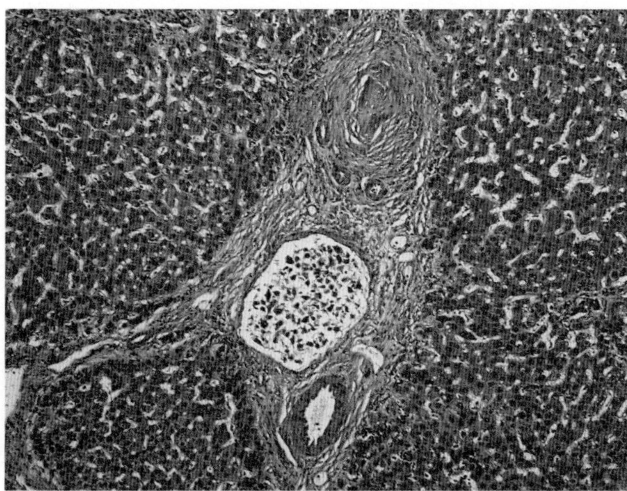

Figure 13.25 Fibro-obliterative lesion. Eventually, no duct remains. A fibrous scar, often round in form, is the only indicator that a bile duct was present.

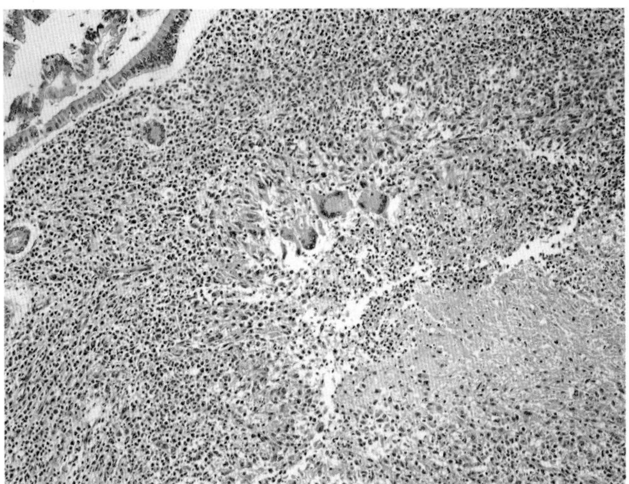

Figure 13.26 Primary sclerosing cholangitis and granulomatous inflammation. Erosion of lining epithelium and bile leakage may occur. Bile in the lower right of the field is associated with an intense polymorphous inflammatory response of lymphocytes, plasma cells, neutrophils, and histiocytes. There is a giant cell reaction to extravasated bile.

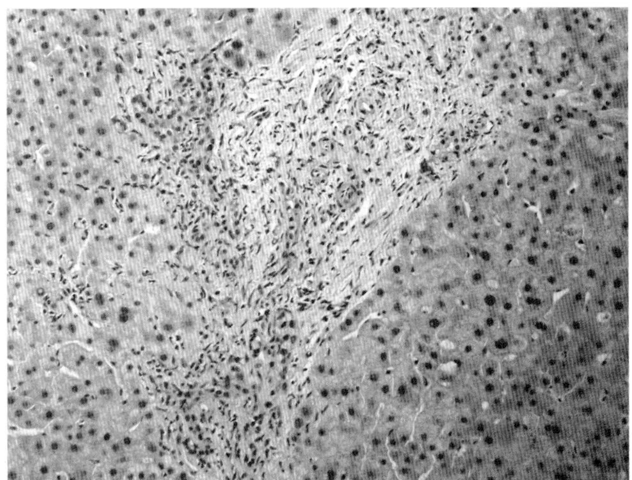

Figure 13.27 Primary sclerosing cholangitis. Typical needle biopsy appearance of portal tract in primary sclerosing cholangitis. There are nonspecific changes of ductular reaction and irregular fibrosis. No bile duct is seen in this portal tract. Although not specific for primary sclerosing cholangitis, the findings are suggestive of a chronic biliary disease.

illustrate the most common findings in biopsy specimens.[4,5,24,25,54]

Stage 1: Peripheral liver biopsies may be essentially normal, with only mild nonspecific changes. There may be a mild ductular proliferation with mild, mixed portal inflammation. The portal inflammation includes lymphocytes, neutrophils, and occasional eosinophils. Fibrosis staging can be challenging as there is portal expansion secondary to inflammation and ductular proliferation. Any portal fibrosis is usually mild. Periportal copper accumulation can be detected in a minority of cases.

Stage 2: There is a diffuse bile ductular reaction along with mild, mixed portal inflammation. The portal tracts show irregular fibrosis imparting a "pulled taffy" appearance (Fig. 13.28). At least focal mild periportal copper accumulation is present most cases.

Stage 3: There is a well-developed ductular reaction, with variable portal-based inflammation. The portal tracts also show variable ductopenia, characterized by an unaccompanied hepatic artery branch. Cholate stasis is common. Trichrome stains show portal–portal bridging fibrosis. Periportal copper accumulation is present in the majority of cases, including some with widespread deposition. Rare cases can show fibro-obliterative duct lesions.

Stage 4: There is cirrhosis with a biliary pattern and associated ductular reaction. Ductopenia is commonly present and is sometimes marked. The lobules show hepatocanalicular cholestasis and cholate stasis. Copper deposition is present in almost all cases and is extensive in many. Fibro-obliterative duct lesions can be found.

Of note, percutaneous needle biopsies and sub capsular wedge biopsies sample the periphery of the liver, which contains predominantly microscopic ducts.[24] Because fibro-obliterative lesions preferentially involve medium bile duct branches, they are often absent in needle biopsies.[24,25,54]

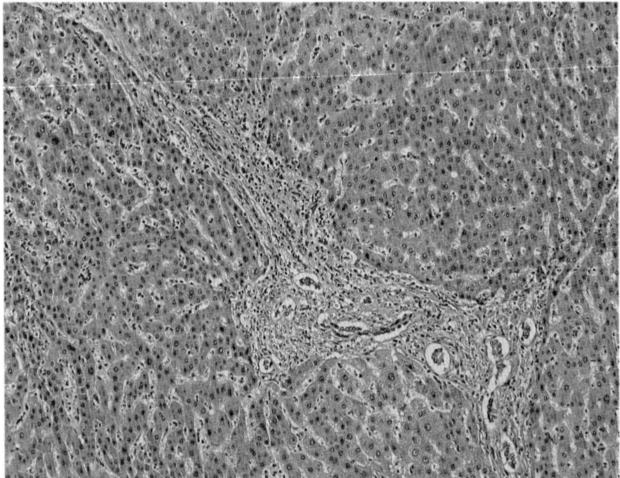

Figure 13.28 Primary sclerosing cholangitis. Portal tracts in primary sclerosing cholangitis often have a jagged and irregular pattern of fibrosis. It appears as though the edges of the tract were pulled in different directions, imparting a "pulled taffy" appearance.

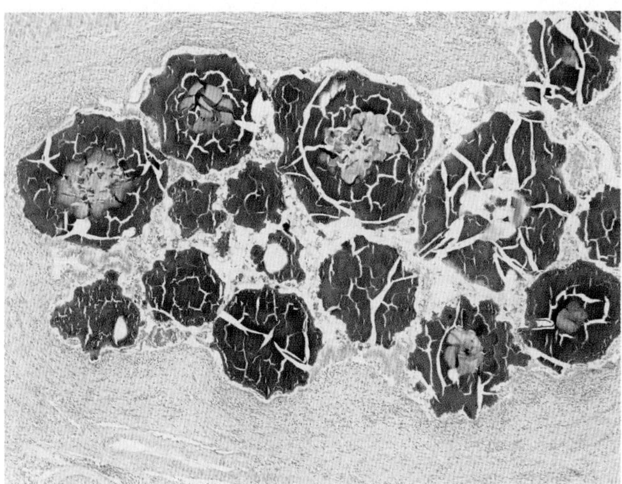

Figure 13.29 Primary sclerosing cholangitis. Bile stasis can lead to the formation of casts and stones within the biliary tree. This duct is filled with bile casts. There is an inflammatory reaction in the adjacent wall.

Explant findings

There is a biliary pattern of fibrosis. Fibro-obliterative duct lesions are typically identified, but may not be present in every section. The large bile ducts are often ectactic and filled with inspissated bile plugs (Fig. 13.29).[58] Bile infarcts and hepatoliths are common.[58] The biliary epithelium may show a variety of metaplastic changes, including mucinous (77%), pyloric (73%), intestinal (26%), and pancreatic acinar (10%) metaplasia.[61] In an extensive study of 100 liver explants with primary sclerosing cholangitis, high grade dysplasia was found in 60% of cases with cholangiocarcinoma and 11% of livers that did not have cholangiocarcinoma.[61]

Immunohistochemistry and special stains

CK7 immunostain can be used to identify interlobular bile ducts in cases with marked portal inflammation, helping to identify ductopenia, as well as intermediate hepatocytes, a marker of chronic cholestatic liver injury. The rhodanine stain for copper may provide support for a chronic biliary disease.

Primary sclerosing cholangitis variants

Small duct primary sclerosing cholangitis

In small duct primary sclerosing cholangitis, which constitutes approximately 5% of all cases, the disease affects only the microscopic ducts.[42] The criteria for diagnosis are: (1) chronic cholestasis (elevated alkaline phosphatase); (2) histologic features compatible with primary sclerosing cholangitis; (3) normal cholangiogram; and (4) exclusion of other causes of chronic biliary disease.[62] Some centers require a history of inflammatory bowel disease.[44] The role of the pathologist is to identify features of chronic biliary disease, including ductular reactions, periportal copper accumulation, ductopenia, and fibrosis. This constellation of features is sufficient to suggest the diagnosis of primary sclerosing cholangitis in the appropriate setting.

Small duct primary sclerosing cholangitis has a better long-term prognosis than large duct primary sclerosing cholangitis, with a longer transplantation free survival and lower risk of cholangiocarcinoma.[62] Approximately 20% of patients will develop large duct primary sclerosing cholangitis over a 7 to 10 year period.[44]

Primary sclerosing cholangitis–autoimmune hepatitis overlap

The diagnosis of primary sclerosing cholangitis–autoimmune hepatitis overlap syndrome is made when serologic and histologic findings of autoimmune hepatitis are present in the setting of cholangiographic changes and/or histologic findings of primary sclerosing cholangitis.[44] The rates of autoimmune hepatitis in patients with primary sclerosing cholangitis vary by study, ranging from 1.4% to 17%, but the disease is more common in the young[51]. Some authors recommend that primary sclerosing cholangitis patients be tested for autoimmune hepatitis when they are under 25 years of age or have transaminase levels greater than 5× upper limit of normal.[42] Likewise, it is suggested that autoimmune hepatitis patients under 25 years of age, or those with alkaline phosphatase levels >2× upper limit of normal, undergo imaging to rule out superimposed primary sclerosing cholangitis.[42]

Portal inflammation may be present in primary sclerosing cholangitis, particularly in early stage disease. However, it is usually mild and interface activity is not a prominent feature.[40] In contrast, when there is an autoimmune hepatitis overlap, the portal inflammation is rich in plasma cells, interface activity is extensive, and lobular necroinflammatory activity is prominent. (Fig. 13.30).

Complications and associated conditions

The clinical course in primary sclerosing cholangitis can be complicated by dominant strictures, cholangitis, and malignancy, including cholangiocarcinoma, colorectal carcinoma, and gallbladder neoplasia.[50,63,64]

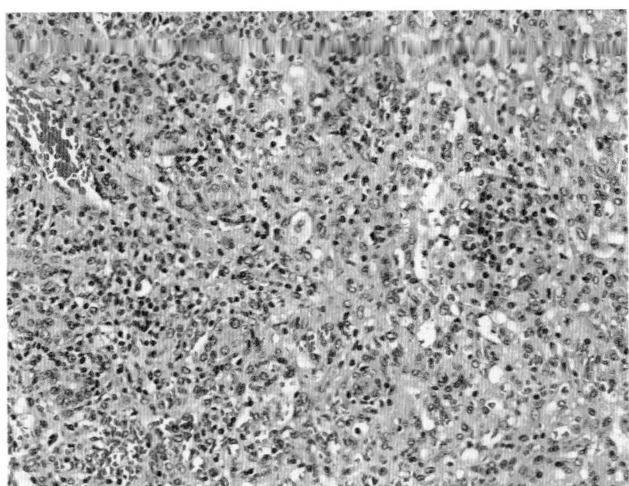

Figure 13.30 Primary sclerosing cholangitis–autoimmune hepatitis overlap. In this case of primary sclerosing cholangitis–autoimmune hepatitis overlap, there is extensive collapse of the lobular parenchyma along the right edge and lower half of the field. Interface activity is so severe that it is impossible to identify the limiting plate and portal inflammation is greater than one typically sees in primary sclerosing cholangitis.

Dominant strictures

Roughly half of patients will develop a dominant stricture, which is defined as an area of stenosis in which the luminal diameter is ≤1.5 mm in the common bile duct or ≤1 mm in the right or left hepatic duct.[50,63] These strictures may induce pruritus, jaundice, and/or bacterial cholangitis.[51,63] In one study, enteric bacteria were cultured from the bile of 40% of primary sclerosing cholangitis patients with a dominant stricture, but in no cases without a stricture.[65] Dominant strictures are treated by endoscopic dilation with or without stent placement in the majority of cases.[44,51]

Cholangiocarcinoma

Primary sclerosing cholangitis is a major risk factor for cholangiocarcinoma, which develops in 10% to 15% of patients.[44,48,66,67] The annual incidence of cholangiocarcinoma is 0.5% to 2% once the diagnosis of primary sclerosing cholangitis has been made.[44,48,67] Cholangiocarcinoma can develop in the absence of advanced fibrosis.[44] In fact, a significant percentage of cholangiocarcinomas (up to 50%) are identified within 1 to 3 years of a primary sclerosing cholangitis diagnosis.[44,51,67] Given the risk of cholangiocarcinoma, patients are often followed with annual imaging studies and serum CA19.9 levels.[42,67]

Inflammatory bowel disease

There is a strong association between primary sclerosing cholangitis and inflammatory bowel disease. The prevalence and incidence rates of co-occurring disease vary globally, from 21% in Japan to 80% in Sweden.[68] In North America and Northern Europe, most studies show a prevalence of inflammatory bowel disease in primary sclerosing cholangitis ranging from 60% to 80%.[49,51,69] Ulcerative colitis constitutes 80% to 89% of inflammatory bowel disease cases, with the remaining divided between Crohn disease and indeterminate colitis.[49,67] When present, Crohn disease typically involves the colon, and Crohn disease restricted to the small bowel is not associated with primary sclerosing cholangitis.[51] The risk of developing primary sclerosing cholangitis in patients with inflammatory bowel disease is significantly lower, at 2.0% to 7.5%.[49,68,70]

Primary sclerosing cholangitis can be diagnosed prior to, concurrent with, or after a diagnosis of inflammatory bowel disease.[51,71] There are reports of primary sclerosing cholangitis occurring after total colectomy for ulcerative colitis, and inflammatory bowel disease arising after liver transplantation for primary sclerosing cholangitis.[51] Given this strong association, it is recommended that all newly diagnosed patients with primary sclerosing cholangitis undergo colonoscopy to rule out superimposed inflammatory bowel disease.[42,51] Similarly, patients with primary sclerosing cholangitis and inflammatory bowel disease should undergo annual colonoscopy for surveillance purposes.[42,51]

Inflammatory bowel disease in the setting of primary sclerosing cholangitis has unique characteristics. Patients are typically younger and disease is often subclinical.[42] In spite of the mild activity, pan-colitis is typical, even for Crohn disease.[51,72] Endoscopically, rectal sparing is common, but histologic examination of the rectum usually demonstrates active disease.[51,72]

Colorectal carcinoma

There is an increased risk of colorectal carcinoma development in patients with primary sclerosing cholangitis + ulcerative colitis, compared to those with ulcerative colitis alone. A meta-analysis has demonstrated a 4× increased risk of developing colorectal carcinoma compared to patients with ulcerative colitis alone.[73] When present, the carcinoma is most commonly located in the proximal colon.[67] Because of the elevated risk of colorectal carcinoma, most clinicians perform surveillance colonoscopy every 1 to 2 years once a patient has been diagnosed with primary sclerosing cholangitis.[42]

Gallbladder neoplasia

Given the increased risk of cholangiocarcinoma in patients with primary sclerosing cholangitis, it is not surprising that primary sclerosing cholangitis patients are also at increased risk for developing gallbladder neoplasia. Mass lesions are found in 3% to 15% of primary sclerosing cholangitis gallbladders.[67] Up to 60% of these may be malignant, so it is recommended that patients undergo annual ultrasound to screen for gallbladder polyps/masses, followed by cholecystectomy if any lesion is identified.[52,74]

Differential diagnosis

There are no histologic features that are pathognomonic for primary sclerosing cholangitis and, as mentioned above, the characteristic fibro-obliterative lesion is typically not present on needle biopsy specimens. The differential includes all entities that have a chronic obstructive biliary disease pattern, including ductular reaction, fibrosis, periportal copper accumulation, and ductopenia. Leading considerations include primary biliary cirrhosis, secondary sclerosing cholangitis, IgG4-related sclerosing cholangitis, drug-induced liver injury, and idiopathic adulthood ductopenia.

Primary biliary cirrhosis

In general, the distinction between primary biliary cirrhosis and primary sclerosing cholangitis is straightforward. Clinically, small duct primary sclerosing cholangitis can cause a diagnostic dilemma given the normal cholangiographic findings. There is typically greater portal inflammation and interface activity in primary biliary cirrhosis than in primary sclerosing cholangitis.[40] While granulomas may rarely be encountered in primary sclerosing cholangitis, they are not directed towards the interlobular bile ducts as is seen in primary biliary cirrhosis. Late stage disease is more problematic, with both showing nonspecific features of chronic biliary disease.[40] When present, onion skin fibrosis and fibrous scars are supportive of a diagnosis of primary sclerosing cholangitis.

Prognosis and treatment

Primary sclerosing cholangitis is a chronic and progressive disorder, with a 12 to 18 year median interval to death or transplantation.[46] Death usually results from malignancy or liver failure.[46] The Mayo Risk Score can be utilized to estimate patient survival, utilizing patient age, bilirubin, albumin, AST, and history of variceal bleeding.[9] Currently, there is no medical therapy to slow the progression of the disease or prevent complications. Treatment is aimed at alleviating symptoms and managing complications, with liver transplant reserved for decompensated cirrhosis.[42,51] There is an 85% 5-year survival after transplantation, and primary sclerosing cholangitis recurs in 20% to 25% of transplant recipients after 5 to 10 years.[51]

13.4 SECONDARY SCLEROSING CHOLANGITIS

Secondary sclerosing cholangitis is a generic term for entities that cause stricture formation, fibrosis, and variable inflammation within the intra- and/or extrahepatic biliary tree.[75] The histologic features typically overlap significantly with those of primary sclerosing cholangitis, including ductular reaction, bile duct injury, irregular fibrosis, periportal copper accumulation, and ductopenia. Common etiologies that cause secondary sclerosing cholangitis are listed in Table 13.3. These entities should be excluded via a combination of clinical and serologic features, imaging studies, and tissue biopsy when indicated, prior to making the diagnosis of primary sclerosing cholangitis. A brief overview of the more common entities is detailed below.

Table 13.3 Causes of secondary sclerosing cholangitis

Mechanism	Etiology
Ischemia	Liver transplantation Intraoperative arterial injury Hepatic arterial chemotherapy Vasculitis Hereditary hemorrhagic telangiectasia Atherosclerosis Critical illness Hypoxia
Mechanical obstruction	Choledocholithiasis Pancreatitis Pancreatobiliary neoplasm Postcholecystectomy common bile duct trauma Portal biliopathy
Infection	Cryptococcus CMV Becteria
Neoplasms	Langerhans histiocytosis Hodgkin lymphoma
Immunologic	Autoimmune pancreatitis Hypereosinophilic syndrome Systemic mastocytosis

Mechanical obstruction

Obstruction anywhere along the extrahepatic biliary tree can lead to histologic features that overlap with primary sclerosing cholangitis. Acute large duct obstruction may be associated with a prominent ductular reaction and portal edema (Fig. 13.31). Unless the process is chronic, there is typically no fibrosis. The histologic changes that result from chronic or repeated obstruction may be impossible to differentiate from primary sclerosing cholangitis (Fig. 13.32). Common etiologies include choledocholithiasis, surgical bile duct trauma (e.g., during cholecystectomy), chronic pancreatitis, abdominal trauma, and pancreatic adenocarcinoma, or cholangiocarcinoma.[76–78]

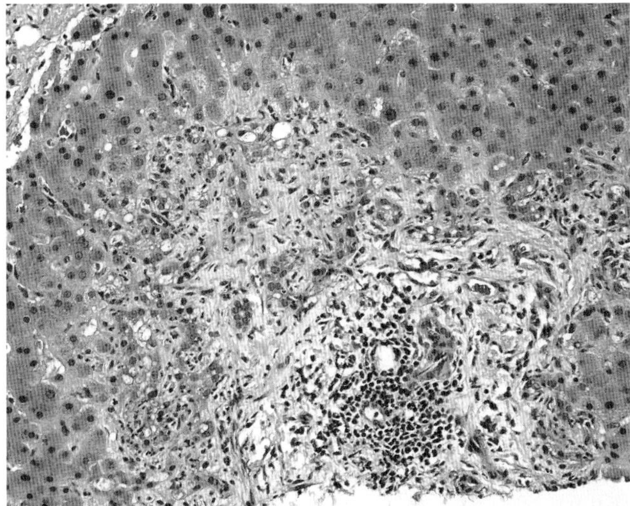

Figure 13.31 Acute large duct obstruction. In acute large duct obstruction, the portal tract is enlarged and no longer has a light eosinophilic tincture because of edema. Structures are loosely organized and not as compact as in chronic processes.

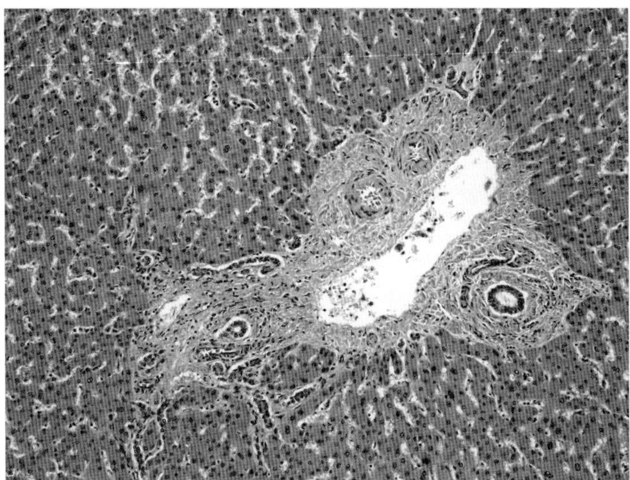

Figure 13.32 Chronic large duct obstruction. In this example of chronic large duct obstruction secondary to a hilar cholangiocarcinoma, nonspecific features of chronic biliary disease, including mild ductular reaction and periportal fibrosis, are seen.

Infectious cholangiopathy

Chronic inflammation due to infection of the biliary tree may result in histologic changes similar to primary sclerosing cholangitis.[79] This pattern of injury typically occurs in patients with congenital (e.g., X-linked hyper IgM syndrome) or acquired immunodeficiency (e.g., AIDS, organ transplantation, etc.).[25,79] AIDS cholangiopathy is the best characterized of these. Although the true incidence is unknown, early studies found bile duct abnormalities in up to 26% of patients with AIDS, typically when the CD4 count fell below 100/mm^3.[80,81] It is much less common in the era of effective antiviral therapy.[7,76,80,81] Bacterial, viral, protozoal, and fungal organisms have all been identified as causal agents.[82] Cryptosporidium and cytomegalovirus (CMV) are the most common.[25,79,80,82]

Ischemic cholangiopathy

Blood to biliary epithelial cells is supplied only by the hepatic artery.[75,83] Compromise anywhere along this vasculature can result in ischemic injury of the bile ducts, with histologic features of sclerosing cholangitis.[83] Liver transplantation–related hepatic artery thrombosis and infusion of chemotherapeutic agents (floxuridine) into the hepatic artery are the best characterized examples of ischemic cholangiopathy.[83,84] However, other reported etiologies include vasculitis, surgical arterial injury, chronic liver rejection, blunt abdominal wounds, hereditary hemorrhagic telangiectasia, atherosclerosis, and trauma (so-called traumatic sclerosing cholangitis).[75,83,85]

Ischemic cholangiopathy preferentially affects the large hilar and/or intrahepatic bile ducts.[84,86] In the setting of liver transplantation, nonanastomotic biliary complications are identified in 2% to 19% of patients.[83] Ischemic cholangiopathy can manifest as focal or circumferential necrosis of the bile duct wall (Fig. 13.33). The bile duct epithelium can be atrophic or demonstrate erosions. Cholangiectases and strictures are often present.[83,84] Superimposed bacterial colonies (56%) or fungal organisms (11%) are frequently found.[86] With intra-arterial chemotherapy-associated damage, the large hilar bile ducts demonstrate fibrous cholangitis, periductal fibrosis, and fibrous cords.[83]

Ischemic injury to the large ducts (hilar or septal intrahepatic) can only be evaluated in explant specimens of patients undergoing transplantation. Needle biopsy findings from the liver periphery are far less specific and typically overlap with those of primary sclerosing cholangitis. In a series of 18 liver allograft

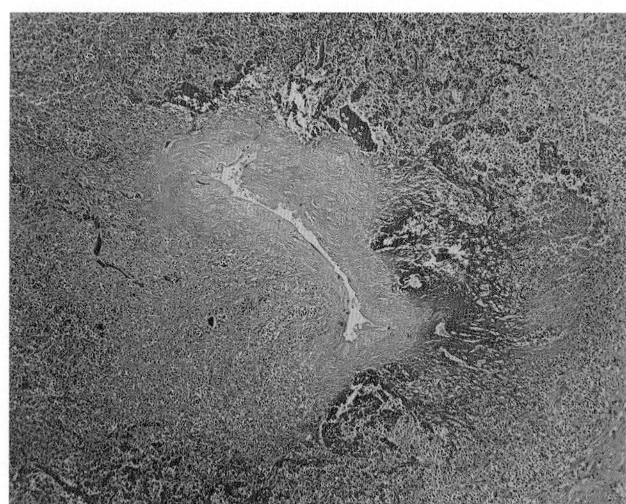

Figure 13.33 Bile duct necrosis. In this hilar section of a patient with hepatic artery thrombosis after liver transplantation, there is extensive necrosis of the bile duct wall. Image courtesy of Dr. Raouf Nakhleh, Mayo Clinic, Florida.

explants with documented bile duct necrosis, intrahepatic biliary abnormalities were identified in only 24% of cases (though the allografts also had other changes reflecting coexisting arterial thrombi).[86] When present, biliary features are typically those of duct obstruction/bile outflow impairment, including edema, ductular reaction, ductopenia, and cholate stasis (Fig. 13.34). Similar changes are found in peripheral biopsies of patients with intra-arterial chemotherapy-associated cholangitis.[83]

The clinical setting is helpful in distinguishing ischemic cholangiopathy from primary sclerosing cholangitis. Biopsy findings of bile flow impairment/obstruction should prompt clinicians to image the biliary tree (endoscopic retrograde cholangiopancreatography (ERCP) or magnetic resonance retrograde cholangiopancreatography (MRCP)) with imaging of hepatic vasculature if strictures are seen.

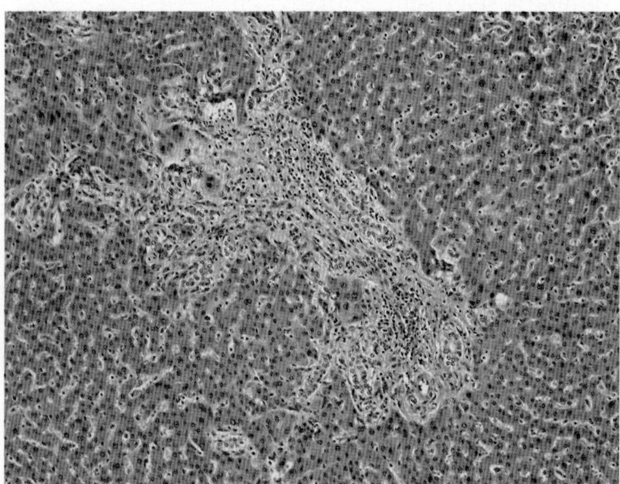

Figure 13.34 Ischemic cholangiopathy. Sections of the periphery of the liver in ischemic cholangiopathy often demonstrate nonspecific biliary changes. In this example, there is ductular reaction and irregular fibrosis.

Portal biliopathy

Portal hypertension in the setting of extrahepatic portal vein obstruction may lead to the development of large collateral vessels—cavernous transformation of the portal vein.[75] These collaterals can compress the adjacent common bile duct, particularly if the obstruction is in the region of the porta hepatis. ERCP has demonstrated biliary abnormalities in 81% to 100% of patients with extrahepatic portal vein obstruction, though the majority of patients are not symptomatic.[87] Biliary injury is thought to occur because of a combination of mechanical compression and ischemic-mediated damage.[75] Needle biopsies can demonstrate nonspecific biliary changes similar to those seen in primary sclerosing cholangitis.[75]

Neoplasms

Langerhans cell histiocytosis and Hodgkin lymphoma can be associated with sclerosing cholangitis.[24,25] The former may result from direct infiltration of the biliary tree by CD1a-positive Langerhans cells.[88,89] Sclerosing cholangitis can occur in nonhepatic forms of Langerhans cell histiocytosis as well.[88,89] Similarly, patients with Hodgkin lymphoma in extrahepatic sites (e.g., lymph nodes) may develop a paraneoplastic secondary sclerosing cholangitis.[90]

13.5 IGG4-RELATED SCLEROSING CHOLANGITIS

Definition

IgG4-related sclerosing cholangitis is a biliary manifestation of IgG4-related disease, which is characterized by dense, lymphoplasmacytic inflammation containing increased numbers of IgG4-positive plasma cells and fibrosis, resulting in the formation of bile duct strictures or an inflammatory pseudotumor.

Clinical features

IgG4-related sclerosing cholangitis preferentially affects elderly men.[59,91,92] In a Mayo Clinic series of 53 patients, 85% were men with a mean age of 62 years at diagnosis.[92] This is similar to the demographics for IgG4-related disease in other organs.[93] An analysis of

235 individuals with IgG4-related disease demonstrated a median age of 67 years and a 4:1 male-to-female ratio.[94] In that series, 91% of patients were 50 years of age or older and bile duct involvement was the 6th most common manifestation, present in 13% of patients. In this subset of individuals, obstructive jaundice was the most common presenting symptom.[95]

The majority of cases arise in the setting of autoimmune pancreatitis (92% in the Mayo Clinic series).[92] Other systemic sites of involvement include the kidney, retroperitoneum, salivary glands, lymph node, and lungs.[92,96–98] Disease restricted to only the biliary tree is very uncommon[59] but has been reported.[99]

At Mayo Clinic, the HISORt criteria (Histology, Imaging, Serum IgG4, Other organ involvement, and Response to steroid therapy) for autoimmune pancreatitis were adapted to diagnose IgG4-related sclerosing cholangitis.[92] Unlike primary biliary cirrhosis and primary sclerosing cholangitis, histologic assessment is the mainstay of diagnosis and the only parameter which, if present, is diagnostic of IgG4-related sclerosing cholangitis, even in isolation.[92,93,96] All other criteria must be present in various combinations, with or without characteristic histology.[92,96]

Because most patients with liver disease (>90%) will have concurrent autoimmune pancreatitis, the pancreas should be examined for disease.[59,88,92,100] In those rare cases without pancreatic involvement, biopsies of the liver, bile duct, or ampulla of Vater may be diagnostic.[59]

Laboratory findings

Elevated serum IgG4 levels are the most sensitive and specific serologic marker, though the test is not diagnostic in isolation. IgG4 is not elevated in all patients with IgG4-related sclerosing cholangitis; conversely, patients with diseases other than IgG4-related sclerosing cholangitis may have elevated serum IgG4 levels.[59,92] For example, approximately 10% of primary sclerosing cholangitis and 15% of cholangiocarcinoma patients will have an elevated IgG4 level.[59]

At the Mayo Clinic, the reference range for serum IgG4 is 8 to 140 mg/dL. Approximately 70% to 80% of patients will have a value greater than 135 to 140.[59,92] In the Mayo Clinic series, the mean serum IgG4 level was markedly elevated at 516 mg/dL, which is very similar to the median observed in another study.[101] However, there was a wide range, from 6 to 2,490 mg/dL. Elevations of serum IgG4 >2× normal range (>280 mg/dL) is highly specific for IgG4-sclerosing cholangitis, as is an IgG4: total IgG ratio of >10%.[59,92]

A variety of nonspecific autoimmune markers may be seen. Elevated serum IgG is the most common, present in 60% of patients.[100] ANA positivity is detected in 40% to 50% of patients, whereas AMA and ANCA are usually negative (<6% positive).[100] In a study by Ghazale et al.,[92] alkaline phosphatase was elevated in 84% of patients and markedly increased (>500 U/L) in roughly one-third. ALT and AST were greater than 3× normal in 62% and 32% of cases, respectively. Other studies have confirmed the frequent elevation of alkaline phosphate.[91]

Imaging findings

Cholangiography reveals strictures, which are usually segmental and long with prestenotic dilatation of the bile duct, and there is frequent involvement of the distal common bile duct.[102] Strictures can show these patterns: (1) isolated distal common bile duct stricture; (2) intra- and extrahepatic duct strictures; (3) liver hilum and distal common bile duct strictures or (4) liver hilum strictures only.[96,103] In the Mayo Clinic series, there was involvement of the distal common bile duct in 70% of cases, with isolated distal common bile duct disease in 51% of cases.[92] Isolated intrahepatic strictures suggestive of primary sclerosing cholangitis were present in 8% of cases.[92] The location of the strictures will affect the differential diagnosis.

Gross findings

IgG4-related sclerosing cholangitis can result in either diffuse wall thickening, strictures of the bile ducts, or form an inflammatory pseudotumor.[59,104]

Microscopic findings

General features

Microscopically, the inflammation in IgG4-related sclerosing cholangitis is primarily portal-based and can be either localized or diffuse.[95,104] There are increased numbers of IgG4-positive plasma cells in conjunction with three additional histologic changes: (1) dense lymphoplasmacytic infiltrates; (2) storiform fibrosis; and (3) obliterative phlebitis (Figs. 13.35, 13.36, and 13.37). In 2012, a consensus paper summarized the histology of IgG4-related disease.[105] In addition to increased numbers of IgG4+ plasma cells (Fig. 13.38), the diagnosis in this consensus paper required the presence of 2 of these 3 features.[105]

Lymphoplasmatyic infiltrates: a mix of lymphocytes and plasma cells, the latter of which can be the most prominent cell type. Eosinophils are frequently present and may be quite numerous in some cases.

Storiform fibrosis: proliferation of spindle cells in a characteristic storiform (cartwheel) pattern.

Obliterative phlebitis: transmural lymphoplasmacytic inflammation of veins, which can result in partial or total venous obliteration.

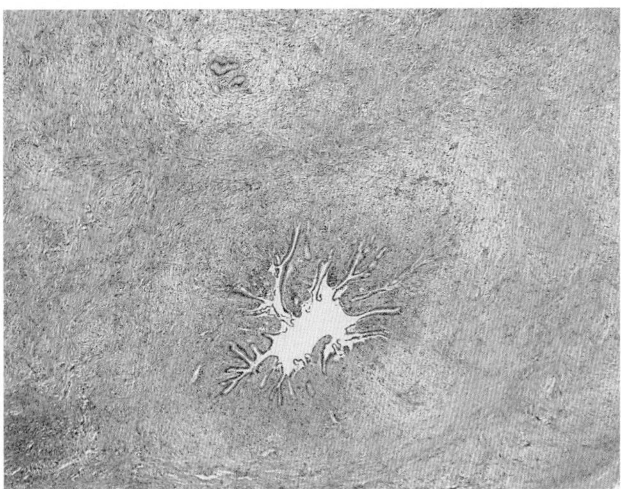

Figure 13.35 IgG4-related sclerosing cholangitis. Hilar section of a liver involved by IgG4-related sclerosing cholangitis. There is transmural and circumferential involvement of the hilar bile duct. A loose spindle cell proliferation diffusely involves and thickens the wall. In the upper half of the field, the storiform pattern of fibrosis is appreciated.

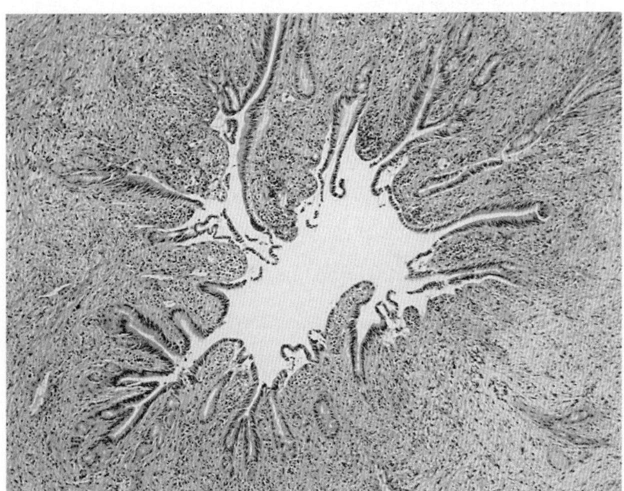

Figure 13.36 IgG4-related sclerosing cholangitis. On higher power examination, the surface epithelium is relatively intact without erosion.

Prominent neutrophilic infiltrates and granulomatous inflammation argue against the diagnosis of IgG4-related disease.[105]

IgG4-related sclerosing cholangitis preferentially affects large ducts, so diagnostic features are best seen in surgical bile duct resections or liver explants.[59] Given the superficial nature of wedge biopsy specimens, the tissue may not contain all of the necessary findings. Similarly, percutaneous liver biopsy can show a variety of patterns, including nonspecific changes (see below).

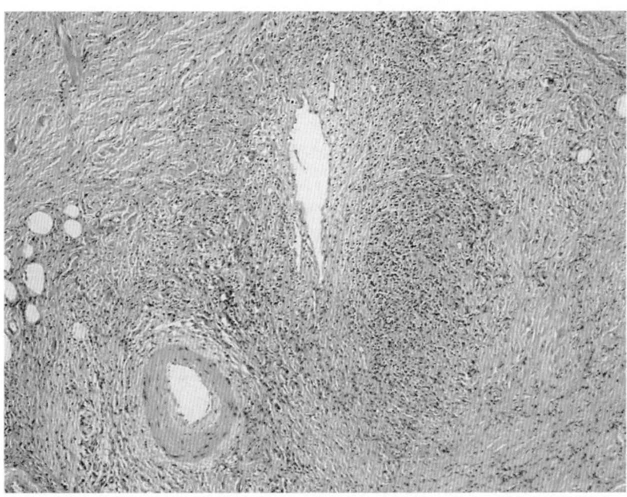

Figure 13.37 IgG4-related sclerosing cholangitis. Phlebitis is present in the center of the field. In some instances, the vein is completely obliterated and can only be appreciated with silver stain.

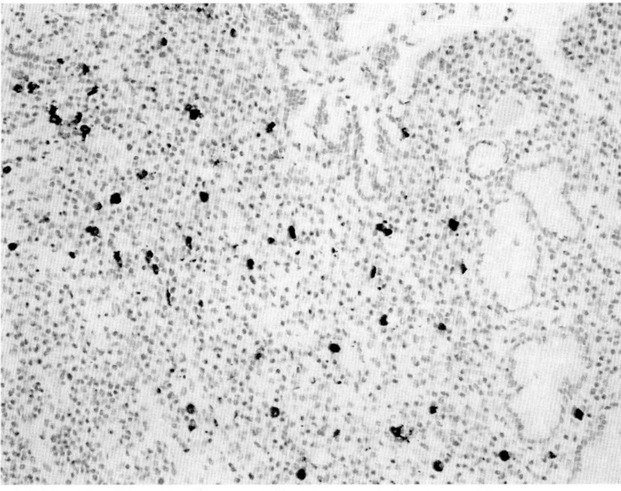

Figure 13.38 IgG4-related sclerosing cholangitis. IgG 4 immunostain demonstrates increased number of IgG4+ plasma cells.

Needle biopsy findings of the liver

The needle biopsy findings will depend on whether there is isolated autoimmune pancreatitis, large duct IgG4-related sclerosing cholangitis, or large and small duct IgG4-related sclerosing cholangitis. Diagnostic levels of IgG4+ plasma cells will only be present if there is small duct involvement.[106]

Liver biopsies of patients with autoimmune pancreatitis demonstrate primarily portal-based disease with features overall that suggest large duct obstruction.[101] Portal infiltrates consist predominately of lymphocytes, along with variably prominent plasma cells and eosinophils.[101,106] Mild, patchy lobular inflammation is also a common finding and in rare cases can be sufficiently striking to suggest viral hepatitis.[101,106] The liver biopsies usually show at least rare IgG4+ plasma cells, though they may not reach the commonly used threshold of >10 IgG4+ plasma cells/hpf.[101,106]

Unlike primary sclerosing cholangitis, there are no reported cases of isolated small duct IgG4-related sclerosing cholangitis (i.e., without involvement of the extrahepatic biliary tree).[59] However, the microscopic intrahepatic ducts can be involved in conjunction with the large ducts in 26% to 30% of cases.[101,106] The frequency of small duct involvement (defined by the presence of >10 IgG4+ cells) increases when intrahepatic biliary strictures are seen on cholangiography.[106]

Small duct involvement is characterized by dense portal-based lymphoplasmacytic infiltrates with >10 IgG4-positive plasma cells/hpf and an IgG4:IgG-positive plasma cell ratio of greater than 40%.[59,105] Neutrophils are not typically seen.[59] Fibroinflammatory nodules, which may represent an intrahepatic form of storiform fibrosis, may be present.[59,91] Ductopenia and obliterative phlebitis are rarely found.[59] In addition, nonspecific changes of chronic biliary disease are common. The biopsies can show a ductular reaction (59% of cases), canalicular cholestasis (51%), periportal fibrosis (94%), and periportal copper accumulation (24%).[101]

Bile duct biopsy

Cytologic sampling of bile duct epithelium will show only benign epithelial cells. However, endoscopic biopsies of the common bile duct and ampulla of Vater can be diagnostic in some instances, showing prominent IgG4+ plasma cells.[107]

Explants and excisional biopsy findings

When available for evaluation, the large ducts affected by IgG4-related sclerosing cholangitis demonstrate features similar to type 1 autoimmune pancreatitis. In the majority of cases, the fibroinflammatory process is transmural, diffuse, and circumferential.[59] The epithelium in the affected bile ducts is usually intact. Inflammation may be greatest along the periphery of the duct.[95,97,104,108]

Gallbladder

The gallbladder may be a site of involvement in IgG4-related disease, particularly in the setting of autoimmune pancreatitis. The most characteristic feature is dense, trans- or extramural inflammation which is greater than that within the overlying mucosa. This pattern has been identified in 35% to 41% of gallbladders from autoimmune pancreatitis patients.[109,110] Other findings include phlebitis, inflammatory nodules, and increased levels of tissue IgG4.[110,111] Although diffuse lymphoplasmacytic chronic cholecystitis, characterized by a dense, superficial infiltrate of lymphocytes and plasma cells may also be identified, it is not specific for IgG4-related disease and is more common in primary sclerosing cholangitis.[109]

Immunohistochemistry and special stains

The identification of IgG4+ plasma cells plays a central role in the diagnosis of IgG4-related sclerosing cholangitis. Commonly used cutoff values for surgical specimens are >50 IgG4-positive plasma cells/hpf and >10 IgG4-positive plasma cells/hpf for biopsy specimens.[105] In most cases, the IgG4:IgG-positive plasma cell ratio will be greater than 40%.[105] Of note, increased IgG4+ plasma cells is neither entirely sensitive nor specific for IgG4-related sclerosing cholangitis, and the diagnosis cannot be made solely based on IgG4 immunostains. Identifying the pertinent histologic features on H&E sections described above are still critical.

Quantification of IgG4+ plasma cells can be challenging. It is recommended that the number of IgG4+ plasma cells be averaged across three 40× fields, choosing the fields based upon the areas with the greatest concentration of staining.[105] The same three fields should be utilized for counting IgG+ plasma cells.[105]

Differential diagnosis

Primary sclerosing cholangitis

As was discussed in the preceding section, 87% of primary sclerosing cholangitis cases demonstrate involvement of both the intra- and extrahepatic biliary tree.[49] For this reason, IgG4-related sclerosing cholangitis with stenosis in the intra- and extrahepatic ducts is the subtype most likely to be confused with primary sclerosing cholangitis.[98] Primary sclerosing cholangitis preferentially affects younger men (average age of onset 40 years old) with a history of inflammatory bowel disease. In contrast, the majority of IgG4-related sclerosing cholangitis patients are older than 60 and do not have inflammatory bowel disease.[91,92,101]

IgG4-related sclerosing cholangitis typically occurs in the setting of extrahepatic disease.[59,94] By cholangiography, the strictures are usually long and segmental with prestenotic dilatation and frequent involvement of the distal common bile duct.[103] In contrast, the strictures of primary sclerosing cholangitis are typically short and band-like with a beaded or pruned tree appearance.[103] Serum IgG4 is helpful and is elevated in 74% to 80% of patients, with half of individuals having a level which is >2× normal.[59,82] However, elevated IgG4 can also be seen in 9% of patients with primary sclerosing cholangitis so this finding cannot be used in isolation.[112]

Evaluation of explants and surgical resection specimens typically does not pose a diagnostic challenge. Primary sclerosing cholangitis is a fibro-obliterative process that shows marked injury to the surface epithelium with concentric periductal fibrosis and fibrous scars. Surface epithelial erosion or ulceration with a granulomatous response is typical.[59,113] In contrast, the inflammation in IgG4-related sclerosing cholangitis is more homogenous and transmural, is not luminal-centric, and surface epithelial injury is rare.[59]

Two studies have demonstrated that there can be elevated numbers of IgG4+ cells in liver explants from primary sclerosing cholangitis patients.[113,114] However, other characteristic features of IgG4-related sclerosing cholangitis (including storiform fibrosis and obliterative phlebitis) are not seen in these livers. One study found that 23% of 98 primary sclerosing cholangitis explants contained elevated IgG4+ plasma cells involving the hilar and large bile ducts, and 74% of these contained moderate-marked lymphoplasmacytic infiltrates.[114] Approximately 22% had elevated serum IgG4 levels. Similarly, another study identified markedly increases numbers of IgG4+ plasma cells (>100/hpf) in 5% of 41 explants from patients with primary sclerosing cholangitis.[113] These changes involved the hilar and large bile ducts.

As outlined in Table 13.4, needle biopsy specimens can distinguish primary sclerosing cholangitis from IgG4-related sclerosing cholangitis, especially when there is small duct involvement by the latter. Because both are chronic biliary diseases, features such as ductular reaction and periportal copper accumulation are not helpful. However, IgG4-related sclerosing cholangitis is associated with greater portal and lobular inflammation, particularly plasma cells and eosinophils.[91] Needle biopsies of these patients contain at least an occasional IgG4+ plasma cell in the majority of cases. They are less commonly found in primary sclerosing cholangitis.[91] Lymphoplasmacytic inflammation with >10 IgG4 + cells/hpf and fibroinflammatory nodules suggest IgG4-related sclerosing cholangitis, whereas ductopenia and fibro-obliterative lesions suggest a diagnosis of primary sclerosing cholangitis.[24,91]

Table 13.4 Needle biopsy findings in primary sclerosing cholangitis and IgG4-related sclerosing cholangitis

	Primary Sclerosing Cholangitis	IgG4-related Sclerosing Cholangitis
Typical inflammatory cells	Lymphocytes, neutrophils	Lymphocytes, plasma cells, eosinophils No neutrophils
Portal inflammation	Minimal-mild	May be prominent
Lobular inflammation	Minimal-mild	May be prominent
Onion-skin fibrosis	Occasionally	Occasionally
Epithelial cell injury	Common	Absent
Ductular reaction	Common	Occasionally
Ductopenia	Common	Absent
Fibrous nodules	Absent	Occasionally
IgG4+ plasma cells	Absent to rare	Common May reach diagnostic threshold

Cholangiocarcinoma

Cholangiocarcinoma is in the clinical differential when there is isolated involvement of the distal common bile duct, liver hilum, or a combination of these two, especially if the IgG4 infiltrate is tumefactive and not diffuse.[98,99,102] Cholangiography may not be able to differentiate IgG4-sclerosing cholangitis from cholangiocarcinoma in these situations. In addition, approximately 15% of patients with cholangiocarcinoma will also have elevated serum IgG4 levels.[59] Given that the strictures are extrahepatic, percutaneous needle biopsy of the liver would only demonstrate nonspecific features of chronic biliary disease, including ductular reaction, fibrosis, and periportal copper accumulation. Endoscopic procedures play a vital role in the final diagnosis, including biliary cytology sampling and bile duct biopsy.[59,98,107]

Pancreatic carcinoma

As with cholangiocarcinoma, pancreatic carcinoma enters the clinical differential diagnosis in cases with isolated common bile duct involvement.[98] A Mayo Clinic series evaluating serum IgG4 in pancreatic carcinoma and autoimmune pancreatitis demonstrated elevated serum IgG4 levels in 10% of pancreatic cancer cases; however, only 1% had IgG4 levels > 280 mg/dL.[92] Identification of malignant cells on fine needle aspiration or biopsy is diagnostic of pancreatic carcinoma.

Prognosis and treatment

The natural history of IgG4-related sclerosing cholangitis is still under investigation. However, there does appear to be a slight risk of cirrhosis (4 of 53 patients in one study).[96] In general, high dose steroids are administered until remission is achieved, followed by a taper, and then monitoring for disease recurrence.[63,104] Relapses are not uncommon. In the Mayo Clinic series, 53% of patients experienced recurrence of disease after withdrawal of therapy.[96] In addition to relapse, there is also a subset of patients who are refractory to high dose steroids. Several studies have shown that Rituximab can lower serum IgG4 concentrations and induce marked clinical improvement in patients who do not respond to conventional steroid therapy.[115,116]

13.6 MISCELLANEOUS DISORDERS

Drug-induced liver injury

Cholestatic forms of drug-induced liver injury can be either acute or chronic. Acute forms can be associated with significant inflammation, termed *cholestatic hepatitis*, or occur in the absence of inflammation, so-called bland cholestasis.[117,118] The latter is rarely confused with chronic cholangiopathies because it is not associated with features of large duct obstruction. Importantly, lobular cholestasis does not occur until late in the course of primary biliary cirrhosis or primary sclerosing cholangitis, at which point significant fibrosis is usually present (stage 3 or 4).[118] An exception to this would be a dominant stricture in the setting of primary sclerosing cholangitis. However, this type of injury would be associated with features of large duct obstruction, including portal edema, mild inflammation, and ductular reaction.

Drug-induced cholestatic hepatitis can overlap histologically with primary biliary cirrhosis, particularly if there is a granulomatous component. However, the granulomas related to drug-induced injury are often not directed toward the interlobular bile ducts, as they are in primary biliary cirrhosis.[118] Serologic studies (positive AMA) and fibrosis would also support a diagnosis of primary biliary cirrhosis.

Chronic drug-induced liver injury is characterized by biochemical abnormalities lasting longer than 3 months and is often associated with significant bile duct injury and ductopenia.[14,118] This type of drug-induced cholangiopathy may be difficult to distinguish from primary biliary cirrhosis and primary sclerosing cholangitis solely on histologic features. However, chronic drug-mediated injury typically lacks florid duct lesions as well as changes of large duct obstruction. Drugs associated with biliary injury include antimicrobials, antipsychotics, neuroleptics, NSAIDs, and amiodarone.[14,118] Clinical history, in conjunction with negative AMA and normal cholangiogram, support the impression of a drug-induced injury.[118]

Graft versus host disease

Liver involvement by graft versus host disease typically occurs in the setting of bone marrow transplantation. Hepatic graft versus host disease is usually associated with systemic disease (skin and gastrointestinal manifestations). Graft versus host disease is divided into acute (<100 days post transplantation) and chronic (>100 days post transplantation) forms. The histologic findings in acute and chronic graft versus host disease overlap significantly.[14]

The histologic hallmark of graft versus host disease is bile duct injury, which is characterized by both nuclear and cytoplasmic alterations (Figs. 13.39, 13.40, and 13.41).[14,119] Unlike in the tubular gut, apoptosis within biliary epithelial cells is unusual or difficult to find.[120] Instead, there is typically nuclear hyperchromasia and cellular disarray with cytoplasmic vacuolization and eosinophilia.[121,122] There is no consensus on a minimum threshold of bile duct injury to diagnose graft versus host disease,[120] but at the practical level the findings should be more than minimal to have diagnostic specificity and clinical relevance.

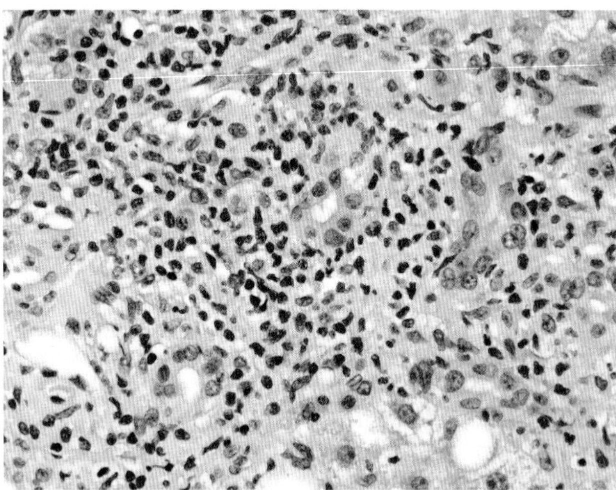

Figure 13.39 Graft versus host disease. Typical example of graft versus host disease characterized by portal-based inflammation with lymphocytic cholangitis and bile duct injury. Bile duct damage is manifested by nuclear disarray, overlapping, and hyperchromasia. Focal cytoplasmic vacuolization is present.

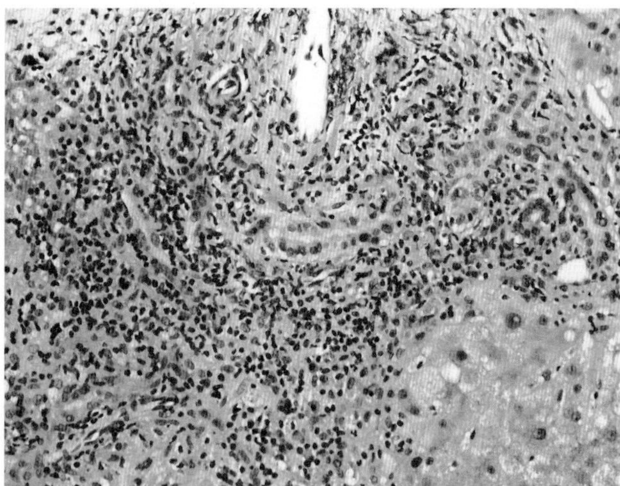

Figure 13.40 Graft versus host disease. In addition to bile duct damage and lymphocytic cholangitis, this field demonstrates portal vein endotheliitis. Though not always present, it is very specific for graft versus host disease.

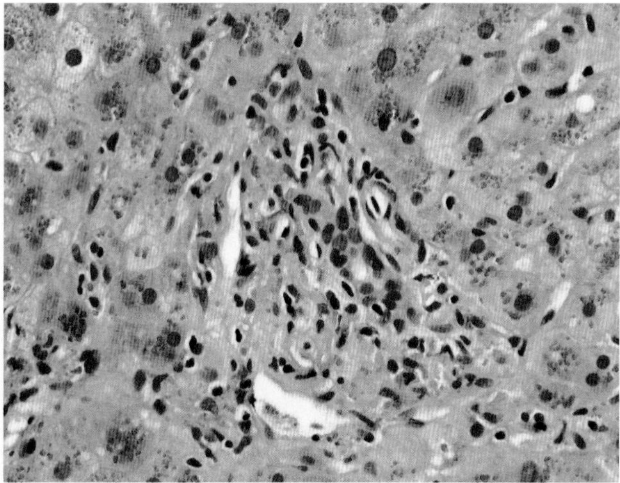

Figure 13.41 Graft versus host disease. In some cases, the portal changes may be very subtle. No expansile infiltrates are present in the portal tract. However, there is lymphocytic cholangitis with mild nuclear hyperchromasia and disarray. In the appropriate setting, the changes are consistent with graft versus host disease.

One study carried out a detailed assessment of hepatic graft versus host disease in 48 biopsy samples.[119] Bile duct injury was present in 98% of specimens. Just over half the cases (52%) demonstrated lymphocytic cholangitis. Importantly, only one-third of cases demonstrated features considered classic for graft versus host disease (bile duct injury with lymphocytic cholangitis and canalicular cholestasis). Although lobular inflammation was present in about three-fourth of biopsies, it was typically mild. However, in 23% of cases it was severe enough to be considered a lobular hepatitis. This hepatitic pattern of graft versus host disease has been reported by others[122] and can be associated with donor lymphocyte infusion,[123] which can be used to treat disease recurrence.

Bile duct injury can eventually lead to ductopenia, which is typically not associated with a ductular reaction (Fig. 13.42). However, a mild ductular reaction can occur in a minority of patients and does not preclude the diagnosis.[119,122] There is conflicting data on the timeline of ductopenia.[119,120] According to the most recent National Institutes of Health (NIH) guidelines, it can be a useful criterion for chronic graft versus host disease.[120] While graft versus host disease is not considered a fibrosing disorder per se, mild portal fibrosis can be seen in around one-third of cases.[119] As with ductopenia, mild fibrosis has been suggested as a possible criterion for chronic graft versus host disease.[120]

Graft versus host disease must be differentiated from infection and drug-induced liver injury.[120] Classic cases of graft versus host disease are relatively straightforward when they show bile duct injury, minimal inflammation, cholestasis, ±ductopenia, and absent ductular reaction in conjunction with cholestatic clinical findings and systemic disease. However, chronic graft versus host disease (>100 days post transplantation) can be more challenging when it presents acutely with marked elevations in transaminase levels and hepatitic histologic changes.[122] In such cases, the typical features of bile duct injury are often present.[122] A clinical history of decreased immunosuppression, well-developed bile duct injury, and extrahepatic disease support the diagnosis of graft versus host disease.[119,122] In some situations it may not

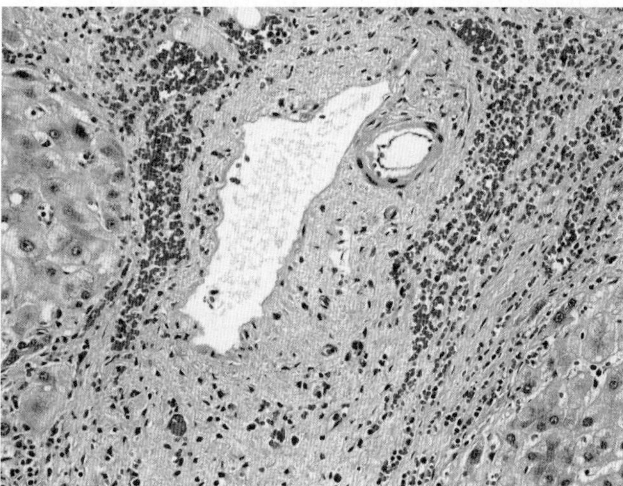

Figure 13.42 Chronic graft versus host. Chronic graft versus host disease may result in ductopenia. No bile duct branch is present in this portal tract. Note the absence of a ductular reaction. Although characteristic of chronic graft versus host disease, a mild ductular reaction may be seen in some cases.

be possible to entirely exclude a drug injury, requiring a descriptive diagnosis with the differential of graft versus host disease versus drug-induced liver injury.

Idiopathic adulthood ductopenia

Idiopathic adulthood ductopenia is a chronic cholestatic disease characterized by the absence of interlobular bile ducts in ≥50% of portal tracts, without an identifiable cause.[3,124] Idiopathic adulthood ductopenia is more common in men than women (M:F, 1.8:1) with a median age of 34 years.[3] Patients present with cholestatic symptoms of jaundice, pruritus, and an elevated alkaline phosphatase.[3]

Idiopathic adulthood ductopenia is uncommon, constituting only 1.2% of 2,082 cases of small duct biliary disease in a Mayo Clinic study.[3] It is a histologic diagnosis, and all other causes of cholangiopathy must be excluded by serologic, radiographic, and pathologic studies. Patients should have an elevated alkaline phosphatase, ductopenia on biopsy, normal imaging, and negative serology for specific diseases (chronic hepatitis C, primary biliary cirrhosis, etc.).[3] In addition, there should be no known exposure to drugs or a history of malignancy that can cause bile duct injury (e.g., Hodgkin disease or Langerhan cell histiocytosis), and no history of inflammatory bowel disease.[3]

Biopsy material from cases of idiopathic adulthood ductopenia show nonspecific chronic biliary disease, including patchy portal inflammation, a mild ductular reaction (may be seen early on in some cases, not present in later disease), hepatocanalicular cholestasis, periportal copper accumulation, and biliary-type fibrosis (Figs. 13.43).[3] By definition, more than half of portal tracts must lack an identifiable interlobular bile duct.[3] Granulomas and neoplastic involvement must be absent.[3]

Idiopathic adulthood ductopenia may represent a final common pathway of several different processes. In younger patients (less than 40 years old), possible etiologies include late-onset nonsyndromic paucity of intrahepatic bile ducts and small duct primary sclerosing cholangitis, in which there is no history of inflammatory bowel disease.[3] In older individuals, resolved autoimmune or viral cholangitis are also possible etiologies.[3]

Segmental cholangiectasia

Segmental cholangiectasia is a rare disorder of uncertain etiology characterized by dilatation of the large intrahepatic bile ducts. It is thought to be related to recurrent pyogenic cholangitis seen in Asian populations.[125] Imaging studies demonstrate ductal dilatation and obstruction which can mimic primary sclerosing cholangitis, IgG-related sclerosing cholangitis, or cholangiocarcinoma.

The clinicopathologic features have also been described in 10 non-Asian patients in the USA.[125] The median age at diagnosis was 70, with an even M:F ratio. There was universal involvement of the left lobe, stones were frequent (70%), and secondary parenchymal atrophy of the left lobe was common (60%). Microscopically, the lesions were characterized by periductal fibrosis and gland hyperplasia with variable inflammation, typically most intense when stones were also present (Fig. 13.44). Concentric onion-skin fibrosis was documented in 30% of cases. Importantly, ductular reaction was absent.

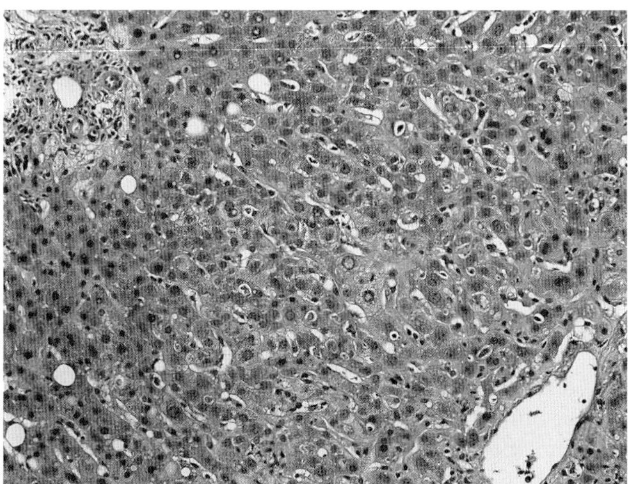

Figure 13.43 Idiopathic adult ductopenia. The portal tract in the left aspect of the field lacks a bile duct, and prominent canalicular cholestasis is present. No features are seen which would suggest a specific etiology.

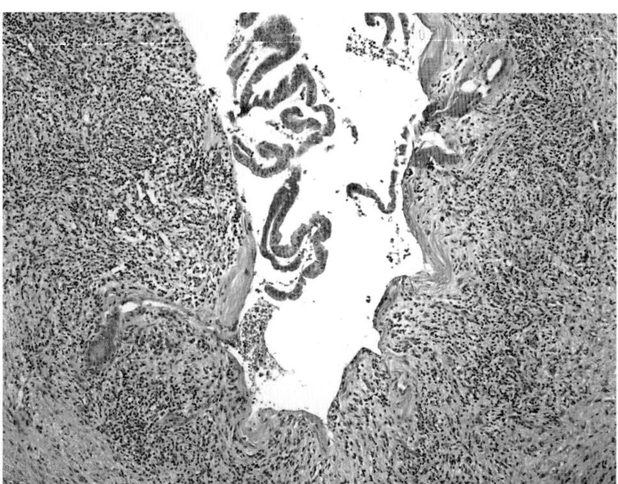

Figure 13.44 Segmental cholangiectasia. Segmental bile duct from the left lobe demonstrating prominent inflammation with erosion of the lining epithelium. There is mild periductal fibrosis. An hepatolith was present in this case.

Cholangiocarcinoma can be excluded by the absence of malignant glands and dysplasia. Segmental cholangiectasia typically occurs in older individuals than primary sclerosing cholangitis. In addition, Zhao et al. identified none of the typical histologic changes of chronic biliary disease in any of their cases, including advanced fibrosis, cholate stasis, fibroobliterative lesions, or ductular reaction.[125] Although a rare IgG4 (+) plasma cell was noted in some cases, diagnostic levels of tissue IgG4 were not present.

REFERENCES

1. Li MK, Crawford JM. The pathology of cholestasis. *Semin Liver Dis*. 2004;24(1):21–42. PubMed PMID: 15085484.
2. Gouw AS, Clouston AD, Theise ND. Ductular reactions in human liver: diversity at the interface. *Hepatology*. 2011;54(5):1853–1863. PubMed PMID: 21983984.
3. Ludwig J. Idiopathic adulthood ductopenia: an update. *Mayo Clin Proc*. 1998;73(3):285–291. PubMed PMID: 9511789.
4. Mounajjed T, Oxentenko AS, Qureshi H, et al. Revisiting the topic of histochemically detectable copper in various liver diseases with special focus on venous outflow impairment. *Am J Clin Pathol*. 2013;139(1):79–86. PubMed PMID: 23270902.
5. Ludwig J, Dickson ER, McDonald GS. Staging of chronic nonsuppurative destructive cholangitis (syndrome of primary biliary cirrhosis). *Virchows Arch A Pathol Anat Histol*. 1978;379(2):103–112. PubMed PMID: 150690.
6. Mendes FD, Kim WR, Pedersen R, et al. Mortality attributable to cholestatic liver disease in the United States. *Hepatology*. 2008;47(4):1241–1247. PubMed PMID: 18318437.
7. Kaplan MM, Gershwin ME. Primary biliary cirrhosis. *N Engl J Med*. 2005;353(12):1261–1273. PubMed PMID: 16177252.
8. Czaja AJ, Carpenter HA. Autoimmune hepatitis with incidental histologic features of bile duct injury. *Hepatology*. 2001;34(4 Pt 1):659–665. PubMed PMID: 11584360.
9. Kim WR, Therneau TM, Wiesner RH, et al. A revised natural history model for primary sclerosing cholangitis. *Mayo Clin Proc*. 2000;75(7):688–694. PubMed PMID: 10907383.
10. Boberg KM, Chapman RW, Hirschfield GM, et al. Overlap syndromes: the International Autoimmune Hepatitis Group (IAIHG) position statement on a controversial issue. *J Hepatol*. 2011;54(2):374–385. PubMed PMID: 21067838.
11. Prince M, Chetwynd A, Newman W, et al. Survival and symptom progression in a geographically based cohort of patients with primary biliary cirrhosis: follow-up for up to 28 years. *Gastroenterology*. 2002;123(4):1044–1051. PubMed PMID: 12360466.
12. Talwalkar JA, Lindor KD. Primary biliary cirrhosis. *Lancet*. 2003;362(9377):53–61. PubMed PMID: 12853201.
13. Lindor KD, Gershwin ME, Poupon R, et al. Primary biliary cirrhosis. *Hepatology*. 2009;50(1):291–308. PubMed PMID: 19554543.
14. Nakanishi Y, Saxena R. Pathophysiology and diseases of the proximal pathways of the biliary system. *Arch Pathol Lab Med*. 2015;139(7):858–866. PubMed PMID: 26125426.
15. Zeman MV, Hirschfield GM. Autoantibodies and liver disease: uses and abuses. *Can J Gastroenterol*. 2010;24(4):225–231. PubMed PMID: 20431809; PubMed Central PMCID: PMC2864616.
16. Rubin E, Schaffner F, Popper H. Primary biliary cirrhosis chronic non-suppurative destructive cholangitis. *Am J Pathol*. 1965;46:387–407. PubMed PMID: 14266218; PubMed Central PMCID: PMC1920366.
17. Scheuer P. Primary biliary cirrhosis. *Proc R Soc Med*. 1967;60(12):1257–1260. PubMed PMID: 6066569; PubMed Central PMCID: PMC1901478.
18. Combes B, Markin RS, Wheeler DE, et al. The effect of ursodeoxycholic acid on the florid duct lesion of primary biliary cirrhosis. *Hepatology*. 1999;30(3):602–605. PubMed PMID: 10462363; NIHMSID: NIHMS515106; PubMed Central PMCID: PMC3935822.
19. Saxena R, Hytiroglou P, Thung SN, et al. Destruction of canals of Hering in primary biliary cirrhosis. *Hum Pathol*. 2002;33(10):983–988. PubMed PMID: 12395370.
20. Lleo A, Maroni L, Glaser S, et al. Role of cholangiocytes in primary biliary cirrhosis. *Semin Liver Dis*. 2014;34(3):273–284. PubMed PMID: 25057951; NIHMSID: NIHMS630454; PubMed Central PMCID: PMC4182310.
21. Khan FM, Komarla AR, Mendoza PG, et al. Keratin 19 demonstration of canal of Hering loss in primary biliary cirrhosis: "minimal change PBC"? *Hepatology*. 2013;57(2):700–707. PubMed PMID: 22911653.
22. Saxena R, Theise N. Canals of Hering: recent insights and current knowledge. *Semin Liver Dis*. 2004;24(1):43–48. PubMed PMID: 15085485.
23. Scheuer PJ. Ludwig Symposium on biliary disorders--part II Pathologic features and evolution of primary biliary cirrhosis and primary sclerosing cholangitis. *Mayo Clin Proc*. 1998;73(2):179–183. PubMed PMID: 9473003.
24. Portmann B, Zen Y. Inflammatory disease of the bile ducts-cholangiopathies: liver biopsy challenge and clinicopathological correlation. *Histopathology*. 2012;60(2):236–248. PubMed PMID: 21668470.

25. Washington MK. Autoimmune liver disease: overlap and outliers. *Mod Pathol.* 2007;20 suppl 1:S15–30. PubMed PMID: 17486048.
26. Nakanuma Y, Ohta G. Quantitation of hepatic granulomas and epithelioid cells in primary biliary cirrhosis. *Hepatology.* 1983;3(3):423–427. PubMed PMID: 6840688.
27. Michieletti P, Wanless IR, Katz A, et al. Antimitochondrial antibody negative primary biliary cirrhosis: a distinct syndrome of autoimmune cholangitis. *Gut.* 1994;35(2):260–265. PubMed PMID: 8307480; PubMed Central PMCID: PMC1374505.
28. Terracciano LM, Patzina RA, Lehmann FS, et al. A spectrum of histopathologic findings in autoimmune liver disease. *Am J Clin Pathol.* 2000;114(5):705–711. PubMed PMID: 11068543.
29. Heathcote EJ. Autoimmune cholangitis. *Clin Liver Dis.* 1998;2(2):303–311, viii–ix. PubMed PMID: 15560034.
30. Chazouillères O, Wendum D, Serfaty L, et al. Primary biliary cirrhosis-autoimmune hepatitis overlap syndrome: clinical features and response to therapy. *Hepatology.* 1998;28(2):296–301. PubMed PMID: 9695990.
31. Gossard AA, Lindor KD. Development of autoimmune hepatitis in primary biliary cirrhosis. *Liver Int.* 2007;27(8):1086–1090. PubMed PMID: 17845536.
32. Daniels JA, Torbenson M, Anders RA, et al. Immunostaining of plasma cells in primary biliary cirrhosis. *Am J Clin Pathol.* 2009;131(2):243–249.
33. Cabibi D, Tarantino G, Barbaria F, et al. Intrahepatic IgG/IgM plasma cells ratio helps in classifying autoimmune liver diseases. *Dig Liver Dis.* 2010;42(8):585–592.
34. Moreira RK, Revetta F, Koehler E, et al. Diagnostic utility of IgG and IgM immunohistochemistry in autoimmune liver disease. *World J Gastroenterol.* 2010;16(4):453–457.
35. Graham RP, Smyrk TC, Zhang L. Evaluation of langerhans cell infiltrate by CD1a immunostain in liver biopsy for the diagnosis of primary biliary cirrhosis. *Am J Surg Pathol.* 2012;36(5):732–736.
36. Kaji K, Nakanuma Y, Sasaki M, et al. Hepatitic bile duct injuries in chronic hepatitis C: histopathologic and immunohistochemical studies. *Mod Pathol.* 1994;7(9):937–945. PubMed PMID: 7892163.
37. Ishak KG. Sarcoidosis of the liver and bile ducts. *Mayo Clin Proc.* 1998;73(5):467–472. PubMed PMID: 9581591.
38. Karagiannidis A, Karavalaki M, Koulaouzidis A. Hepatic sarcoidosis. *Ann Hepatol.* 2006;5(4):251–256. PubMed PMID: 17151576.
39. Murphy JR, Sjogren MH, Kikendall JW, et al. Small bile duct abnormalities in sarcoidosis. *J Clin Gastroenterol.* 1990;12(5):555–561. PubMed PMID: 2229999.
40. Ferrell L. Liver pathology: cirrhosis, hepatitis, and primary liver tumors Update and diagnostic problems. *Mod Pathol.* 2000;13(6):679–704. PubMed PMID: 10874674.
41. Toy E, Balasubramanian S, Selmi C, et al. The prevalence, incidence, and natural history of primary sclerosing cholangitis in an ethnically diverse population. *BMC Gastoenterol.* 2011;11:83.
42. Lindor KD, Kowdley KV, Harrison ME. ACG clinical guideline: primary sclerosing cholangitis. *Am J Gastroenterol.* 2015;110(5):646–659; quiz 660. PubMed PMID: 25869391.
43. Boonstra K, Beuers U, Ponsioen CY. Epidemiology of primary sclerosing cholangitis and primary biliary cirrhosis: a systematic review. *J Hepatol.* 2012;56(5):1181–1188. PubMed PMID: 22245904.
44. Eaton JE, Talwalkar JA, Lazaridis KN, et al. Pathogenesis of primary sclerosing cholangitis and advances in diagnosis and management. *Gastroenterology.* 2013;145(3):521–536. PubMed PMID: 23827861; NIHMSID: NIHMS505873; PubMed Central PMCID: PMC3815445.
45. Molodecky NA, Kareemi H, Parab R, et al. Incidence of primary sclerosing cholangitis: a systematic review and meta-analysis. *Hepatology.* 2011;53(5):1590–1599. PubMed PMID: 21351115.
46. Silveira MG, Lindor KD. Primary sclerosing cholangitis. *Can J Gastroenterol.* 2008;22(8):689–698. PubMed PMID: 18701947; PubMed Central PMCID: PMC2661291.
47. Broomé U, Olsson R, Lööf L, et al. Natural history and prognostic factors in 305 Swedish patients with primary sclerosing cholangitis. *Gut.* 1996;38(4): 610–615. PubMed PMID: 8707097; PubMed Central PMCID: PMC1383124.
48. Feuerstein JD, Tapper EB. Primary sclerosing cholangitis: an update. *OA Hepatology.* 2013;1(1):6.
49. Lee YM, Kaplan MM. Primary sclerosing cholangitis. *N Engl J Med.* 1995;332(14):924–933. PubMed PMID: 7877651.
50. Krones E, Graziadei I, Trauner M, et al. Evolving concepts in primary sclerosing cholangitis. *Liver Int.* 2012;32(3):352–369. PubMed PMID: 22097926.
51. Chapman R, Fevery J, Kalloo A, et al. Diagnosis and management of primary sclerosing cholangitis. *Hepatology.* 2010;51(2):660–678. PubMed PMID: 20101749.
52. Said K, Glaumann H, Bergquist A. Gallbladder disease in patients with primary sclerosing cholangitis. *J Hepatol.* 2008;48(4):598–605. PubMed PMID: 18222013.
53. Brandt DJ, MacCarty RL, Charboneau JW, et al. Gallbladder disease in patients with primary sclerosing cholangitis. *AJR Am J Roentgenol.* 1988;150(3):571–574. PubMed PMID: 3277348.

54. Burak KW, Angulo P, Lindor KD. Is there a role for liver biopsy in primary sclerosing cholangitis? *Am J Gastroenterol.* 2003;98(5):1155–1158. PubMed PMID: 12809842.
55. Chapman RW, Arborgh BA, Rhodes JM, et al. Primary sclerosing cholangitis: a review of its clinical features, cholangiography, and hepatic histology. *Gut.* 1980;21(10):870–877. PubMed PMID: 7439807; PubMed Central PMCID: PMC1419383.
56. Hov JR, Boberg KM, Karlsen TH. Autoantibodies in primary sclerosing cholangitis. *World J Gastroenterol.* 2008;14(24):3781–3791. PubMed PMID: 18609700; PubMed Central PMCID: PMC2721433.
57. Vitellas KM, Keogan MT, Freed KS, et al. Radiologic manifestations of sclerosing cholangitis with emphasis on MR cholangiopancreatography. *Radiographics.* 2000;20(4):959–975; quiz 1108–1109, 1112. PubMed PMID: 10903686.
58. Carrasco-Avino G, Schiano TD, et al. Primary sclerosing cholangitis: detailed histologic assessment and integration using bioinformatics highlights arterial fibrointimal hyperplasia as a novel feature. *Am J Clin Pathol.* 2015;143(4): 505–513. PubMed PMID: 25780002.
59. Zen Y, Kawakami H, Kim JH. IgG4-related sclerosing cholangitis: all we need to know. *J Gastroenterol.* 2016;51(4):295–312. PubMed PMID: 26817943.
60. Ludwig J, Colina F, Poterucha JJ. Granulomas in primary sclerosing cholangitis. *Liver.* 1995;15(6):307–312. PubMed PMID: 8609810.
61. Lewis JT, Talwalkar JA, Rosen CB, et al. Precancerous bile duct pathology in end-stage primary sclerosing cholangitis, with and without cholangiocarcinoma. *Am J Surg Pathol.* 2010;34(1):27–34. PubMed PMID: 19898228.
62. Björnsson E, Olsson R, Bergquist A, et al. The natural history of small-duct primary sclerosing cholangitis. *Gastroenterology.* 2008;134(4):975–980. PubMed PMID: 18395078.
63. Björnsson E, Lindqvist-Ottosson J, Asztely M, et al. Dominant strictures in patients with primary sclerosing cholangitis. *Am J Gastroenterol.* 2004;99(3):502–508. PubMed PMID: 15056092.
64. Hirschfield GM, Karlsen TH, Lindor KD, et al. Primary sclerosing cholangitis. *Lancet.* 2013;382(9904): 1587–1599. PubMed PMID: 23810223.
65. Pohl J, Ring A, Stremmel W, et al. The role of dominant stenoses in bacterial infections of bile ducts in primary sclerosing cholangitis. *Eur J Gastroenterol Hepatol.* 2006;18(1):69–74. PubMed PMID: 16357622.
66. Khaderi SA, Sussman NL. Screening for malignancy in primary sclerosing cholangitis (PSC). *Curr Gastroenterol Rep.* 2015;17(4):17. PubMed PMID: 25786901.
67. Razumilava N, Gores GJ, Lindor KD. Cancer surveillance in patients with primary sclerosing cholangitis. *Hepatology.* 2011;54(5): 1842–1852. PubMed PMID: 21793028; NIHMSID: NIHMS312954; PubMed Central PMCID: PMC3205332.
68. Broomé U, Bergquist A. Primary sclerosing cholangitis, inflammatory bowel disease, and colon cancer. *Semin Liver Dis.* 2006;26(1):31–41. PubMed PMID: 16496231.
69. Bambha K, Kim WR, Talwalkar J, et al. Incidence, clinical spectrum, and outcomes of primary sclerosing cholangitis in a United States community. *Gastroenterology.* 2003;125(5):1364–1369. PubMed PMID: 14598252.
70. Loftus EV Jr, Harewood GC, Loftus CG, et al. PSC-IBD: a unique form of inflammatory bowel disease associated with primary sclerosing cholangitis. *Gut.* 2005;54(1):91–96. PubMed PMID: 15591511; PubMed Central PMCID: PMC1774346.
71. Sinakos E, Samuel S, Enders F, et al. Inflammatory bowel disease in primary sclerosing cholangitis: a robust yet changing relationship. *Inflamm Bowel Dis.* 2013;19(5):1004–1009. PubMed PMID: 23502353.
72. Joo M, Abreu-e-Lima P, Farraye F, et al. Pathologic features of ulcerative colitis in patients with primary sclerosing cholangitis: a case-control study. *Am J Surg Pathol.* 2009;33(6):854–862. PubMed PMID: 19295408.
73. Soetikno RM, Lin OS, Heidenreich PA, et al. Increased risk of colorectal neoplasia in patients with primary sclerosing cholangitis and ulcerative colitis: a meta-analysis. *Gastrointest Endosc.* 2002;56(1):48–54. PubMed PMID: 12085034.
74. Buckles DC, Lindor KD, Larusso NF, et al. In primary sclerosing cholangitis, gallbladder polyps are frequently malignant. *Am J Gastroenterol.* 2002;97(5):1138–1142. PubMed PMID: 12014717.
75. Abdalian R, Heathcote EJ. Sclerosing cholangitis: a focus on secondary causes. *Hepatology.* 2006;44(5):1063–1074. PubMed PMID: 17058222.
76. Gossard AA, Angulo P, Lindor KD. Secondary sclerosing cholangitis: a comparison to primary sclerosing cholangitis. *Am J Gastroenterol.* 2005;100(6):1330–1333. PubMed PMID: 15929765.
77. Geraghty JM, Goldin RD. Liver changes associated with cholecystitis. *J Clin Pathol.* 1994;47(5):457–460. PubMed PMID: 8027400; PubMed Central PMCID: PMC502026.
78. Afroudakis A, Kaplowitz N. Liver histopathology in chronic common bile duct stenosis due to chronic alcoholic pancreatitis. *Hepatology.* 1981;1(1):65–72. PubMed PMID: 7286890.
79. Imam MH, Talwalkar JA, Lindor KD. Secondary sclerosing cholangitis: pathogenesis, diagnosis, and management. *Clin Liver Dis.* 2013;17(2):269–277. PubMed PMID: 23540502.

80. Bouche H, Housset C, Dumont JL, et al. AIDS-related cholangitis: diagnostic features and course in 15 patients. *J Hepatol*. 1993;17(1):34–39. PubMed PMID: 8445217.
81. Chen XM, Keithly JS, Paya CV, et al. Cryptosporidiosis. *N Engl J Med*. 2002;346(22): 1723–1731. PubMed PMID: 12037153.
82. Gao Y, Chin K, Mishriki YY. AIDS cholangiopathy in an asymptomatic, previously undiagnosed late-stage HIV-positive patient from Kenya. *Int J Hepatol*. 2011;2011:465895. PubMed PMID: 21994858; PubMed Central PMCID: PMC3170813.
83. Batts KP. Ischemic cholangitis. *Mayo Clin Proc*. 1998;73(4):380–385. PubMed PMID: 9559044.
84. Ludwig J, Batts KP, MacCarty RL. Ischemic cholangitis in hepatic allografts. *Mayo Clin Proc*. 1992;67(6):519–526. PubMed PMID: 1434878.
85. Deltenre P, Valla DC. Ischemic cholangiopathy. *Semin Liver Dis*. 2008;28(3):235–246. PubMed PMID: 18814077.
86. Krishna M, Keaveny AP, Genco PV, et al. Clinicopathological review of 18 cases of liver allografts lost due to bile duct necrosis. *Transplant Proc*. 2005;37(5):2221–2223. PubMed PMID: 15964383.
87. Chattopadhyay S, Nundy S. Portal biliopathy. *World J Gastroenterol*. 2012;18(43):6177–6182. PubMed PMID: 23180936; PubMed Central PMCID: PMC3501764.
88. Hatemi I, Baysal B, Senturk H, et al. Adult Langerhans cell histiocytosis and sclerosing cholangitis: a case report and review of the literature. *Hepatol Int*. 2010;4(3):653–658. PubMed PMID: 21063491; PubMed Central PMCID: PMC2940001.
89. Kaplan KJ, Goodman ZD, Ishak KG. Liver involvement in Langerhans' cell histiocytosis: a study of nine cases. *Mod Pathol*. 1999;12(4):370–378. PubMed PMID: 10229501.
90. Abedi SH, Ghassami M, Molaei M, et al. Secondary sclerosing cholangitis and Hodgkin's lymphoma. *Clin Med Insights Case Rep*. 2015;8:83–87. PubMed PMID: 26380560; PubMed Central PMCID: PMC4560457.
91. Deshpande V, Sainani NI, Chung RT, et al. IgG4-associated cholangitis: a comparative histological and immunophenotypic study with primary sclerosing cholangitis on liver biopsy material. *Mod Pathol*. 2009;22(10):1287–1295. PubMed PMID: 19633647.
92. Ghazale A, Chari ST, Zhang L, et al. Immunoglobulin G4-associated cholangitis: clinical profile and response to therapy. *Gastroenterology*. 2008;134(3):706–715. PubMed PMID: 18222442.
93. Stone JH, Zen Y, Deshpande V. IgG4-related disease. *N Engl J Med*. 2012;366(6):539–551. PubMed PMID: 22316447.
94. Inoue D, Yoshida K, Yoneda N, et al. IgG4-related disease: dataset of 235 consecutive patients. *Medicine*. 2015;94(15):e680. PubMed PMID: 25881845; PubMed Central PMCID: PMC4602507.
95. Björnsson E, Chari ST, Smyrk TC, et al. Immunoglobulin G4 associated cholangitis: description of an emerging clinical entity based on review of the literature. *Hepatology*. 2007;45(6):1547–1554. PubMed PMID: 17538931.
96. Ohara H, Okazaki K, Tsubouchi H, et al. Clinical diagnostic criteria of IgG4-related sclerosing cholangitis 2012. *J Hepatobiliary Pancreat Sci*. 2012;19(5):536–542. PubMed PMID: 22717980.
97. Kamisawa T, Nakajima H, Egawa N, et al. IgG4-related sclerosing disease incorporating sclerosing pancreatitis, cholangitis, sialadenitis and retroperitoneal fibrosis with lymphadenopathy. *Pancreatology*. 2006;6(1–2):132–137. PubMed PMID: 16327291.
98. Nakazawa T, Naitoh I, Hayashi K, et al. Diagnosis of IgG4-related sclerosing cholangitis. *World J Gastroenterol*. 2013;19(43):7661–7670. PubMed PMID: 24282356; PubMed Central PMCID: PMC3837265.
99. Graham RP, Smyrk TC, Chari ST, et al. Isolated IgG4-related sclerosing cholangitis: a report of 9 cases. *Hum Pathol*. 2014;45(8):1722–1729.
100. Zen Y, Nakanuma Y. IgG4 cholangiopathy. *Int J Hepatol*. 2012;2012:472376. PubMed PMID: 21994885; PubMed Central PMCID: PMC3170733.
101. Umemura T, Zen Y, Hamano H, et al. Immunoglobin G4-hepatopathy: association of immunoglobin G4-bearing plasma cells in liver with autoimmune pancreatitis. *Hepatology*. 2007;46(2):463–471. PubMed PMID: 17634963.
102. Nakazawa T, Ohara H, Sano H, et al. Schematic classification of sclerosing cholangitis with autoimmune pancreatitis by cholangiography. *Pancreas*. 2006;32(2):229. PubMed PMID: 16552350.
103. Nakazawa T, Ohara H, Sano H, et al. Cholangiography can discriminate sclerosing cholangitis with autoimmune pancreatitis from primary sclerosing cholangitis. *Gastrointest Endosc*. 2004;60(6):937–944. PubMed PMID: 15605009.
104. Zen Y, Harada K, Sasaki M, et al. IgG4-related sclerosing cholangitis with and without hepatic inflammatory pseudotumor, and sclerosing pancreatitis-associated sclerosing cholangitis: do they belong to a spectrum of sclerosing pancreatitis? *Am J Surg Pathol*. 2004;28(9):1193–1203. PubMed PMID: 15316319.
105. Deshpande V, Zen Y, Chan JK, et al. Consensus statement on the pathology of IgG4-related disease. *Mod Pathol*. 2012;25(9):1181–1192. PubMed PMID: 22596100.

106. Naitoh I, Zen Y, Nakazawa T, et al. Small bile duct involvement in IgG4-related sclerosing cholangitis: liver biopsy and cholangiography correlation. *J Gastroenterol*. 2011;46(2):269–276. PubMed PMID: 20821235.
107. Kawakami H, Zen Y, Kuwatani M, et al. IgG4-related sclerosing cholangitis and autoimmune pancreatitis: histological assessment of biopsies from Vater's ampulla and the bile duct. *J Gastroenterol Hepatol*. 2010;25(10):1648–1655. PubMed PMID: 20880174.
108. Nakazawa T, Ohara H, Sano H, et al. Clinical differences between primary sclerosing cholangitis and sclerosing cholangitis with autoimmune pancreatitis. *Pancreas*. 2005;30(1):20–25. PubMed PMID: 15632695.
109. Abraham SC, Cruz-Correa M, Argani P, et al. Lymphoplasmacytic chronic cholecystitis and biliary tract disease in patients with lymphoplasmacytic sclerosing pancreatitis. *Am J Surg Pathol*. 2003;27(4):441–451.
110. Wang WL, Farris AB, Lauwers GY, et al. Autoimmune pancreatitis-related cholecystitis: a morphologically and immunologically distinctive form of lymphoplasmacytic sclerosing cholecystitis. *Histopathology*. 2009;54(7):829–836.
111. Leise MD, Smyrk TC, Takahashi N, et al. IgG4-associated cholecystitis: another clue in the diagnosis of autoimmune pancreatitis. *Dig Dis Sci*. 2011;56(5):1290–1294.
112. Mendes FD, Jorgensen R, Keach J, et al. Elevated serum IgG4 concentration in patients with primary sclerosing cholangitis. *Am J Gastroenterol*. 2006;101(9):2070–2075. PubMed PMID: 16879434.
113. Zen Y, Quaglia A, Portmann B. Immunoglobulin G4-positive plasma cell infiltration in explanted livers for primary sclerosing cholangitis. *Histopathology*. 2011;58(3):414–422. PubMed PMID: 21348891.
114. Zhang L, Lewis JT, Abraham SC, et al. IgG4+ plasma cell infiltrates in liver explants with primary sclerosing cholangitis. *Am J Surg Pathol*. 2010;34(1):88–94. PubMed PMID: 20035148.
115. Hart PA, Topazian MD, Witzig TE, et al. Treatment of relapsing autoimmune pancreatitis with immunomodulators and rituximab: the Mayo Clinic experience. *Gut*. 2013;62(11):1607–1615. PubMed PMID: 22936672.
116. Khosroshahi A, Bloch DB, Deshpande V, et al. Rituximab therapy leads to rapid decline of serum IgG4 levels and prompt clinical improvement in IgG4-related systemic disease. *Arthritis Rheum*. 2010;62(6):1755–1762. PubMed PMID: 20191576.
117. Padda MS, Sanchez M, Akhtar AJ, et al. Drug-induced cholestasis. *Hepatology*. 2011;53(4):1377–1387. PubMed PMID: 21480339; NIHMSID: NIHMS284311; PubMed Central PMCID: PMC3089004.
118. Ramachandran R, Kakar S. Histological patterns in drug-induced liver disease. *J Clin Pathol*. 2009;62(6):481–492. PubMed PMID: 19474352.
119. Quaglia A, Duarte R, Patch D, et al. Histopathology of graft versus host disease of the liver. *Histopathology*. 2007;50(6):727–738. PubMed PMID: 17493237.
120. Shulman HM, Cardona DM, Greenson JK, et al. NIH Consensus development project on criteria for clinical trials in chronic graft-versus-host disease: II The 2014 Pathology Working Group Report. *Biol Blood Marrow Transplant*. 2015;21(4):589–603. PubMed PMID: 25639770; NIHMSID: NIHMS666262; PubMed Central PMCID: PMC4359636.
121. Shulman HM, Kleiner D, Lee SJ, et al. Histopathologic diagnosis of chronic graft-versus-host disease: National Institutes of Health Consensus Development Project on Criteria for Clinical Trials in Chronic Graft-versus-Host Disease: II Pathology Working Group Report. *Biol Blood Marrow Transplant*. 2006;12(1):31–47. PubMed PMID: 16399567.
122. Strasser SI, Shulman HM, Flowers ME, et al. Chronic graft-versus-host disease of the liver: presentation as an acute hepatitis. *Hepatology*. 2000;32(6):1265–1271. PubMed PMID: 11093733.
123. Akpek G, Boitnott JK, Lee LA, et al. Hepatitic variant of graft-versus-host disease after donor lymphocyte infusion. *Blood*. 2002;100(12):3903–3907.
124. Ludwig J, Wiesner RH, LaRusso NF. Idiopathic adulthood ductopenia A cause of chronic cholestatic liver disease and biliary cirrhosis. *J Hepatol*. 1988;7(2):193–199. PubMed PMID: 3057064.
125. Zhao L, Hosseini M, Wilcos R, et al. Segmental cholangiectasia clinically worrisome for cholangiocarcinoma: comparison with recurrent pyogenic cholangitis. *Hum Pathol*. 2015;46: 426–433. PubMed PMID: 25600951

14 Pediatric cholestatic liver disease

Marcela Salomao, MD

14.1 INTRODUCTION

Pediatric cholestatic liver diseases are a heterogeneous group of illnesses, including infections, metabolic disorders, congenital malformations, and many others.[1] Liver biopsy interpretation is challenging because major histologic findings commonly overlap and clinicopathologic correlation is almost always required for a final diagnosis. (Fig. 14.1). This chapter will provide a pattern recognition-based approach to describe pediatric diseases associated with cholestasis, with an emphasis on key histopathologic features and common diagnostic pitfalls.

14.2 BILIARY ATRESIA

Introduction

Biliary atresia is an inflammatory and fibrosing disease of extrahepatic bile ducts and represents an important cause of neonatal cholestasis. Early diagnosis is crucial to prevent progression to biliary cirrhosis. Biliary atresia cases are almost always treated with hepatoportoenterostomy (or Kasai procedure), a technique named after its creator, surgeon Morio Kasai, that aims at restoring the bile flow to the small bowel, hence slowing progression to cirrhosis.[2] The procedure yields variable results, with most patients progressing to biliary cirrhosis and ultimately requiring liver transplantation.[3] In fact, biliary atresia is the most common indication for liver transplantation in pediatric patients.

Liver biopsy evaluation plays a key role in the diagnosis of biliary atresia. Awareness about the early changes in the disease and the possible pitfalls is critical in the histologic evaluation of these cases.

Epidemiology

In the United States, biliary atresia occurs at a frequency of 1 in 15,000 live births with seasonal clustering of the disease and higher rates in nonwhite infants.[4] European and Asian studies have demonstrated rates ranging from 1:6,000 in Taiwan to 1:20,000 live births in France, but no seasonal variation was identified.[5–7] Female gender, advanced maternal age, and multiparity are associated with slightly increased

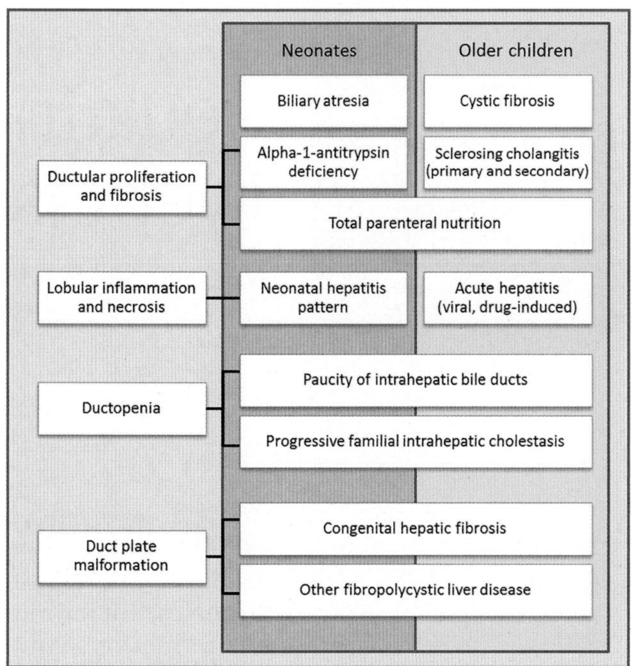

Figure 14.1 Differential diagnosis and key histologic features of cholestasis in neonates and older children.

risk for the disease.[8,9] Splenic malformation and other syndromic features are present in about 10% of cases. Reports of familial biliary atresia are exceptionally rare[10] and studies of twin infants showed discordance of presentation.[11,12]

Classification

Biliary atresia can be broadly classified as nonsyndromic (or perinatal), syndromic (or embryonic), and cystic. Nonsyndromic biliary atresia accounts for 80% of cases and is not typically associated with other malformations. Syndromic biliary atresia represents about 10% of cases and encompasses a heterogeneous group of patients, who present with early onset jaundice and, many times, absent extrahepatic biliary tree. Macroscopic splenic malformations are classically described in syndromic biliary atresia, a condition named biliary atresia-splenic malformation syndrome. Biliary atresia-splenic malformation syndrome typically occurs together with other malformations, including situs inversus, intestinal malrotations, portal vein anomalies, and cardiac defects. The syndrome occurs more frequently in females, has a higher association with maternal diabetes, and has a worse outcome following Kasai procedure.[13,14] Syndromic cases are often referred to as "early" or "embryonic" forms and nonsyndromic biliary atresia as "late" or "perinatal," presuming that timing of disease in syndromic cases is different than nonsyndromic biliary atresia. More recent studies have demonstrated that this temporal classification may be too simplistic and therefore should be avoided until studies with better definitions and better group homogeneity are made available.[15] The cystic variant of biliary atresia represents 8% of patients and is characterized by cystic dilatation of the atretic biliary remnants. Some cases can be detected prenatally, and jaundice may occur early or late. Cystic biliary atresia appears to have a better prognosis than syndromic and nonsyndromic cases.[16]

Etiology and pathogenesis

Biliary atresia is a multifactorial disease, and its exact etiology remains unclear. Recent studies suggest that developmental, environmental, and immune elements play a role in the disease. Infectious etiologies have been proposed but never confirmed, whereas the clustering of biliary atresia cases in Australia livestock suggests that toxins can lead to the development of disease.[17,18] Mutations in the *CFC1* gene have been associated with biliary atresia-splenic malformation cases.[19]

Clinical presentation

Jaundice is the first and most important manifestation of biliary atresia, occurring anywhere from birth to 8 weeks of age. In most cases, infants are born at full term and are healthy in the first weeks of life. Acholic stools and dark urine may be present, but are often unrecognized by parents. Patients who present later in the course of disease often have hepatosplenomegaly. Conjugated hyperbilirubinemia (>2 mg/dL) and extremely high levels of γ-glutamyl transpeptidase (GGT) are typical. Recent studies show that conjugated bilirubin levels are slightly elevated in the asymptomatic early stages of disease and suggest that serum bilirubin concentrations or stool color cards can be useful as newborn screening tools.[20]

Imaging findings

When the diagnosis of biliary atresia is suspected, abdominal ultrasound is performed to rule out anatomical anomalies, such as choledochal cysts, polycystic liver/kidney disease, Caroli disease, and tumors. In biliary atresia, ultrasonographic evaluation demonstrates an absent or abnormal gallbladder. When present, portal hypertension can usually be identified on ultrasound. Other possible findings include an absent common bile duct, the "triangular cord" sign (triangular echogenic density present immediately above the porta hepatis), and an abnormal gallbladder shape.[21]

Following abdominal ultrasound, hepatobiliary scintigraphy is performed to evaluate the patency of the extrahepatic biliary tree using a technetium-labeled iminodiacetic acid analogous compound as a marker. Absent excretion of the marker into the bowel strongly supports the diagnosis of biliary atresia. This test is found to be 100% sensitive and 93% specific when patients are pretreated with phenobarbital.[22] Magnetic resonance cholangiography is another imaging modality of high diagnostic accuracy.[23]

Liver biopsy is performed in nearly all infants with suspected biliary atresia. The main purpose of the biopsy is to confirm the diagnosis of biliary tract obstruction by histology and to exclude diseases that may mimic biliary atresia. Following scans and liver biopsy, patients undergo intraoperative cholangiogram, the gold standard for the diagnosis of biliary atresia. The presence of biliary obstruction on intraoperative cholangiogram confirms the diagnosis of biliary atresia and is usually followed by hepatoportoenterostomy at the time of examination.

Histopathologic features

On liver biopsies, the histologic findings of biliary atresia are not entirely specific, requiring correlation with clinical and laboratorial findings. Microscopically, there is marked cholestasis in the form of canalicular, hepatocellular, and ductular bile accumulation. Features of large bile duct obstruction are almost always present, including portal edema, fibrosis, and ductular proliferation (Figs. 14.2 and 14.3). Mild neutrophilic infiltrates typically accompany the proliferating bile ductules. In addition, the lobular parenchyma may show centrilobular hepatocyte swelling with or without features of cholate stasis, namely periportal hepatocellular swelling, cytoplasmic rarefaction, and Mallory–Denk bodies. Periportal accumulation of copper-binding protein is sometimes present. Extramedullary hematopoiesis is often seen and needs to be differentiated from inflammation. The presence of significant inflammation, apoptosis, or confluent necrosis should raise the possibility of an alternative diagnosis, such as neonatal hepatitis (Table 14.1). Giant cell transformation of hepatocytes, a feature classically described in neonatal hepatitis, can occur in biliary atresia (Fig. 14.2). Liver biopsies performed at earlier stages will demonstrate less conspicuous findings and may be harder to differentiate from other processes (Fig. 14.4). Later, portal-based fibrosis

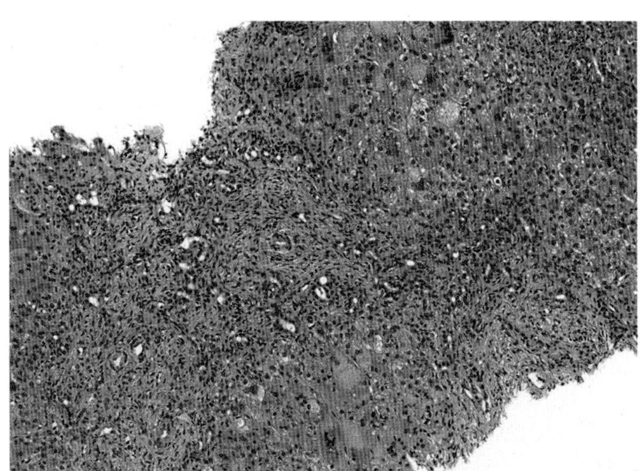

Figure 14.2 Biliary atresia. Portal tracts are expanded by fibrosis and ductular proliferation. Note multinucleated giant hepatocytes (**upper center**; **lower center**).

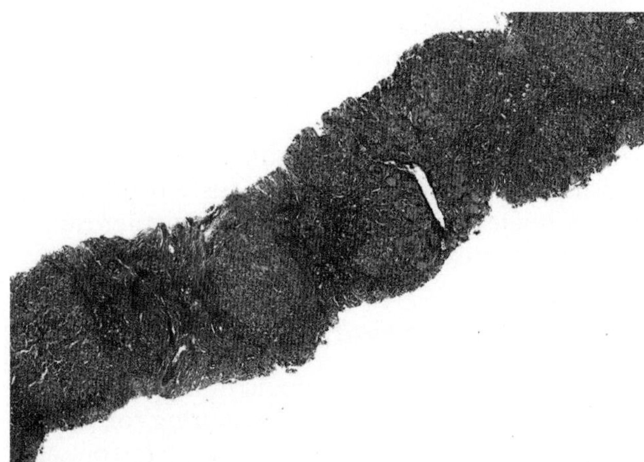

Figure 14.3 Biliary atresia. Masson-trichrome stain demonstrates extensive bridging fibrosis in a 16-week-old patient.

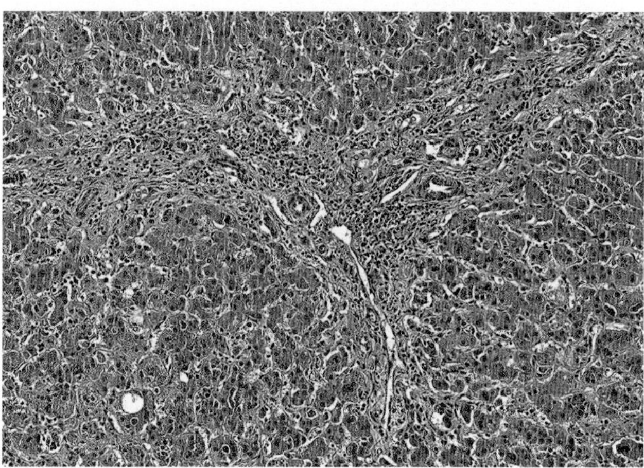

Figure 14.4 Biliary atresia. At earlier stages, cholestasis and minimal portal changes may be the only findings. This biopsy was obtained at 9 weeks of age.

Table 14.1 Clinical and histopathologic features of biliary atresia and neonatal hepatitis syndrome

Histology	
Biliary atresia	Neonatal hepatitis
Ductular proliferation	Lobular inflammation
Portal-based fibrosis	Confluent necrosis
Absence of lobular inflammation/apoptosis	
Absence of confluent necrosis	
Clinical Features	
Elevated GGT	GGT normal or mildly elevated
Nonexcreting IDA scan	Normal imaging of biliary tree
Normal A1AT phenotype	
No history of TPN	

Abbreviations: A1AT, α-1-antitrypsin; GGT, γ-glutamyl transpeptidase; IDA, technetium-labeled diisopropyl iminodiacetic acid; TPN, total parenteral nutrition.

can progress to bridging and nodularity. The loss of native bile ducts also occurs in the later stages of disease.[24] Occasionally, bile duct plate malformations may be present and have been reported to predict a worse clinical outcome.[25]

Typically, a Kasai procedure is performed at the time of intraoperative cholangiogram. In this procedure, a loop of small intestine is anastomosed to the hepatic hilum, after the biliary remnant and portal fibrous plate have been resected. The resected specimen that results from a Kasai procedure consists of a fibrotic/atrophic segment of the extrahepatic bile duct (Fig. 14.5). Proper orientation of the specimen by the surgeon and the pathologist is a key step in the evaluation of a Kasai specimen. The proximal aspect of the specimen contains the portal plate and surrounding liver parenchyma. Distally, the specimen contains a segment of common hepatic duct, the cystic duct, and gallbladder, and finally a segment of common bile duct. The gallbladder is typically smaller than normal and might not have a lumen. Sampling should include the portal plate and consecutive sections of the extrahepatic biliary tree, including the gallbladder remnant. Sections of the atretic bile duct demonstrate partial to total luminal occlusion by fibrosis and variable inflammation (Fig. 14.6). Evaluation of the portal plate is recommended because the presence of large-caliber bile ducts (150 to 200 μm) within the portal plate is associated with a better clinical prognosis, while

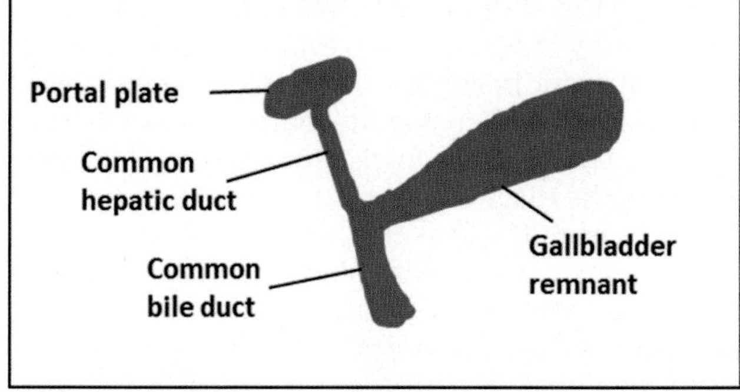

Figure 14.5 Kasai specimen. The components of a Kasai specimen that should be sampled for microscopic examination.

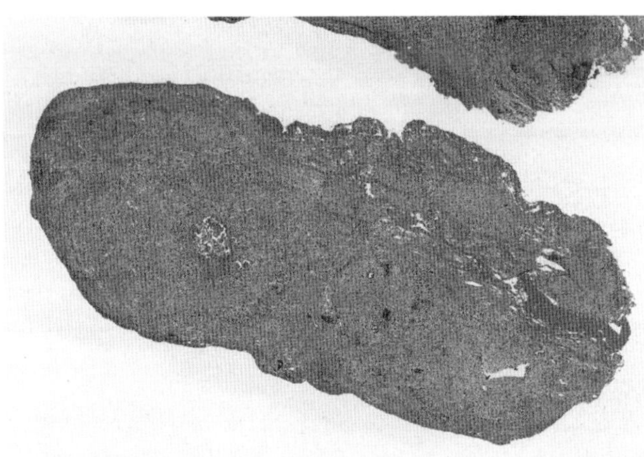

Figure 14.6 Kasai specimen. Cross-section of partially occluded bile duct with fibrosis, chronic inflammation and inspissated luminal bile.

scant small bile ducts in the portal plate sections are associated with a worse prognosis and lower survival (Fig. 14.7).[26,27,28]

Explant specimens from patients who have failed a Kasai procedure and proceeded to liver transplantation will show a shrunken and cirrhotic liver with the typical features of biliary cirrhosis. Histologically, incomplete nodule formation can confer a "geographic" appearance. Features of large bile duct obstruction are present throughout the specimen. At this stage, inflammation, injury, and loss of interlobular bile ducts may be present. Prolonged cholestasis will result in cholate stasis. Extramedullary hematopoiesis and giant multinucleated hepatocytes are less common, unless liver transplantation occurs at an early stage of disease. Hepatocellular carcinoma is a rare complication, reported in less than 1% of biliary atresia patients.[29] Large regenerative nodules are described in patients that have undergone Kasai procedure and may mimic hepatocellular neoplasms.[30]

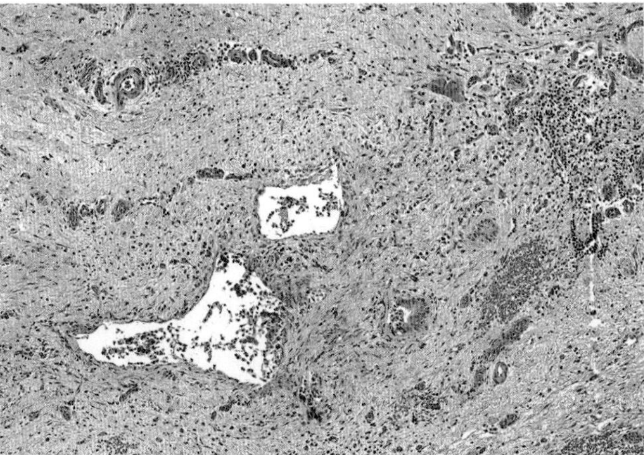

Figure 14.7 Kasai specimen. Sampling of hepatic plate will demonstrate the degree of bile duct patency. In this example, denuded medium-sized bile ducts are present.

Differential diagnosis

The differential diagnosis should include diseases that can mimic biliary atresia both clinically and histologically (Fig. 14.1). As biliary atresia is managed surgically, the correct diagnosis is critical to avoid unnecessary procedures. Ductular proliferation, well-established portal fibrosis, and the absence of sinusoidal fibrosis are the most predictive diagnostic features of biliary atresia.[31] It is important to remember that early in the disease (less than 6 to 8 weeks), these findings may not have developed, and the liver biopsy may need to be repeated. Scant biopsy samples may also lack diagnostic features of biliary atresia, and a minimum of 10 portal tracts should be required for adequate assessment. Of note, liver biopsies of patients with α-1-antitrypsin (A1AT) deficiency and total parenteral nutrition (TPN)-related hepatopathy may be identical to early changes of biliary atresia. In order to exclude these possibilities, the pathologist should be aware of the clinical history, and if needed, suggest further testing, because A1AT globules are typically not evident in liver biopsies of neonates. More recently, ultrastructural analysis of cases originally diagnosed as biliary atresia identified a subset of patients with anomalous canalicular microvilli and abnormalities in villin expression. These have been postulated as a novel cause of cholestatic liver disease mimicking biliary atresia.[32]

Complications

The natural history of untreated biliary atresia is characterized by death within the first 2 years of life. Biliary cirrhosis develops early in the course of disease. Approximately half of patients treated with a Kasai procedure will improve, whereas the other half will require liver transplantation. Following liver transplantation, prognosis is favorable, and long-term survival is approximately 85% at 10 years.[33]

14.3 NEONATAL HEPATITIS

Neonatal hepatitis syndrome is a cholestatic syndrome characterized by hepatocellular injury occurring in the neonatal period. A number of possible etiologies has been associated with the neonatal hepatitis pattern, including infections, inborn errors of metabolism, anatomical defects, and many others (Table 14.2). Among infectious etiologies, TORCH infections, especially *Cytomegalovirus*, remain an important

Table 14.2 Etiology of neonatal hepatitis

Etiology
Infections
TORCH infections (congenital Toxoplasmosis, Others such as syphilis, varicella-zoster, parvovirus B19, Rubella, Cytomegalovirus, Herpes simplex), viral hepatitis B and C, HHV-6, HIV, bacterial infections, listeria, and tuberculosis
Metabolic disorders
α-1-Antitrypsin deficiency, galactosemia, tyrosinemia, fructosemia, glycogen storage disorder type IV, Niemann–Pick disease Types A and C, Gaucher disease, Wolman disease, inborn errors of bile acid metabolism, Zellweger syndrome, citrullinemia Type II, mitochondrial DNA depletion syndrome, panhypopituitarism, hypothyroidism, and Dubin–Johnson syndrome
Immune-mediated diseases
ABO incompatibility, neonatal lupus erythematosus, and neonatal hepatitis with neonatal hemolytic anemia
Idiopathic

cause.[34] Other considerations include sepsis (*Escherichia coli*) and other viral processes (*Coxsackievirus*, *Echovirus*, *Herpesvirus*, and *Adenovirus*). The syndrome is more commonly described in male infants and is associated with prematurity and low-birth weight.[35] Clinically, not all patients will have noticeable jaundice, but conjugated hyperbilirubinemia is consistently present.

When evaluating a liver biopsy, it is key to exclude biliary atresia as this distinction directly affects patient management and outcome.

Histologically, neonatal hepatitis is characterized by cholestasis, prominent giant cell transformation of hepatocytes, and extramedullary hematopoiesis (Figs. 14.8 and 14.9). Portal and lobular inflammation and lobular apoptosis are helpful diagnostic findings, but are not always present (Fig. 14.10). Portal tracts may have inflammation and mild fibrosis. Significant ductular proliferation and advanced fibrosis are typically absent. Small, "hypoplastic" interlobular bile ducts were described in about one-third of cases and can be easily mistaken for ductopenia.[36] CK7 immunohistochemistry is useful in delineating native bile ducts and ductular proliferation. A minority of cases show massive/submassive necrosis, characterized by extensive parenchymal loss and collapse of the reticulin framework, in a pattern most commonly associated with gestational alloimmune disease (neonatal hemochromatosis, see

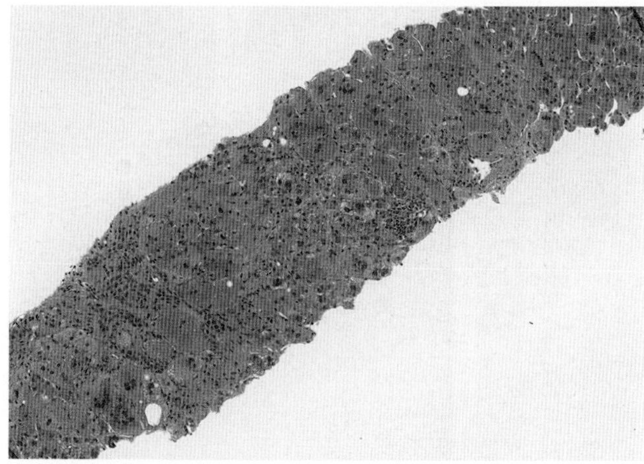

Figure 14.8 Neonatal hepatitis. Prominent giant cell transformation of hepatocytes and extramedullary erythropoiesis.

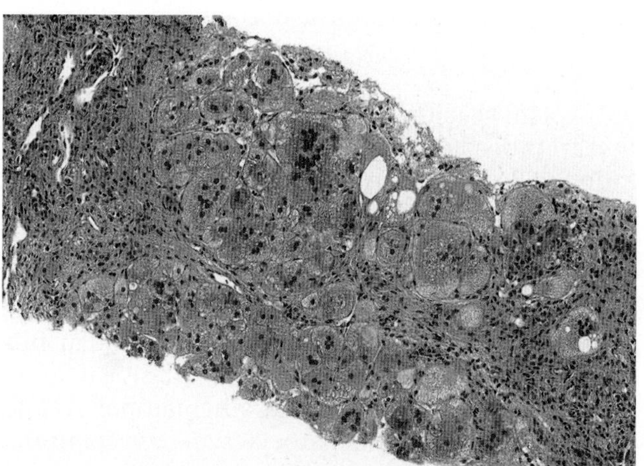

Figure 14.9 Neonatal hepatitis. Multinucleated giant hepatocytes predominate in this centrilobular region. Note the lack of significant ductular proliferation and portal fibrosis.

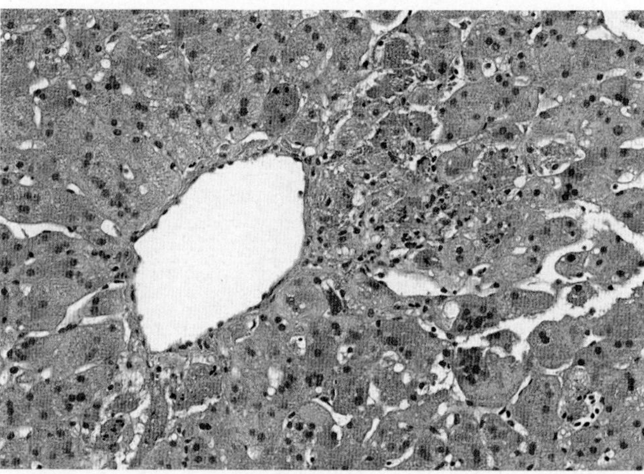

Figure 14.10 Neonatal hepatitis. Lobular inflammation and apoptosis.

Chapter 17), viral hepatitis B and certain metabolic disorders. A diligent search for viral cytopathic effect is important in identifying infectious hepatitis, and immunohistochemical studies may be useful in this setting.

Following a histologic diagnosis of neonatal hepatitis, patients usually undergo further testing. Patients found to have viral diseases may benefit from antiviral therapy, whereas cases of tyrosinemia, defects in bile acid synthesis, and hypopituitarism can be managed with appropriate pharmacotherapy. Idiopathic neonatal hepatitis still accounts for 25% of cases.[34,37,38] Higher mortality rates are seen in patients with severe inflammation in the biopsy, prolonged jaundice, acholic stools, familial disease, and unremitting hepatosplenomegaly.[39]

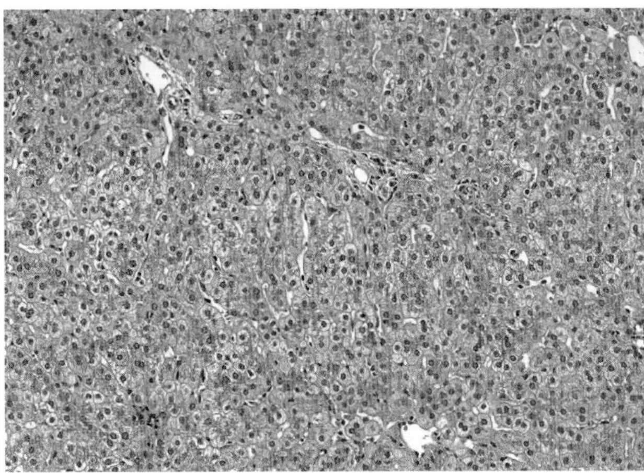

Figure 14.11 Paucity of intrahepatic bile ducts. Mild canalicular cholestasis and ductopenia without significant fibrosis or ductular proliferation.

14.4 PAUCITY OF INTRAHEPATIC BILE DUCTS

Syndromic paucity of intrahepatic bile ducts (Alagille syndrome)

As described by Alagille and colleagues,[40,41] this disease, also known as arteriohepatic dysplasia, is characterized by bile duct loss, cholestatic liver injury, and distinct extrahepatic malformations, including congenital heart disease, dysmorphic facies (inverted triangle with broad forehead and pointy chin, mild hypertelorism, and deep-set eyes), posterior embryotoxon in the eye, butterfly-shaped vertebrae, and renal abnormalities.[42,43] Nonsyndromic cases are also described and include a vast number of diseases discussed later in this chapter.

Alagille syndrome affects 1:30,000 live births and is classified into two types: Alagille syndrome 1 and Alagille syndrome 2. Alagille syndrome 1 accounts for over 90% of cases and is caused by *JAGGED1* gene mutations.[44] The gene is located on chromosome 20p12 and encodes the ligand for Notch-1 receptor. Alagille syndrome 1 can have an autosomal dominant inheritance pattern with high penetrance and variable expression, whereas approximately 70% of cases are sporadic.[45,46] Alagille syndrome 2 affects a very small proportion of cases, is associated with more severe renal disease, and is caused by mutations in the *NOTCH2* gene.[47]

In addition to extrahepatic malformations, a number of liver anomalies have been reported, including portal vein hypoplasia, hypoplasia of the extrahepatic biliary tree, and hypoplasia of the gallbladder. Endoscopic retrograde cholangiopancreatography (ERCP) may show narrowing of the biliary ducts and decreased arborization of the biliary tree.[48]

Microscopically, the disease is characterized by cholestasis and, by definition, loss of more than 50% of the bile ducts (Fig. 14.11). However, ductopenia may not be well developed before 6 months of age and its absence does not preclude the diagnosis.[49] Ductular proliferation is not typical. Cases presenting early may show giant cell transformation and, over time, cholate stasis. Portal fibrosis tends to be absent or mild, and progression to cirrhosis is rare.[40,50]

The differential diagnosis for Alagille syndrome includes other diseases associated with ductopenia. The clinical history of extrahepatic congenital malformations, including the typical facies, helps guide the diagnosis. Although a lack of CD10 canalicular staining by immunohistochemistry is described an Alagille syndrome, its diagnostic utility is limited by the physiologic loss of CD10 staining seen in healthy children younger than 2 years.[51]

The prognosis of patients with Alagille syndrome is better if jaundice resolves early. About one-fourth of patients die from severe cardiac or liver disease.[43] Liver transplantation can be an option in patients who develop liver failure, intractable pruritus, or severe growth delay.

Nonsyndromic paucity of intrahepatic bile ducts

Similarly to Alagille syndrome, this group of diseases presents with cholestasis and ductopenia, but lacks the classical congenital abnormalities. These cases are classified under the term "nonsyndromic paucity of intrahepatic bile ducts." Table 14.3 lists the disease processes implicated in this group.

Table 14.3 Etiology of nonsyndromic paucity of intrahepatic bile ducts

Infections: congenital CMV, syphilis, rubella
Metabolic: cystic fibrosis, α-1-antitrypsin deficiency, disorders of bile acid synthesis, Zellweger syndrome, mitochondrial disorders
Drug toxicity: antibiotics, carbamazepine
Chromosomal: trisomy 17, trisomy 18, trisomy 21, Turner syndrome
Chronic diseases: graft-versus-host disease, chronic rejection, Langerhans cell histiocytosis, sclerosing cholangitis
Idiopathic

14.5 PROGRESSIVE FAMILIAL INTRAHEPATIC CHOLESTASIS

Progressive familial intrahepatic cholestasis (PFIC) consists of three autosomal recessive diseases (referred to as PFIC1, PFIC2, and PFIC3) characterized by intrahepatic cholestasis that most commonly presents in infancy or early childhood. Each form of PFIC is caused by mutations in different canalicular proteins, which are involved in the transport or formation of bile: familial intrahepatic cholestasis Type 1 (FIC1), bile salt export pump (BSEP), and multidrug resistance protein 3 (MDR3) mutations are described in PFIC1, 2, and 3, respectively.

PFIC was first described in Amish kindred.[52] Clinically, it manifests with cholestasis, conjugated hyperbilirubinemia and high plasma bile acids. A distinctive finding in PFIC1 and PFIC2 is low (or normal) serum GGT. On liver biopsy, the three diseases can be indistinguishable as they share many histologic findings, including cholestasis, portal inflammation, ductular proliferation and fibrosis. Luckily, there are some unique histologic findings that correlate with each entity. Table 14.4 lists helpful clinical and histopathologic features that may help differentiate one type from another.

Progressive familial intrahepatic cholestasis type 1

PFIC Type 1 (PFIC1) is caused by a mutation in the *ATP8B1* gene, resulting in diminished expression of FIC1, a protein also deficient in benign, recurrent, intrahepatic cholestasis (BRIC).[53] Currently, PFIC1 and BRIC are grouped under the term FIC1 deficiency. Clinically, PFIC1 presents with persistent cholestasis, resulting in intractable pruritus and jaundice. FIC1 protein is also expressed in the pancreas, and its deficiency may cause pancreatitis in a minority of cases. Serum bile acid levels are high, and GGT levels are

Table 14.4 Comparison of features in PFIC

	PFIC1 (FIC1 deficiency)	PFIC2 (BSEP deficiency)	PFIC3 (MDR3 deficiency)
Mutated gene	*ATP8B1*	*ABCB11*	*ABCB4*
Clinical manifestations	Presents at birth Extrahepatic symptoms Low/normal GGT	Presents at birth No extrahepatic symptoms Low/normal GGT Progression to cirrhosis within 1 year	Presents later (1 mo–20 yr) High GGT
Histology	Cholestasis Late portal inflammation and fibrosis Small hepatocytes	Cholestasis Hepatitic features (giant cells, lobular inflammation, and hepatocyte necrosis) Early fibrosis, duct loss Late ductular proliferation	Cholestasis Early ductular proliferation Early portal fibrosis
Complications	Steatohepatitis Cirrhosis within 2–3 yr	HCC, cholangiocarcinoma, pancreatic tumors	Cirrhosis within 5 mo–20 yr
		Cirrhosis within 6 mo–10 yrs	
		Recurs after liver transplantation	

Abbreviations: PFIC, progressive familial intrahepatic cholestasis; GGT, γ-glutamyl transpeptidase.

low or normal. Electron microscopy evaluation shows a distinct granular appearance of the bile, described as Byler bile.[54]

The liver biopsy shows canalicular cholestasis and smaller hepatocytes with higher nucleous–cytoplasm ratio, resembling hepatobiliary hepatocytes.[55] Bile duct paucity is not a characteristic finding, but may be seen with progression of the disease. Compared to PFIC Type 2 (PFIC2), PFIC1 shows a slower progression to cirrhosis, which usually occurs after 3 years of life. The diagnosis of PFIC1 can be established by electron microscopy and/or genetic studies. Treatment options include partial external biliary diversion and liver transplantation. Steatosis and steatohepatitis are a common complication in liver allografts and may be related to malnutrition or impaired intestinal absorption of bile acids.[56]

Progressive familial intrahepatic cholestasis type 2

PFIC2 is caused by a mutation in the *ABCB11* gene, which is located on chromosome 2q24-31, resulting in deficient expression of BSEP in hepatocytes.[57] The disease manifests early in the neonatal period with jaundice and pruritus. High bile acid levels and low serum GGT are characteristic of this disease. In contrast to PFIC1, transaminases may be more significantly elevated. Serum α-feto protein levels can also be elevated.

The histologic features are quite variable in PFIC2 (Figs. 14.12, 14.13, and 14.14).[58] Cholestasis is always present. In infants, the liver biopsy may demonstrate giant multinucleated hepatocytes. Some cases show features of neonatal hepatitis, including necroinflammation, hepatocellular swelling, and giant cell transformation. Cholestasis is both hepatocellular and canalicular and tends to involve predominantly centrilobular areas. Ductular proliferation and bile duct paucity appear later in the course of disease. PFIC2 patients typically progress to cirrhosis rapidly, with many individuals having cirrhosis within as early as 6 months. Ductopenia and prominent hepatocellular CK7 immunostaining (intermediate hepatocytes) may be seen in the cirrhotic livers (Fig. 14.15).[59] Patients who develop cirrhosis are known to carry more aggressive genotypes.[60]

By immunohistochemistry, the absence of canalicular BSEP expression supports the diagnosis. However, the presence of BSEP staining does not exclude BSEP deficiency because complete BSEP loss occurs only in the setting of protein-truncating mutations.[57] In the remaining cases, BSEP staining may be normal (Fig. 14.16). In such cases, genotype analysis may provide a more definitive diagnosis.

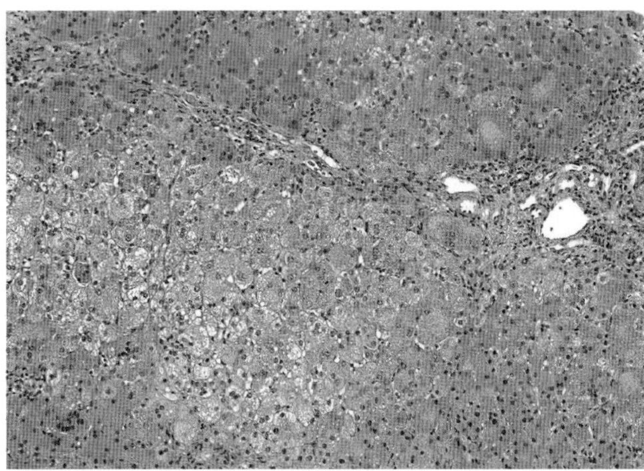

Figure 14.13 Progressive familial intrahepatic cholestasis 2. Lobular inflammation and apoptosis.

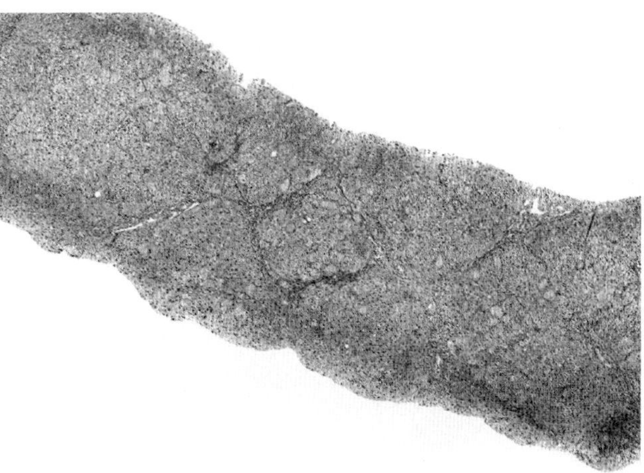

Figure 14.14 Progressive familial intrahepatic cholestasis 2. Masson-trichrome stain demonstrating bridging fibrosis

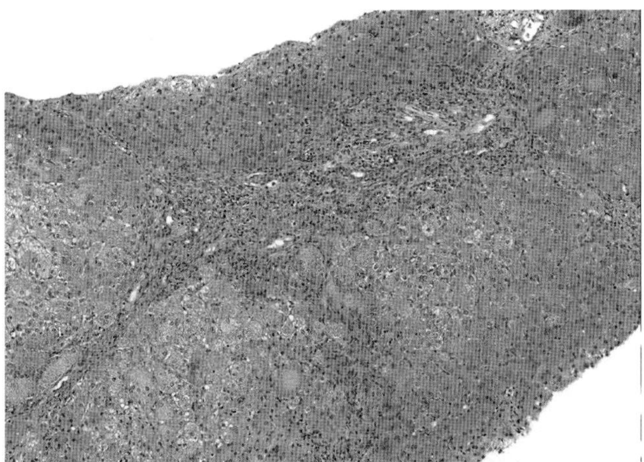

Figure 14.12 Progressive familial intrahepatic cholestasis 2. Mild portal inflammation, ductular proliferation, and periportal fibrosis. Note multinucleated giant hepatocytes (**lower center**).

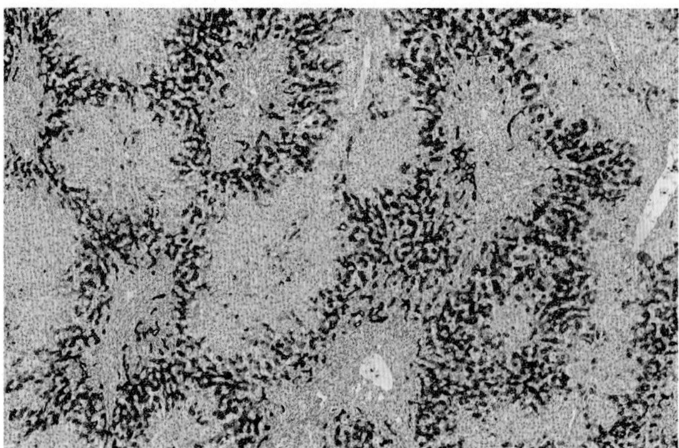

Figure 14.15 Progressive familial intrahepatic cholestasis 2. CK7 immunohistochemistry demonstrates bile duct paucity, which can occur in progressive familial intrahepatic cholestasis 1 and 2. Note the bile ductular proliferation and intermediate hepatobiliary cells.

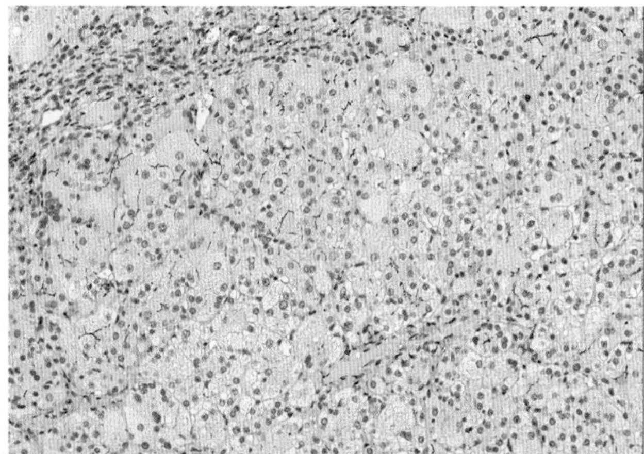

Figure 14.16 Progressive familial intrahepatic cholestasis 2. BSEP immunohistochemistry shows patchy canalicular staining of hepatocytes.

Treatment options are similar to those offered to PFIC1 patients. Hepatocellular carcinoma and cholangiocarcinoma are known complications of PFIC2. Hepatocellular carcinoma occurs in young patients and has been described as early as 2 years of age.[61] Interestingly, PFIC2 cases managed with liver transplantation can recur, and recurrence has been associated with the development of autoantibodies against normal donor-derived BSEP.[62,63]

Progressive familial intrahepatic cholestasis type 3

PFIC Type 3 (PFIC3) is caused by mutations in the *ABCB4* gene, which encodes MDR3, a flippase responsible for bile secretion. MDR3 deficiency has also been implicated in other liver diseases, including intrahepatic cholestasis of pregnancy and drug-induced cholestasis. PFIC3 presents with jaundice, hepatomegaly, and acholic stools. Unlike PFIC1 and PFIC2, this disease tends to present later in life, anywhere from 1 month to over 20 years of age, and presents with GGT elevation.[64] Microscopically, liver biopsies obtained early in the disease may show ductular proliferation and portal fibrosis (Fig. 14.12). Cholestasis tends to predominate in hepatocytes, but canalicular and ductular cholestasis can also be present. Ductopenia is not a feature of PFIC3. Recently, MDR3 immunohistochemistry has become available. Similarly to PFIC2, complete loss of MDR3 expression correlates with truncating mutations of *ABCB4* gene, and normal MDR3 expression may be seen with other mutations.[65] Genetic testing is helpful in establishing the diagnosis. Varying presentations and progression of disease have been associated with specific mutations, with truncating mutations causing earlier presentation and quicker progression to cirrhosis.[66] Treatment options include ursodeoxycholic acid and liver transplantation.

14.6 FIBROPOLYCYSTIC DISEASES

Fibropolycystic diseases are a complex group of inherited cystic diseases affecting the liver and the kidneys. The family of hereditary polycystic diseases involving the liver includes autosomal recessive polycystic kidney disease, autosomal dominant polycystic kidney disease, and polycystic liver disease without kidney involvement. The degree of organ insult varies significantly among individuals, and the same disease can manifest exclusively in the liver or kidneys, or both.

Congenital dilatations of biliary system/ choledochal cysts

Choledochal cysts are congenital dilatations of the biliary system. They are infrequent in the Western countries,[67] but common in Asia, especially Japan, with a 1:1,000 incidence rate. Choledochal cysts are classified into five types according to their distribution along the biliary tree (Table 14.5).[68–70] The exact pathogenesis is unclear, but an abnormal pancreatobiliary junction is present in up to 80% of patients with biliary tract cysts and appears to play a role in the development of choledochal cysts.[71] Even though Caroli disease is sometimes classified as a Type V congenital dilatation, its relationship to choledochal cysts is not established. Instead, a strong association with congenital hepatic

Table 14.5 Choledochal cyst classification

Type IA	Cystic dilation of extrahepatic duct
Type IB	Focal segmental dilation of extrahepatic duct
Type IC	Fusiform dilation of entire extrahepatic bile duct
Type II	Diverticulum of common bile duct
Type III	Cyst/choledochocele of the common bile duct within the duodenal wall
Type IVA	Combined intrahepatic and extrahepatic duct dilation
Type IVB	Multiple extrahepatic bile duct dilations
Type V	Multiple intrahepatic bile duct dilations (Caroli disease)

From Todani T, Watanabe Y, Toki A, et al. Classification of congenital biliary cystic disease: special reference to type Ic and IVA cysts with primary ductal stricture. *J Hepatobiliary Pancreat Surg.* 2003;10(5):340–344.

fibrosis and renal fibrocystic lesions suggests that this entity belongs to this distinct subgroup.

Most choledochal cysts are identified during the first decade of life, and 25% are diagnosed in adulthood.[72] Jaundice is the most common presentation. The classic triad of pain, a mass in the right lower quadrant, and jaundice occur in a minority of patients, mostly in children. The diagnosis is established with imaging studies of the biliary tree.

Liver biopsies demonstrate cholestasis and bile duct obstructive features. In resected cysts, Intestinal metaplasia is a common finding and appears to be associated with the duration of disease.[73] Complete surgical resection is curative in most cases; however, involvement of intrahepatic biliary tree or pancreas can pose a bigger challenge to surgeons. The most common complications are infections (e.g., ascending cholangitis and liver abscesses) and perforations. Secondary biliary cirrhosis, pancreatitis, and malignancies can occur in long standing cases, and early diagnosis is important to avoid such complications. The risk of malignancy is 20 to 30 times higher than the general population, including pediatric patients.[74,75] Cholangiocarcinomas are most frequently reported, but squamous cell carcinomas and anaplastic carcinomas do occur. Careful gross and histologic examination of resection specimens is required to exclude the possibility of early carcinomas.

Caroli disease and congenital hepatic fibrosis

Caroli disease

Caroli disease is defined as congenital segmental dilatations of intrahepatic bile ducts. The majority of cases occur in combination with congenital hepatic fibrosis, the so-called Caroli syndrome.[76,77] The mechanism of disease is not well understood, but an association with autosomal recessive polycystic kidney disease suggests that defects in primary cilia and centromere complex might be implicated in the pathogenesis.[78] The distribution of disease within the liver is variable, but the left lobe is more frequently involved. The clinical presentation depends on the degree of liver and kidney involvement. Children may present with abdominal pain, pruritus, and hepatomegaly. Elevation of alkaline phosphatase and conjugated bilirubin levels is typical, and the diagnosis can be established with imaging studies of the biliary tree.

Gross examination of liver specimens with Caroli disease reveals saccular segmental dilatations of large bile ducts. Altered bile flow and recurrent episodes of ascending cholangitis may result in bile duct ulceration, abscess formation, and fibrosis. Features of biliary tract obstruction can be seen, with or without features of congenital hepatic fibrosis.

Liver transplantation has recently emerged as a potentially curative option for patients with advanced disease.[79] Cases that are not eligible for transplantation are managed with supportive measures. Over time, impaired bile drainage results in stone formation and acute cholangitis, sometimes complicated by liver abscesses and sepsis. Antibiotic therapy is used to manage infections. In patients with Caroli syndrome, portal hypertension can be managed with shunting procedures. Similarly to choledochal cysts, there is an increased risk of cholangiocarcinoma, and specimens should be extensively sampled.

Congenital hepatic fibrosis

Congenital hepatic fibrosis is an autosomal recessive disease resulting from defective remodeling of the bile ductal plate.[80] It has been regarded as a less severe variant of autosomal recessive polycystic kidney disease, occurring generally in children and adolescents. As mentioned earlier, this condition may or may not occur in combination with Caroli disease. Patients may present anywhere from early in the neonatal period to late childhood. Clinically, a combination of

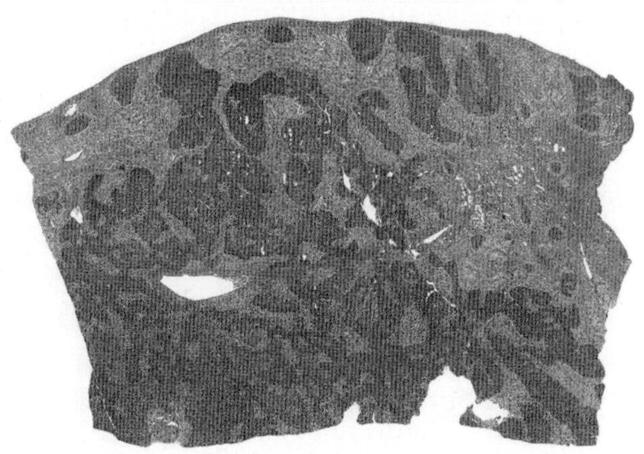

Figure 14.17 Congenital hepatic fibrosis. Irregular pattern of fibrosis and "jigsaw" appearance.

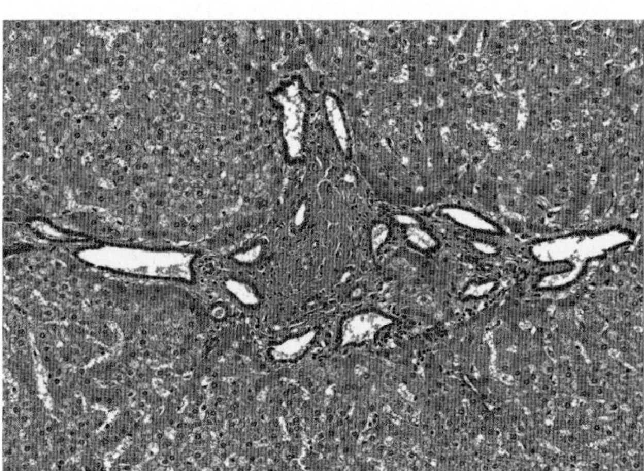

Figure 14.19 Congenital hepatic fibrosis. Ductal plate malformations.

acute cholangitis and portal hypertension is seen in most patients. Kidney involvement may be present, and displayed as medullary tubular ectasia.

Gross examination of congenital hepatic fibrosis explants demonstrates enlarged and firm livers with a distinctive reticular pattern of fibrosis. Histologically, portal areas are diffusely expanded by fibrosis. Broad fibrous bands bridge adjacent portal structures forming a characteristic "jigsaw" pattern (Fig. 14.17). Portal veins may be inconspicuous. Multiple cross sections of small, serpentine bile ducts are seen within the fibrosed portal areas (Fig. 14.18). Occasionally, ductal plate malformations are present (Fig. 14.19). Cholestasis and inflammation are not frequently seen, but can occur with acute cholangitis and obstruction, normally in the setting of Caroli syndrome. The diagnosis of congenital hepatic fibrosis is particularly challenging in liver biopsies, where it can mimic cirrhosis. The presence of portal chronic inflammation and the absence of abnormal ductal structures should point toward the diagnosis of cirrhosis, whereas ductal plate malformations and dense fibrosis indicate congenital hepatic fibrosis (Fig. 14.20).

Autosomal recessive polycystic kidney disease

Autosomal recessive polycystic kidney disease affects 1:10,000 live births.[81] The disease is divided into four subtypes depending on the time of presentation: perinatal, neonatal, infantile, and juvenile.[82] The neonatal type is the most common presentation of the disease, whereas perinatal autosomal recessive polycystic kidney disease is the most severe form,

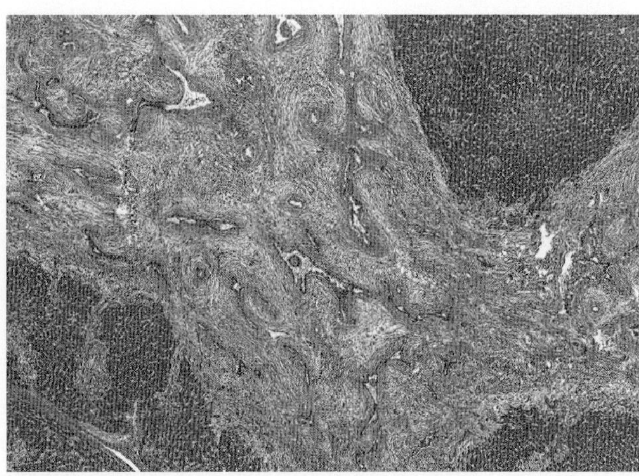

Figure 14.18 Congenital hepatic fibrosis. Numerous cross sections of bile ducts are seen within the edematous and fibrotic portal areas.

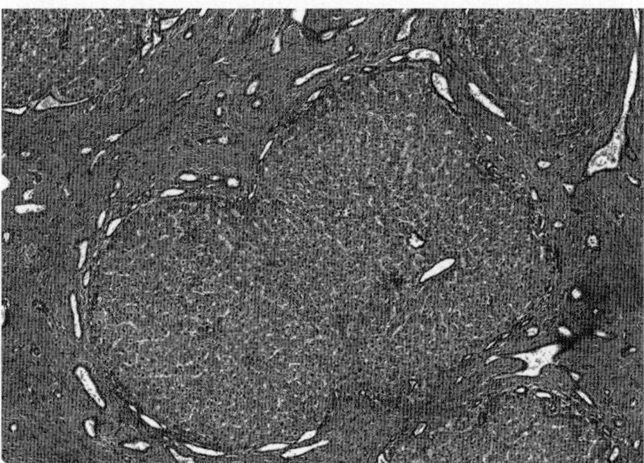

Figure 14.20 Congenital hepatic fibrosis. The pattern of fibrosis can mimic cirrhosis. The presence of ductal plate malformations and absence of inflammation favors the diagnosis of congenital hepatic fibrosis.

resulting in perinatal death in the majority of cases. Neonatal autosomal recessive polycystic kidney disease manifests early in the neonatal period with large echogenic kidneys. Patients have hypertension and kidney dysfunction and progress to end-stage renal disease within the first decade of life, often requiring renal transplantation. Pyelonephritis is common. Liver involvement by neonatal autosomal recessive polycystic kidney disease includes cystic dilatation of bile ducts, fibrosis, and recurrent acute cholangitis. Infantile and juvenile forms of the disease are characterized by chronic renal failure and portal hypertension.

Grossly, the liver may be normal to mildly enlarged. Microscopically, interlobular bile ducts are either absent or greatly reduced in number. A distinctive ductal plate surrounding the edges of portal areas is seen with markedly prominent and irregular ducts. Cysts are not typically seen. In some cases, evidence of acute cholangitis may be present. This pattern can resemble congenital hepatic fibrosis. However, in autosomal recessive polycystic kidney disease, the distribution of ducts within the ductal plate tend to be more continuously circumferential. In addition, interlobular bile ducts are often present in congenital hepatic fibrosis.

Autosomal dominant polycystic kidney disease

Autosomal dominant polycystic kidney disease is characterized by cysts and tissue abnormalities affecting multiple organs.[83] It is one of the most common hereditary disorders worldwide and affects approximately 1 in 1,000 live births. The disease is characterized by liver and kidney cysts that develop over time. Liver manifestations are rare in children. The degree of liver involvement by cysts correlates with female gender and the number of pregnancies.[84] Patients present with upper abdominal pain and are found to have an enlarged liver. The disease is managed by supportive therapy. Liver and combined liver/kidney transplantation can be offered in end stage cases. Cholangiocarcinoma and infections remain the most important complications in autosomal dominant polycystic kidney.

Gross examination of liver in autosomal dominant polycystic kidney reveals a massively enlarged liver with diffuse replacement of the parenchyma by cystic structures (Fig. 14.21). Histologically, the cysts are lined by a cuboidal simple epithelium. Epithelial attenuation can be seen in large cysts; cyst rupture is associated with ulceration, fibrosis, and abscess formation (Fig. 14.22). In some areas, numerous bile duct hamartomas (von Meyenburg complexes) are seen and are thought to correlate with degree of liver involvement.[85] Careful gross and microscopic examination is important to evaluate for possible cholangiocarcinoma.

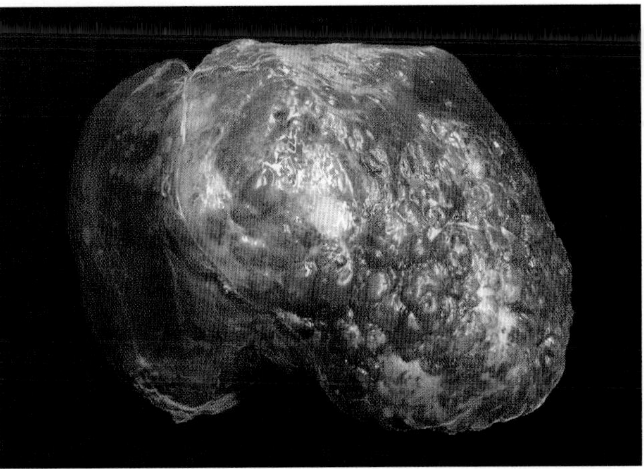

Figure 14.21 Autosomal dominant polycystic kidney disease. Liver explant demonstrates numerous cystic lesions affecting predominantly the left lobe.

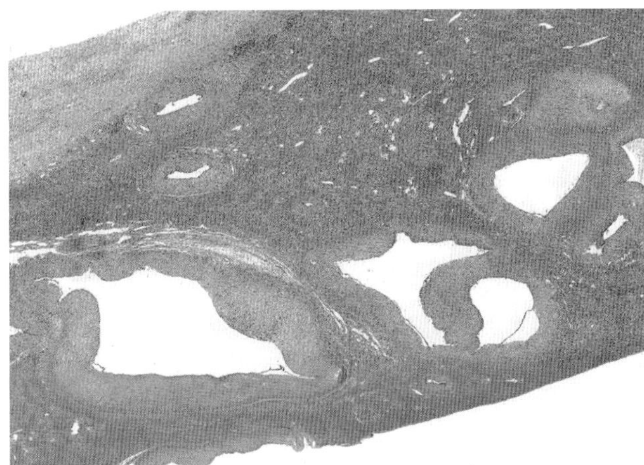

Figure 14.22 Autosomal dominant polycystic kidney disease. Hepatic cysts are lined by benign cuboidal epithelium and may be associated with fibrosis, rupture, and hemorrhage.

14.7 CYSTIC FIBROSIS

Cystic fibrosis is the most common autosomal recessive disease, affecting about 1:2,500 live births in the Caucasian population. It affects the pancreas, bronchial and intestinal glands, the sweat glands, and the biliary tree. It is caused by mutations in the cystic fibrosis transmembrane regulator (*CFTR*) gene, which encodes a protein named CFTR, which is responsible for the regulation of chloride ions across cellular membranes.[86,87] Disruption in CFTR expression results in abnormally viscous mucus, causing occlusion of affected airways, pancreatic ducts, and bile ducts. Clinically severe liver involvement in cystic fibrosis is uncommon, affecting only 5% of patients developing significant disease.[88,89]

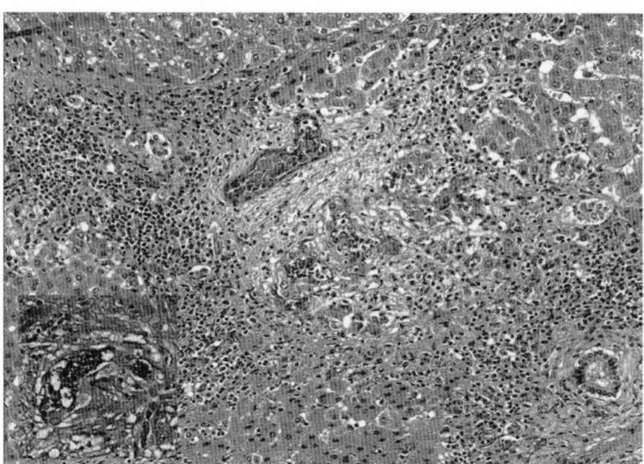

Figure 14.23 Cystic fibrosis. Portal inflammation, ductular proliferation, and acute "chemical" cholangitis. *Inset*: The presence of Periodic acid–Schiff-positive inspissated material occluding bile duct lumen is pathognomonic of cystic fibrosis.

Abnormal liver function tests are seen in up to 50% of patients.[90] Clinically, the disease may present as transient neonatal cholestasis and meconium ileus. Older children will have hepatosplenomegaly and abnormal liver enzymes, predominantly transaminases and alkaline phosphatase.

The most common histopathologic change is macrovesicular steatosis, present in more than 50% of cases.[91] Portal fibrosis and ductular proliferation can be seen. In some cases, sampling of intrahepatic bile ducts may demonstrate mucus accumulation. This is appreciated as inspissated eosinophilic secretions within dilated bile ducts or ductules (Fig. 14.23). Periodic acid–Schiff-positive, diastase-resistant material within bile duct lumina is strongly suggestive of cystic fibrosis, but often absent in biopsy specimens. Features of acute cholangitis may be focally present and are typically regarded as a chemical reaction to the inspissated secretions.

Focal biliary fibrosis, also known as focal biliary cirrhosis, is present in about 25% of children older than 1 year and 70% of adults older than 24 years of age.[92] This lesion results from the coalescence of fibrotic portal tracts with entrapment of several hepatic lobules. The term focal biliary fibrosis is used to describe a macroscopic lesion consisting of small scars within the hepatic parenchyma. In addition, hypoplastic gallbladders are present in up to one-third of patients. See also Chapter 18 for more information.

14.8 TOTAL PARENTERAL NUTRITION OR INTESTINAL FAILURE-ASSOCIATED LIVER DISEASE

Cholestatic disease is a common complication of total parenteral nutrition (TPN). The condition was, recently named intestinal failure-associated liver disease and accounts for up to 20% of neonatal cholestasis cases.[1] The etiology of TPN-associated liver disease is not clear. Some studies suggest that inappropriate quantities (excess or deficiency) of certain nutrients may induce liver disease. However, the disease cannot be attributed to one cause and is considered a multifactorial process.

The indication for TPN in pediatric patients ranges from extreme prematurity, to short bowel syndrome following necrotizing enterocolitis, to congenital malformations, such as intestinal atresia. Rare conditions impairing intestinal absorption, including microvillus inclusion disease and tufting enteropathy are also treated with TPN. In premature neonates, TPN will cause elevations of serum conjugated bilirubin and GGT. The abnormalities typically resolve upon repair of intestinal function. More severe diseases requiring prolonged TPN are associated with a higher incidence and severity of liver disease. In these patients, conjugated hyperbilirubinemia persists for months, and biliary cirrhosis is a serious potential complication.

Microscopically, mild cases of TPN-associated liver disease show hepatocellular and canalicular cholestasis, ductular proliferation, and mild portal fibrosis. Extramedullary hematopoiesis may be seen.[93] These features can resemble biliary atresia. Prolonged TPN causes progressive liver disease with portal inflammation and fibrosis. Hemosiderin and lipofuscin are often seen in liver specimens from patients on TPN.[94] Improvement of cholestasis and regression of mild fibrosis have been described following cessation of TPN therapy. Cases with advanced fibrosis may not regress completely and require liver transplantation. Older patients, typically adolescents, may present with the adult-pattern of TPN-induced liver injury, characterized by cholestasis, macrovesicular steatosis, and portal fibrosis. Steatohepatitis can also be present.[95] Combined liver and small intestinal transplantation can improve survival in some patients. A study of chronologic progression of TPN-associated liver disease indicates that cholestasis may be seen as early as 10 days after initiation of therapy, followed by ductular proliferation within a few weeks of therapy, and significant fibrosis after 3 months. Cirrhosis can develop as early as 5 months, but is usually not found until there has been at least 1 year of TPN.[94] See also Chapter 19 for more information.

REFERENCES

1. Stormon MO, Dorney SF, Kamath KR, et al. The changing pattern of diagnosis of

infantile cholestasis. *J Paediatr Child Health.* 2001;37(1):47–50.
2. Kasai M, Watanabe I, Ohi R. Follow-up studies of long term survivors after hepatic portoenterostomy for "noncorrectible" biliary atresia. *J Pediatr Surg.* 1975;10(2):173–182.
3. Altman RP, Lilly JR, Greenfeld J, et al. A multivariable risk factor analysis of the portoenterostomy (Kasai) procedure for biliary atresia: twenty-five years of experience from two centers. *Ann Surg.* 1997;226(3):348–353; discussion 53–55.
4. Yoon PW, Bresee JS, Olney RS, et al. Epidemiology of biliary atresia: a population-based study. *Pediatrics.* 1997;99(3):376–382.
5. Hsiao CH, Chang MH, Chen HL, et al. Universal screening for biliary atresia using an infant stool color card in Taiwan. *Hepatology.* 2008;47(4):1233–1240.
6. Houwen RH, Kerremans II, van Steensel-Moll HA, et al. Time-space distribution of extrahepatic biliary atresia in The Netherlands and West Germany. *Z Kinderchir.* 1988;43(2):68–71.
7. Chardot C, Carton M, Spire-Bendelac N, et al. Epidemiology of biliary atresia in France: a national study 1986-96. *J Hepatol.* 1999;31(6):1006–1013.
8. Shneider BL, Brown MB, Haber B, et al. A multicenter study of the outcome of biliary atresia in the United States, 1997 to 2000. *J Pediatr.* 2006;148(4):467–474.
9. Strickland AD, Shannon K. Studies in the etiology of extrahepatic biliary atresia: time-space clustering. *J Pediatr.* 1982;100(5):749–753.
10. Lachaux A, Descos B, Plauchu H, et al. Familial extrahepatic biliary atresia. *J Pediatr Gastroenterol Nutr.* 1988;7(2):280–283.
11. Fallon SC, Chang S, Finegold MJ, et al. Discordant presentation of biliary atresia in premature monozygotic twins. *J Pediatr Gastroenterol Nutr.* 2013;57(4):e22–e23.
12. Smith BM, Laberge JM, Schreiber R, et al. Familial biliary atresia in three siblings including twins. *J Pediatr Surg.* 1991;26(11):1331–1333.
13. Davenport M, Tizzard SA, Underhill J, et al. The biliary atresia splenic malformation syndrome: a 28-year single-center retrospective study. *J Pediatr.* 2006;149(3):393–400.
14. Davenport M, Caponcelli E, Livesey E, et al. Surgical outcome in biliary atresia: etiology affects the influence of age at surgery. *Ann Surg.* 2008;247(4):694–698.
15. Davenport M. A challenge on the use of the words embryonic and perinatal in the context of biliary atresia. *Hepatology.* 2005;41(2):403–404; author reply 4–5.
16. Caponcelli E, Knisely AS, Davenport M. Cystic biliary atresia: an etiologic and prognostic subgroup. *J Pediatr Surg.* 2008;43(9):1619–1624.
17. Caton AR, Druschel CM, McNutt LA. The epidemiology of extrahepatic biliary atresia in New York State, 1983-98. *Paediatr Perinat Epidemiol.* 2004;18(2):97–105.
18. Lorent K, Gong W, Koo KA, et al. Identification of a plant isoflavonoid that causes biliary atresia. *Sci Transl Med.* 2015;7(286):286ra67.
19. Davit-Spraul A, Baussan C, Hermeziu B, et al. CFC1 gene involvement in biliary atresia with polysplenia syndrome. *J Pediatr Gastroenterol Nutr.* 2008;46(1):111–112.
20. Wang KS. Newborn screening for biliary atresia. *Pediatrics.* 2015;136(6):e1663–1669.
21. Park WH, Choi SO, Lee HJ, et al. A new diagnostic approach to biliary atresia with emphasis on the ultrasonographic triangular cord sign: comparison of ultrasonography, hepatobiliary scintigraphy, and liver needle biopsy in the evaluation of infantile cholestasis. J Pediatr Surg. 1997;32(11): 1555–1559.
22. Kwatra N, Shalaby-Rana E, Narayanan S, et al. Phenobarbital-enhanced hepatobiliary scintigraphy in the diagnosis of biliary atresia: two decades of experience at a tertiary center. *Pediatr Radiol.* 2013;43(10):1365–1375.
23. Huang CT, Lee HC, Chen WT, et al. Usefulness of magnetic resonance cholangiopancreatography in pancreatobiliary abnormalities in pediatric patients. *Pediatr Neonatol.* 2011;52(6):332–336.
24. Landing BH, Wells TR, Ramicone E. Time course of the intrahepatic lesion of extrahepatic biliary atresia: a morphometric study. *Pediatr Pathol.* 1985;4(3–4):309–319.
25. Arii R, Koga H, Arakawa A, et al. How valuable is ductal plate malformation as a predictor of clinical course in postoperative biliary atresia patients? *Pediatr Surg Int.* 2011;27(3):275–277.
26. Mirza Q, Kvist N, Petersen BL. Histologic features of the portal plate in extrahepatic biliary atresia and their impact on prognosis–a Danish study. *J Pediatr Surg.* 2009;44(7):1344–1348.
27. Baerg J, Zuppan C, Klooster M. Biliary atresia–a fifteen-year review of clinical and pathologic factors associated with liver transplantation. *J Pediatr Surg.* 2004;39(6):800–803.
28. Tan CE, Davenport M, Driver M, et al. Does the morphology of the extrahepatic biliary remnants in biliary atresia influence survival? A review of 205 cases. *J Pediatr Surg.* 1994;29(11):1459–1464.
29. Hadzic N, Quaglia A, Portmann B, et al. Hepatocellular carcinoma in biliary atresia: King's College Hospital experience. *J Pediatr.* 2011;159(4):617–622.e1.

30. Sharma S, Das P, Dattagupta S, et al. Liver and portal histopathological correlation with age and survival in extra hepatic biliary atresia. *Pediatr Surg Int.* 2011;27(5):451–461.
31. Russo P, Magee JC, Boitnott J, et al. Design and validation of the biliary atresia research consortium histologic assessment system for cholestasis in infancy. *Clin Gastroenterol Hepatol.* 2011;9(4):357–362.e2.
32. Phillips MJ, Azuma T, Meredith SL, et al. Abnormalities in villin gene expression and canalicular microvillus structure in progressive cholestatic liver disease of childhood. *Lancet.* 2003;362(9390):1112–1119.
33. Bassett MD, Murray KF. Biliary atresia: recent progress. *J Clin Gastroenterol.* 2008;42(6):720–729.
34. Deutsch J, Smith AL, Danks DM, et al. Long term prognosis for babies with neonatal liver disease. *Arch Dis Child.* 1985;60(5):447–451.
35. Balistreri WF. Neonatal cholestasis. *J Pediatr.* 1985;106(2):171–184.
36. Torbenson M, Hart J, Westerhoff M, et al. Neonatal giant cell hepatitis: histological and etiological findings. *Am J Surg Pathol.* 2010;34(10):1498–1503.
37. Chang MH, Hsu HC, Lee CY, et al. Neonatal hepatitis: a follow-up study. *J Pediatr Gastroenterol Nutr.* 1987;6(2):203–207.
38. Suita S, Arima T, Ishii K, et al. Fate of infants with neonatal hepatitis: pediatric surgeons' dilemma. *J Pediatr Surg.* 1992;27(6):696–699.
39. Roberts EA. Neonatal hepatitis syndrome. *Semin Neonatol.* 2003;8(5):357–374.
40. Alagille D, Odievre M, Gautier M, et al. Hepatic ductular hypoplasia associated with characteristic facies, vertebral malformations, retarded physical, mental, and sexual development, and cardiac murmur. *J Pediatr.* 1975;86(1):63–71.
41. Alagille D, Estrada A, Hadchouel M, et al. Syndromic paucity of interlobular bile ducts (Alagille syndrome or arteriohepatic dysplasia): review of 80 cases. *J Pediatr.* 1987;110(2):195–200.
42. Russo PA, Ellis D, Hashida Y. Renal histopathology in Alagille's syndrome. *Pediatr Pathol.* 1987;7(5–6):557–568.
43. Emerick KM, Rand EB, Goldmuntz E, et al. Features of Alagille syndrome in 92 patients: frequency and relation to prognosis. *Hepatology.* 1999;29(3):822–829.
44. Yuan ZR, Kohsaka T, Ikegaya T, et al. Mutational analysis of the Jagged 1 gene in Alagille syndrome families. *Hum Mol Genet.* 1998;7(9):1363–1369.
45. Crosnier C, Driancourt C, Raynaud N, et al. Mutations in JAGGED1 gene are predominantly sporadic in Alagille syndrome. *Gastroenterology.* 1999;116(5):1141–1148.
46. Spinner NB, Colliton RP, Crosnier C, et al. Jagged1 mutations in alagille syndrome. *Hum Mutat.* 2001;17(1):18–33.
47. McDaniell R, Warthen DM, Sanchez-Lara PA, et al. NOTCH2 mutations cause Alagille syndrome, a heterogeneous disorder of the notch signaling pathway. *Am J Hum Genet.* 2006;79(1):169–173.
48. Morelli A, Pelli MA, Vedovelli A, et al. Endoscopic retrograde cholangiopancreatography study in Alagille's syndrome: first report. *Am J Gastroenterol.* 1983;78(4):241–244.
49. Dahms BB, Petrelli M, Wyllie R, et al. Arteriohepatic dysplasia in infancy and childhood: a longitudinal study of six patients. *Hepatology.* 1982;2(3):350–358.
50. Kahn EI, Daum F, Markowitz J, et al. Arteriohepatic dysplasia. II. Hepatobiliary morphology. *Hepatology.* 1983;3(1):77–84.
51. Byrne JA, Meara NJ, Rayner AC, et al. Lack of hepatocellular CD10 along bile canaliculi is physiologic in early childhood and persistent in Alagille syndrome. *Lab Invest.* 2007;87(11):1138–1148.
52. Clayton RJ, Iber FL, Ruebner BH, et al. Byler disease. Fatal familial intrahepatic cholestasis in an Amish kindred. *Am J Dis Children (1960).* 1969;117(1):112–124.
53. Bull LN, van Eijk MJ, Pawlikowska L, et al. A gene encoding a P-type ATPase mutated in two forms of hereditary cholestasis. *Nat Genet.* 1998;18(3):219–224.
54. Bull LN, Carlton VE, Stricker NL, et al. Genetic and morphological findings in progressive familial intrahepatic cholestasis (Byler disease [PFIC-1] and Byler syndrome): evidence for heterogeneity. *Hepatology.* 1997;26(1):155–164.
55. Alissa FT, Jaffe R, Shneider BL. Update on progressive familial intrahepatic cholestasis. *J Pediatr Gastroenterol Nutr.* 2008;46(3):241–252.
56. Miyagawa-Hayashino A, Egawa H, Yorifuji T, et al. Allograft steatohepatitis in progressive familial intrahepatic cholestasis type 1 after living donor liver transplantation. *Liver Transpl.* 2009;15(6):610–618.
57. Strautnieks SS, Byrne JA, Pawlikowska L, et al. Severe bile salt export pump deficiency: 82 different ABCB11 mutations in 109 families. *Gastroenterology.* 2008;134(4):1203–1214.
58. Evason K, Bove KE, Finegold MJ, et al. Morphologic findings in progressive familial intrahepatic cholestasis 2 (PFIC2): correlation with genetic and immunohistochemical studies. *Am J Surg Pathol.* 2011;35(5):687–696.
59. Ernst LM, Spinner NB, Piccoli DA, et al. Interlobular bile duct loss in pediatric cholestatic disease is associated with aberrant cytokeratin 7 expression by hepatocytes. *Pediatr Dev Pathol.* 2007;10(5):383–390.

60. Pawlikowska L, Strautnieks S, Jankowska I, et al. Differences in presentation and progression between severe FIC1 and BSEP deficiencies. *J Hepatol*. 2010;53(1):170–178.
61. Knisely AS, Strautnieks SS, Meier Y, et al. Hepatocellular carcinoma in ten children under five years of age with bile salt export pump deficiency. *Hepatology*. 2006;44(2):478–486.
62. Jara P, Hierro L, Martinez-Fernandez P, et al. Recurrence of bile salt export pump deficiency after liver transplantation. *N Engl J Med*. 2009;361(14):1359–1367.
63. Siebold L, Dick AA, Thompson R, et al. Recurrent low gamma-glutamyl transpeptidase cholestasis following liver transplantation for bile salt export pump (BSEP) disease (posttransplant recurrent BSEP disease). *Liver Transpl*. 2010;16(7):856–863.
64. Wendum D, Barbu V, Rosmorduc O, et al. Aspects of liver pathology in adult patients with MDR3/ABCB4 gene mutations. *Virchows Arch*. 2012;460(3):291–298.
65. Gordo-Gilart R, Andueza S, Hierro L, et al. Functional analysis of ABCB4 mutations relates clinical outcomes of progressive familial intrahepatic cholestasis type 3 to the degree of MDR3 floppase activity. *Gut*. 2015;64(1):147–155.
66. Jacquemin E. Role of multidrug resistance 3 deficiency in pediatric and adult liver disease: one gene for three diseases. *Semin Liver Dis*. 2001;21(4):551–562.
67. Lipsett PA, Pitt HA, Colombani PM, et al. Choledochal cyst disease. A changing pattern of presentation. *Ann Surg*. 1994;220(5):644–652.
68. Todani T, Watanabe Y, Narusue M, et al. Congenital bile duct cysts: classification, operative procedures, and review of thirty-seven cases including cancer arising from choledochal cyst. *Am J Surg*. 1977;134(2):263–269.
69. Todani T, Watanabe Y, Toki A, et al. Classification of congenital biliary cystic disease: special reference to type Ic and IVA cysts with primary ductal stricture. *J Hepatobiliary Pancreat Surg*. 2003;10(5):340–344.
70. Savader SJ, Benenati JF, Venbrux AC, et al. Choledochal cysts: classification and cholangiographic appearance. *AJR Am J Roentgenol*. 1991;156(2):327–331.
71. Yamashiro Y, Miyano T, Suruga K, et al. Experimental study of the pathogenesis of choledochal cyst and pancreatitis, with special reference to the role of bile acids and pancreatic enzymes in the anomalous choledocho-pancreatico ductal junction. *J Pediatr Gastroenterol Nutr*. 1984;3(5):721–727.
72. Komi N, Takehara H, Kunitomo K, et al. Does the type of anomalous arrangement of pancreaticobiliary ducts influence the surgery and prognosis of choledochal cyst? *J Pediatr Surg*. 1992;27(6):728–731.
73. Komi N, Tamura T, Tsuge S, et al. Relation of patient age to premalignant alterations in choledochal cyst epithelium: histochemical and immunohistochemical studies. *J Pediatr Surg*. 1986;21(5):430–433.
74. Soreide K, Soreide JA. Bile duct cyst as precursor to biliary tract cancer. *Ann Surg Oncol*. 2007;14(3):1200–1211.
75. Lee SE, Jang JY, Lee YJ, et al. Choledochal cyst and associated malignant tumors in adults: a multicenter survey in South Korea. *Arch Surg*. 2011;146(10):1178–1184.
76. Summerfield JA, Nagafuchi Y, Sherlock S, et al. Hepatobiliary fibropolycystic diseases. A clinical and histological review of 51 patients. *J Hepatol*. 1986;2(2):141–156.
77. Desmet VJ. Congenital diseases of intrahepatic bile ducts: variations on the theme "ductal plate malformation". *Hepatology*. 1992;16(4):1069–1083.
78. Hildebrandt F. Genetic kidney diseases. *Lancet*. 2010;375(9722):1287–1295.
79. Millwala F, Segev DL, Thuluvath PJ. Caroli's disease and outcomes after liver transplantation. *Liver Transpl*. 2008;14(1):11–17.
80. Desmet VJ. What is congenital hepatic fibrosis? *Histopathology*. 1992;20(6):465–477.
81. McDonald RA, Avner ED. Inherited polycystic kidney disease in children. *Semin Nephrol*. 1991;11(6):632–642.
82. Blyth H, Ockenden BG. Polycystic disease of kidney and liver presenting in childhood. *J Med Genet*. 1971;8(3):257–284.
83. Gabow PA. Autosomal dominant polycystic kidney disease. *N Engl J Med*. 1993;329(5):332–342.
84. Everson GT, Taylor MR. Management of polycystic liver disease. *Curr Gastroenterol Rep*. 2005;7(1):19–25.
85. Melnick PJ. Polycystic liver; analysis of seventy cases. *AMA Arch Pathol*. 1955;59(2):162–172.
86. Kerem B, Rommens JM, Buchanan JA, et al. Identification of the cystic fibrosis gene: genetic analysis. *Science*. 1989;245(4922):1073–1080.
87. Riordan JR, Rommens JM, Kerem B, et al. Identification of the cystic fibrosis gene: cloning and characterization of complementary DNA. *Science*. 1989;245(4922):1066–1073.
88. Colombo C, Battezzati PM, Crosignani A, et al. Liver disease in cystic fibrosis: a prospective study on incidence, risk factors, and outcome. *Hepatology*. 2002;36(6):1374–1382.
89. Psacharopoulos HT, Howard ER, Portmann B, et al. Hepatic complications of cystic fibrosis. *Lancet*. 1981;2(8237):78–80.

90. Lamireau T, Monnereau S, Martin S, et al. Epidemiology of liver disease in cystic fibrosis: a longitudinal study. *J Hepatol*. 2004;41(6):920–925.
91. Craig JM, Haddad H, Shwachman H. The pathological changes in the liver in cystic fibrosis of the pancreas. *AMA J Dis Child*. 1957;93(4):357–369.
92. Oppenheimer EH, Esterly JR. Pathology of cystic fibrosis review of the literature and comparison with 146 autopsied cases. *Perspect Pediatr Pathol*. 1975;2:241–278.
93. Mullick FG, Moran CA, Ishak KG. Total parenteral nutrition: a histopathologic analysis of the liver changes in 20 children. *Mod Pathol*. 1994;7(2):190–194.
94. Cohen C, Olsen MM. Pediatric total parenteral nutrition. Liver histopathology. *Arch Pathol Lab Med*. 1981;105(3):152–156.
95. Bowyer BA, Fleming CR, Ludwig J, et al. Does long-term home parenteral nutrition in adult patients cause chronic liver disease? *JPEN J Parenter Enteral Nutr*. 1985;9(1):11–17.

15 Drug effects

Michael S. Torbenson, MD

15.1 OVERVIEW

The acronym DILI, which stands for "drug-induced liver injury", is commonly used in the literature on drug reactions. In the United States, the most common categories of drugs associated with DILI in adults are acetaminophen, antibiotics, central nervous system agents, antihypertensive agents, and antidiabetic agents.[1] Dietary supplements are also important causes of DILI, being found in about 10% of cases.[1] In contrast to adults, the most common agents causing DILI in children are antibiotics and central nervous system agents.[2] DILI can be broadly classified by the main mechanism of injury: direct toxin, allergic (hypersensitivity) drug reaction, or an idiosyncratic drug reaction. Idiosyncratic drug reactions are the most common type seen in routine surgical pathology, as allergic reactions and direct toxins are often readily identified by clinical findings and laboratory testing.

When evaluating a liver biopsy for a possible drug reaction, one of the most important points to remember is that essentially no findings are pathognomonic for a drug reaction. In addition, there can be a wide range of histological findings for any given single drug. Tamoxifen-associated DILI nicely illustrates this point, being associated with acute hepatitis, massive liver necrosis, peliosis hepatitis, steatosis, steatohepatitis, and cholestasis.[3] Although some medications tend to have a typical pattern of injury, the findings in DILI overall tend to be neither very sensitive nor specific, and it is unwise to rely solely on memorizing a few or even many patterns that are illustrated in books or review articles. Instead, the best approach is to have a high degree of suspicion and to consider drug reactions in your differential in all cases, but especially in those cases that have patterns of injury that do not fit for the known clinical and serological findings. In fact, histological patterns that "just don't fit" for other entities can often be a useful clue to DILI.

When correlating the histological findings with the patient's mediations, the goal is to identify medications that are the most likely to have caused the injury, but it's not uncommon to have multiple potentially offending agents. In this setting, the overall pattern of injury can provide some guidance, but is not foolproof because of the variability of injury patterns for any one drug and the large degree of overlap seen with different DILI causing agents. Thus, correlation with other clinical findings is often critical, including prior reactions to drugs in the same class and temporal associations. In general, the most straightforward temporal associations are with direct toxins such as acetaminophen because toxicity is dose-dependent and based on both recent usage and the amount of intake. In contrast, for idiosyncratic drug reactions, a compatible exposure history includes only that the drug is in current usage or was recently discontinued. Most idiosyncratic drug reactions occur within the first several weeks following exposure, a very helpful observation, but there are exceptions where a drug is used for months to years before hepatic injury develops.

Resources for the patterns of DILI associated with drugs are numerous. Books can be an excellent starting point, but the list of potential agents for any given pattern of injury seems to be ever growing, so other important resources include searching PubMed or commercial databases. Another helpful resource is the LiverTox website, http://livertox.nlm.nih.gov/, a free resource hosted by the NIDDK and the NLM of the United States.

A diagnosis of DILI is made by identifying a compatible history of drug exposure, finding compatible histological findings, and excluding other potential causes. However, in most idiosyncratic DILI cases, the diagnosis should be considered as "most consistent with" a drug reaction and not a proven drug reaction, as subsequent testing can sometimes identify other causes. As an example, both acute hepatitis E and acute hepatitis C can closely mimic drug reactions and are sometimes only retrospectively identified, after a presumed diagnosis of DILI has been made based on the then available clinical and histological findings.[1,4]

15.2 ISOLATED HYPERAMMONEMIA

Isolated elevations in serum ammonia can result from drug toxicity to the liver, in particular valproic acid[5] or infusion of high-dose 5-fluorouracil for chemotherapy.[6] The liver biopsy often looks essentially normal, other than minimal fatty change (Fig. 15.1). The differential includes urea cycle defects[7] or portosystemic shunts,[8] but the clinical findings in these entities are distinct.

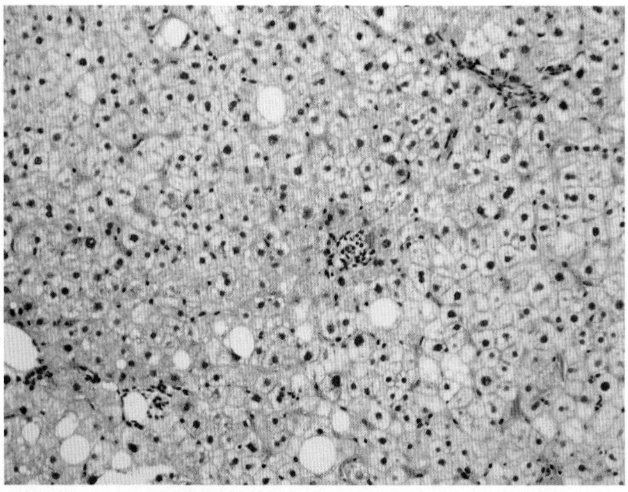

Figure 15.1 Isolated hypermoniaemia. This patient was taking valoproic acid. The liver biopsy shows minimal fat and inflammation but is otherwise essentially normal in appearance.

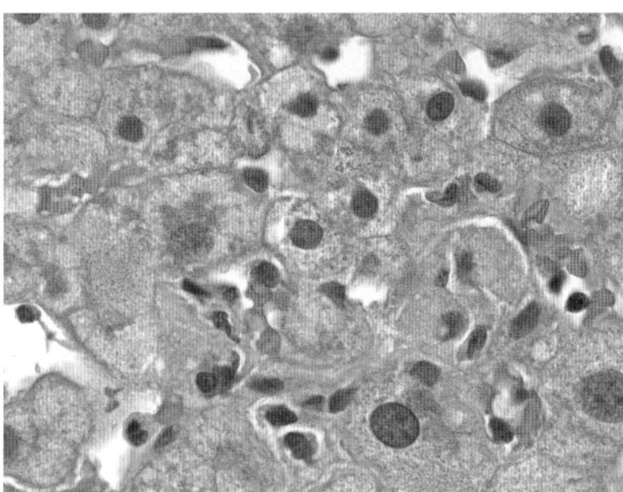

Figure 15.2 Resolving hepatitis. The clinical history was that of previously elevated enzymes that were significantly lower at the time of biopsy. The liver biopsy shows only minimal inflammation, but numerous pigmented Kupffer cells are present in the lobules.

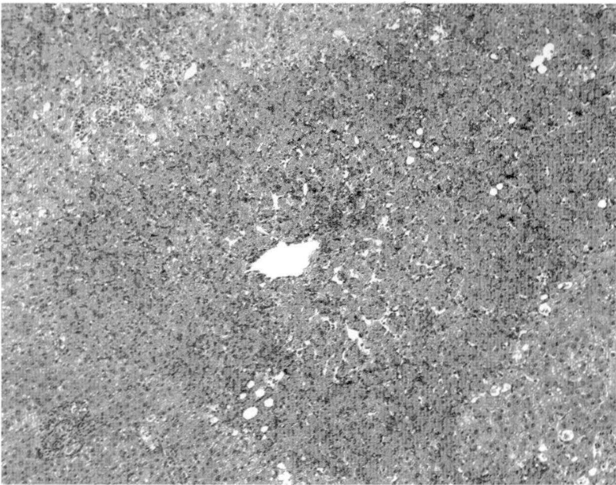

Figure 15.3 Acetaminophen toxicity. There is extensive hepatocellular necrosis in Zone 3, with sparing of the Zone 1 hepatocytes. Inflammation is minimal.

15.3 RESOLVING PATTERN OF HEPATITIS

In most cases of idiosyncratic DILI, the hepatitic injury diminishes after stopping the drug, but the liver enzymes may take months to completely normalize. DILI with significant cholestasis tends to resolve more slowly than cases that are purely hepatitic. This clinical situation, of improved but persistent biochemical abnormalities despite stopping a drug, can often prompt a liver biopsy. Biopsies in this setting typically show a resolving hepatitis pattern, but sometimes can show findings that suggest an alternative diagnosis to DILI. The resolving hepatitis pattern, like most patterns, is not etiologically specific, but the histological differential always includes resolving DILI. The main finding is in the lobules, with a mild prominence in Kupffer cells, often small Kupffer cell aggregates that are easiest to seen on periodic acid–Schiff (PAS)-D stains, and minimal lobular inflammation (Fig. 15.2). Rare acidophil bodies may be present, and patchy minimal cholestasis can also be present. The portal tracts often show minimal to mild lymphocytic inflammation and scattered ceroid-laden macrophages.

15.4 DIRECT TOXINS

Direct toxins by definition lead to liver injury in a reproducible and dose-dependent fashion. The most common cause is acetaminophen, but other causes include mushroom poisoning and miscellaneous household and industrial chemicals.

Toxins cause direct hepatocyte necrosis with little inflammation. In most cases, the necrosis tends to have a Zone 3 pattern (Fig. 15.3). The dead hepatocytes are typically a deep eosinophilic color and lose their nuclei. Although the hepatocytes in Zone 3 will be dead, the Kupffer cells and endothelial cells in the same areas are often still intact and present in their normal locations. When there is severe injury, the necrosis is often panacinar, and no zonation will be evident. Other zonal patterns of necrosis are less common. A Zone 1 pattern of necrosis has been associated with toxic injury from phosphorous, ferrous sulfate, and cocaine.[9,10] Hepatitis A, while not a toxic injury, can rarely show a Zones 1 and 2 pattern of necrosis with sparing of Zone 3 (Fig. 15.4). A Zone 2 pattern of necrosis has been associated with Beryllium toxicity. With any of these patterns, those hepatocytes that survive often show mild small- and medium-sized droplet fatty change and cholestasis. Depending on the time interval between injury and biopsy, a reactive bile ductular proliferation can also be seen in later biopsies. At these later time points, the liver can also show mild portal inflammation and mild Kupffer cell hyperplasia. The Kupffer cells and the proliferating bile ductules can also show significant reactive iron accumulation.

Acetaminophen toxicity

Acetaminophen toxicity is the most common etiology of direct liver injury, causing up to 50% of cases of acute liver failure in the United States and the United Kingdom.[11,12] Acetaminophen toxicity tends to have very high serum alanine aminotransferase levels (ALT; median ALT levels of about 4,000 IU/L) with relative low

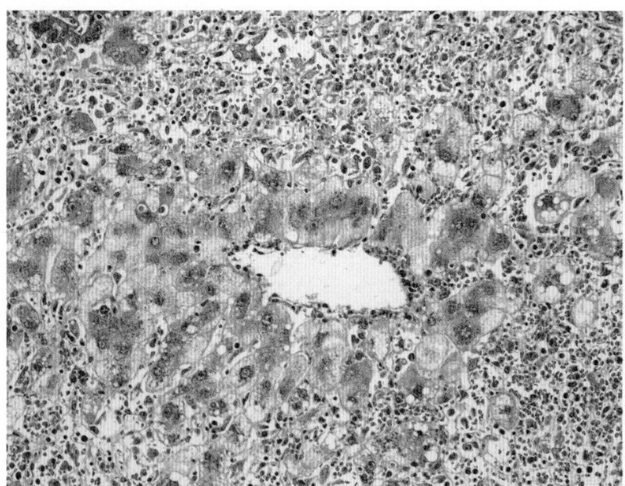

Figure 15.4 Acute hepatitis A. The liver shows extensive necrosis in Zones 1 and 2, with sparing of Zone 3 hepatocytes.

bilirubin (median levels of about 4 mg/dL). This stands in contrast to idiosyncratic DILI which tends to have lower ALT levels (median of approximately 500 IU/L) but higher bilirubin levels (median around 20 mg/dL).

Toxicity occurs both with intentional overdose as part of suicide attempts (approximately 40% of cases) and with unintentional overdoses. Unintentional overdoses most commonly occur when there is significant alcohol use or in the setting of chronic pain, with patients using medications that contain both narcotics and acetaminophen.[11] In general, hepatic injury requires an exposure of more than 7.5 g, with severe injury seen at levels of 15 to 25 g. However, these general toxic thresholds can be lowered by the coexistence of fatty liver disease,[13] chronic alcohol consumption,[11] sleep apnea,[14] or use of drugs that stimulate the P-450 enzyme system, including carbamazepine, dimetidine, isoniazid, and phenytoin.[11] Treatment for acetaminophen toxicity with *N*-acetylcysteine is very effective when given within the first 24 hours of presentation.

15.5 ALLERGIC TYPE DRUG REACTIONS

Allergic drug reactions in general are rarely biopsied because the clinical findings tend to be easily recognized, including hives, wheezing, and peripheral eosinophilia. However, in some cases, the clinical findings can be mild or obscured by other comorbid conditions, leading to a liver biopsy in order to evaluate elevated liver enzymes. In these cases, the drug exposure is typically recent, usually within the preceding few days or weeks.

The main biopsy findings are increased eosinophils in the portal tract, lobules, and often the sinusoids. Both the portal inflammation and the lobules also commonly show mild lymphocytic inflammation, and occasional apoptotic bodies are found in the lobules.

Eosinophil-rich inflammation is the main histological finding in allergic DILI of the liver. However, diagnoses of drug reactions can be wrong when they are based solely on finding eosinophils in the biopsy because eosinophils are a common component of many other inflammatory conditions of the liver, including viral hepatitis, autoimmune hepatitis, acute cellular rejection, and primary biliary cirrhosis. In some of these cases, the eosinophils can even be focally prominent, for example, with a small cluster of cells in a portal tract. However, eosinophils are not the dominant finding in these cases, lacking the diffuse nature and density of eosinophils seen in an allergic type drug reaction. In addition, an eosinophilic drug reaction will lack the histological changes that typify these other diseases. Finally, the differential also includes a peripheral eosinophilia without an eosinophil-rich hepatitis. In these cases, the eosinophils are essentially all located in the sinusoids, and there is minimal or absent lobular injury.

DRESS syndrome

Rare drug reactions develop a cluster of severe systemic conditions called the DRESS syndrome, an acronym that stands for "drug reaction with eosinophilia and systemic symptoms." The DRESS syndrome typically develops three weeks or more after starting the triggering medication and can have a mortality of up to 10%.[15] Symptoms can last for weeks after discontinuing the triggering medication. The symptoms tend to include a core set of findings consisting of a fever greater than 38°C, rash, lymphadenopathy in at least two locations, and peripheral blood findings of eosinophilia, thrombocytopenia, and either lymphocytosis or lymphopenia. The lymphocytes also commonly show cytological atypia. The liver is involved in about 80% of cases, with primarily aspartate aminotransferase (AST) and ALT elevations. Biopsies show marked portal and lobular eosinophilia (Fig. 15.5). The list of drugs that can lead to the DRESS syndrome grows continually, but in one comprehensive review of the literature,[16] the most common reported drugs were carbamazepine (27% of cases), allopurinol (11%), lamotrigine (6%), phenobarbital (6%), nevirapine (5%), phenytoin (4%), and abacavir (3%), with many more drugs at lower frequencies.

15.6 IDIOSYNCRATIC DRUG REACTIONS

Idiosyncratic drug reactions are the most common form of DILI encountered in surgical pathology. This

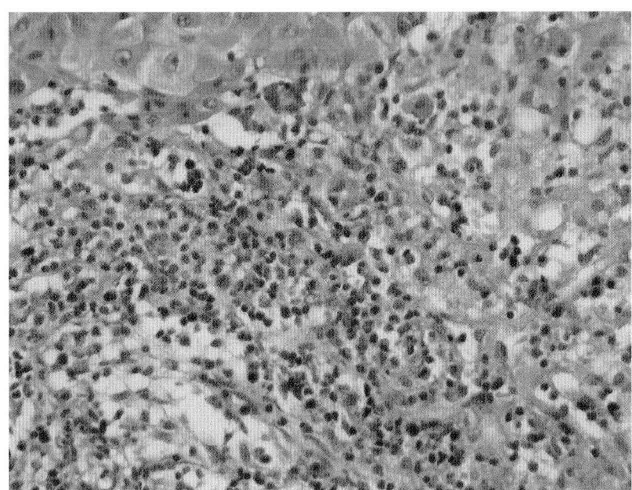

Figure 15.5 DRESS. The portal tracts are filled with eosinophils.

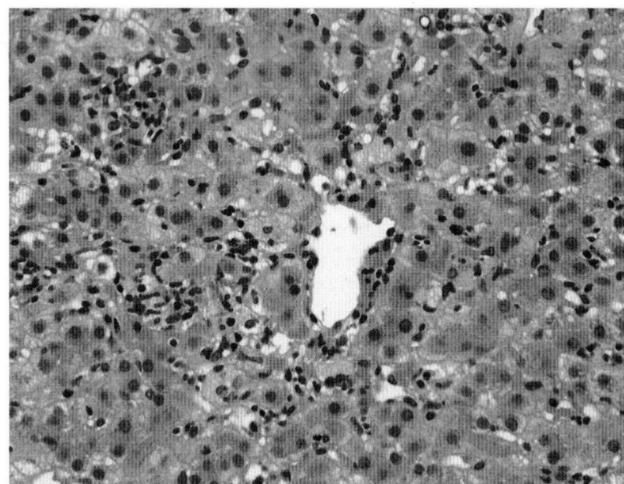

Figure 15.6 Hepatitic drug reaction. This drug reaction resulted from a herbal remedy.

type of DILI by definition is not dose related and cannot be predicted on an individual level, making the diagnosis a clinical challenge. A diagnosis of idiosyncratic DILI requires exclusion of viral hepatitis (A, B, C, and E) and autoimmune hepatitis. Several broad histological patterns are seen with idiosyncratic DILI, which are described in more detail later. These patterns are not exclusive, and a biopsy can show elements of more than one of these patterns.

Of note, idiosyncratic drug reactions are rarely if ever the cause of significant fibrosis. If a biopsy does show convincing fibrosis, then other causes of chronic hepatitis are more likely. Identifying a drug reaction superimposed upon another form of known chronic hepatitis, such as chronic hepatitis C, can be very challenging. These cases are approached by looking for findings atypical for the known underlying liver disease and by correlating histology with the laboratory and clinical findings. For example, an individual with known chronic hepatitis C who has long term but relative stable elevations in liver enzymes may present with a sudden increase in AST and ALT, suggesting a superimposed injury. A biopsy of the liver in this setting might show marked lobular hepatitis, further supporting the likelihood of a superimposed injury, because the vast majority of chronic hepatitis C biopsies show mild to moderate lobular inflammation.

Hepatic pattern

The hepatitic pattern is a common pattern with DILI and shows lobular and portal inflation that can range from mild to marked. Most herbal remedies also tend to show this pattern of injury (Fig. 15.6). The lobular hepatitis can be panacinar or can show a Zone 3 accentuation (Fig. 15.7). Zone 3 necrosis is common with more severe grades of lobular hepatitis. In some cases, there can be extensive necrosis with few surviving hepatocytes (Fig. 15.8). The inflammation is predominately T cells but there can be B cell aggregates in the portal tracts. Lobular cholestasis is common when there is moderate to marked lobular hepatitis. The inflammation in the portal tracts commonly includes occasional plasma cells, neutrophils, and eosinophils. Interface activity is typically present when there is moderate to marked portal inflammation.

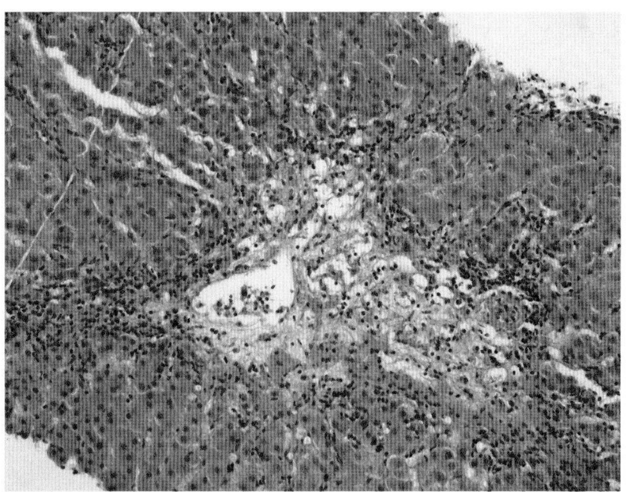

Figure 15.7 Hepatitic drug reaction. The lobular hepatitis in this drug reaction (Atorvastatin) shows a clear Zone 3 accentuation with Zone 3 hepatocyte necrosis.

The differential for a hepatic pattern of DILI is primarily acute viral hepatitis and autoimmune hepatitis. There are no histological findings that will reliably separate these three possibilities, and a diagnosis of DILI is based on excluding other causes and having exposure to a plausible drug candidate. Histological findings such as prominent plasma cells,

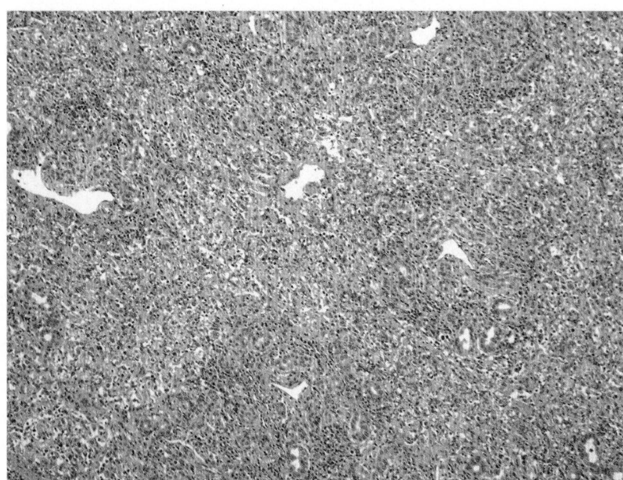

Figure 15.8 Hepatitic drug reaction. This severe drug reaction (Isoniazid [INH]) has led to the death of nearly all of the hepatocytes, with residual inflammation and ductular proliferation in the portal tracts.

interface activity, or Zone 3 accentuated inflammation are not etiologically specific and can be seen in all three of these entities. To reinforce this point, several drugs can cause DILI with a plasma cell-rich hepatitic pattern, one that often cannot be reliably separated from autoimmune hepatitis based on histological findings (Fig. 15.9). The most common of these are minocycline (acne), methyldopa (hypertension), clometacin (anti-inflammatory), and nitrofurantoin (urinary tract infections) (Table 15.1). Further complicating the workup of these cases, the DILI can start soon after beginning the medication or can start after several years of taking the medication. Furthermore, these drugs can also be associated with elevated serum antinuclear antibody (ANA) and/or antismooth muscle

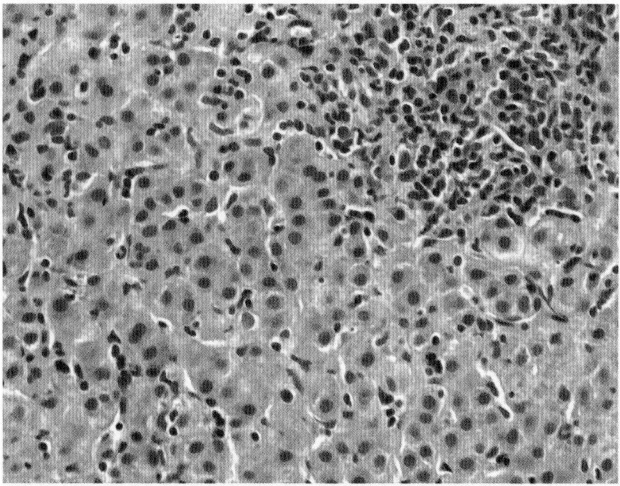

Figure 15.9 Plasma cell-rich drug reaction. This case (minocycline) histologically looks like autoimmune hepatitis.

Table 15.1 Drugs associated with both an autoimmune hepatitis like pattern of injury on histology plus positive autoantibody serology

Drug	Comments
Strongest association	
Atorvastatin (Lipitor)[41]	Statin used to lower cholesterol
Clometacin[42]	NSAID
Diclofenac[43]	NSAID
Dihydralizine[44]	Antihypertensive
Halothane[45]	Inhalational general anesthetic
Infliximab[46,47]	Antibody against tumor necrosis factor α
Interferon[48,49]	Liver transplant setting
Isoniazid[45]	Tuberculosis treatment
Methyldopa[50]	Antihypertensive
Minocycline[51]	Antibiotic
Nitrofurantoin[51]	Antibiotic
Oxyphenisatin[52]	Herbal laxative
Propylthiouracil[53]	Treatment for hyperthyroid disease
Tienilic acid[54]	Diuretic
Other reports	
Benzbromarone[55]	Xanthine oxidase inhibitor, used to treat gout
Black Cohosh[56]	Herbal remedy
Cefaclor[55]	Antibiotic
Cephalexin[51]	Antibiotic
Loxoprofen sodium hydrate[55]	NSAID
Ofloxacin[55]	Antibiotic
Ornidazole[57]	Anti-protozoan
Prometrium[51]	Progesterone
Pemoline[58]	Simulant used to treat attention-deficit hyperactivity disorder and narcolepsy
Rosuvastatin (Crestor)[59]	Statin
Simvastatin[41]	Statin

antibody (ASMA) titers. Thus, potentially offending drugs need to be stopped as part of the clinical management before a diagnosis of either drug reaction or autoimmune hepatitis is secured. The presence of fibrosis strongly favors autoimmune hepatitis over one of these drug reactions. However, care must be taken to not over interpret expansion of the portal tracts by inflammation as portal fibrosis. Likewise, the Kupffer cell hyperplasia that accompanies many drug reactions can mimic pericellular fibrosis, whereas Zone 3 necrosis or bridging necrosis can mimic central vein fibrosis or bridging fibrosis, respectively.

Granulomatous pattern

The differential for granulomas of the liver is broad, and most cases do not represent DILI. Instead, the most common causes of hepatic granulomas are idiopathic, sarcoidosis, infection, or primary biliary cirrhosis.[17] Nonetheless, DILI is an important part of the differential. In most cases of DILI, the granulomas are part of a hepatitic pattern, accompanied by mild to moderate lymphocytic inflammation of the portal tracts and lobules, although occasionally the main pattern of injury is granulomas. The granulomas can be well formed and epithelioid or can be loose and ill defined. The granulomas are not associated with fibrosis (which suggests sarcoidosis when present) and do not show necrosis (which suggests infection when present). The granulomas can be in the portal tracts or the lobules or the bile ducts, but their location does not provide a strong clue to DILI as the etiology.

As is generally true for all cases of DILI, a diagnosis of DILI with granulomatous inflammation is one of exclusion. Stains should be performed to examine for fungal and acid fast bacterial infections. Beyond organism stains, there are no immunohistochemical stains that will identify the etiology of a granuloma. All granulomas should be polarized for foreign material and serum testing for antimitochondrial antibodies is important. Other findings that would favor primary biliary cirrhosis over DILI include florid duct lesions, bile duct loss, or fibrosis.

Cholangitic pattern

The cholangitic pattern is most commonly seen with antibiotics and shows duct inflammation, bile duct injury, reactive epithelial changes, and apoptotic duct epithelial bodies. The inflammation in the portal tracts is often mixed, with predominately lymphocytes and occasional neutrophils, eosinophils, and/or plasma cells. The bile ducts also show reactive changes and can be infiltrated by lymphocytes and neutrophils.

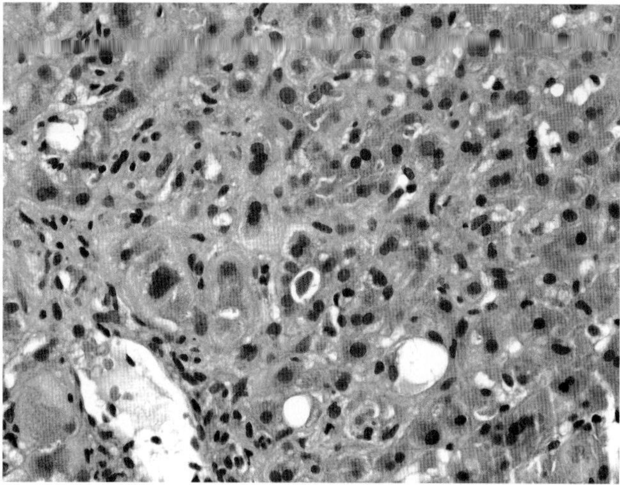

Figure 15.10 Bland lobular cholestasis pattern. This drug reaction (androgens) shows a canalicular cholestasis pattern, nuclear pleomorphism, and relative little inflammation.

Cholestatic pattern

This pattern refers to cases with lobular cholestasis that do not have significant inflammation and do not show changes of downstream biliary tract disease, a pattern also called bland lobular cholestasis. The cholestasis is often mild to moderate and may show a Zone 3 predominance in some cases. The bile can be in the hepatocyte cytoplasm or in the bile canaliculi. In contrast, bile is only seen in the bile ducts proper or the proliferating ductules, when the cholestasis is severe. This pattern of injury can be seen with a wide range of medications but the classic examples are oral contraceptives or anabolic steroids (Fig. 15.10). Of note, drug-induced lobular cholestasis can persist for several months after discontinuing the drug. In other cases, DILI can initially show a mixed hepatitic and cholestatic pattern, with significant inflammation and lobular cholestasis. When the medication is stopped, the inflammation disappears more rapidly than the cholestasis, and there is a window of time when biopsies show a bland lobular cholestatic pattern.

The differential for the bland lobular cholestasis pattern of injury includes sepsis, heart failure, hypothyroidism, and individuals critically ill from multiple organ failure. The explanation for the liver dysfunction is generally known in these clinical settings, so biopsies are rarely performed.

Ductopenic pattern

This pattern of drug injury (Fig. 15.11 and Table 15.2) can be subtle but shows reduced numbers of bile ducts or total loss of bile ducts. The diagnostic approach to ductopenia is similar to that for chronic rejection. Any loss of large- or medium-sized bile ducts (septal

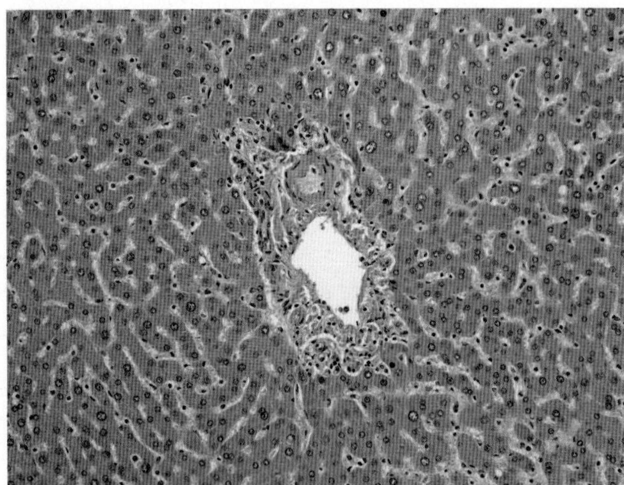

Figure 15.11 Ducteopenic pattern. This portal tract has no bile duct.

sized and larger) is abnormal. For the smaller branches of the biliary tree, 50% or more of the smaller portal tracts should be missing bile ducts to confidently make this diagnosis. Correlation with the serum alkaline phosphatase levels is important because the levels invariably are substantially elevated when there is established ductopenia. Another useful clue can be examination of the bile ducts that still remain because they commonly show atrophy and reactive changes. Inflammation of the remaining bile ducts can also be seen, but is often absent. Immunostains for cytokeratin can help identify bile duct loss. A CK7 stain can both identify bile duct loss and highlight intermediate hepatocytes, which are typically present with chronic cholestasis. The biopsy may also have other changes, including nonspecific portal lymphocytic inflammation, fatty change, and lobular cholestasis. In contrast, the following findings are typically absent with DILI-induced ductopenia, and if present suggest alternative etiologies for the bile duct loss: florid duct lesions, granulomas associated with the bile ducts, bile ductular reaction, bile duct duplication, onion skinning fibrosis, fibro-obliterative duct lesions, significant portal fibrosis, bridging fibrosis, or cirrhosis.

Fatty pattern

DILI that leads to fatty change usually causes a macrovesicular pattern of steatosis, but drugs that cause mitochondrial injury can lead to microvesicular steatosis. In terms of macrovesicular steatosis, an estimated 2% of all cases of nonalcoholic fatty liver disease result from DILI.[3] There are many different drugs that can cause steatosis (Table 15.3). Most drugs cause steatosis and not steatohepatitis, but amiodarone

Table 15.2 Causes of DILI associated with ductopenia

Drug	Comments
Antibiotics	
Amoxicillin/clavulanic acid[60]	Antibiotic
Azithromycin[61]	Antibiotic
Ciprofloxacin[62]	Antibiotic
Flucloxacillin[63]	Antibiotic
fluoroquinolone[64]	Antibiotic
Itraconazole[65]	Antifungal
Meropenem[66]	Antibiotic
Moxifloxacin[67]	Antibiotic
Nevirapine[68]	Reverse transcriptase inhibitor
Terbinafine[69]	Antifungal
Thiabendazole[70]	Antifungal
Trimethoprim-sulfamethoxazole[71]	Antibiotic
NSAIDs	
Ibuprofen[72]	NSAID
Naproxen[73]	NSAID
Tenoxicam[74]	NSAID
Others	
Anabolic steroids[75]	
Carbamazepine[76]	Used to treat epilepsy
Chlorpromazine (Thorazine)[77]	Antipsychotic
Gold salt therapy[78]	Has been used to treat rheumatoid arthritis
Interferon therapy[79]	
Tibolone and St Johns Wort[80]	Synthetic hormone and herbal remedy
Total parenteral nutrition[81]	Up to 25% of cases in one study
Valproic acid[82]	Used to treat epilepsy

Table 15.3 Drugs associated with a macrovesicular steatosis

Drug	Comments
Amiodarone	Antiarrhythmic medication
Cannabis	Limited data; strength of association unclear but may be strongest in the setting of HCV[83]
Glucocorticoids	
Irinotecan	Chemotherapeutic, commonly used in colon cancer
Methotrexate	
Nucleoside reverse transcriptase inhibitors	HIV treatment
Oxaliplatin	Chemotherapeutic, commonly used in colon cancer
Perihexline	Anti-anginal agent
Protease inhibitors	HIV treatment, can be associated with lipodystrophy
Tamoxifen	Estrogen receptor antagonist. 30%–40% of breast cancer patients under treatment will develop fatty liver disease in the first 2 years of therapy[84]

This table is not comprehensive (see also Table 15.7 and Chapter 16).

and irinotecan are two well-known exceptions, causing steatosis, ballooned hepatocytes, and Mallory hyaline. The diagnosis of DILI requires exclusion of other diseases, including the metabolic syndrome, alcohol-related injury, Wilson disease, celiac disease, protein malnutrition, and cystic fibrosis.

Amiodarone

Amiodarone therapy is a recognized risk for fatty liver disease, which develops in up to 4% of individuals on chronic therapy.[18,19] The risk for fatty liver disease is driven more by the duration of therapy and total accumulated dose, and less by the current dosage, with most cases having at least a year of use before developing fatty liver disease.[3] Amiodarone is one of the rare drugs that can become very concentrated in the liver, contributing up to 1% of the wet weight of the liver in severe cases.[3] Amiodarone also has a very long half-life, which can lead to ongoing liver injury despite stopping the medication. The pattern of injury seen on biopsy is typically mild to moderate macrovesicular steatosis with disproportionately

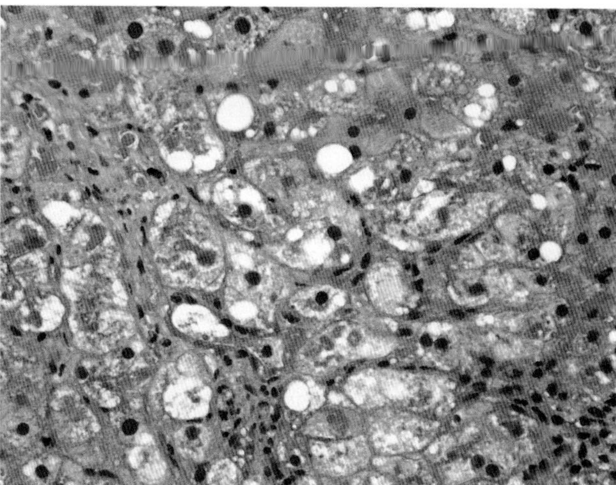

Figure 15.12 Amioadarone DILI. The hepatocytes show mild steatosis and marked ballooning with striking Mallory hyaline.

marked hepatocellular ballooning and Mallory hyaline (Fig. 15.12). The injured cells are often surrounded by many neutrophils, which is also known as neutrophilic satellitosis. In some cases, the fat can even be minimal, despite abundant hepatocyte ballooning. The portal and lobular inflammation is generally mild. The marked ballooning and Mallory hyaline can suggest alcoholic liver disease.[20] Cholestasis and granulomas are uncommon but have been reported.[21,22]

Phospholipidiosis

In addition to steatohepatitis, some drugs can also cause Kupffer cell hyperplasia and enlargement with foamy appearing cytoplasm, a finding called phospholipidosis (Figs. 15.13 and 15.14). Phospholipidosis can be

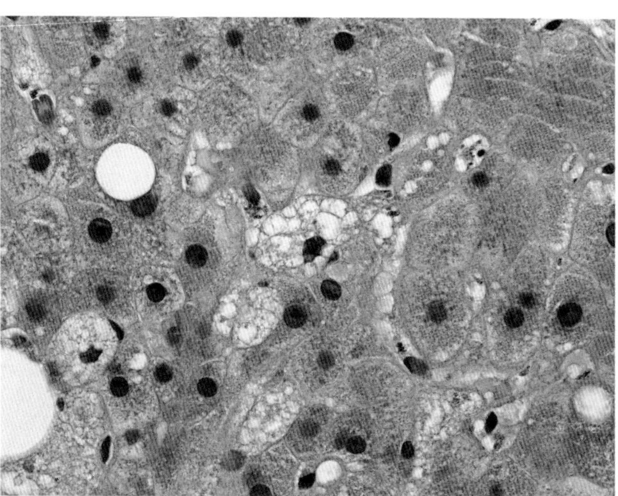

Figure 15.13 Phospholipidosis. At low power, the Kupffer cells are prominent, with a bubbly cytoplasmic quality.

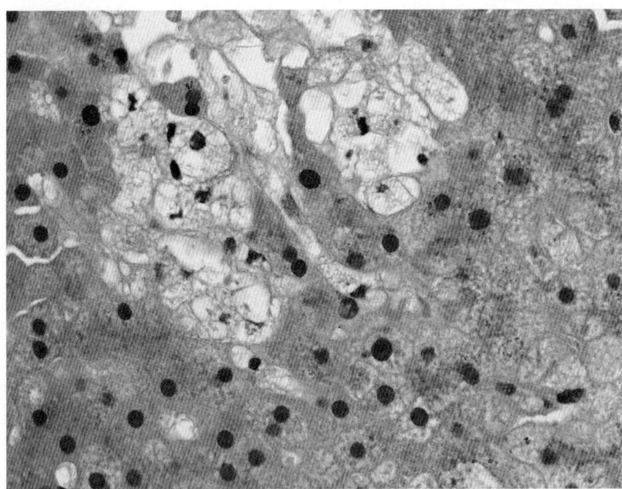

Figure 15.14 Phospholipidosis. At higher power, the Kupffer cells are filled with numerous vacuoles of various sizes.

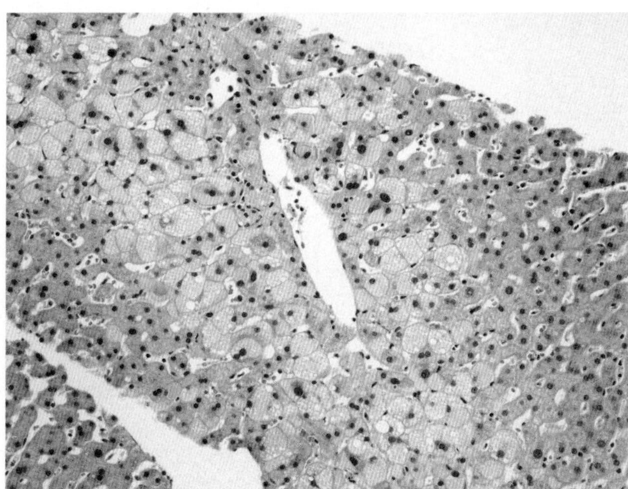

Figure 15.15 Microvesicular steatosis. The hepatocytes cytoplasm is filled with numerous tiny droplets of fat. In this case, a Zone 3 predominance is evident.

accompanied by steatosis, but can also be an isolated finding. Although the list is long,[23] some examples of drugs that can cause phospholipidosis include amiodarone, perhexiline maleate, and diethylaminoethoxyhexestrol. The degree of phospholipidosis will vary from subtle to well developed. In some cases, the findings can be sufficiently prominent to suggest a storage disorder such as Niemann–Pick disease. The phospholipidosis results from the accumulation of lamellar inclusions in the lysosomes.

DILI in the setting of other risk factors for fatty liver disease

In addition to drugs that can cause de novo fatty liver disease, some drugs are thought to contribute to liver injury primarily by exacerbating the fatty liver disease in individuals who already have major risk factors, such as the metabolic syndrome. Examples of these drugs include estrogens, tamoxifen, methotrexate, and nifedipine. At a practical level, the pathologist cannot distinguish the relative role of DILI versus, for example, the metabolic syndrome in any given biopsy. Thus, the best approach is to fully report the amount of fat, the degree of ongoing injury (lobular inflammation, balloon cells, and/or apoptotic bodies), and the fibrosis stage, including in a note that the biopsy findings do not reliably separate drug effect from other causes of fatty liver disease.

Microvesicular steatosis

Microvesicular steatosis results from medications that impair mitochondrial function, including valproic acid, tetracycline, and zivodine. The hepatocytes have numerous tiny vacuoles that fill their cytoplasm (Fig. 15.15). This change diffusely affects the hepatocytes in most cases, though there can be some zonal accentuation, most commonly in Zone 3, with relative sparing of Zone 1. Of note, finding scattered hepatocytes with medium or larger sized fat droplets is still consistent with a diagnosis of microvesicular steatosis, as long as the predominant pattern is microvesicular steatosis. The most common diagnostic pitfall is misinterpreting the small- and medium-sized droplets of fat in conventional steatohepatitis (Fig. 15.16) as microvesicular steatosis, but comparison to reference images almost always clarifies this part of the differential. The differential includes two additional entities. First, ordinary fatty

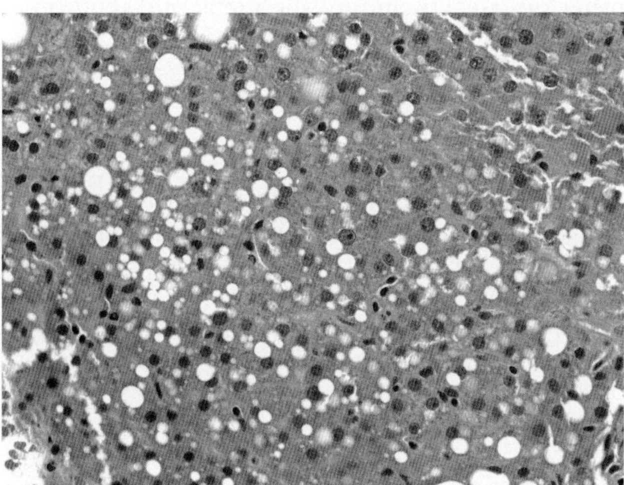

Figure 15.16 Intermediate-sized fat droplets (not microvesicular steatosis). Conventional fatty liver disease from the metabolic syndrome, with scattered intermediate size fat droplets.

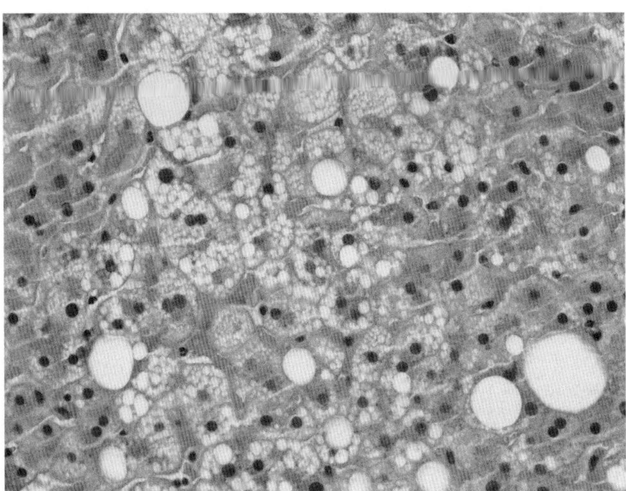

Figure 15.17 Microvesicular steatosis in conventional fatty liver disease. A small discrete focus of microvesicular steatosis is seen with macrovesicular steatosis in the background.

liver disease can occasionally have small and discrete, well-delineated foci of microvesicular steatosis (Fig. 15.17). This change is considered to be part of conventional fatty liver disease and does not indicate either a drug effect or widespread mitochondrial injury from other causes. Secondly, alcoholic hepatitis can rarely have a pattern of injury with diffuse microvesicular steatosis, a pattern called acute alcohol foamy degeneration. The clinical history of alcohol use will help make the diagnosis in most cases.

15.7 MEDICATIONS ASSOCIATED WITH FIBROSIS

Fibrosis is not part of the typical injury pattern in most cases of DILI. However, a small number of medications are recognized for their ability to cause fibrosis. It is also true that a much longer list of drugs has been associated with liver fibrosis, mostly in case reports and small case series, but it is often unclear if the medication actually caused the fibrosis, because many individuals have comorbidities that could also explain the fibrosis, such as the metabolic syndrome. Registry-based studies also fall into this category, reporting possible associations with fibrosis that are difficult to validate. As one example, a registry-based study found cryptogenic cirrhosis in 0.7% of individuals after long-term follow-up for a drug-induced hepatitis.[24]

On the other hand, there are medications that have strong causal links to fibrosis, two of which are discussed further below. Given this, it may very well be that other medications cause fibrosis, but actual causation needs to be demonstrated. Otherwise, there is a risk of making life-improving drugs less available to those who may need them, based on spurious associations. In this regard, a history of taking a drug that can cause fibrosis does not always mean the drug caused the fibrosis in that specific case. In this setting, the clinical work up can be incomplete when fibrosis is ascribed too quickly to a drug reaction, potentially missing other important underlying liver diseases. For this reason, each liver biopsy has to be evaluated on its own merits, incorporating the clinical and laboratory context.

Methotrexate

Methotrexate is an important medicine used to manage some chronic autoimmune conditions, including psoriasis, rheumatoid arthritis, and Crohn disease. Methotrexate is also used to treat some cancers, but in that setting the fibrosis risk is less often clinically relevant. When methotrexate is used for chronic medical conditions, liver biopsies are sometimes performed at baseline and after the introduction of methotrexate to monitor for fibrosis, though biopsies for this purpose tend to be much less common now because of the widespread availability of noninvasive markers of fibrosis. With methotrexate use, factors that increase the risk for fibrosis include mainly the cumulative dose and the presence of other chronic liver diseases, such as fatty liver disease or alcohol-related liver disease. The dosage regiment also affects fibrosis risk, with the older practice of daily use having a greater risk then the modern usage of weekly dosing, supplemented with folate.

Methotrexate use is frequently stopped when there is moderate portal fibrosis or bridging fibrosis. Historically, data suggested a frequency of cirrhosis of about 20% after 5 to 10 years of daily use. With modern dosage, advanced fibrosis or cirrhosis appears to be rare, though methotrexate can likely be a cofactor when other risk factors are present, such as steatohepatitis from the metabolic syndrome.

Histologically, biopsies can show either or both portal fibrosis and pericellular fibrosis (Fig. 15.18). A classification schema for methotrexate injury is available,[25] as shown in Table 15.4, but is primarily used in research settings. In clinical practice, the most common approach is to stage the fibrosis using the local go-to system, such as the Ishak, Batts–Ludwig, or METAVIR staging system. Other histological findings can include mild to focally moderate portal lymphocytic inflammation, fatty change, and hepatocyte nuclear pleomorphism. Of note, other clinical risk factors for fatty liver disease are commonly present, such as the metabolic syndrome. In this setting, the biopsy findings do not distinguish methotrexte effect from ordinary fatty liver disease.

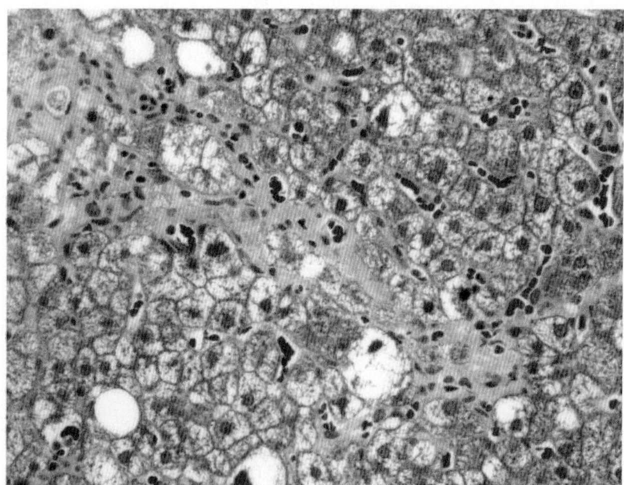

Figure 15.18 Methotrexate injury. The Trichrome stain shows pericellular fibrosis.

Hypervitaminosis A

Vitamin A excess most commonly occurs as a result of ingesting too much preformed vitamin A in the form of vitamins, dietary supplements, or rarely the livers of certain animals such as moose or polar bear. In contrast, hypervitaminosis A generally does not occur from ingesting too many vegetables rich in β carotenes because the conversion of β carotenes to vitamin A is tightly regulated. The degree to which topical Retin-A is a risk factor is controversial.

Hypervitaminosis A toxicity can be either acute or chronic. Acute toxicity results from either a single or a few very high doses of vitamin A, usually >100 times the RDA of 3,000 IU for men and 2,300 IU for women.[26] With acute toxicity, clinical signs and symptoms typically develop within days to weeks and can include severe headache, nausea, vertigo, blurred vision, muscle pain, and skin desquamation with alopecia. In contrast, chronic exposure usually results from at least 6 months of taking doses of >10 the RDA of vitamin A. In this setting, the clinical diagnosis is often hard to make, and the patient's history may be complicated by many other possible conditions that have been explored by the clinical team. Patients can present with a wide range of initial clinical symptoms (Table 15.5), but the most common presentation is unexplained mild but persistent elevations in AST and ALT. Of note, a history of excess vitamin A intake is frequently missed on early patient visits and only revealed on repeat taking of the patient's history, with focused questions on possible exposures to vitamin A. Blood testing for vitamin A (retinol) can also be a source of confusion for both clinicians and pathologists. Vitamin A blood testing is useful to detect vitamin A deficiency, and when elevated, can be consistent with excess intake, but normal serum levels of vitamin A do not exclude vitamin A toxicity. This is because a large proportion of vitamin A circulates as esters bound to plasma proteins and thus may not be detected in routinely used serum tests.[27]

In most cases, the liver biopsy appears almost normal at first because the enlarged and lipid laden stellate cells are easily missed. However, once you see one engorged stellate cell, then others are more easily found (Fig. 15.19). The stellate cells are enlarged with cytoplasm that is filled with small lipid vacuoles, giving the cytoplasm a bubbly appearance. There is typically no strong zonal pattern. The lobules usually

Table 15.4 Grading schema for methotrexate toxicity

Grade	Histological description
1	Normal Mild steatosis Mild nuclear variability Mild portal inflammation Allowed fibrosis is not specified, typically none
2	Moderate to marked steatosis Moderate to marked nuclear variability Moderate to marked portal inflammation Allowed fibrosis is not specified, typically none or minimal portal fibrosis
3	3A: "mild" fibrosis[a]. 3B: "moderate to severe" fibrosis[a].
4	Cirrhosis
	Suggested clinical implications
1	Can continue to receive methotrexate therapy
2	Can continue to receive methotrexate therapy
3A	Can continue to receive methotrexate therapy but should have a repeat liver biopsy after approximately 6 mo of continued therapy.
3B	Should not be given further methotrexate therapy. However, exceptional circumstances may require continued methotrexate therapy with careful follow-up.
4	Should not be given further methotrexate therapy. However, exceptional circumstances may require continued methotrexate therapy with careful follow-up.

[a]The original paper did not provide histologically meaningful definitions for the fibrosis. By common practice, portal fibrosis is classified as 3A and bridging fibrosis as 3B.
From Roenigk HH Jr, Auerbach R, Maibach HI, et al. Methotrexate in psoriasis: revised guidelines. *J Am Acad Dermatol*. 1988;19(1, pt 1):145–156, with permission from the American Academy of Dermatology.

Table 15.5 Clinical and laboratory features in chronic vitamin A excess
Clinical manifestations
Anorexia
Ascites
Bone pain
Cheilosis (painful drying and cracking at the corners of the mouth)
Dry skin
Fatigue
Gingivitis
Headache
Hepatomegaly
Muscle pain
Pleural effusions
Unexplained fevers
Unexplained liver enzymes elevations

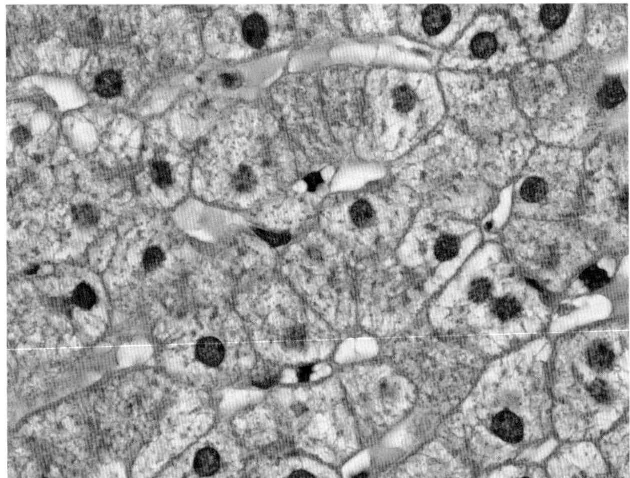

Figure 15.19 Stellate cell hyperplasia. Stellate cells are enlarged by numerous small cytoplasmic vacuoles that indent the nuclei. Three of them are present in this image.

show no or minimal inflammatory changes, as do the portal tracts. Nodular regenerative hyperplasia can occasionally be seen.[28] There is usually no fibrosis, but when present there will be a pericellular pattern. Typically, years to decades of chronic exposure to excess vitamin A are needed to develop fibrosis.[28]

The differential for stellate cell hyperplasia is primarily cytoplasmic vacuolization of Kupffer cells, which is

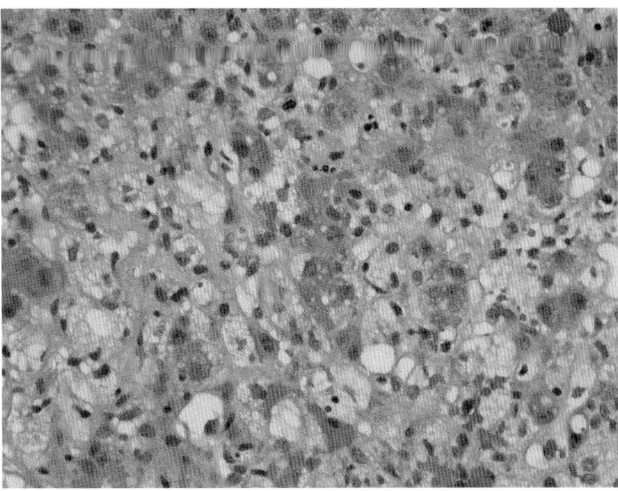

Figure 15.20 Kupffer cell hyperplasia. The liver is cholestatic, and the resulting Kupffer cell hyperplasia was initially misdiagnosed as stellate cell hyperplasia.

common in cholestatic livers (Fig. 15.20). This finding has been misinterpreted as stellate cell hyperplasia both in clinical practice and in the literature. A CD68 immunostain can help identify these mimics as foamy Kupffer cells. In addition, Kupffer cell hyperplasia is typically more diffuse and striking than is stellate cell hyperplasia. There are currently no specific immunostains to highlight stellate cells in human tissue. Although not necessary for diagnosis, immunostains for smooth muscle actin often highlight sinusoidal cells when there is stellate cell hyperplasia (Fig. 15.21), a nonspecific finding that tends to be more sensitive than specific. If there is no stellate cell hyperplasia on the hematoxylin and eosin, then smooth muscle actin staining should not be interpreted in isolation as evidence for hypervitaminosis A.

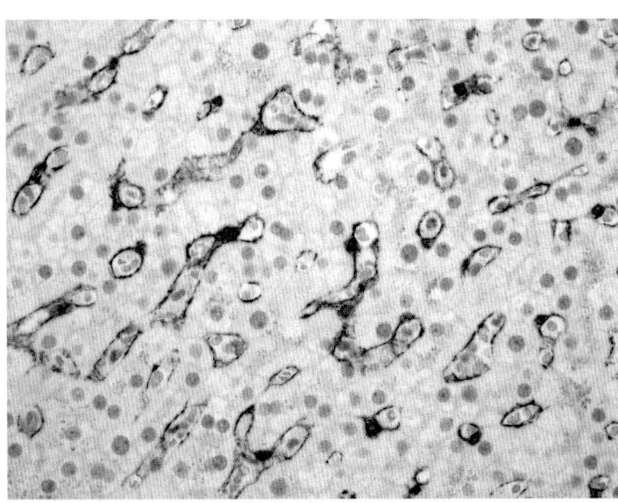

Figure 15.21 Kupffer cell hyperplasia, smooth muscle actin immunostain. The stellate cells are highlighted.

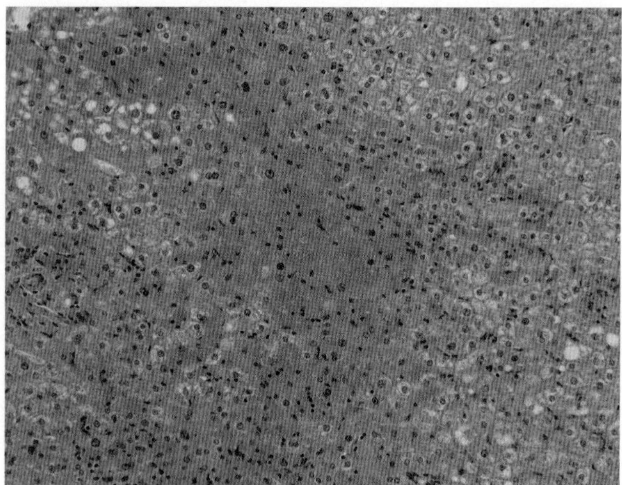

Figure 15.22 Sinusoidal obstructive syndrome. The sinusoids show patchy but striking dilatation and congestion (oxaliplatin).

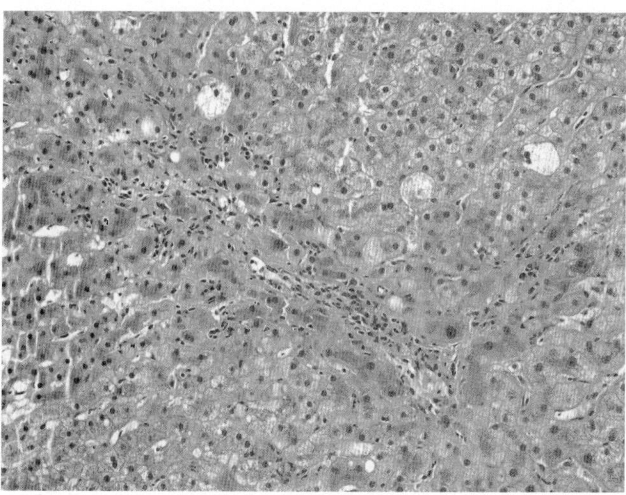

Figure 15.23 Hepatitic pattern. A Zone 3 pattern of hepatitis is seen (Ipilimumab).

15.8 CHEMOTHERAPY-RELATED CHANGES

Chemotherapy can lead to three main patterns of injury: vascular, fatty liver disease, or a hepatitis pattern of injury.

The most common pattern of vascular injury results from damage to the sinusoidal endothelial cells, a finding called sinusoidal obstructive syndrome or veno-occlusive disease. This pattern of injury is most strongly associated with oxaliplatin and is most evident in resection specimens of metastatic colon adenocarcinoma to the liver. In these cases, the background liver can show marked Zone 3 sinusoidal dilatation and congestion (Fig. 15.22) and occasionally nodular regenerative hyperplasia.[29–31] In more severe cases, the Zone 3 congestion will connect central veins to central veins, a pattern called "bridging congestion". Zone 3 hepatocyte atrophy is also commonly present, but is usually mild. In some cases, the central veins will show partial or complete occlusion by loose collagen. This pattern of injury is not associated with significant portal or lobular inflammation, bile duct injury, or obstructive type biliary changes.

A second drug-induced pattern of injury is that of fatty liver disease, with moderate to marked steatosis and sometimes active steatohepatitis, a pattern of injury sometimes referred to as CASH, for chemotherapy-associated steatohepatitis. This pattern is associated with irinotecan and to a lesser degree with oxaliplatin.[30] Many affected individuals also have risk factors for the metabolic syndrome,[31] and there probably is a synergistic effect between the chemotherapy and the metabolic syndrome.

Finally, some of the monoclonal antibody therapies can induce a hepatitis pattern of DILI. The best known is Ipilimumab, a monoclonal antibody that blocks the action of CTLA-4, a receptor that downregulates the immune system. By blocking CTLA-4, the immune system can be more active against the tumor. Ipilimumab therapy, however, can also induce a hepatitic pattern of DILI, with either a panlobular hepatitis or a Zone 3 predominate hepatitis (Fig. 15.23).[32,33] Like most drug reactions, the inflammation is predominately CD8 positive T cells. The lobules can also show Kupffer cell hyperplasia with the formation of loose granulomas, especially with more severe inflammation. As another example, infliximab, a monoclonal antibody against TNF-α, can on rare occasions induce an autoimmune like hepatitis pattern on biopsy and can also induce serum ANA and ASMA autoantibodies.[34] Finally, many of these antibodies also serve as immunomodulators and can indirectly cause liver damage by reactivation of hepatitis B. One example is rituximab, a monoclonal antibody that targets CD20.[35]

15.9 VASCULAR CHANGES ASSOCIATED WITH DILI

Common vascular changes include chemotherapy-induced sinusoidal obstructive change and nodular regenerative hyperplasia, which are discussed earlier. Less common patterns of injury include peliosis hepatis and vascular thrombosis. Drugs associated with peliosis hepatitis include androgens (Fig. 15.24), estrogens, azathioprine, and corticosteroids. Herbal remedies most often cause a hepatitic pattern of injury, but can also cause a veno-occlusive pattern of injury (Fig. 15.25).

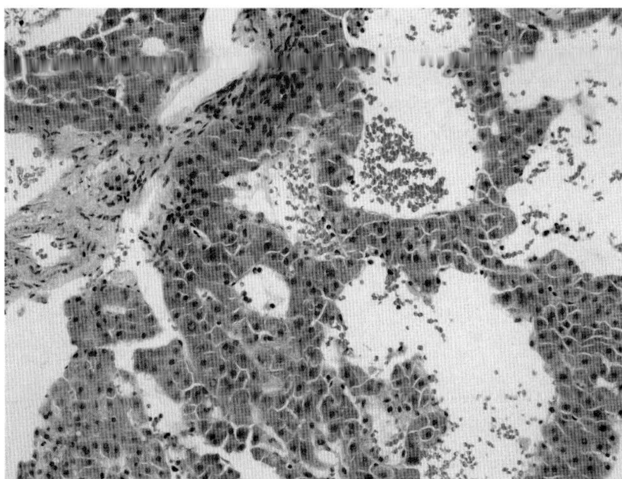

Figure 15.24 Peliosis hepatis. This case resulted from androgen use.

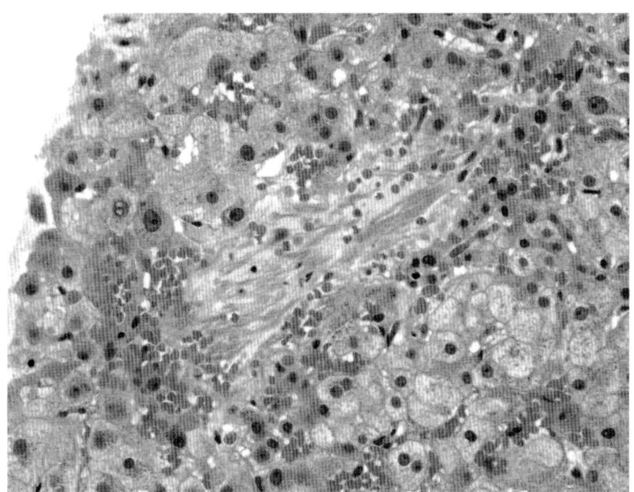

Figure 15.25 Veno-occlusive disease. This case resulted from use of a herbal remedy.

15.10 CYTOPLASMIC CHANGES INCLUDING INCLUSIONS

Some cases of DILI manifest as cytoplasmic changes in the hepatocytes without significant inflammation, fatty change, cholestasis, or fibrosis. This pattern of injury tends to be a milder form of DILI, associated with mild enzyme elevations and no risk for fibrosis. In fact, sometimes these findings are referred to as adaptive changes instead of DILI. These patterns share in common a drug-induced smooth endoplasmic reticulum proliferation. In the first pattern, which is also called "induced" hepatocytes, the hepatocytes show a diffuse gray homogenous change to the cytoplasm without well-developed inclusions (Fig. 15.26). Two drugs commonly associated with this pattern are phenobarbital and barbiturates.[36] The cytoplasmic changes can be variable, with milder cases often showing Zone 3 accentuation.

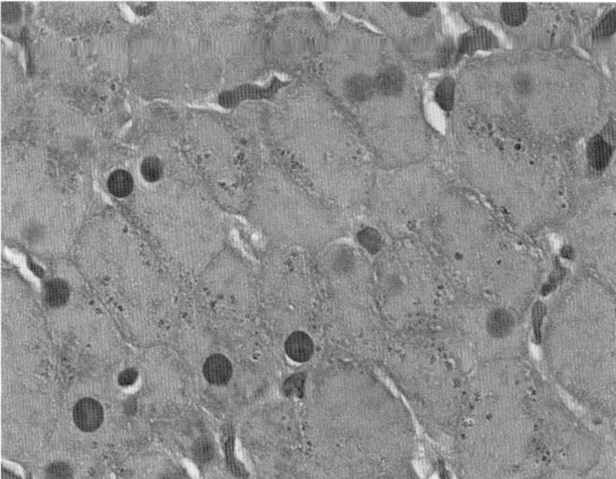

Figure 15.26 Induced hepatocytes. The hepatocytes show diffuse amphophilic change in the cytoplasm that results from smooth endoplasmic reticulum proliferation, pushing lipofuschin to the edge of the hepatocytes (phenobarbital).

A second major pattern has been described as "two-tone" hepatocytes because hepatocytes have two distinct cytoplasmic colors (Figs. 15.27 and 15.28). About half of the cytoplasm typically shows the normal cytoplasmic color, whereas the other half shows the distinctive homogenous gray color of smooth endoplasmic reticulum proliferation. The endoplasmic reticulum proliferation can affect either the cytoplasm next to the bile canaliculi or it can be perisinusoidal.

In the third pattern, the smooth endoplasmic reticulum proliferation leads to distinctive round

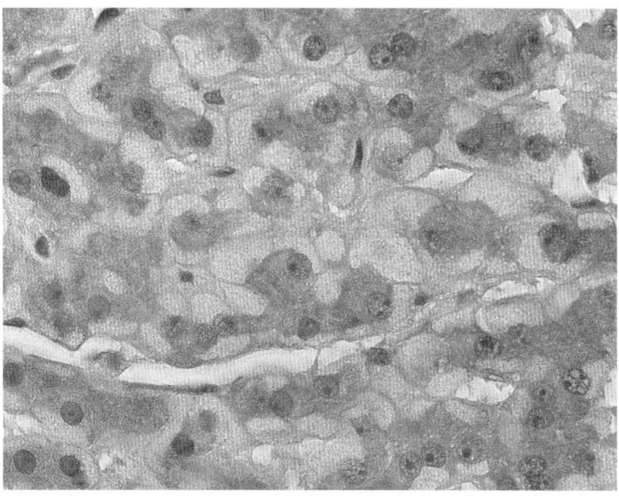

Figure 15.27 Two-tone hepatocytes. The hepatocyte cytoplasm has two distinct colors.

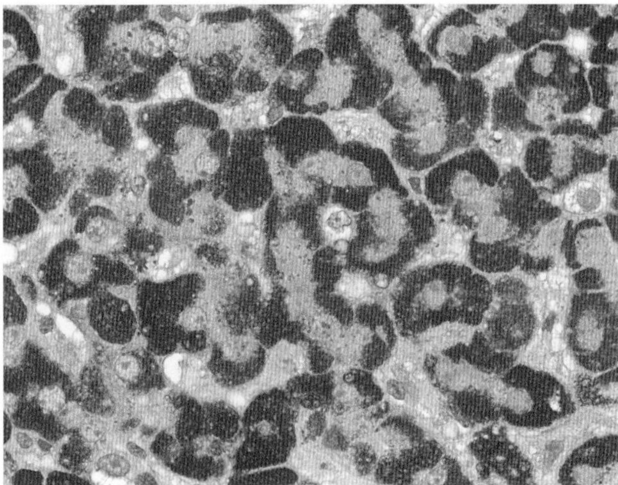

Figure 15.28 Two-tone hepatocytes, periodic acid–Schiff (PAS) stain. The two tones of the hepatocyte cytoplasm are brought out by a PAS stain.

hepatocyte inclusions (Fig. 15.29). This pattern is called "glycogen pseudoground glass" because it closely resembles the ground glass changes seen in some cases of long standing chronic hepatitis B infection.[37] In addition to the smooth endoplasmic reticulum proliferation, the inclusions are rich in glycogen so can be highlighted by a PAS stain. The glycogen has an abnormal pattern by electron microscopy, but the reasons for this change remain unknown.[37–39] The ground glass-like changes can be persistent on subsequent biopsies but to date there is no evidence that this pattern of DILI leads to fibrosis. Liver enzyme elevations are generally mild, and the biopsy shows no significant inflammation or cholestasis, with the exception of when this pattern occurs in the setting of other concomitant disease processes.

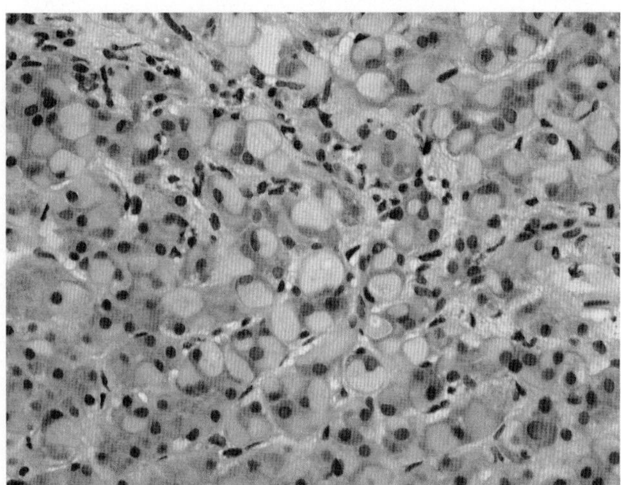

Figure 15.29 Glycogen psuedoground glass. The hepatocytes show distinct amphophilic inclusions in the cytoplasm.

Table 15.6 Differential for pseudoground glass inclusions in hepatocytes

Type of inclusion	Staining properties
Glycogen pseudoground glass	PAS+ diastase sensitive; colloidal iron negative
Cyanamide	PAS+ diastase sensitive
Fibrinogen	PAS–; Fibrinogen+; PTAH+; C3, C4 positive ±
Type IV glycogen storage disease	PAS+ partially diastase sensitive; colloidal iron negative
LaFora bodies	PAS+ diastase resistant; colloidal iron positive
Uremia	PAS+

The diastase reaction can vary between labs, so the results may vary. PAS stains are useful when they are negative, suggesting fibrinogen storage disease.
Abbreviation: PAS, periodic acid–Schiff.

To date, most cases of hepatocytes with pseudoground glass change have been reported in immunosuppression individuals who are on numerous medications, although no single drug or class of drugs has been identified as the cause. In rare cases, glycogen pseudoground glass can be seen in individuals on single medications who do not have documented immunosuppression, but this subset of cases has not been well studied. The histological differential for the glycogen pseudoground glass inclusions is primarily the ground glass changes associated with late stage chronic hepatitis B infection. Immunostains for hepatitis B surface antigen will sort this out. Serological findings are also helpful to rule in chronic hepatitis B, but negative HBsAg serology does not completely exclude hepatitis B infection[40] and immunostains should be performed. The larger differential also includes other drug effects such as cyanamide, genetic disorders such as Lafora bodies or fibrinogen storage disease, and reactive changes associated with uremia (Table 15.6). In most cases, the clinical situations are sufficiently distinct that these possibilities can be readily ruled out.

15.11 GLYCOGENIC HEPATOPATHY

Finally, DILI can also manifest as glycogenosis of the liver, with the hepatocytes showing abundant pale cytoplasm as a result of glycogen accumulation (Fig. 15.30). Corticosteroids are the most common

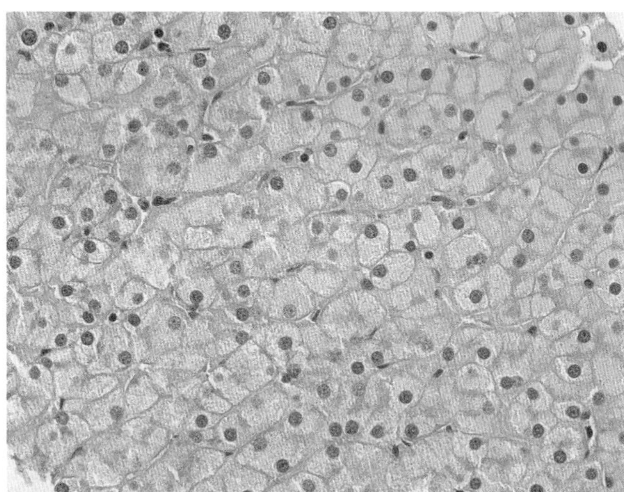

Figure 15.30 Hepatic glycogenosis. The hepatocytes are enlarged and pale, filled with glycogen (corticosteroids).

cause of this pattern of DILI. The differential for this pattern is primarily glycogenic hepatopathy resulting from poorly controlled diabetes mellitus.

REFERENCES

1. Chalasani N, Fontana RJ, Bonkovsky HL, et al. Causes, clinical features, and outcomes from a prospective study of drug-induced liver injury in the United States. *Gastroenterology*. 2008;135(6):1924–1934. e1–4.
2. Molleston JP, Fontana RJ, Lopez MJ, et al. Characteristics of idiosyncratic drug-induced liver injury in children: results from the DILIN prospective study. *J Pediatr Gastroenterol Nutr*. 2011;53(2):182–189.
3. Farrell GC. Drugs and steatohepatitis. *Semin Liver Dis*. 2002;22(2):185–194.
4. Davern TJ, Chalasani N, Fontana RJ, et al. Acute hepatitis E infection accounts for some cases of suspected drug-induced liver injury. *Gastroenterology*. 2011;141(5):1665–16672 e1–9.
5. Wadzinski J, Franks R, Roane D, et al. Valproate-associated hyperammonemic encephalopathy. *J Am Board Fam Med*. 2007;20(5):499–502.
6. Nott L, Price TJ, Pittman K, et al. Hyperammonemia encephalopathy: an important cause of neurological deterioration following chemotherapy. *Leuk Lymphoma*. 2007;48(9):1702–1711.
7. Acikalin A, Dişel NR, Direk EÇ, et al. A rare cause of postpartum coma: isolated hyperammonemia due to urea cycle disorder. *Am J Emerg Med*. 2015;34(7):1324.e3–1324.e4.
8. Belenky A, Igov I, Konstantino Y, et al. Endovascular diagnosis and intervention in patients with isolated hyperammonemia, with or without ascites, after liver transplantation. *J Vasc Interv Radiol*. 2009;20(2):259–263.
9. Pestaner JP, Ishak KG, Mullick FG, et al. Ferrous sulfate toxicity: a review of autopsy findings. *Biol Trace Elem Res*. 1999;69(3):191–198.
10. Ramachandran R, Kakar S. Histological patterns in drug-induced liver disease. *J Clin Pathol*. 2009;62(6):481–492.
11. Yoon E, Babar A, Choudhary M, et al. Acetaminophen-induced hepatotoxicity: a comprehensive update. *J Clin Transl Hepatol*. 2016;4(2):131–142.
12. Jacschke H. Acetaminophen: dose-dependent drug hepatotoxicity and acute liver failure in patients. *Dig Dis*. 2015;33(4):464–471.
13. Michaut A, Moreau C, Robin MA, et al. Acetaminophen-induced liver injury in obesity and nonalcoholic fatty liver disease. *Liver Int*. 2014;34(7):e171–179.
14. Savransky V, Reinke C, Jun J, et al. Chronic intermittent hypoxia and acetaminophen induce synergistic liver injury in mice. *Exp Physiol*. 2009;94(2):228–239.
15. Lopez-Rocha E, Blancas L, Rodríguez-Mireles K, et al. Prevalence of DRESS syndrome. *Rev Alerg Mex*. 2014;61(1):14–23.
16. Cacoub P, Musette P, Descamps V, et al. The DRESS syndrome: a literature review. *Am J Med*. 2011;124(7):588–597.
17. Drebber U, Kasper HU, Ratering J, et al. Hepatic granulomas: histological and molecular pathological approach to differential diagnosis—a study of 442 cases. *Liver Int*. 2008;28(6):828–834.
18. Lewis JH, Ranard RC, Caruso A, et al. Amiodarone hepatotoxicity: prevalence and clinicopathologic correlations among 104 patients. *Hepatology*. 1989;9(5):679–685.
19. Kum LC, Chan WW, Hui HH, et al. Prevalence of amiodarone-related hepatotoxicity in 720 Chinese patients with or without baseline liver dysfunction. *Clin Cardiol*. 2006;29(7):295–299.
20. Lewis JH, Mullick F, Ishak KG, et al. Histopathologic analysis of suspected amiodarone hepatotoxicity. *Hum Pathol*. 1990;21(1):59–67.
21. Rigas B, Rosenfeld LE, Barwick KW, et al. Amiodarone hepatotoxicity. A clinicopathologic study of five patients. *Ann Intern Med*. 1986;104(3):348–351.
22. Chang CC, Petrelli M, Tomashefski JF Jr, et al. Severe intrahepatic cholestasis caused by amiodarone toxicity after withdrawal of the drug: a case report and review of the literature. *Arch Pathol Lab Med*. 1999;123(3):251–256.
23. Reasor MJ, Hastings KL, Ulrich RG. Drug-induced phospholipidosis: issues and future directions. *Expert Opin Drug Saf*. 2006;5(4):567–583.

24. Bjornsson E, Davidsdottir L. The long-term follow-up after idiosyncratic drug-induced liver injury with jaundice. *J Hepatol.* 2009;50(3):511–517.
25. Roenigk HH Jr, Auerbach R, Maibach HI, et al. Methotrexate in psoriasis: revised guidelines. *J Am Acad Dermatol.* 1988;19(1, pt 1):145–156.
26. Penniston KL, Tanumihardjo SA. The acute and chronic toxic effects of vitamin A. *Am J Clin Nutr.* 2006;83(2):191–201.
27. Miksad R, de Lédinghen V, McDougall C, et al. Hepatic hydrothorax associated with vitamin a toxicity. *J Clin Gastroenterol.* 2002;34(3):275–279.
28. Geubel AP, De Galocsy C, Alves N, et al. Liver damage caused by therapeutic vitamin A administration: estimate of dose-related toxicity in 41 cases. *Gastroenterology.* 1991;100(6):1701–1709.
29. Morris-Stiff G, White AD, Gomez D, et al. Nodular regenerative hyperplasia (NRH) complicating oxaliplatin chemotherapy in patients undergoing resection of colorectal liver metastases. *Eur J Surg Oncol.* 2014;40(8):1016–1020.
30. Vauthey JN, Pawlik TM, Ribero D, et al. Chemotherapy regimen predicts steatohepatitis and an increase in 90-day mortality after surgery for hepatic colorectal metastases. *J Clin Oncol.* 2006;24(13):2065–2072.
31. Ryan P, Nanji S, Pollett A, et al. Chemotherapy-induced liver injury in metastatic colorectal cancer: semiquantitative histologic analysis of 334 resected liver specimens shows that vascular injury but not steatohepatitis is associated with preoperative chemotherapy. *Am J Surg Pathol.* 2010;34(6):784–791.
32. Johncilla M, Misdraji J, Pratt DS, et al. Ipilimumab-associated hepatitis: clinicopathologic characterization in a series of 11 cases. *Am J Surg Pathol.* 2015;39(8):1075–1084.
33. Kleiner DE, Berman D. Pathologic changes in ipilimumab-related hepatitis in patients with metastatic melanoma. *Dig Dis Sci.* 2012;57(8):2233–2240.
34. Germano V, Picchianti D, Baccano G, et al. Autoimmune hepatitis associated with infliximab in a patient with psoriatic arthritis. *Ann Rheum Dis.* 2005;64(10):1519–1520.
35. Civan J, Hann HW. Giving rituximab in patients with occult or resolved hepatitis B virus infection: are the current guidelines good enough? *Expert Opin Drug Saf.* 2015;14(6):865–875.
36. Jezequel AM, Librari ML, Mosca P, et al. Changes induced in human liver by long-term anticonvulsant therapy functional and ultrastructural data. *Liver.* 1984;4(5):307–317.
37. Wisell J, Boitnott J, Haas M, et al. Glycogen pseudoground glass change in hepatocytes. *Am J Surg Pathol.* 2006;30(9):1085–1090.
38. O'Shea AM, Wilson GJ, Ling SC, et al. Lafora-like ground-glass inclusions in hepatocytes of pediatric patients: a report of two cases. *Pediatr Dev Pathol.* 2007;10(5):351–357.
39. Bejarano PA, Garcia MT, Rodriguez MM, et al. Liver glycogen bodies: ground-glass hepatocytes in transplanted patients. *Virchows Arch.* 2006;449(5):539–545.
40. Torbenson M, Thomas DL. Occult hepatitis B. *Lancet Infect Dis.* 2002;2(8):479–486.
41. Alla V, Abraham J, Siddiqui J, et al. Autoimmune hepatitis triggered by statins. *J Clin Gastroenterol.* 2006;40(8):757–761.
42. Islam S, Mekhloufi F, Paul JM, et al. Characteristics of clometacin-induced hepatitis with special reference to the presence of anti-actin cable antibodies. *Autoimmunity.* 1989;2(3):213–221.
43. Scully LJ, Clarke D, Barr RJ. Diclofenac induced hepatitis. 3 cases with features of autoimmune chronic active hepatitis. *Dig Dis Sci.* 1993;38(4):744–751.
44. Bourdi M, Gautier JC, Mircheva J, et al. Anti-liver microsomes autoantibodies and dihydralazine-induced hepatitis: specificity of autoantibodies and inductive capacity of the drug. *Mol Pharmacol.* 1992;42(2):280–285.
45. Czaja AJ. Drug-induced autoimmune-like hepatitis. *Dig Dis Sci.* 2011;56(4):958–976.
46. Doyle A, Forbes G, Kontorinis N. Autoimmune hepatitis during infliximab therapy for Crohn's disease: a case report. *J Crohns Colitis.* 2011;5(3):253–255.
47. Efe C. Drug induced autoimmune hepatitis and TNF-alpha blocking agents: is there a real relationship? *Autoimmun Rev.* 2013;12(3):337–339.
48. Fiel MI, Agarwal K, Stanca C, et al. Posttransplant plasma cell hepatitis (de novo autoimmune hepatitis) is a variant of rejection and may lead to a negative outcome in patients with hepatitis C virus. *Liver Transpl.* 2008;14(6):861–871.
49. Fiel MI, Schiano TD. Plasma cell hepatitis (de-novo autoimmune hepatitis) developing post liver transplantation. *Curr Opin Organ Transplant.* 2012;17(3):287–292.
50. Shalev O, Mosseri M, Ariel I, et al. Methyldopa-induced immune hemolytic anemia and chronic active hepatitis. *Arch Intern Med.* 1983;143(3):592–593.
51. Bjornsson E, Talwalkar J, Treeprasertsuk S, et al. Drug-induced autoimmune hepatitis: clinical characteristics and prognosis. *Hepatology.* 2010;51(6):2040–2048.
52. Dietrichson O. Chronic active hepatitis. Aetiological considerations based on clinical and serological studies. *Scand J Gastroenterol.* 1975;10(6): 617–624.
53. Maggiore G, Larizza D, Lorini R, et al. Propylthiouracil hepatotoxicity mimicking

autoimmune chronic active hepatitis in a girl. *J Pediatr Gastroenterol Nutr*. 1989;8(4):547–548.
54. Lecoeur S, Andre C, Beaune PH. Tienilic acid-induced autoimmune hepatitis: anti-liver and-kidney microsomal type 2 autoantibodies recognize a three-site conformational epitope on cytochrome P4502C9. *Mol Pharmacol*. 1996;50(2):326–333.
55. Sugimoto K, Ito T, Yamamoto N, et al. Seven cases of autoimmune hepatitis that developed after drug-induced liver injury. *Hepatology*. 2011;54(5):1892–1893.
56. Guzman G, Kallwitz ER, Wojewoda C, et al. Liver injury with features mimicking autoimmune hepatitis following the use of black Cohosh. *Case Rep Med*. 2009;2009:918156.
57. Ersoz G, Vardar R, Akarca US, et al. Ornidazole-induced autoimmune hepatitis. *Turk J Gastroenterol*. 2011;22(5):494–499.
58. Sterling MJ, Kane M, Grace ND. Pemoline-induced autoimmune hepatitis. *Am J Gastroenterol*. 1996;91(10):2233–2234.
59. Wolters LM, Van Buuren HR. Rosuvastatin-associated hepatitis with autoimmune features. *Eur J Gastroenterol Hepatol*. 2005;17(5):589–590.
60. Chawla A, Kahn E, Yunis EJ, et al. Rapidly progressive cholestasis: an unusual reaction to amoxicillin/clavulanic acid therapy in a child. *J Pediatr*. 2000;136(1):121–123.
61. Juricic D, Hrstic I, Radic D, et al. Vanishing bile duct syndrome associated with azithromycin in a 62-year-old man. *Basic Clin Pharmacol Toxicol*. 2010;106(1):62–65.
62. Bataille L, Rahier J, Geubel A. Delayed and prolonged cholestatic hepatitis with ductopenia after long-term ciprofloxacin therapy for Crohn's disease. *J Hepatol*. 2002;37(5):696–699.
63. Eckstein RP, Dowsett JF, Lunzer MR. Flucloxacillin induced liver disease: histopathological findings at biopsy and autopsy. *Pathology*. 1993;25(3):223–228.
64. Orman ES, Conjeevaram HS, Vuppalanchi R, et al. Clinical and histopathologic features of fluoroquinolone-induced liver injury. *Clin Gastroenterol Hepatol*. 2011;9(6):517–523 e3.
65. Adriaenssens B, Roskams T, Steger P, et al. Hepatotoxicity related to itraconazole: report of three cases. *Acta Clin Belg*. 2001;56(6):364–369.
66. Schumaker AL, Okulicz JF. Meropenem-induced vanishing bile duct syndrome. *Pharmacotherapy*. 2010;30(9):953.
67. Robinson W, Habr F, Manlolo J, et al. Moxifloxacin associated vanishing bile duct syndrome. *J Clin Gastroenterol*. 2010;44(1):72–73.
68. Kochar R, Nevah MI, Lukens FJ, et al. Vanishing bile duct syndrome in human immunodeficiency virus: nevirapine hepatotoxicity revisited. *World J Gastroenterol*. 2010;16(26):3335–3338.
69. Anania FA, Rabin L. Terbinafine hepatotoxicity resulting in chronic biliary ductopenia and portal fibrosis. *Am J Med*. 2002;112(9):741–742.
70. Groh M, Blanche P, Calmus Y, et al. Thiabendazole-induced acute liver failure requiring transplantation and subsequent diagnosis of polyarteritis nodosa. *Clin Exp Rheumatol*. 2012;30(1 suppl 70):S107–S109.
71. Yao F, Behling CA, Saab S, et al. Trimethoprim-sulfamethoxazole-induced vanishing bile duct syndrome. *Am J Gastroenterol*. 1997;92(1):167–169.
72. Alam I, Ferrell LD, Bass NM. Vanishing bile duct syndrome temporally associated with ibuprofen use. *Am J Gastroenterol*. 1996;91(8):1626–1630.
73. Ali S, Pimentel JD, Ma C. Naproxen-induced liver injury. *Hepatobiliary Pancreat Dis Int*. 2011;10(5):552–556.
74. Trak-Smayra V, Cazals-Hatem D, Asselah T, et al. Prolonged cholestasis and ductopenia associated with tenoxicam. *J Hepatol*. 2003;39(1):125–128.
75. Capra F, Nicolini N, Morana G, et al. Vanishing bile duct syndrome and inflammatory pseudotumor associated with a case of anabolic steroid abuse. *Dig Dis Sci*. 2005;50(8):1535–1537.
76. Ramos AM, Gayotto LC, Clemente CM, et al. Reversible vanishing bile duct syndrome induced by carbamazepine. *Eur J Gastroenterol Hepatol*. 2002;14(9):1019–1022.
77. Chlumska A, Curík R, Boudová L, et al. Chlorpromazine-induced cholestatic liver disease with ductopenia. *Cesk Patol*. 2001;37(3):118–122.
78. Basset C, Vadrot J, Denis J, et al. Prolonged cholestasis and ductopenia following gold salt therapy. *Liver Int*. 2003;23(2):89–93.
79. Dousset B, Conti F, Houssin D, et al. Acute vanishing bile duct syndrome after interferon therapy for recurrent HCV infection in liver-transplant recipients. *N Engl J Med*. 1994;330(16):1160–1161.
80. Etogo-Asse F, Boemer F, Sempoux C, et al. Acute hepatitis with prolonged cholestasis and disappearance of interlobular bile ducts following tibolone and Hypericum perforatum (St. John's wort). Case of drug interaction? *Acta Gastroenterol Belg*. 2008;71(1):36–38.
81. Naini BV, Lassman CR. Total parenteral nutrition therapy and liver injury: a histopathologic study with clinical correlation. *Hum Pathol*. 2012;43(6):826–833.
82. Gokce S, Durmaz O, Celtik C, et al. Valproic acid-associated vanishing bile duct syndrome. *J Child Neurol*. 2010;25(7):909–911.
83. Hezode C, Zafrani ES, Roudot-Thoraval F, et al. Daily cannabis use: a novel risk factor of steatosis severity in patients with chronic hepatitis C. *Gastroenterology*. 2008;134(2):432–439.
84. Larrain S, Rinella ME. A myriad of pathways to NASH. *Clin Liver Dis*. 2012;16(3):525–548.

16

Fatty liver disease: alcoholic and nonalcoholic

Maxwell L. Smith, MD

16.1 INTRODUCTION

This chapter covers the spectrum of fatty liver disease from simple steatosis to severely active steatohepatitis. The chapter begins with general definitions and discussion germane to most cases of steatosis and steatohepatitis, regardless of the etiology. This is followed by a review of specific diseases, including alcoholic liver disease, nonalcoholic fatty liver disease (NAFLD), drug-induced fatty liver disease, Wilson disease, overlap diseases, and diffuse microvesicular steatosis.

16.2 DEFINITIONS

Simply defined, fatty liver disease is the accumulation of lipid droplets in the cytoplasm of hepatocytes. Steatosis is divided into macrovesicular and microvesicular steatosis based on the size of the fat droplets. Macrovesicular steatosis contains large centrally located fat droplets that displace the nucleus to the periphery of the hepatocyte (Fig. 16.1), whereas microvesicular steatosis involves small droplets of lipid not displacing the nucleus. Also of note, there is a diagnostic distinction between true microvesicular steatosis and simply smaller droplets of steatosis, which are seen in the majority of cases of macrovesicular steatosis. For this reason, authors sometimes use the term mixed large-droplet and small-droplet steatosis in the setting of typical fatty liver disease (alcoholic, nonalcoholic, and others) (Fig. 16.2), but reserve the term microvesicular steatosis for cases of diffuse microvesicular steatosis (Table 16.1). The mixed pattern is considered to be part of the normal findings in macrovesicular steatosis and should not be confused with microvesicular steatosis. The distinction is important because there are significant differences in the differential diagnosis between macrovesicular steatosis and diffuse microvesicular steatosis (Table 16.2). True microvesicular steatosis shows diffuse involvement of the hepatocyte cytoplasm by small droplets of lipid, giving the cytoplasm a bubbly appearance (Fig. 16.3). This pattern of injury is much less common than macrovesicular steatosis. Whereas steatosis is the accumulation of lipid in the cytoplasm, steatohepatitis includes the presence of active injury such as lobular inflammation and ballooning degeneration of hepatocytes.

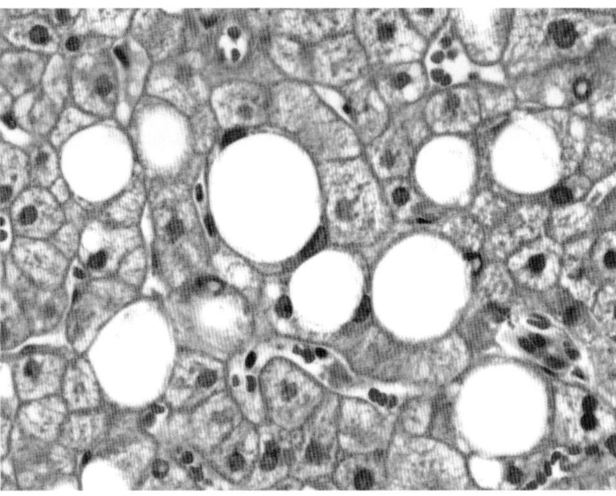

Figure 16.1 Steatosis seen in fatty liver disease. Large-droplet steatosis with single large cytoplasmic fat droplets displacing the hepatocyte nucleus to the periphery of the cell. Also called macrovesicular steatosis.

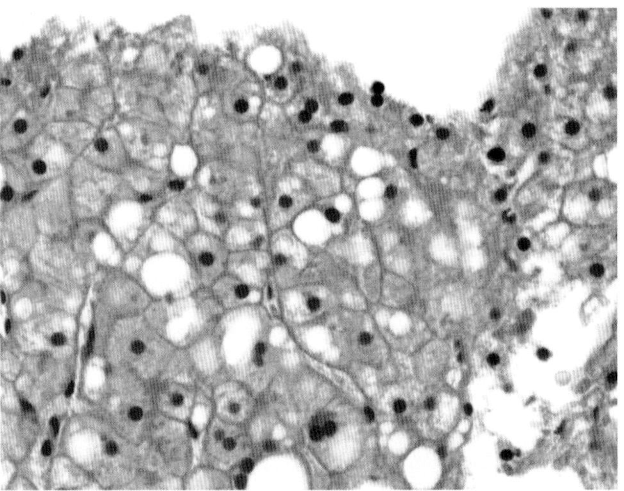

Figure 16.2 Steatosis seen in fatty liver disease. Small-droplet steatosis seen in routine fatty liver disease is characterized by smaller cytoplasmic fat droplets that may be multiple and do not displace the nucleus to the periphery. Over time, these droplets coalesce and will become large droplets.

16.3 GENERAL PATHOLOGIC APPROACH

The recognition of steatosis is straightforward in practice. Identifying the etiology of the steatosis requires clinical and serologic correlation. If no clinical data are available, a descriptive diagnosis with a differential is often as far as the pathologist can go (Table 16.3). One of the major distinctions to make is between the presence of steatosis alone and the presence of a superimposed steatohepatitis. Compared to steatohepatitis, steatosis alone is considered a benign disease that will not progress to cirrhosis and has a lower risk for hepatocellular carcinoma (HCC). In contrast, steatohepatitis is a progressive fibrotic liver disease that can lead to cirrhosis and increased risk for HCC. Although this is a useful dichotomy for clinical management, in reality

Table 16.1 Definitions in fatty liver disease

Term	Definition
Steatosis	Accumulation of lipid in the cytoplasm of hepatocytes
Steatohepatitis	Presence of steatosis with evidence of hepatocyte injury, usually in the form of inflammation and ballooning degeneration
Microvesicular steatosis	Diffuse involvement of hepatocyte cytoplasm by small lipid droplets giving a "bubbly" appearance. Nucleus is not displaced
Macrovesicular steatosis	Large lipid droplets in the cytoplasm of hepatocytes, displacing the nucleus to the periphery, usually singular
Small-droplet steatosis	Term used to describe the small droplets of lipid seen in the setting of macrovesicular steatosis. Not a distinct entity
Large-droplet steatosis	Synonym for macrovesicular steatosis
Ballooning hepatocyte	Swollen hepatocytes (greater than 2–3× normal) with voluminous clear to rarified cytoplasm and small bits of eosinophilic material *but without* lipid droplets. Many balloon cells contain Mallory hyaline
Mallory hyaline	Clumped or ropy appearing eosinophilic material often seen in the setting of ballooning hepatocytes. Represents clumped and damaged cytoskeleton components

there is a spectrum of biologic disease ranging from simple steatosis to active steatohepatitis.

Distinguishing simple steatosis from steatohepatitis

Lobular inflammation and hepatocellular injury are the key features distinguishing simple steatosis from steatohepatitis.[1] Either extreme of the spectrum of steatosis and steatohepatitis is easy to recognize. The key questions become how much steatosis is sufficient to be called abnormal, what are the criteria for ballooning degeneration, and how much inflammation should be required. A definitive diagnosis of steatohepatitis requires both steatosis and hepatocyte injury.

By generally accepted definition, the normal liver may show up to less than 5% macrovesicular steatosis

Table 16.2 Differential diagnosis of fatty liver disease

Macrovesicular steatosis	Microvesicular steatosis
Alcohol Nonalcoholic • Metabolic syndrome (obesity, diabetes, growth hormone deficiency) Drug reaction[a] Infection • Hepatitis C virus Genetic diseases • Wilson disease • Tyrosinemia • Lipodystrophy • Cystic fibrosis • Prader–Willi syndrome • Turner syndrome Small bowel disease (malabsorption) • Crohn disease • Celiac disease • Surgical resection	Drug reaction[a] Toxin exposure • Alcohol (foamy degeneration) • Arsenic • Insect sting • Industrial solvents Genetic diseases • Wolman disease • Ornithine transcarbamylase deficiency (can also show macrovesicular steatosis) Mitochondrial • Alper syndrome • Pearson syndrome • Oxidative phosphorylation deficiency • Navaho neuropathy Mitochondrial depletion syndrome Acute fatty liver disease of pregnancy Surviving hepatocytes following massive injury (ischemia, necrosis)

Selected data from Hautekeete ML, Degott C, Benhamou JP. Microvesicular steatosis of the liver. *Acta Clin Belg*. 1990;45:311–326; Krieeman JM, Misdraji J, Corey KE. Secondary causes of nonalcoholic fatty liver disease. *Therap Adv Gastroenterol*. 2012;5:199–207.
[a]See Table 16.7.

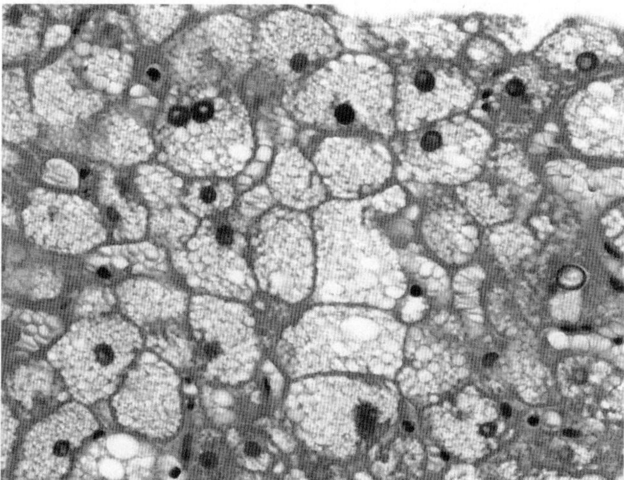

Figure 16.3 Microvesicular steatosis. True microvesicular steatosis characterized by innumerable fine lipid droplets filling the hepatocyte cytoplasm giving it a foamy appearance. Because of the fine cytoplasmic vacuoles, often the cell membranes appear accentuated.

Table 16.3 Sample reports, assuming the pathologist *does not have clinical history*

Simple steatosis
Liver, needle core biopsy: Predominantly macrovesicular steatosis involving approximately 50% of hepatocytes (see comment). Negative for fibrosis. Comment: Steatosis is a nonspecific pattern of injury seen in a variety of settings including alcohol, obesity, diabetes, metabolic syndrome, and drug reactions. There is no evidence of an active steatohepatitis.
Active steatohepatitis with steatosis, inflammation, and ballooning degeneration
Liver, needle core biopsy: Macrovesicular steatosis involving 75% of hepatocytes with moderate lobular inflammation and ballooning degeneration, consistent with a severely active steatohepatitis (NAS grade: 7/8) (see comment) Bridging fibrosis with early architectural distortion (NAS fibrosis stage: 3/4) Comment: Overall, the histopathological changes are most consistent with an active steatohepatitis. Steatohepatitis is a nonspecific pattern of injury seen most commonly in the setting of morbid obesity, diabetes, insulin resistance, and alcohol abuse. However, there is a broad differential diagnosis, including drug reaction, genetic abnormalities, metabolic conditions, and malnutrition. An etiology is often identified clinically.

Abbreviation: NAS, nonalcoholic fatty liver disease activity score.

(Fig. 16.4). In this setting, the steatosis is often randomly distributed and may have both small and large droplets of fat. Vary rarely, in severe alcoholic hepatitis, the degree of steatosis may approach this lower limit of normal. However, in this setting, there also tends to be diffuse ballooning degeneration, Mallory hyaline formation, and neutrophilic inflammation suggesting the underlying disease process.

Ballooning degeneration is described as swollen hepatocytes (usually greater than 2 to 3× normal size) with voluminous clear to rarified cytoplasm and small bits of eosinophilic material (Fig. 16.5). The eosinophilic material represents degenerated cytoskeleton filaments. This material can coalesce and form large ropy structures of Mallory hyaline (Fig. 16.6). Balloon cells do not have lipid droplets and must be distinguished from swollen hepatocytes with a single large fat droplet. This is best done by looking at high power for the fine fragments of cytoskeletal remnants that would not be seen within a large fat droplet. If a case has steatosis, lobular inflammation, and pericellular fibrosis, it is more likely to show ballooning when compared with cases lacking these other features. Despite this clear definition of ballooning degeneration, there will be cells that everyone will agree show ballooning but other cells will generate

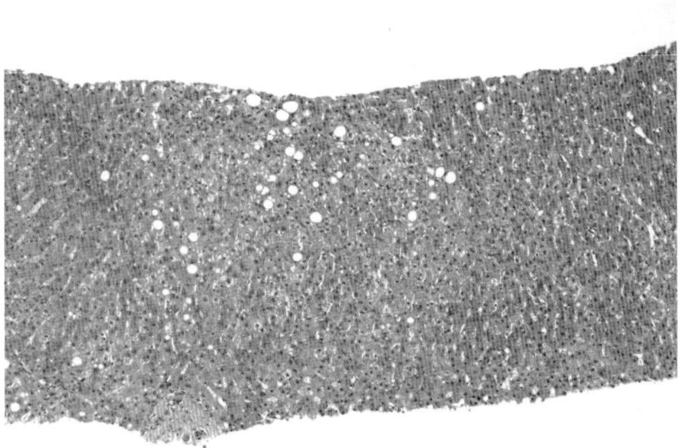

Figure 16.4 Minimal macrovesicular steatosis. This liver biopsy from a patient with autoimmune hepatitis showed minimal steatosis (less than 5%). It is not necessary to comment on this degree of steatosis in the report.

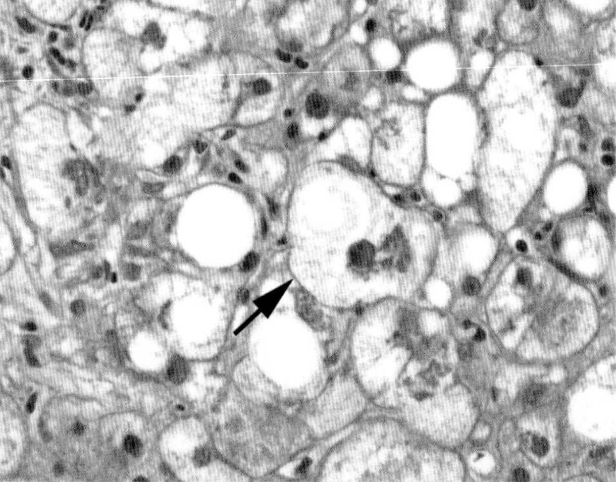

Figure 16.5 Hepatocyte ballooning. Hepatocyte with ballooning degeneration characterized by cytoplasmic swelling, rarefication, lack of fat droplets, and small fragments of eosinophilic material (*arrow*). Nearly everyone would agree this represent ballooning degeneration.

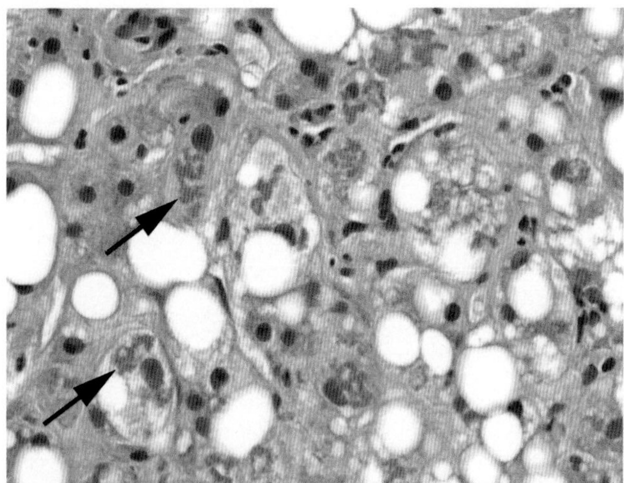

Figure 16.6 Mallory hyaline. Mallory hyaline is characterized by large ropy eosinophilic cytoplasmic inclusions representing coalesced cytoskeleton filaments (*arrows*). These are often seen in the cytoplasm of ballooning hepatocytes.

disagreement. The hepatocytes that are the most likely to cause disagreement usually have one or more of the above features missing (Fig. 16.7). Some cells are only slightly swollen and have some cytoplasmic clearing but lack Mallory hyaline. In these equivocal settings, a trichrome stain may be useful because the ballooning cells are usually surrounded by delicate pericellular fibrosis (Fig. 16.8). A periodic acid–Schiff (PAS) with diastase stain can highlight scattered ceroid laden macrophages that may be used as an indirect marker for past foci of hepatocyte injury (Figs. 16.9 and 16.10), but this can occur in any type of hepatitic injury. Other conditions that can lead to swollen and rarefied hepatocytes include cholestatic conditions (sepsis, duct obstruction, and drug reaction) and conditions associated with increased glycogen deposition (glycogenic hepatopathy and anorexia nervosa).

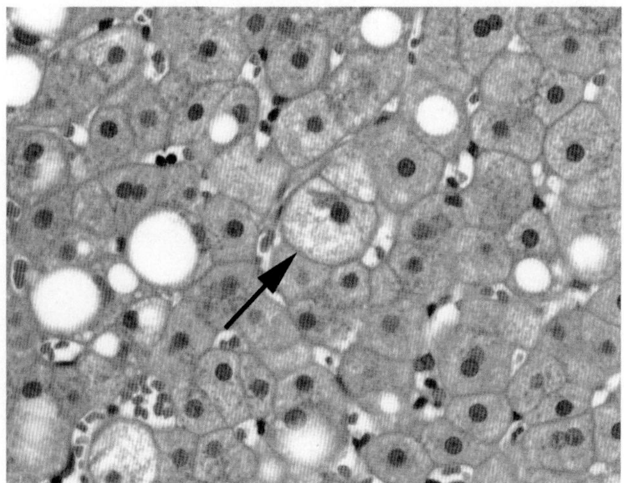

Figure 16.7 Equivocal hepatocyte ballooning. This cell shows mild swelling and some cytoplasmic rarefication (*arrow*). Is this a hepatocyte undergoing ballooning degeneration? Not everyone will agree. It may not be prudent to base a diagnosis of steatohepatitis on only a single cell with this morphology.

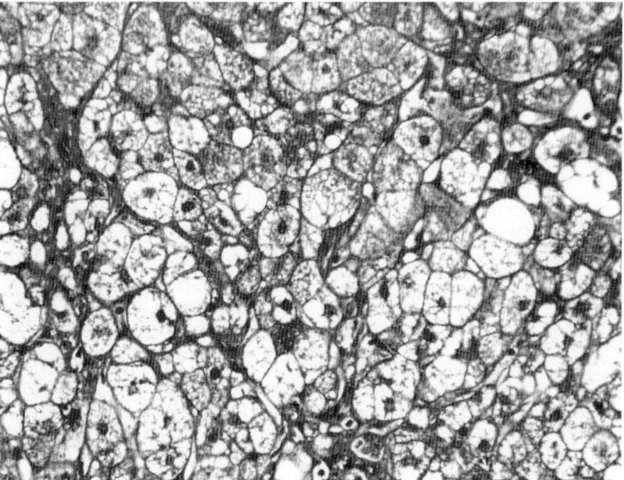

Figure 16.8 Pericellular fibrosis. Ballooning hepatocytes with "chicken-wire" pericellular fibrosis (trichrome stain).

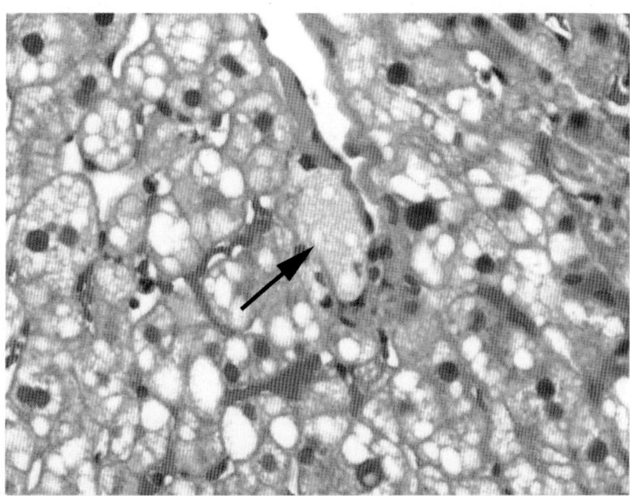

Figure 16.9 Ceroid laden macrophages. These are Kupffer cells that reside in the sinusoidal spaces and are responsible for phagocytizing dead hepatocytes (*arrow*). They are recognized as gray to brown cells with abundant foamy cytoplasm.

Lobular inflammation is a characteristic feature of steatohepatitis. In steatohepatitis, the inflammation is predominantly lymphocytic but rarely can show neutrophils, most commonly in the setting of alcohol or drug effects (Figs. 16.11 and 16.12). The inflammation consists of scattered clusters of cells or single cells scattered throughout the lobule, but can be more prominent in areas of hepatocyte injury or ballooning degeneration. Taking all of the features together, one can often appreciate a component of lobular disarray and injury in steatohepatitis that is

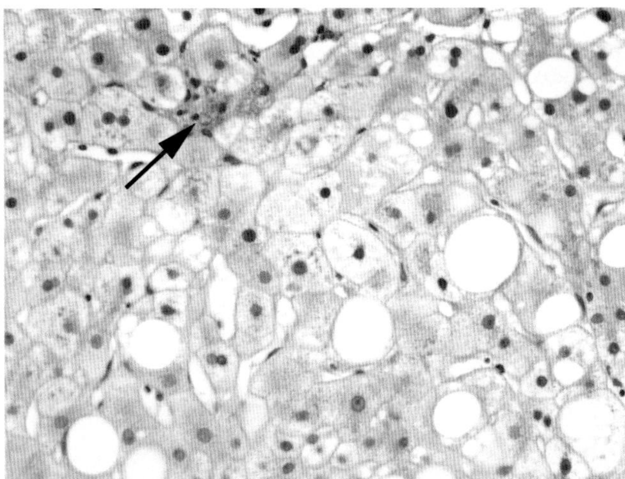

Figure 16.10 Ceroid laden macrophages. PAS with diastase stains can highlight ceroid laden macrophages in the sinusoidal spaces. Some use the presence of ceroid laden macrophages as indirect evidence of hepatocyte ballooning degeneration in fatty liver disease. PAS, periodic acid–Schiff.

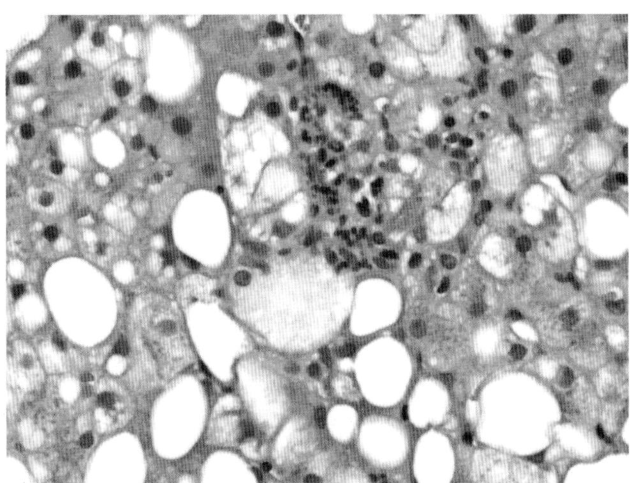

Figure 16.11 Lobular inflammation in steatohepatitis. Clusters of neutrophils can be seen to the right of a few ballooning hepatocytes in this cases of alcoholic steatohepatitis.

missing in steatosis alone. Sometimes this low-power gestalt approach can be a helpful supplement to individual criteria scrutinized at medium or high power.

Estimating the degree of steatosis

Pathologists may spend a significant amount of time perseverating over the exact percentage of steatosis on liver biopsies. The perceived *quantitative* percentage score given in each case may drive this behavior. In reality, the reproducibility of this quantitative scoring process is poor, and pathologists tend to overestimate the degree of steatosis when compared with morphometric studies.[2] It is best to think of the scoring in terms of mild, moderate, and severe steatosis, based on the estimated fat percentage as 5% to 33%, 34% to 67%, and >67%, respectively. Overall fat percentage should be estimated at low power using a 4× or 10× objective. The percentage being estimated was originally defined as the percent of hepatocytes with macrovesicular (large droplet) steatosis.[1] However, several other studies have used the surface area of fat within the biopsy. Either approach works fine and should lead to the same final fat score. Studies have shown improved estimation of steatosis using guideline images.[3] Examples of mild, moderate, and severe steatoses are shown in Figures 16.13, 16.14, and 16.15 for reference, respectively.

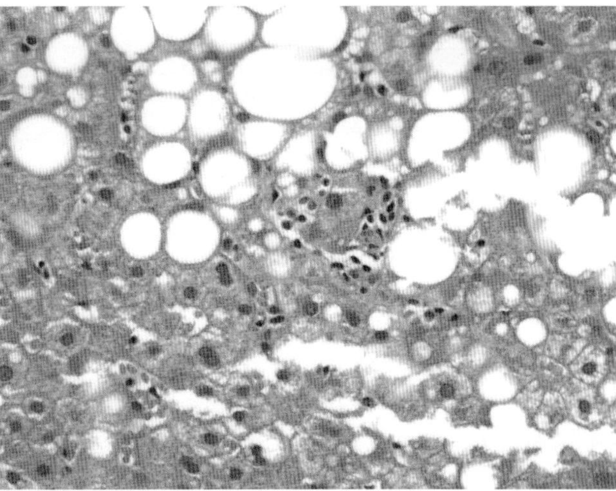

Figure 16.12. Lobular inflammation in steatohepatitis. This case of nonalcoholic steatohepatitis has a lymphocytic lobular infiltrate.

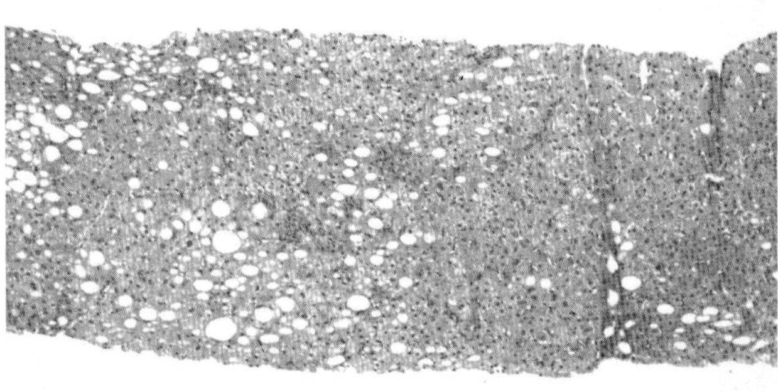

Figure 16.13 Mild steatosis. Estimating the amount of fat in liver biopsies can be challenging and is best done by thinking about it in terms of mild moderate or severe amount of fat. Mild steatosis has more than 5% but less than 33%.

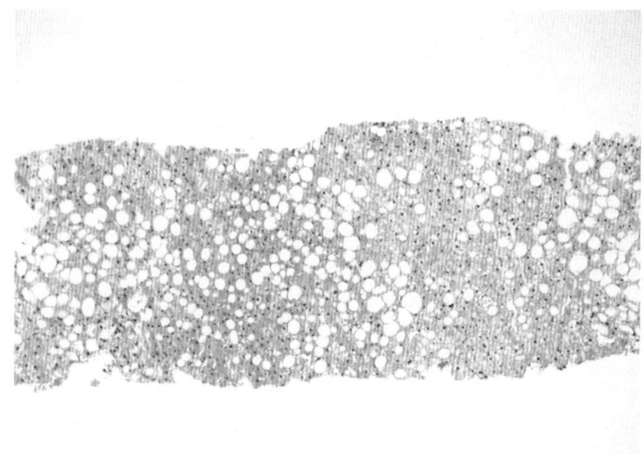

Figure 16.14 Moderate steatosis. Moderate steatosis has more than 34% but less than 66%.

Table 16.4 Nonalcoholic fatty liver disease activity score[4]

Score	Steatosis	Ballooning hepatocytes	Lobular inflammation
0	<5%	None	None
1	6%–33%	Few[a]	Less than 2 foci per 20× field
2	34%–66%	Many	2–4 foci per 20× field
3	67%–100%		Greater than 4 foci per 20× field

Scores are summed for a total of 8.
[a]Including definitive but sparse ballooned hepatocytes.
From Kleiner DE, Brunt EM, Van Natta M, et al. Design and validation of a histological scoring system for nonalcoholic fatty liver disease. *Hepatology*. 2005;41:1313–1321.

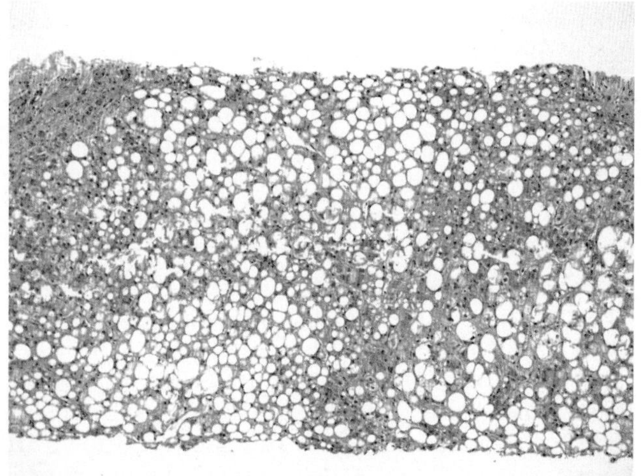

Figure 16.15 Severe steatosis. Severe steatosis shows more than 67% macrovesicular steatosis.

Grading activity in steatohepatitis

The nonalcoholic fatty liver disease activity score (NAS) was introduced in 2005 as a way to grade the degree of activity in cases of nonalcoholic steatohepatitis[4] (Table 16.4). Only features with high interobserver agreement (kappa values ranging from 0.5 to 0.79) and those independently associated with a diagnosis of nonalcoholic steatohepatitis were included in the NAS. The features include steatosis (scored 0 to 3), ballooning degeneration (scored 0 to 2), and lobular inflammation (scored 0 to 3). The scoring system is based on the unweighted sum of all three scores and thus ranges from 0 to 8. There is general agreement that most biopsies with NAS scores of 0 to 2 *do not* represent nonalcoholic steatohepatitis, whereas biopsies with NAS scores of 5 to 8 *do* represent nonalcoholic steatohepatitis.[4] Biopsies with NAS scores of 3 or 4 may represent simple steatosis or nonalcoholic steatohepatitis depending on the presence or absence of all three histologic features. Other grading systems have been developed but the NAS is the most widely used.

Grading systems should not take the place of thorough histologic assessment in the reporting of liver biopsies with fatty change. Many have argued strongly that scoring systems were developed for clinical trials and have less of a role in the clinical record.[5] Scoring systems do have advantages in that they assure assessment and reporting of all of the pertinent features associated with fatty liver disease. They also provide standard criteria for reporting and for communication with clinicians. Although the NAS was developed for cases of NAFLD, in common practice it is often applied to all biopsies with fatty disease, because the etiology is rarely known at the time of sign-out (Table 16.3). The decision to use a scoring system, regardless of the disease process, should be made in conjunction with input from the clinicians ordering the liver biopsy.

Staging fibrosis in steatohepatitis

In 1999, Brunt et al.[1] proposed a fibrosis staging system for NAFLD to take into account the unique centrilobular and subsinusoidal patterns of fibrosis (other synonyms include sinusoidal fibrosis and pericellular fibrosis) seen in nonalcoholic steatohepatitis. The staging system was revised in 2005 and incorporated into the NAS staging system, with modifications of the Stage 1 fibrosis to include a substage with portal fibrosis alone

(Table 16.5).[4] Histologic examples of the four fibrosis stages are shown in Figures 16.16, 16.17, 16.18, and 16.19. Note that even fine subsinusoidal fibrosis that bridges from central to portal or central to central regions is sufficient for Stage 3 fibrosis. This fibrosis staging system is quite helpful as the majority of the other fibrosis staging systems were developed for chronic viral hepatitis and do not take into account the unique fibrosis patterns seen in early stages of steatohepatitis associated fibrosis. Similar to the NAS grade, the NAS stage is often applied to all cases because the etiology is often unknown at the time of sign-out.

Table 16.5 Nonalcoholic steatohepatitis clinical research network fibrosis staging system[a]

Stage	Description
0	No fibrosis
1a	Mild pericellular fibrosis requiring trichrome stain to recognize
1b	Moderate pericellular fibrosis recognized on the H&E stain
1c	Portal fibrosis alone
2	Periportal fibrosis (any) and pericellular fibrosis (any)
3	Bridging fibrosis
4	Cirrhosis

[a]Sometimes referred to the "Brunt" fibrosis staging system.
Abbreviation: H&E, hematoxylin and eosin.
Reprinted by permission from Macmillan Publishers Ltd: Brunt EM, Janney CG, Di Bisceglie AM, Neuschwander-Tetri BA, Bacon BR. Nonalcoholic steatohepatitis: a proposal for grading and staging the histological lesions. *Am J Gastroenterol*. 1999;94:2467–2474.

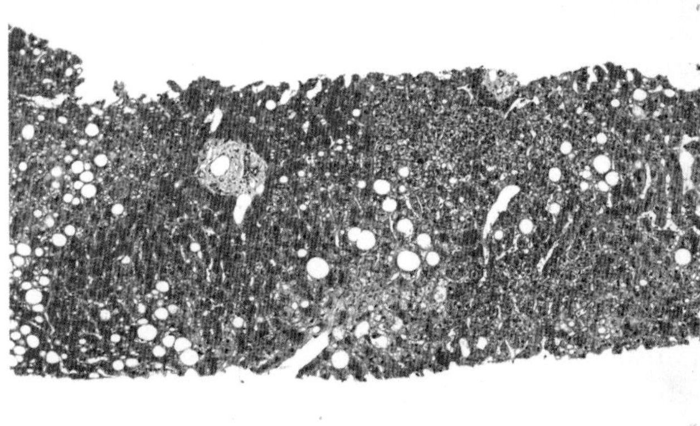

Figure 16.16 Fibrosis Stage 1a. Stage 1a fibrosis shows fine early subsinusoidal fibrosis in zone 3 and normal appearing portal areas.

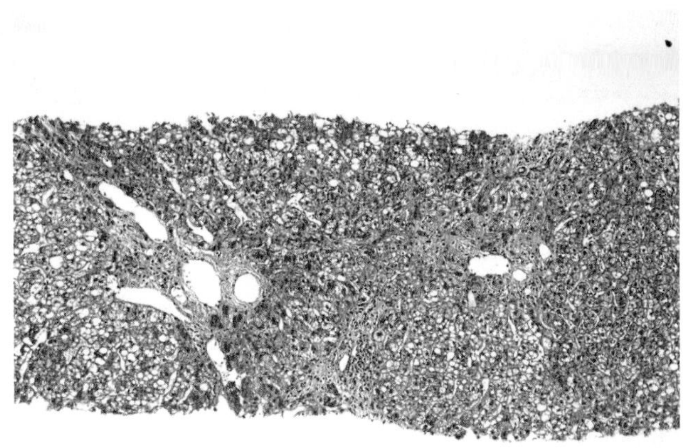

Figure 16.17 Fibrosis Stage 2. Stage 2 fibrosis shows portal, focal periportal, and Zone 3 subsinusoidal fibrosis but no definite bridging fibrosis.

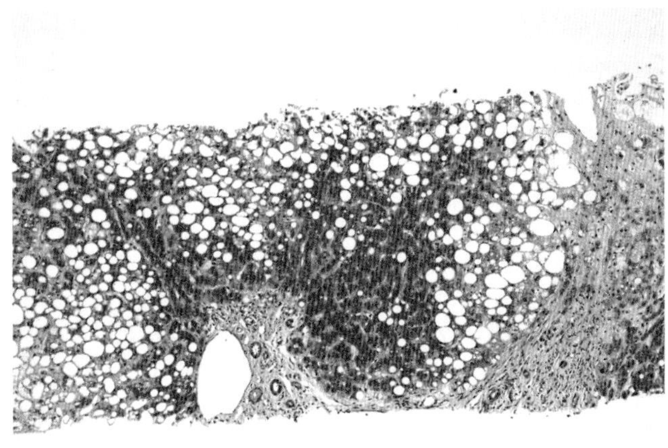

Figure 16.18 Fibrosis Stage 3. Stage 3 fibrosis is seen, with clear bridging fibrosis and some early architectural distortion.

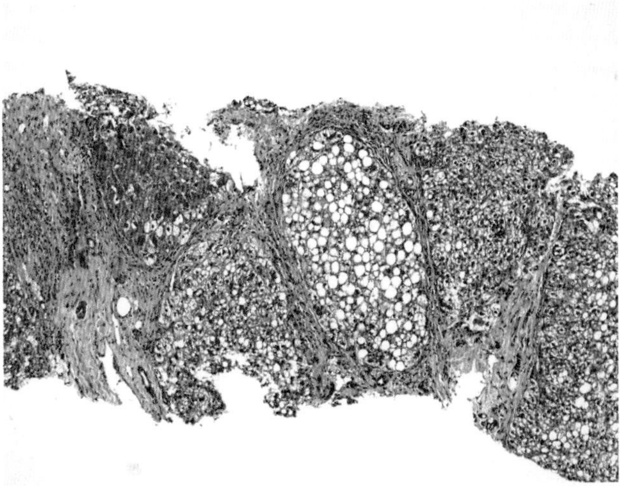

Figure 16.19 Fibrosis Stage 4. Stage 4 fibrosis is seen, with clear regenerative nodules.

16.4 ALCOHOLIC FATTY LIVER DISEASE

Clinical features

Alcohol-associated liver disease may be encountered in anyone exposed to excessive amounts of alcohol because alcohol is a direct hepatotoxin. The exact amount of alcohol required to induce liver disease is variable from one person to the other because of genetic susceptibility, comorbid conditions, and exposure to other hepatotoxins. As low as 40 g/day of alcohol for men and 20 g/day for women has been reported to increase risk of fibrosis. Nearly everyone who has excessive exposure will develop steatosis, which is reversible, whereas approximately 30% of individuals will develop steatohepatitis, with an increased risk of fibrosis, cirrhosis, and HCC. Excessive alcohol may affect several other organ systems, including the nervous system, gastrointestinal system, and cardiovascular system. Patients with cirrhosis secondary to alcohol can show any of the typical consequences of cirrhosis, including portal hypertension, splenomegaly, esophageal varices, and ascites.

Laboratory findings

Alcohol-related liver disease causes elevations of both aspartate transaminase (AST) and alanine transaminase (ALT); however, AST is usually increased at least 2× the ALT. The levels of alkaline phosphatase (ALP) are usually only mildly elevated, whereas γ glutamyltransferase (GGT) can show marked elevations. Although there are many exceptions, an AST to ALT ratio of greater than 2, along with an elevated GGT out of proportion to the ALP, can raise the possibility of alcohol as an etiology. In advanced disease, there may be synthetic dysfunction with low albumin and a prolonged international normalized ratio.

Imaging

Imaging studies can be useful in establishing the presence and distribution of steatosis. Ultrasound is widely used as a noninvasive method but has low sensitivity for lower amounts of fat. Ultrasound cannot detect fat levels below 15% to 20%. Magnetic resonance imaging (MRI) is more sensitive in quantifying the amount of fat (Figs. 16.20 and 16.21). Hepatic fat content can also be estimated with multi-echo gradient-recalled-echo MRI, known as Liver Imaging of Phase-related signal Oscillation and Quantification (LIPO-Quant). Most of the time, the fat accumulation occurs diffusely throughout the liver. However, in a minority of cases, the fat accumulates in particular areas; a phenomenon termed focal fatty infiltration. The medial segment of the left lobe of the liver is a common site and this can mimic a mass lesion. There are no imaging studies that can reliably distinguish steatosis from steatohepatitis.[6] There has been significant recent interest in the use of transient elastography for noninvasive means of fibrosis monitoring. However, both steatosis and active inflammation decrease the accuracy of transient elastography, limiting its usefulness in the setting of alcoholic liver disease.[7]

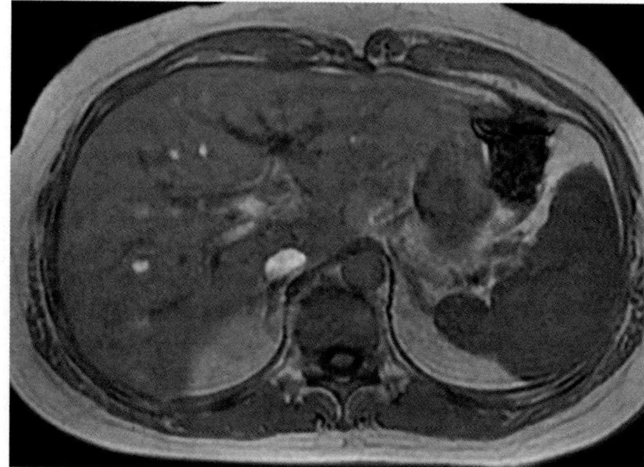

Figure 16.20 Steatosis and MRI, T1 in phase. Evaluation of fat content by MRI involves the comparison of the T1-weighted images in phase and out of phase (see below). MRI, magnetic resonance imaging.

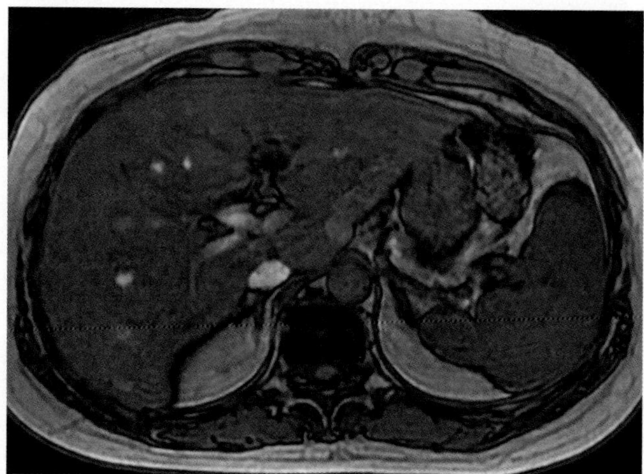

Figure 16.21 Steatosis and MRI, T1 out of phase. A drop of greater than 10% in signal intensity is abnormal. Note the change in signal intensity in this case that showed 20% fat on biopsy. MRI, magnetic resonance imaging.

Gross findings

The presence of steatosis imparts a yellow appearance to the gross specimen, both on needle core biopsy and explant specimens. There is a direct correlation

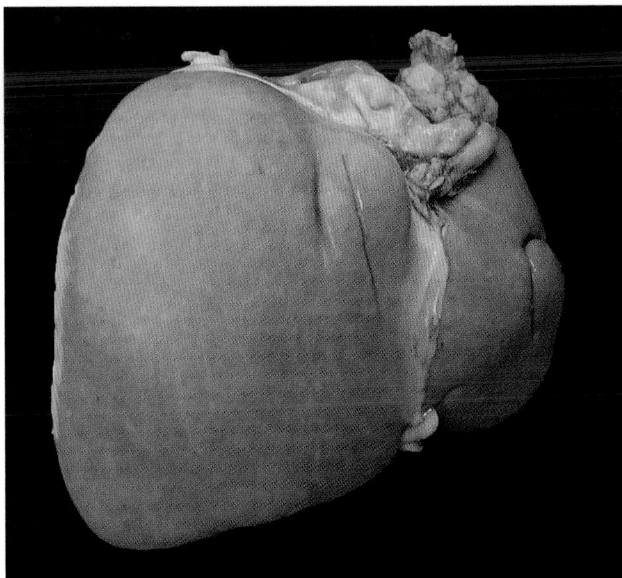

Figure 16.22 Fatty liver disease, gross. Characteristic swollen and yellow appearance of fatty liver disease. This was an organ harvest from a patient with risk factors for nonalcoholic fatty liver disease. The biopsy showed moderate large-droplet steatosis but no steatohepatitis or fibrosis. Photo courtesy of Dr. Amit Mathur, Transplantation Surgery, Mayo Clinic Arizona.

between the percent of steatosis and the degree of yellow color (Fig. 16.22). In early alcohol-related liver disease, the liver is often swollen and enlarged. In cirrhosis secondary to alcohol, the liver disease appears similar to end stage cirrhotic livers from other etiologies. The nodularity with active disease is classically micronodular, but in many cases is mixed micro- and macronodular (Fig. 16.23).

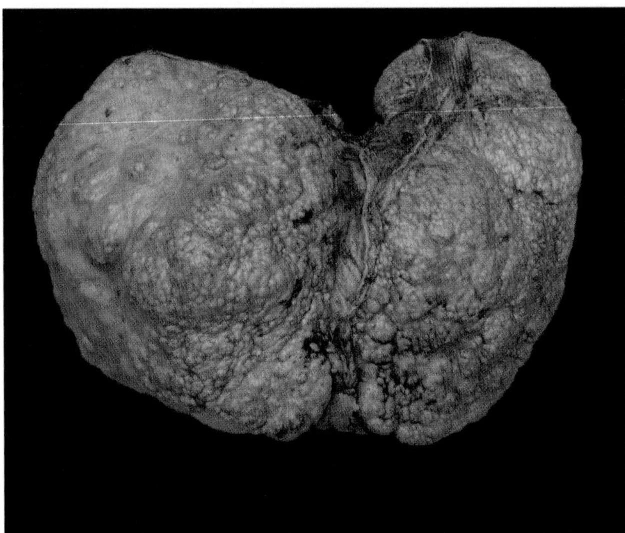

Figure 16.23 Fatty liver disease and cirrhosis, gross. Cirrhotic liver in end stage liver disease secondary to alcoholic liver disease. Note the nodular surface and slight yellow color to the regenerative nodules.

Microscopic findings

The histologic findings in alcohol-related liver disease range from simple steatosis to steatohepatitis to "burned out" cirrhosis with little or no fat. The steatosis is most often in the form of macrovesicular steatosis. Because the enzymes involved in the metabolism of alcohol are more prevalent in the centrilobular regions, the steatosis tends to begin in Zone 3 (Fig. 16.24). With increasing alcohol exposure, the steatosis involves the entire lobule. Cases routinely have a component of small droplet steatosis because fat droplets begin small and over time coalesce to form the larger droplets of fat.

Even in simple steatosis, megamitochondria may be encountered. Megamitochondria are enlarged and abnormally shaped mitochondria seen in the setting of many different liver diseases including both alcohol and NAFLD (Fig. 16.25).

Steatohepatitis shows the three key features of steatosis, ballooning degeneration, and lobular inflammation. If there is clinical documentation of alcohol exposure, the findings are termed alcohol-related steatohepatitis. As discussed earlier, recognition of a ballooned hepatocyte can be challenging. However, compared to nonalcohol steatohepatitis, alcohol-related steatohepatitis typically shows more abundant ballooning degeneration with more robust Mallory hyaline formation. Some florid cases of alcoholic steatohepatitis may have more ballooning hepatocytes than actual steatosis (Fig. 16.26). Ballooned cells are swollen hepatocytes with a cleared out or rarified cytoplasm. The cytoskeletal structures may coalesce creating Mallory hyaline structures.

Although the inflammatory cell infiltrates are commonly mixed and predominately lymphocytic,

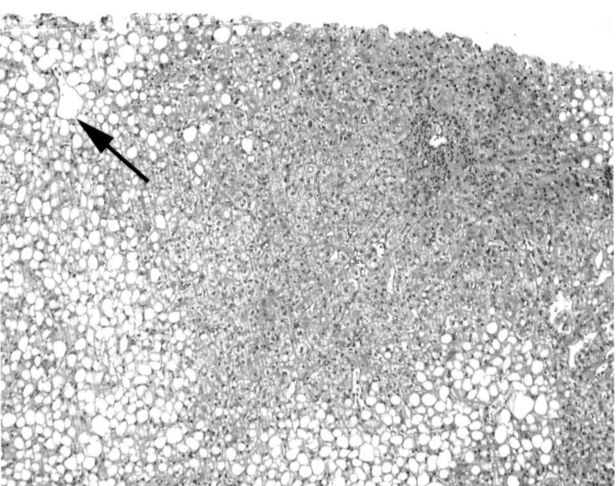

Figure 16.24 Zone 3 steatosis. The fat shows a distinct Zone 3 distribution. Note the portal tract in the upper right without Zone 1 steatosis. A central vein is surrounded by steatosis (*arrow*).

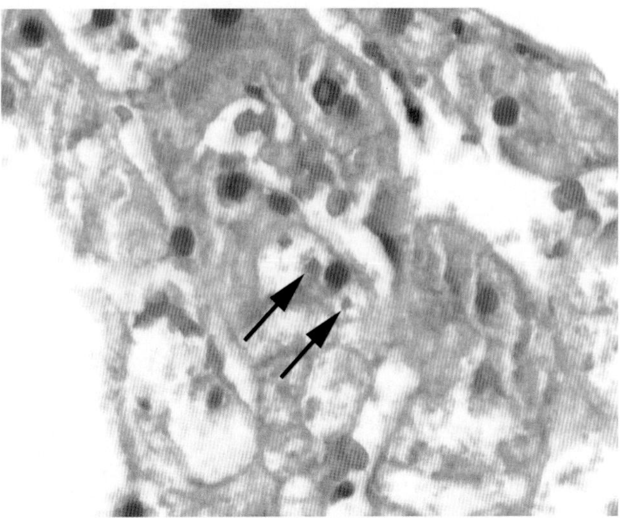

Figure 16.25 Megamitochondria. Megamitochondria are characterized by globular eosinophilic cytoplasmic inclusions, often in swollen hepatocytes.

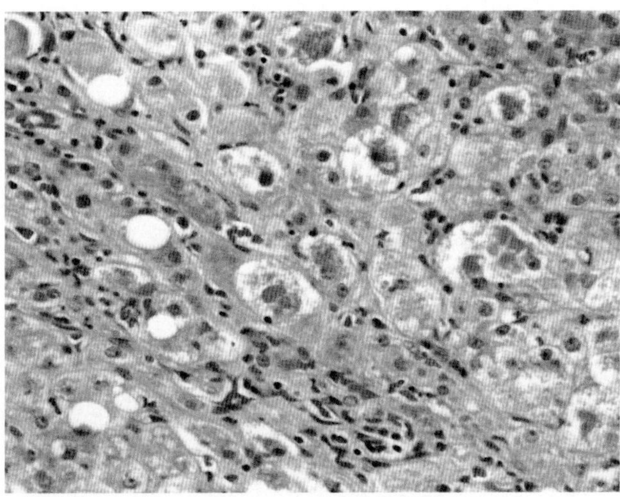

Figure 16.26 Alcoholic steatohepatitis. Florid case of alcoholic steatohepatitis shows relatively minimal steatosis, despite the extensive ballooning degeneration, inflammation, and Mallory hyaline.

neutrophils can sometimes be a dominant finding in alcohol-related steatohepatitis.[8] In more severely active cases, there may be small aggregates of neutrophils in the lobules. Some cases show rings of neutrophils surrounding ballooning hepatocytes that have Mallory hyaline, a finding referred to as neutrophil satellitosis (Fig. 16.27).

As the inflammation and hepatocellular injury continues over time, progressive fibrosis occurs, usually beginning in the centrilobular region. The early fibrosis deposition occurs in a subsinusoidal distribution, creating the so-called "chicken-wire" or "arachnoid" pattern of fibrosis (Figs. 16.28 and 16.29). Perivenular fibrosis may be prominent as well, sometime occluding

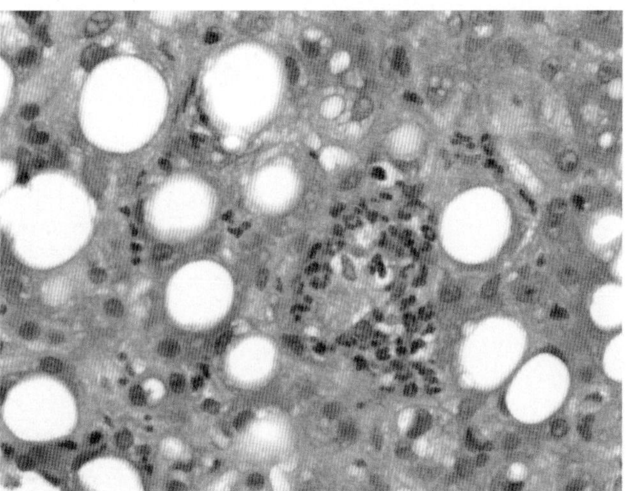

Figure 16.27 Neutrophilic statellitosis. Neutrophilic inflammation surrounds a hepatocyte with ballooning degeneration.

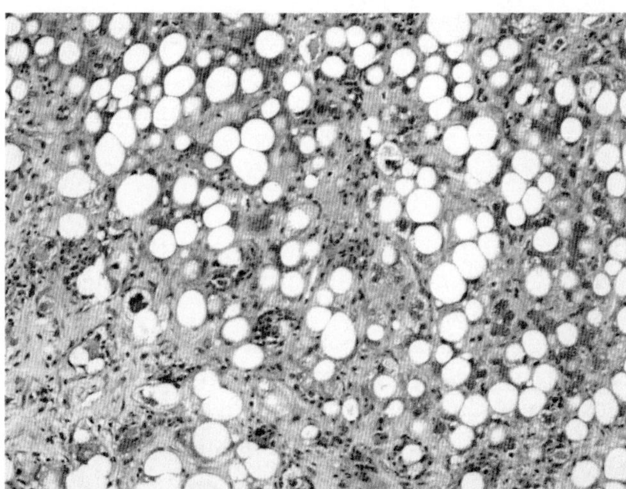

Figure 16.28 Subsinusoidal fibrosis. Fine but diffuse subsinusoidal fibrosis creating a "chicken-wire" or "arachnoid" pattern of blue fibrosis on trichrome staining.

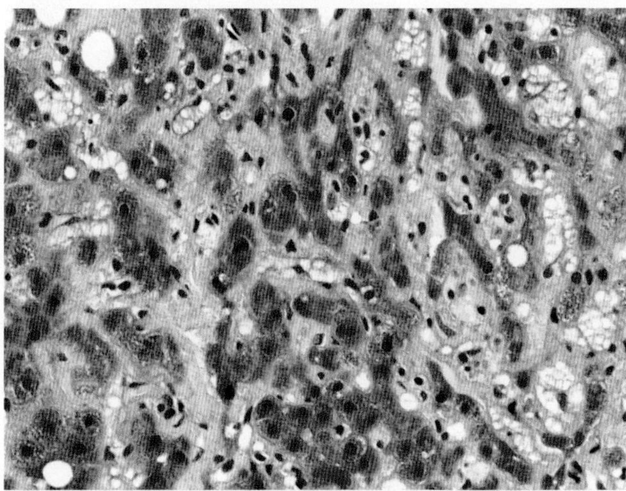

Figure 16.29 Subsinusoidal fibrosis. Marked subsinusoidal fibrosis is seen.

the central veins. Overtime, the fibrosis extends to the portal regions (portal to central bridging) and to other central regions (central to central bridging) with progressive architectural distortion and eventual nodule formation indicative of cirrhosis. Even in cirrhotic livers, there is commonly evidence of a subsinusoidal pattern of fibrosis. The cirrhosis of alcohol-related liver disease is classically described as micronodular when there is ongoing injury, but with abstinence, the liver commonly shows a mixed micro- and macronodular pattern of cirrhosis. There is a potential for significant regression of cirrhosis should the patient abstain from alcohol.[9]

Lipogranulomas may be seen in both alcohol-related steatosis and steatohepatitis and represents a reaction pattern to extravasated lipid. They consist of collections of histiocytes with foamy cytoplasm and are commonly associated with mild chronic inflammation and focal fibrosis (Fig. 16.30). Lipogranulomas are most often seen in the lobules but may be portal based as well. Lipogranulomas are not specific to alcohol-related liver disease and may be seen in NAFLD as well as other causes of steatosis.

Alcoholic foamy degeneration is a rare histologic finding that may be associated with increased alcohol exposure, either binge drinking or heavy drinking following a period of abstinence. Patients usually have quite elevated AST and ALT levels, and the ratio of 2 commonly found with alcohol exposure may *not* be present. Despite the marked enzyme elevations, the biopsy shows only focal inflammation that is mostly portal based. The lobules show minimal inflammation with extensive true microvesicular change imparting a "foamy" appearance to the biopsy (Fig. 16.31). This often has a Zone 3 distribution. Occasional single necrotic hepatocytes and focal macrovesicular steatosis may be present as well. The differential diagnosis for diffuse microvesicular steatosis is discussed later.

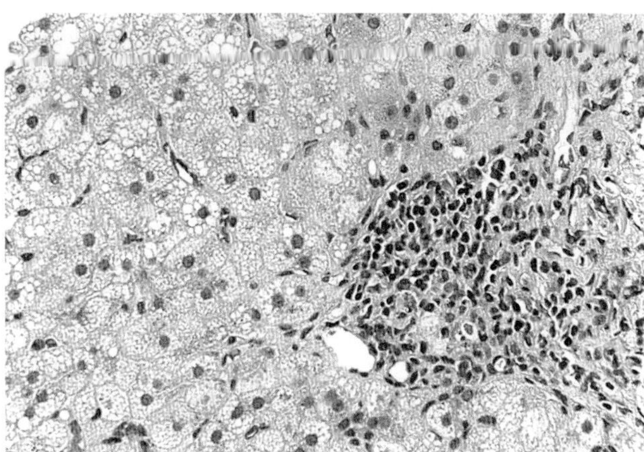

Figure 16.31 Alcoholic foamy degeneration. Alcoholic foamy degeneration is seen in this biopsy of a patient with alcoholic liver disease and chronic hepatitis C (which accounts for the portal based infiltrate).

A subset of patient with acute alcoholic liver disease may show central confluent hepatocyte necrosis with obliteration of the central veins and prominent neutrophilic inflammation (Fig. 16.32). This rare constellation of findings has been called central sclerosing hyaline necrosis and can be seen in alcohol-related liver disease but is generally not found in nonalcohol-related fatty liver disease.

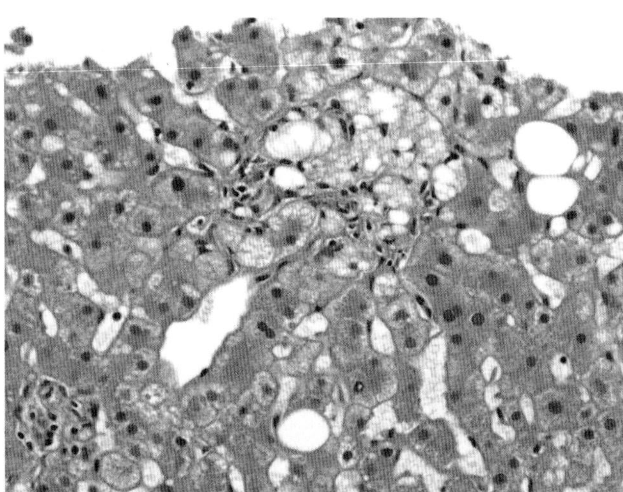

Figure 16.30 Lipogranuloma. Lipogranulomas are collections of foamy histiocytes and inflammation along with droplets of fat. These are thought to be a response to extracellular fat and may be seen in the lobules or portal areas.

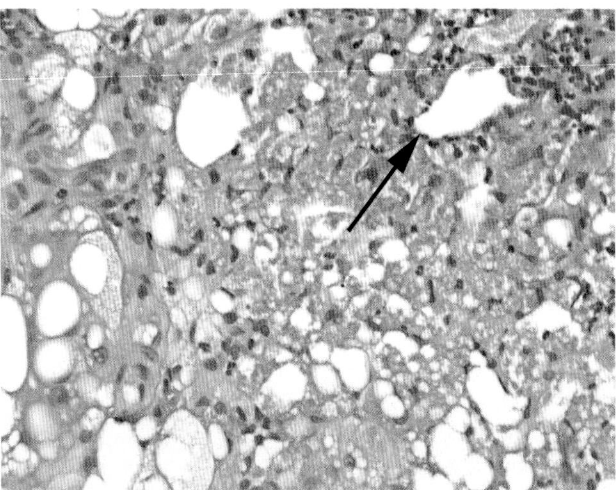

Figure 16.32 Alcoholic central hyaline necrosis. This patient had an extensive history of alcohol abuse but was admitted following several days of heavy binge drinking. Note the confluent hepatocyte necrosis on the right side of the image, surrounding a central vein (*arrow*).

Immunohistochemistry and special stains

Liver biopsies for alcohol-related fatty liver disease rarely need additional work-up aside from the standard nonneoplastic stains of iron, PAS with diastase, and trichrome. A trichrome stain is useful in demonstrating the early delicate subsinusoidal fibrosis seen in early stages of fibrosis. Rare small globules of PAS positive, diastase resistant material may be seen in alcohol-related liver disease and should not be confused with α-1-antitrypsin deficiency. Mallory hyaline can be demonstrated with CK8, ubiquitin, and Cam 5.2 stains, but these are not necessary clinically.

Ultrastructural findings

Ultrastructural studies play no role in the routine work-up of alcohol-related fatty liver disease specimens.

Molecular genetic findings

Molecular studies play no role in the routine work-up of alcohol-related fatty liver disease specimens.

Differential diagnosis

Unfortunately, the histologic findings seen in alcohol-related fatty liver disease are not specific and without a clinical history of alcohol exposure, it is nearly impossible to make a definitive diagnosis based on the histology alone. That being said, there are several features that are more commonly seen with alcohol-related fatty liver disease than with NAFLD (Table 16.6), including the following: neutrophils, intense neutrophilic lobular inflammation, prominent megamitochondria, central sclerosing hyaline necrosis, cholestasis, abundant Mallory hyaline, and obliterative fibrosis of the central vein.[10–15] The classic case of acute alcoholic steatohepatitis will show mild steatosis, marked ballooning degeneration, abundant Mallory hyaline, numerous neutrophils, and a background of subsinusoidal fibrosis. Although the differential diagnosis is quite long (Table 16.2), primary considerations include adverse drug reactions (amiodarone, methotrexate, and others) and Wilson disease, if the patient is young. This constellation of findings (marked ballooning, abundant Mallory hyaline, and numerous neutrophils) is not seen in all cases of alcohol-related fatty liver disease, but when present suggests alcoholic steatohepatitis.

In specimens that show cirrhosis without significant steatosis or steatohepatitis, some pathologists may be tempted to use the presence of prominent subsinusoidal fibrosis as a clue to an etiology of

Table 16.6 Histologic features comparing alcoholic steatohepatitis and nonalcoholic fatty steatohepatitis from the metabolic syndrome[a]

Features	Alcoholic steatohepatitis	Nonalcoholic steatohepatitis
Neutrophils in lobules	More common	Rare
Canalicular cholestasis	May be present	Rare without additional coexisting disease process
Cholangiolitis	May be present	Rare without additional coexisting disease process
Steatosis	lower grade	More common and severe
Glycogenated nuclei	Less common	More common
Mallory hyaline	More common	Less common
Obliterative fibrosis of the central vein	More striking	Less striking
Sclerosing hyaline necrosis	More common	Less common
Megamitochondria	More common	Less common
Ballooning hepatocytes	May be diffuse	Rarely diffuse
Lobular lymphocytic inflammation	Most commonly mild	Most commonly mild
Portal inflammation	Usually mild	Usually mild

[a]However, there are no specific features to distinguish between these two entities.
Data from Refs. 10–15.

alcohol-related cirrhosis. However, this finding is not very sensitive because the subsinusoidal fibrosis often diminishes or disappears with abstinence or reduced alcohol consumption. Nor is this finding specific, also being present with other causes of fatty liver disease, with drug effects, and with vascular outflow disease.

Prognosis and treatment

The only treatment for alcohol-related disease, aside from transplantation, is abstinence of alcohol. A complete histologic reversal of the nonfibrotic changes and some component of cirrhosis regression have been documented following abstinence. Although there is some variability, the steatosis seems to regress within the first few weeks, whereas the inflammation and ballooning degeneration may take 2 to 3 months.[15] Mallory hyaline may be present for longer periods of time. For patients with cirrhosis and clinical evidence of liver failure, transplantation may be an option. Most liver transplant centers require complete abstinence from alcohol for at least 6 months prior to consideration, in addition to psychiatric evaluation. Because of this time period, explanted livers often no longer have histologic evidence of alcoholic steatohepatitis. Ongoing steatohepatitis raises the possibility of more recent alcohol exposure.

A number of histologic features have been associated with a poor prognosis in alcohol-related liver disease including the following: severe steatosis on initial biopsy, mixed micro- and macrovesicular steatosis,[16] steatohepatitis and cirrhosis,[17] cholestasis,[18] and the presence of severe acute steatohepatitis.[19] The prognosis of alcohol-related liver disease seems to depend on the frequency and amount of alcohol exposure following diagnosis. Patients who continue to drink following diagnosis have a significantly decreased survival.[20]

16.5 NONALCOHOLIC FATTY LIVER DISEASE

Clinical features

Nonalcoholic fatty liver disease (NAFLD) is the most common chronic liver disease in the United States and is on the rise,[12,21] with a current prevalence estimated between 11% and 30%.[21,22] The term NAFLD includes simple steatosis and the progressive fibrosing disease, nonalcoholic steatohepatitis. NAFLD is seen in the setting of the metabolic syndrome. The metabolic syndrome includes five abnormal metabolic conditions that increase risk for NAFLD and includes abdominal obesity, elevated triglycerides, low high-density lipoprotein cholesterol (HDL), high blood pressure, and high fasting blood sugar levels. As many of these conditions are on the rise, it is not surprising that NAFLD is also increasing. Approximately 20% to 30% of NAFLD patients go on to develop nonalcoholic steatohepatitis. Most patients with NAFLD are asymptomatic. Some patients with nonalcoholic steatohepatitis will present with abdominal pain and fatigue.

Laboratory findings

Patients with NAFLD show elevated AST and ALT that may fluctuate over time. Patients with nonalcoholic steatohepatitis tend to show higher levels of enzyme elevation. The AST to ALT ratio is typically around 1. The transaminitis is usually in the 1.5 to 2 times normal range. ALP and GGT may also be mildly elevated. Most patients with NAFLD will also show elevated cholesterol, low HDL, and elevated fasting blood sugars. There are no specific laboratory markers, and a definitive diagnosis requires a liver biopsy.

Between 20% and 30% of patients with NAFLD will have autoantibodies in the serum.[23–25] This is often an indication for biopsy to help distinguish between NAFLD, autoimmune hepatitis, or both conditions. These autoantibodies are typically low titer and are most commonly antinuclear antibody and antismooth muscle antibody. If the presence of autoantibodies is known, it is helpful to the clinical service to specifically mention the presence or absence of histologic features of autoimmune hepatitis.

Imaging

Ultrasound is commonly used for the identification of steatosis and is quite sensitive when there is moderate to severe fat. However with less than 15% to 20% fat, the sensitivity drops off dramatically.[26] Other imaging studies, such as MRI, are more sensitive at lower fat content levels. There are no imaging studies that can reliably distinguish steatosis from steatohepatitis. As mentioned with alcohol-related liver disease, the presence of steatosis and inflammation decreases the accuracy of transient elastography, rendering it less helpful in NAFLD cases.[7]

Gross findings

As the degree of steatosis increases, the gross specimen will be increasingly yellow in color. As the disease progresses and more fibrosis develops, the explant and resection specimens will show increasing fibrosis, architectural distortion, nodularity, and eventually cirrhosis.

Microscopic findings

The basic histologic features of NAFLD are similar to those of alcohol-related liver disease. The disease

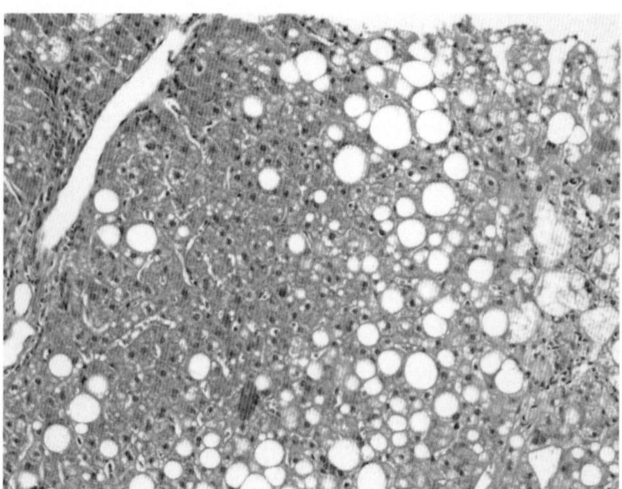

Figure 16.33 Nonalcoholic steatohepatitis. A typical case of nonalcoholic steatohepatitis showing centrilobular steatosis, lobular inflammation, and ballooning degeneration (**far right**).

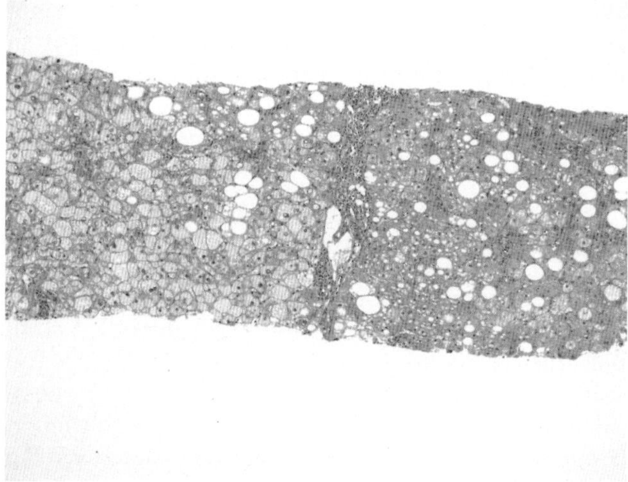

Figure 16.34 Patch of microvesicular steatosis. A patch of microvesicular steatosis is seen in this biopsy that otherwise showed typical nonalcoholic steatohepatitis. Note the foamy appearance of the hepatocytes on the left side of the biopsy.

shows a macrovesicular pattern of steatosis, though occasional small, well-demarcated patches of true microvesicular steatosis may be encountered in about 10% of cases. The fat can have a Zone 3 pattern, a Zone 1 pattern, an azonal pattern, or can be diffusely found throughout the lobules. A Zone 1 pattern tends to be somewhat more common in children, but overall the zonation pattern has no clinical significance. In NAFLD without nonalcoholic steatohepatitis, there is no inflammation or evidence of other forms of active hepatocellular injury. Portal inflammation is usually minimal to mild.

The diagnosis of nonalcoholic steatohepatitis is based on finding steatosis (at least 5%) plus evidence of active injury, including ballooning degeneration and lobular inflammation. The lobular inflammation is primarily lymphocytic but can also rarely include neutrophils (Fig. 16.33). The first part of this chapter reviewed challenges related to the identification of these features. As a general rule, the extent of ballooned hepatocytes and Mallory hyaline is less in nonalcoholic steatohepatitis when compared with alcohol-related liver disease. The small patches of true microvesicular steatosis mentioned previously are more often encountered in cases with marked steatosis, active steatohepatitis, and fibrosis[27] (Fig. 16.34).

Several other nonspecific histologic findings may be present in both steatosis and nonalcoholic steatohepatitis. Lipogranulomas may be encountered (Fig. 16.30) but are usually not mentioned in the pathology diagnosis as they have no clinical significance and can lead to confusion among the clinical team, who can mistake the term for traditional granulomas. Secondly, almost all cases show some component of portal-based inflammation, which is primarily lymphocytic but can include occasional plasma cells and histiocytes. This infiltrate should avoid the bile ducts. If there is a component of lymphocytic cholangitis, a chronic biliary disease should be further investigated. Similarly if the portal-based infiltrate is dense and out of proportion to the degree of lobular activity (ballooning and inflammation), the possibility of a superimposed chronic hepatitis should be considered. The relationship between chronic hepatitis C and steatosis is discussed later.

As hepatocytes die, their remnants are engulfed by Kupffer cells in the sinusoids. As the cellular components are digested, the cytoplasm of the Kupffer cells often takes on a finely vacuolated appearance and a grayish color. These are referred to as ceroid laden macrophages and can be highlighted by a PAS with diastase stain. Finding multiple ceroid laden macrophages in the lobules can sometimes provide indirect evidence supporting a component of active lobular injury, and thus a diagnosis of nonalcoholic steatohepatitis.

Multiple abnormal arterial changes have been described in the setting of steatosis and nonalcoholic steatohepatitis. As the centrilobular region undergoes fibrosis, arterioles may grow into the fibrotic areas, creating fibrotic structures with arterioles reminiscent of portal tracts (Fig. 16.35). This can make the initial architectural evaluation of the liver biopsy difficult, especially in smaller samples, like transjugular needle core biopsies. Some cases may also show a proliferation of small arterioles within the portal tracts (Fig. 16.36). This finding is of uncertain clinical significance but suggests a possible response to chronic hypoxic states, like obstructive sleep apnea. Occasional unpaired arteries may also be encountered in the lobules and

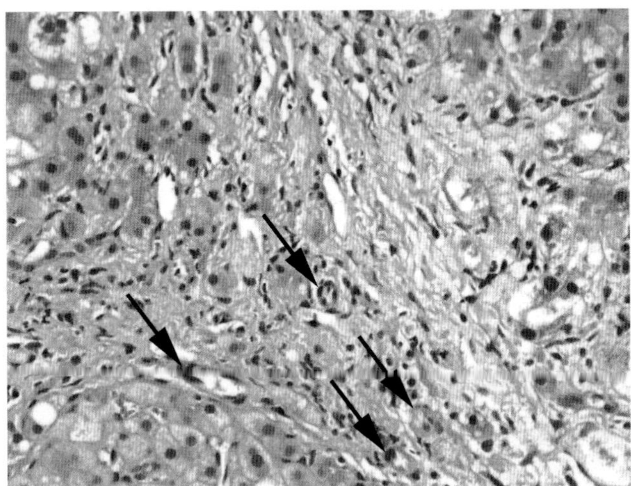

Figure 16.35 Arteriolization in Zone 3. Centrilobular region with fibrosis and an ingrowth of arterioles (*arrows*) simulating a portal area.

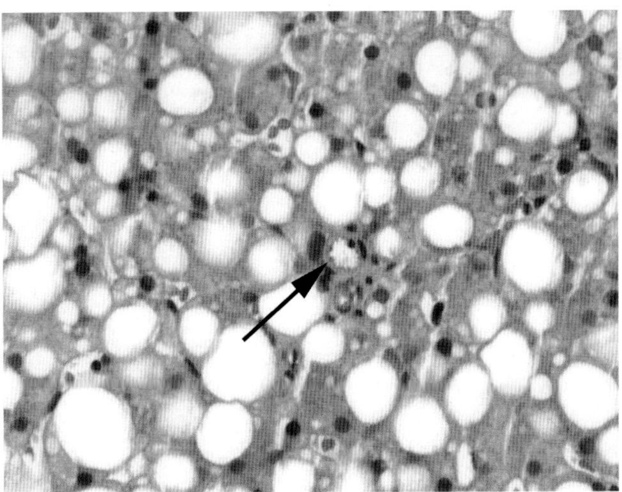

Figure 16.37 Arteriolization of the lobules. Unpaired artery in the lobule (*arrow*).

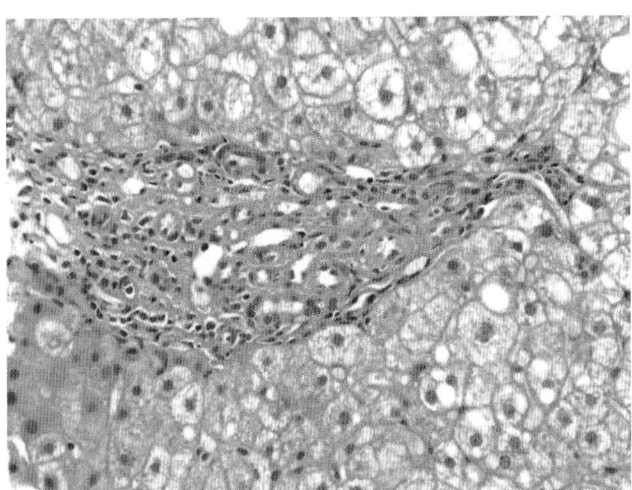

Figure 16.36 Arteriolization in a portal tract. A portal tract shows numerous arteriole profiles in a case of nonalcoholic steatohepatitis.

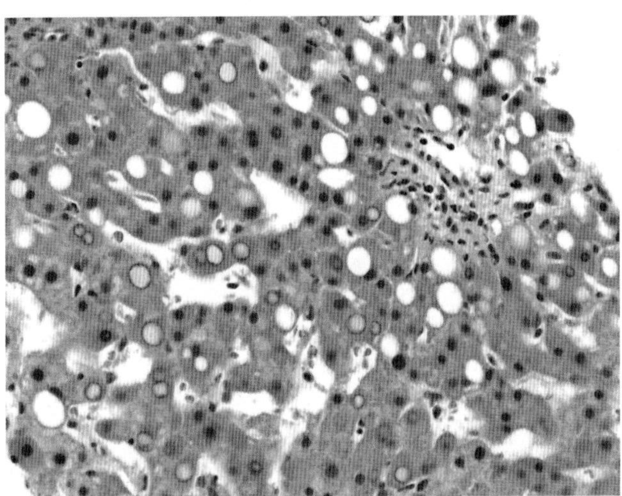

Figure 16.38 Nuclear glycogenation. Extensive nuclear glycogenation. Note the clearing of the nucleus with compression of the chromatin to the periphery.

this can lead to confusion with hepatic mass lesions (Fig. 16.37).

Glycogenation of hepatocyte nuclei is a common but nonspecific finding in steatosis and steatohepatitis, seen in approximately half of the cases (Fig. 16.38). Histologically, glycogen nuclei show a distinctive clearing of the chromatin of the nucleus. The finding may be present in both alcohol- and nonalcohol-related fatty liver diseases as well as other conditions such as glycogenic hepatopathy and glycogen storage diseases. Glycogen nuclei may be more common in diabetic patients.[28] In addition to glycogenated nuclei, small patches of hepatocytes may also be encountered with marked glycogen accumulation in their cytoplasm. This is characterized by cell swelling with rarefication of the cytoplasm. Although not necessary, the glycogen can be confirmed by PAS and PAS with diastase stains. These small patches seen in fatty liver disease must be distinguished from diffuse glycogenic hepatopathy seen in the setting of poorly controlled diabetes. Patients with glycogenic hepatopathy often present with diabetic ketoacidosis, markedly elevated liver function tests, and right upper quadrant pain. The histologic changes in glycogenic hepatopathy are readily reversible with improved glycemic control.

Increasing rates of childhood obesity are fueling an epidemic of childhood fatty liver disease. Although the basic histologic features are similar, cases of pediatric NAFLD show some unique features including less prominent lobular inflammation, less frequent

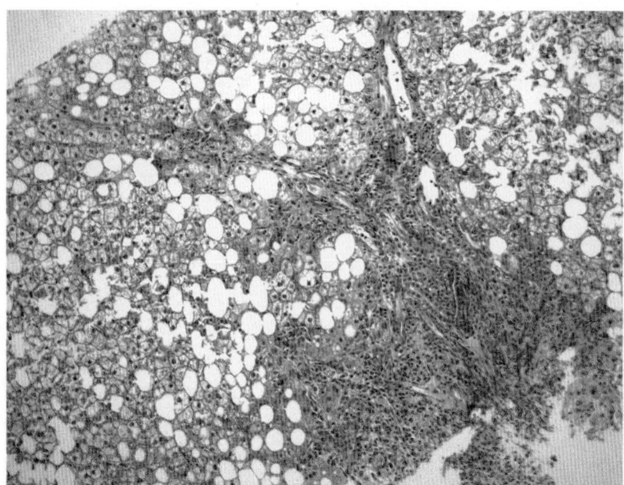

Figure 16.39 Nonalcoholic steatohepatitis in children. Periportal steatosis and portal-based fibrosis (Trichrome stain).

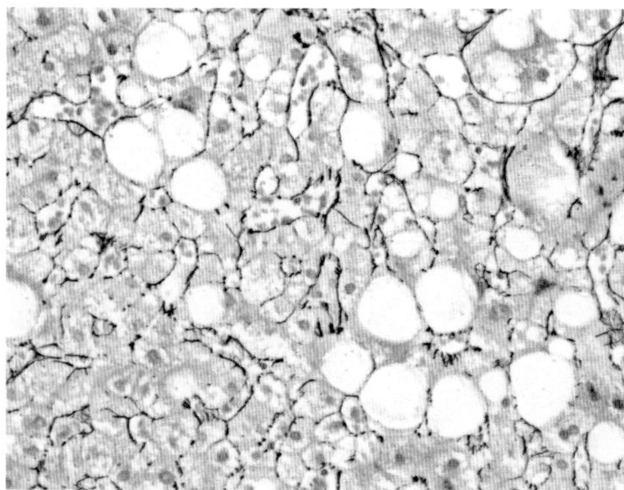

Figure 16.40 Reticulin stain in fatty liver disease. Disruption of the reticulin framework in marked steatosis (**lower right**). This is a pitfall in the use of reticulin staining to evaluate for hepatocellular carcinoma.

ballooned hepatocytes, more frequent Zone 1 distribution of the steatosis, and more frequent portal-based fibrosis[29] (Fig. 16.39).

Immunohistochemistry and special stains

Biopsies for fatty liver disease are evaluated by hematoxylin and eosin and a variety of other stains. A trichrome stain is essential in evaluating for fibrosis. The very early subsinusoidal or pericellular fibrosis seen in steatohepatitis may be missed without a stain for fibrosis. The PAS with diastase stain can be useful in excluding α-1 antitrypsin deficiency. Some cases of steatohepatitis may show rare small PAS positive diastase resistant globules in hepatocytes, but this should not be confused with the large and numerous globules seen in α-1 antitrypsin deficiency. Iron is not a component of fatty liver disease, but increased hepatocellular iron from other sources may speed the development of fibrosis and should be mentioned in the report.

Many centers perform a reticulin stain on every liver biopsy because it helps to evaluate the architecture of the hepatic plates. Loss of the reticulin framework is a classic histologic feature of HCC.[30] However, similar loss of the reticulin framework can be focally encountered in cases of fatty liver disease[31] (Fig. 16.40). There is a correlation between increasing amounts of steatosis and increasing loss of reticulin. No correlation is seen between the loss of the reticulin framework and the amount of inflammation and fibrosis. This is an important pitfall to be aware of when evaluating steatotic biopsies and considering the possibility of a mass lesion. Mallory hyaline can be highlighted with immunohistochemical stains for CK8, ubiquitin, and Cam 5.2 but this is not necessary in routine practice.

Ultrastructural findings

Ultrastructural studies play no role in the routine work-up of fatty liver disease specimens. In young children without the metabolic syndrome, ultrastructural studies are sometimc useful to help rule out inborn errors of metabolism.

Molecular genetic findings

Molecular studies play no role in the routine work-up of fatty liver disease specimens in adults. In children, molecular studies can be useful when an inborn error of metabolism is suspected.

Differential diagnosis

The differential diagnosis for steatosis and steatohepatitis is provided in Table 16.2. Because of the prevalence the metabolic syndrome, alcohol use, and chronic hepatitis C, these entities are often the major considerations. Most cases require clinical correlation to identify the exact etiology. Table 16.6 presents the histologic differences between alcohol and nonalcoholic liver disease. Overall, the histologic changes tend to be more severe in active alcohol-related liver disease compared to nonalcohol-related fatty liver disease. However, there are no findings that allow a specific diagnosis based solely on morphology. As an example, both canalicular cholestasis and ductular reactions are more common in alcohol versus nonalcohol-related fatty liver disease. However, these histologic changes may be seen if a patient with NAFLD has superimposed conditions such as a drug reaction, hepatic decompensation, or duct obstruction. For these reasons, a descriptive diagnosis with a prioritized differential is often rendered (Table 16.3). The clinician often has the information necessary to clarify the etiology and suggests a treatment strategy; the pathologist has provided valuable data regarding the pattern of injury, the disease activity, and the amount of fibrosis.

Drug reactions are also in the differential, including drugs such as Methotrexate and Amiodarone. Wilson disease can also present with fatty liver disease, and a high index of suspicion is needed in younger patients. Finally, a variety of hepatocellular mass lesions may show steatosis and steatohepatitis,[32] and caution should be used when interpreting a small fragmented biopsy targeted at a mass lesion, to be sure there are true portal tracts and central veins prior to rendering a diagnosis of steatohepatitis.

Prognosis and treatment

Steatosis alone does not increase the risk for hepatic fibrosis but does increase the risk for nonalcoholic steatohepatitis. Nonalcoholic steatohepatitis on the other hand is a progressive fibrotic disease. The prognosis of nonalcoholic steatohepatitis depends on the ability to modify the underlying causes of the steatohepatitis and on the degree of hepatic fibrosis. For this reason, the liver biopsy plays a significant role in defining the prognosis of patients with nonalcoholic steatohepatitis. As the fibrosis progresses to cirrhosis, several studies have shown that the degree of steatosis actually decreases.[33] It is generally accepted that the majority of cases of cryptogenic cirrhosis in patients with the metabolic syndrome actually represent end stage nonalcoholic steatohepatitis. Patients with cirrhosis are at increased risk of developing HCC, but the risk may be less than other causes of cirrhosis, especially chronic hepatitis C.[34]

The treatment of nonalcoholic steatohepatitis is targeted at modifying risk factors of the underlying metabolic syndrome. This is done with optimal blood sugar control, weight loss, and increased exercise. High doses of vitamin E (800 IU) have been shown to decrease the degree of steatosis and lobular inflammation in patients without diabetes.[35] There was no observed change in the fibrosis score. In the same study, Pioglitazone also showed some potential benefits in the secondary outcomes.[35] Because of the synergistic effects, other drugs/medications associated with steatosis and steatohepatitis, including alcohol, should be avoided.

16.6 DRUG-INDUCED FATTY LIVER DISEASE

An extensive list of drugs, medications, and supplements associated with fatty liver disease is provided in Table 16.7. Drug-induced fatty liver disease is also discussed in more detail in Chapter 15. The histologic features of drug-induced fatty liver disease can be broken down into three basic patterns: simple steatosis, active steatohepatitis, and diffuse microvesicular steatosis. Simple steatosis and steatohepatitis are the most commonly encountered patterns and most medications that cause fatty liver disease can produce either pattern. Amiodarone and methotrexate can create a histologic appearance of active steatohepatitis indistinguishable from that seen in the metabolic syndrome or alcoholic steatohepatitis (Fig. 16.41). The injury caused by these drugs can also progress to fibrosis and cirrhosis if not discontinued. Diffuse microvesicular steatosis is a distinctive finding with a long list of offending agents (Fig. 16.42). This pattern is often seen in the setting of lactic acidosis, hepatomegaly, and hepatic failure, and is associated with mitochondrial toxicity. Table 16.2 highlights the differential diagnosis for microvesicular steatosis (see discussion later).

The diagnosis of drug-induced fatty liver disease should not be made based on the histological findings alone and requires clinical and serologic correlation. Even with all of the available data, documenting causation remains a challenge. A variety of causality scoring methods have been proposed. In general, one must consider the following features: temporal relationship between organ dysfunction and exposure, exclusion of other causes (including toxicology analysis), an agent with known potential to cause the pattern of injury, and improvement of the liver injury after removal of the offending agent.

16.7 WILSON DISEASE

Wilson disease is an autosomal recessive disease in which patients have a defective copper transport mechanism, resulting in the accumulation of toxic copper levels at multiple sites. The disease usually presents in children and young adults. The liver can be a primary organ of involvement in Wilson disease, and histologic analysis reveals a variety of patterns of injury. Some cases may be quite reminiscent of an active steatohepatitis, with robust lobular inflammation and marked ballooning degeneration[29] (Fig. 16.43). Mallory hyaline and glycogenated nuclei may be commonly seen. Occasionally, the deposits of copper can be seen as faint, gray, stippled cytoplasmic granules. Copper stains will highlight the copper but a negative copper

Table 16.7 Drugs and supplements associated with fatty liver disease

Routine fatty liver disease	Diffuse microvesicular steatosis
• Mixed large- and small-droplet steatoses • With or without inflammation and ballooning degeneration	• Patients often have lactic acidosis • Mitochondrial dysfunction
Amiodarone	Amineptine
Corticosteroids	Amiodarone[43]
Isonizid	Azathioprine
L-Asparginase[44]	Calcium hopantenate
Methotrexate	Camphor
Naproxen	Chloroform[45]
Perhexiline maleate	Demeclocycline
Raloxifene	D-Nucleoside analogues • Fialuridine • Didanosine • Stavudine Zidovudine
Risperidone	• Ibuprofen
Steroid hormones (estrogen, testosterone)	Jinbuhuan
Sulfasalazine	Ketoprofen
Tomoxifen	L-Asparginase[44]
Valproic acid	Linezolid[46]
	Margosa oil
	Pennyroyal oil
	Piroxicam
	Pirprofen
	Syo-saiko-to
	Tetracycline
	Tolmetin
	Urethane
	Valproic Acid[47]
	Vitamin A
	Warfarin

Data from Refs. 48, 49.

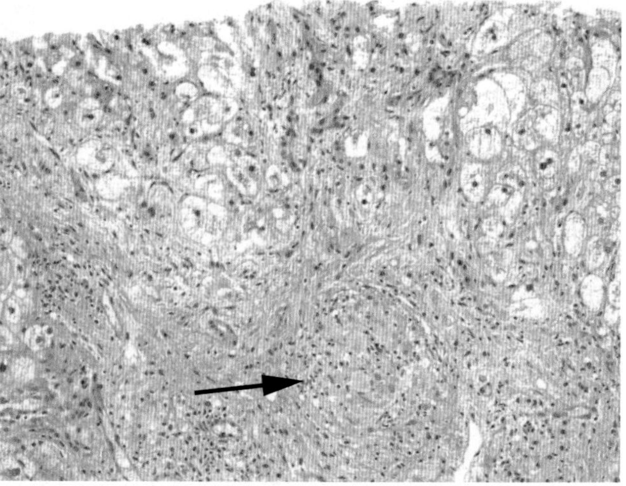

Figure 16.41 Steatohepatitis, drug induced. Steatohepatitis in a patient on Amiodarone. Note the granuloma (*arrow*) that may or may not be present in Amiodarone drug reactions.

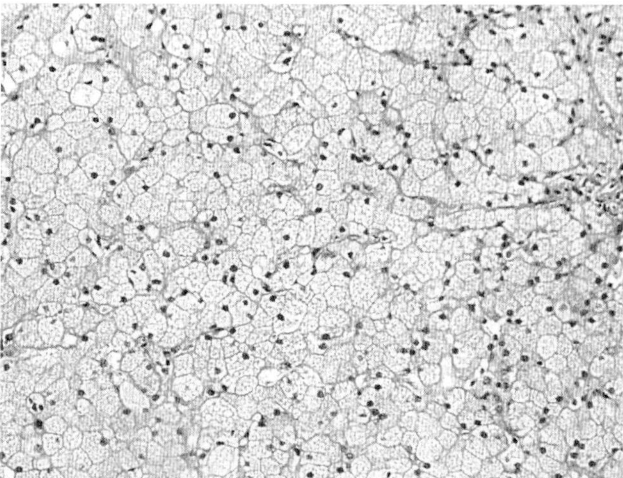

Figure 16.42 Steatohepatitis, drug induced. Tetracycline-induced diffuse microvesicular steatosis.

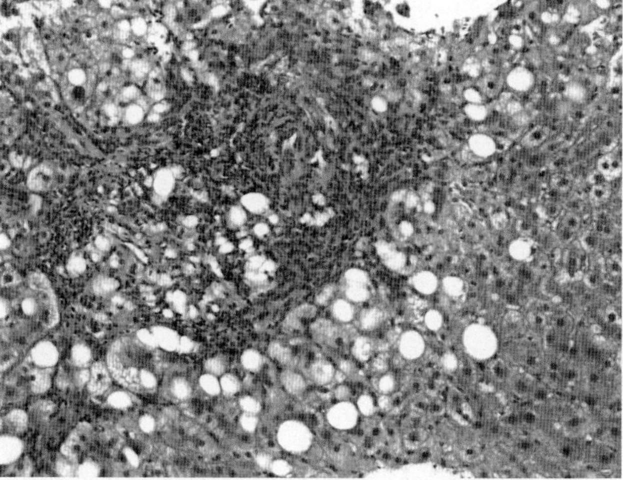

Figure 16.43 Wilson disease with fatty liver disease. Steatohepatitis in a patient with Wilson disease. Note the prominent portal-based inflammation that is more than typically seen in cases of nonalcoholic fatty liver disease alone.

stain does not exclude the diagnosis of Wilson disease. Quantitative copper testing and genetic testing can help establish the diagnosis. In some cases, especially in younger aged individuals, distinguishing Wilson disease from other forms of fatty liver disease can be quite difficult, and it remains the pathologists job to suggest Wilson disease as a possibility for an otherwise unexplained steatohepatitis.

16.8 OVERLAP DISEASES

Hepatitis C virus infection can be associated with steatosis and even steatohepatitis (Figs. 16.44 and 16.45). Hepatitis C genotype 3a has the strongest association,[36] though the mechanism is unknown. In most cases, these individuals also have some or all of the risk factors for the metabolic syndrome, and there may be a synergistic effect between the metabolic syndrome and the virus in causing fatty liver disease. The steatosis and steatohepatitis in chronic hepatitic C show similar findings to that of the metabolic syndrome and alcohol use, without any unique findings to differentiate between these possibilities. Despite the challenges in distinguishing the specific etiology, finding either concurrent steatosis or steatohepatitis should always be included in the reporting of liver biopsy specimens. This alerts the clinicians to evaluate the patient for metabolic syndrome risk factors and recommend appropriate lifestyle modifications, including alcohol abstinence. Regardless of the etiology, concurrent steatohepatitis can speed the progression of fibrosis in patients with chronic hepatitis C.[37] Pericellular fibrosis, if present, should be mentioned in addition to the fibrosis stage of the chronic hepatitis C.

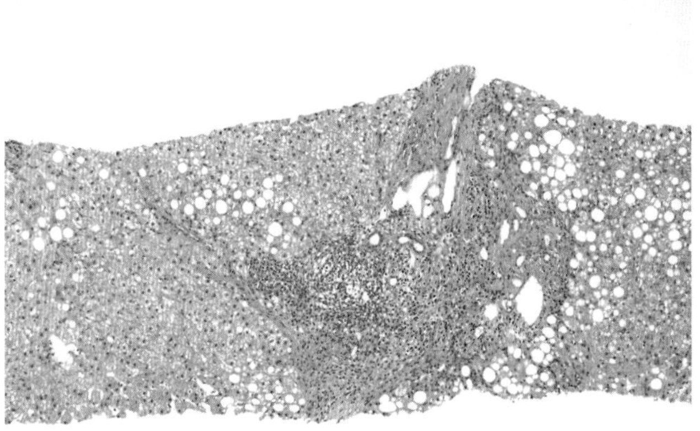

Figure 16.44 Hepatitis C virus with fatty liver disease. Steatosis with classic lymphoid aggregates in the portal areas.

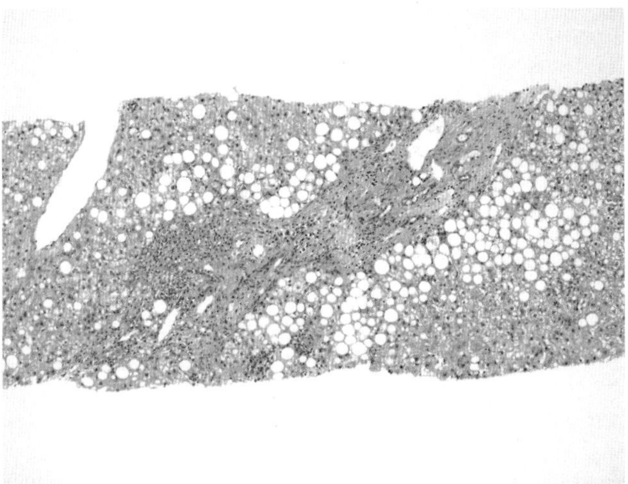

Figure 16.45 Hepatitis C virus with fatty liver disease. In this case of chronic hepatitis C, the steatosis shows a distinct zone 1 distribution.

Active steatohepatitis has been identified in the setting of a number of other chronic liver diseases, including primary biliary cirrhosis (6.2%), α-1 antitrypsin deficiency (7.9%), hemochromatosis (2.2%), chronic hepatitis B virus infection (3.4%), autoimmune hepatitis (1.6%), and drug-induced liver disease (2.4%).[38] In most cases, this is likely related to the concurrence of both diseases.

The pathologist must remain diligent and complete a detailed histologic analysis of the biopsy for secondary forms of liver disease, even in the setting of an active steatohepatitis (Fig. 16.46). Hepatocellular

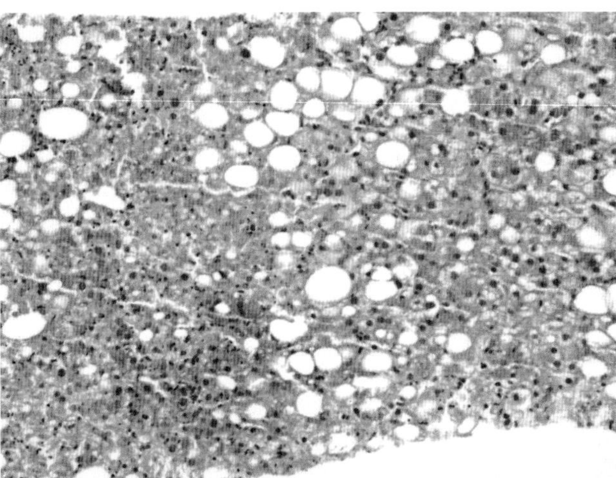

Figure 16.46 Fatty liver disease plus other findings. This patient had many risk factors for both alcoholic and nonalcoholic steatohepatitis. However, the biopsy not only showed an active steatohepatitis but also geographic areas of dirty necrosis suspicious for an acute viral infection. Immunohistochemical stains confirmed herpes simplex virus infection.

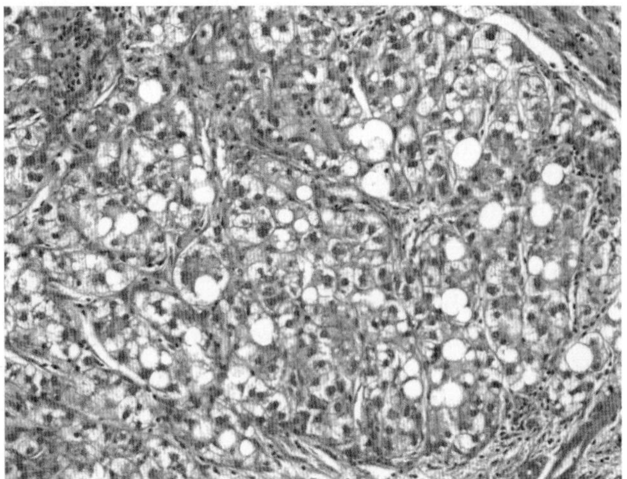

Figure 16.47 Steatohepatitic variant of hepatocellular carcinoma. There is marked cytological atypia and thickened hepatic plates.

neoplasms that can show steatosis include the steatohepatitic subtype of HCC (Fig. 16.47), hepatocellular adenomas (Fig. 16.48), and less commonly focal nodular hyperplasia. If the biopsy is small and fragmented and no clinical history of a mass lesion is provided to the pathologist, it can be very easy to miss-interpret the steatohepatitic subtype of HCC as active steatohepatitis, because these tumors can show extensive ballooning degeneration, lobular inflammation, and steatosis. In most cases, close inspection reveals the characteristic features of the HCC, including increased nuclear density, pleomorphism, thickened hepatic plates, unpaired arteries, and endothelialization of the sinusoids. Similarly, hepatocellular adenomas, in particular the HNF1α mutated subtype and the inflammatory subtype, may have a significant component of steatosis, and close inspection for the background portal tracts and central veins is required to exclude a lesion with aberrant architecture.

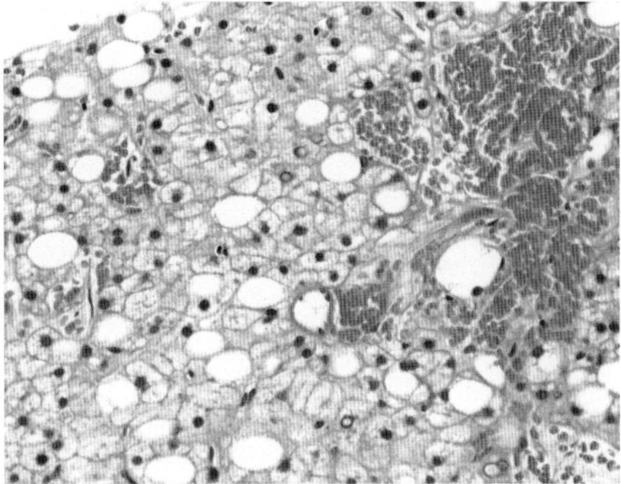

Figure 16.48 Inflammatory type adenoma with steatosis. In addition to the steatosis, there is hemorrhage and unpaired arteries.

16.9 MICROVESICULAR STEATOSIS

True microvesicular steatosis is characterized by diffuse involvement of the hepatocytes with small lipid droplets filling the cytoplasm. The hepatocyte nucleus usually retains its central location within the cell. These features impart a diffuse "bubbly" appearance to the cells (Fig. 16.2). Initial publications describing this condition advocated the use of oil red O staining to help identify this lesion. However, the histologic findings are relatively distinct on routine H&E staining, and small lipid droplets are encountered in normal control patient specimens with oil red O staining. For these reasons, standard H&E staining is recommended. Ballooning degeneration and lobular inflammation are typically absent.

Diffuse microvesicular steatosis is an uncommon finding in liver biopsies and when identified, a broad differential diagnosis should be considered (Table 16.2). Most of the implicated diseases are associated with mitochondrial metabolism defects. Although all of these conditions are rare, the commonly encountered are adverse drug reactions (discussed above), alcohol-related foamy liver disease (discussed above), and fatty liver disease of pregnancy. Distinct patches of microvesicular steatosis may be encountered in otherwise typical cases of NAFLD.[27] Microvesicular steatosis can also be found in the surviving hepatocytes adjacent to areas of massive hepatocellular injury.

Acute fatty liver disease of pregnancy is a rare syndrome characterized by microvesicular steatosis on liver biopsy (Fig. 16.49). The steatosis may be mostly

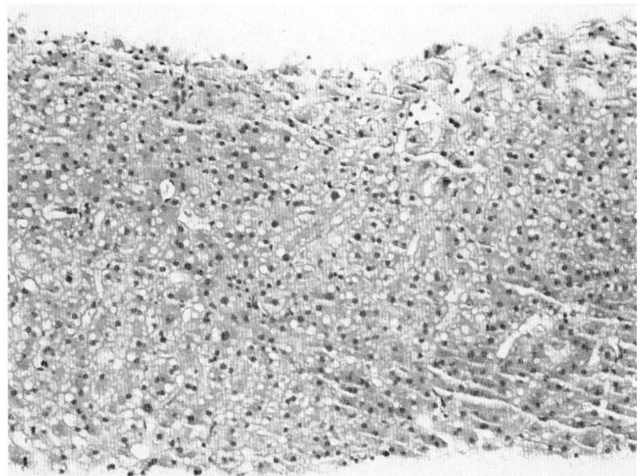

Figure 16.49 Acute fatty liver of pregnancy. Diffuse microvesicular steatosis without necroinflammatory activity.

centrilobular or may be diffuse. Other changes include variable hepatocyte swelling, cholestasis, and minimal to mild lobular inflammation. Megamitochondria are often prominent. Delivery of the fetus is the most effective treatment, and histologic resolution occurs rapidly, often within weeks.[39,40]

REFERENCES

1. Brunt EM, Janney CG, Di Bisceglie AM, et al. Nonalcoholic steatohepatitis: a proposal for grading and staging the histological lesions. *Am J Gastroenterol*. 1999;94:2467–2474.
2. Hall AR, Dhillon AP, Green AC, et al. Hepatic steatosis estimated microscopically versus digital image analysis. *Liver Int*. 2013;33:926–935.
3. Hall AR, Green AC, Luong TV, et al. The use of guideline images to improve histological estimation of hepatic steatosis. *Liver Int*. 2014;34: 1414–1427.
4. Kleiner DE, Brunt EM, Van Natta M, et al. Design and validation of a histological scoring system for nonalcoholic fatty liver disease. *Hepatology*. 2005;41:1313–1321.
5. Brunt EM, Kleiner DE, Behling C, et al. Misuse of scoring systems. *Hepatology*. 2011;54:369–370; author reply 370–371.
6. Mehta SR, Thomas EL, Bell JD, et al. Non-invasive means of measuring hepatic fat content. *World J Gastroenterol*. 2008;14:3476–3483.
7. Yoshioka K, Kawabe N, Hashimoto S. Transient elastography: applications and limitations. *Hepatol Res*. 2008;38:1063–1068.
8. Jaeschke H. Neutrophil-mediated tissue injury in alcoholic hepatitis. *Alcohol*. 2002;27:23–27.
9. Wanless IR, Nakashima E, Sherman M. Regression of human cirrhosis. Morphologic features and the genesis of incomplete septal cirrhosis. *Arch Pathol Lab Med*. 2000;124:1599–1607.
10. Itoh S, Yougel T, Kawagoe K. Comparison between nonalcoholic steatohepatitis and alcoholic hepatitis. *Am J Gastroenterol*. 1987;82:650–654.
11. Diehl AM, Goodman Z, Ishak KG. Alcohollike liver disease in nonalcoholics. A clinical and histologic comparison with alcohol-induced liver injury. *Gastroenterology*. 1988;95:1056–1062.
12. Neuschwander-Tetri BA, Caldwell SH. Nonalcoholic steatohepatitis: summary of an AASLD Single Topic Conference. *Hepatology*. 2003;37:1202–1219.
13. Morita Y, Ueno T, Sasaki N, et al. Comparison of liver histology between patients with non-alcoholic steatohepatitis and patients with alcoholic steatohepatitis in Japan. *Alcohol Clin Exp Res*. 2005;29:277S–281S.
14. Nonomura A, Enomoto Y, Takeda M, et al. Clinical and pathological features of non-alcoholic steatohepatitis. *Hepatol Res*. 2005;33:116–121.
15. Yip WW, Burt AD. Alcoholic liver disease. *Semin Diagn Pathol*. 2006;23:149–160.
16. Teli MR, Day CP, Burt AD, et al. Determinants of progression to cirrhosis or fibrosis in pure alcoholic fatty liver. *Lancet*. 1995;346:987–990.
17. Chedid A, Mendenhall CL, Gartside P, et al. Prognostic factors in alcoholic liver disease. VA Cooperative Study Group. *Am J Gastroenterol*. 1991;86:210–216.
18. Nissenbaum M, Chedid A, Mendenhall C, et al. Prognostic significance of cholestatic alcoholic hepatitis. VA Cooperative Study Group #119. *Dig Dis Sci*. 1990;35:891–896.
19. Haber PS, Warner R, Seth D, et al. Pathogenesis and management of alcoholic hepatitis. *J Gastroenterol Hepatol*. 2003;18:1332–1344.
20. Powell WJ Jr, Klatskin G. Duration of survival in patients with Laennec's cirrhosis. Influence of alcohol withdrawal, and possible effects of recent changes in general management of the disease. *Am J Med*. 1968;44:406–420.
21. Younossi ZM, Stepanova M, Afendy M, et al. Changes in the prevalence of the most common causes of chronic liver diseases in the United States from 1988 to 2008. *Clin Gastroenterol Hepatol*. 2011;9:524–530 e1; quiz e60.
22. Browning JD, Szczepaniak LS, Dobbins R, et al. Prevalence of hepatic steatosis in an urban population in the United States: impact of ethnicity. *Hepatology*. 2004;40:1387–1395.
23. Adams LA, Lindor KD, Angulo P. The prevalence of autoantibodies and autoimmune hepatitis in patients with nonalcoholic fatty liver disease. *Am J Gastroenterol*. 2004;99:1316–1320.
24. Cotler SJ, Kanji K, Keshavarzian A, et al. Prevalence and significance of autoantibodies in patients with non-alcoholic steatohepatitis. *J Clin Gastroenterol*. 2004;38:801–804.
25. Vuppalanchi R, Gould RJ, Wilson LA, et al. Clinical significance of serum autoantibodies in patients with NAFLD: results from the nonalcoholic steatohepatitis clinical research network. *Hepatol Int*. 2012;6:379–385.
26. Ryan CK, Johnson LA, Germin BI, et al. One hundred consecutive hepatic biopsies in the workup of living donors for right lobe liver transplantation. *Liver Transpl*. 2002;8:1114–1122.
27. Tandra S, Yeh MM, Brunt EM, et al. Presence and significance of microvesicular steatosis in nonalcoholic fatty liver disease. *J Hepatol*. 2011;55:654–659.
28. Abraham S, Furth EE. Receiver operating characteristic analysis of glycogenated nuclei in

liver biopsy specimens: quantitative evaluation of their relationship with diabetes and obesity. *Hum Pathol*. 1994;25:1063–1068.

29. Brunt EM. Pathology of fatty liver disease. *Mod Pathol*. 2007;20 suppl 1:S40–S48.
30. International Consensus Group for Hepatocellular NeoplasiaThe International Consensus Group for Hepatocellular N. Pathologic diagnosis of early hepatocellular carcinoma: a report of the international consensus group for hepatocellular neoplasia. *Hepatology*. 2009;49:658–664.
31. Singhi AD, Jain D, Kakar S, et al. Reticulin loss in benign fatty liver: an important diagnostic pitfall when considering a diagnosis of hepatocellular carcinoma. *Am J Surg Pathol*. 2012;36:710–715.
32. Salomao M, Yu WM, Brown RS Jr, et al. Steatohepatitic hepatocellular carcinoma (SH-HCC): a distinctive histological variant of HCC in hepatitis C virus-related cirrhosis with associated NAFLD/ NASH. *Am J Surg Pathol*. 2010;34:1630–1636.
33. Adams LA, Sanderson S, Lindor KD, et al. The histological course of nonalcoholic fatty liver disease: a longitudinal study of 103 patients with sequential liver biopsies. *J Hepatol*. 2005;42: 132–138.
34. Hui JM, Kench JG, Chitturi S, et al. Long-term outcomes of cirrhosis in nonalcoholic steatohepatitis compared with hepatitis C. *Hepatology*. 2003;38:420–427.
35. Sanyal AJ, Chalasani N, Kowdley KV, et al. Pioglitazone, vitamin E, or placebo for nonalcoholic steatohepatitis. *N Engl J Med*. 2010;362:1675–1685.
36. Monto A, Alonzo J, Watson JJ, et al. Steatosis in chronic hepatitis C: relative contributions of obesity, diabetes mellitus, and alcohol. *Hepatology*. 2002;36:729–736.
37. Adinolfi LE, Gambardella M, Andreana A, et al. Steatosis accelerates the progression of liver damage of chronic hepatitis C patients and correlates with specific HCV genotype and visceral obesity. *Hepatology*. 2001;33:1358–1364.
38. Brunt EM, Ramrakhiani S, Cordes BG, et al. Concurrence of histologic features of steatohepatitis with other forms of chronic liver disease. *Mod Pathol*. 2003;16:49–56.
39. Reyes H, Sandoval L, Wainstein A, et al. Acute fatty liver of pregnancy: a clinical study of 12 episodes in 11 patients. *Gut*. 1994;35:101–106.
40. Rolfes DB, Ishak KG. Acute fatty liver of pregnancy: a clinicopathologic study of 35 cases. *Hepatology*. 1985;5:1149–1158.
41. Hautekeete ML, Degott C, Benhamou JP. Microvesicular steatosis of the liver. *Acta Clin Belg*. 1990;45:311–326.
42. Kneeman JM, Misdraji J, Corey KE. Secondary causes of nonalcoholic fatty liver disease. *Therap Adv Gastroenterol*. 2012;5:199–207.
43. Puli SR, Fraley MA, Puli V, et al. Hepatic cirrhosis caused by low-dose oral amiodarone therapy. *Am J Med Sci*. 2005;330:257–261.
44. Bodmer M, Sulz M, Stadlmann S, et al. Fatal liver failure in an adult patient with acute lymphoblastic leukemia following treatment with L-asparaginase. *Digestion*. 2006;74:28–32.
45. Lionte C. Lethal complications after poisoning with chloroform--case report and literature review. *Hum Exp Toxicol*. 2010;29:615–622.
46. De Bus L, Depuydt P, Libbrecht L, et al. Severe drug-induced liver injury associated with prolonged use of linezolid. *J Med Toxicol*. 2010;6:322–326.
47. Scheffner D, Konig S, Rauterberg-Ruland I, et al. Fatal liver failure in 16 children with valproate therapy. *Epilepsia*. 1988;29:530–542.
48. Lewis JH, Ahmed M, Shobassy A, et al. Drug-induced liver disease. *Curr Opin Gastroenterol*. 2006;22:223–233.
49. Arundel C, Lewis JH. Drug-induced liver disease in 2006. *Curr Opin Gastroenterol*. 2007;23:244–254.

17

Iron overload and liver pathology

Vishal S. Chandan, MD, and Michael S. Torbenson, MD

17.1 INTRODUCTION

The medical community has recognized that iron accumulation causes liver disease for several hundred years, but for the first 100 plus years, progress was slow in understanding the epidemiology, biology, and disease manifestations of iron overload. However, since the early 1970s, progress has been rapid, with key new insights into the genetic causes and mechanisms of iron overload as well as the normal physiology of iron metabolism. A basic understanding of normal iron metabolism helps considerably in understanding the genetic causes of iron overload, so normal iron physiology is reviewed briefly later.

Correlation with serum findings is also important. In most cases of iron overload, both the serum ferritin and the serum transferrin saturation levels are elevated. Serum ferritin levels above 1,000 μg/L and/or transferrin saturation levels of 45% or greater are widely used clinically as surrogate markers for excess body iron stores. Interestingly, there are four relatively rare conditions where these two markers do not rise in parallel, with transferrin saturation levels that remain low or normal despite significantly elevated ferritin levels: ferroportin disease, African iron overload, hereditary hyperferritinemia, and aceruloplasminemia.

17.2 OVERVIEW OF NORMAL IRON METABOLISM

A liter of healthy blood contains 0.5 g of iron, and the healthy adult body contains a total of 3 to 5 g of iron (for comparison, a USA nickel weighs 5 g). About 20 mg of iron are needed daily for ordinary physiologic functions. Most of this iron is obtained by recycling the iron found in aged and damaged red blood cells. The rest of the iron comes from dietary sources, with 1 to 2 mg needed per day. Iron is naturally present in many foods and is also a common food additive. Dietary iron can be either heme iron from meat or nonheme iron from a variety of sources, including both plants and meat.

In normal physiology, iron is important for heme synthesis, oxidative phosphorylation, DNA synthesis, and a number of other metabolic processes. Nonetheless, too much iron can generate free oxygen radicals, which are highly toxic to cells. To prevent this, the body tightly regulates iron levels in the blood and tissues. Iron levels in the body are regulated almost exclusively by controlling iron absorption in the small intestine.

Iron absorption

The major proteins and cells involved in iron metabolism are presented in Table 17.1 for quick reference. Most iron is absorbed in the duodenum and proximal jejunum. Once iron is absorbed into enterocytes, it can have several fates. If the body has sufficient iron stores, then the iron remains within the cytoplasm of the enterocytes. When the enterocytes naturally undergo apoptosis at the end of their lifespan, the iron is lost within the fecal stream, preventing iron overload. In contrast, if the body needs iron, iron is transported out of the enterocyte by ferroportin, with some help by accessory proteins including ceruloplasmin and hephaestin, and enters the blood stream, where

Table 17.1 Important proteins and cells that play a role in iron metabolism

Protein or cells	Notes
Proteins	
DMT-1	Dimetal transporter-1. Transports iron from gut lumen into enterocyte cytoplasm
Ferritin	Protein with an enormous capacity to bind iron and a major physiologic storage form of iron; located in the cell cytoplasm of hepatocytes, enterocytes, and Kupffer cells. Elevated serum ferritin levels are one of the most widely used surrogates for iron overload. Testing is highly sensitive (normal levels rule out iron overload) but not very specific. Ferritin levels are also used to guide phlebotomy therapy
Ferroportin	Transports iron from inside cells out to the blood (principally enterocytes and macrophages, also hepatocytes)
Hemojuvelin	Interacts with important signaling pathways (BMP, SMAD) that have hepcidin as a downstream target. Without hemojuvelin, these signaling pathways do not activate hepcidin gene synthesis in a normal fashion
Transferrin	Binds and transports iron in blood. Elevated saturation levels are (>45%) suggest increased iron stores
HFE	Mutations are the most common cause of genetic hemochromatosis. Interacts with transferrin receptor 1 and regulates hepcidin levels
Cells	
Enterocytes	Absorption and short-term storage of iron
Hepatocytes	Major producer of ferritin and hepcidin and is the major organ for storing iron in the form of ferritin
Macrophages	Scavenges old/damage red blood cells. Another major cell type for storage of iron in the form of ferritin
Other	
Hemosiderin	Abnormal deposits of iron

it is bound by transferrin and circulates within the blood. In healthy individuals, the blood contains much more transferrin protein than iron, and the transferrin proteins are approximately 30% saturated with iron. As blood iron levels increase, the excess transferrin proteins buffer the excess iron to help prevent toxicity. Saturation levels of 45% and above are associated with excess body iron stores.

Iron movement from blood into cells

Individual cells have mechanisms to determine if they have sufficient iron stores within their cytoplasm to meet their needs. If iron is needed, cells increase expression of transferrin receptors. There are two transferrin receptors: transferrin receptor 1 is present on the membrane of all nucleated cells, whereas receptor 2 is primarily found on hepatocytes and macrophages. These membrane receptors take iron into the cells through receptor-mediated endocytosis.

Iron storage

Excess iron in hepatocytes and macrophages is incorporated into ferritin molecules for storage. Ferritin can hold up to 4,500 atoms of iron per ferritin protein complex. Serum ferritin levels above 1,000 µg/L are widely used as a surrogate marker for excess body iron stores. Ferritin in the liver is not visible on Perls stain in most cases, but occasionally ferritin is seen as a faint blue blush in the hepatocyte cytoplasm. The iron in ferritin can be rapidly accessed to meet physiologic needs. If body iron levels are excessive over a sufficiently long period of time, hemosiderin deposits develop.

Hemosiderin deposits are granular and golden brown on hematoxylin and eosin (H&E) stains. They are made of iron, degraded ferritin, and small amounts of various proteins. In contrast to ferritin, the iron in hemosiderin is not readily available for biologic needs. Hemosiderin in both genetic and nongenetic iron overload is identical on H&E and Perls iron stain, but they differ significantly in both the metal composition and the organic components.[1]

The central role of hepcidin in regulation of iron levels

When blood iron levels are low, iron is released from the ferritin stored in enterocytes, hepatocytes, and macrophages into the blood. When blood levels are adequate or high, hepcidin prevents these cells from releasing iron into the blood. Hepcidin accomplishes this in part by degrading ferroportin,[2] which is the key protein involved in transporting iron out of cells into the blood. In contrast, hepcidin levels decline in response to low iron levels, allowing increased release of iron into the blood from enteric cells, hepatocytes, and macrophages. Hepcidin (encoded by *HAMP*) is an acute phase reactant produced by hepatocytes[3] and biliary epithelium.[4] Because it is an acute phase reactant, hepcidin levels can be elevated in a variety of inflammatory and infectious conditions, leading to anemia of chronic disease.

Hepcidin plays a central role in all known forms of genetic hemochromatosis, with each mutation leading to impaired hepcidin production or function.[5,6] The loss of production or function of hepcidin in turn gradually leads to excess iron absorption, with subsequent iron deposition in the liver and other organs. The major causes of genetic hemochromatosis are discussed individually below and are summarized in Table 17.2.

In contrast to hemochromatosis that results from loss of hepcidin function, rare mutations have also been described that increase hepcidin function, with clinical manifestations of congenital refractory anemia.[7] Increased expression of hepcidin (with subsequent development of anemia) has also been reported in a hepatic adenoma.[8] Similarly, hepatic adenomas occurring in individuals with Type 1a glycogen storage disease are often associated with anemia that resolves after the adenoma is resected,[9] implying hepcidin is overexpressed by the adenomas. In contrast, hepatocellular carcinomas tend to have lower levels of hepcidin expression.[10]

17.3 HEMOCHROMATOSIS

History of hemochromatosis as a disease

Armand Trousseau (1801 to 1867), a French internist, reported the syndrome of liver cirrhosis, pancreas fibrosis, and cutaneous hyperpigmentation in 1865,[11] shortly before his own death from pancreas carcinoma. However, it appears that he did not recognize the role of iron in the disease process. Another French physician, Troisier, described a case of "diabète bronzé et cirrhose pigmentaire" in 1871 and both confirmed the observation of Trousseau and demonstrated iron in various tissues.[12] In fact, Troisier's triad of diabetes, skin hyperpigmentation, and cirrhosis became the working definition for hemochromatosis for many decades. Another milestone occurred in 1935 when Sheldon, an English gerontologist, reviewed the literature of 300+ cases of hemochromatosis and concluded that iron accumulation was likely the result of increased absorption.[13] Other physicians and scientists before and after Sheldon's seminal paper thought the iron accumulation in hemochromatosis might be secondary to hemorrhage or other sources of tissue injury. Sheldon's paper also suggested hemochromatosis had a genetic

Table 17.2 Summary of genetic iron diseases involving the liver

Disease	Gene (protein)	Inheritance	Primary ethnicity	Onset	Principal iron location
Hemochromatosis Type 1	*HFE*	Recessive	Northern European	Late	Hepatocytes > Kupffer cells
Juvenile hemochromatosis Type 2A	*HFE2* (also known as *HJV*)	Recessive	European	Early	Hepatocytes > Kupffer cells
Juvenile hemochromatosis Type 2B	*HAMP* (hepcidin)	Recessive	European	Early	Hepatocytes > Kupffer cells
TFR2-associated hemochromatosis	*TFR2*	Recessive	European Asian	Late	Hepatocytes > Kupffer cells
Hemochromatosis	*SCL11A2* (DMT-1)	Recessive	European	Early	Hepatocytes > Kupffer cells
Ferroportin disease	*SLC40A1* (ferroportin, loss of function mutation)	Dominant	Pan-ethnic	Late	Kupffer cells > hepatocytes
Ferroportin associated hemochromatosis (previously referred to as ferroportin disease type B)	*SLC40A1* (ferroportin, activating mutation)	Dominant	Pan-ethnic	Late	Hepatocytes > Kupffer cells
Hypotransferrinemia	*TF* (Transferrin)	Recessive	European Asian	Early	Kupffer cells > hepatocytes
Hypoceruloplasminemia	*CP* (Ceruloplasmin)	Recessive	European Asian	Late	

basis. A genetic link was subsequently confirmed in 1975 by Simon and colleagues in a study that demonstrated a link between the clinical hemochromatosis phenotype and a human leukocyte antigen-A locus on chromosome 6p, with an inheritance pattern most consistent with an autosomal recessive disease.[14] The specific gene causing most forms of hemochromatosis was discovered in 1996[15] and eventually named *HFE*, with the H shorthand for "high" and "FE" for iron. Subsequent studies identified cases of iron overload that were not caused by *HFE* mutations, leading to a gradual recognition of additional genes important in iron metabolism. The discovery of Hepcidin (coded by *HAMP*) by several groups in 2000[16] and 2001[3,17] eventually led to a unifying mechanism for iron genetic iron overload disease: impairment of hepcidin function.

17.4 *HFE* MUTATIONS

Clinical and epidemiologic findings

More than 37 *HFE* mutations have been reported,[18] but C282Y and H63D mutations are by far the most numerically and clinically important. C282Y mutations are strongly linked to northern European genetic ancestry,[18] whereas H63D mutations have a wider ethnic distribution.[19] Approximately 35% of individuals with northern European ancestry will have an *HFE* mutation (Table 17.3). In contrast, other ethnic groups have much lower frequencies of *HFE* mutations (Table 17.4).

The normal HFE protein is expressed principally in cells that traffic iron, such as duodenal crypt cells,

Table 17.3 *HFE* mutations in northern European populations

Genetic status	Population (percent affected)
C282Y heterozygote	9
C282Y homozygote	0.5
H63D heterozygote	22
H63D homozygote	2.0
C282Y/H63D compound heterozygote	2.0
Wild/wild	65

From Hanson, E.H., G. Imperatore, and W. Burke, HFE gene and hereditary hemochromatosis: a HuGE review. Human Genome Epidemiology. *Am J Epidemiol*, 2001. 154(3): p. 193–206, by permission of Johns Hopkins Bloomberg School of Public Health.

Table 17.4 *HFE* mutations in other populations

Genetic status	Hispanic (% affected)	Black (% affected)	Pacific islander (% affected)	Asian (% affected)
C282Y heterozygote	3	2	2	0.1
C282Y homozygote	0.06	0.01	0.00	0.00
C282Y/H63D compound heterozygote	0.39	0.13	0.00	0.00

Data from Crownover, B.K. and C.J. Covey, Hereditary hemochromatosis. *Am Fam Physician*, 2013. 87(3): p. 183–90.

hepatocytes, and Kupffer cells. Mutations in the *HFE* gene make the HFE protein unstable by disrupting disulfide bonds that are important for HFE binding to b2-microglobulin. The mutations also impair a key signaling pathway in hepcidin synthesis, known as the bone morphogenic protein signaling pathway.

Homozygous C282Y mutations in the *HFE* gene account for 81% of clinical genetic hemochromatosis cases, whereas compound C282Y and H63D mutations are seen in 5% of cases.[20] Homozygosity for H63D mutations appears to lead to iron overload principally in the setting of other chronic liver diseases. Other mutations, such as S65C, have also been linked to iron accumulation[21,22] but their role in iron overloading is less clear.[23] S65C mutations appear to be enriched in populations from Britanny, France.[20] It seems likely that H63D, S65C, and other mutations play a synergistic role for excess iron accumulation in the setting of other disease processes or genetic polymorphisms, but by themselves are insufficient drivers of iron overload and do not directly cause hemochromatosis. They can contribute to iron overload disease when inherited along with a C282Y mutation. Individuals with C282Y mutations are at much higher risk for iron accumulation than individuals with H63D mutations and C282Y homozygotes have greater risk for iron accumulation than C282Y heterozygotes. An important point, however, is that there is great phenotypic variation, even for individuals who are homozygous for C282Y mutations. In fact, a meta-analysis found that the overall clinical disease penetrance of C282Y homozygosity was only 13.5%.[20] Disease penetrance was higher when defined as having at least mild iron on liver biopsy, at 42% for C282Y homozygous men and 19% for homozygous women.[20] The tremendous variation in disease penetrance appears to result from gender, environmental factors, dietary factors, and genetic polymorphisms.[24]

Morbidity and mortality with *HFE*-related hemochromatosis

Individuals with *HFE* hemochromatosis are at increased risk for liver cirrhosis and for hepatocellular carcinoma.[25–28] Heart failure and diabetes also contribute to morbidity and mortality because of iron deposition in the heart and the pancreatic islet cells. Cardiovascular disease continues to be an important cause of morbidity and mortality even after liver transplantation.[29] Also of note, a significant proportion of the diabetes risk may result from genetic changes that cosegregate with *HFE* mutations, but are not directly related to iron overload in the islet cells.[30] Joint disease can affect both heterozygote and homozygote individuals with *HFE* mutations. The second and third metacarpal-phalange joints and the interphalangeal joints can develop arthropathy because of iron deposits in the cartilage and synovial cells. Infections with *Vibrio vulnificus*, a virulent bacterium that is highly dependent on iron, are also increased in individuals with iron overload.[30] Infection can be caused by eating undercooked seafood, especially from the Gulf of Mexico.

Clinical indications for liver biopsy in individuals with *HFE* mutations

The European Association for the Study of the Liver (EASL) guidelines recommend liver biopsies in C282Y homozygous individuals to assess the degree of fibrosis when serum ferritin levels are above 1,000 μg/L, or there are elevated aspartate aminotransferase (AST) levels, hepatomegaly, or age over 40 years. The American Association for the Study of Liver Diseases (AASLD) guidelines are broadly similar and recommend biopsies to stage fibrosis for C282Y homozygotes or compound heterozygotes when ferritin is >1,000 μg/L or there are elevated serum levels of AST or alanine aminotransferase (ALT).

Impact of *HFE* mutations on other chronic diseases

As noted previously, the disease penetrance of *HFE* mutations is influenced by complex genetic, environmental, and dietary variables.[24] In this regard, several other chronic liver diseases can affect *HFE* penetrance, including chronic viral hepatitis C and B, alcohol-related liver disease, nonalcoholic fatty liver disease (NAFLD), and α-1-antitrypsin deficiency. Although the data are incomplete and substantially mixed, the general trend suggests that *HFE* mutations predispose to iron accumulation in other chronic liver diseases and become increasingly penetrant as fibrosis progresses. As one example, cirrhotic livers with both α-1-antitrypsin deficiency and marked iron overload are enriched for *HFE* mutations.[21] There are many negative studies that found no association between iron accumulation and fibrosis stage in other chronic liver diseases, most likely reflecting the difficulty of identifying a modest effect in the very complex setting of clinical cohort studies, where it is very difficult to adequately control for all of the factors that have been reported to influence both iron status as well as fibrosis risk.

17.5 JUVENILE HEMOCHROMATOSIS (USUALLY CHILDREN/EARLY ONSET)

Juvenile hemochromatosis is a rare cause of hemochromatosis. There are two subtypes. Subtype 2A results from mutations in *HFE2*, which encodes the protein hemojuvelin. Subtype 2B results from mutations in *HAMP*, which codes for hepcidin. Overall, Type 2A is more common than Type 2B.[31,32] Hemojuvelin disease typically presents with impotence or amenorrhea and not with liver or joint disease. Cardiomyopathy is also common at presentation. In the liver, there can be marked hepatocellular iron overload. The disease tends to be more aggressive than *HFE*-related hemochromatosis, typically running a rapidly progressive clinical course.[33] G320V mutations are the most common mutation in juvenile hemochromatosis, found in 80% to 90% of cases, but about 30 total mutations in *HFE2* have been reported to date. Juvenile hemochromatosis caused by *HAMP* mutations also has marked hepatocellular iron overload and typically runs a severe clinical course. Approximately 12 different mutations have been reported to date. Hypogonadism and cardiac disease are prominent clinical manifestations.

17.6 TRANSFERRIN RECEPTOR GENE 2 (USUALLY ADULTS/LATE ONSET)

This rare form of genetic iron overload was historically called type 3 hemochromatosis and was initially described in Italian patients with systemic iron overload who were negative for *HFE* mutations.[34] Subsequent studies identified mutations in the *TFR2* gene,[35] with about 20 mutations identified to date. The disease has a variable clinical course, but there can be marked hepatocellular iron deposition and systemic iron overload. Also of note, in the general asymptomatic adult population, polymorphisms in *TRF2* are common and can lead to mild increases in blood iron levels without overt iron overload disease.[36]

17.7 DMT-1 MUTATIONS (USUALLY OLDER CHILDREN)

This very rare disease is caused by mutations in the *SCL11A2* gene. Few cases have been reported, and data are quite limited.[37,38] Children present with severe microcytic anemia. Iron accumulation is primarily in hepatocytes and can be marked, but biopsies may be negative for iron in very young children.

17.8 FERRITIN MUTATIONS

Ferritin has both light and heavy chains, encoded by *FTL* and *FTH* genes. Very rare mutations in both genes have been reported. In general, mutations affecting the ferritin genes are associated with high serum ferritin levels but low transferrin saturation levels.

Mutations in the ferritin light chain gene, *FTL*, lead to both the hereditary hyperferritinemia cataract syndrome and to hereditary neuroferritinopathy. Individuals affected by the hereditary hyperferritinemia cataract syndrome have elevated serum ferritin levels with early onset cataract formation. Individuals with hereditary neuroferritinopathy have iron accumulation in the central nervous system, particularly the basal ganglia, which leads to neurodegenerative dysfunction. There is very little published data on liver histology, but there appears to be no iron accumulation in either of the diseases caused by *FTL* mutations, though the hepatocytes in hereditary neuroferritinopathy can have pale nuclear inclusions on H&E that stain light blue on Perls iron stain.[39,40] Mutations in the heavy gene, *FTH1*, do lead to iron accumulation and there can be moderate iron overload with a Zone 1 predominant pattern.[41] Iron can also accumulate in the splenic macrophages.[41]

17.9 TRANSFERRIN MUTATIONS

Mutations in the transferrin gene, *TF*, are very rare. A complete or nearly complete absence of transferrin protein leads to clinically significant disease in childhood.[42–44] The disease appears to be autosomal recessively inherited.[45] Individuals have very low or absent transferrin levels, severe hypochromic microcytic anemia, and marked hepatic iron overload.[42–45] Histologic descriptions are scant, but marked iron deposition is seen in both hepatocytes and Kupffer cells.[46,47]

In contrast, heterozygosity for *TF* mutations can lead to haploinsufficiency in terms of red blood cell production, but only leads to liver iron overload if other genetic mutations, such as *HFE*, are also present.[48]

17.10 CERULOPLASMIN MUTATIONS (CHILDREN AND ADULTS)

Ceruloplasmin, encoded by the *CP* gene, is the major protein for transporting copper in the blood. However, it also plays a role in iron metabolism, and inactivating mutations can lead to marked iron overload in the liver, pancreatic islet cells (leading to diabetes), and brain (leading to ataxia and dementia).[49,50] Aceruloplasminemia shows a wide age range at presentation, from late teenage years to elderly. Overall, most cases are diagnosed in later years, when individuals present with neurologic symptoms. However, younger individuals can present with anemia, mild liver enzyme elevations, or with blood iron test abnormalities.[51,52] In general, blood testing shows elevated serum ferritin levels, but low serum iron levels and low transferrin saturation. In the liver, iron accumulation is found predominately in hepatocytes and to a lesser degree in Kupffer cells. In the lobules, the hepatic iron deposition tends to have a panlobular distribution and pericanalicular pattern.[53–57]

17.11 FERROPORTIN DISEASE

Ferroportin disease is a classic example of hereditary iron overload, where the iron accumulation can predominately affect Kupffer cells. Ferroportin disease was initially described by Pietrangelo et al. (1999), when they reported an Italian family with an autosomal dominant inheritance pattern of hemochromatosis (in contrast to the recessive inheritance of *HFE* mutations).[58] Subsequent studies in Italian and Dutch families showed mutations in the *SLC40A1* gene.[59,60] Affected individuals have marked serum ferritin levels without elevations of the transferrin saturation, at least early in the course of the disease. Affected individuals were often anemic but had other classic findings of iron overload disease including iron deposits in multiple organ systems, leading to hepatic fibrosis, arrhythmias, and diabetes.

In contrast to most cases of genetic hemochromatosis, transferrin saturation levels in ferroportin disease Type A do not become elevated until much later in the disease course. Ferroportin disease also stands out for its dominant inheritance pattern, and both of these findings can be important clues to the diagnosis. There is substantial phenotypic variability in ferroportin disease, and the disease is divided into two subtypes. Both result from mutations in the *SLC40A1* gene, but one has loss of function (Ferroportin disease) and has one gain of function (Ferroportin associated hemochromatosis, formerly called ferroportin disease type 2). With loss of function, ferroportin is no longer able to export iron from Kupffer cells. With gain of function, ferroportin retains its ability to export iron but is less sensitive to inhibition by hepcidin. Histologically, iron deposits in Kupffer cells predominate over that of hepatocytes in the ferroportin disease (Figs. 17.1 and 17.2), whereas hepatic iron is also seen in ferroportin associated hemochromatosis. Clinically, both types have milder disease than seen with *HFE* mutations, with ferroportin associated hemochromatosis having more iron overload than ferroportin disease.

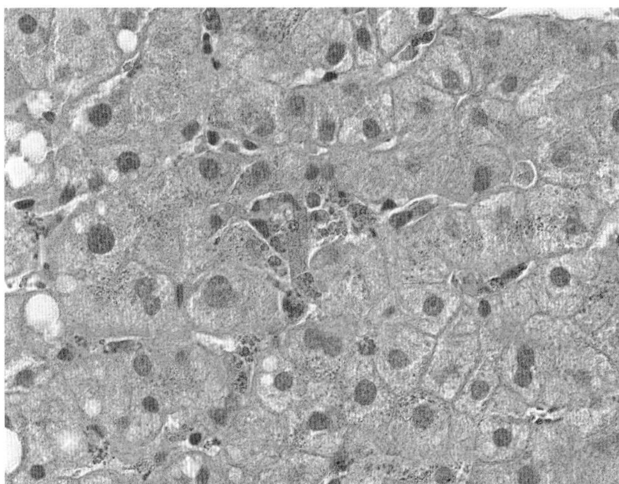

Figure 17.1 Ferroportin disease. The Kupffer cells show iron deposits.

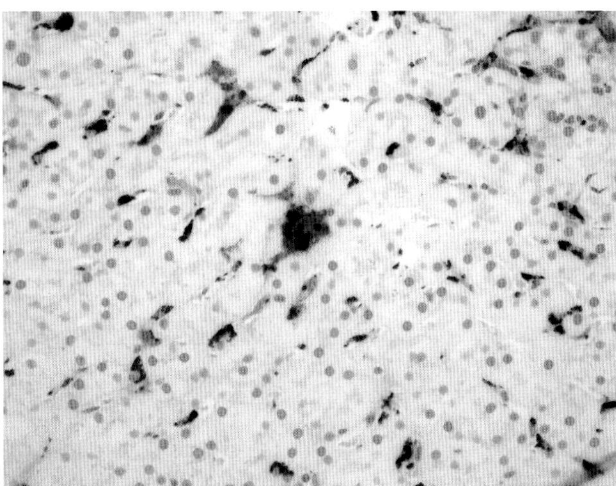

Figure 17.2 Ferroportin disease, Perls iron stain. There are iron deposits in Kupffer cells as well as occasional larger sideronecrotic deposits.

17.12 NEONATAL HEMOCHROMATOSIS (NEONATES)

Neonatal hemochromatosis was first described in 1957 by Cottier in a report of newborn siblings with advanced liver fibrosis, hepatic iron deposition, and extrahepatic iron deposits in the pancreas, thyroid, and myocardium, but with no iron deposits in the spleen or the lymph nodes.[61] Although these findings resembled genetic hemochromatosis, it became clear over time that neonatal hemochromatosis is fundamentally different than other genetic iron-related diseases. Instead of mutations in genes regulating iron metabolism, studies have found that neonatal hemochromatosis is an alloimmune[62] or autoimmune[63] gestational disease, where maternal antibodies cross the placenta, bind to a liver antigen, and activate fetal compliment, leading to in utero liver injury.[64] Maternal serum autoantibodies, such as antinuclear antibody, are seen in about 50% of cases.[65] The target of the immune attack has not been identified to date.

The affected newborn typically presents with hypoglycemia, coagulopathy, and massive liver failure at birth or within the first few days of life. In many cases, there is late second-term or third-term fetal loss. Despite the massive liver necrosis, AST and ALT levels can be normal or only mildly elevated. The relative low levels of AST and ALT do not appear to be due to hepatocyte depletion, and the mechanism remains unknown. Very high serum α-fetoprotein (AFP) levels can be a clue to the diagnosis of neonatal hemochromatosis because AFP levels are typically greater than 100,000 ng/mL and can be as high as 800,000 ng/mL (the healthy neonate typically has values less than 80,000 ng/mL). Other common fetal findings include intrauterine growth retardation, olighydraminios, and hydrops. In newborns, the placenta often shows hydrops on gross examination.[65] Histologically, the placenta can show chronic villitis and intervillitis. Vasculopathy, deciduitis, and chorioamniotis are typically absent.[65]

The liver can be grossly atrophic or enlarged, depending on the degree of necrosis (which leads to atrophy) versus inflammation and cholestasis (which leads to enlargement). On biopsy of the liver or on postmortem examination, the histology can range from massive liver necrosis with almost no residual hepatocytes, to a severely damaged liver with regenerative nodules of postnecrotic cirrhosis. The remaining hepatocytes are often inflamed, cholestatic, and commonly show giant cell transformation (Fig. 17.3). Cholestasis and giant cell transformation tend to be more striking in neonates, but can be absent or mild in fetuses. The fibrosis also varies depending on the length of survival after the liver insult. In early cases, fibrosis can be absent, whereas in later cases cirrhosis can develop (Fig. 17.4). Trichrome stains typically demonstrate diffuse lobular and portal fibrosis. The hepatocytes have moderate to marked iron accumulation (Fig. 17.5), with course granules of iron that are qualitatively similar to that seen in adult hemochromatosis. However, as fibrosis progresses, there can be less iron in the hepatocytes. In fact, one large study found an inverse association between the levels of iron and the degree of fibrosis.[65] Also of note, iron can be absent in cases of massive necrosis with no residual hepatocytes. The Kupffer cells generally have mild or no iron accumulation.

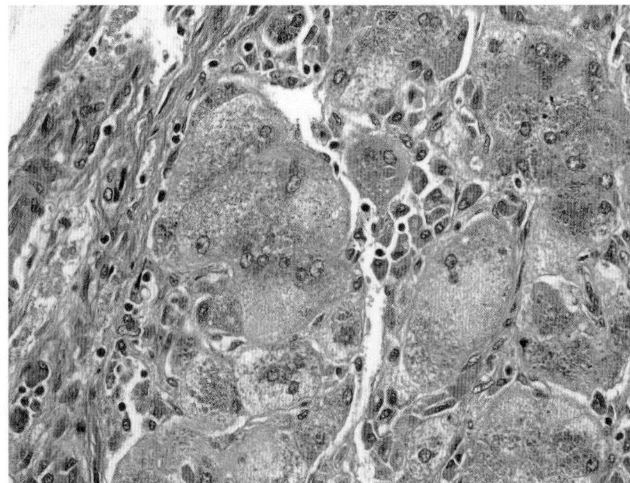

Figure 17.3 Neonatal hemochromatosis. This case shows a giant cell hepatitis pattern.

Extrahepatic iron deposits are key findings in the diagnosis of neonatal hemochromatosis, with the caveat that extrahepatic iron can be absent in the youngest of fetuses. For example, one study found

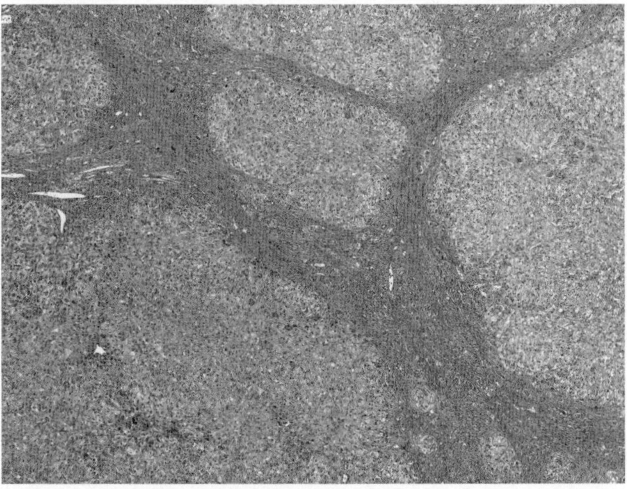

Figure 17.4 Neonatal hemochromatosis. This case shows cirrhosis.

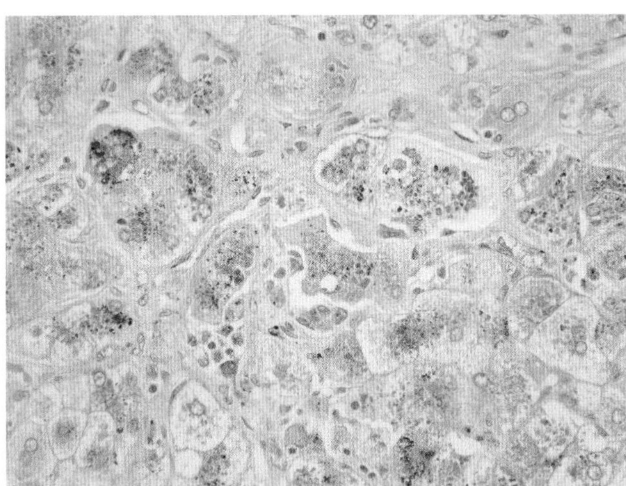

Figure 17.5 Neonatal hemochromatosis. The hepatocytes show moderate iron accumulation (same case as in image 3).

no extrahepatic iron in several cases with death at 27 weeks of gestation.[65] In addition, the patterns of extrahepatic iron deposition are now recognized to be more heterogeneous than previously thought. Thus, it is important to perform iron studies on sections from multiple different organ systems. The best places to look are (in approximate order): pancreas acini, thyroid follicles, renal tubules, myocardium, minor salivary glands, and other epithelium (Brunner glands, stomach, thymus, trachea, etc.).[64] Lip biopsies can be helpful when they are positive,[66] but negative results are noninformative. Negative results are often a result of not sampling the minor salivary glands. However, in other well-documented cases, the minor salivary glands are negative for iron, despite the presence of extrahepatic iron in other organ systems.[65] This observation underscores the need to stain multiple tissues for iron. Other autopsy findings can include renal tubular dysgenesis and, in a small subset of cases, myofibromas in the heart and lung.[65]

The prognosis is poor unless the disease is quickly recognized. Treatment revolves around supportive care and removing the maternal antibody through plasmapheresis. Although data are limited, there are no significant medical sequelae for children who survive. If an infant is affected by this disease, there is about a 90% chance that subsequent pregnancies in the mother will likewise be affected.[62] Prevention of disease in subsequent pregnancies is approached by treatment with IV Ig during gestation, which is typically given from about the 18th week of gestation until delivery.

The differential for the liver findings includes mitochondrial cytopathies such as DGUOK mutations, which can lead to elevated serum iron studies as well as histologic findings of massive liver injury and advanced fibrosis.[67] However, iron stains in the liver and extrahepatic tissues are negative.[67]

17.13 AFRICAN IRON OVERLOAD DISEASE

African iron overload (formerly called Bantu siderosis) was first described in 1929, based on autopsies that showed marked iron overload predominately in men from rural sub-Saharan Africa.[68] Subsequent studies suggested that the excess iron could be coming from traditional beer, which was brewed in iron pots or drums.[69,70] However, more recent studies show some individuals who do not drink traditional beer still get the disease.[71] Thus, African iron overload appears to have both dietary and genetic components.[72] The liver shows a full range of patterns of iron deposits, from predominately hepatocellular, to predominately Kupffer cells, to mixed patterns. This observation, along with the clinical findings, suggests that African iron overload, as currently construed, is likely a mixture of different diseases. Despite the association with traditional beer, fatty liver disease is rarely seen.

17.14 MORE TO COME

There are still cases of hepatic iron overload that do not have the mutations described earlier. For example, in a study from Brazil, one-third of cases with marked iron overload did not have the typical mutations discussed earlier.[73]

17.15 DETECTION OF IRON IN THE LIVER

History of iron stains

In 1704, Heinrich Diesbach (a color maker) and Johann Konrad Dippel (a physician) developed a dark blue pigment that was called "Berliner blau." This color was subsequently used for the uniforms of the Prussian army and became widely known as "Prussian Blue." This basic dye method was used over a century later by Rudolph Virchow, who in 1847 reported that hemosiderin deposits in areas of hemorrhage were positive for the Prussian Blue reaction, and the blue pigment could be seen by light microscopy. Twenty years later, a German pathologist, Perls, created a more practical formulation for the stain and showed that iron could be detected in a variety of tissues.

The basic chemistry of Perls Prussian Blue is that iron in the ferric state will react with hydrochloric acid to form ferric ferrocyanide, an insoluble blue compound (Prussian Blue) that can be seen histologically. The distribution and density of blue staining correlates well with tissue iron concentrations. The stain is not sensitive for very low levels of iron but is easy to perform and is reproducible, and there is no evidence that the very low levels of iron missed by Perls iron stains are clinically relevant.

Iron grading systems

In 1962, Scheur proposed one of the first grading systems for evaluating iron in liver biopsies using the Perls iron stain. Many additional iron grading systems have been proposed over the years. They vary in their approach, but all provide semiquantitative data on the extent of iron accumulation. Some systems are based on the zonation of iron distribution, some on the lowest magnification that discernible granules can be seen, and some on the percent of hepatocytes positive for iron. Is one system clearly the best for clinical care? Probably not, or at least not that has been demonstrated to date. In the end, iron accumulation that reaches the moderate and marked levels has the greatest clinical relevance and all grading systems capture those cases well. A numerical system is important in research studies because it allows statistical comparison of groups. However, for routine clinical care, using descriptors in the pathology report for the results of Perls iron stains (e.g., "mild," "moderate," etc.) and the localization of the iron (e.g., hepatocellular vs Kupffer cell) is sufficient, and a numerical grade is not necessary. But there are many reasonable grading systems to choose from if you prefer. A modified Scheuer's system (shown in Table 17.5) is one useful and popular system, whereas another popular system is based on the percent of hepatocytes positive on iron stain (Table 17.6).

Table 17.5 Modified Scheuer's grading system for iron in the liver

Grade	Description
0	Iron granules absent or Iron granules barely seen at 400×
1	Iron granules resolved at 250×
2	Iron granules resolved at 100×
3	Iron granules resolved at 25×
4	Iron deposits resolved at 10× or Iron deposits visible without magnification

From Turlin, B. and Y. Deugnier, Evaluation and interpretation of iron in the liver. *Semin Diagn Pathol*, 1998. 15(4): p. 237–45.

Table 17.6 Schema for evaluating iron in the liver (similar to that of LeSage)

Grade	Description	Hepatocytes	Lobular Kupffer cells
0	None	None	None
1	Minimal	<5%	<5%
2	Mild	5–30%	5–30%
3	Moderate	31–60%	31–60%
4	Marked	>60%	>60%

From LeSage, G.D., et al., Hemochromatosis: genetic or alcohol-induced? *Gastroenterology*, 1983. 84(6): p. 1471–7.

Quantitative measurement of hepatic iron concentrations

Hepatic iron concentrations measured in fresh liver tissues or in paraffin-embedded tissues are equivalent.[74] Thus, paraffin-embedded tissues are preferred for ease of transport of material. In addition, it allows direct visualization of the tissue and assures that the tissue is representative, preventing submission of tissue that is largely composed of collapsed/fibrotic stroma. The normal adult liver has between 10 and 36 μmol iron/g dry weight of liver. As a frame of reference, excess iron accumulation has been classified as mild (up to 150 μmol iron/g dry weight of liver), moderate (151 to 300), and marked (>301).[75]

Hepatic iron index

In 1986, Bassett et al. published a seminal article that used a hepatic iron index to separate genetic hemochromatosis from alcohol-related iron deposition.[76] The hepatic iron index adjusts the total iron concentration for age, based on the observation that hepatic iron concentrations tend to increase steadily with age in individuals with genetic hemochromatosis, but not in individuals with "secondary" alcohol-related iron overload. Subsequent studies extended the use of the hepatic iron index to separate genetic hemochromatosis from any cause of secondary liver siderosis. A hepatic iron index greater than 1.9 was interpreted as consistent with genetic hemochromatosis. Today, the advances in genetic testing for hemochromatosis make the hepatic iron index largely of historical interest, and the diagnostic role for the hepatic iron index is gone. However, quantitative iron levels remain useful in managing individuals on iron depletion therapy, regardless of the underlying cause of disease.

17.16 HISTOLOGIC FINDINGS

One common question is whether an iron stain is the "standard of care" for evaluating a medical liver biopsy. There is little or no data on this point, but routine iron stains are performed by many medical centers. One reasonable alternative approach in resource limited environments could be a careful examination of the H&E stain first, followed by ordering stains on that subset of cases with H&E findings that suggest iron overload, or on those cases with significantly elevated serum ferritin (>1,000) or transferrin saturation levels (>45%). Certainly, minimal iron overload would be missed, as well as many cases of mild iron overload. However, it seems likely that all cases with moderate or marked iron accumulation would be identified, and moderate and marked levels of iron overload have the best established clinical relevance.

Ferritin is not seen in most liver biopsies, including normal and diseased tissues. However, in a subset of cases with elevated serum ferritin levels, ferritin may be seen as a light, diffuse, blue blush in the hepatocyte or Kupffer cell cytoplasm. In contrast, hemosiderin forms brown granular deposits on H&E stains (Fig. 17.6) and bright blue granular deposits on iron stain (Fig. 17.7). Residual brown granular material is often seen on iron stains and represents lipofuschin in most cases.

In genetic hemochromatosis, the iron deposits often cluster around the bile canaliculi (Fig. 17.8). In addition, iron classically accumulates first within Zone 1 hepatocytes (Fig. 17.9). A clear gradient in the amount of iron between Zone 1 and Zone 3 hepatocytes can often be seen, even with advanced iron accumulation. However, a Zone 1 distribution of iron can be seen in other nonhemochromatosis conditions, and a diagnosis of hemochromatosis should not be based on a zonal pattern alone. The Zone 1 predominate pattern of iron deposition reflects dysregulation of hepcidin, but this could be either through mutations or through reduced hepcidin production from other causes. As a caveat, cases with both HFE iron overload and α-1 antitrypsin deficiency can sometimes have a band of hepatocytes in Zone 1 immediately adjacent to the portal tracts/fibrous bands that have little or no iron but lots of α-1 antitrypsin deficiency globules (Figs. 17.10 and 17.11). Hepatocyte death leads over time to redistribution of iron into Kupffer cells and portal macrophages. In practice, even mild hepatocellular iron is often accompanied by patchy mild Kupffer cell iron.

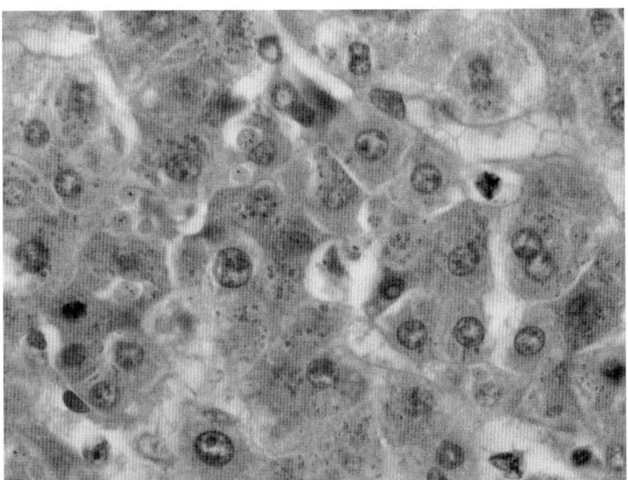

Figure 17.6 Hemosiderin, H&E. This biopsy is from an individual homozygous for *HFE* C282Y mutations. The hemosiderin deposits are granular and golden brown.

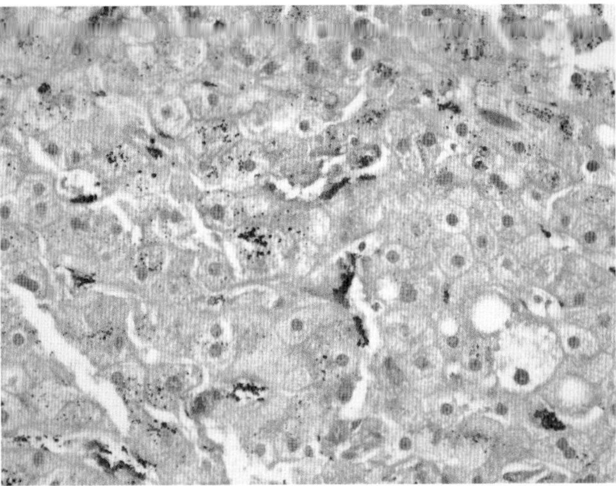

Figure 17.7 Hemosiderin, Perls iron stain. This biopsy is from a patient with a bone marrow transplant and numerous blood transfusions. Both Kupffer cell and hepatocellular iron deposits are seen.

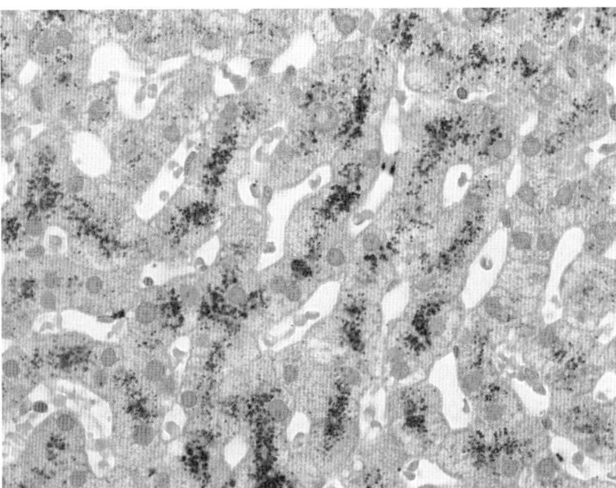

Figure 17.8 Pericanalicular iron deposits, Perls iron stain. Pericanalicular iron deposits are common but not are diagnostic of *HFE* mutations. This biopsy is from an individual homozygous for *HFE* C282Y mutations.

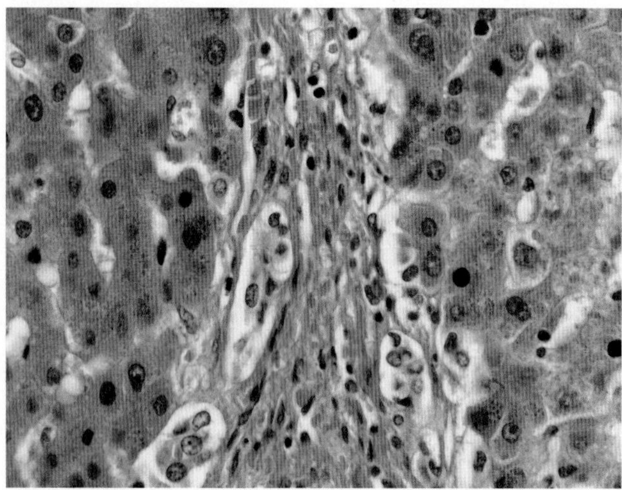

Figure 17.9 Zone 1 iron deposits, Perls iron stain. Hemosiderin can have a Zone 1 pattern of hepatocellular deposition in cases with *HFE* mutations. Pigment is clearly seen in the Zone 1 hepatocytes but rapidly tapers in this case. This biopsy is from an individual homozygous for *HFE* C282Y mutations.

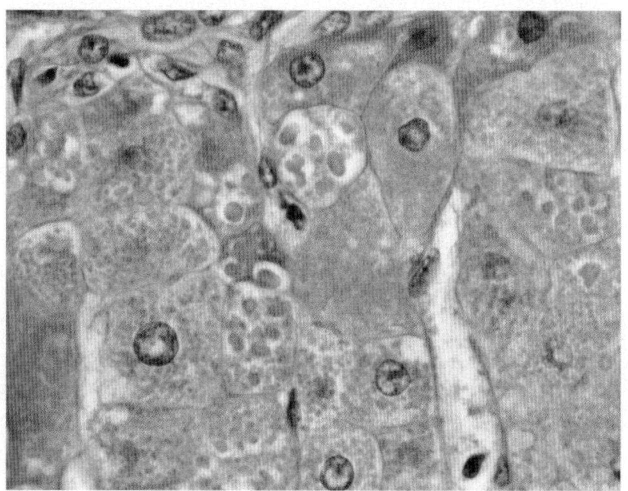

Figure 17.10 *HFE* homozygous C82Y mutations and α-1-antitrypsin deficiency. These two diseases cooccurred in this case. The Zone 1 hepatocytes contain α-1-antitrypsin deficiency globules.

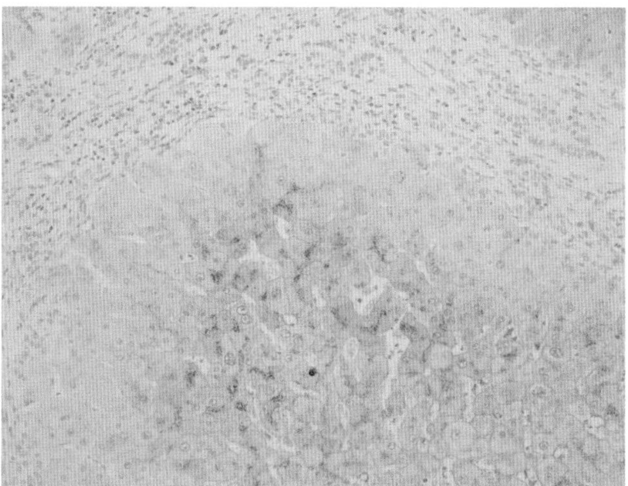

Figure 17.11 *HFE* homozygous C82Y mutations and α-1-antitrypsin deficiency. The iron deposits show relative sparing of the Zone 1 hepatocytes (same case as earlier).

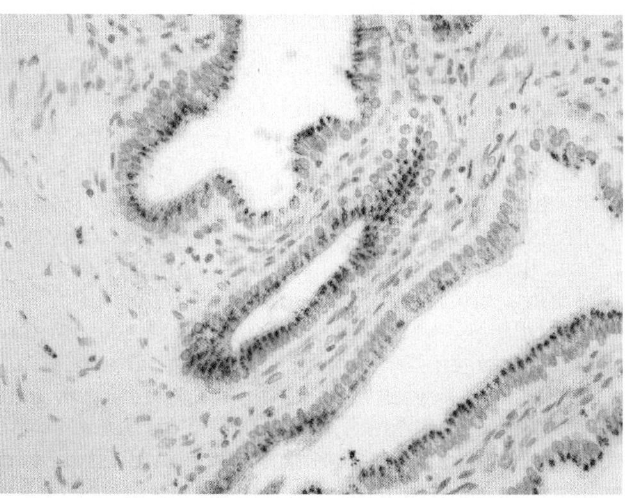

Figure 17.12 Iron in bile duct, Perls iron stain. Iron can be seen in the bile duct epithelium. This biopsy is from an individual homozygous for *HFE* C282Y mutations.

Iron can also be deposited in the epithelium of the bile duct proper (Fig. 17.12). At times, this finding has been interpreted as highly suggestive or even diagnostic of *HFE* mutations. However, this pattern of iron deposition can also be seen in cases that have marked iron overload but lack *HFE* mutations, so should not be over interpreted. In addition, iron is commonly seen in proliferating bile ductules in areas of subacute parenchymal collapse (Fig. 17.13). This finding has no association with genetic hemochromatosis.

When iron overload results from transfusion-dependent anemias or similar causes, iron is classically first deposited in Kupffer cells and with time there is involvement of the hepatocytes. However, in practice, most cases show a mixed hepatocellular and Kupffer cell iron staining pattern. Iron can also be seen in some cases either exclusively in portal endothelial cells (Fig. 17.14) or in a combination of endothelial, hepatocyte, and Kupffer cell iron accumulation. There has not been any specific linkage of endothelial iron accumulation to a disease process or genetic mutation at this time.

Rare liver biopsies can show nuclear staining of hepatocytes on Perls iron stain. This finding can be associated with eosinophilic to pale inclusions visible on H&E stain in individuals with neuroferritinopathy, a movement disorder that is caused by iron deposits in the basal ganglia. In other rare cases, focal nuclear

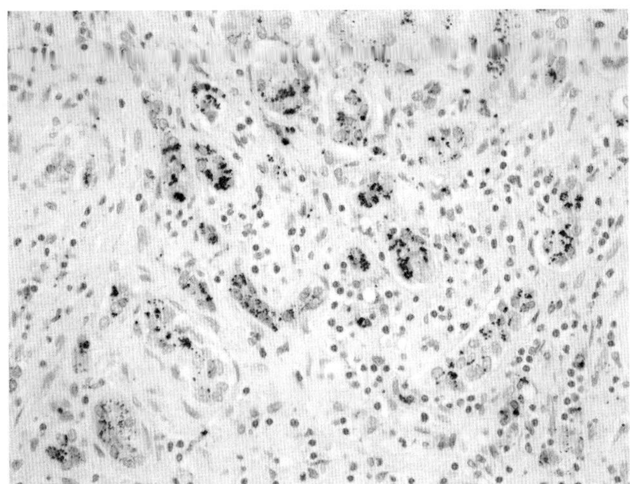

Figure 17.13 Bile ductular proliferation with iron accumulation, Perls iron stain. In this cirrhotic liver with an area of parenchymal collapse, the proliferating ductules show striking iron deposits, but the rest of the liver had only minimal iron deposits.

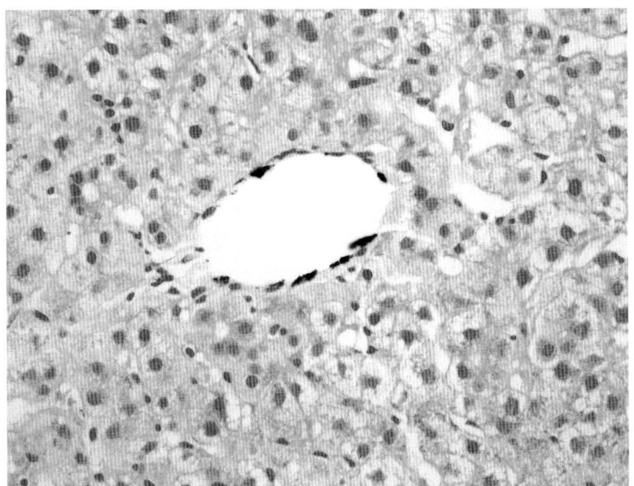

Figure 17.14 Endothelial iron, Perls iron stain. Endothelial iron deposits are often seen in the setting of Kupffer cell/macrophage iron as well as hepatic iron. Occasionally, the deposits only are seen in endothelial cells, as in this case. The clinical significance of isolated endothelial iron is currently unclear.

staining is seen on the Perls iron stain (Fig. 17.15) without the nuclear inclusions or other clinical findings to suggest neuroferritinopathy. In these latter cases, the number of positive nuclei is very small, and the significance is unclear.

Genetic testing

When should the pathology or autopsy report raise the possibility of genetic hemochromatosis? There is no formal data on this question, but one approach is to raise the possibility of genetic iron overload as

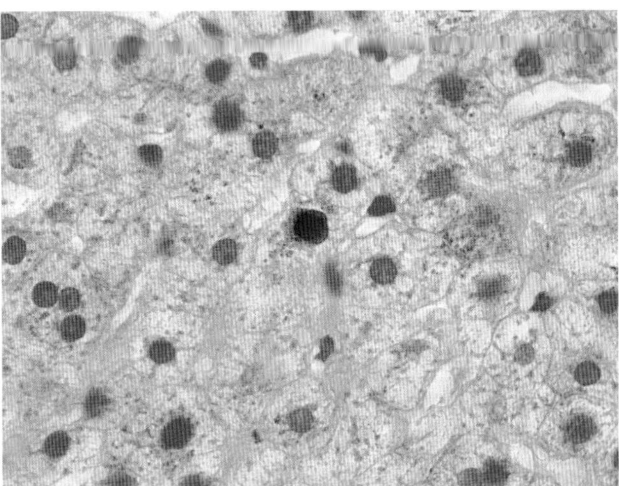

Figure 17.15 Focal nuclear staining, Perls iron stain. This staining pattern can be rarely observed, but is of unknown significance.

outlined below and summarized in Table 17.7. Mild iron accumulation in the liver (either hepatic, Kupffer cells, or mixed) in the setting of another known chronic liver disease is both the most commonly encountered pattern and the pattern least likely to be associated with genetic hemochromatosis.

Situations to strongly consider additional testing

1. Neonatal hemochromatosis (while not genetic in the fetus/neonate) should be considered in any biopsy or autopsy of a neonate or stillbirth with marked liver injury/necrosis and extracellular iron deposits.
2. Hepatocellular iron accumulation in noncirrhotic livers that is more than patchy and minimal and is not explained by other disease processes (transfusion-dependent anemia, etc.), when the individuals are less than 40. It can also be helpful to check the clinical history for heart disease or impotence or amenorrhea.
3. Moderate or marked hepatocellular iron in any noncirrhotic liver without a history of transfusion-dependent anemia, even with chronic liver disease from viral hepatitis, autoimmune hepatitis, alcoholic hepatitis, or NAFLD.
4. Marked iron accumulation in cirrhotic livers. One exception may be when alcoholic liver disease is thought to be the main cause of the cirrhosis or a major contributor to cirrhosis.
5. Kupffer cell iron deposits, or mixed hepatocyte and Kupffer cell iron deposits, in an individual with normal or low transferrin saturation levels suggests ferroportin disease. A parental history of liver disease can also be an important clue.

Table 17.7 Grades of hepatocellular iron: reasonable situations to suggest additional testing for genetic iron overload, when there is no history of multiple blood transfusions

Iron grade	Other findings
Marked	All ages, all fibrosis stages. ETOH-related cirrhosis is a possible exception
Moderate	All noncirrhotic livers of any age
Mild	Only if young, noncirrhotic, and no chronic liver disease on biopsy (e.g., hepatitis, NAFLD, etc.)

Although pathology findings can suggest genetic hemochromatosis, there are no pathognomonic histologic findings, and genetic testing is needed for a definite diagnosis.

Obtaining genetic testing

Mutation testing for *HFE* is widely available by commercial laboratories and universities. Testing for non-*HFE* mutations is less widely available and often requires some phone calls or internet searching to find a provider.

17.17 CLINICOPATHOLOGIC SIGNIFICANCE OF IRON OVERLOAD IN DIFFERENT DISEASE SETTINGS

Iron in explanted livers

Iron accumulates in livers that are cirrhotic from many underlying diseases. In a classic study, Ludwig et al. studied iron levels in 447 liver explants.[77] Marked iron overload was seen in hereditary hemochromatosis (100% of cases), α-1 antitrypsin deficiency (28%), cryptogenic cirrhosis (19%), alcohol cirrhosis (14%), chronic hepatitis B cirrhosis (18%), chronic hepatitis C cirrhosis (7%), primary biliary cirrhosis (1%), and primary sclerosing cholangitis (1%).

Marked iron accumulation in liver explants can be clinically relevant even when not associated with *HFE* mutations. For example, one study[78] found that patients with significant iron in their explanted livers had decreased survival regardless of whether there was an *HFE* mutation, with heart failure and infection the major causes of death. Several studies have shown that iron overload in the heart is present in a subset of individuals with marked iron overload in their explanted livers, despite negative *HFE* mutations.[79,80] These individuals have an increased risk for posttransplant heart failure.

When grossing the explanted liver, parenchymal foci with decreased iron deposition (even subcentimeter foci) should be sampled to evaluate for carcinoma (Fig. 17.16). These "iron free foci" are often associated with dysplastic nodules or with fully developed hepatocellular carcinoma (Fig. 17.17) or cholangiocarcinoma (Fig. 17.18).

Iron in donor liver biopsies

Iron stains are positive in approximately 20% of deceased donors (Fig. 17.19) and about 10% of living related donors, almost always with mild iron deposition.[81,82] The significance, if any, of these mild iron deposits remains unknown, though it is clear that there is no major clinical consequence.

Rarely, inadvertent donor livers homozygous for *HFE* mutations have been transplanted. The clinical course can be surprisingly variable, with some cases leading to progressive iron overload in the liver allograft,[83] whereas in other cases the liver allograft does not accumulate additional iron and may actually lose iron.[84] These disparate findings highlight the variable penetrance of *HFE* mutations and the important role for other genetic and environmental factors.

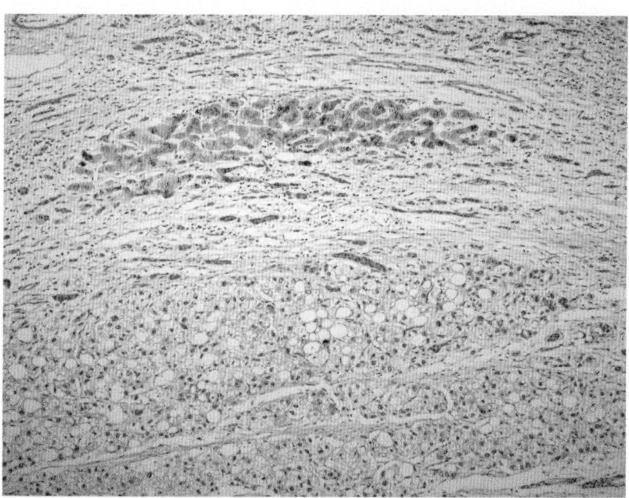

Figure 17.16 Hepatocellular carcinoma. This hepatocellular carcinoma shows no iron staining (**bottom** of image), whereas the background cirrhotic liver shows abundant hepatocellular iron.

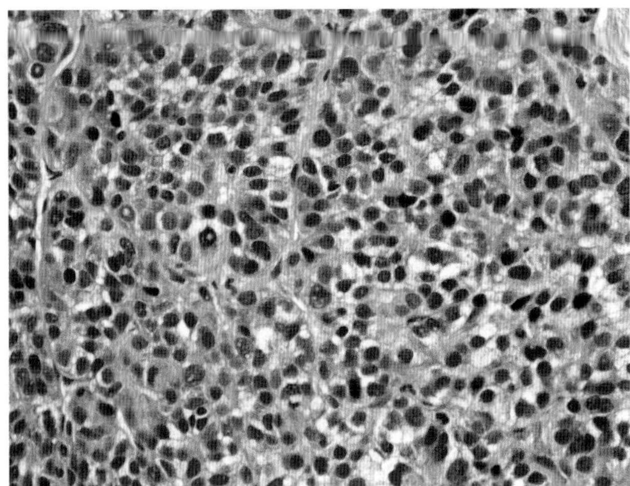

Figure 17.17 Hepatocellular carcinoma. This patient was treated for hemochromatosis by phlebotomy over many years, but developed hepatocellular carcinoma.

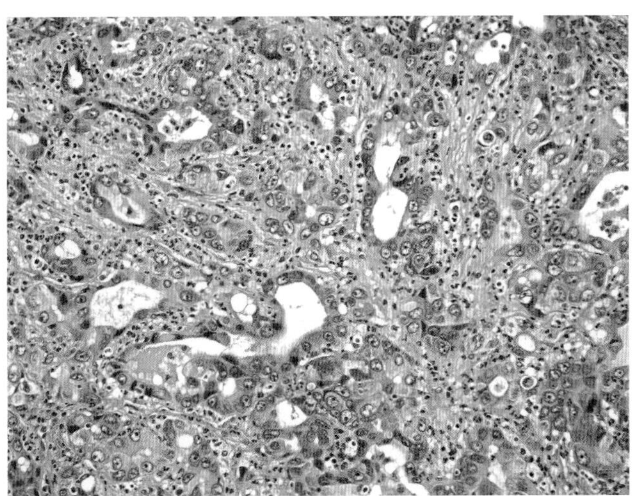

Figure 17.18 Cholangiocarcinoma. The patient had a history of homozygous C282Y *HFE* mutations

Iron in liver tissues with chronic hepatitis C and chronic hepatitis B virus infection

A large body of literature has investigated the significance of iron in liver biopsies of individuals with chronic hepatitis C and B. Iron deposits, including both hepatocellular and reticuloendothelial iron, are seen in a median of 30% of liver biopsies performed to stage and grade chronic hepatitis C and hepatitis B, with a reported range of 5% to 48%.[85–90] The wide range presumably reflects differences in gender, viral genotypes, and the proportion of cirrhotic livers in the cohort. In the majority of cases, the iron deposits are mild, occasionally moderate, and only very rarely severe. Although the data on iron as a risk factor for

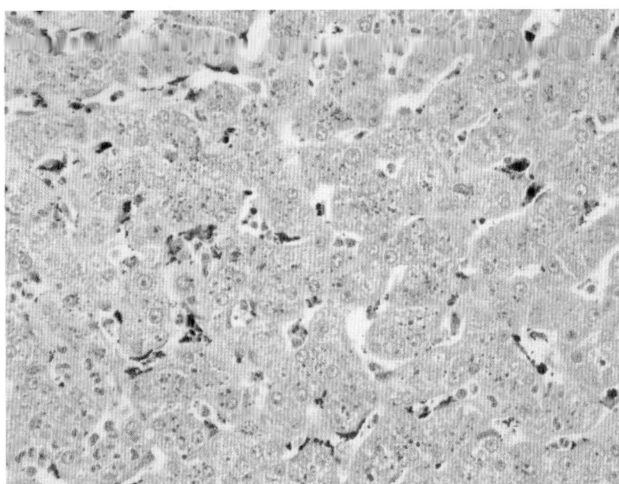

Figure 17.19 Donor liver biopsy, Perls iron stain. Patchy iron deposits are seen in both the hepatocytes and Kupffer cells. The posttransplant course was unremarkable. A liver biopsy 5 months later still showed significant iron.

fibrosis progression are substantially mixed, a reasonable distillation is as follows: mild or greater iron accumulation most likely has a small but measurable impact on fibrosis progression. However, other known risk factors for fibrosis progression, such as viral genotype, duration of infection, gender, etc., have stronger and more consistent impacts on fibrosis than do iron accumulation. The risk for fibrosis progression and iron accumulation can be further stratified by the extent of iron accumulation, with moderate and marked iron levels have the greatest risk.

Iron in non-alcoholic fatty liver disease

Hepatic iron deposition in NAFLD is seen in 30% to 40% of liver biopsies. As with chronic viral hepatitis, the siderosis is mild in most cases and may involve either or both of the hepatic and Kupffer cell compartments. Moderate iron accumulation is much less common, and marked iron accumulation is rare. The role of iron in fibrosis progression remains under studied. One major study from the NASH-Clinical Research Network found that reticuloendothelial iron, but not hepatocellular iron, was associated with increased fibrosis.[91]

Iron overload and liver carcinoma

There is a high risk for hepatocellular carcinoma in individuals with *HFE* hemochromatosis and marked iron accumulation. The risk is greatest in the setting of cirrhosis, but hepatocellular carcinomas can occasionally arise in noncirrhotic livers,[92] including those with non-*HFE*-related iron overload.[93] The risk was previously estimated to be as high as 200 fold, but more recent data suggest a lower, but still elevated, risk.[94] Precursor lesions include iron free foci. Most liver carcinomas in genetic hemochromatosis are hepatocellular carcinomas, but cholangiocarcinomas can also occur.[95]

Furthermore, iron in the liver is associated with an increased risk for hepatocellular carcinoma regardless of the underlying cause of liver disease. In a massive study of over 5,000 explanted livers, iron deposits were associated with hepatocellular carcinoma, even after adjusting for underlying liver disease.[96] In the setting of cirrhosis from chronic hepatitis C, liver iron increases the risk for hepatocellular carcinoma and long-term phlebotomy can reduce that risk.[97]

17.18 ACQUIRED IRON OVERLOAD

Transfusion-dependent anemias

Hepatic siderosis is common in liver biopsies of patients with various hematologic disorders including sickle cell disease and thalassemia, as well as other causes of transfusion-dependent anemia (Fig. 17.20), such as chronic renal failure and renal dialysis (Fig. 17.21). Liver biopsies in individuals with bone marrow transplants also commonly show excess iron accumulation. In all of these conditions, iron is classically located primarily in the Kupffer cells and/or portal macrophages early in the course of the disease, but some degree of hepatocellular iron accumulation is also common. In time, hepatocellular iron accumulation can reach high levels.

Sideroblastic anemias

Sideroblastic anemia is not a single disease, but is a heterogeneous group of disorders characterized by anemia with ringed sideroblasts in the bone marrow. The sideroblast is an erythroid precursor that has increased deposition of mitochondrial iron (Fig. 17.22) and is found in the bone marrow, but not the liver. The disease can be either acquired or hereditary. Although the mechanism is not clear, the liver can show marked hepatocellular iron accumulation with a Zone 1 predominant pattern of staining (Fig. 17.23).

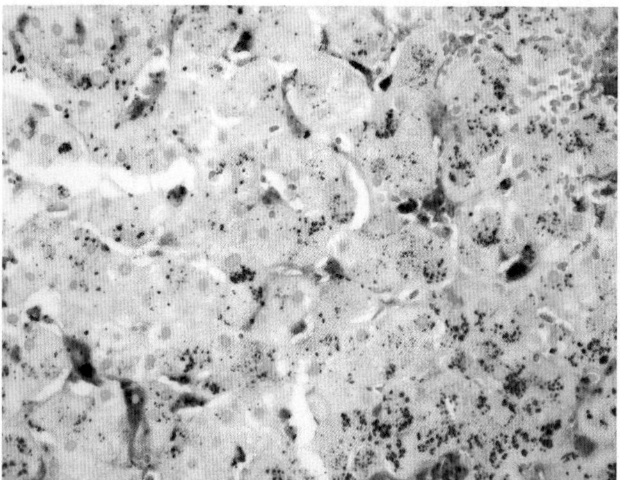

Figure 17.20 Secondary mixed hepatocellular and Kupffer cell iron, Perls iron stain. Iron deposits are seen in both the hepatocytes and Kupffer cells, in this case resulting from transfusion-dependent anemia

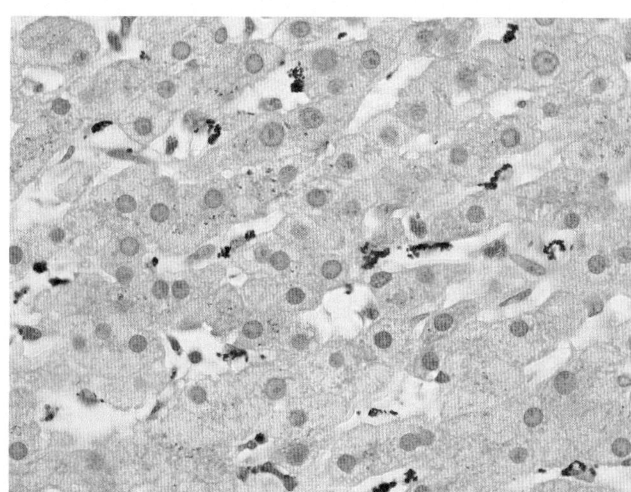

Figure 17.21 Secondary Kupffer cell iron, Perls iron stain. Diffuse Kupffer cell iron deposition is seen in this case from an individual on renal dialysis.

Glucose 6-phoshphatase dehydrogenase deficiency

Glucose 6-phoshphatase dehydrogenase deficiency is an inherited X linked recessive disorder characterized by hemolytic anemia that is triggered by exposure to infection, chemicals, or other substances. The enzyme glucose 6-phoshphatase dehydrogenase is important

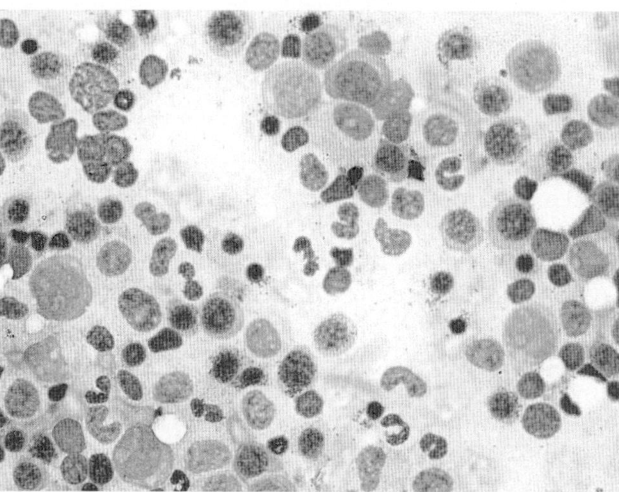

Figure 17.22 Ringed sideroblasts.

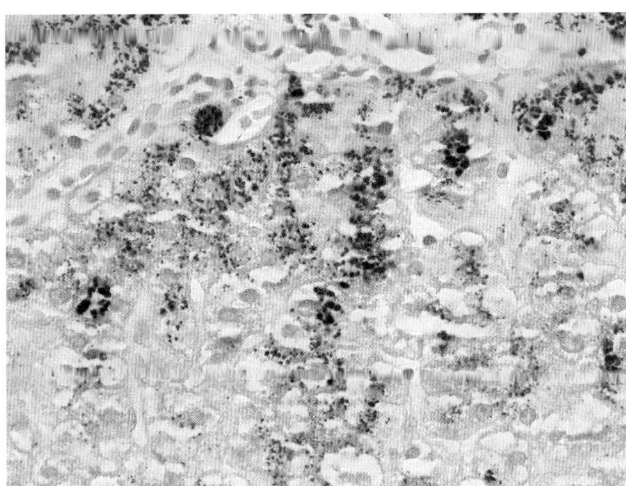

Figure 17.23 Sideroblastic anemia. A Zone 1 predominant patter of iron accumulation is seen.

in red blood cell synthesis, and mutations lead to a defective enzyme. Symptoms are only seen in males and often present as a hemolytic crises. However, rare cases have also been reported in association with neonatal cholestasis.[98] Liver biopsies in adults typically show predominately Kupffer cell or mixed iron accumulation (Fig. 17.24).

Porphyria cutanea tarda

Porphyria cutanea tarda is a genetic disease caused by mutations that lead to a deficiency in heme synthesis. The disease is sporadic in about 80% of cases, whereas the remaining 20% will have family histories consistent with inherited disease. Porphyria cutanea tarda can be precipitated by chronic hepatitis C infection or alcohol use and is also associated with *HFE* gene mutations. Naturally, the biopsy findings in porphyria cutanea tarda will vary depending on the precipitating factors, e.g., chronic hepatitis C, alcohol, etc. Iron accumulation is common in the periportal hepatocytes as well portal macrophages. In the lobules, there can be small granuloma-like aggregates of pigment and iron laden macrophages.[99] The hepatocytes may also contain needle-shaped crystals that are very subtle and nearly impossible to see on H&E stains.

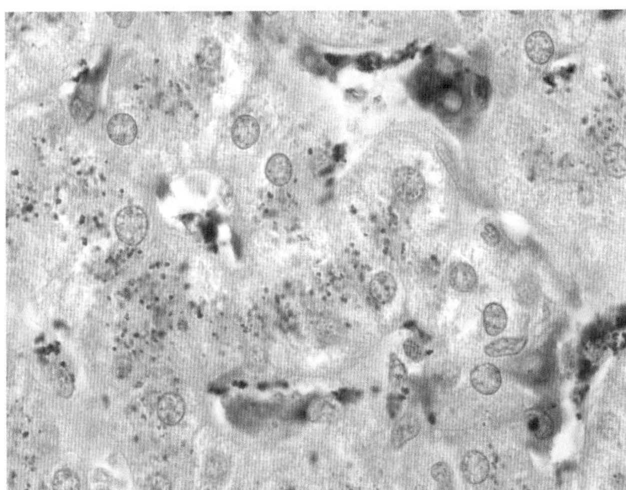

Figure 17.24 Glucose 6 phosphate deficiency, Perls iron stain. Mixed hepatocellular and Kupffer cell iron accumulation are seen.

Excess iron intake

Hepatic siderosis secondary to excess dietary intake is unusual, but rare cases do occur. Many but not all individuals will also have mutations in genes known to predispose to hemochromatosis, including *HFE* and *TFR2*.[100]

REFERENCES

1. Ward RJ, O'Connell MJ, Dickson DP, et al. Biochemical studies of the iron cores and polypeptide shells of haemosiderin isolated from patients with primary or secondary haemochromatosis. *Biochim Biophys Acta.* 1989;993(1):131–133.
2. Nemeth E, Tuttle MS, Powelson J, et al. Hepcidin regulates cellular iron efflux by binding to ferroportin and inducing its internalization. *Science.* 2004;306(5704):2090–2093.
3. Pigeon C, Ilyin G, Courselaud B, et al. A new mouse liver-specific gene, encoding a protein homologous to human antimicrobial peptide hepcidin, is overexpressed during iron overload. *J Biol Chem.* 2001;276(11):7811–7819.
4. Strnad P, Schwarz P, Rasenack MC, et al. Hepcidin is an antibacterial, stress-inducible peptide of the biliary system. *PLoS One.* 2011;6(1):e16454.
5. Pietrangelo A. Hepcidin in human iron disorders: therapeutic implications. *J Hepatol.* 2011;54(1):173–181.
6. Pietrangelo A. Hemochromatosis: an endocrine liver disease. *Hepatology.* 2007;46(4):1291–1301.
7. Finberg KE, Heeney MM, Campagna DR, et al. Mutations in TMPRSS6 cause iron-refractory iron deficiency anemia (IRIDA). *Nat Genet.* 2008;40(5):569–571.
8. Chung A, Leo K, Wong G, et al. Giant hepatocellular adenoma presenting with chronic iron deficiency anemia. *Am J Gastroenterol.* 2006;101(9):2160–2162.
9. Wang DQ, Carreras CT, Fiske LM, et al. Characterization and pathogenesis of anemia in glycogen storage disease type Ia and Ib. *Genet Med.* 2012;14(9):795–799.

10. Kijima H, Sawada T, Tomosugi N, et al. Expression of hepcidin mRNA is uniformly suppressed in hepatocellular carcinoma. *BMC Cancer*. 2008;8:167.
11. Trousseau A. Glycosurie, diabete sucre. *Clin Med Hotel Paris*. 1865;2:663–698.
12. Troisier M. Diabete sucre. *Bull Soc Anat Paris*. 1871;16:231–235.
13. Sheldon JH. *Haemochromatosis*. Oxford Medical Publications. London: Oxford University Press H Milford; 1935:xii, 382 p., 1 l.
14. Simon M, Pawlotsky Y, Bourel M, et al. Letter: idiopathic hemochromatosis associated with HL-A 3 tissular antigen. *Nouv Presse Med*. 1975;4(19):1432.
15. Feder JN, Gnirke A, Thomas W, et al. A novel MHC class I-like gene is mutated in patients with hereditary haemochromatosis. *Nat Genet*. 1996;13(4):399–408.
16. Krause A, Neitz S, Mägert HJ, et al. LEAP-1, a novel highly disulfide-bonded human peptide, exhibits antimicrobial activity. *FEBS Lett*. 2000;480(2–3):147–150.
17. Park CH, Valore EV, Waring AJ, et al. Hepcidin, a urinary antimicrobial peptide synthesized in the liver. *J Biol Chem*. 2001;276(11):7806–7810.
18. Hanson EH, Imperatore G, Burke W. HFE gene and hereditary hemochromatosis: a HuGE review. Human Genome Epidemiology. *Am J Epidemiol*. 2001;154(3):193–206.
19. Settin A, El-Bendary M, Abo-Al-Kassem R, et al. Molecular analysis of A1AT (S and Z) and HFE (C282Y and H63D) gene mutations in Egyptian cases with HCV liver cirrhosis. *J Gastrointestin Liver Dis*. 2006;15(2):131–135.
20. EASL clinical practice guidelines for HFE hemochromatosis. *J Hepatol*. 2010;53(1):3–22.
21. Lam M, Torbenson M, Yeh MM, et al. HFE mutations in alpha-1-antitrypsin deficiency: an examination of cirrhotic explants. *Mod Pathol*. 2010;23(5):637–643.
22. Mura C, Raguenes O, Ferec C. HFE mutations analysis in 711 hemochromatosis probands: evidence for S65C implication in mild form of hemochromatosis. *Blood*. 1999;93(8): 2502–2505.
23. Pedersen P, Milman N. Genetic screening for HFE hemochromatosis in 6,020 Danish men: penetrance of C282Y, H63D, and S65C variants. *Ann Hematol*. 2009;88(8):775–784.
24. Rochette J, Le Gac G, Lassoued K, et al. Factors influencing disease phenotype and penetrance in HFE haemochromatosis. *Hum Genet*. 2010;128(3):233–248.
25. Fargion S, Mandelli C, Piperno A, et al. Survival and prognostic factors in 212 Italian patients with genetic hemochromatosis. *Hepatology*. 1992;15(4):655–659.
26. Milman N, Pedersen P, á Steig T, et al. Clinically overt hereditary hemochromatosis in Denmark 1948-1985: epidemiology, factors of significance for long-term survival, and causes of death in 179 patients. *Ann Hematol*. 2001;80(12):737–744.
27. Niederau C, Fischer R, Pürschel A, et al. Long-term survival in patients with hereditary hemochromatosis. *Gastroenterology*. 1996;110(4):1107–1119.
28. Wojcik JP, Speechley MR, Kertesz AE, et al. Natural history of C282Y homozygotes for hemochromatosis. *Can J Gastroenterol*. 2002;16(5):297–302.
29. Yu L, Ioannou GN. Survival of liver transplant recipients with hemochromatosis in the United States. *Gastroenterology*. 2007;133(2):489–495.
30. Barton JC. Hemochromatosis and iron overload: from bench to clinic. *Am J Med Sci*. 2013;346(5):403–412.
31. Papanikolaou G, Samuels ME, Ludwig EH, et al. Mutations in HFE2 cause iron overload in chromosome 1q-linked juvenile hemochromatosis. *Nat Genet*. 2004;36(1):77–82.
32. Lee PL, Beutler E, Rao SV, et al. Genetic abnormalities and juvenile hemochromatosis: mutations of the HJV gene encoding hemojuvelin. *Blood*. 2004;103(12):4669–4671.
33. Pietrangelo A. Hereditary hemochromatosis: pathogenesis, diagnosis, and treatment. *Gastroenterology*. 2010;139(2):393–408, 408 e1–2.
34. Camaschella C, Fargion S, Sampietro M, et al. Inherited HFE-unrelated hemochromatosis in Italian families. *Hepatology*. 1999;29(5):1563–1564.
35. Camaschella C, Roetto A, Calì A, et al. The gene TFR2 is mutated in a new type of haemochromatosis mapping to 7q22. *Nat Genet*. 2000;25(1):14–15.
36. Pichler I, Minelli C, Sanna S, et al. Identification of a common variant in the TFR2 gene implicated in the physiological regulation of serum iron levels. *Hum Mol Genet*. 2011;20(6):1232–40.
37. Iolascon A, Camaschella C, Pospisilova D, et al. Natural history of recessive inheritance of DMT1 mutations. *J Pediatr*. 2008;152(1):136–139.
38. Iolascon A, d'Apolito M, Servedio V, et al. Microcytic anemia and hepatic iron overload in a child with compound heterozygous mutations in DMT1 (SCL11A2). *Blood*. 2006;107(1):349–354.
39. Wong K, Barbin Y, Chakrabarti S, et al. A point mutation in the iron-responsive element of the L-ferritin in a family with hereditary hyperferritinemia cataract syndrome. *Can J Gastroenterol*. 2005;19(4):253–255.
40. Mancuso M, Davidzon G, Kurlan RM, et al. Hereditary ferritinopathy: a novel mutation, its cellular pathology, and pathogenetic insights. *J Neuropathol Exp Neurol*. 2005;64(4):280–294.

41. Kato J, Fujikawa K, Kanda M, et al. A mutation, in the iron-responsive element of H ferritin mRNA, causing autosomal dominant iron overload. *Am J Hum Genet.* 2001;69(1):191–197.
42. Knisely AS, Gelbart T, Beutler E. Molecular characterization of a third case of human atransferrinemia. *Blood.* 2004;104(8):2607.
43. Beutler E, Gelbart T, Lee P, et al. Molecular characterization of a case of atransferrinemia. *Blood.* 2000;96(13):4071–4074.
44. Aslan D, Crain K, Beutler E. A new case of human atransferrinemia with a previously undescribed mutation in the transferrin gene. *Acta Haematol.* 2007;118(4):244–247.
45. Athiyarath R, Arora N, Fuster F, et al. Two novel missense mutations in iron transport protein transferrin causing hypochromic microcytic anaemia and haemosiderosis: molecular characterization and structural implications. *Br J Haematol.* 2013;163(3):404–407.
46. Hossainy NM. Late diagnosis of a rare disease. *BMJ Case Rep.* 2009;2009.
47. Hamill RL, Woods JC, Cook BA. Congenital atransferrinemia. A case report and review of the literature. *Am J Clin Pathol.* 1991;96(2):215–218.
48. Beaumont-Epinette MP, Delobel JB, Ropert M, et al. Hereditary hypotransferrinemia can lead to elevated transferrin saturation and, when associated to HFE or HAMP mutations, to iron overload. *Blood Cells Mol Dis.* 2015;54(2):151–154.
49. Harris ZL, Takahashi Y, Miyajima H, et al. Aceruloplasminemia: molecular characterization of this disorder of iron metabolism. *Proc Natl Acad Sci U S A.* 1995;92(7):2539–2543.
50. Yoshida K, Furihata K, Takeda S, et al. A mutation in the ceruloplasmin gene is associated with systemic hemosiderosis in humans. *Nat Genet.* 1995;9(3):267–272.
51. Meral Gunes A, Sezgin Evim M, Baytan B, et al. Aceruloplasminemia in a Turkish adolescent with a novel mutation of ceruloplasmin gene: the first diagnosed case from Turkey. *J Pediatr Hematol Oncol.* 2014;36(7):e423–e425.
52. Doyle A, Rusli F, Bhathal P. Aceruloplasminaemia: a rare but important cause of iron overload. *BMJ Case Rep.* 2015;2015.
53. Kono S, Suzuki H, Takahashi K, et al. Hepatic iron overload associated with a decreased serum ceruloplasmin level in a novel clinical type of aceruloplasminemia. *Gastroenterology.* 2006;131(1):240–245.
54. Rusticeanu M, Zimmer V, Schleithoff L, et al. Novel ceruloplasmin mutation causing aceruloplasminemia with hepatic iron overload and diabetes without neurological symptoms. *Clin Genet.* 2014;85(3):300–301.
55. Bethlehem C, van Harten B, Hoogendoorn M. Central nervous system involvement in a rare genetic iron overload disorder. *Neth J Med.* 2010;68(10):316–318.
56. Hofmann WP, Welsch C, Takahashi Y, et al. Identification and in silico characterization of a novel compound heterozygosity associated with hereditary aceruloplasminemia. *Scand J Gastroenterol.* 2007;42(9):1088–1094.
57. Perez-Aguilar F, Burguera JA, Benlloch S, et al. Aceruloplasminemia in an asymptomatic patient with a new mutation. Diagnosis and family genetic analysis. *J Hepatol.* 2005;42(6):947–949.
58. Pietrangelo A, Montosi G, Totaro A, et al. Hereditary hemochromatosis in adults without pathogenic mutations in the hemochromatosis gene. *N Engl J Med.* 1999;341(10):725–732.
59. Montosi G, Donovan A, Totaro A, et al. Autosomal-dominant hemochromatosis is associated with a mutation in the ferroportin (SLC11A3) gene. *J Clin Invest.* 2001;108(4):619–623.
60. Njajou OT, Vaessen N, Joosse M, et al. A mutation in SLC11A3 is associated with autosomal dominant hemochromatosis. *Nat Genet.* 2001;28(3):213–214.
61. Cottier H. A hemochromatosis similar disease in newborn. *Schweiz Med Wochenschr.* 1957;87(2):39–43.
62. Lopriore E, Mearin ML, Oepkes D, et al. Neonatal hemochromatosis: management, outcome, and prevention. *Prenat Diagn.* 2013;33(13):1221–1225.
63. Smyk DS, Mytilinaiou MG, Grammatikopoulos T, et al. Primary biliary cirrhosis-specific antimitochondrial antibodies in neonatal haemochromatosis. *Clin Dev Immunol.* 2013;2013:642643.
64. Whitington PF. Neonatal hemochromatosis: a congenital alloimmune hepatitis. *Semin Liver Dis.* 2007;27(3):243–250.
65. Collardeau-Frachon S, Heissat S, Bouvier R, et al. French retrospective multicentric study of neonatal hemochromatosis: importance of autopsy and autoimmune maternal manifestations. *Pediatr Dev Pathol.* 2012;15(6):450–470.
66. Smith SR, Shneider BL, Magid M, et al. Minor salivary gland biopsy in neonatal hemochromatosis. *Arch Otolaryngol Head Neck Surg.* 2004;130(6):760–763.
67. Pronicka E, Węglewska-Jurkiewicz A, Taybert J, et al. Post mortem identification of deoxyguanosine kinase (DGUOK) gene mutations combined with impaired glucose homeostasis and iron overload features in four infants with severe progressive liver failure. *J Appl Genet.* 2011;52(1):61–66.
68. Gordeuk VR, McLaren CE, MacPhail AP, et al. Associations of iron overload in Africa with hepatocellular carcinoma and tuberculosis:

Strachan's 1929 thesis revisited. *Blood*. 1996;87(8):3470–3476.
69. Walker AR, Arvidsson UB. Iron overload in the South African Bantu. *Trans R Soc Trop Med Hyg*. 1953;47(6):536–548.
70. Bothwell TH, Bradlow BA. Siderosis in the Bantu. A combined histopathological and chemical study. *Arch Pathol*. 1960;70:279–292.
71. Moyo VM, Gangaidzo IT, Gomo ZA, et al. Traditional beer consumption and the iron status of spouse pairs from a rural community in Zimbabwe. *Blood*. 1997;89(6):2159–2166.
72. Gordeuk V, Mukiibi J, Hasstedt SJ, et al. Iron overload in Africa. Interaction between a gene and dietary iron content. *N Engl J Med*. 1992;326(2):95–100.
73. Bittencourt PL, Carnevale Marin ML, Alves Couto C, et al. Analysis of HFE and non-HFE gene mutations in Brazilian patients with hemochromatosis. *Clinics*. 2009;64(9):837–841.
74. Olynyk JK, O'Neill R, Britton RS, et al. Determination of hepatic iron concentration in fresh and paraffin-embedded tissue: diagnostic implications. *Gastroenterology*. 1994;106(3):674–677.
75. Deugnier Y, Turlin B. Pathology of hepatic iron overload. *World J Gastroenterol*. 2007;13(35):4755–4760.
76. Bassett ML, Halliday JW, Powell LW. Value of hepatic iron measurements in early hemochromatosis and determination of the critical iron level associated with fibrosis. *Hepatology*. 1986;6(1):24–29.
77. Ludwig J, Hashimoto E, Porayko MK, et al. Hemosiderosis in cirrhosis: a study of 447 native livers. *Gastroenterology*. 1997;112(3):882–888.
78. Kowdley KV, Brandhagen DJ, Gish RG, et al. Survival after liver transplantation in patients with hepatic iron overload: the national hemochromatosis transplant registry. *Gastroenterology*. 2005;129(2):494–503.
79. Fenton H, Torbenson M, Vivekanandan P, et al. Marked iron in liver explants in the absence of major hereditary hemochromatosis gene defects: a risk factor for cardiac failure. *Transplantation*. 2009;87(8):1256–1260.
80. O'Glasser AY, Scott DL, Corless CL, et al. Hepatic and cardiac iron overload among patients with end-stage liver disease referred for liver transplantation. *Clin Transplant*. 2010;4(5):643–651.
81. Minervini MI, Ruppert K, Fontes P, et al. Liver biopsy findings from healthy potential living liver donors: reasons for disqualification, silent diseases and correlation with liver injury tests. *J Hepatol*. 2009;50(3):501–510.
82. Ryan CK, Johnson LA, Germin BI, et al. One hundred consecutive hepatic biopsies in the workup of living donors for right lobe liver transplantation. *Liver Transpl*. 2002;8(12):1114–1122.
83. Dwyer JP, Sarwar S, Egan B, et al. Hepatic iron overload following liver transplantation of a C282y homozygous allograft: a case report and literature review. *Liver Int*. 2011;31(10):1589–1592.
84. Adams PC, McAlister V, Chakrabarti S, et al. Is serum hepcidin causative in hemochromatosis? Novel analysis from a liver transplant with hemochromatosis. *Can J Gastroenterol*. 2008;22(10):851–853.
85. Gehrke SG, Stremmel W, Mathes I, et al. Hemochromatosis and transferrin receptor gene polymorphisms in chronic hepatitis C: impact on iron status, liver injury and HCV genotype. *J Mol Med*. 2003;81(12):780–787.
86. Thorburn D, Curry G, Spooner R, et al. The role of iron and haemochromatosis gene mutations in the progression of liver disease in chronic hepatitis C. *Gut*. 2002;50(2):248–252.
87. Negro F, Samii K, Rubbia-Brandt L, et al. Hemochromatosis gene mutations in chronic hepatitis C patients with and without liver siderosis. *J Med Virol*. 2000;60(1):21–27.
88. Sebastiani G, Vario A, Ferrari A, et al. Hepatic iron, liver steatosis and viral genotypes in patients with chronic hepatitis C. *J Viral Hepat*. 2006;13(3):199–205.
89. Pirisi M, Scott CA, Avellini C, et al. Iron deposition and progression of disease in chronic hepatitis C. Role of interface hepatitis, portal inflammation, and HFE missense mutations. *Am J Clin Pathol*. 2000;113(4):546–554.
90. Valenti L, Pulixi EA, Arosio P, et al. Relative contribution of iron genes, dysmetabolism and hepatitis C virus (HCV) in the pathogenesis of altered iron regulation in HCV chronic hepatitis. *Haematologica*. 2007;92(8):1037–1042.
91. Nelson JE, Wilson L, Brunt EM, et al. Relationship between the pattern of hepatic iron deposition and histological severity in nonalcoholic fatty liver disease. *Hepatology*. 2011;53(2):448–457.
92. Britto MR, Thomas LA, Balaratnam N, et al. Hepatocellular carcinoma arising in non-cirrhotic liver in genetic haemochromatosis. *Scand J Gastroenterol*. 2000;35(8):889–893.
93. Chung H, Kudo M, Kawasaki T, et al. Hepatocellular carcinoma associated with secondary haemochromatosis in non-cirrhotic liver: a case report. *Hepatol Res*. 2003;26(3):254–258.
94. Kowdley KV. Iron, hemochromatosis, and hepatocellular carcinoma. *Gastroenterology*. 2004.;27(5 suppl 1):S79–86.
95. Morcos M, Dubois S, Bralet MP, et al. Primary liver carcinoma in genetic hemochromatosis reveals a broad histologic spectrum. *Am J Clin Pathol*. 2001;116(5):738–743.

96. Ko C, Siddaiah N, Berger J, et al. Prevalence of hepatic iron overload and association with hepatocellular cancer in end-stage liver disease: results from the National Hemochromatosis Transplant Registry. *Liver Int.* 2007;27(10):1394–1401.
97. Kato J, Miyanishi K, Kobune M, et al. Long-term phlebotomy with low-iron diet therapy lowers risk of development of hepatocellular carcinoma from chronic hepatitis C. *J Gastroenterol.* 2007;42(10):830–836.
98. Mizukawa B, George A, Pushkaran S, et al. Cooperating G6PD mutations associated with severe neonatal hyperbilirubinemia and cholestasis. *Pediatr Blood Cancer.* 2011;56(5):840–842.
99. Lefkowitch JH, Grossman ME. Hepatic pathology in porphyria cutanea tarda. *Liver.* 1983;3(1):19–29.
100. Barton JC, Lee PL, West C, et al. Iron overload and prolonged ingestion of iron supplements: clinical features and mutation analysis of hemochromatosis-associated genes in four cases. *Am J Hematol.* 2006;81(10):760–767.
101. Crownover BK, Covey CJ. Hereditary hemochromatosis. *Am Fam Physician.* 2013;87(3):183–190.
102. Turlin B, Deugnier Y. Evaluation and interpretation of iron in the liver. *Semin Diagn Pathol.* 1998;15(4):237–245.
103. LeSage GD, Baldus WP, Fairbanks VF, et al. Hemochromatosis: genetic or alcohol-induced? *Gastroenterology.* 1983;84(6):1471–1477.

18 Wilson disease and other inherited metabolic diseases of liver

Lizhi Zhang, MD

18.1 INTRODUCTION

Metabolic dysfunction of liver can be due to several causes. Congenital deficiency of a specific enzyme or enzymes is the most important etiology in this group of diseases. Inherited disorders of liver metabolism can essentially involve any metabolic pathway, which results in abnormalities in the synthesis or catabolism of carbohydrates, proteins, or lipids; the metabolism of copper, iron, amino acids, or vitamins; bile acid synthesis and metabolism; detoxification; coagulation cascade; and urea cycle. These diseases can lead to hepatocyte injury and liver structural damage, but some may present with severe functional abnormalities without obvious structural changes. Abnormal accumulations of metabolites in the liver are often revealed by histopathologic examination and may provide diagnostic clues. These changes are summarized in Table 18.1 for quick reference.

In this chapter, Wilson disease and other inherited metabolic diseases are discussed, with a focus on entities that are mostly commonly encountered in the practice of surgical pathology. Of note, there are many additional genetic diseases that can involve liver but are not covered in this chapter due to limited space. Comprehensive reviews of the rare entities that are not covered in this chapter are available in most cases through a PubMed search.

18.2 DISORDERS OF COPPER METABOLISM

Wilson disease

Definition

Wilson disease is an autosomal recessive genetic disorder of copper metabolism owing to mutations in the Wilson disease gene (*ATP7B*), leading to copper accumulation in the liver and brain, resulting in liver disease and neurologic or psychiatric symptoms.

Clinical features

The estimated prevalence of Wilson disease is 1 in 30,000, with a corresponding carrier frequency of 1 in 90 in most populations.[1] Neurologic and psychiatric signs can include movement disorders, rigid dystonia, and depression. Overall, approximately 40% of individuals with Wilson disease will manifest clinically primarily with liver disease, especially in children and younger adults, typically between 5 to 35 years old. However, initial presentation as severe liver disease has been reported in children <2 years old and in older adults.[2,3] The clinical presentation of liver disease varies significantly and may include recurrent jaundice because of acute or chronic hemolysis, acute self-limited hepatitis, autoimmune hepatitis, fulminant hepatic failure, chronic liver disease with portal hypertension, or fatty liver disease. Kayser–Fleischer rings owing to copper deposition in Descemet's membrane of the cornea can be observed in 50% to 90% cases.

Laboratory findings

Mildly elevated liver transaminase and bilirubin levels are present in most patients but can be significantly elevated in cases of acute liver failure. Alkaline phosphatase levels may be low in individuals presenting with acute liver failure. With disease progression, liver synthetic function can be affected and manifested as low albumin levels or prolonged prothrombin times. The AST (aspartate aminotransferase):ALT (alanine aminotransferase) ratio is commonly >2.2, but this finding is not very specific.

Laboratory tests can be used to evaluate for Wilson disease. Serum ceruloplasmin levels are low (<0.2 g/L) in over 90% of cases, but can be normal in patients with significant active liver inflammation because ceruloplasmin is an acute phase protein. Serum copper levels are usually low because ceruloplasmin, the main copper carrier protein, is also low. In addition, 24-hour urine level above 100 μg confirms Wilson disease, although levels above 40 μg strongly suggest Wilson disease. However, these tests are not entirely specific. For example, elevated urine copper levels sometimes occur in autoimmune hepatitis and cholestatic liver disease.[4]

Quantitative liver copper analysis is also useful in diagnosing Wilson disease, in which the hepatic copper concentration is usually >250 μg/g dry weight. Copper levels can also be elevated in chronic cholestatic liver disease, though usually the levels are considerably lower. Finally, some individuals with early Wilson disease can have moderately elevated copper levels that are less than 250 μg/g dry weight.

Imaging

Imaging findings of liver in Wilson disease vary with the form and degree of liver diseases, but may include fatty change, fulminant liver necrosis, or cirrhosis.

Gross findings

Explanted livers typically show established cirrhosis. The cirrhosis commonly has a micronodular pattern but can be mixed or even macronodular. In cases with fulminant liver failure, the liver may keep its normal shape and surface texture, but in most cases the necrosis will also lead to shrinkage of liver with a wrinkled capsular surface.

Microscopic findings

The pathologic changes in the liver are believed to result from toxic effects of copper accumulation. In precirrhotic livers, the histologic findings can range from almost normal liver parenchyma to massive necrosis. The histopathologic changes can be categorized into the following patterns:

"Almost normal" liver pattern. In this pattern, the liver shows minimal to mild nonspecific changes. These changes can include variable combinations of minimal to mild portal lymphocytic inflammation, minimal to absent steatosis, rare apoptotic cells, moderate hepatocyte nuclear anisonucleosis, focal hepatocyte nuclear glycogenation, mild Kupffer cell hyperplasia, and no fibrosis (Fig. 18.1).

Acute hepatitis pattern. In this pattern, affected individuals typically present clinically with acute hepatitis and sometimes with liver failure. The liver biopsy shows marked inflammation with hepatocyte necrosis. The portal tracts show marked inflammation composed of lymphocytes and plasma cells. Interface hepatitis can be prominent and there can be a brisk bile ductular proliferation. The lobular parenchyma has significant necroinflammatory activity and variable degrees of necrosis (Fig. 18.2). The hepatocytes are swollen with ballooning degenerations. Copper deposition may be identified in hepatocytes and, when there is massive or submassive necrosis, in the Kupffer cells or portal macrophages.[5] Macrovesicular steatosis can be present but is not a predominant feature. Mild cholestasis and fibrosis can also be seen. This pattern is often indistinguishable from autoimmune hepatitis.

Fatty liver disease pattern. In this pattern, the findings can range from steatosis to steatohepatitis. Hepatyoctes with nuclear glycogenation are common. When there is steatohepatitis, the biopsy shows macrovesicular steatosis, hepatocytes with ballooning degeneration, Mallory body formation, and occasional apoptotic cells (Fig. 18.3). Fibrosis can also be found in some cases.

Chronic hepatitis pattern. The findings in this pattern are similar to those of chronic hepatitis due to other etiologies (Fig. 18.4). Some changes can mimic autoimmune hepatitis. The portal tracts are expanded by lymphocytes, occasional plasma cells, variable degrees of bile ductular proliferation, and fibrosis. Interface activity can be prominent. The lobules also show variable inflammation with spotty necrosis. Steatosis can be present in variable degrees. Advanced fibrosis can be present.

Cryptogenic cirrhosis pattern. In this pattern, the liver biopsy shows established cirrhosis with minimal or mild inflammatory activity (Fig. 18.5). The fibrotic septa may be thin or wide, containing mild nonspecific inflammation and mild bile ductular proliferation. Mild steatosis can be present and ballooned hepatocytes with Mallory hyaline can be prominent in a subset of cases. The lobules usually lack significant inflammation, besides scattered apoptotic cells. The hepatocytes may be enlarged and show oncocytic changes with prominent granular eosinophilic cytoplasm because of increased number of mitochondria. Giant cell transformation is occasionally seen, especially in the setting of cholestasis. The copper deposits can be readily seen in periseptal hepatocytes using Rhodanine copper stain, but the distribution of copper is variable, with some nodules being loaded with copper and others having only minimal copper or no copper (Fig. 18.6).

Immunohistochemistry and special stains

There are several stains that can be used to identify copper, including Orcein, Timm silver, Rhodanine, Victoria blue, and rubeanic acid. Rhodanine is the most commonly used stain because of its reliability, reproducibility, a linear relationship with tissue copper concentration, and simple and fast staining techniques. Orçein and Victoria blue stains are not specific for copper, as they detect copper-associated proteins in lysosomes, which may or may not contain copper. The Timm silver sulfide and rubeanic acid stains are more sensitive than Rhodanine but are not widely used. The Timm silver sulfide stain needs a longer (24-hour) deparrafination time, and rubeanic acid requires a 72-hour incubation to reach the best results.[6,7]

Copper deposits on the Rhodanine stain are seen as small red-brown granules in the cytoplasm of hepatocytes and tend to have a zone 1 distribution (Fig. 18.6), but the copper deposition can be panlobular when there is marked copper accumulation.[8] The Rhodanine copper stain is very helpful but is neither entirely sensitive nor specific in isolation for diagnosing Wilson disease. This is because early in the course of Wilson disease, the copper in the hepatocytes is located in the cytosol and not the lysosomes and the Rhodanine stain only detects lysosomal deposits. Therefore, a negative copper stain cannot rule out Wilson disease. If Wilson disease is clinical suspected, quantitative copper analysis should be performed on the liver biopsy.

In addition, the Rhodanine stain is positive in chronic cholestatic liver disease. Copper is normally excreted in the bile and cholestatic conditions can lead over time to copper deposits in the hepatocytes, though the deposits tend to be more focal and milder than seen in Wilson disease. Cirrhotic livers can also have nonspecific copper accumulation, but again the copper deposition tends to be focal and mild.[9]

Ultrastructural findings

On ultrastructural examination, the mitochondria show variable numbers and sizes, dense matrix with occasional vacuolated granules, crystal inclusions, enlarged intercristal spaces, and separation of the outer from the inner membranes. Other alterations include increased numbers of peroxisomes, lipofusion granules, multivesicular bodies, and lipid droplets.[5,10]

Molecular genetic findings

Wilson disease is inherited in an autosomal recessive manner. Heterozygotes may have mild biochemical abnormalities in copper metabolism but most of them have no clinically significant disease. Although more than 300 disease-causing mutations of *ATP7B* have been identified, only a small number of mutations are responsible for most cases in a specific population. For example, in Western populations, the H1069Q mutation is present in approximately 50% of cases, but it is rare in Chinese populations, who tend to have the R778L mutation. The mutations can be detected using targeted mutation analysis or whole gene sequencing. Identification of two disease-causing mutations establishes the diagnosis of Wilson disease. However, genetic testing for clinical diagnosis is often difficult because of the large number of mutations and the fact that not all mutations are disease-causing. If disease-causing mutations are detected in an index case, then subsequent targeted mutation analysis can be very helpful for screening the extended family.

Differential diagnosis

There are no specific histopathologic patterns for Wilson disease. Therefore, the possibility of Wilson disease is considered in essentially

Table 18.1 Inclusions, Deposits, or Crystals in Live of Common Genetic Disorders

Disorders	Deposit component	Location of inclusions	Light microscopic features	Electron microscopic features	Special stains	Mimickers
Wilson disease	Copper	Hepatocytes; rare in Kupffer cells and macrophages	Not visible	Prominent mitochondria with variable number and size, dense matrix, occasional vacuolated granules, crystal inclusions, and separation of the outer from the inner membranes	Rhodanine (most commonly used), Orcein, Timm silver, Victoria blue, and rubeanic acid	Lipofuscin
Hereditary Hemochromatosis	Iron	Hepatocytes; also in Kupffer cells, biliary epithelial and endothelial cells	Dark brown rusty pigments	Electron-dense ferritin cores and siderosomes	Prussian blue stain, with pericanalicular pattern	Lipofuscin, Dubin–Johnson pigments, bile, hemosiderin
Glycogen storage disease (GSD)	Glycogen	Hepatocytes	Swollen hepatocytes with pale-staining cytoplasm and prominent cell membrane; Light eosinophilic ground glass inclusions in type IV	Abundant glycogen rosettes in all types; monoparticulate glycogen in enlarged lysosomes in type II; nonmembrane bound, randomly oriented fibrillary material in type IV	PAS and digested by diastase	Glycogenic hepatopathy; Lafora bodies and hepatitis B inclusions for type IV; Pseudoground glass inclusions
Lafora disease	Insoluable glycogen in the form of polyglucosan	Hepatocytes	Homogeneously eosinophilic or ground glass Lafora bodies with round or oval shape and distinct border surrounded by a halo	Nonmembrane bound fibrillary and granular material	PAS, colloidal iron, Lugol iodine stains	Inclusions in type IV GSD, hepatitis B; Pseudoground ground glass inclusions; Lafora body-like inclusions related to cyanamide or 6-thioguanine
Mucopolysac-charidosis	Glycosamino-glycans	Hepatocytes and Kupffer cells	Hepatocytes and Kupffer cells with rarified cytoplasm or numerous small- to medium-sized cytoplasmic vacuoles.	Membrane bound vacuoles in the hepatocytes and Kupffer cells	Colloidal iron stains with greenish-blue cytoplasmic staining; weakly positive of PAS and PASD	GSD, microvesicular steatosis

(continued)

Table 18.1 Inclusions, Deposits, or Crystals in Liver of Common Genetic Disorders (*continued*)

Disorders	Deposit component	Location of inclusions	Light microscopic features	Electron microscopic features	Special stains	Mimickers
α-1-Antitrypsin deficiency	α-1-Antitrypsin	Hepatocytes	Eosinophilic globules with variable size in periportal hepatocytes	Amorphous finely granular or fibrillary deposits in endoplasmic reticulum	PASD; bright red on Trichrome stain; α-1-Antitrypsin immunostain	Megamitochondria, Globular amyloid, fibrin globules
Afibrinogen	Fibrinogen	Hepatocytes	Round or polygonal light eosinophilic inclusions with a dark core, irregular outline, and a clear halo. The cytoplasm filled with fine globules with ground-glass appearance.	Dilated cisterns of rough endoplasmic reticulum filled with densely packed tubular structures arranged in curved bundles with a fingerprint-like pattern	Fibrinogen immunostain; PTAH; PAS	α-1-Antitrypsin globules, hepatitis B ground glass or pseudoground ground glass inclusions
Gaucher disease	Glycocerebroside	Kupffer cells and macrophages	Amphophilic or faintly stained, striated, and wrinkled-paper appearance	Spindle or rod-shaped inclusions surrounded by a limiting membrane with internal tubular structures on cross section	PAS or Trichrome stains	GSD inclusions, Lafora bodies, pseudo-Gaucher cells in patients with hematologic malignancy or anemia
Niemann–Pick disease	Sphingomyelin	Kupffer cells, macrophages, and hepatocytes	Hypertrophied Kupffer cells with foamy or microvesicular cytoplasm in sinusoidal spaces; hepatocytes less foamy than Kupffer cells	Dense mixed lipid lysosomes containing centrically laminated myelin-like inclusions	Oil red O, Luxal fast blue, or Baker acid hematin stains on frozen sections. PAS stain is variable positive or negative	Lipid-laden foamy cells in other disorders. Gaucher cells, cystine crystals
Cholesterol storage disease	Cholesteryl ester	Kupffer cells and hepatocytes; may also in biliary epithelial and endothelial cells	Kupffer cells and macrophages with foamy cytoplasm, marked microvesicular steatosis in hepatocytes, and brilliant silver birefringent crystals in frozen sections.	Peripheral vacules or large central cholesterol ester clefts in Kupffer cells; lipid droplets and occasional crystal clefts in hepatocytes	PASD	GSD, microvesicular steatosis, Gaucher cells, Niemann–Pick disease

Table 18.1 Inclusions, Deposits, or Crystals in Live of Common Genetic Disorders (*continued*)

Disorders	Deposit component	Location of inclusions	Light microscopic features	Electron microscopic features	Special stains	Mimickers
Porphyria cutanea tarda	Uroporphyrin	Hepatocytes	Needle-shaped crystals with variable lengths; birefringent under polarized light best seen in unstained paraffin sections	Needle-shaped crystals with alternating areas of differing electron density	Ferric ferricyanide reduction test on unstained paraffin sections	Cystine crystals; may be overlooked in cases with heavy iron overload.
Erythropoietic protoporphyria	Protoporphyrin	Hepatocytes, Kupffer cells, and canaliculi	Dark brown pigments within the biliary canaliculi and macrophages; red to orange Maltese cross shape of birefringent crystalline pigment under polarized light	Crystal-containing vacuoles arranged in a "star-burst" pattern in cytoplasm and canaliculi	N/A	Bile plugs, Dubin–Johnson pigments, large iron deposits
Cystinosis	Cystine	Kupffer cells	Cystine crystals with a brilliant silvery birefringence under polarized light	Hexagonal crystalline structures	N/A	Gaucher cells, Niemann–Pick disease
Dubin–Johnson syndrome	Polymers of epinephrine metabolites	Hepatocytes	Coarsely granular dark brown pigments	Dense particles within lysosomes in a background of more homogenous moderately dense granular material, often associated with lipid droplets	Fontana–Masson	Lipofuscin, hemosiderosis, bile

all liver biopsies when working up the etiology of unexplained liver disease, especially in children and younger adults. Several patterns can raise suspicion for Wilson disease, including fatty liver disease in younger individuals with no risk factors, cryptogenic cirrhosis in young or middle aged adults with no risk factors, or an acute unexplained hepatitis or acute liver failure in young individuals. Even in cases where the clinical and pathological findings suggest autoimmune hepatitis, clinicians should still be reminded to rule out Wilson disease.

Prognosis and treatment

If left untreated, Wilson disease tends to become progressively worse and can eventually be fatal. With early detection and treatment, most patients can live relatively normal lives. The main therapy for Wilson disease is chelating agents such as D-penicillamine and trientine to increase the removal of copper from the body or to prevent the absorption of copper from the diet. Liver transplantation is indicated in cases with fulminant liver failure or advanced fibrosis. Liver

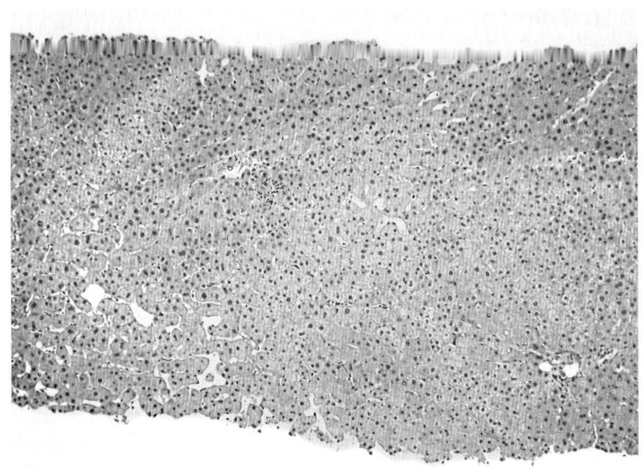

Figure 18.1 Wilson disease. Almost normal liver pattern.

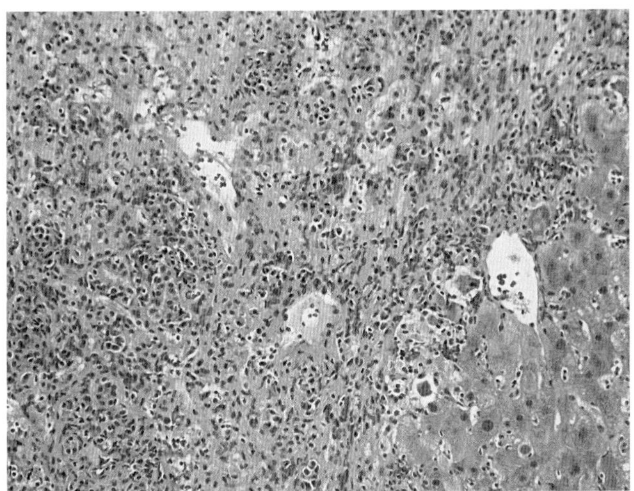

Figure 18.2 Wilson disease. Autoimmune hepatitis–like pattern with marked lymphoplasmacytic infiltrate, interface activity, and necrosis.

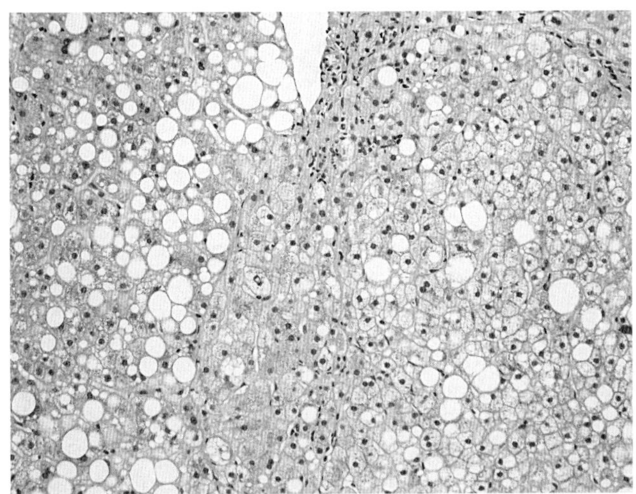

Figure 18.3 Wilson disease. Fatty liver changes.

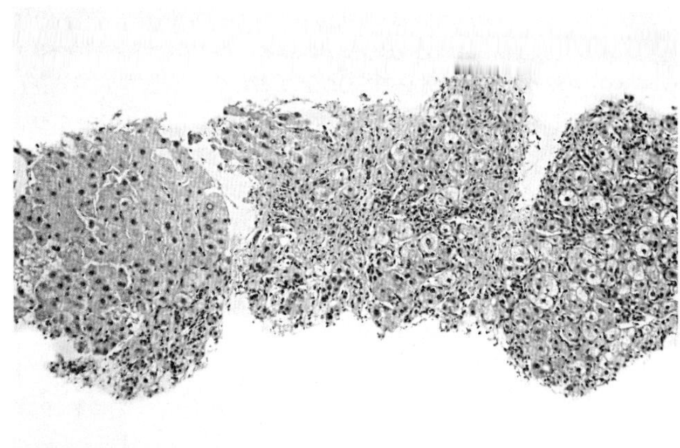

Figure 18.4 Wilson disease. Chronic hepatitis changes.

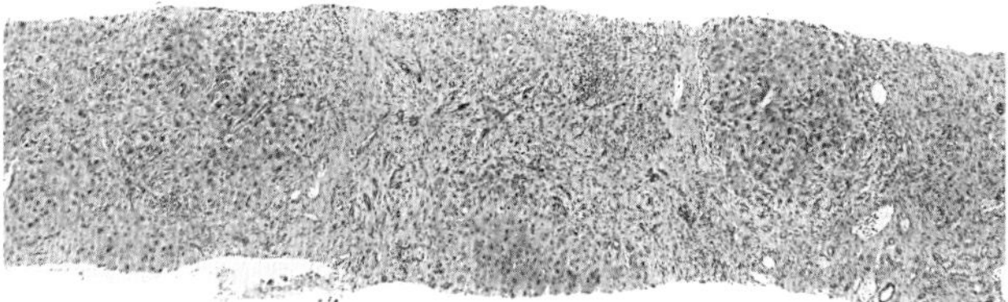

Figure 18.5 Wilson disease. Cirrhotic liver with no specific morphologic features.

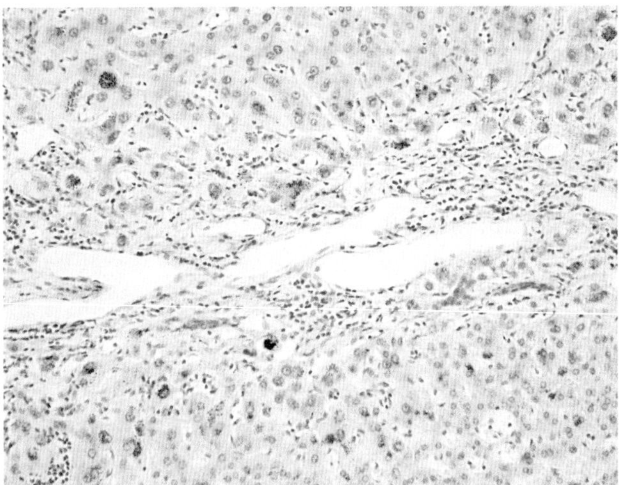

Figure 18.6 Wilson disease. Marked copper accumulation in periportal hepatocytes demonstrated by a Rhodanine stain.

transplantation is not recommended in those cases with severe neuropsychiatric illness, as its benefit in this setting is uncertain.

Other copper metabolic disorders

Besides Wilson disease, there are several other copper overload disorders not related to *ATP7B* mutations, including Indian childhood cirrhosis,

Tyrolean infantile cirrhosis, and idiopathic copper toxiocosis. Most individuals with these diseases present before the age of 2 years with histories of progressive lethargy, increased infections, and hepatomegaly. The etiology of these diseases is still not fully understood and both genetic defects in copper metabolism and excessive copper intake may have roles in the excess copper accumulation. The histologic changes in the liver appear to be similar in these diseases, though published descriptions remain sparse. Essentially all cases are diagnosed at the cirrhotic stage and characteristically have a micronodular pattern composed of very tiny nodules. The lobules typically show marked hepatocyte ballooning degeneration, abundant Mallory body formation, and scattered acidophil bodies. Steatosis is typically absent. The inflammation is mild and composed of lymphocytes, histiocytes, neutrophils, and a few plasma cells. Cholestasis can be prominent. The copper accumulation starts in periportal hepatocytes and then extends to the entire lobules and is typically marked and diffuse by the time the liver is cirrhotic. In addition to cirrhosis, the trichrome stains can show marked central vein fibrosis and marked pericellular fibrosis.

18.3 ENDOPLASMIC RETICULUM STORAGE DISEASES

Endoplasmic reticulum storage diseases are a group of inborn errors of metabolism affecting secretory proteins, resulting in hepatocellular storage and plasma deficiency of the corresponding protein. The abnormal proteins cannot be transferred from the rough endoplasmic reticulum to the smooth endoplasmic reticulum, leading to hepatocellular accumulation. Diseases include α-1-antitrypsin deficiency, afibrinogenaemia or hypofibrinogenaemia, α-1-antichymotrypsin deficiency, and antithrombin III deficiency.

α-1-Antitrypsin deficiency

Definition

α-1-Antitrypsin deficiency is a genetic disorder caused by defective production of α-1-antitrypsin (A1AT) by liver cells, leading to accumulation of abnormal A1AT protein in hepatocytes and decreased A1AT levels in the blood.

Clinical features

α-1-Antitrypsin deficiency is an uncommon but not rare disease, and it has been estimated that 1 in 3,000 to 5,000 individuals carry mutations in the *SERPINA1* gene. α-1-Antitrypsin deficiency is underdiagnosed because not every individual with mutations will develop clinically significant disease.[11] The clinical presentation depends on the degree of α-1-antitrypsin deficiency, which is associated with different mutations in the *SERPINA1* gene. Over 100 alleles of *SERPINA1* have been identified. The allelic genotypes have historically been determined by migration of the α-1-antitrypsin protein using gel electrophoresis. The normal phenotype is designated as PiM (Pi = protease inhibitor). The most common deficiency variants are PiS and PiZ. The most prevalent carrier phenotypes (not associated with disease in most cases) are PiMS and PiMZ, whereas the most common deficiency phenotypes (disease causing) are PiSS, PiSZ, and PiZZ, along with other rare deficiency alleles such as Mmalton, Mduarte, and null.[12,13] Most individuals with α-1-antitrypsin deficiency have symptoms that manifest primarily in the respiratory system, with the development of emphysema during their thirties or forties. Cigarette smoking can accelerate disease progression.

Approximately 10% of PiZ individuals develop clinically significant liver disease with variable presentations. There is a distinct bimodal distribution of liver diseases in α-1-antitrypsin deficiency. It is the most common genetic cause of liver disease in neonates and children, which manifests as neonatal hepatitis and cholestatic jaundice. The prognosis of α-1-antitrypsin deficiency is generally excellent during children and adolescence, and most of them recover and have minimal or no liver disease by adulthood. Adults with α-1-antitrypsin deficiency, especially male patients, may have chronic liver disease, typically presenting in their 50s. They may present with asymptomatic abnormal liver enzymes, advanced cirrhosis, or hepatocellular carcinoma.

The association between heterozygosity of A1AT alleles and risk of developing chronic liver disease is controversial. It is generally accepted that heterozygosity of A1AT alleles does not increase the risk of liver disease in childhood, but approximately 10% adults with PiMZ phenotype will develop chronic liver disease.[14]

Laboratory findings

Serum A1AT levels are used to screen for α-1-antitrypsin deficiency. The serum A1AT levels correlate broadly with the genotype, but the serum levels alone cannot establish a diagnosis of α-1-antitrypsin deficiency. The serum levels of A1AT are typically as follows: PiMS (80% of normal), PiMZ (60%), PiSS (60%), PiSZ (40%), and PiZZ (15%).

Neonates with PiZ who develop neonate hepatitis and jaundice can have markedly elevated liver enzymes and hyperbilirubinemia. Approximately 50% of clinically well PiZ infants have mildly abnormal liver enzymes in the neonatal period, but most resolve during follow-up, with fewer than 10% of individuals having persistence of mildly abnormal liver enzymes.[15] Adults may present with asymptomatic abnormal liver enzymes which are indistinguishable from other common causes of chronic liver diseases.

Imaging

Imaging studies may show hepatomegaly or changes associated with cirrhosis or hepatocellular carcinoma. Chest imaging studies show changes of emphysema or chronic obstructive pulmonary disease.

Gross findings

In cirrhotic livers removed for transplantation, α-1-antitrypsin deficiency usually shows either a micronodular or a mixed micro- and macronodular pattern of cirrhosis.

Microscopic findings

The finding of intracytoplasmic round or oval eosinophilic globules in periportal hepatocytes is characteristic of α-1-antitrypsin deficiency. It should be noted that the presence of α-1-antitrypsin globules in hepatocytes does not always correlate with clinical deficiency or with the presence of liver disease. The globules are eosinophilic on hematoxylin and eosin (H&E) sections and are bright red on trichrome stain (Figs. 18.7 and 18.8). The globules are best seen using periodic acid–Schiff (PAS) stain with diastase (PASD), which shows bright magenta globules (Fig. 18.9). The globules are only in the hepatocytes and can be patchy in the early phases of the disease. They are not always recognizable on H&E examination, and routine PASD stains are helpful to ensure the globules are not missed (Figs. 18.10 and 18.11). Although they are typically in periportal hepatocytes, the hepatocytes in all the zones can be affected in severe cases. In rare cases with the null phenotype, there are no globules in the hepatocytes because there is no production of the protein and there generally is no liver disease. The globules are absent or difficult to detect in infants less than 3 months of age, and the diagnosis of α-1-antitrypsin deficiency will depend on serum or genetic tests. Infants with clinical disease may exhibit liver injury resembling neonatal hepatitis, cholestatic hepatitis, or

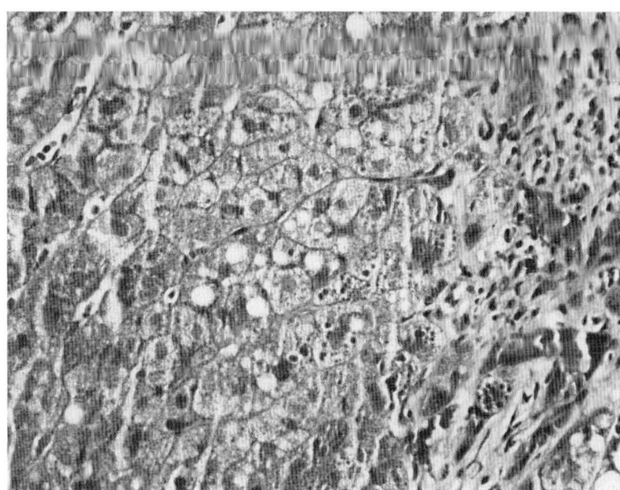

Figure 18.8 α-1-Antitrypsin deficiency. Bright red globules on Trichrome stain.

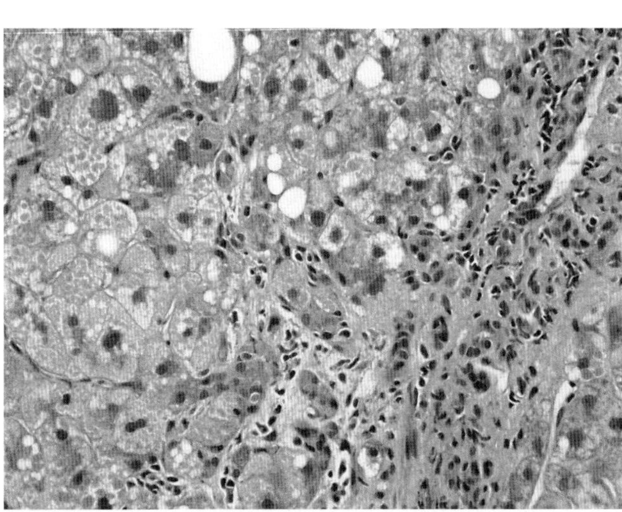

Figure 18.7 α-1-Antitrypsin deficiency. Round intracytoplasmic α-1-antitrypsin globules in variable sizes seen on H&E section as eosinophilic globules.

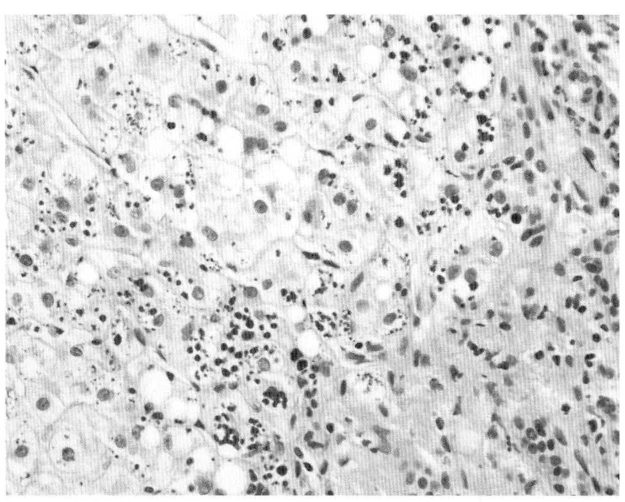

Figure 18.9 α-1-Antitrypsin deficiency. Bright magenta PAS-positive globules with diastase resistance.

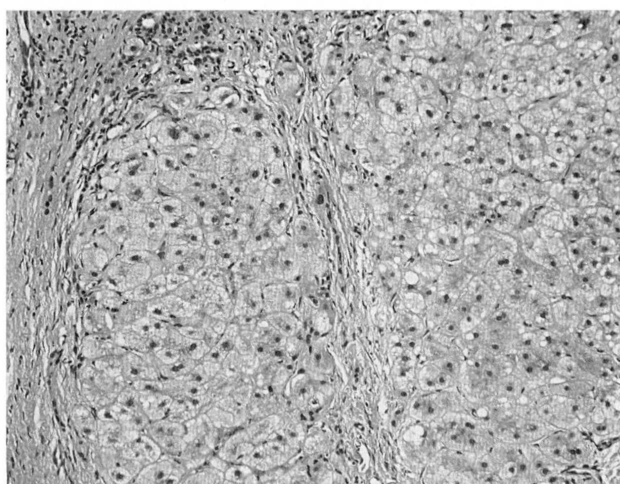

Figure 18.10 α-1-Antitrypsin deficiency. The globules may not be recognizable on routine H&E section.

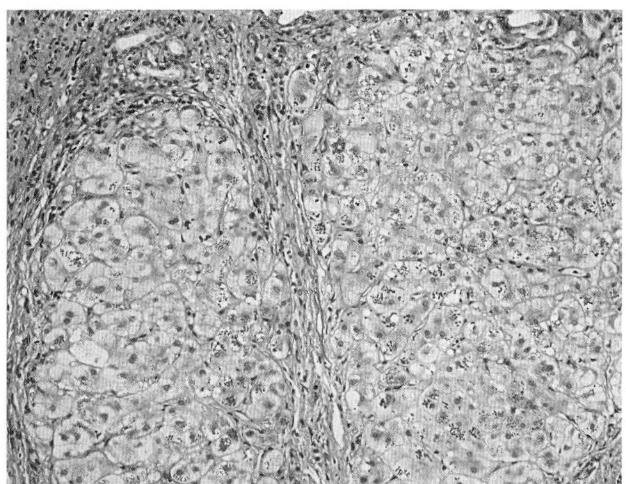

Figure 18.11 α-1-Antitrypsin deficiency. The globules are readily revealed by PASD stain in the same case showed in Figure 18.10.

extrahepatic biliary atresia. The liver biopsy can show marked cholestasis, bile ductular proliferation, mild portal and lobular inflammation, periportal steatosis, and occasional giant cell transformation (Fig. 18.12). Variable degrees of fibrosis are often present and occasional cases may have bridging fibrosis or even cirrhosis in the initial biopsy, which is indicative of rapid progression of liver disease.

In adults affected with PiZ, the pathologic findings of liver are usually nonspecific, besides the presence of A1AT globules. The number and size of the globules increases with age. The portal tracts may contain mild inflammation and mild bile ductular proliferation, whereas interface hepatitis and lobular necroinflammatory activity are minimal or absent. Mild steatosis is common. Variable fibrosis is present and cirrhosis can develop in about 15% of patients (Fig. 18.13).

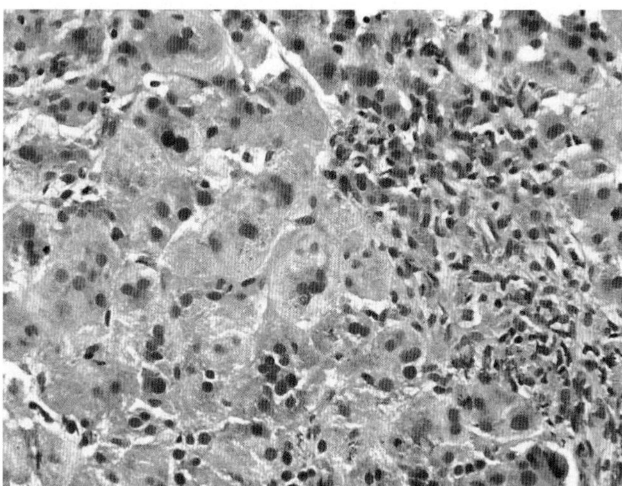

Figure 18.12 Neonatal α-1-Antitrypsin deficiency. Presented with neonatal giant cell hepatitis with cholestasis, small foci of hematopoiesis, mild portal inflammation, and ductopenia. No α-1-antitrypsin globules present.

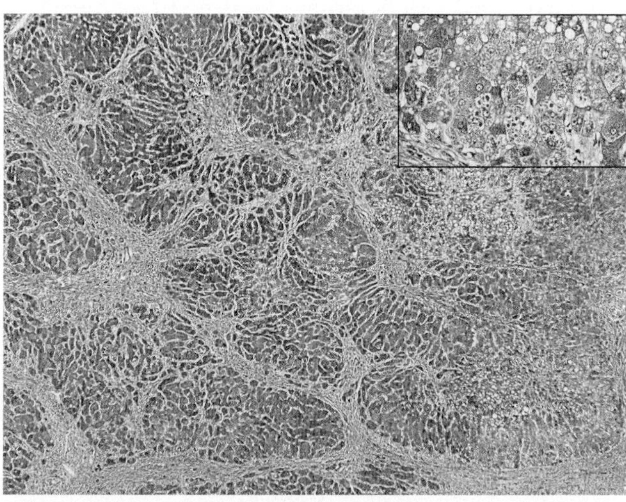

Figure 18.13 α-1-Antitrypsin deficiency. Established cirrhosis owing to α-1-antitrypsin deficiency in adults (inset, high magnification showing bright red α-1-antitrypsin globules in hepatocytes).

Cirrhosis is the major driver of risk for hepatocellular carcinoma in α-1-antitrypsin deficiency, but both cholangiocarcinoma and combined hepatocellular carcinoma-cholangiocarcinoma have been reported in patients with PiZ but without cirrhosis.[16]

Immunohistochemistry and special stains

PASD stains are routinely performed on medical liver biopsy specimens. The A1AT globules are strongly PASD-positive. Of note, there are many intracytoplasmic globules or inclusions that can mimic globules, which are discussed in the differential diagnosis section.

Immunostains for A1AT globules can be useful in certain circumstances, such as in infants when A1AT globules have not become apparent or when PASD-positive globules are focal or have unusual shapes or distribution. The A1AT globules are strongly positive by immunostain and are typically present in periportal hepatocytes (Figs. 18.14 and 18.15). The larger globules may show more intense positive staining at their periphery. Normal hepatocytes will also show granular diffuse cytoplasmic staining, so to be positive, there should be strongly staining of distinct globules. There is no correlation between immunostaining patterns and either A1AT serum concentrations or the phenotypes.[17]

Ultrastructural findings

Electron microscopy shows characteristic amorphous A1AT deposits primarily in dilated smooth endoplasmic reticulum and also in the rough endoplasmic reticulum. The deposits have a finely granular or fibrillary appearance, but there are no distinct patterns or structures. The findings in early A1AT accumulation can appear as less dense deposits or barely detectable deposits in dilated smooth endoplasmic reticulum.[18]

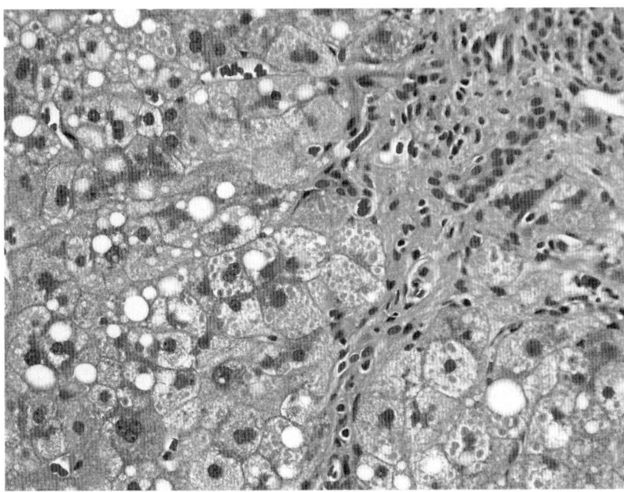

Figure 18.14 α-1-Antitrypsin deficiency. Eosinophilic globulesin periportal hepatocytes.

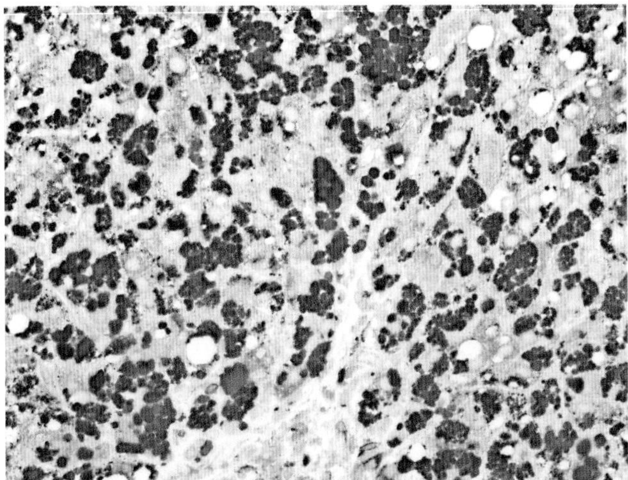

Figure 18.15 α-1-Antitrypsin blobules. Confirmed by an immunohistochemical stain showing intense cytoplasmic staining and darker globules.

Molecular genetic findings

α-1-Antitrypsin deficiency is inherited in an autosomal codominant manner, caused by mutations in the *SERPINA1* gene, which is located on the long arm of chromosome 14. There are more than 100 allelic variations/mutations of the *SERPINA1* gene, but the most important is a missense mutation in exon 5 that produces the allele "Z." The nonmutated *SERPINA1* corresponds to the "M" allele and produce normal A1AT. Genetic testing for α-1-antitrypsin deficiency targets the mutated region of *SERPINA1*using either DNA amplification and sequencing or hybridization by allele-specific oligonucleotides probes.

Differential diagnosis

Of note, PASD-positive globules in hepatocytes are not pathognomonic for clinical disease, as they can be found in genetic A1AT heterozygotes and homozygotes who lack clinical disease. In addition, very rare cases have been reported of individuals with a normal PiM phenotype developing A1AT globules during acute inflammation or severe illness, because of overproduction and high plasma levels of A1AT.[19,20]

In addition, there are many eosinophilic inclusions in hepatocytes that can mimic A1AT globules on H&E. Mega-mitochondria are frequently seen in liver biopsies. They tend to be randomly distributed, oval-shaped, single or few numbers in the cells and are PASD-negative (Fig. 18.16). Lipofuscin has fine

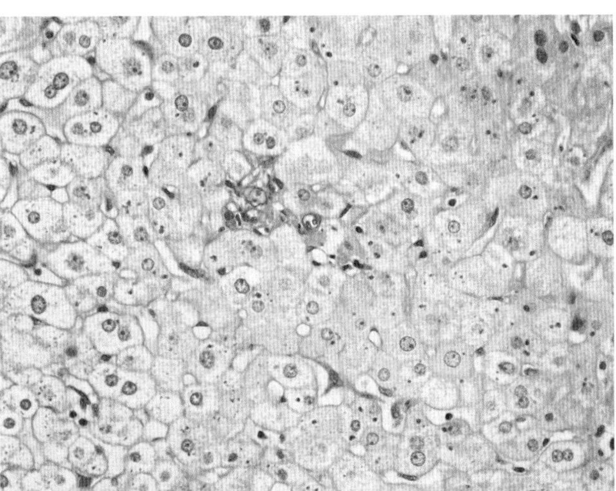

Figure 18.16 Megamitochondria (PASD stain), mimicking α-1-antitrypsin globules.

granular particles but the granules are smaller than A1AT globules, are not eosinophilic on H&E and are reddish brown color on PASD stains (Fig. 18.17). Macrophages can contain large granules, mimicking A1AT globules on PASD stain (Fig. 18.18). Immunoglobulin globules are round and eosinophilic on H&E staining and can be highlighted by immunoglobulin G (IgG) or immunoglobulin M (IgM) immunostains (Fig. 18.19). In most cases, these result from elevated serum immunoglobulin levels, so are found in autoimmune hepatitis, primary biliary cirrhosis, and other conditions associated with high serum immunoglobulin levels. The fibrin globules seen in fibrinogen storage disease are often larger than A1AT globules and are PASD-negative. They sometimes will contain dark cores and can be highlighted by phosphotungstic acid hematoxylin (PTAH) stains (Fig. 18.20) or immunostains for fibrinogen.

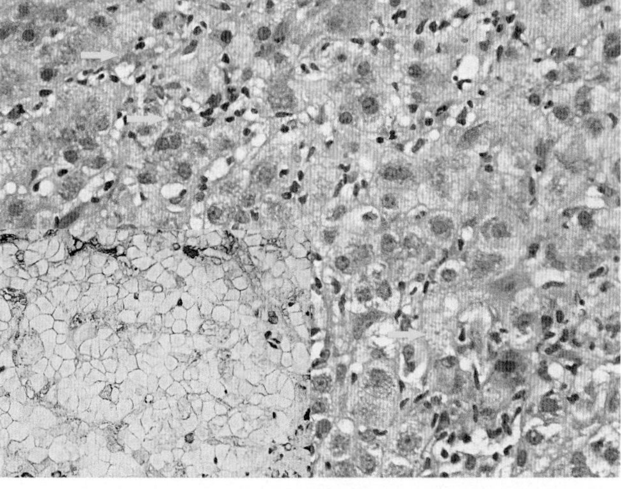

Figure 18.19 IgG globules (*arrows*) in macrophages in autoimmune hepatitis (inset, IgG immunohistochemistry).

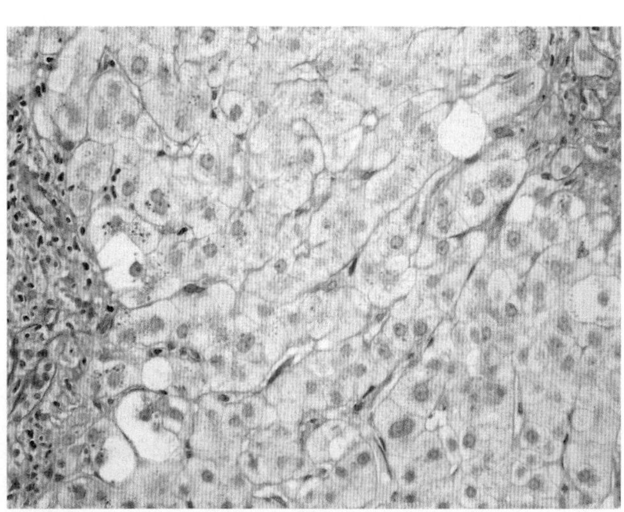

Figure 18.17 Lipofuscin (PASD stain).

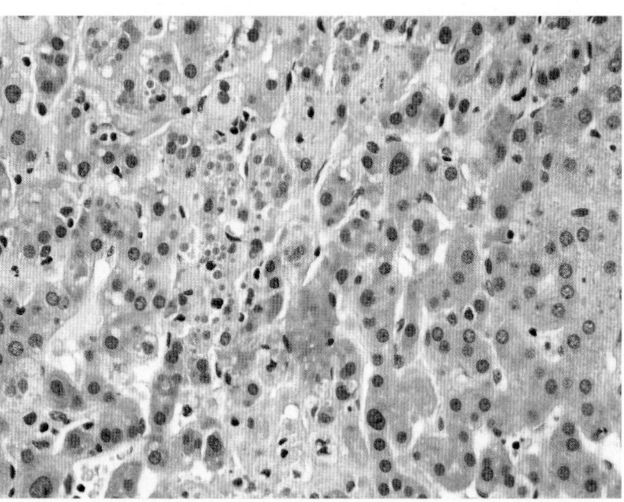

Figure 18.20 Afibrinogenemia. Cytoplasmic inclusions of abnormal fibrinogens surrounded by a clear halo with a pink core.

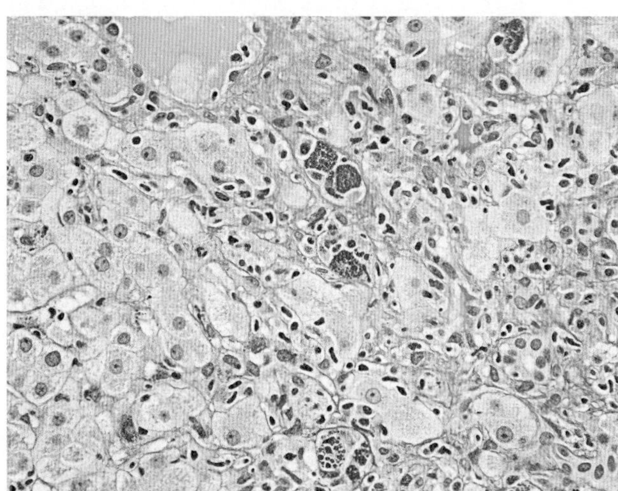

Figure 18.18 Ceroid-laden macrophages (PASD stain).

Prognosis and treatment

Patients with lung disease can receive augmentation therapy using intravenous infusions of A1AT, which is derived from donated human plasma. However, augmentation therapy is not used to treat liver disease. Instead, treatment of liver disease focuses on alleviating the symptoms of the disease. For example, ursodeoxycholic acid (UDCA) can improve symptoms for some affected children. Liver transplantation can correct the genetic abnormality and treat cirrhosis.

Afibrinogenaemia and hypofibrinogenaemia

Afibrinogenemia and hypofibrinogenemia are rare inherited disorders caused by mutations in any one of three fibrinogen genes located on chromosome

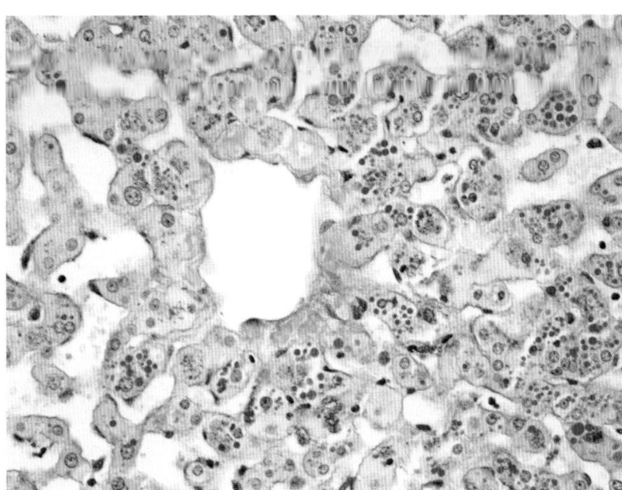

Figure 18.21 Afibrinogenemia. Weaker PASD staining of the inclusions.

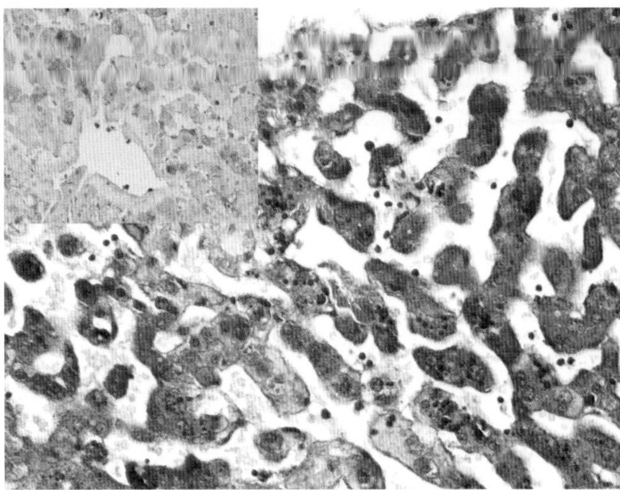

Figure 18.22 Afibrinogenemia. Abnormal fibrinogens stained black with phosphotungstic acid hematoxylin (PTAH) stain (inset, inclusions negative for α-1-antitrypsin immunohistochemistry).

4, *FGA, FGB,* and *FGG*. In afibrinogenemia, the fibrinogen levels are less than 0.1 g/L and manifests clinically primarily as bleeding, which can range from mild to severe. Patients with hypofibrinogenemia are usually asymptomatic, with no spontaneous bleeding episode, or have mild bleeding. Both can also be associated with thrombosis. Laboratory testing shows abnormal coagulation tests with low or absence of fibrinogen. Replacement of the fibrinogen is the main treatment.

Mutations in *FGG* are associated with storage of fibrinogen in the rough endoplasmic reticulum of hepatocytes, leading to liver disease of variable severity. Affected individuals may have elevated liver enzymes or present with cryptogenic cirrhosis.[21,22] The cytoplasmic inclusions of abnormal fibrinogen are round or polygonal with irregular outlines (Fig. 18.20). The globules are often surrounded by a clear halo with a dark pink core. The globules are eosinophilic or weakly stained on H&E sections and are either weakly positive or negative on PAS stain (Fig. 18.21). The globules can be detected with PTAH stain (Fig. 18.22) or immunostain for fibrinogen. Electron microscopy shows dilated rough endoplasmic reticulum filled with densely packed tubular structures arranged in curved bundles with a fingerprint-like pattern.[22]

18.4 DISORDERS OF CARBOHYDRATE METABOLISM

Glycogen storage diseases are inherited disorders of glycogen metabolism caused by defects in the processing of glycogen synthesis or the breakdown of glycogen within liver, muscles, and other cell types. Most cases are inherited in an autosomal recessive manner. There are at least 11 types of glycogen storage disease, which are classified based on the enzyme deficiency and the affected tissue. The estimated incidence of glycogen storage disease is 1 in 20,000 to 43,000 live births and the most common type is IX.[23]

Types I, III, VI, IX, and XI, primarily involve liver with abnormal accumulations of glucose within the hepatocytes. Many of the different glycogen storage diseases have common findings at clinical presentation, including hepatomegaly, hypoglycemia, short stature, and recurrent infections. As an exception, glycogen storage disease types II and IV typically are not associated with hypoglycemia at presentation.

The hepatocytes in glycogen storage disease will show glycogenosis or steatosis or both. The cases with glycogenosis can either show diffuse changes affecting all of the hepatocytes or show a mosaic pattern with admixed hepatocytes that show less striking glycogen accumulation. The affected hepatocytes are swollen and pale-staining with prominent cell membranes and often have prominent glycogenated or pyknotic nuclei. Glycogen storage diseases types III, IV, and VI are the most likely to develop liver fibrosis, but fibrosis can also be seen in types I and IX.[24] The abnormal glycogen accumulation can be highlighted by PAS stains, but the diagnosis of glycogen accumulation is based on the H&E findings and not the PAS stain, as even hepatocytes in the normal liver can be strongly PAS-positive. In addition, the diagnosis of glycogen storage disease and the specific subtype cannot be established by histology alone. Instead, a diagnosis is based on the combination of clinical findings, biochemical profiles, enzyme activity assay results, histologic findings, and genetic testing.

Glycogen storage diseases

Glycogen storage disease type 0

Glycogen storage disease type 0 is due to glycogen synthase deficiency. In fact, type 0 is not a true glycogen storage disease because there is a marked decrease in liver glycogen content. Individuals with type 0 glycogen storage disease present typically in the first year of life with fasting hypoglycemia but no hepatomegaly. The liver typically shows macrovesicular steatosis with no glycogenosis. PAS stains can show diminished glycogen in hepatocytes.[25]

Glycogen storage disease types Ia/b

Type I glycogen storage disease is caused by deficiency of either glucose-6 phosphatase (type Ia) or glucose-6-phoshate translocase (type Ib). In type 1b, the defective translocase doesn't allow entry of substrate glucose-6-phosphate into the endoplasmic reticulum. Both subtypes present with hypoglycemia and hepatomegaly shortly after birth. Lactic acidosis, hyperlipidemia, hyperuricemia, and slightly elevated liver transaminase levels are common. Type Ib also has distinct features of recurrent infections, neutropenia, neutrophil dysfunction, and the development of inflammatory bowel disease resembling ulcerative colitis or Crohn's disease.[26,27] Microscopically, the hepatocytes are typically swollen with pale-staining cytoplasm, have prominent cell membranes, and have prominent glycogenated nuclei (Figs. 18.23 and 18.24).[24] Some cases will also show macrovesicular steatosis. Unusual findings including localized peliosis hepatis and Mallory body formation in the perivenular hepatocytes.[28] Portal fibrosis may be present in some cases.

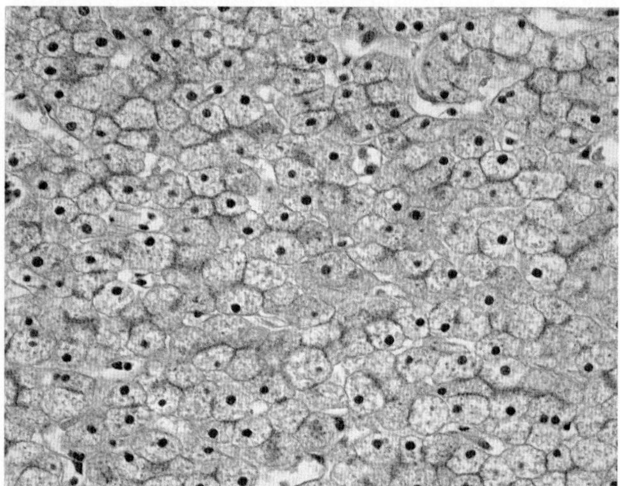

Figure 18.23 Glycogen storage disease type I. Diffusely enlarged hepatocytes with pale-staining cytoplasm and centrally located pyknotic nuclei.

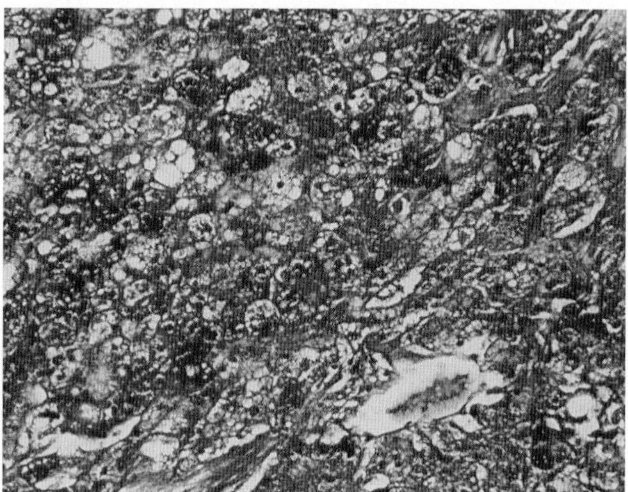

Figure 18.24 Glycogen storage disease type I. PAS stain confirming abundant glycogen.

Hepatic adenomas can develop at any age but typically occur during or after puberty, with a reported prevalence ranging from 22% to 75%.[29] Most of the adenomas are of the inflammatory subtype.[30] They can also be β-catenin activated and have a risk for malignant transformation.[31] Hepatocellular carcinoma has been reported in children younger than 1 year of age.[32]

Glycogen storage disease type II

Type II glycogen storage disease, also known as Pompe disease, is due to acid maltase deficiency. This type primarily involves the muscular system and the main clinical features are cardiomyopathy and muscular hypotonia. Although the enzyme is also deficient in the liver, hepatomegaly and hypoglycemia usually are not present. The liver typically shows marked glycogenosis with no fibrosis. Of note, electron microscopy in type II glycogen storage disease shows a distinct pattern of glycogen accumulation, with monoparticulate glycogen in enlarged lysosomes.[33]

Glycogen storage disease type III

Type III glycogen storage disease, also known as Forbes disease or Cori disease, results from a deficiency of glycogen debranching enzyme. There are four subtypes are IIIa and IIIb and the two major subtypes. Type IIIa (80% of cases) affects both the liver and muscle, whereas type IIIb (15% of cases) affects only the liver. Patients typically present with hepatomegaly, hypoglycemia, and short stature. The liver biopsy shows marked hepatocellular glycogenosis, with rarefied cytoplasm and centrally or eccentrically located pyknotic nuclei. Portal fibrosis is often present and some cases can progress to cirrhosis, increasing the risk for hepatocellular carcinoma.[34]

Glycogen storage disease type IV

Type IV glycogen storage disease, also known as Andersen disease, is caused by a deficiency of glycogen branching enzyme, leading to the accumulation of amylopectin-like polysaccharides in affected tissues. The clinical presentations vary significantly depending on which tissues develop polysaccharide accumulation. In the classic hepatic form, affected individuals present with failure to thrive and hepatosplenomegaly and the disease can rapidly progress to cirrhosis, which is often present by age 5.[35] However, a variant of type IV glycogen storage disease has been reported with liver involvement that is either nonprogressive or slowly progressive. In these cases, there is hepatosplenomegaly and mildly elevated transaminases, but there is no further progression of disease and liver enzymes may return to normal.[36]

Type IV glycogen storage disease is the only glycogen storage disease with characteristic findings under light microscopy. The hepatocytes show distinctive ground glass type inclusions (Fig. 18.25). The inclusions are PAS-positive and are commonly partially diastase resistant because they are composed of amylopectin-like material, not glycogen (Fig. 18.26). However, the PAS with diastases results will also depend on how aggressively the slide is digested. The inclusions can be digested by pectinase or amylase.[37] This cytoplasmic finding is not seen in any of the other glycogens storage diseases, but chronic hepatitis B infection (Fig. 18.27), drug induced glycogen psuedoground glass changes (Fig. 18.28), and Lafora disease (Fig. 18.29) should be excluded. The inclusions in type IV glycogen storage disease are typically found in periportal hepatocytes, but they can also be found in other zones. On ultrastructural examination, the inclusions are composed of nonmembrane bound, randomly oriented fibrillary material with abundant glycogen rosettes. Fibrosis

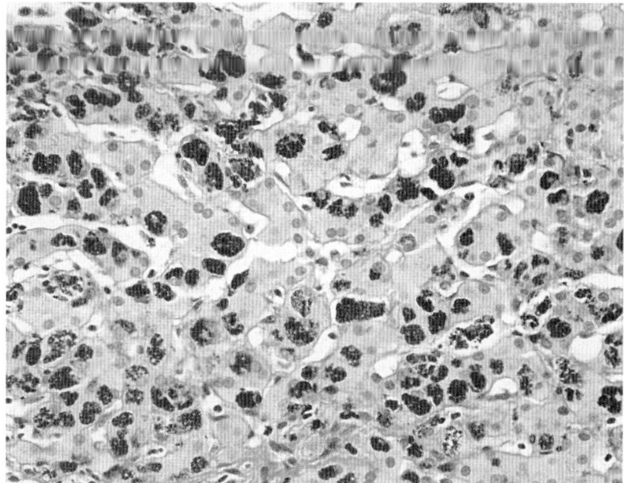

Figure 18.26 Glycogen storage disease type IV. The inclusions resistant to diastase digestion because they are composed of amylopectin-like material but not typical glycogen (PASD stain).

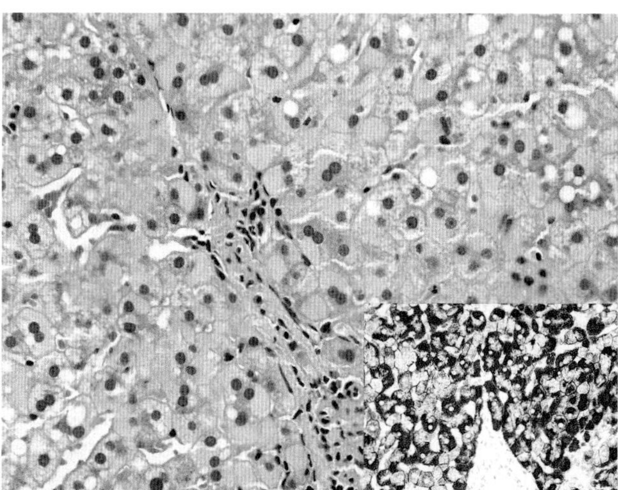

Figure 18.27 Hepatitis B ground-glass inclusions (inset showing hepatitis B surface antigen immunohistochemistry).

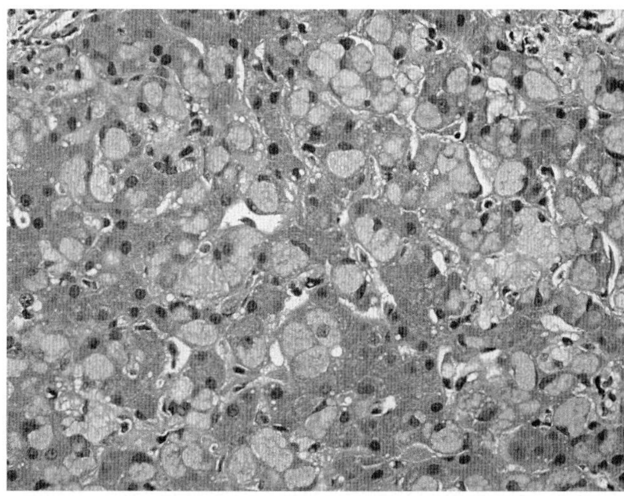

Figure 18.25 Glycogen storage disease type IV. Light eosinophilic or pale ground-glass inclusions in hepatocytes.

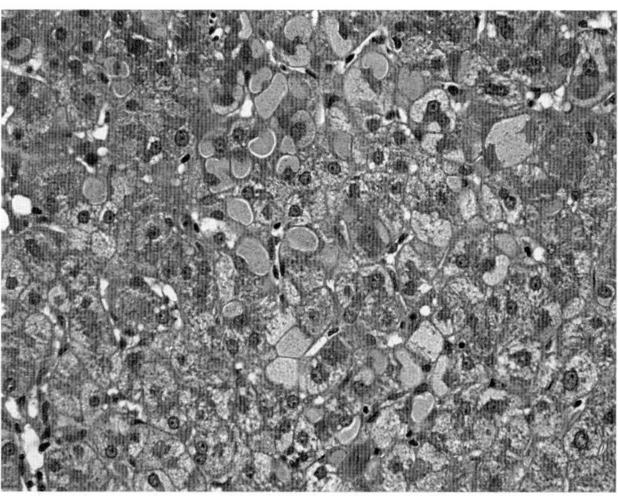

Figure 18.28 Pseudoground-glass inclusions, mimicking glycogen storage disease type IV inclusions.

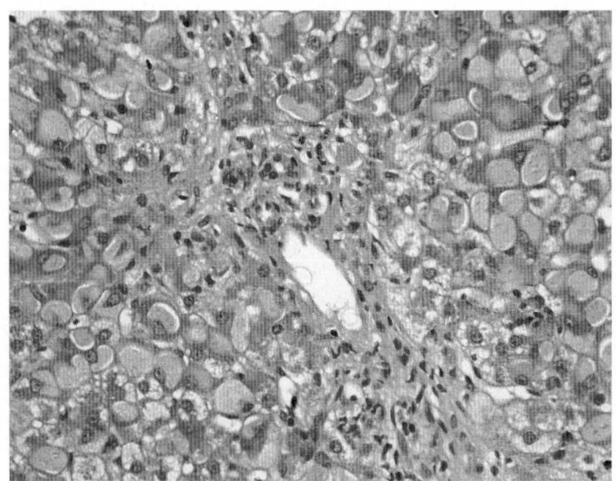

Figure 18.29 Inclusions in Lafora disease. Lafora bodies, distinct round and oval eosinophilic inclusions surrounded by a halo in periportal hepatocytes.

is common in type IV glycogen storage disease and some cases may develop cirrhosis.

Glycogen Storage Disease Type VI

Type VI glycogen storage disease, also known as Hers disease, is a rare form of glycogen storage disease caused by phosphorylase deficiency. Phosphorylase deficiency affects only the liver. Affected infants present primarily with hepatomegaly, growth retardation and mild to moderate hypoglycemia, but the clinical course is typically benign with symptom remission as children grow up.[37] The hepatocytes show glycogenosis and there may be mild steatosis, minimal inflammation, and advanced fibrosis. Electron microscopy shows less compact glycogen accumulation than other types of glycogen storage disease. Rare cases of focal nodular hyperplasia, hepatic adenomas, and hepatocellular carcinoma have been reported.[38]

Glycogen Storage Disease Type IX

Type IX glycogen storage disease is caused by a deficiency of glycogen phosphorylase kinase and can be inherited in both an autosomal recessive and X-linked pattern. Affected individuals may present with hypoglycemia, hepatomegaly, and failure to thrive in the first year of life, but the clinical course is benign and most symptoms resolve by adulthood.[39] The hepatocytes can show marked glycogenosis. Rare cases may develop fibrosis or cirrhosis.

Glycogen Storage Disease Type XI

Type XI glycogen storage disease is also known as Fanconi–Bickel syndrome and results from defective function of GLUT2, leading to impaired utilization of glucose and galactose because there is defective transport of these monosaccharides across the cell membranes. Patients usually present between the ages of 3 to 10 months with fasting hypoglycemia, postprandial hyperglycemia, proximal renal tubular dysfunction, and hypergalactosemia. Affected individuals typically have hepatomegaly (not present in all patients), marked growth retardation, and a round "moon" face. In addition, fat deposits develop in the shoulders and abdomen.[40] The liver biopsy typically shows a mixed pattern with both macrovesicular steatosis and glycogenosis.

Lafora disease

Lafora disease, also known as Lafora progressive myoclonic epilepsy, is an autosomal recessive fatal genetic disorder caused by mutations in either the *EPM2A* gene or *NHLRC1* gene, which code for the proteins laforin and malin respectively. These mutations lead to insufficiently branched glycogen, which is poorly soluble and precipitates out as polyglucosan bodies, also known as Lafora bodies.

Affected individuals present in later childhood or adolescence with seizures, myoclonus, and ataxia. They quickly progress to severe dementia. Rarely, individuals can first present with abnormal liver tests and quickly develop liver failure requiring liver transplantation.[41] Lafora bodies can be detected in the hepatocytes of asymptomatic patients, a finding that sometimes can first suggest the diagnosis. The Lafora bodies are found in hepatocytes and histologically resemble the inclusions in type IV glycogen storage disease. On H&E sections, the round or oval Lafora bodies are found in periportal hepatocytes and are seen as homogeneously eosinophilic inclusions with distinct borders, often surrounded by a halo (Figs. 18.29 and 18.30). The Lafora bodies are PAS-positive.

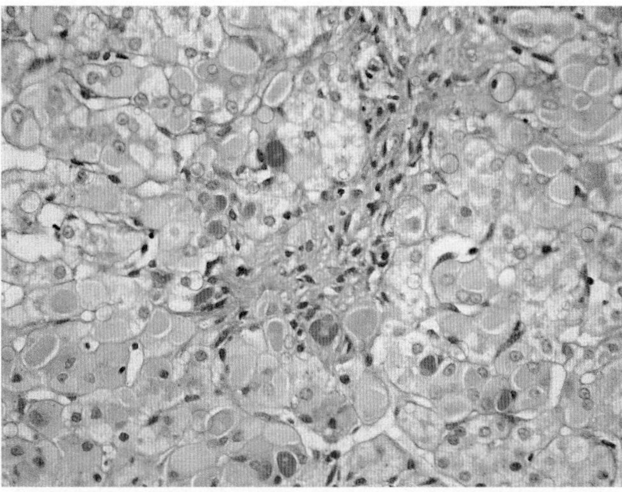

Figure 18.30 Lafora bodies partially digested by diastase (PASD stain).

They are also positive when stained with colloidal iron and Lugol iodine, whereas the inclusions in type IV glycogen storage disease are negative on colloidal iron stains. The histologic differential also includes ground-glass changes in hepatitis B and various drug reactions,[42,43] but the clinical settings are very distinct and in most cases the final diagnosis is evident based on the combined clinical and histologic findings. On electron microscopy, Lafora bodies are composed of nonmembrane bound fibrillary and granular material.

18.5 MUCOPOLYSACCHARIDOSIS

The mucopolysaccharidosis are a group of rare metabolic disorders caused by defective activity of various lysosomal enzymes that break down glycosaminoglycans, leading to abnormal accumulation of glycosaminoglycans in the liver and other tissues. Most of these diseases are inherited in an autosomal recession manner, with rare diseases inherited as X-linked disorders. There are at least eight distinct subtypes of mucopolysaccharidosis, including Hunter syndrome, Hurler syndrome, Scheie syndrome, Hurler–Scheie syndrome, Marquio syndrome, Sanfilippo syndrome, Marteauz–Lamy syndrome, and Sly syndrome. Each subtype has specific gene mutation leading to a deficiency of the corresponding lysosomal enzyme levels or activity.

The liver in affected individuals is enlarged and firm and can show a yellowish or grayish color. Microscopically, the hepatocytes can be swollen with rarified cytoplasm that resembles glycogenosis, but will be PAS weak or negative. In other cases, the hepatocytes and Kupffer cells can show numerous small- to medium-sized cytoplasmic vacuoles. Rare cases may have advanced fibrosis.

The mucopolysaccharides are often removed from the tissue by routine processing for histology, but some cases will have residual material that can be highlighted by colloidal iron stains, showing greenish-blue cytoplasmic staining.[44] If mucopolysaccharidosis is clinically suspected before the biopsy, special fixatives for the liver specimen can help preserve the glycosaminoglycans, such as Lindsay's dioxane picrate solution or adding a 10% solution of acetyl trimethylammonium bromide to the formalin fixative. Electron microscopy shows characteristic membrane-bound vacuoles in the hepatocytes and Kupffer cells.

18.6 DISORDERS OF LIPID AND LIPOPROTEIN METABOLISM

There are numerous disorders of lipid and lipoprotein metabolism and some can lead to abnormal deposits in the liver. Gaucher disease and Niemann–Pick disease are the most common of these, though the overall incidences of these disorders is rare.

Gaucher disease

Definition

Gaucher disease is the most common lysosomal storage disease and is caused by mutations in the acid β-glucosidase *(GBA)* gene, leading to accumulation of glucocerebroside in certain organs.

Clinical features

The estimated incidence of Gaucher disease is about one in 20,000 live births. There are three distinct types of Gaucher disease and each type has been linked to particular mutations of the gene *GBA*. Type I is the most common and is also called *nonneuropathic*. This type occurs mainly in Ashkenazi Jews. The main symptoms of type I Gaucher disease are splenomegaly and bone erosions. Type II Gaucher disease is characterized by neurologic problems in young children with progressive hepatosplenomegaly and mental retardation. Most affected individuals die within their childhood. Type III Gaucher disease also affects the central nervous system, but develops more slowly and most patients can survive into their early adulthood.[45]

Laboratory findings

Enzyme tests can confirm the diagnosis by measuring glucocerebrosidase activity in peripheral blood leukocytes. Testing that shows less than 15% of normal activity is diagnostic. Mild elevations of liver transaminases and alkaline phosphatase are very common.

Imaging

Imaging studies reveal significant enlargement of the spleen and liver, as well as bone abnormalities.

Gross findings

The liver is typically significantly enlarged and firm. Rare cases may progress to cirrhosis.

Microscopic findings

The histologic hallmark of Gaucher disease is the presence of Gaucher cells. Gaucher cells are histiocytes containing abundant deposits of glycocerebroside, leading to a characteristic appearance of amphophilic or faintly stained, striated, and wrinkled-paper-like cytoplasm (Fig. 18.31). The striated cytoplasm of Gaucher cells are best seen on trichrome or PAS/PASD stains

(Fig. 18.32). In the liver, Kupffer cells and macrophages in the portal tracts are affected. The hepatocytes are spared of deposits, probably because of biliary excretion of glucocerebroside and that exogenous glycolipids are mainly handled by the mononuclear phagocytes. The distribution of Gaucher cells can be zonal or focal, with zone 3 being the most affected area.[46] The cells are significantly enlarged and can measure up to 100 µm in diameter. On the other hand, the nuclei of Gaucher cells are pyknotic and either eccentrically or centrally located.

The enlarged Gaucher cells can block the movement of blood through the sinusoidal spaces. This change, along with perisinusoidal fibrosis, can result in portal hypertension. Rare cases may also progress to bridging fibrosis and cirrhosis, with extensive replacement of the liver parenchyma by Gaucher cells.[46,47]

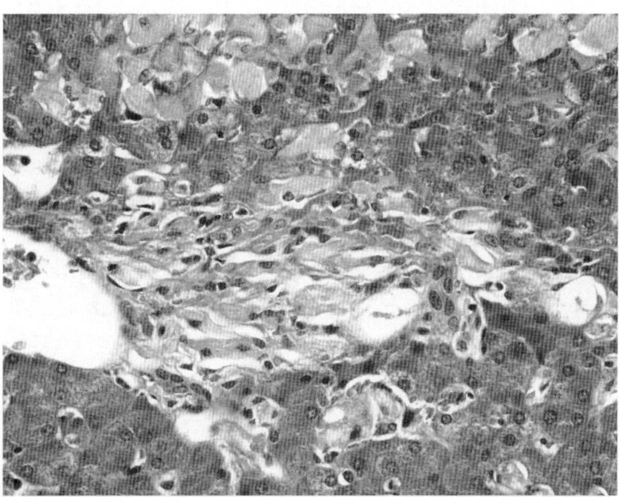

Figure 18.31 Gaucher disease. Gaucher cells in sinusoids and portal tract, showing characteristic amphophilic striated cytoplasm.

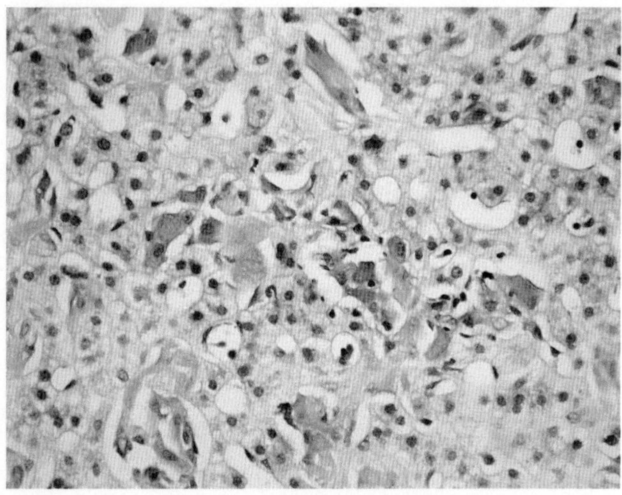

Figure 18.32 Gaucher cells (PASD stain).

Immunohistochemistry and special stains

Gaucher cells are positive for histiocytic immunomarkers such as CD68. The striated cytoplasm of Gaucher cells are best seen on trichrome or PAS/PASD stains. The phenylphosphate Mx acid phosphatase reaction can reveal markedly increased acid phosphatase activity.

Ultrastructural findings

Electron microscopy of Gaucher cells reveals a variable size and number of Gaucher bodies in the cytoplasm of Kupffer cells. The characteristic findings are spindle or rod-shaped inclusions surrounded by a limiting membrane, with internal tubular structures evident on cross section.[48]

Molecular genetic findings

Gaucher disease is inherited in an autosomal recessive manner. Six *GBA* mutations (N370S, c.84insG, L444P, IVS2+1g>a, V394L, and R496H) have been identified that account for most disease alleles. Type I Gaucher disease has been linked to homozygous N370S mutations; Type II Gaucher disease is associated with one or two L444P mutations; and Type III Gaucher disease is also because of one or two mutated alleles of L444P, but is associated with a mild phenotype, thought to reflect the presence of additional but protective polymorphisms. The mutations are usually detected using full gene sequencing, but specific mutation analysis for individual *GBA* mutations is used when mutations are known for a specific family.

Differential diagnosis

The differential diagnosis includes other storage diseases of the liver. Glycogen storage diseases affect the hepatocytes and will not have Gaucher cells (Fig. 18.25). Likewise, Lafora disease affects the hepatocytes only (Fig. 18.29). The Kupffer cells are affected in Niemann–Pick disease but have foamy or microvesicular cytoplasm (see Fig. 18.37) instead of the wrinkled-paper appearance of Gaucher cells. The macrophages in cystinosis contain brilliant, silver, birefringence cysteine crystals under polarized light (see Figs. 18.44 and 18.45). Pseudo-Gaucher cells have been observed in the liver of patients with hematologic malignancies or anemia, such as the intracellular crystal formation of paraproteins and/or immunoglobulins (usually kappa light chains) in crystal-storing histiocytosis (Figs. 18.33 and 18.34).[49] Distinguishing pseudo-Gaucher cells from true Gaucher cells may need electron microscopic examination, which will show a microfibrillary ultrastructure in pseudo-Gaucher cells and the characteristic spindle or rod-shaped inclusions with tubular structures seen

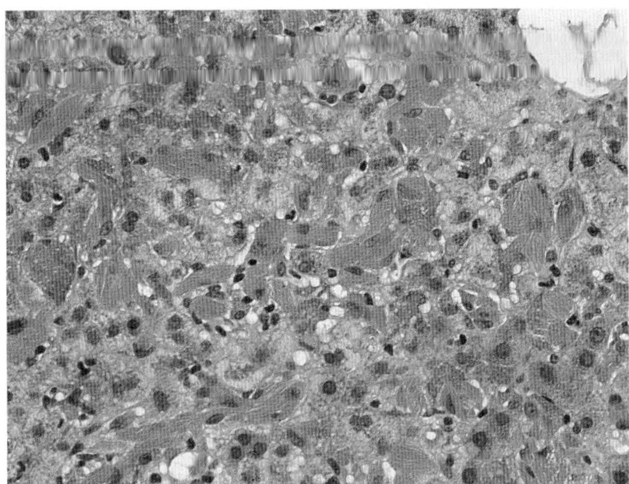

Figure 18.33 Pseudo-Gaucher cells in crystal-storing histiocytosis.

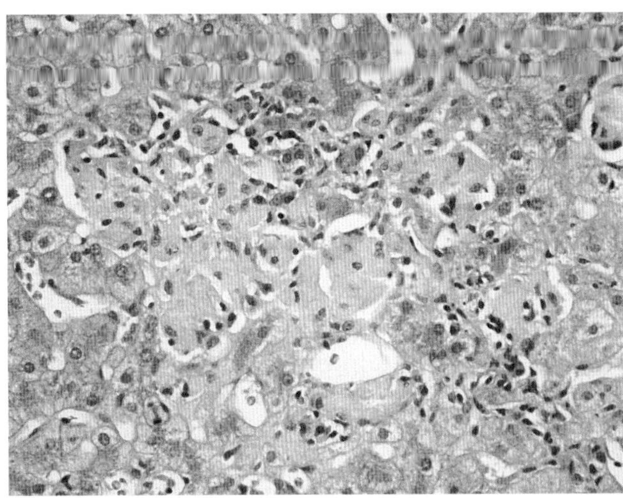

Figure 18.35 Fabry disease. Kupffer cells with pale-staining cytoplasm.

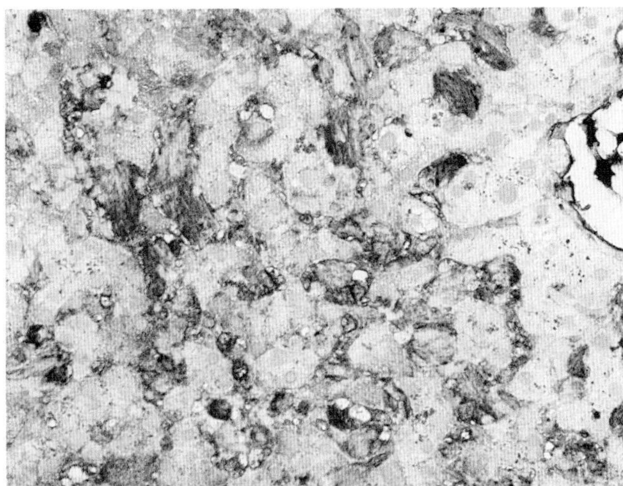

Figure 18.34 Pseudo-Gaucher cells. The accumulation of immunoglobulin kappa light chains confirmed by an immunohistochemical stain.

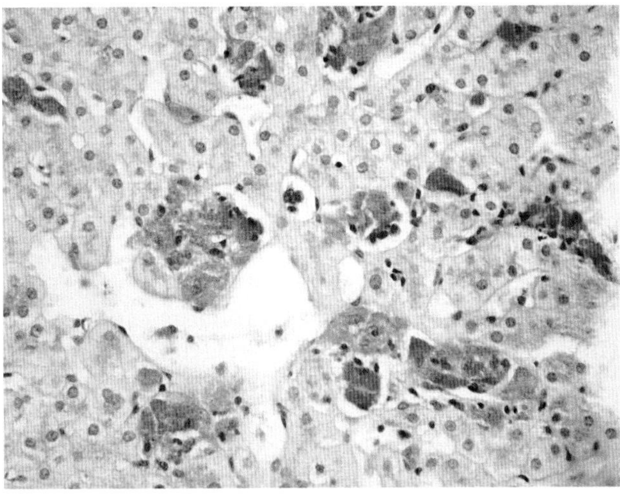

Figure 18.36 Fabry disease. Kupffer cells with granular appearance on PASD stain.

in true Gaucher cells. In Fabry disease, which is a rare X-linked inherited α-galactosidase A deficiency, accumulation of globotriaosylceramide in Kupffer cells and macrophages may mimic Gaucher cells. However, the cytoplasmic deposits in Fabry disease have a granular appearance on both H&E and PASD stains (Figs. 18.35 and 18.36), rather than striated cytoplasm of Gaucher cells.

Prognosis and treatment

Gaucher disease can be treated with enzyme replacement therapy using intravenous recombinant glucocerebrosidase, which can reduce liver and spleen size and improve skeletal abnormalities in type I and most type III Gaucher disease, but cannot improve neurologic symptoms. Glucosylceramide synthase inhibitors have been approved for treatment of adults with mild-to-moderate type I Gaucher disease for whom enzyme replacement therapy is not a therapeutic option.

Niemann–Pick disease

Definition

Niemann–Pick disease is a group of inherited severe metabolic disorders owing to a deficiency of acid sphingomyelinase, leading to sphingomyelin accumulation in lysosomes in cells (Niemann–Pick disease types A and B) and defects in cholesterol metabolism leading to the accumulation of unesterified cholesterol and other lipids in lysosomes (Niemann–Pick disease type C).

Clinical features

The estimated incidence of Niemann–Pick disease types A and B is about 1 in 250,000, whereas the incidence of Niemann–Pick disease type C is estimated to be 1 in 150,000. The classical form of the disease is Niemann–Pick disease type A, where hepatosplenomegaly develops within the first few months of life and becomes progressively massive. The disease also manifests clinically by developmental delays followed by regression, loss of motor function, deterioration of intellectual capabilities, spasticity and rigidity, and total loss of ability to interact with the environment. The clinical presentation and course in patients with Niemann–Pick disease type B disease is milder and more variable. Niemann–Pick disease type C is both genetically and clinically different from Niemann–Pick disease types A or and B, and is characterized primarily by progressive neurologic disease, but other symptoms such as hepatosplenomegaly can also be seen.

Laboratory findings

Measurement of acid sphingomyelinase activity in peripheral white blood cells or in cultured fibroblasts can confirm the diagnosis of Niemann–Pick disease types A and B. Detection of cholesterol esterification and staining for unesterified cholesterol using the Filipin test in cultured fibroblasts can confirm the diagnosis of Niemann–Pick disease type C. Liver transaminases may be elevated in some cases. Niemann–Pick disease type B typically has reduced high-density lipoprotein, elevated total cholesterol and low-density lipoprotein-cholesterol levels, and hypertriglyceridemia.

Imaging

Imaging studies usually show marked hepatomegaly. A typical reticulonodular pattern of infiltration may be seen on chest imaging.

Microscopic findings

The characteristic morphologic finding in Niemann–Pick disease is the presence of large Kupffer cells and macrophages with foamy or microvesicular cytoplasm (Fig. 18.37). These cells are less prominent in the livers of Niemann–Pick disease type C, but are more obvious in bone marrow specimens, showing sea-blue histiocytes. In the liver, the Kupffer cells show marked hyperplasia with cytoplasm containing very small vacuoles that are uniform in size, giving a mulberry-like in appearance. The Kupffer cell nuclei are generally small and either eccentrically or centrally located. The hepatocytes also contain

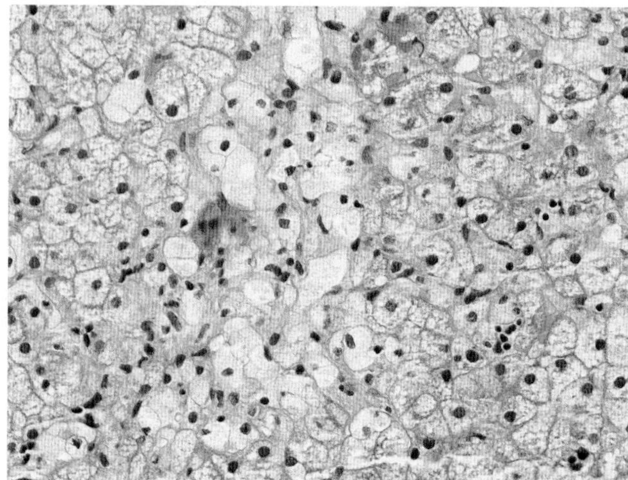

Figure 18.37 Niemann–Pick disease. Hypertrophied Kupffer cells with foamy or microvesicular cytoplasm.

sphingomyelin.[50] Their cytoplasm initially is less foamy than Kupffer cells, but eventually can become indistinguishable from Kupffer cells. Other pathologic changes include cholestasis, giant cell transformation, and atrophy of liver cells. Variable degrees of fibrosis can occur and rare cases can progress to cirrhosis.[50,51]

Immunohistochemistry and special stains

The Kupffer cells and macrophages are positive for histiocytic markers such as CD68. On frozen sections, the lipid content can be stained with Oil red O, Luxal fast blue, or Baker acid hematin stains. PAS stains can also highlight the Kupffer cells in negative relief, staining pale against the strong positivity in the background of hepatocytes (Fig. 18.38).

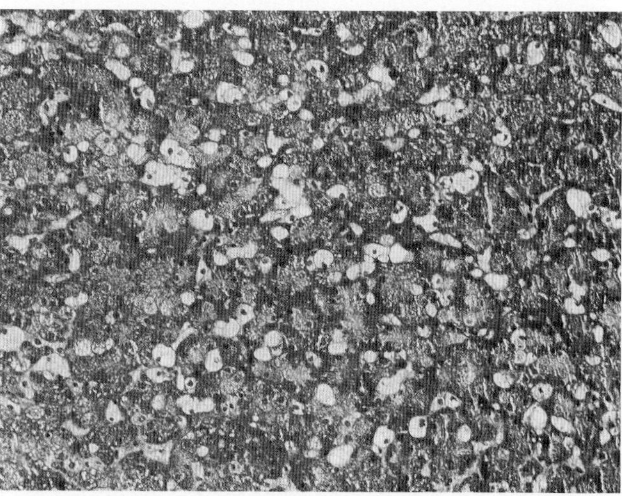

Figure 18.38 Niemann–Pick disease. Pale-stained distinct foamy histiocytes in a background of strong PAS-positive hepatocytes.

Ultrastructural findings

Electron microscopy shows that the foamy Kupffer cells have dense, lipid filled lysosomes containing centrally laminated myelin-like inclusions.

Molecular genetic findings

Niemann–Pick disease is inherited in an autosomal recessive pattern. Genetic testing such as sequencing or deletion/duplication analysis can detect four common mutations in the *SMPD1* gene for Niemann–Pick disease types A and B and mutations in *NPC1* or *NPC2* genes for Niemann–Pick disease type C.

Differential diagnosis

The differential diagnosis includes other storage diseases of liver. The foamy macrophages are not pathognomonic for Niemann–Pick disease. Histologically similar lipid-laden foamy cells can be seen in patients with Wolman disease, Xanthoma disseminatum (Fig. 18.39), cholesterol ester storage disease (Fig. 18.40), lipoprotein lipase deficiency, and some patients with GM1 gangliosidosis type 2. Gaucher cells can be readily recognized by their wrinkled-paper appearance (Fig. 18.31), in contrast to the foamy or microvesicular cytoplasm in the macrophages of Niemann–Pick disease. The macrophages in cystinosis containing cystine crystals can be recognized under polarized light, showing a brilliant silvery birefringence (see Figs. 18.44 and 18.45).

Prognosis and treatment

There are no specific treatments for Niemann–Pick disease. Type A has an extremely poor prognosis, whereas Types B and C have a better prognosis. Liver transplantation has been attempted with limited success.[52] Statins are used in Niemann–Pick disease type B to control cholesterol levels. Miglustat has been tried to treat Niemann–Pick disease type C with progressive neurologic manifestations. Enzyme replacement and gene therapy are under investigation.

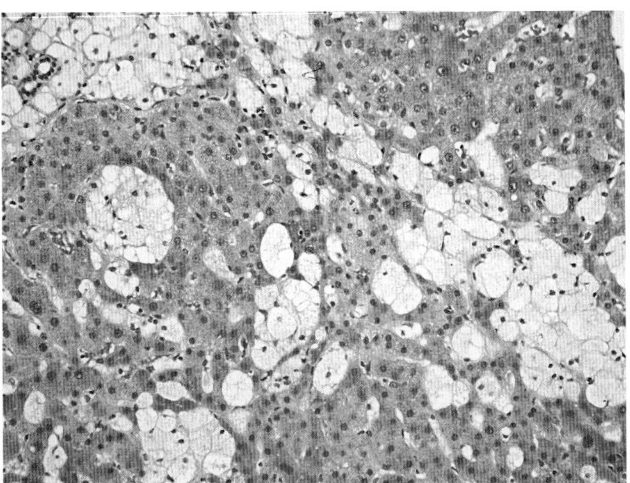

Figure 18.39 Xanthoma disseminatum. Diffuse foamy histiocytic infiltrate is indistinguishable from foamy Kupffer cells in Niemann–Pick disease.

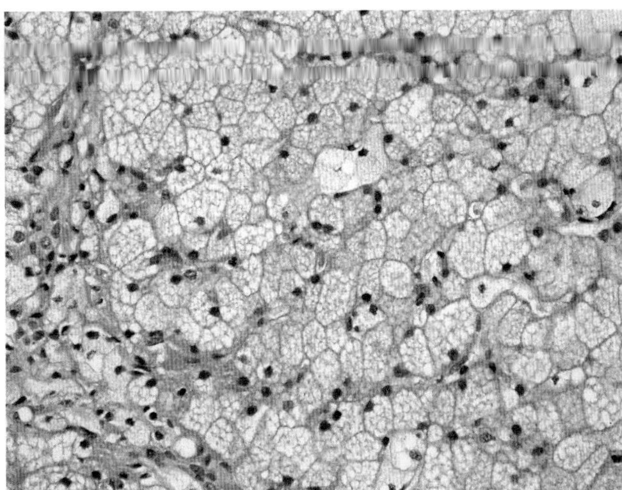

Figure 18.40 Cholesteryl ester storage disease. Hypertrophied Kupffer cells and portal macrophages with foamy cytoplasm and diffuse microvesicular steatosis in hepatocytes.

Cholesterol ester storage disease

Cholesteryl ester storage disease is an autosomal recessive lysosomal storage disorder caused by deficient lysosomal acid lipase activity owing to different mutations of the *LIPA* gene, resulting in accumulation of cholesteryl esters in the liver, spleen, and macrophages. The severe form of cholesteryl ester storage disease is known as Wolman disease in infants, in which cases the enzyme activity is very low or absent, leading to failure to thrive, malabsorption, ascites, hepatosplenomegaly and early, rapid death. The milder forms of cholesteryl ester storage disease can present at any age with hepatosplenomegaly and/or lipid retention. Liver biopsy can be diagnostic for cholesteryl ester storage disease. The characteristic histologic findings include hypertrophied Kupffer cells and portal macrophages with PASD-positive foamy cytoplasm, marked microvesicular steatosis in hepatocytes, and classic brilliant silver birefringent cholesteryl ester crystals in frozen sections (Figs. 18.40 and 18.41). Fat accumulation can also be seen in biliary epithelial and endothelial cells.[53] Fibrosis can range from mild pericellular and portal fibrosis to micronodular cirrhosis.[54] Electron microscopy shows peripheral vacuoles in Kupffer cells or large central cholesterol ester clefts. The hepatocytes contain lipid droplets and only occasional crystal clefts.[55]

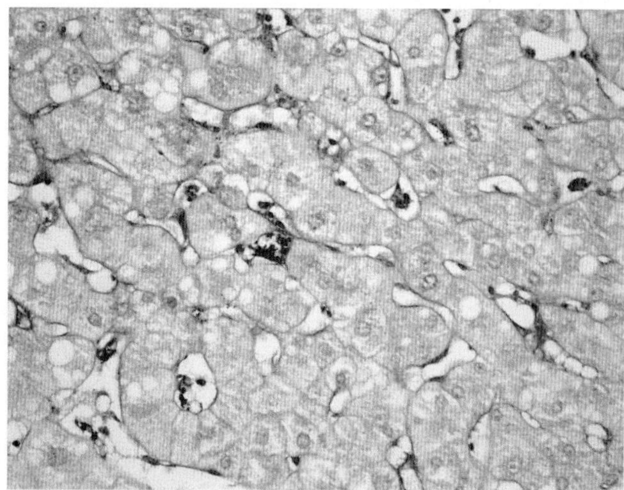

Figure 18.41 Cholesteryl ester storage disease. The foamy Kupffer cells and macrophages are PASD-positive.

18.7 DISORDERS OF AMINO ACID METABOLISM

Tyrosinemia

Definition

Hereditary tyrosinemia, often referred as type I tyrosinemia, is caused by a deficiency of fumarylacetoacetate hydrolase (FAH), an enzyme responsible for the degradation of the amino acid tyrosine, leading to accumulation of the toxic metabolite succinylacetone and resulting in liver and renal damage.

Clinical features

The estimated prevalence of hereditary tyrosinemia is about 1 in 100,000 births.[56] Affected infants usually present with failure to thrive and hepatomegaly. Some infants may have acute onset symptoms with vomiting and diarrhea and rapidly progress to bloody stools, lethargy, and jaundice. A distinctive cabbage-like odor may be appreciated. Most patients also have renal tubular defects and about a third of survivors develop hepatocellular carcinoma.[57]

Laboratory findings

Liver function tests and bilirubin levels are elevated, reflecting liver damage. α-Fetoprotein levels are also commonly increased. Quantitation of plasma amino acids shows selective increases in tyrosine and methionine levels. Urinalysis may show an alkaline pH, glycosuria, proteinuria, and generalized aminoaciduria. Normocytic anemia and leukocytosis are uniformly present in tyrosinemia.

Imaging

Imaging studies usually show hepatomegaly in early stages of the disease. Cirrhosis and hepatocellular carcinoma are common in survivors beyond 2 years old. Imaging studies often do not reliably differentiate large regenerative nodules from hepatocellular carcinoma.

Gross findings

The liver is generally firm and enlarged with a yellow color. The cirrhotic liver can show a micronodular, macronodular, or mixed pattern. In fulminate disease, the liver can be shrunken and brown.

Microscopic findings

The histopathologic changes evolve with disease progression. In early or acute onset disease, the liver typically shows vary degrees of fatty change, marked lobular cholestasis, "pseudoacinar" or "pseudoglandular" arrangement of liver cells, occasional giant cell transformation, variable sidersosis, and extramedulary hematopoiesis. The hepatocytes often show ballooning.[58] Advanced fibrosis is commonly present early on and there can small regenerative nodules, a pattern which has been referred to as the micronodular phase.[59] The fibrotic septa usually contain a bile ductular proliferation and mild chronic inflammation. In a matter of a few months, the initial micronodular cirrhosis progresses through a mixed cirrhotic pattern to the final pattern of macronodular cirrhosis (Figs. 18.42 and 18.43).[59] Variable degrees of steatosis are present within the nodules. Dysplastic nodules with low grade and high grade dysplasia are common. Some cases can be difficult to distinguish from well differentiated hepatocellular carcinoma.[60]

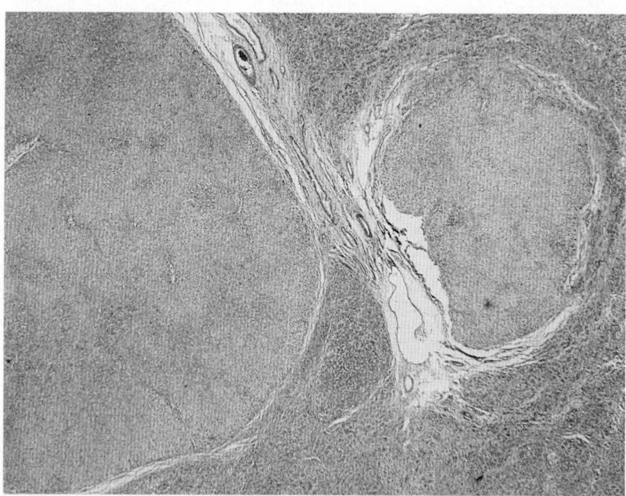

Figure 18.42 Tyrosinemia. Formation of regenerative nodules in variable sizes.

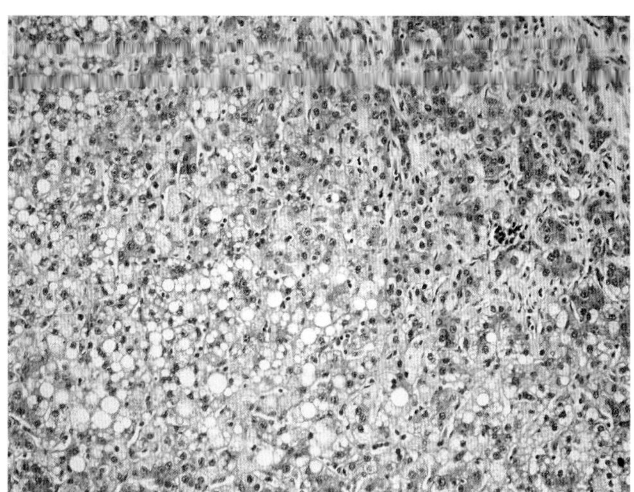

Figure 18.43 Tyrosinemia. Marked fatty changes, hepatocanalicular cholestasis, "pseudoacinar" arrangement of liver cells, and foci of extramedulary hematopoiesis.

Immunohistochemistry and special stains

Immnunostains are of limited use in diagnosing tyrosinemia. Trichrome stains reveal advanced fibrosis.

Ultrastructural findings

Electron microscopy shows nonspecific changes including fat in the hepatocytes, cholestasis, increased numbers and pleomorphic mitochondria, and enlarged peroxisomes containing small lipid droplets.

Molecular genetic findings

Tyrosinemia type 1 is an autosomal recessive disease. Sequencing of the entire coding region or deletion/duplication analysis of *FAH* gene can confirm the diagnosis.

Differential diagnosis

The overall morphologic features of tyrosinemia in infants are nonspecific. The biopsy can show a neonatal hepatitis–like pattern or hepatitis-like pattern.

Prognosis and treatment

If untreated, patients with tyrosimemia die within childhood. Currently, many patients are detected prior to clinical decompensation by newborn screening. The management incudes a low-protein diet, nitisinone, and liver transplantation.

Cystinosis

Definition

Cystinosis is a rare lysosomal storage disease characterized by the abnormal accumulation of the amino acid cysteine in different organs and tissues, especially the kidneys and eyes, leading to organ dysfunction.

Clinical findings

Cystinosis affects approximately 1 in 100,000 to 200,000 newborns. Three distinct types of cystinosis are recognized: nephropathic cystinosis, intermediate cystinosis, and ocular cystinosis. Nephropathic cystinosis is characterized by poor growth and kidney problems in infants (sometimes called renal Fanconi syndrome). Intermediate cystinosis has the same symptoms as nephropathic cystinosis, but patients present at a later age. Ocular cystinosis presents with photophobia due to cystine crystals in the cornea, with no growth impairment or kidney malfunction. Hepatomegaly is common in cystinosis. Rarely, individuals can develop cholestatic liver disease or noncirrhotic portal hypertension owing to the combination of massive crystal accumulation within Kupffer cells and sinusoidal fibrosis.[61]

Laboratory findings

Liver enzymes are usually normal in cystinosis despite the presence of hepatomegaly. Abnormal serum and urine electrolyte tests indicate renal dysfunction. The diagnosis of cystinosis can be confirmed by measuring cystine levels in polymorphonuclear leukocytes or cultured fibroblasts.

Gross findings

The liver is usually noncirrhotic, markedly enlarged, and firm owing to massive crystal accumulation within the Kuppfer cells.

Microscopic findings

There is limited data on the morphologic changes seen in liver biopsies in long-term cystinosis, being described mostly in rare case reports. However, massive accumulation of cystine, predominantly in Kupffer cells, is a characteristic finding found in all cases, along with intense sinusoidal fibrosis and hepatocyte atrophy (Fig. 18.44). The cystine crystals have a brilliant, silvery, birefringence under polarized light (Fig. 18.45). Numerous enlarged and fat-laden Ito cells have also been described. The liver shows no significant inflammation. The obstruction of the sinusoids can lead to noncirrhotic portal hypertension.[61,62] Other changes include cholestatic liver disease that can suggest sclerosing cholangitis.[63]

Immunohistochemistry and special stains

Immunostains or special stains are of limited use in diagnosing cystinosis.

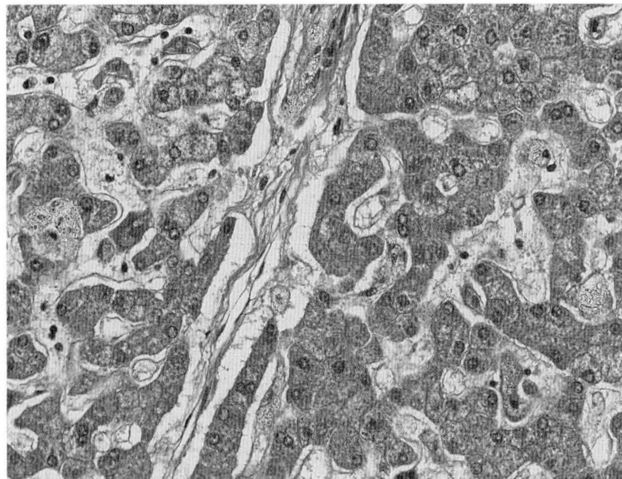

Figure 18.44 Cystinosis. Accumulation of cystine crystals in Kupffer cells.

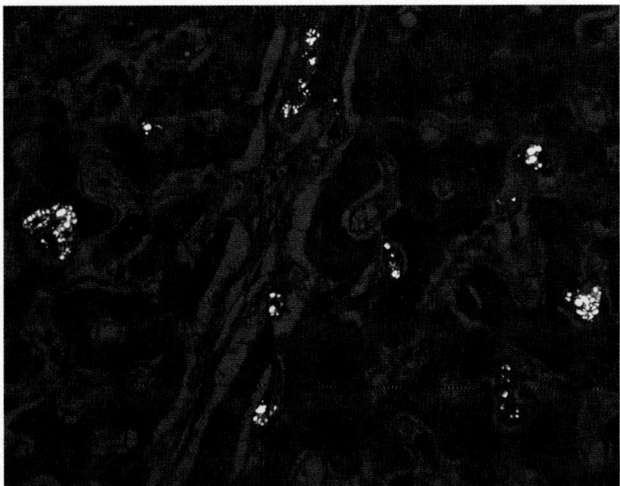

Figure 18.45 Cystinosis. Brilliant silvery birefringence of cystine crystals under polarized light.

Ultrastructural findings

Electron microscopy of the liver shows characteristic hexagonal crystalline structures in the Kupffer cells or spaces left behind after crystals dissolved during processing.

Molecular genetic findings

Cystinosis is inherited in an autosomal recessive manner and is caused by mutations in the *CTNS* gene, located on chromosome 17, which codes for cystinosin. A diagnosis of cystinosis can be confirmed by genetic testing for mutations or deletions in this gene.

Differential diagnosis

Morphologically, the differential diagnosis includes other lysosome storage disease such as Gaucher disease or Niemann–pick disease.

Prognosis and treatment

Besides symptomatic management, Cysteamine is the only drug specific for cystinosis that can slow the progression of cystinosis by removing cystine from cells. Renal transplantation is eventually required in patients with end stage renal disease.

Urea cycle disorders

The urea cycle is a series of biochemical steps in detoxification of ammonia produced by amino acid metabolism. Urea cycle disorders are caused by genetic defects of enzymes involving this pathway. Liver is the only organ expressing all six enzymes in the urea cycle, and these enzymes are: *N*-acetylglutamate synthase, carbamoyl phosphate synthetase, ornithine transcarbamylase, argininosuccinate synthetase, argininosuccinate lyase, and arginase. All the defects of these enzymes in urea cycle disorders are inherited in an autosomal recessive manner except for ornithine transcarbamylase, which is inherited in an X-linked manner and is also the most common type.[64]

Urea cycle disorders are rare, with an overall prevalence estimated at 1:35,000 newborns. Hyperammonemia and encephalopathy are the main features of affected individuals, although the age of onset and severity of clinical symptoms vary between the different types of urea cycle disorders. Neonates with a severe urea cycle disorder are normal at birth but rapidly develop cerebral edema, lethargy, anorexia, seizures, and coma. Severe urea cycle disorders are also thought to account for some cases of sudden infant death syndrome. In milder forms of urea cycle disorders, which are because of partial deficiencies of these enzymes or arginase deficiency, the clinical presentations are subtle and mild, and the first clinical episode may not occur until months or decades. The elevations of plasma ammonia concentration and symptoms are usually triggered by illness or stress. The symptoms may include vomiting, nausea, hyperactive behavior, neurologic or psychiatric abnormalities. Elevated plasma ammonia levels and abnormal blood and urine metabolites are used to diagnose urea cycle disorders, and measurement of specific enzyme activities or molecular genetic tests can establish the diagnosis.

A spectrum of histopathologic changes of liver in urea cycle disorders have been described in a number of reports, ranging from normal liver, to nonspecific changes and to cirrhosis (Fig. 18.46).[65–70] There are no specific features for a particular enzyme deficiency in urea cycle disorder. Abnormal glycogen accumulation is very common in urea cycle disorders, although some cases may be mild. The hepatocytes are swelling with appearance resembling glycogen storage diseases or glycogenic hepatopathy. It is often

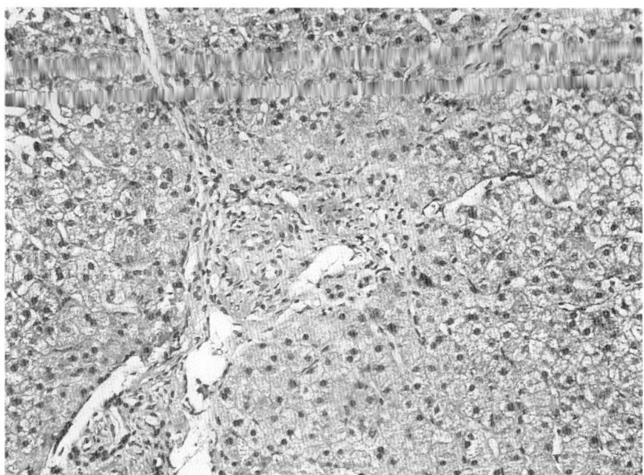

Figure 18.46 Urea cycle disorders. Liver biopsy from a 37-year-old male with carbamoyl phosphate synthetase deficiency showing minimal changes and mild portal fibrosis.

accompanied by megamitochondria and nuclear glycogenation. Other changes including steatosis, cholestasis, mild inflammation, focal necrosis, or nodular regenerative hyperplasia are also observed. Fibrosis is variable and progresses slowly. Most cases typically present with portal fibrosis, and the late onset cases may develop thin septal fibrosis.[68] Established cirrhosis rarely occurs, especially in individuals with argininosuccinate synthetase 1 or argininosuccinate lyase deficiencies.[69,70] Of note, hepatocellular carcinoma has been associated with urea cycle disorders in adults without cirrhosis.[71]

18.8 DISORDERS OF PORPHYRIN METABOLISM

The porphyrias are a group of rare diseases caused by a deficiency of the enzymes that metabolize porphyrin, leading to excessive accumulation of porphyrin and its precursors. Two disorders of porphyrin metabolism affecting the liver are discussed in this section: porphyria cutanea tarda and erythropoietic protoporphyria.

Porphyria cutanea tarda

Definition

Porphyria cutanea tarda is the most common subtype of the porphyritic diseases and results from mutations in the *UROD* gene, which in turn leads to deficiency of the heme synthetic enzyme uroporphyrinogen decarboxylase. The lack of this enzyme results in skin sensitivity to sunlight and liver enzyme abnormalities.

Clinical features

The estimated prevalence of porphyria cutanea tarda is about 1 in 10,000. Approximately 80% of all cases of porphyria cutanea tarda are sporadic and 20% are familial. Familial cases of porphyria cutanea tarda that result from heterozygous *UROD* gene mutations may remain latent or have mild manifestations in adults, but individuals with homozygous mutations or those with compound heterozygous mutations can have severe symptoms that begin in early childhood, leading to the clinical condition known as hepatoerythropoietic porphyria. The main symptoms are skin erosions and blisters after sunlight exposure, which results from increased mechanical fragility. Liver enzyme abnormalities are common but usually mild. The liver disease becomes active after exposure to environmental or infectious agents or when there is coexisting conditions such as iron overload, ethanol intake, or hepatitis C infection. A few patients may progress to cirrhosis and some of these will develop hepatocellular carcinoma.

Laboratory findings

Patients with porphyria cutanea tarda have high levels of uroporphyrinogen in the urine. High levels of porphyrins can also be found in serum or plasma. The fecal coproporphyrin fraction is often elevated. Uroporphyrinogen decarboxylase enzyme activity can be measured in red blood cells and this can both help to confirm the diagnosis and determine patterns of inheritance in familial cases. Because porphyria cutanea tarda is often triggered by viral hepatitis or hemochromatosis, a thorough evaluation of hematologic and iron profiles and screening for hepatitis virus is required in all new diagnoses of porphyria cutanea tarda.

Imaging

Imaging studies can show hepatomegaly, advanced fibrosis or cirrhosis, or hepatocellular carcinoma in patients with long-standing disease.

Gross findings

The liver is generally enlarged and may have patchy gray discoloration (Fig. 18.47). Cirrhosis and hepatocellular carcinoma can be seen in patients with long-standing disease.

Microscopic findings

The characteristic histologic finding is the needle-shaped crystals with variable lengths owning to the accumulation of uroporphyrin in the cytoplasm of hepatocytes a finding believed to be unique to porphyria cutanea tarda. The crystals show red autofluorescence and are

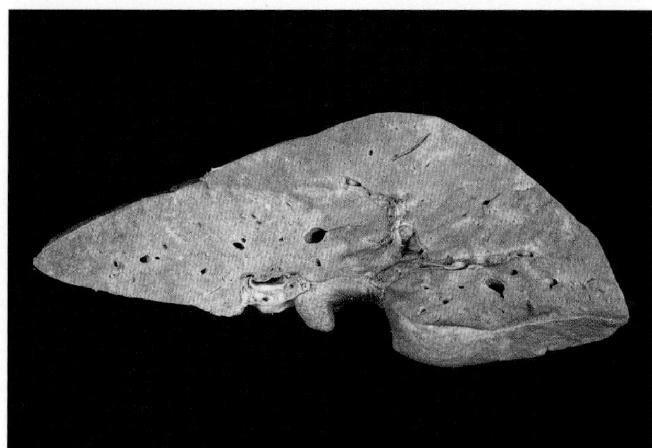

Figure 18.47 Porphyria cutanea tarda. Liver explant of Porphyria cutanea tarda showing enlargement and patchy gray discoloration and vague nodularity.

birefringent under polarized light. It is not easy to identify the crystals on route histologic examination. One study demonstrated that the crystals are best seen by light microscopy in unstained paraffin sections because the crystals can be removed during tissue staining (Fig. 18.48).[72] The liver pathology generally shows nonspecific reactive changes including mild steatosis, focal hepatocyte necrosis with ceroid-laden macrophage, and periductal lymphocyte aggregates. Iron overload is very common and most cases show mild to moderate hepatic siderosis with a zone 1 pattern. Of note, over 20% of individuals with porphyria cutanea tarda will also have homozygous or compound heterozygous mutations in the *HFE* gene. In these cases, iron overload can be much more dramatic.[73] In addition, up to 50% of cases will have coexisting hepatitis B or hepatitis C infection and the biopsies will also show changes of chronic hepatitis.[74] Overall, a third of patients with porphyria cutanea tarda will eventually progress to cirrhosis[72] and a subset of these will develop hepatocellular carcinoma. Individuals with porphyria cutanea tarda plus an additional coexisting disease are at the highest risk for cirrhosis and carcinoma.

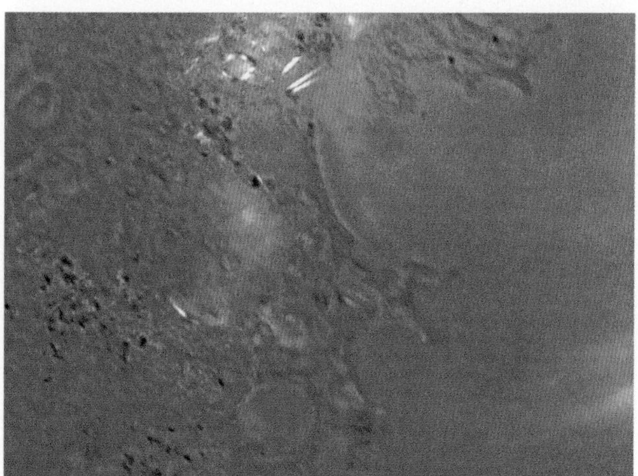

Figure 18.48 Porphyria cutanea tarda. Needle-shaped crystal in the hepatocytes, revealed on unstained slide with polarized light (×1,000). Note the brownish iron pigments in the background.

Immunohistochemistry and special stains

Immunohistochemistry is of limited use in porphyria cutanea tarda. The ferric ferricyanide reduction test is reported to stain the crystals when using unstained paraffin sections.[75] Perls iron stains are useful to evaluate for iron overload.

Ultrastructural findings

Electron microscopy can show needle-shaped crystals with alternating areas of differing electron density.

Molecular genetic findings

Mutation analysis of *UROD* gene is the standard for diagnosis of familial porphyria cutanea tarda. *HFE* genetic testing should also be considered, especially when there is significant iron overload.

Differential diagnosis

The differential diagnosis includes other types of crystal inclusions in the liver, but the needle-shaped intracytoplasmic crystals are unique for porphyria cutanea tarda, though they are difficult to be revealed. Although the crystals can help establish a diagnosis of porphyria cutanea tarda, the histologic findings do not distinguish familial cases from sporadic cases. Familial porphyria cutanea tarda generally shows significantly higher amount of uroporphyrin crystals than sporadic porphyria cutanea tarda.[76] The crystals can be easily missed in cases with heavy iron overload.

Prognosis and treatment

The treatment of porphyria cutanea tarda is directed to specific symptoms, including patient education to avoid sunlight, alcohol use, and estrogen use. Therapeutic phlebotomy is the standard treatment to reduce iron and porphyrin levels in the liver. Complete remission may be achieved but relapse is still possible.

Erythropoietic protoporphyria

Definition

Erythropoietic protoporphyria is a form of porphyria that results from a deficiency of ferrochelatase, which is caused by mutations of the *FECH* gene.

Clinical features

Erythropoietic protoporphyria is a rare disease, with an estimated prevalence of 1 in 75,000 to 1 in 200,000. Disease results from the accumulation of high levels of protoporphyrin in the erythrocytes, plasma, skin, and liver. The first presentation in childhood is commonly with acute photosensitivity of the skin. Liver disease results from the accumulation of insoluble protoporphyrin in the bile canaliculi and occurs in about 5% to 20% of patients. In some cases, the liver disease can progress to cirrhosis. Patients can also develop cholelithiasis.

Laboratory findings

A diagnosis can be supported by finding increased levels of protoporphyrin in the feces and demonstrating an excess of free protoporphyrin in erythrocytes. Mildly abnormal liver enzyme tests are relatively common. In rare cases, patients may have acute liver failure with significantly abnormal liver tests.

Imaging

Imaging studies may reveal cholelithiasis and cirrhosis for end stage cases.

Gross findings

Macroscopically, the liver usually has a black color that results from diffuse protoporphyrin deposits (Fig. 18.49). Under Wood's lamp, the liver shows a red fluorescence due to protoporphyrin.

Microscopic findings

Liver biopsies in cases of erythropoietic protoporphyria show protoporphyrin deposits, which are seen as a brown pigment within the bile canaliculi, Kupffer cells, and portal macrophages (Fig. 18.50). Using polarized light, the pigment will show the characteristic red to orange Maltese cross shape of birefringent crystalline deposits (Fig. 18.51). Variable amounts of fibrosis can be observed.[77,78] Inflammation is typically absent to mild.

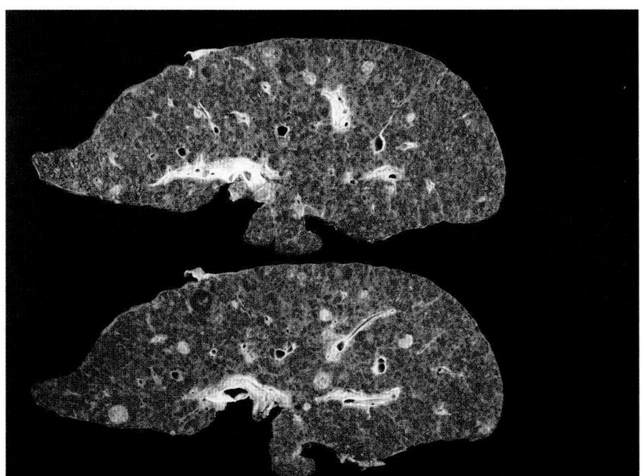

Figure 18.49 Erythropoietic protoporphyria. Liver explant with patchy black discoloration, cirrhosis, and many macroregenerative nodules.

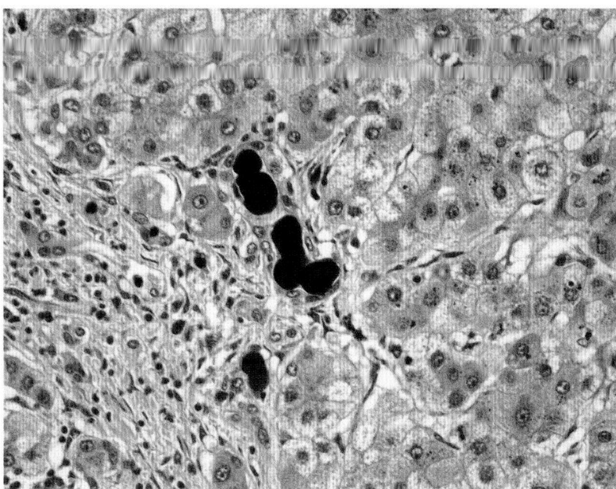

Figure 18.50 Erythropoietic protoporphyria. Brown protoporphyrin deposits in biliary canaliculi, bile ductules, hepatocytes, and macrophage cells.

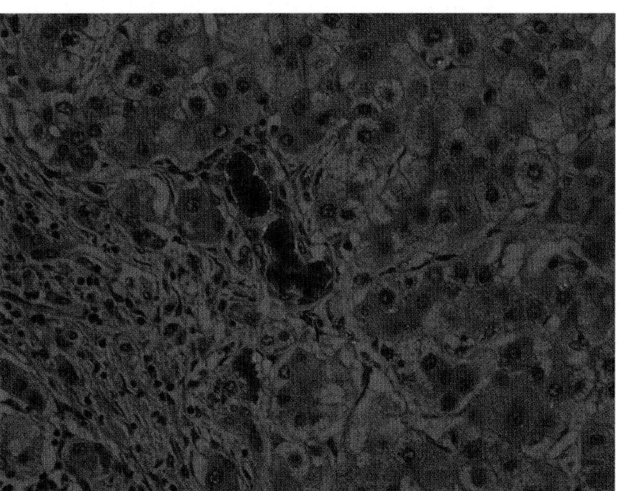

Figure 18.51 Erythropoietic protoporphyria. Characteristic red to orange Maltese cross shape of birefringent crystalline pigment deposits under polarized light.

Immunohistochemistry and special stains

Immunostains or special stains are of limited use in diagnosing erythropoietic protoporphyria.

Ultrastructural findings

Electron microscopy shows characteristic crystal-containing vacuoles.[77] The crystals can be arranged in a "star-burst."

Molecular genetic findings

Genetic testing can detect mutations in the *FECH* gene, which encodes the enzyme ferrochelatase. About 96% of affected individuals are compound heterozygotes, while the remaining 4% of families have two loss-of-function *FECH* mutations.

Differential diagnosis

Other pigments in liver biopsy specimens can potentially mimic protoporphyrin deposits, such as bile, but the characteristic red to orange Maltese cross pattern of birefringent crystalline under polarized light is unique for erythropoietic protoporphyria.

Prognosis and treatment

There is no cure for erythropoietic protoporphyria. Symptoms can usually be managed by limiting exposure to daytime sun and fluorescent lights. Several nonsurgical therapies have been adopted to protect the liver and to prevent progressive hepatocellular fibrosis. However, none of these treatments have unequivocally proven to be effective. Liver transplantation is necessary for end stage liver disease. Of note, erythropoietic protoporphyria liver disease can reoccur in the allograft because liver transplantation does not correct the constitutional deficiency of ferrochelatase.

18.9 DISORDERS OF MITOCHONDRIA

Genetic disorders of mitochondria can be caused by either mutations in the mitochondrial DNA (mtDNA) or mutations in genes located in nuclear DNA that encode mitochondrial proteins. Most mutations lead to dysfunction of the mitochondrial respiratory chain. Mutations in mtDNA are either sporadic or familial. When familial, they are exclusively maternally inherited, as mtDNA is largely acquired from the egg and not the sperm during fertilization. In contrast, mutations in nuclear DNA are autosomally inherited.[79]

Mitochondrial diseases can be classified in various ways, for example according to the clinical presentations or based on whether the mutations are in mtDNA or nuclear DNA. However, they remain a clinically heterogeneous group of diseases and the correlation between genotype and phenotype is poor. Affected individuals may have a very wide range of clinical presentations, often with confusing signs and symptoms. Neurologic symptoms are common, including encephalopathy, seizures, dementia, migraines, stroke-like episodes, ataxia, and spasticity. Other findings can include myopathy and exercise intolerance, cardiomyopathy, deafness, optic atrophy, and diabetes mellitus. Diagnosing mitochondrial diseases is very challenging and patients with complex neurologic symptoms or progressive multisystem disorders should be evaluated for a mitochondrial disorder, including physical and neurologic examination, family history, biochemical and histologic findings, and molecular genetic testing. The treatment for mitochondrial diseases is still very limited, being primarily focused on supportive care and prevention of complications.

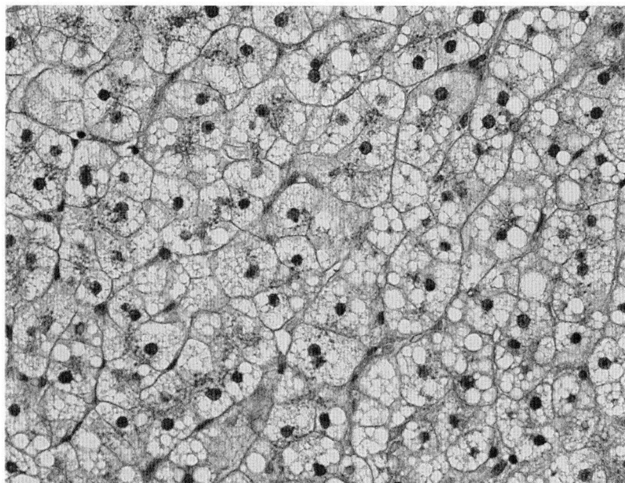

Figure 18.52 Mitochondrial hepatopathy. Diffuse microvesicuclar steatosis.

A subset of the mitochondrial diseases involves the liver. In these cases, the clinical presentations can include neonatal acute liver failure, cholestasis, lactic acidosis, chronic liver failure, and cirrhosis.[80] Histologically, the liver typically show diffuse microvesicuclar steatosis (Fig. 18.52), along with variable degrees of hepatocyte ballooning, cholestasis, and bile ductular proliferation.[81–83] Other findings include increased hepatocellular iron deposition, oncocytic changes of the hepatocytes owing to increased numbers of mitochondria, or adenoma-like nodules in a noncirrhotic liver. Fibrosis can develop and may progress to micronodular cirrhosis. Hepatocellular carcinomas have also been reported in livers that progress to cirrhosis.[83]

18.10 DISORDERS OF BILE ACID METABOLISM

Bile acids are synthesized by hepatocytes and play a key role in excretion of bile, assisting in the absorption of fat and fat soluble vitamins in the small intestine, and regulating lipid, cholesterol, glucose, and energy homeostasis.[84] Primary bile acid synthesis disorders are a group of rare metabolic disorders caused by congenital deficiencies of enzymes important for synthesizing two key bile acids known as cholic acid and chenodeoxycholic acid. At least nine defects have been described in the literatures, including Δ4-3-oxosteroid-5β-reductase deficiency, 7α-hydroxylase deficiency, 3β-hydroxy-Δ5-C27-steroid dehydrogenase deficiency, sterol 27-hydroxylase deficiency, α-methylacyl-CoA racemase deficiency, and Zellweger syndrome.[83]

The diagnosis of a primary bile acid synthesis disorder is established by analyses of serum, urine, or bile using methods such as fast atom bombardment, electrospray ionization tandem, or gas chromatography-mass spectrometry. In some cases, genetic testing can also identify mutations in specific genes, confirming a diagnosis of primary bile acid synthesis disorder. Affected individuals usually present with a neonatal cholestasis pattern of injury, but with normal GGT levels and normal or low serum bile acid concentrations. The age of onset, clinical presentations, and rate of progression can vary greatly with the underlying specific defect. Primary bile acid synthesis disorders should be suspected in infants or young children who have jaundice or cholestatic liver disease with an unknown cause, or who have fat soluble vitamin deficiencies and growth failure. Early diagnosis is important, because the majority of patients respond well to bile acid replacement therapy. Individuals who do not respond can progress to cirrhosis and liver transplantation may be required.

Liver biopsies are frequently performed to evaluate for neonatal cholestasis. There are no specific morphologic features that can make the diagnosis of primary bile acid synthesis disorders. Instead, the liver usually shows nonspecific neonatal hepatitis with giant cell transformation, marked lobular cholestasis, bile plugs, pseudoacinar transformation, and extramedullary hematopoiesis (Fig. 18.53).[86] The hepatocytes may show ballooning and feathery degeneration because of the cholate stasis. The portal tracts can show mild to moderate nonspecific inflammation. There may be mild bile ductular proliferation, but should be no paucity of interlobular bile ducts. Variable degrees of fibrosis can be present and may progress to cirrhosis if there is no response to treatment. The differential diagnosis includes other causes of neonatal hepatitis or cholestatic liver disease, but the normal GGT levels can provide a helpful clue to the possible diagnosis of a primary bile acid synthesis disorder.

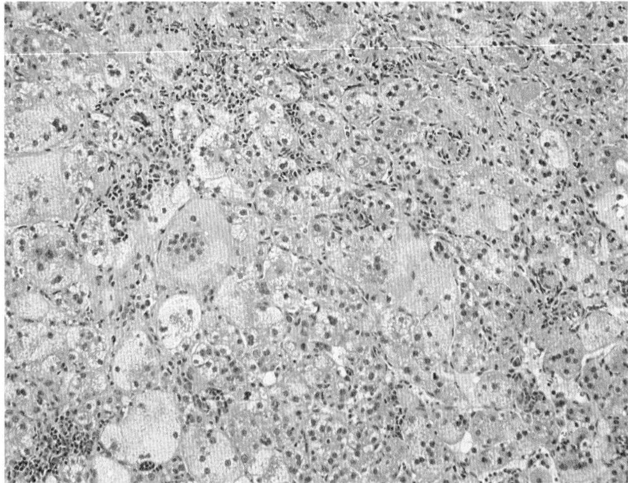

Figure 18.53 Δ4-3-oxosteroid-5β-reductase deficiency. The liver shows nonspecific neonatal hepatitis with giant cell transformation, cholestasis, pseudoacinar transformation, and extramedullary hematopoiesis.

18.11 DISORDERS OF BILIRUBIN METABOLISM

Inherited disorders of bilirubin metabolism, also referred as hereditary hyperbilirubinemia, are caused by defective bilirubin transport or conjugation by the hepatocytes. Affected individuals usually present with asymptomatic jaundice and elevated unconjugated or conjugated serum bilirubin levels.

Dubin–Johnson syndrome

Dubin–Johnson syndrome is a rare autosomal recessive disorder caused by impairment of bilirubin secretions that results from mutations in the canalicular multispecific organic anion transporter (*cMOAT*) gene, also called the multidrug resistance protein 2 (*MRP2*) or *ABCC2*.[87] Dubin–Johnson syndrome is characterized by nonpruritic jaundice associated with conjugated hyperbilirubinemia, normal liver transaminases, a unique pattern of urinary excretion of coproporphyrins, and pigment deposition in liver.[88] The total bilirubin serum levels are usually in the range of 2 to 5 mg/dL, but may go as high as 25 mg/dL. The diagnosis of Dubin–Johnson syndrome can be confirmed by demonstrating the unique pattern of urinary excretion of coproporphyrins. The total level of coproporphyrins in urine is normal, but the ratio of coproporphyrin I to coproporphyrin III is increased, with isomer I $>$ 80% in affected patients (normally 25%). Dubin–Johnson syndrome is a benign disorder and does not require any specific treatment.

The liver in Dubin–Johnson syndrome is characterized by a diffuse deposition of coarsely granular dark brown pigment in the hepatocytes, usually most prominent in zone 3 (Fig. 18.54). The pigments are composed of polymers of epinephrine metabolites,[89] but not bile. The liver appears gray to almost black grossly. The pigments have melanin-like features and are positive on Fontana–Masson stain (Fig. 18.55) and variably positive on PAS stain. The degree of pigment deposition can range considerably. In addition, the pigments can also disappear in certain situations, such as acute viral

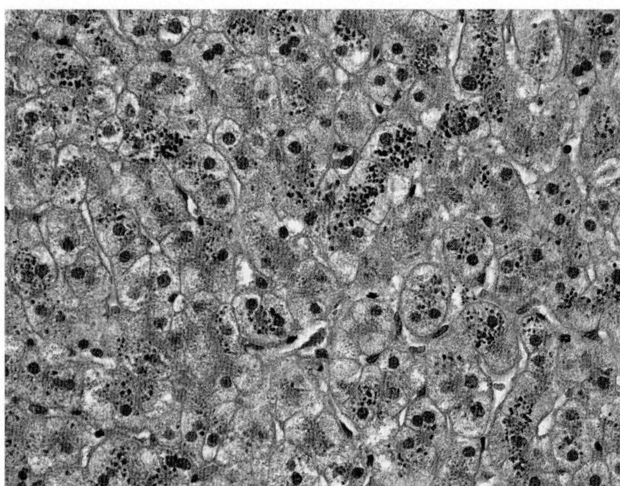

Figure 18.54 Dubin–Johnson syndrome. Diffuse deposition of coarsely granular dark brown pigments in liver cells.

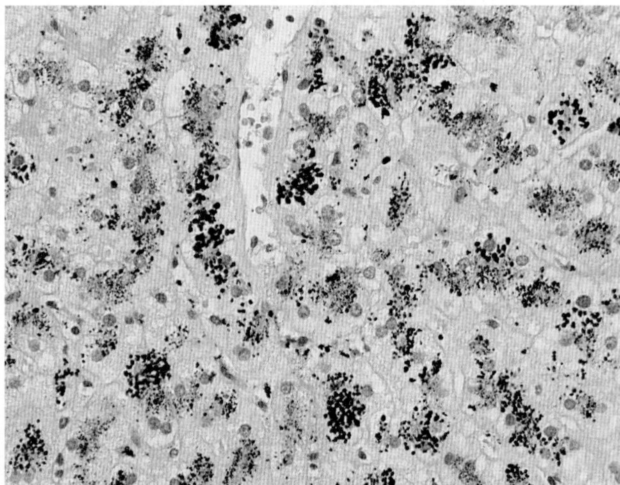

Figure 18.55 Dubin–Johnson syndrome. The pigments positive on Fontana–Masson stain.

hepatitis, but they will slowly reaccumulate once the acute injury has resolved.[90] The Kupffer cells can also show hyperplasia and contain pigments that originated from dying hepatocytes. Outside of the pigment deposition, the liver in Dubin–Johnson syndrome typically does not show other significant morphologic changes. Of note, lipofuscin on liver biopsy, even when heavy, should not be the sole basis for diagnosing Dubin–Johnson syndrome, as there can be significant histologic overlap with other causes of lipofuscin deposits.

Crigler–Najjar syndrome and Gilbert syndrome

Both the Crigler–Najjar syndrome and the Gilbert syndrome are characterized by unconjugated hyperbilirubinemia, both of which result from defects in bilirubin conjugation because of genetic alterations of the uridine diphosphate-glucuronosyl transferase 1A1 gene (*UGT1A1*).[91] Both syndromes are inherited in an autosomal recessive manner. A single normal *UGT1A1* allele is sufficient to maintain a normal plasma bilirubin concentration, so heterozygotes do not have disease.

Affected individuals can present with either a severe form known as type I Crigler–Najjar syndrome or with milder forms known as Gilbert syndrome and type II Crigler–Najjar syndrome. In type I Crigler–Najjar syndrome, UGT1A1 enzyme activity is completely or nearly completely lost and the serum bilirubin levels range from 20 to 50 mg/dL. Jaundice is present from the first days of life and the risk of kernicterus is very high, which can lead to death. Liver transplantation is currently the only cure.

In Crigler–Najjar syndrome type II, UGT1A1 enzyme activity is <10% of normal, but the activity can be induced by lifelong phenobarbital therapy. The serum bilirubin levels are lower than type I, ranging from 7 to 20 mg/dL. The clinical course is generally benign, although bilirubin-induced brain damage can occur in rare cases. Gilbert syndrome is the most common genetic bilirubin disorder with an estimated incidence of 3% to 10% of the population. There are more than100 *UGT1A1* mutations that can lead to Gilbert syndrome. The most common genetic change is the addition of an extra dinucleotide sequence, TA, to the promoter TATA box of *UGT1A1*. The UGT1A1 enzyme activity is about 20% to 30% of normal and the only abnormal finding is mild elevations of the serum bilirubin levels, ranging from 1 to 5 mg/dL. Gilbert syndrome is a benign condition and no specific treatment is necessary.

In Crigler–Najjar syndrome type I, the liver typically shows lobular cholestasis without other changes. The lobular cholestasis can range considerably and in some cases the liver can appear essentially normal.[92] In contrast, the liver often looks essentially normal in Gilbert syndrome and type II Crigler–Najjar syndrome. There can be minimal nonspecific inflammation in the portal tracts and lobules. Increased lipofuscin pigments in zone 3 hepatocytes is seen in about 1/3 of biopsies in patients with Gilbert syndrome.[93] However, when individuals with Gilbert syndrome or type II Crigler–Najjar syndrome have other illnesses, such as infections, hemolysis, or medication induced liver injury, then the lobules can also show cholestasis. An immunohistochemical staining for UGT can detect decreased expression level of the enzyme in hepatocytes, but is not widely available.[94]

Rotor syndrome

Rotor syndrome is caused by reductions of bilirubin reuptake by hepatocytes and removed from the body owing to mutations in both *SLCO1B1* and *SLCO1B3* genes, which lead to proteins that are abnormally short, nonfunctional, or absent. These proteins are known as organic anion transporting polypeptides 1B1 and 1B3 (OATP1B1 and OATP1B3).[95,96] Rotor syndrome shares many clinical features with Dubin–Johnson syndrome such as nonitching jaundice and elevation of conjugated bilirubin, but the liver has no pigments or other obvious morphologic abnormalities.

18.12 OTHER GENETIC DISORDERS

Cystic fibrosis

Definition

Cystic fibrosis is a genetic disorder caused by the mutations of the gene cystic fibrosis transmembrane conductance regulator (*CFTR*), leading to thickened secretions that affect mostly the lungs but also the pancreas, liver, kidney, and intestine.

Clinical features

Cystic fibrosis is most common among individuals of Northern European ancestry and affects about one out of every 3,000 newborns, with about one in 25 people being carriers of one mutated allele.[97] The symptoms and severity of cystic fibrosis can vary. Some individuals have serious problems from birth, while others only have mild symptoms that don't lead to medical presentation until they grow up. Affected children present mainly with salty-tasting skin, poor growth and poor weight gain, bowel obstruction due to meconium ileus, exocrine and endocrine pancreatic dysfunction, and accumulation of thick, sticky mucus leading to frequent lung infections. Males can be infertile owing to congenital absence of the vas deferens.

Liver involvement is common in cystic fibrosis. In fact, liver disease is considered the third most common cause of death in cystic fibrosis patients, after lung disease and complications related to organ transplantation.[98] The clinical manifestations of liver disease varies but can include neonatal cholestasis, cholelithiasis, isolated elevation of liver enzymes, hepatic steatosis, hepatic fibrosis, focal or multilobular cirrhosis with or without portal hypertension. Only a small number of patients develop cirrhosis, but certain mutations have been linked to a higher risk of progressing to end-stage liver disease.[99]

Laboratory findings

The sweat chloride test is a standard test used to diagnose cystic fibrosis. If sweat chloride concentration is 60 mmol/L or greater, cystic fibrosis can be diagnosed; a result between 40 to 59 mmol/L is equivocal and further testing is required.

Intermittently elevated liver enzyme levels are common in cystic fibrosis but the levels do not always correlate well with the severity of the liver injury. Transient elevation of liver enzymes may be seen during pulmonary exacerbation, hypoxemia, and antibiotic treatment. Chronic elevations of GGT and alkaline phosphatase are more common because of obstructive biliary disease. Liver disease should be suspected if any liver enzyme is more than 1.5 times the upper limit of normal on two occasions measured at least six months apart.[100]

Imaging

Ultrasonography with Doppler is commonly used to evaluate for liver disease and can demonstrate hepatosplenomegaly, cholelithiasis, diffuse fatty change, cirrhosis, and microgallbladder. MRI and MRCP are useful in detecting pancreatobiliary abnormalities, including cholelithiasis, strictures, and/or dilatation of the intra- and extrahepatic bile ducts.

Gross findings

The liver may show focal biliary cirrhosis, which is characterized by focal areas of scarring with fine nodularity interspersed between normal liver parenchyma. In time, full cirrhosis can develop, usually with a macronodular pattern.

Microscopic findings

Hepatic steatosis is the most common finding in cystic fibrosis. The steatosis is macrovesicular and can range from mild to marked. The steatosis is believed to be multifactorial, resulting from malnutrition, essential fatty acid deficiency, and oxidative stress. Steatohepatitis can be seen but is uncommon. In some cases, the portal veins can appear atrophic or even missing and there can be an associated nodular regenerative hyperplasia in the liver parenchyma.

Biliary tract disease is also a common finding but can be very focal. In one biopsy core there can be normal portal tracts, while another core shows significant bile ductular proliferation, mixed lymphocytic and neutrophilic inflammation, and portal fibrosis. Bile duct plugs with granular eosinophilic materials can strongly suggest cystic fibrosis, but they are found in only a minority of cases (Fig. 18.56). Focal biliary fibrosis (Fig. 18.57) can progress to fully established cirrhosis in some cases. Rare cases of hepatocellular carcinoma and cholangiocarcinoma have been reported.[101]

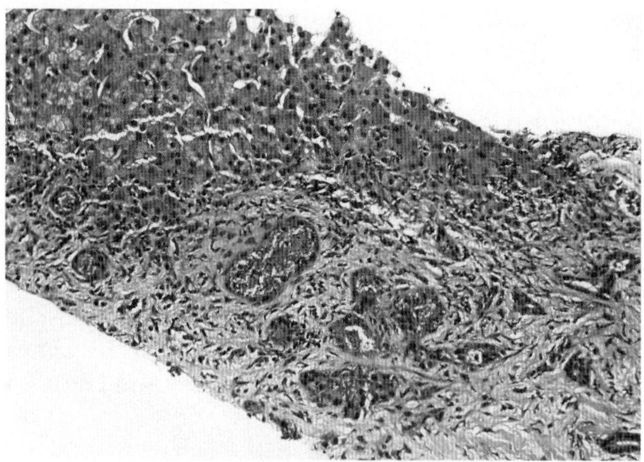

Figure 18.56 Cystic fibrosis. Granular eosinophilic secretions in bile ducts in a portal tract with chronic inflammation, marked bile ductular proliferation and fibrosis.

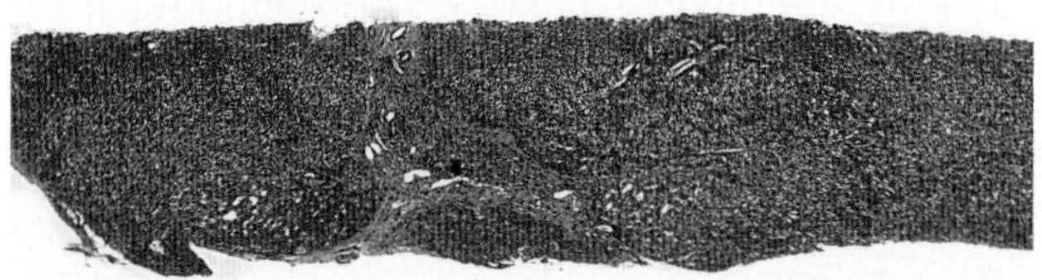

Figure 18.57 Cystic fibrosis. Focal biliary cirrhosis, note the unaffected portal tracts at the right (Trichrome stain).

Immunohistochemistry and special stains

Immunostains are of limited use in diagnosing cystic fibrosis. The bile duct plugs are PAS-positive. Trichrome stains are used to evaluate fibrosis. Copper stains can be positive in cases with chronic biliary injury and CK7 immunostains can highlight intermediate hepatocytes.

Ultrastructural findings

Electron microscopy usually shows nonspecific changes including hypertrophy of the smooth endoplasmic reticulum and the Golgi apparatus.[102]

Molecular genetic findings

The *CFTR* gene is located at the q31.2 locus of chromosome 7, which is 230,000 base pairs long and produces a protein that is 1,480 amino acids long. More than 2,000 mutations of the *CFTR* gene have been discovered, and these can be divided into six classes based on their impact on CFTR protein function. The most common mutation is ΔF508, i.e., the deletion of three nucleotides—CTT that in turns leads to a deletion of phenylalanine at position 508 of CFTR protein. ΔF508 accounts for 70% cystic fibrosis cases and is found in >90% of cases in North America. A number of different molecular genetic testing approaches for the *CFTR* gene have been developed and are used to confirm the diagnosis or to screen carriers in high risk populations, including specific site testing (ΔF508), a panel of multiple site mutations, or full *CFTR* gene sequence analysis.

Differential diagnosis

Cystic fibrosis can present with cholestasis in neonates. Other disorders causing neonate cholestasis such as biliary atresia, infection, TPN, or other metabolic disorders need to be ruled out. In cases that show predominately fatty liver disease, other causes of fatty liver disease need to be excluded including alcoholic liver disease, the metabolic syndrome, and Wilson disease.

Prognosis and treatment

There is no cure for cystic fibrosis. Instead, clinical care focuses on management of complications related to portal hypertension and cirrhosis. UDCA is recommended for every patient with cystic fibrosis and may have a protective role in preventing cirrhosis. A small subset of patients require liver transplantation or multiple organ transplantation.[103]

Chronic granulomatous disease

Chronic granulomatous disease is a rare genetically heterogeneous immunodeficiency disorder that affects the abilities of phagocytes to kill intracellular pathogens leading to recurrent or persistent infections and granuloma formation. Chronic granulomatous disease is caused by mutations of one of five genes that encode the subunits of the phagocytic NADPH oxidase: *CYBA*, *CYBB*, *NCF1*, *NCF2*, and *NCF4* genes. These mutations lead to little or no function or no production of the protein. The most common type (80%) of chronic granulomatous disease involves the *CYBB* gene on chromosome X and thus affects boys. Symptoms typically occur in the first 2 years of life, but onset is occasionally delayed into the second decade of life. The patients present with recurrent pyogenic infections. Skin infections are usually the earliest signs. About one third of patients can have liver abscesses and some patients may develop noncirrhotic portal hypertension.[104]

The diagnosis of chronic granulomatous disease can be established using laboratory tests. The nitroblue tetrazolium (NBT) test is the most widely used screening test for chronic granulomatous disease. This test depends upon the direct reduction of NBT to the insoluble blue compound formazan by NADPH oxidase. Neutrophils in chronic granulomatous disease patients are unable to reduce oxidized NBT to insoluble blue formazan. The dihydrorhodamine test is similar, in which DHR is oxidized by superoxide radicals to rhodamine in cells. An additional test, called the cytochrome C reduction assay, can directly measure the production of superoxide by a patient's phagocytes. Once the diagnosis of chronic granulomatous disease is established, genetic testing can be used to determine the underlying mutations.

Abnormal liver enzyme elevations are common in chronic granulomatous disease but are usually mild and transient. However, about half of patients may have persistent mildly to moderately elevated alkaline phosphatase levels.[105]

Liver abscesses are the main liver manifestation of chronic granulomatous disease. Over a third of patients with chronic granulomatous disease will have liver abscesses at some point. The abscesses can also be multifocal. Most of liver abscesses are either polymicrobial or due to *Staphylococcus* species. Fungal infections including *Candida*, *Aspergillus*, and *Cryptococcus* species are not uncommon.[105] The liver abscesses are usually multiloculated with irregularly shaped and variably sized cysts. The abscess shows abundant neutrophils and necrotic debris surrounded by connective tissue containing epithelioid macrophages, mixed inflammatory cells, and remnants of portal areas.

Besides abscesses, several other pathologic changes have also been observed.[105] Portal and/or lobular inflammatory is present in essentially all cases, while non-necrotizing granulomas are present in most cases. Abnormalities of the portal and central veins or both are common, being found in 60% to 80% of livers with chronic granulomatous disease. These changes are sometimes best seen on trichrome stains and show narrowing or complete obliteration of portal and/or central veins. The venopathy in chronic granulomatous disease liver is believed to be related to the liver abscesses.[105] Nodular regenerative hyperplasia is seen in about a third of cases, most likely reflecting the venopathy. Advanced fibrosis typically does not occur in chronic granulomatous disease.

Bile duct injury has been described in a subset of cases. The injured bile ducts have narrowed lumens with periductal concentric fibrosis, edema, and lymphocytic inflammation, mimicking the changes found in primary sclerosing cholangitis, but fibrobliterative duct lesions are rare and extensive ductopenia does not typically develop. Acute cholangitis is also observed in a small number of cases.

Chronic granulomatous disease was initially known as *fatal granulomatous disease of childhood* because affected children usually died within their first decade. Currently, early diagnosis and treatment has significantly improved the prognosis. With modern treatment, including aggressive and prolonged administration of antibiotics, immunomodulation, and hematopoietic stem cell transplantation, the mortality rate has been fallen to under 3% and the average survival time is at least 40 years.[106]

REFERENCES

1. Olivarez L, Caggana M, Pass KA, et al. Estimate of the frequency of Wilson's disease in the US Caucasian population: a mutation analysis approach. *Ann Hum Genet.* 2001;65(pt 5):459–463.
2. Beyersdorff A, Findeisen A. Morbus Wilson: case report of a two-year-old child as first manifestation. *Scand J Gastroenterol.* 2006;41(4):496–497.
3. Ala A, Borjigin J, Rochwarger A, et al. Wilson disease in septuagenarian siblings: raising the bar for diagnosis. *Hepatology.* 2005;41(3):668–670.
4. Roberts EA, Schilsky ML, Division of G, et al. A practice guideline on Wilson disease. *Hepatology.* 2003;37(6):1475–1492.
5. Davies SE, Williams R, Portmann B. Hepatic morphology and histochemistry of Wilson's disease presenting as fulminant hepatic failure: a study of 11 cases. *Histopathology.* 1989;15(4):385–394.
6. Pilloni L, Lecca S, Van Eyken P, et al. Value of histochemical stains for copper in the diagnosis of Wilson's disease. *Histopathology.* 1998;33(1):28–33.
7. Thornburg LP, Beissenherz M, Dolan M, et al. Histochemical demonstration of copper and copper-associated protein in the canine liver. *Vet Pathol.* 1985;22(4):327–332.
8. Faa G, Nurchi V, Demelia L, et al. Uneven hepatic copper distribution in Wilson's disease. *J Hepatol.* 1995;22(3):303–308.
9. Mounajjed T, Oxentenko AS, Qureshi H, et al. Revisiting the topic of histochemically detectable copper in various liver diseases with special focus on venous outflow impairment. *Am J Clin Pathol.* 2013;139(1):79–86.
10. Sternlieb I. Mitochondrial and fatty changes in hepatocytes of patients with Wilson's disease. *Gastroenterology.* 1968;55(3):354–367.
11. Stoller JK, Brantly M. The challenge of detecting alpha-1 antitrypsin deficiency. *COPD.* 2013;10 suppl 1:26–34.
12. de Serres FJ, Blanco I, Fernandez-Bustillo E. Genetic epidemiology of alpha-1 antitrypsin deficiency in North America and Australia/New Zealand: Australia, Canada, New Zealand and the United States of America. *Clin Genet.* 2003;64(5):382–397.
13. Brantly M, Nukiwa T, Crystal RG. Molecular basis of alpha-1-antitrypsin deficiency. *Am J Med.* 1988;84(6A):13–31.

14. Graziadei IW, Joseph JJ, Wiesner RH, et al. Increased risk of chronic liver failure in adults with heterozygous alpha1-antitrypsin deficiency. *Hepatology*. 1998;28(4):1058–1063.
15. Sveger T. Liver disease in alpha1-antitrypsin deficiency detected by screening of 200,000 infants. *N Engl J Med*. 1976;294(24): 1316–1321.
16. Zhou H, Fischer HP. Liver carcinoma in PiZ alpha-1-antitrypsin deficiency. *Am J Surg Pathol*. 1998;22(6):742–748.
17. Theaker JM, Fleming KA. Alpha-1-antitrypsin and the liver: a routine immunohistological screen. *J Clin Pathol*. 1986;39(1):58–62.
18. Yunis EJ, Agostini RM Jr, Glew RH. Fine structural observations of the liver in alpha-1-antitrypsin deficiency. *Am J Pathol*. 1976;82(2):265–286.
19. Iezzoni JC, Gaffey MJ, Stacy EK, et al. Hepatocytic globules in end-stage hepatic disease: relationship to alpha1-antitrypsin phenotype. *Am J Clin Pathol*. 1997;107(6):692–697.
20. Carlson J, Eriksson S, Hagerstrand I. Intra- and extracellular alpha1-antitrypsin in liver disease with special reference to Pi phenotype. *J Clin Pathol*. 1981;34(9):1020–1025.
21. Brennan SO, Wyatt J, Medicina D, et al. Fibrinogen brescia: hepatic endoplasmic reticulum storage and hypofibrinogenemia because of a gamma284 Gly-->Arg mutation. *Am J Pathol*. 2000;157(1):189–196.
22. Brennan SO, Davis RL, Conard K, et al. Novel fibrinogen mutation gamma314Thr-->Pro (fibrinogen AI duPont) associated with hepatic fibrinogen storage disease and hypofibrinogenaemia. *Liver Int*. 2010;30(10):1541–1547.
23. Applegarth DA, Toone JR, Lowry RB. Incidence of inborn errors of metabolism in British Columbia, 1969-1996. *Pediatrics*. 2000;105(1):e10.
24. Gogus S, Kocak N, Ciliv G, et al. Histologic features of the liver in type Ia glycogen storage disease: comparative study between different age groups and consecutive biopsies. *Pediatr Dev Pathol*. 2002;5(3):299–304.
25. Laberge AM, Mitchell GA, van de Werve G, et al. Long-term follow-up of a new case of liver glycogen synthase deficiency. *Am J Med Genet A*. 2003;120A(1):19–22.
26. Yamaguchi T, Ihara K, Matsumoto T, et al. Inflammatory bowel disease-like colitis in glycogen storage disease type 1b. *Inflamm Bowel Dis*. 2001;7(2):128–132.
27. Couper R, Kapelushnik J, Griffiths AM. Neutrophil dysfunction in glycogen storage disease Ib: association with Crohn's-like colitis. *Gastroenterology*. 1991;100(2):549–554.
28. Itoh S, Ishida Y, Matsuo S. Mallory bodies in a patient with type Ia glycogen storage disease. *Gastroenterology*. 1987;92(2):520–523.
29. Miller JH, Gates GF, Landing BH, et al. Scintigraphic abnormalities in glycogen storage disease. *J Nucl Med*. 1978;19(4):354–358.
30. Sakellariou S, Al-Hussaini H, Scalori A, et al. Hepatocellular adenoma in glycogen storage disorder type I: a clinicopathological and molecular study. *Histopathology*. 2012;60(6B):E58–65.
31. Calderaro J, Labrune P, Morcrette G, et al. Molecular characterization of hepatocellular adenomas developed in patients with glycogen storage disease type I. *J Hepatol*. 2013;58(2):350–357.
32. Bianchi L. Glycogen storage disease I and hepatocellular tumours. *Eur J Pediatr*. 1993;152 suppl 1:S63–70.
33. Baudhuin P, Hers HG, Loeb H. An electron microscopic and biochemical study of type Ii glycogenosis. *Lab Invest*. 1964;13:1139–1152.
34. Demo E, Frush D, Gottfried M, et al. Glycogen storage disease type III-hepatocellular carcinoma a long-term complication? *J Hepatol*. 2007;46(3):492–498.
35. Andersen DH. Familial cirrhosis of the liver with storage of abnormal glycogen. *Lab Invest*. 1956;5(1):11–20.
36. Greene HL, Brown BI, McClenathan DT, et al. A new variant of type IV glycogenosis: deficiency of branching enzyme activity without apparent progressive liver disease. *Hepatology*. 1988;8(2):302–306.
37. Hers HG. Enzymatic studies of hepatic fragments; application to the classification of glycogenoses. *Rev Int Hepatol*. 1959;9(1):35–55.
38. Manzia TM, Angelico R, Toti L, et al. Glycogen storage disease type Ia and VI associated with hepatocellular carcinoma: two case reports. *Transplant Proc*. 2011;43(4):1181–1183.
39. Willems PJ, Gerver WJ, Berger R, et al. The natural history of liver glycogenosis due to phosphorylase kinase deficiency: a longitudinal study of 41 patients. *Eur J Pediatr*. 1990;149(4):268–271.
40. Saltik-Temizel IN, Coskun T, Yuce A, et al. Fanconi-Bickel syndrome in three Turkish patients with different homozygous mutations. *Turk J Pediatr*. 2005;47(2):167–169.
41. Gomez-Garre P, Gutierrez-Delicado E, Gomez-Abad C, et al. Hepatic disease as the first manifestation of progressive myoclonus epilepsy of Lafora. *Neurology*. 2007;68(17):1369–1373.
42. Ng IO, Sturgess RP, Williams R, et al. Ground-glass hepatocytes with Lafora body like inclusions—histochemical, immunohistochemical

and electronmicroscopic characterization. *Histopathology*. 1990;17(2):109–113.

43. O'Shea AM, Wilson GJ, Ling SC, et al. Lafora-like ground-glass inclusions in hepatocytes of pediatric patients: a report of two cases. *Pediatr Dev Pathol*. 2007;10(5):351–357.
44. Resnick JM, Whitley CB, Leonard AS, et al. Light and electron microscopic features of the liver in mucopolysaccharidosis. *Hum Pathol*. 1994;25(3):276–286.
45. Nagral A. Gaucher disease. *J Clin Exp Hepatol*. 2014;4(1):37–50.
46. James SP, Stromeyer FW, Chang C, et al. Liver abnormalities in patients with Gaucher's disease. *Gastroenterology*. 1981;80(1):126–133.
47. Lachmann RH, Wight DG, Lomas DJ, et al. Massive hepatic fibrosis in Gaucher's disease: clinico-pathological and radiological features. *QJM*. 2000;93(4):237–244.
48. Hibbs RG, Ferrans VJ, Cipriano PR, et al. A histochemical and electron microscopic study of Gaucher cells. *Arch Pathol*. 1970;89(2):137–153.
49. Stenzel P, Weeks DA. Abundant hepatic Gaucher-like cells following chemotherapy and bone marrow transplantation for hematologic malignancy: report of two cases. *Int J Surg Pathol*. 2013;21(1):89–92.
50. Thurberg BL, Wasserstein MP, Schiano T, et al. Liver and skin histopathology in adults with acid sphingomyelinase deficiency (Niemann-Pick disease type B). *Am J Surg Pathol*. 2012;36(8):1234–1246.
51. Tassoni JP Jr, Fawaz KA, Johnston DE. Cirrhosis and portal hypertension in a patient with adult Niemann-Pick disease. *Gastroenterology*. 1991;100(2):567–569.
52. Coelho GR, Praciano AM, Rodrigues JP, et al. Liver transplantation in patients with Niemann-Pick disease—single-center experience. *Transplant Proc*. 2015;47(10):2929–2931.
53. Di Bisceglie AM, Ishak KG, Rabin L, et al. Cholesteryl ester storage disease: hepatopathology and effects of therapy with lovastatin. *Hepatology*. 1990;11(5):764–772.
54. Bernstein DL, Hulkova H, Bialer MG, et al. Cholesteryl ester storage disease: review of the findings in 135 reported patients with an underdiagnosed disease. *J Hepatol*. 2013;58(6):1230–1243.
55. Lake BD, Patrick AD. Wolman's disease: deficiency of E600-resistant acid esterase activity with storage of lipids in lysosomes. *J Pediatr*. 1970;76(2):262–266.
56. Schulze A, Lindner M, Kohlmuller D, et al. Expanded newborn screening for inborn errors of metabolism by electrospray ionization-tandem mass spectrometry: results, outcome, and implications. *Pediatrics*. 2003;111(6, pt 1):1399–1406.
57. Weinberg AG, Mize CE, Worthen HG. The occurrence of hepatoma in the chronic form of hereditary tyrosinemia. *J Pediatr*. 1976;88(3):434–438.
58. Russo P, O'Regan S. Visceral pathology of hereditary tyrosinemia type I. *Am J Hum Genet*. 1990;47(2):317–324.
59. Dehner LP, Snover DC, Sharp HL, et al. Hereditary tyrosinemia type I (chronic form): pathologic findings in the liver. *Hum Pathol*. 1989;20(2):149–158.
60. Jaffe R. Liver transplant pathology in pediatric metabolic disorders. *Pediatr Dev Pathol*. 1998;1(2):102–117.
61. Klenn PJ, Rubin R. Hepatic fibrosis associated with hereditary cystinosis: a novel form of noncirrhotic portal hypertension. *Mod Pathol*. 1994;7(8):879–882.
62. Rossi S, Herrine SK, Navarro VJ. Cystinosis as a cause of noncirrhotic portal hypertension. *Dig Dis Sci*. 2005;50(7):1372–1375.
63. Cornelis T, Claes K, Gillard P, et al. Cholestatic liver disease in long-term infantile nephropathic cystinosis. *J Gastroenterol Hepatol*. 2008;23(8, pt 2):e428–431.
64. Braissant O. Current concepts in the pathogenesis of urea cycle disorders. *Mol Genet Metab*. 2010;100 suppl 1:S3–S12.
65. Badizadegan K, Perez-Atayde AR. Focal glycogenosis of the liver in disorders of ureagenesis: its occurrence and diagnostic significance. *Hepatology*. 1997;26(2):365–373.
66. LaBrecque DR, Latham PS, Riely CA, et al. Heritable urea cycle enzyme deficiency-liver disease in 16 patients. *J Pediatr*. 1979;94(4):580–587.
67. Zimmermann A, Bachmann C, Baumgartner R. Severe liver fibrosis in argininosuccinic aciduria. *Arch Pathol Lab Med*. 1986;110(2):136–140.
68. Yaplito-Lee J, Chow CW, Boneh A. Histopathological findings in livers of patients with urea cycle disorders. *Mol Genet Metab*. 2013;108(3):161–165.
69. Gucer S, Asan E, Atilla P, et al. Early cirrhosis in a patient with type I citrullinaemia (CTLN1). *J Inherit Metab Dis*. 2004;27(4):541–542.
70. Marble M, McGoey RR, Mannick E, et al. Living related liver transplant in a patient with argininosuccinic aciduria and cirrhosis: metabolic follow-up. *J Pediatr Gastroenterol Nutr*. 2008;46(4):453–456.
71. Wilson JM, Shchelochkov OA, Gallagher RC, et al. Hepatocellular carcinoma in a research subject with ornithine transcarbamylase deficiency. *Mol Genet Metab*. 2012;105(2):263–265.

72. Cortes JM, Oliva H, Paradinas FJ, et al. The pathology of the liver in porphyria cutanea tarda. *Histopathology*. 1980;4(5):471–485.
73. Bulaj ZJ, Phillips JD, Ajioka RS, et al. Hemochromatosis genes and other factors contributing to the pathogenesis of porphyria cutanea tarda. *Blood*. 2000;95(5):1565–1571.
74. Gisbert JP, Garcia-Buey L, Pajares JM, et al. Prevalence of hepatitis C virus infection in porphyria cutanea tarda: systematic review and meta-analysis. *J Hepatol*. 2003;39(4):620–627.
75. Fakan F, Chlumska A. Demonstration of needle-shaped hepatic inclusions in porphyria cutanea tarda using the ferric ferricyanide reduction test. *Virchows Arch A Pathol Anat Histopathol*. 1987;411(4):365–368.
76. Siersema PD, Rademakers LH, Cleton MI, et al. The difference in liver pathology between sporadic and familial forms of porphyria cutanea tarda: the role of iron. *J Hepatol*. 1995;23(3):259–267.
77. MacDonald DM, Germain D, Perrot H. The histopathology and ultrastructure of liver disease in erythropoietic protoporphyria. *Br J Dermatol*. 1981;104(1):7–17.
78. Rademakers LH, Cleton MI, Kooijman C, et al. Early involvement of hepatic parenchymal cells in erythrohepatic protoporphyria? An ultrastructural study of patients with and without overt liver disease and the effect of chenodeoxycholic acid treatment. *Hepatology*. 1990;11(3):449–457.
79. Koopman WJ, Willems PH, Smeitink JA. Monogenic mitochondrial disorders. *N Engl J Med*. 2012;366(12):1132–1141.
80. Lee WS, Sokol RJ. Liver disease in mitochondrial disorders. *Semin Liver Dis*. 2007;27(3):259–273.
81. Bioulac-Sage P, Parrot-Roulaud F, Mazat JP, et al. Fatal neonatal liver failure and mitochondrial cytopathy (oxidative phosphorylation deficiency): a light and electron microscopic study of the liver. *Hepatology*. 1993;18(4):839–846.
82. Ducluzeau PH, Lachaux A, Bouvier R, et al. Depletion of mitochondrial DNA associated with infantile cholestasis and progressive liver fibrosis. *J Hepatol*. 1999;30(1):149–155.
83. Scheers I, Bachy V, Stephenne X, et al. Risk of hepatocellular carcinoma in liver mitochondrial respiratory chain disorders. *J Pediatr*. 2005;146(3):414–417.
84. Lefebvre P, Cariou B, Lien F, et al. Role of bile acids and bile acid receptors in metabolic regulation. *Physiol Rev*. 2009;89(1):147–191.
85. Sundaram SS, Bove KE, Lovell MA, et al. Mechanisms of disease: inborn errors of bile acid synthesis. *Nat Clin Pract Gastroenterol Hepatol*. 2008;5(8):456–468.
86. Bove KE, Daugherty CC, Tyson W, et al. Bile acid synthetic defects and liver disease. *Pediatr Dev Pathol*. 2000;3(1):1–16.
87. Tsujii H, Konig J, Rost D, et al. Exon-intron organization of the human multidrug-resistance protein 2 (MRP2) gene mutated in Dubin-Johnson syndrome. *Gastroenterology*. 1999;117(3):653–660.
88. Dubin IN. Chronic idiopathic jaundice; a review of fifty cases. *Am J Med*. 1958;24(2):268–292.
89. Swartz HM, Sarna T, Varma RR. On the natural and excretion of the hepatic pigment in the Dubin-Johnson syndrome. *Gastroenterology*. 1979;76(5 Pt 1):958–964.
90. Ware A, Eigenbrodt E, Naftalis J, et al. Letter: Dubin-Johnson syndrome and viral hepatitis. *Gastroenterology*. 1974;67(3):560–561.
91. Erlinger S, Arias IM, Dhumeaux D. Inherited disorders of bilirubin transport and conjugation: new insights into molecular mechanisms and consequences. *Gastroenterology*. 2014;146(7):1625–1638.
92. Kaufman SS, Wood RP, Shaw BW Jr, et al. Orthotopic liver transplantation for type I Crigler-Najjar syndrome. *Hepatology*. 1986;6(6):1259–1262.
93. Barth RF, Grimley PM, Berk PD, et al. Excess lipofuscin accumulation in constitutional hepatic dysfunction (Gilbert's syndrome). Light and electron microscopic observations. *Arch Pathol*. 1971;91(1):41–47.
94. Debinski HS, Lee CS, Dhillon AP, et al. UDP-glucuronosyltransferase in Gilbert's syndrome. *Pathology*. 1996;28(3):238–241.
95. van de Steeg E, Stranecky V, Hartmannova H, et al. Complete OATP1B1 and OATP1B3 deficiency causes human Rotor syndrome by interrupting conjugated bilirubin reuptake into the liver. *J Clin Invest*. 2012;122(2):519–528.
96. Rotor AB ML, Florentin A. Familial nonhemolytic jaundice with direct van den Bergh reaction. *Acta Med Phil*. 1948;5.
97. O'Sullivan BP, Freedman SD. Cystic fibrosis. *Lancet*. 2009;373(9678):1891–1904.
98. Siano M, De Gregorio F, Boggia B, et al. Ursodeoxycholic acid treatment in patients with cystic fibrosis at risk for liver disease. *Dig Liver Dis*. 2010;42(6):428–431.
99. Castaldo G, Fuccio A, Salvatore D, et al. Liver expression in cystic fibrosis could be modulated by genetic factors different from the cystic fibrosis transmembrane regulator genotype. *Am J Med Genet*. 2001;98(4):294–297.
100. Sokol RJ, Durie PR. Recommendations for management of liver and biliary tract disease in cystic fibrosis. Cystic Fibrosis Foundation

Hepatobiliary Disease Consensus Group. *J Pediatr Gastroenterol Nutr*. 1999;28(suppl 1): S1–13.

101. Perdue DG, Cass OW, Milla C, et al. Hepatolithiasis and cholangiocarcinoma in cystic fibrosis: a case series and review of the literature. *Dig Dis Sci*. 2007;52(10):2638–2642.
102. Lindblad A, Hultcrantz R, Strandvik B. Bile-duct destruction and collagen deposition: a prominent ultrastructural feature of the liver in cystic fibrosis. *Hepatology*. 1992;16(2):372–381.
103. Mendizabal M, Reddy KR, Cassuto J, et al. Liver transplantation in patients with cystic fibrosis: analysis of United Network for Organ Sharing data. *Liver Transpl*. 2011;17(3):243–250.
104. Feld JJ, Hussain N, Wright EC, et al. Hepatic involvement and portal hypertension predict mortality in chronic granulomatous disease. *Gastroenterology*. 2008;134(7):1917–1926.
105. Hussain N, Feld JJ, Kleiner DE, et al. Hepatic abnormalities in patients with chronic granulomatous disease. *Hepatology*. 2007;45(3):675–683.
106. Seger RA. Modern management of chronic granulomatous disease. *Br J Haematol*. 2008;140(3):255–266.

19

Liver involvement in systemic diseases

Lizhi Zhang, MD

19.1 INTRODUCTION

Just as primary liver disease can affect other organ systems in the body, the liver may be affected in many systemic diseases. The patterns of liver involvement vary considerably. For example, the liver can be directly involved by systemic diseases that lead to grossly evident changes readily seen on imaging studies, such as metastatic tumors. In other cases, findings are seen only by microscopy. For example, mild nonspecific reactive changes or nonspecific reactive hepatitis is common in the liver of individuals with systemic disease. In other cases, specific morphological features are found. Systemic diseases can also rarely present with acute liver failure requiring liver transplantation. Finally, systemic disease at times can present with only abnormal liver enzyme elevation, without recognizable histological changes.

19.2 INTESTINAL FAILURE–ASSOCIATED LIVER DISEASE

Definition

Intestinal failure–associated liver disease (IFALD) is defined as hepatobiliary complications because of a consequence of medical or surgical managements for intestinal failure, in which parenteral nutrition plays a central role in the pathogenesis. This term is used by some authors as replacement for the term parenteral nutrition–associated liver disease because of the recognition that many other patient-dependent and treatment-related factors contribute to the pathogenesis of IFALD.[1]

Clinical features

IFALD was recognized shortly after total parenteral nutrition (TPN) was widely used in the late 1960s.[2] IFALD is the most common complication of neonates and infants with intestinal failure receiving TPN. The disease manifestations differ in infants versus older children and adults, but biliary sludging and cholecystitis (acalculous and calculus) frequently occur in both.

Neonates who receive TPN usually present with early abnormal liver enzyme tests with no clinical symptoms, but jaundice can develop about 2 weeks after starting TPN. Hepatic dysfunction, hepatic fibrosis, and splenomegaly gradually progress with the duration of TPN treatment. In infants receiving TPN, the reported incidences of IFALD varies widely from 15% to 85%.[3–5] The incidence correlates inversely with the gestational age and birth weight and is also related to the underlying disease and duration of treatment. The incidence of cholestasis is 50% in infants with birth weight <1,000 g but falls to 7% if birth weight is >1,500 g.[6] The highest incidence of IFALD occurs in infants <34 weeks of gestation and <2,000 g body weight.[7] A prolonged length of TPN increases the overall incidence of liver injury, with cholestasis occurring in 85% of infants who are on TPN >100 days.

IFALD can also develop in older children and adults following TPN, but its incidence is much lower. The clinical presentations are also different from those seen in infants and usually are less severe. After 9 to 12 days of TPN therapy, mildly elevated liver transaminase and alkaline phosphatase levels are observed in 54% to 68% of adult patients, and serum bilirubin levels are elevated in 21% of patients.[8] Abnormal liver enzyme elevations in adults are usually self-limited. Patients who develop infections while on TPN are at greater risk of developing steatosis and intrahepatic cholestasis. Patients on long-term TPN therapy may present with persistent elevations in liver tests and steatohepatitis.[9]

The pathogenesis of IFALD remains poorly understood and is believed to be multifactorial. Known associations include prematurity, low birth weight, duration of TPN, short bowel syndrome, and the frequency of infection. A lack of enteral feeding results in gut mucosal atrophy, and this in turn leads to a disruption of enterohepatic circulation, which is also considered to play an important mechanistic role.[10]

Laboratory findings

Laboratory findings are not specific for IFALD. Elevated conjugated bilirubin levels are usually the earliest sign but may not be significantly elevated in adults with early-phase disease. IFALD is often associated with elevated liver transaminases, alkaline phosphatase levels, and γ-glutamyl transpeptidase (GGT) levels. Total bilirubin levels persistently >5.8 mg/dL for at least 2 to 4 weeks are a marker of severe IFALD.

Elevated liver transaminase levels are commonly observed within the first 2 to 3 weeks of TPN therapy. Typically, this is a transient increase and self-limited in adult patients. However, liver transaminase levels are not sensitive or specific indicators of hepatic dysfunction. In a study of long-term TPN patients, a significant correlation between TPN duration and the serum alkaline phosphatase was observed, although TPN duration and aspartate transaminase (AST) and alanine transaminase (ALT) levels were not correlated.[11] A fall in albumin or prolonged coagulation is a late sign of hepatic dysfunction, whereas thrombocytopenia suggests splenomegaly secondary to portal hypertension from advanced hepatic fibrosis or cirrhosis.

Imaging

Ultrasound of the liver may demonstrate hepatomegaly, a contracted gallbladder, biliary sludge, or gallstones. Splenomegaly may be seen in cases with portal hypertension from cirrhosis.

Gross findings

Explanted livers of end-stage IFALD typically appear shrunken and cirrhotic, with regenerative nodules of various sizes and greenish discoloration because of chronic cholestasis (Fig. 19.1).

Microscopic findings

There are no specific histological features in IFALD. The liver shows a wide range of morphological changes, with some differences in infants versus older children and adults.[12] The severity of liver injury is related to the length of TPN therapy. Patients with >6 weeks of TPN are more likely to have significant cholestasis and fibrosis.

Cholestasis is the most common finding in both infants and adults. Perivenular hepatocanalicular cholestasis can occur a few days to a few weeks after starting TPN. With disease progression, features of chronic cholestasis can be observed, such as hepatocyte feathery degeneration, cholestatic rosettes, and bile infarcts (Fig. 19.2). Bile plugs can be present in the interlobular bile ducts. Inflammation in the portal tracts and the lobular parenchyma is usually mild and nonspecific. Hepatocellular injury is more severe in infants and can show extensive ballooning and feathery degeneration. Steatosis is more commonly

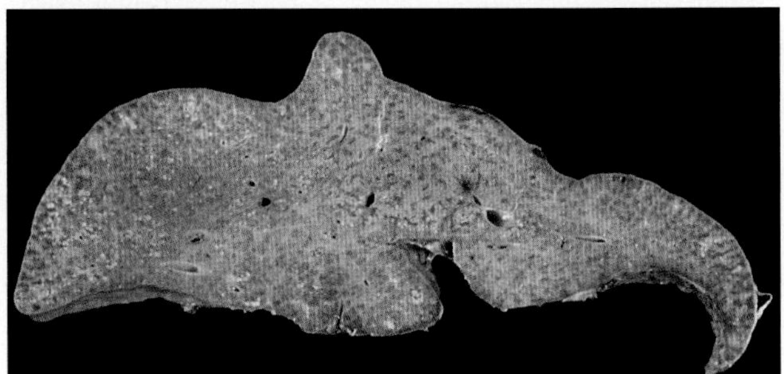

Figure 19.1 Intestinal failure–associated liver disease (IFALD). A liver explant because of IFALD. The liver appears atrophic with cirrhosis and green discoloration.

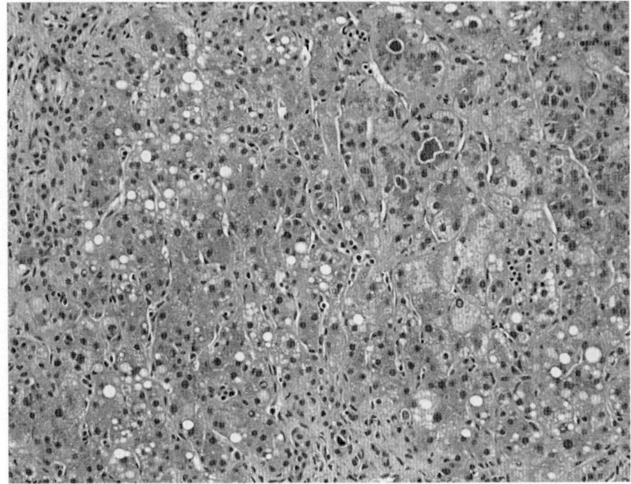

Figure 19.2 Neonatal intestinal failure–associated liver disease. Chronic cholestasis with hepatocyte feathery degeneration, cholestatic rosettes, bile plugs, rare acidophil bodies, mild steatosis, and extramedullary hematopoiesis.

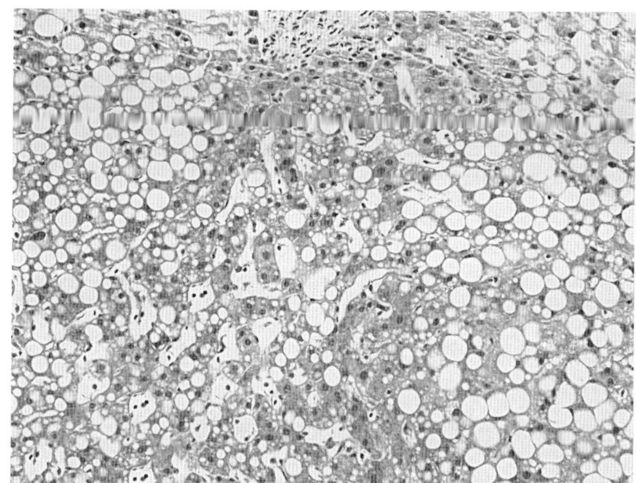

Figure 19.3 Adult intestinal failure–associated liver disease. Note the marked fatty change.

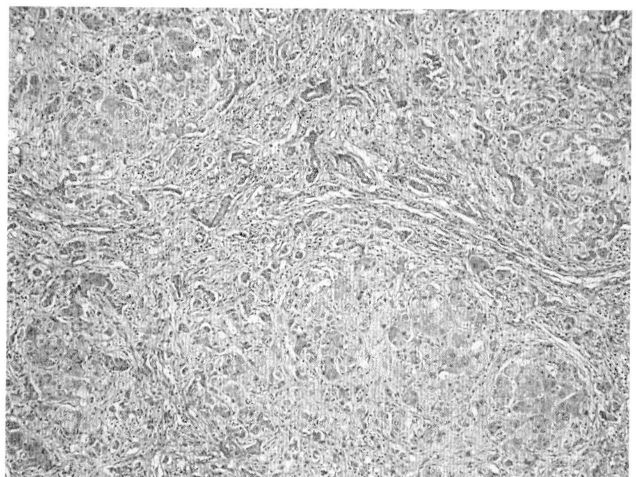

Figure 19.4 Biliary cirrhosis in intestinal failure–associated liver disease.

found in older children and adults, typically seen as mild periportal macrovesicular steatosis (Fig. 19.3). Steatohepatitis can develop after long-term TPN and progress to cirrhosis in a small number of patients.[13] Ductopenia is frequently seen but is not accompanied by a bile ductular reaction. This ductopenic pattern of injury may have a different mechanism from that of bile sludge or bile duct obstruction, which can also lead to biliary obstructive changes and eventually to biliary cirrhosis with ductopenia (Fig. 19.4).[3,12]

Hepatic fibrosis occurs in essentially all cases of IFALD and is related to the length of treatment. Liver function tests and bilirubin level are not correlated with the degree of fibrosis. Fibrosis is common even after the cholestasis has resolved. Serial liver biopsy may be necessary for staging purposes in cases of long-term IFALD. Portal fibrosis often occurs early in the course of IFALD and may progress rapidly.

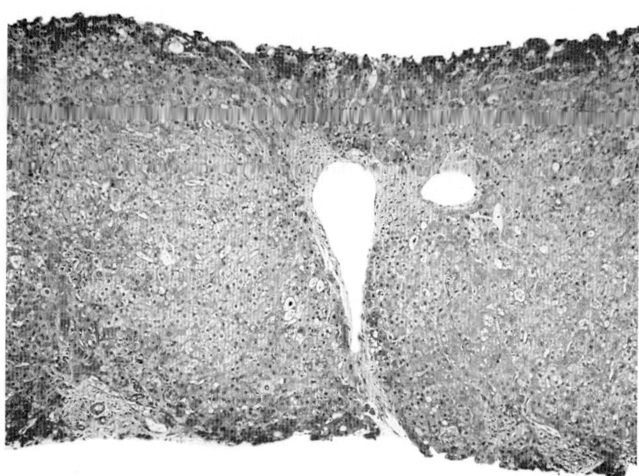

Figure 19.5 Early stage of intestinal failure–associated liver disease, showing perivenular fibrosis.

Progression to cirrhosis is more likely in infants. One study showed that 34% of infants developed cirrhosis, whereas none of 36 patients older than 1 year had cirrhosis.[12] Perivenular fibrosis is also observed in early-stage disease, which is a distinctive feature of IFALD that separates it from other causes of biliary cirrhosis (Fig. 19.5).[12]

Immunohistochemistry and special stains

Immunohistochemical and special stains are mainly used for evaluating hepatic fibrosis (i.e., trichrome stain) and to exclude entities in the differential diagnosis, such as infection or inherited liver diseases.

Ultrastructural findings

Electron microscopy is mainly used as needed to exclude metabolic liver diseases. If there is a specific clinical suspicion or histologic features suggestive of metabolic diseases, a portion of liver biopsy tissue should be saved in glutaraldehyde for electron microscopy.

Molecular genetic findings

Molecular genetic testing is mainly used to exclude genetic/metabolic liver diseases if there is specific clinical suspicion or histological features suggestive of those diseases.

Differential diagnosis

The diagnosis of IFALD requires the exclusion of other causes of liver injury, especially other cholestatic liver diseases. Of course, a clinical history of intestinal failure and TPN therapy is essential to establish the diagnosis of IFALD in the first place.

There are no specific histological features found in IFALD. In neonates, biliary atresia should be excluded. Biliary atresia shows histologic evidence of extrahepatic bile duct obstruction, with a prominent bile ductular reaction, often with bile plugs in dilated ductules, portal edema, fibrosis, and in time variable loss of intrahepatic bile ducts. The differential for IFALD also includes nonobstructive causes of cholestasis, such as neonatal hepatitis, which can be either idiopathic or because of a variety of causes, such as infection or metabolic liver diseases. Giant cell transformation is a typical feature in neonatal hepatitis but also can be seen in cases of IFALD, especially in neonates. Marked portal and lobular inflammation and liver necrosis are uncommon findings in IFALD, but they can be observed when there is superimposed injury, such as viral hepatitis. In adults, preexisting steatosis or steatohepatitis cannot be reliably distinguished from IFALD-induced steatosis based on histology alone. The steatosis in IFALD often shows a zone 1 pattern, but so does steatosis in the setting of the metabolic syndrome in children. However, the clinical settings are sufficiently distinct that this is rarely a problem.

Prognosis and treatment

IFALD usually is progressive as long as TPN is continued. The cholestasis and liver dysfunction tend to improve after TPN is discontinued but may persist in some cases.[14] Some patients are at higher risk for liver failure or death. Studies have shown that the maximum conjugated bilirubin is a risk factor for infants younger than 2 months of age with IFALD: 17% of individuals with conjugated bilirubin >2 mg/dL died or went on to liver transplantation versus 38% of those with a maximum conjugated bilirubin >10 mg/dL.[15] Another study showed that 36% of infants with short bowel syndrome went on to liver failure when they had a total bilirubin >6 mg/dL at 3 to 6 months of age.[16]

The most important clinical management goal in IFALD is to promote enteral feedings in order to reduce the dependence on parenteral nutrition. In premature infants with mild cholestasis, liver dysfunction usually improves after discontinuation of TPN. Optimization of TPN composition may reduce the risk of IFALD, such as avoiding excess total energy and excess macronutrients, lipid reduction strategies, and fish oil-based fat emulsions. Ursodeoxycholic acid has been shown to improve liver function tests, but the long-term efficacy of this drug has not been established. Prevention of infection or sepsis is also very important, because these are an important risk factor for IFALD and also one of the leading causes of death. Despite these therapies, a significant number of IFALD patients progress to liver failure and require liver transplantation for their end-stage liver disease. IFALD patients with short bowel syndrome are a major indication for combined liver–small bowel transplantation.[12]

19.3 LIVER IN ENDOCRINE DISORDERS

Glycogenic hepatopathy (Mauriac syndrome)

Definition

Glycogenic hepatopathy (GH) is a pathologic overloading of hepatocytes with glycogen mainly in poorly controlled type 1 diabetic patients. GH can be part of the Mauriac syndrome when it is accompanied by growth retardation and cushingoid features.

Clinical features

GH was first described by Pierre Mauriac in a 10-year-old type 1 diabetic patient as part of a constellation of findings, including growth retardation, hepatomegaly, cushingoid features, hypercholesterolemia, delayed puberty, and glycogen accumulation in hepatocytes.[17]

GH typically occurs in children and younger adults with poorly controlled type 1 diabetes.[18] They present with abdominal pain, hepatomegaly, diabetic ketoacidosis, elevated serum glucose and hemoglobin A1c (HbA1c) levels, elevated liver transaminase levels, and hypercholesterolemia. Many of the findings described in the Mauriac syndrome, such as growth retardation and cushingoid features, are uncommon today, probably because of better glycemic control.[18–20] Mechanistically, a combination of three main factors lead to deposition of glycogen in hepatocytes: elevated glucose levels, fluctuated insulin levels, and decreased glycogen phosphorylase activity in the hepatocyte.[19]

Laboratory findings

All patients have elevated serum glucose levels. Ketoacidosis and elevated HbA1c levels are frequently present, which indicate poor long-term glycemic control. Essentially, all patients have hepatomegaly and elevated transaminase levels, which in some cases can be greater than 10 times the upper limit of normal. Modest serum alkaline phosphatase elevations are common. Hyperbilirubinemia is rare. Most patients also have moderate hypercholesterolemia. Adult GH patients tend to have higher ALT and lower albumin levels than pediatric patients.[20]

Imaging

Hepatomegaly is a common finding in GH on imaging.

Microscopic findings

The key finding is diffuse hepatocyte swelling with pale cytoplasm and accentuation of the cell membranes because of excessive accumulation of glycogen (Fig. 19.6). The sinusoids often appear compressed by the swollen hepatocytes. Nuclear glycogenation is often present. Portal and lobular inflammation is essentially absent; if there is any inflammation, it is usually minimal. Steatosis is absent in most cases but can be mild in a small number of patients.[18] Giant mitochondria are commonly found (Fig. 19.6). GH does not induce liver fibrosis. Focal pericellular and periportal fibrosis can be seen, but this usually represents prior or concurrent injury from other liver disease, such as steatohepatitis.[18]

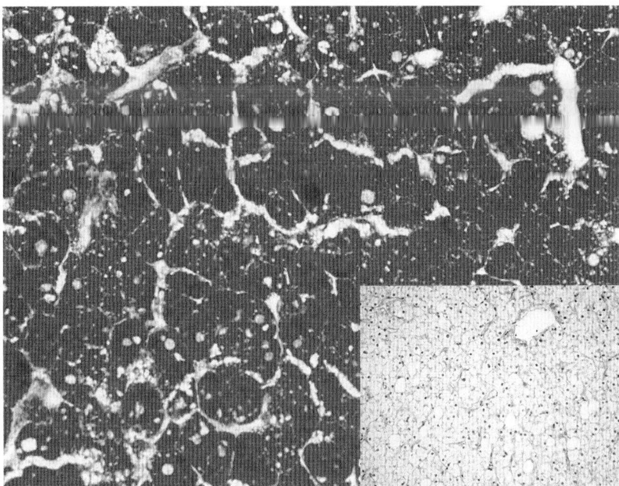

Figure 19.7 Glycogenic hepatopathy. Diffuse and strong periodic acid–Schiff (PAS) staining confirming excessive accumulation of glycogen in hepatocytes (inset, glycogen completely removed after diastase digestion, periodic acid–Schiff with diastase [PASD] stain).

Immunohistochemistry and special stains

Periodic acid–Schiff (PAS) stains show abundant cytoplasmic glycogen deposits, which are removed by diastase digestion (Fig. 19.7). However, hepatocytes in even normal liver biopsies are strongly PAS positive, so the diagnosis of GH is based on hematoxylin–eosin (H&E) findings. A trichrome stain is used to evaluate for liver fibrosis.

Ultrastructural findings

Electron microscopy shows marked glycogen accumulation in the hepatocytes.

Molecular genetic findings

Molecular genetic testing is of limited utility in GH but may be used to exclude genetic/metabolic liver diseases in pediatric patents if there is specific clinical suspicion. However, this is rare if ever needed because of the strong association between GH and poorly controlled diabetes.

Differential diagnosis

Mild GH can be overlooked on liver biopsy when the changes are subtle, with preserved liver architecture and lack of inflammation, steatosis, or fibrosis. The

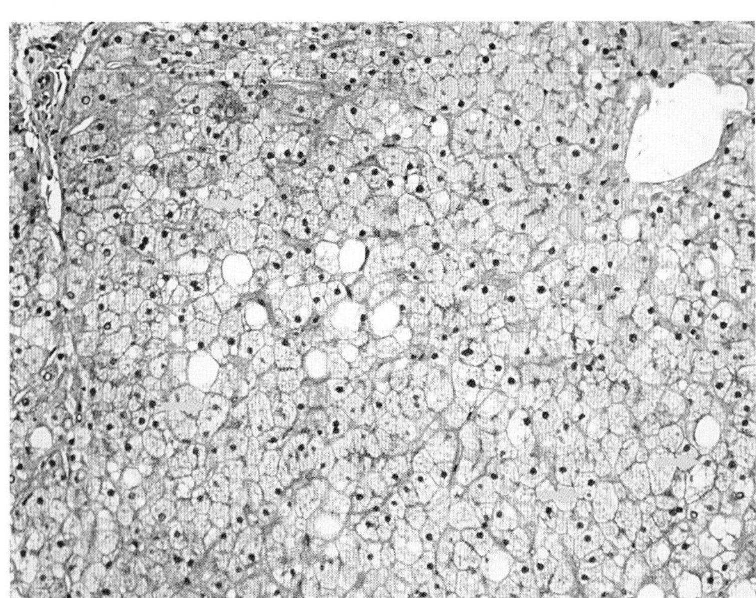

Figure 19.6 Glycogenic hepatopathy. Diffuse hepatocyte swelling by pale-staining cytoplasm and accentuation of the cell membrane, mimicking plant cells. Megamitochondria in some hepatocytes (*arrows*).

diagnosis is made by careful attention to the hepatocytes, which show abundant pale or clear cytoplasm and often show prominent cell membranes. PAS stains are strongly positive in both GH and the normal liver, and there is no quantitative method to distinguish normal glycogen content from excessive glycogen accumulation. The clinical and laboratory findings provide important clues to the diagnosis, because essentially all cases of GH occur in the setting of poorly controlled blood sugars with hepatomegaly and elevated liver enzymes.

Inherited glycogen storage diseases can have similar morphological findings of hepatocytes enlarged by glycogen accumulation, but inherited glycogen storage diseases can be easily distinguished from GH by the different clinical settings.

In some cases, hepatocytes can appear swollen because of artifacts, such as improper fixation or dry tissue, but they usually do not have pale-staining cytoplasm. Hepatocytes can also become enlarged because of intracytoplasmic inclusions, for example, with hepatitis B infection, but hepatitis B inclusions have a ground-glass appearance with distinct cytoplasmic inclusions and not a uniform cytoplasmic swelling. Pseudoground glass inclusions can also develop in hepatocytes as a drug effect.[21] These cases show distinct inclusion that have a distinct grayish to pink appearance and do not affect all hepatocytes. Diffuse microvesicular steatosis can mimic GH at low power, but high power examination will show tiny droplets of fat in microvesicular steatosis, and the hepatocytes are not strongly PAS positive.

Other cause of glycogenic hepatopathy

Short-term, high-dose steroid therapy can lead to GH,[22] although high-dose steroid therapy can lead to the full picture of hepatomegaly, elevated transaminases elevations, and GH on biopsy. Rarely, patients with type 2 diabetes can also develop GH if their blood sugars are poorly controlled[23,24] and occasionally when blood sugar levels appear to be well controlled.[25] Although counterintuitive, malnutrition can also lead to GH. For example, a 22-year-old patient with anorexia nervosa presented with abnormal liver enzymes and was found to have GH.[26] The liver enzyme elevations improved after nutritional therapy. Finally, clinical diagnosis of dumping syndrome can be associated with a hyperglycemic–hyperinsulinemic state and with GH on liver biopsy.[27]

Prognosis and treatment

GH results from poor glycemic control in most cases, but this does not lead to adverse long-term outcomes related to liver (e.g., fibrosis or necrosis). Some patients can have fluctuations of liver transaminases on follow up, especially if glycemic control remains a challenge.[18,20,28]

Type 2 diabetes

Liver involvement in type 2 diabetes covers a wide spectrum of liver diseases, ranging from mildly abnormal liver enzymes to cryptogenic cirrhosis. The most common chronic liver disease associated with diabetes is nonalcoholic fatty liver disease. The prevalence of nonalcoholic fatty liver disease in patients with type 2 diabetes is estimated at 34% to 74%.[29–31] The details of nonalcoholic fatty liver disease are further discussed in Chapter 16.

Diabetic hepatosclerosis

Recently, an additional pattern of liver injury was described in long-standing diabetic patients, termed "diabetic hepatosclerosis."[32] This injury pattern is characterized by dense sinusoidal fibrosis, even though the livers are non-cirrhotic in the traditional sense (Fig. 19.8). Alkaline phosphatase elevations are common. Hepatosclerosis can be an independent finding that is not accompanied by nonalcoholic fatty liver disease or GH. Most cases of diabetic hepatosclerosis have evidence of microvascular complications that leads to damage in multiple organs, suggesting that hepatosclerosis is result of microangiopathic disease of the liver. An autopsy study has found a prevalence of 12% in diabetic patients.[33] Indeed, diabetic

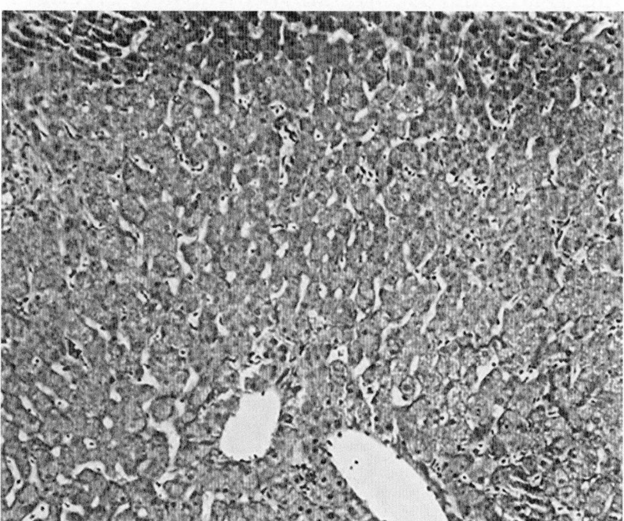

Figure 19.8 Diabetic hepatosclerosis. Diffuse sinusoidal fibrosis in a long-standing diabetic patient. Note the absence of liver plate atrophy or sinusoidal dilation, which makes it different from perisinusoidal fibrosis caused by venous outflow impairment.

microangiopathy in the liver has been associated with hepatosclerosis in a recent study.[34]

Thyroid disease

Hepatic dysfunction is often observed in hyperthyroidism, which can range from mild abnormal liver function tests to severe cholestasis and acute liver failure.[35–37] Elevated alkaline phosphatase levels are common and transaminases can also elevate, but they usually normalize when patients become euthyroid. The liver pathology in hyperthyroidism is mild and nonspecific but can include mild steatosis, mild to moderate cholestasis, mild lobular inflammatory inflammation with some eosinophils, and Kupffer cell hyperplasia. In patients who died of thyrotoxicosis, severe liver injury can occur, such as fatty liver, necrosis, venous congestion, and cirrhosis.[38] Autoimmune liver diseases, such as primary biliary cirrhosis or autoimmune hepatitis, can also be found in patients with thyroid disease, for example, co-occurring in about 10% of patients with Grave disease.[39]

Hypothyroid disease can be associated with mild elevations in liver enzymes, which normalize after hormone replacement therapy. The liver biopsy findings are usually normal or show minimal changes.[40] Hypothyroidism in infants and children may lead to cholestatic liver disease, leading to liver biopsy to rule out other pediatric cholestatic liver diseases. Hypothyroidism is also associated with nonalcoholic fatty liver disease.[41]

Hypopituitary disease

Hypopituitary disease can be a part of inherited syndromes or secondary to parenchymal loss, for example, following pituitary surgery. In infants, congenital hypopituitarism can manifest as cholestasis and/or neonatal giant cell hepatitis (Fig. 19.9).[42] There is growing evidence that adult hypopituitary patients can develop a similar phenotype as that of the metabolic syndrome, with central obesity, diabetes, and nonalcoholic fatty liver disease.[43] A study has shown that growth hormone replacement therapy in patients with hypopituitary disease can significantly improve the liver function tests and the histological changes of nonalcoholic fatty liver disease.[44]

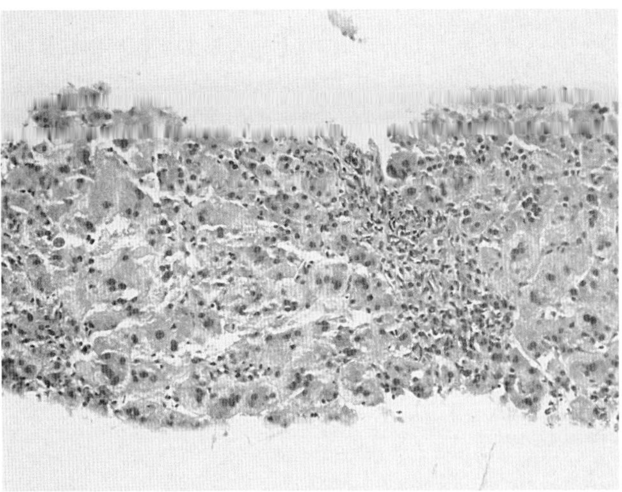

Figure 19.9 Liver in congenital hypopituitarism showing neonatal giant cell hepatitis with cholestasis.

19.4 LIVER IN GASTROINTESTINAL DISEASES

Inflammatory bowel disease

Hepatobiliary involvement is common in inflammatory bowel disease. Abnormal liver function tests are present in up to 30% of patients with inflammatory bowel disease but do not appear to correlate with disease activity.[45] Primary sclerosing cholangitis is one of the more common hepatobiliary complications of inflammatory bowel disease, particularly in patients with ulcerative colitis. The association of primary sclerosing cholangitis with inflammatory bowel disease and its manifestation are discussed in more detail in Chapter 13. Most of the medications used in the treatment of inflammatory bowel disease have been associated with a variety of liver injuries, including sulfasalazine, thiopurines, methotrexate, and biological agents. However, the overall incidence of serious complications is low. The general topic of medication-associated liver injury is also discussed in more detail in Chapter 15. The hepatobiliary complications also somewhat differ in ulcerative colitis versus Crohn's disease (Table 19.1).

In general, the liver can show a range of findings in individuals with inflammatory bowel disease, including minimal to mild nonspecific reactive hepatitis. In these cases, the inflammation may be a result of inflammatory changes in the intestine with increased mucosal permeability, leading to increased antigens in the portal circulation and secondary mild liver inflammation. Steatosis is also a common finding in the livers of inflammatory bowel disease patients, with a prevalence of up to 35%.[46] The liver shows macrovesicular steatosis, and the extent of fatty liver changes can correlate with the severity of the colitis, especially in ulcerative colitis.[47] Granulomas with mild inflammatory changes are rare and are predominantly seen in Crohn's disease (Fig. 19.10). Approximately 3% of patients with granulomatous hepatitis have Crohn's disease, but it also has been suggested that granulomatous

Table 19.1 Liver and Biliary Disorders in Inflammatory Bowel Disease

	Ulcerative Colitis	Crohn's Disease
Common	Primary sclerosing cholangitis (PSC) Small-duct PSC Medication-associated liver injury Steatosis Cholangiocarcinoma	Gallstones Medication-associated liver injury Steatosis
Less common	Gallstones	PSC Small-duct PSC Cholangiocarcinoma
Rare	Portal vein thrombosis Liver abscesses Granulomatous hepatitis Amyloidosis	Portal vein thrombosis Liver abscesses Granulomatous hepatitis Amyloidosis

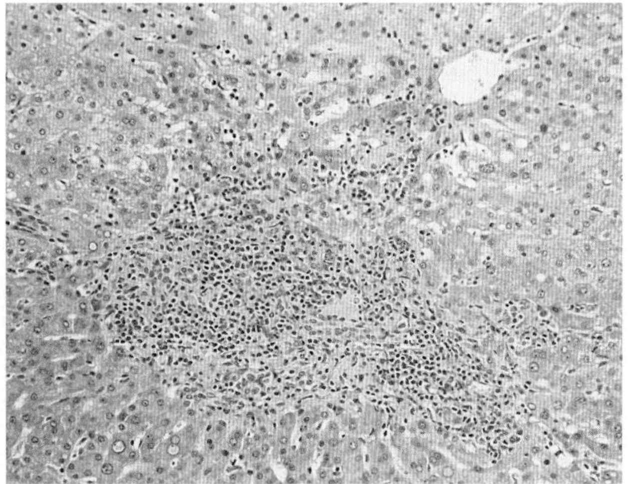

Figure 19.10 Liver in Crohn's disease showing mild portal and lobular nonspecific inflammation.

hepatitis in some cases can be secondary to treatment with sulfasalazine.[48] If the patient is under active immunomodulatory therapy, the biopsy should be carefully examined for cytomegalovirus (CMV) and other opportunistic infections. Finally, approximately 2% to 5% of inflammatory bowel disease patients with hepatobiliary involvement will develop cirrhosis, primarily because of primary sclerosing cholangitis.[49]

Celiac disease

Celiac disease is an autoimmune disorder seen in genetically predisposed people that is induced by a reaction to dietary gluten. Although primarily affecting the small bowel, celiac disease is a multisystem illness that can potentially involve other organs, including the hepatobiliary system. Approximately 30% to 40% of individuals with celiac disease will at some point have elevated transaminases or alkaline phosphatase levels.[50,51] In addition, studies have shown that up to 10% of unexplained elevations of liver enzymes will eventually prove to result from celiac disease.[52]

Transaminases are typically mildly elevated but can occasionally be seen in the several hundreds.[53] Mild elevations of antinuclear antibody and anti-smooth muscle antibody can be observed in about 10% of celiac disease patients. Liver enzymes will normalize following gluten-free diet in most cases, although the normalization often takes several months and may take up to a year.

If gluten restriction does not lead to normalized liver tests, then the possibility of other autoimmune liver disorders needs to be ruled out, such as autoimmune hepatitis, primary biliary cirrhosis, and primary sclerosing cholangitis, because they share common genetic factors and immunopathogenesis. Overall, approximately 3% to 7% of individuals with autoimmune hepatitis or primary biliary cirrhosis are found to have celiac disease, although the association was as high as 63% in one study.[54–56] An association with primary sclerosing cholangitis is less clearly established. The histological findings of the associated liver autoimmune disorders are the same as those in patients without celiac disease.

The histological changes in celiac disease are typically very mild and consist mostly of nonspecific portal and lobular chronic inflammation, Kupffer cell hyperplasia, focal ductular proliferation, and often some mild fatty change. This pattern has been referred as celiac hepatitis (Fig. 19.11). Steatosis is often associated with celiac disease, but it is unclear if the fatty change results from coexisting metabolic syndrome or is directly related to the celiac disease. A recent large epidemiological study has shown that individuals with celiac disease have nearly a threefold increased risk of nonalcoholic fatty liver disease compared with the general population.[57] Portal venopathy and nodular regenerative hyperplasia have also been described in patients with celiac disease.[58,59] In general, the mild inflammatory changes of celiac disease are not associated with fibrosis. Advanced fibrosis or cirrhosis can be seen but, in most cases, appears to be related to coexisting autoimmune liver disease or steatohepatitis.

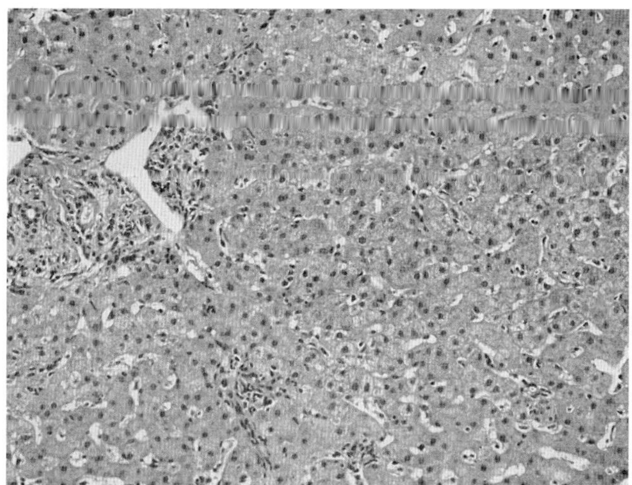

Figure 19.11 Liver in Celiac disease showing mild nonspecific portal and lobular chronic inflammation, Kupffer cell hyperplasia, and focal bile ductular proliferation.

19.5 LIVER IN SYSTEMIC AUTOIMMUNE DISEASES

Systemic autoimmune diseases have been associated with liver injury in general, but there are different prevalence, mechanisms, clinical significance, and liver pathology findings among the different diseases. The common features include mild elevation of liver enzymes with nonspecific histology, although rare cases can also present with fulminant hepatitis. Drug-induced liver injury also needs to be ruled out before considering an association between systemic autoimmune disease and liver dysfunction.

Rheumatoid arthritis

Rheumatoid arthritis is a systemic autoimmune disorder characterized by symmetric polyarticular joint involvement. Abnormal liver enzymes have been reported in up to 80% of patients with rheumatoid arthritis. Elevated alkaline phosphatase and GGT levels are the predominant biochemical abnormality.[60,61] Although rheumatoid arthritis involves bone damage, it has been shown that the predominant source of alkaline phosphatase is the liver. The increase in the liver isoenzyme levels of alkaline phosphatase has been shown to correlate with the clinical activity of rheumatoid arthritis.[62,63]

The liver histology is usually normal or shows minor alterations, such as variations in nuclear size, congestion, or mild steatosis. Some cases may present with mild nonspecific reactive hepatitis.[64,65] Nodular regenerative hyperplasia has also been reported in a small number of patients with rheumatoid arthritis. Nodular regenerative hyperplasia is more commonly seen in the Felty syndrome, in which rheumatoid arthritis patients also have splenomegaly and neutropenia. It has been reported that nearly 50% of patients with Felty syndrome have nodular regenerative hyperplasia and portal hypertension.[66] Nodular regenerative hyperplasia in rheumatoid arthritis and Felty syndrome is believed to be associated with rheumatoid vasculitis.[67] Lipogranulomas have been found in 56% of liver biopsies in rheumatoid arthritis patients, which is thought to be related to treatment, because these granulomas contain gold particles.[68] Rheumatoid nodules, the pathognomonic feature of rheumatoid arthritis in skin and other organ sites, are rarely reported in the liver.[69] Rheumatoid nodules are typically large and show a central area of necrosis/fibrosis surrounded by a middle layer of histiocyte-rich inflammation that can show palisading and often has multinucleated giant cells. An outer layer shows chronic inflammation with lymphocytes and plasma cells as well as areas that look like granulation tissue.

Methotrexate is one of the most commonly used drugs in the treatment of rheumatoid arthritis. Liver biopsy is recommended if patients have other significant risk factors for liver disease (alcohol use, chronic viral hepatitis, diabetes, or obesity) or 6 of 12 liver transaminases or serum albumin tests are abnormal in any year. Methotrexate-induced liver histologic changes include steatosis, steatohepatitis, focal necrosis, anisonucleosis, fibrosis, and cirrhosis (Fig. 19.12). If advanced fibrosis or cirrhosis is present on the liver biopsy, then halting methotrexate is typically recommended. Methotrexate also has synergistic effect with other risk factors of steatohepatitis, such as alcohol consumption, and can further aggravate steatohepatitis.

Systemic lupus erythematosus

Systemic lupus erythematosus is a systemic autoimmune disease in which the liver can also be affected. Overall, 25% to 50% of systemic lupus erythematosus patients have abnormal liver enzymes.[70] The histological changes of the liver in systemic lupus erythematosus are extremely variable and can range from normal or minimal changes to cirrhosis. Liver involvement in systemic lupus erythematosus has been classified into three major patterns: (1) lupus hepatitis or systemic lupus erythematosus-associated hepatitis; (2) co-occurrence with other autoimmune liver diseases, such as autoimmune hepatitis and primary biliary cirrhosis; and (3) liver injury due to non-autoimmune etiologies, for example, drug-induced liver damage, viral hepatitis, or thrombotic liver disease, among others.[71]

Lupus hepatitis refers to a mild, subclinical liver injury directly associated with systemic lupus erythematosus. Although it is still controversial whether

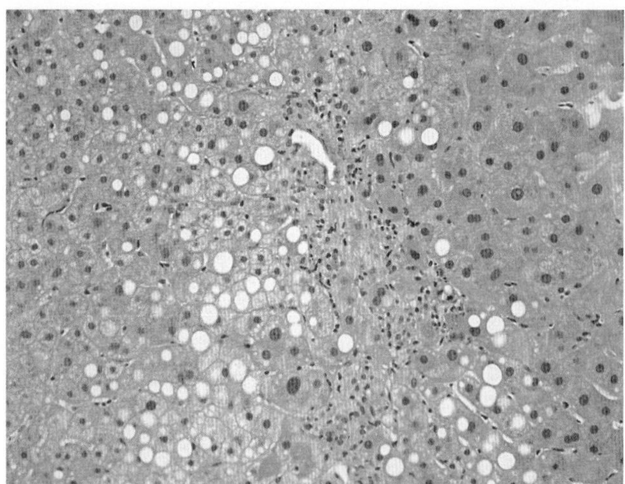

Figure 19.12 Methotrexate-induced liver changes in rheumatoid arthritis, including mild steatosis, focal zone 3 necrosis, and anisonucleosis.

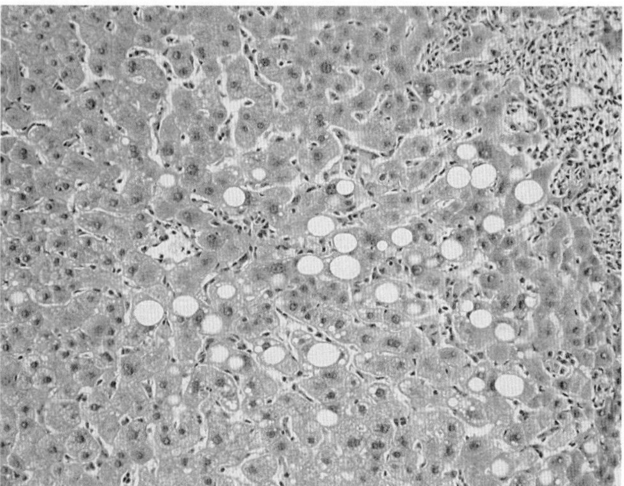

Figure 19.13 Lupus hepatitis presented as mild panacinar hepatitis. Note the mild steatosis and many plasma cells in the portal tract.

the hepatic dysfunction is attributed to lupus itself, recent studies have shown that autoantibodies to ribosomal P proteins (anti-ribosomal P), a highly specific marker for systemic lupus erythematosus, are associated with hepatic enzyme abnormalities in patients with systemic lupus erythematosus.[72] The prevalence of lupus hepatitis is about 10%.[73] However, lupus hepatitis is essentially a diagnosis of exclusion. On biopsy, lupus hepatitis shows a very mild nonspecific reactive hepatitis. The inflammation is mainly in the lobules, with lymphocytic inflammation and occasional acidophil bodies. Portal inflammation is absent or very mild. Lupus hepatitis is not associated with either severe or progressive liver injury (Fig. 19.13).

Patients with lupus can also have other autoimmune liver diseases, such as autoimmune hepatitis or primary biliary cirrhosis, which have different autoimmune pathogenesis from systemic lupus erythematosus. Autoimmune hepatitis has been reported in 15% to 20% of patients with systemic lupus erythematosus and abnormal liver enzymes; primary biliary cirrhosis is less frequent.[74] Autoimmune hepatitis overlaps clinically with lupus hepatitis, including shared features, such as hypergammaglobulinemia, positive autoantibodies, and response to steroid treatment. Liver biopsy findings can help distinguish these two possibilities. Autoimmune hepatitis is characterized by moderate to marked portal lymphoplasmacytic infiltrates, brisk lobular activity, interface activity, hepatic rosette formation, and often shows fibrosis. On the other hand, the presence of very mild lobular inflammation and patchy mild portal inflammation without a prominence of plasma cells is more compatible with lupus hepatitis.[75] Systemic lupus erythematosus can also rarely co-occur with primary biliary cirrhosis. In these cases, the typical features of primary biliary cirrhosis will be found. There also can be shared serological markers. One study found that serological markers of systemic lupus erythematosus, anti-dsDNA and anti-ribosomal-P antibodies, were detected in 22% and 5% of primary biliary cirrhosis patients, respectively.[76]

Non-autoimmune–mediated liver injury in patients with systemic lupus erythematosus can present with a wide spectrum of changes. Macrovesicular steatosis and nonalcoholic fatty liver disease are commonly seen in liver biopsy, in many cases related to corticosteroid treatment. Drug-induced hepatotoxicity tends to occur at higher rates in patients with lupus erythematosus patients, when compared with patients without systemic lupus erythematosus.[77] Analgesic drugs and nonsteroidal anti-inflammatory drugs (NSAIDs) are commonly used to treat systemic lupus erythematosus and can cause hepatitis, fulminant hepatic failure, and cholestasis. Methotrexate can lead to chronic liver injury and is discussed in Chapter 15. Other medications, such as thiopurine analogues and anti-tumor necrosis factor agents, can also cause mild liver injury. Nodular regenerative hyperplasia has been reported in association with systemic lupus erythematosus, resulting from hepatic circulation disorders caused by vascular diseases, such as vasculitis of the intrahepatic arteries, occlusion of intrahepatic small vessels in association with antiphospholipid antibodies, and portal vein thrombosis.[78]

IgG4-related systemic disease

IgG4-related systemic disease is a recently recognized autoimmune multi-organ fibroinflammatory disease.[79,80] This disease is discussed in more detail in Chapter 13 but is also briefly reviewed here. Autoimmune pancreatitis is the prototype of IgG4-related systemic disease. Patients with IgG4-related systemic disease typically have elevated serum IgG4 levels, tissue infiltration with abundant IgG4-positive plasma cells that is commonly associated with storiform fibrosis, multiple organ involvement, and response to corticosteroid treatment.

Many different manifestations of hepatobiliary involvement by IgG4-related systemic disease have been described, including IgG4-associated sclerosing cholangitis, IgG4 hepatopathy, and IgG4-associated inflammatory pseudotumors.[81–84] The extrahepatic bile ducts are the most commonly involved extrapancreatic site in patients with IgG4-associated autoimmune pancreatitis, with a reported frequency ranging from 71% to 100%. Bile duct involvement can present clinically either as a bile duct stricture or as a local tumefactive growth, and both presentations can mimic neoplasms. In fact, distinguishing IgG4-associated sclerosing cholangitis from primary sclerosing cholangitis and cholangiocarcinoma can be challenging in clinical practice.

Histologically, IgG4-associated sclerosing cholangitis differs from primary sclerosing cholangitis by the presence of obliterative phlebitis, transmural lymphoplasmacytic infiltrates, fibrosis with a storiform pattern, and markedly increased IgG4-positive plasma cells (Figs. 19.14 and 19.15). In contrast, primary sclerosing cholangitis shows bile duct injury and inflammation without markedly increased plasma cells. Biopsies from cholangiocarcinoma are characterized by high-grade cytological atypia, infiltrative growth patterns, and architectural changes of malignant glands.

Unfortunately, biopsy tissue obtained via endoscopic retrograde cholangiopancreatography is usually small and superficial and seldom reveals the

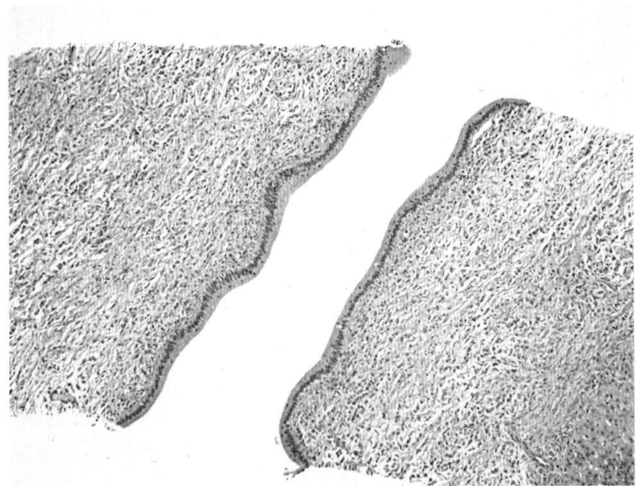

Figure 19.14 IgG4-associated sclerosing cholangitis. Periductal lymphoplasmacytic infiltrate and storiform fibrosis.

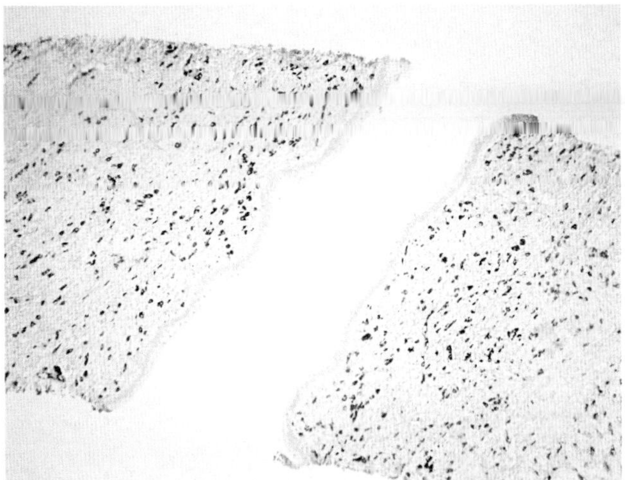

Figure 19.15 IgG4-associated sclerosing cholangitis. Numerous IgG4 positive plasma cells.

defined histopathological features of IgG4-associated sclerosing cholangitis. The biliary epithelial cells in the cytology or small biopsy material can also be very atypical for a variety of reasons, such as stenting, marked inflammation, or crush artifact. Even when present, increased IgG4-positive plasma cells are not entirely specific for IgG4-associated sclerosing cholangitis in this setting, because increased IgG4 plasma cells can also be observed in about 25% of primary sclerosing cholangitis biopsies, as well as cases of cholangiocarcinoma.[85] Therefore, correlation with other findings is necessary to establish the diagnosis of IgG4-associated sclerosing cholangitis, including clinical presentation, imaging, serum IgG4 level, and evidence of other organ involvement.

IgG4-related systemic disease can also involve the liver parenchyma and intrahepatic bile ducts, in most cases associated with IgG4-related autoimmune pancreatitis. In liver biopsies, the histological changes are usually mild and nonspecific, including mild portal and lobular inflammation, changes of large bile duct obstruction, and mild fibrosis. IgG4-positive plasma cell infiltrates are slightly increased and typically are seen in the portal tracts.[82] However, in some cases, the characteristic findings of IgG4-related systemic disease can also be seen, including portal-based inflammatory nodules composed of lymphocytes, plasma cells, and eosinophils, admixed with fibroblasts showing somewhat of a storiform fibrosis pattern. Immunostain also shows increased IgG4-positive plasma cells (Figs. 19.16 and 19.17).[86] This histologic appearance is very similar to other organs in IgG4-related systemic disease, although obliterative phlebitis is often absent in liver biopsies.

Inflammatory pseudotumors of the liver are a heterogeneous group of mass-forming liver lesions. A subset of inflammatory pseudotumors corresponds

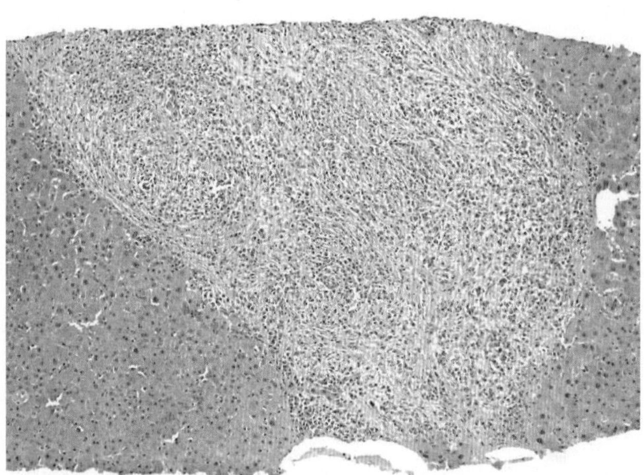

Figure 19.16 IgG4-related systemic disease involving liver. Nodular expansion of portal tracts by lymphoplasmacytic infiltrate and fibrosis.

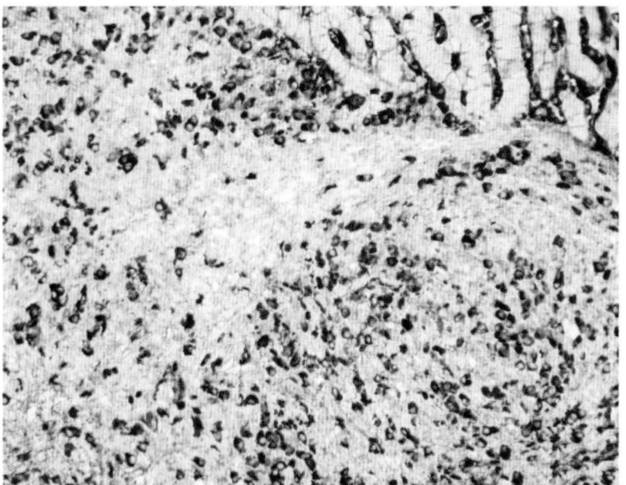

Figure 19.17 IgG4-related systemic disease involving liver. Numerous IgG4 positive plasma cells.

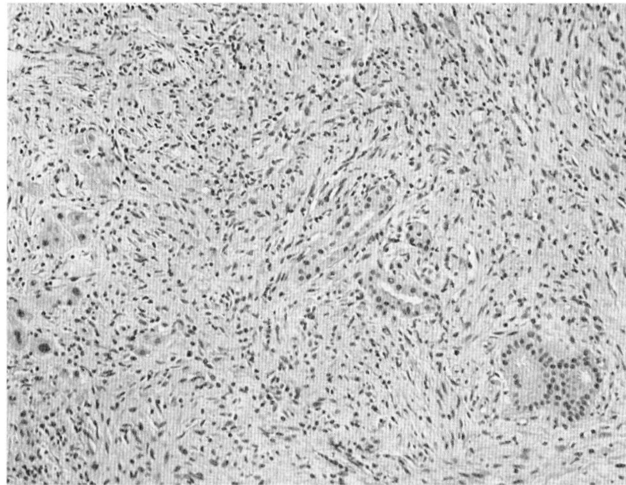

Figure 19.18 IgG4-related systemic disease involving liver, presented as an inflammatory pseudotumor.

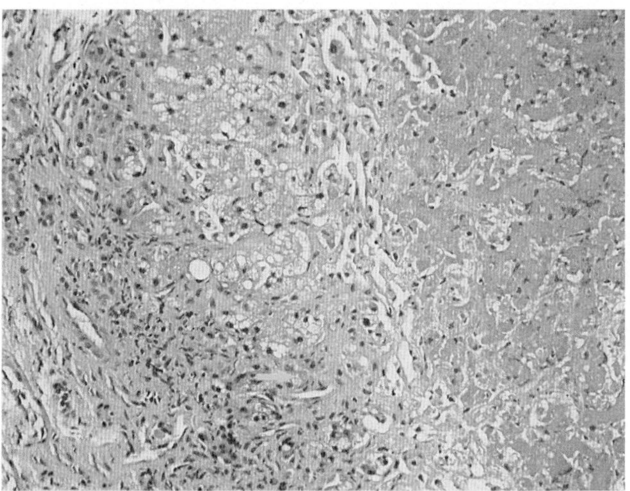

Figure 19.19 Liver in sepsis. The portal tract contains mild inflammation and bile ductular proliferation. There is bland necrosis and cholangiolar cholestasis (*arrow*). The hepatocytes also show cholestasis injury.

to IgG4-related systemic disease involving the liver (Fig. 19.18). These cases are often found around the hepatic hilum, mimicking cholangiocarcinoma. Microscopically, these inflammatory pseudotumors characteristically show features of IgG4-related systemic diseases, with diffuse lymphoplasmacytic infiltration, obliterative phlebitis, storiform fibrosis, and numerous IgG4-positive plasma cells.[81]

19.6 LIVER CHANGES IN SEPSIS

In sepsis, the liver plays a major role in host defense through metabolic, inflammatory, and immunological controls. However, the liver itself can suffer damage if these controls are not adequate, which can contribute to multiple organ failure and death. Sepsis usually exhibits a mixed hepatic and cholestatic pattern of liver enzyme elevations.[87]

Liver biopsies in septic patients can show a variety of changes. The most common finding is macrovesicular steatosis, and some cases have moderate to severe fatty liver changes. Bacterial toxins, hypoxia, drug effects, or TPN can all contribute to the development of fatty liver changes in sepsis.[88] In addition to steatosis, there are three other common patterns of injury. In some cases, varying degrees of all three of these patterns can be seen (Fig. 19.19).

The first pattern of liver injury shows "hepatitic" type changes with portal/lobular inflammation and/or centrilobular necrosis. The portal tracts usually show mixed inflammatory infiltrates but can be plasma cell rich. The lobules typically have numerous apoptotic cells. The second pattern is characterized by different combinations of hepatocanalicular and cholangiolar cholestasis with generally mild bile ductular reactions, cholangitis, or cholangiolitis. The liver in patients with shock from causes other than sepsis also can have this finding. The third pattern is mainly because of ischemic injury secondary to prolonged hypotension. There is bland lobular necrosis that begins in zone 3 and can extend to involve larger panacinar area, depending on the degree and duration of hypotension.

19.7 LIVER CHANGES IN SYSTEMIC HYPERTENSION

Systemic hypertensive–related changes are more commonly evident in the larger vessels and thus are more likely to be seen in resection or autopsy specimens, compared with liver biopsies. However, hepatic arteriolosclerosis in the smaller arteries can be observed in peripheral needle biopsies of the liver in some individuals with severe hypertension, particularly when there is co-occurrence with diabetes. The arteries show significant intimal thickening and hyaline change (Fig. 19.20).[34]

19.8 SHOCK LIVER

Shock liver results from insufficient blood flow and oxygen supply to liver. It typically occurs in critically ill patients with hemodynamic instability/shock. Clinically, the laboratory tests vary from a mild elevation of serum transaminases and bilirubin levels to an abrupt onset of strikingly high serum transaminases. The abnormal liver function tests can improve quickly after correcting the hemodynamic instability. Microscopic changes of liver are those of

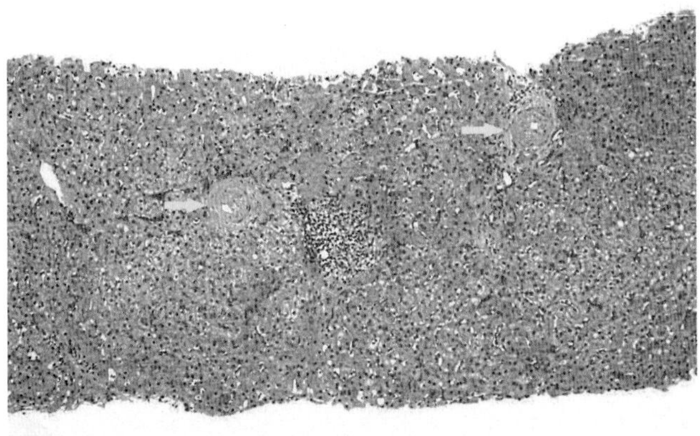

Figure 19.20 Arteriolosclerosis of hepatic arterioles in systemic hypertension. Marked thickening with hyalinization of arteriole wall in the portal tracts (arrows).

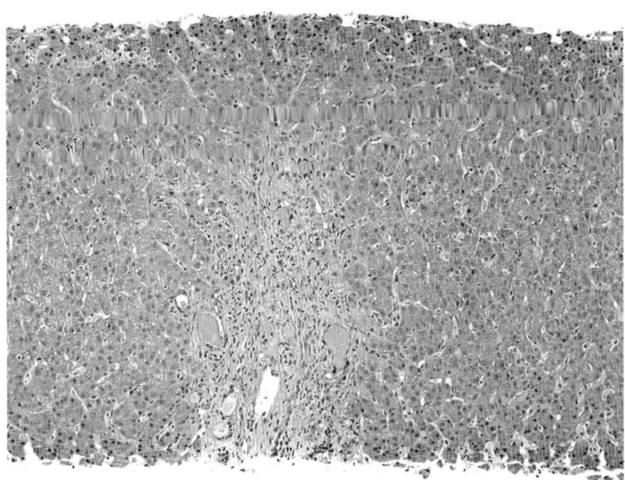

Figure 19.21 Shock liver showing marked cholangiolar cholestasis with mild inflammation and rare acidophil bodies.

ischemic hepatitis, characterized by necrosis of zone 3 hepatocytes without significant inflammation. The necrosis may extend to zone 2 or even be panacinar if the ischemia is severe or persistent. Cholestasis is commonly present in shock liver and can be lobular, cholangiolar, or both (Fig. 19.21). Other findings can include sinusoidal dilation, zone 3 hemorrhage, and variable degrees of fatty changes. If patients survive and recover from the shock, the liver functions tests and the liver histology can be restored to normal.

19.9 AMYLOIDOSIS

Definition

Amyloidosis is a systemic disorder characterized by the extracellular deposition of amyloid protein in many organs. The liver is one of the most commonly involved organs.

Basic classification of amyloidosis

Amyloidosis is generally classified based on the chemical composition of the amyloid fibrils and their precursor protein. About 60 amyloid proteins have been identified so far, and at least, 36 of those have been associated with human diseases. The five most common systemic forms of amyloid seen in liver pathology specimens are amyloid light chain (AL), acquired amyloidosis (AA), $\beta_{2\ microglobulin}$ amyloidosis ($A\beta_2M$), and two types of transthyretin amyloidosis (ATTR). Four of these are nonhereditary, and one is hereditary.

1. Primary or myeloma-related amyloidosis is caused by plasma cell dyscrasia, multiple myeloma, B-cell lymphoma, or Waldenström disease. Precursor

proteins of this type of amyloid are the κ or λ immunoglobulin light chains derived from plasma cells. Heavy chain deposition is associated with heavy chain disease, a pattern that is much less common than AL disease.

2. AA is also known as secondary or reactive amyloidosis and is caused by long-standing chronic inflammation. Serum amyloid A (SAA) protein is an acute phase reactant produced during inflammation, which is the precursor protein of this type of amyloid.
3. $A\beta_2M$ amyloidosis is seen in the setting of renal failure and dialysis. The precursor protein is β_2-microglobulin, and high serum levels develop over time because the protein is not removed by dialysis.
4. ATTR amyloidosis is found in individuals older than 80 years with normal, wild-type precursor protein transthyretin (TTR).
5. Hereditary ATTR amyloidosis, caused by more than 80 autosomal dominant point mutations of *TTR,* leads to familial amyloid polyneuropathies.

Clinical features

Hepatic involvement is common in amyloidosis. Autopsy studies have shown that 55% to 95% of patients with amyloidosis have hepatic involvement.[89] Up to 90% of individuals with AL amyloid and up to 60% with AA amyloid have liver involvement.[90] The clinical presentation of amyloidosis depends on the site of amyloid accumulation. Hepatic amyloid deposition is associated usually with mild and nonspecific presentations, including hepatomegaly and elevated alkaline phosphatase levels, along with symptoms of fatigue, weight loss, and anorexia. Advanced fibrosis and portal hypertension are rare.

Laboratory findings

Elevated serum alkaline phosphatase levels are the most frequent abnormal test in hepatic amyloidosis. One study showed that 86% of patients had an elevated alkaline phosphatase, of which 61% had values of 500 units/L or more.[91] The serum transaminase was more than twice the upper limit of normal in 37% of patients.

Imaging

Hepatomegaly is a common finding on imaging, but it is not correlated with the amount of amyloid deposition in the liver. Hepatic amyloidosis can show heterogeneous echogenicity by ultrasound. Computed tomography (CT) scans show diffuse or focal regions of decreased parenchymal attenuation. Magnetic resonance imaging (MRI) studies usually demonstrate significantly increased signal intensity on T1-weighted images without significantly altered signal intensity on T2-weighted images.

Gross findings

Gross specimens of hepatic amyloidosis are occasionally encountered at autopsy and liver transplant. The liver in AL or AA amyloid disease is usually enlarged with pale yellow material within the liver tissue, which gives a characteristic "waxy" appearance to the cut surface (Fig. 19.22). Livers with hereditary ATTR amyloidosis can be grossly normal.

Microscopic findings

In most cases, amyloidosis is diagnosed on tissue taken from the fat, kidney, intestine, or bone marrow. The liver is usually not biopsied in individuals with known amyloidosis because of the risk for bleeding or liver rupture, although many biopsies are performed safely. However, in the setting of difficult or nonspecific clinical presentations, new diagnoses of amyloid continue to be made on liver biopsy. Amyloid in the liver has the same morphological features as it does elsewhere, that is, deposition of acellular eosinophilic amorphous material (Figs. 19.23 and 19.24). The amount of amyloid deposits varies significantly. Some cases may have massive deposition with significant hepatocyte atrophy, whereas other cases can show very mild, subtle, and easily missed deposits (Figs. 19.25 and 19.26). Amyloid can be seen in the sinusoids, in the portal tracts, or in hepatic artery walls, and most cases have mixed patterns of deposition.

Some studies have suggested that different patterns of amyloid deposition can provide clues to distinguishing AA and non-AA type amyloidosis. For example, the predominant pattern of AA amyloidosis

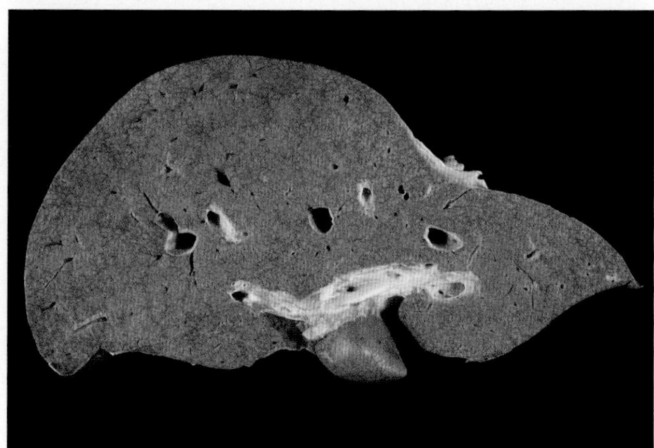

Figure 19.22 Hepatic amyloidosis. The liver is enlarged with pale yellow color and "waxy" appearance.

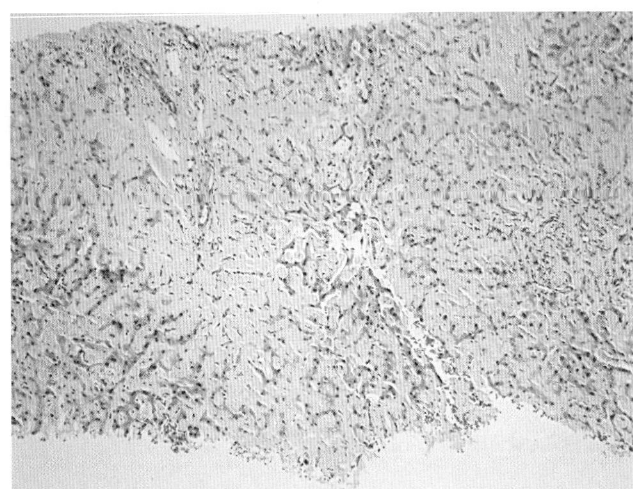

Figure 19.23 Hepatic amyloidosis. Amyloid light chain (AL)-type amyloidosis, diffuse deposition of light eosinophilic chunky material in sinusoids, portal tracts, and vascular wall. Note the significant loss of liver parenchyma.

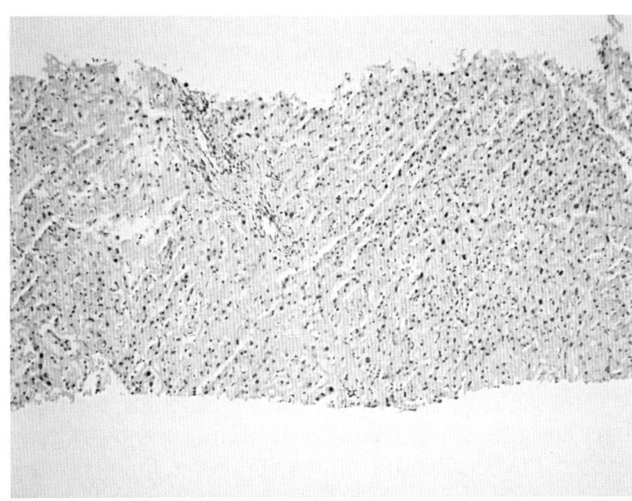

Figure 19.24 Hepatic amyloidosis. Amyloid deposition demonstrated by a Congo red stain in a red-orange color.

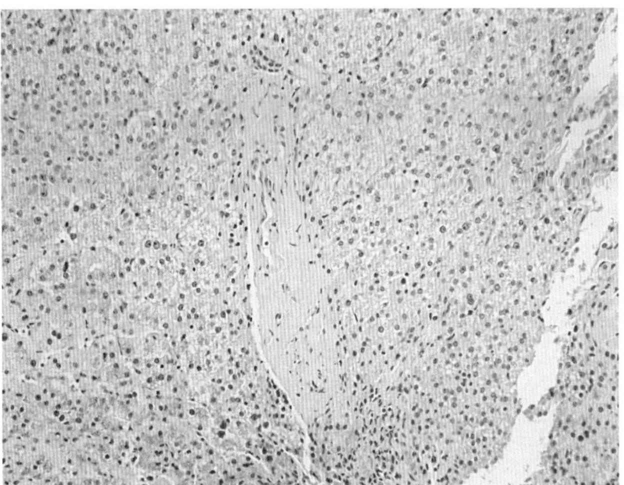

Figure 19.25 Hepatic amyloidosis. Acquired amyloidosis (AA)-type amyloidosis, subtle amyloid deposition may be easily overlooked.

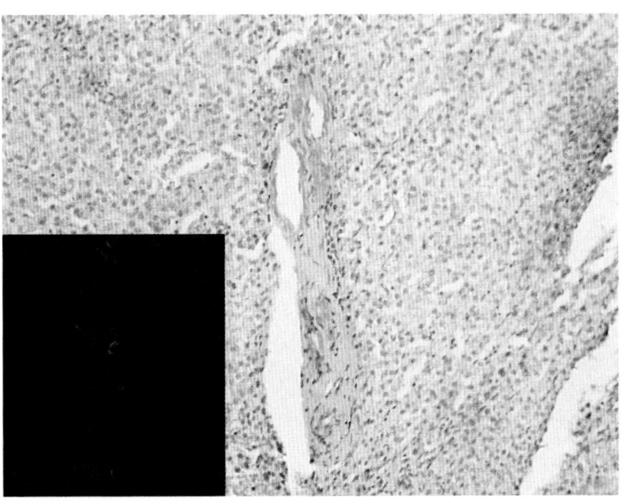

Figure 19.26 Hepatic amyloidosis. A Congo red stain can confirm amyloid (inset showing apple green birefringence under polarization).

shows deposits primarily in the blood vessels of the portal tracts, whereas AL amyloidosis usually shows a "sinusoidal" pattern, with amyloid being heavily deposited along the hepatic sinusoids as well as in the portal stroma.[92,93] In some familial cases, the amyloid is seen exclusively or predominately in the small arterioles. Although these patterns can be seen, most cases show a mixed pattern of amyloid deposits, and the amyloid distribution pattern is not used clinically to subtype amyloid.

In contrast to most forms of hepatic amyloidosis, the morphological findings in globular amyloid are highly specific for leukocyte chemotactic factor–associated amyloidosis (LECT2) (Figs. 19.27, 19.28, and 19.29).[94] LECT2 amyloidosis most commonly presents clinically with renal failure but also can be first observed in liver biopsy specimens. Most patients are elderly, and there is a strong association with Mexican heritage. Other ethnic associations include Native Americans, Sudanese, and Punjabis. Globular amyloid has distinct features on H&E, with large round eosinophilic globular deposits within the hepatocytes and to a lesser degree the reticuloendothelial cells. In some cases, the amyloid deposits tend to be concentrated zone 3 hepatocytes. The pattern and distribution of hepatic amyloid deposits are summarized in Table 19.2. Rarely, AL type amyloid can show a focal globular like pattern when sinusoidal deposits are cut in cross section, but linear amyloid deposits are the still the prominent pattern in AL amyloid. Immunostain for LECT2 can confirm the diagnosis (Fig. 19.29).

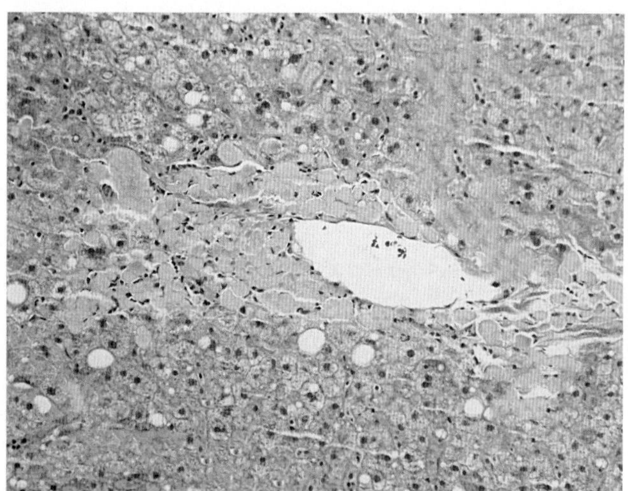

Figure 19.27 Global form hepatic amyloidosis. Globular amyloid in perivenular area.

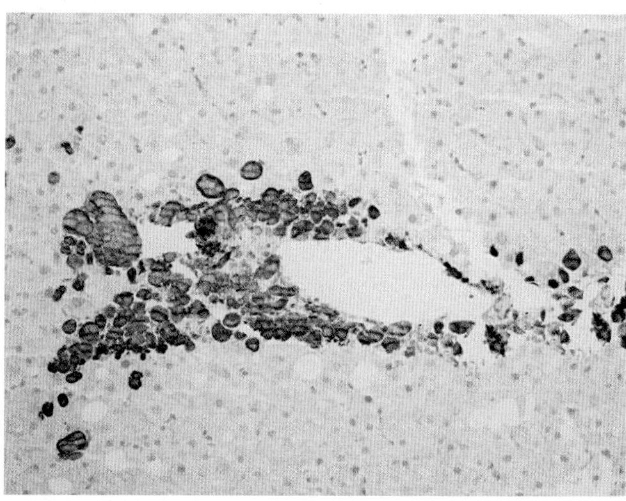

Figure 19.29 Global form hepatic amyloidosis. An immunostain of leukocyte chemotactic factor (leukocyte chemotactic factor–associated amyloidosis, LECT2).

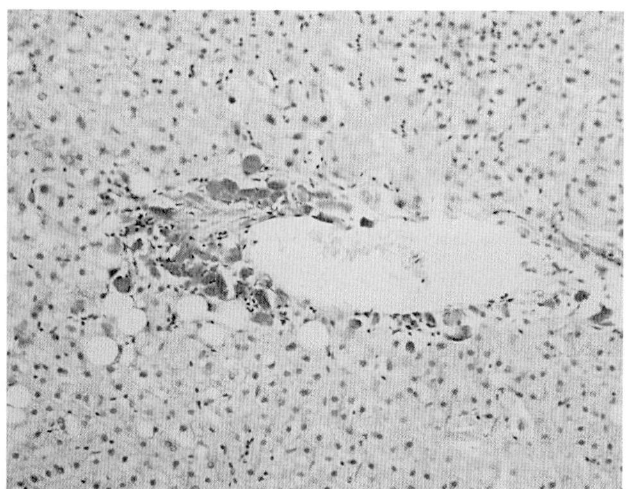

Figure 19.28 Global form hepatic amyloidosis, confirmed by a Congo red stain.

Immunohistochemistry and special stains

A Congo red stain is the most commonly used stain to confirm the presence of amyloid deposits. By routine light microscopy, the amyloid deposits should demonstrate a distinctive red-orange color (Figs. 19.24, 19.26, and 19.28). Polarization will then demonstrate "apple green" birefringence (Fig. 19.26). Interpretation of Congo red stain stains can sometimes be tricky. The globular amyloid in LECT2 can be less congophilic on Congo red stain, with only faint birefringence. Some false-negative Congo red stains may be because of technique failure, such as inappropriate thickness of the slide (the Congo red, stain should be performed on 10 μm thick sections, instead of the usual 4 μm for light microscopy). Other cause of false-negative birefringence includes having the lights in the room too bright, not turning up the light source on the microscope to full light, or not removing the internal, built-in filters on the microscope.

Table 19.2 Pattern and Distribution of Common Types of Hepatic Amyloid Deposits

Amyloid Type	Fibril Protein Precursor	Pattern	Distribution
	Immunoglobulin light chains	Linear, rare cases with focal globular	Mixed, may be parenchymal predominant
	Serum amyloid A	Linear	Predominant vascular, some mixed
ATTR	Normal or variant transthyretin	Linear	Predominant vascular
ALECT2	Leukocyte chemotactic factor 2	Globular, may have focal linear	Mixed, including intracellular distribution
AFib	Fibrinogen α-chain	Linear	Predominant vascular
AApoA1	Apolipoprotein A1	Linear	Mixed

If the amyloid-like material is truly negative on Congo red stain, other similar diseases need be considered, including Waldenström macroglobulinemia (associated with deposits of IgM heavy chains) or light chain deposition disease (associated with deposits of light chains that are Congo red negative).

Immunohistochemistry is mainly used for amyloid typing. Positive staining for κ- or λ-light chains indicates AL amyloidosis; positive staining for TTR indicates familial or senile amyloidosis; positive staining for SSA component occurs with AA amyloidosis; positive staining for LECT2 of globular amyloid indicates LECT2 amyloidosis (Fig. 19.29). However, the interpretation of these immunostains is often difficult because of high background staining.

Because of the challenges with subtyping the amyloid using immunostains, other methods have been developed. Laser microdissection with mass spectrometry has proven to be a very sensitive and specific method for identifying all types of amyloid. Mass spectrometry in most cases is the preferred method for amyloid typing, as the results have a specificity of 100% and sensitivity of 98%.[95] In addition, the mass spectrometry method is very useful because it uses formalin-fixed paraffin-embedded tissue instead of fresh tissue, frozen tissue, or other specially stored tissue samples. Mass spectrometry also can be helpful in histologically difficult cases, such as those with equivocal Congo red staining or less common forms of amyloid.[96]

Ultrastructural findings

Electron microscopy can also be used to identifying amyloid deposits, which are characterized by straight, unbranching fibrils 8 to 10 nm in width. Immunoelectron microscopy combines immunohistochemistry and electron microscopy to confirm amyloidosis with very high sensitivity and specificity but is not routinely used in clinical practice.

Molecular genetic findings

There are many types of hereditary or familial amyloidosis. Three types of genetic abnormalities have been identified in amyloidogenic proteins: polymorphisms, variant molecules, and genetically determined posttranslational modifications. Although important for understanding the biology of amyloid, molecular genetic testing is of limited utility for clinical care.

Differential diagnosis

The differential diagnosis for hepatic amyloid is primarily extracellular deposits that can look somewhat similar on H&E. Collagen deposits, for example, can mimic amyloid on H&E, especially when artifacts are present, such as because of poor fixation or crush effect. Overall, collagen fibers tend to be brighter and more eosinophilic than amyloid on H&E. Trichrome stains will show strong staining of collagen, whereas amyloid tends to be negative or very weakly staining. Congo red stains are also help differentiate collagen from amyloid. In contrast to amyloid, collagen is not congophilic. In addition, under polarizing light, the collagen shows a silvery white birefringence instead of "apple green" birefringence. The normal portal tracts serve as a built-in reference point for demonstrating the silvery white birefringence of collagen. Elastosis can also mimic amyloid on the H&E but is not congophilic and shows no birefringence.

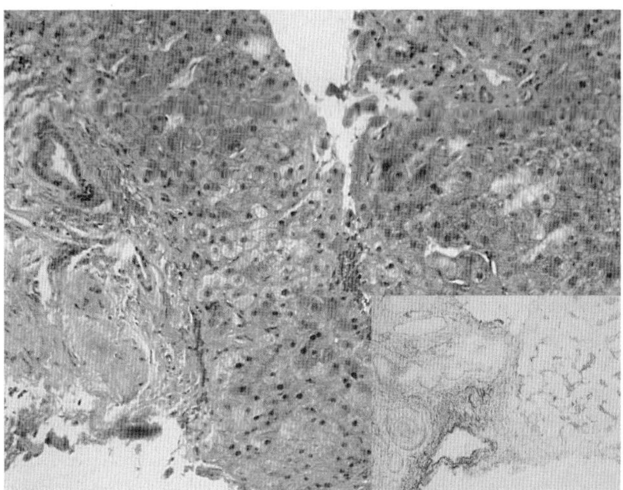

Figure 19.30 Light chain deposition disease resembling amyloidosis. Light chain deposits negative for Congo red stain and revealed by diffuse κ-light chain immunostain (inset).

The differential also includes the closely related process of light chain deposition disease. Light chain deposition disease is typically associated with renal disease, but the liver is the most common site of extrarenal involvement and can occasionally be the first clinical manifestation. Light chain deposits in the liver resemble amyloid, with a strong sinusoidal deposition pattern. Depending on the disease stage, the deposits can range from very subtle to diffuse and heavy (Fig. 19.30), but in all cases, the deposits are negative on Congo red stain. On ultrastructural examination, they show finely granular electron-dense deposits, rather than a fibrillar structures seen in amyloid. The monoclonal light chains are usually κ-light chain restricted (if they are λ restricted, classical amyloid disease is more likely). Waldenström macroglobulinemia is associated with deposits of IgM heavy chains, which can closely resemble amyloid but is also Congo red negative.

Treatment and prognosis

The treatment of amyloidosis varies depending on the underlying disease. For example, in AA amyloidosis, therapy is aimed at the underlying infectious or inflammatory disorder. In AL amyloidosis, therapy focuses on the underlying plasma cell dyscrasia. For the hereditary forms of amyloidosis, in which the mutant amyloid precursor protein is produced by the liver (e.g., TTR, apolipoprotein A-I, and fibrinogen Aa), liver transplantation may be an effective therapy to prevent further deposition of amyloid and may also lead to regression of established deposits.[97] Patients with sporadic or undiagnosed hereditary amyloidosis who present with end-stage organ failure may benefit from combined hepatorenal or hepatocardiac transplantation. In general, the presence of hepatic amyloidosis is an indicator of poor prognosis because it reflects relatively severe systemic disease. One study showed that the median survival in patients with hepatic amyloidosis was 9 months.[91]

19.10 LIVER CHANGES IN HEMOTOLOGICAL DISEASE

Langerhans histiocytosis

Liver involvement occurs in about 20% of both adult and pediatric patients with Langerhans histiocytosis and is an indicator of worse prognosis.[98,99] Isolated liver involvement by Langerhans histiocytosis has also been reported.[100] Liver involvement usually manifests as elevated liver enzymes and hepatomegaly, but tumor-like lesions or cystic lesions can also occur. The biliary tree is frequently involved, which results in sclerosing cholangitis pattern on imaging.

Histologically, Langerhans cells can be very subtle but show abundant eosinophilic cytoplasm and grooved nuclei with indented nuclear membranes. Immunoreactivity for CD1a, Langrin, or S100 can confirm the presence of Langerhans histiocytosis. Langerhans cells can form granulomatous small nodules or discrete mass lesions. Langerhans histiocytosis also frequently involves the biliary tree, leading to a sclerosing cholangitis pattern of injury. When florid, the bile ducts are surrounded and infiltrated by Langerhans cells, often with a background of mixed inflammation including numerous eosinophils. The bile duct epithelium is often damaged or totally denuded (Figs. 19.31 and 19.32). Secondary changes that result from the bile duct injury are common, including bile ductular reaction, ductopenia, chronic cholestasis, and positive copper stain in periportal hepatocytes. Periductal concentric fibrosis or "onion-skin" like fibrosis can also be found. The fibrosis can progress

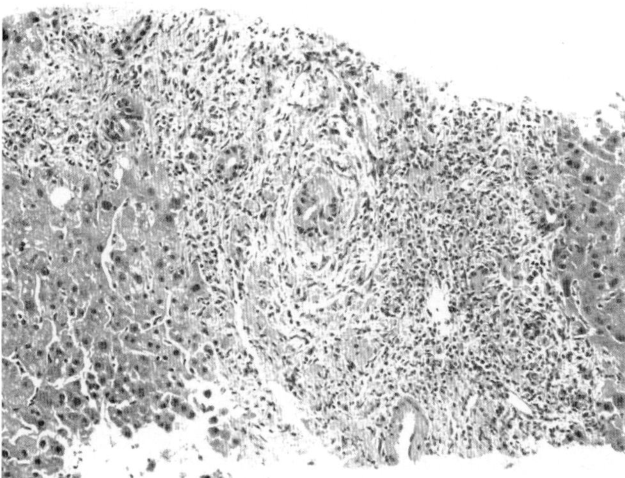

Figure 19.31 Langerhans histiocytosis. Portal expansion with many eosinophils in the background and bile duct destruction.

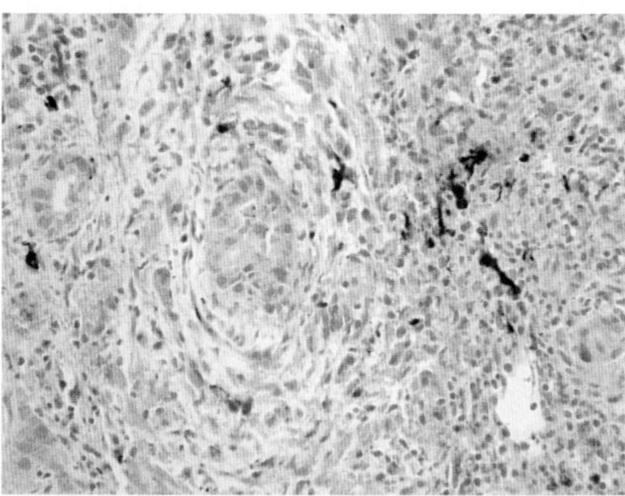

Figure 19.32 Langerhans histiocytosis. Langerhans cell infiltrate highlighted by a CD1a immunostain.

over time to a biliary pattern of cirrhosis and require liver transplantation.

The sclerosing cholangitis seen in Langerhans histiocytosis can mimic primary sclerosing cholangitis in both imaging studies and by histology. Extrahepatic manifestation of Langerhans histiocytosis, when present, can indicate the proper diagnosis. In cases without a history, immunostains for Langerhans cells will help establish the diagnosis of Langerhans histiocytosis.

Mastocytosis

Mastocytosis is a myeloproliferative disorder characterized by mast cell hyperplasia involving many organ systems (see also Chapter 30). Liver involvement in mastocytosis occurs in about 60% of cases.[101] Affected individuals can present with hepatosplenomegaly

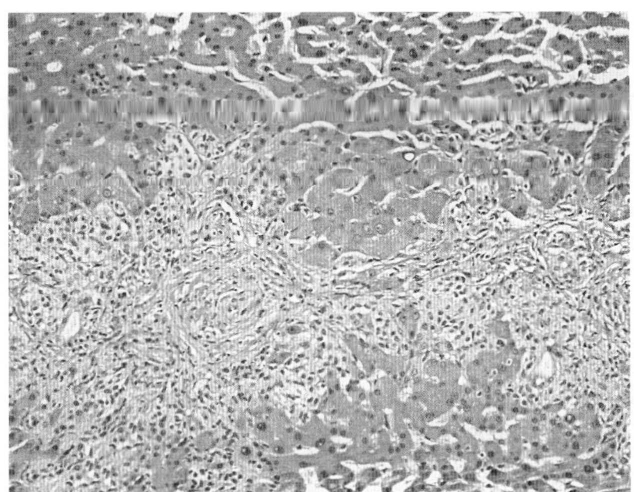

Figure 19.33 Mastocytosis. Mast cell infiltration in portal and periportal area, accompanied with eosinophils and bile duct injury.

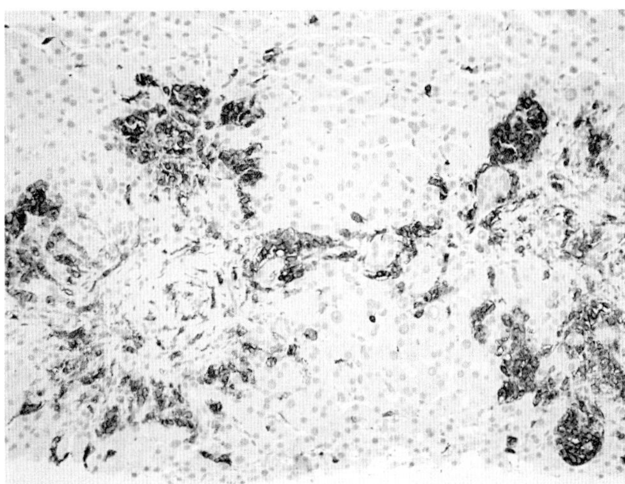

Figure 19.34 Mastocytosis. KIT immunostain showing numerous and small aggregates of mast cells.

and elevated liver enzymes, predominately alkaline phosphatase and GGT levels.

When there are elevated liver enzymes, mast cell infiltration is commonly seen on liver biopsy. The mast cells are predominantly located in the portal tracts and may form small aggregates or have a periductal accentuation, with bile duct injury that can suggest sclerosing cholangitis (Figs. 19.33 and 19.34).[102] Eosinophilic infiltrates often accompany the mast cells and sometimes can obscure the mast cells. Dense infiltrates of eosinophils can serve as a diagnostic clue for mastocytosis. The portal inflammation also includes small lymphocytes, histiocytes, and plasma cells. Portal fibrosis is frequently seen, especially with more extensive mast cell infiltration, but progression to cirrhosis is rare. Vascular injury can lead to portal venopathy or veno-occlusive disease, often associated with a nodular regenerative hyperplasia pattern in the lobules. Mast cells can be identified using special stains, including toluidine blue, chloroacetate esterase stains, KIT, and tryptase. KIT immunostain is the most commonly used stain when evaluating for mast cell disease, followed by tryptase immunostain as needed. Of note, almost all livers with inflammatory disease of any sort will contain a few mast cells. However, the mast cell infiltrates will be striking in cases of mast cell disease, with sheets of mast cells in the portal tracts and patchy aggregates in the sinusoids. CD25 immunostains are also performed, because neoplastic mast cells are CD25 positive, whereas normal/reactive mast cells are negative.[103]

Extramedullary hematopoiesis

Extramedullary hematopoiesis in the liver is normal in newborns up to 5 weeks after birth and can persist in the presence of neonatal hepatitis or anemia. Extramedullary hematopoiesis can also occur in adult livers, where it is usually a focal and incidental finding. However, associations in adults can include anemia, myeloproliferative disorders, or systemic infections. Erythroid and myeloid precursors are usually found in the sinusoids. In more striking cases, rarely seen outside of the pediatric setting, myeloid precursors can also be found in the portal tracts. Erythroid precursors can resemble lymphocytes, but they usually have scant cytoplasm and form small clusters with more discrete and hyperchromatic nuclei than lymphocytes. Megakaryocytes can also appear within sinuses with no accompanying erythroid and myeloid precursors. Megakaryocytes sometimes can look atypical and bizarre-shaped, and it is important not to misinterpret them as malignant tumor cells (Fig. 19.35). Rarely, extramedullary hematopoiesis can have a nodular appearance and mimic a tumor on imaging.[104]

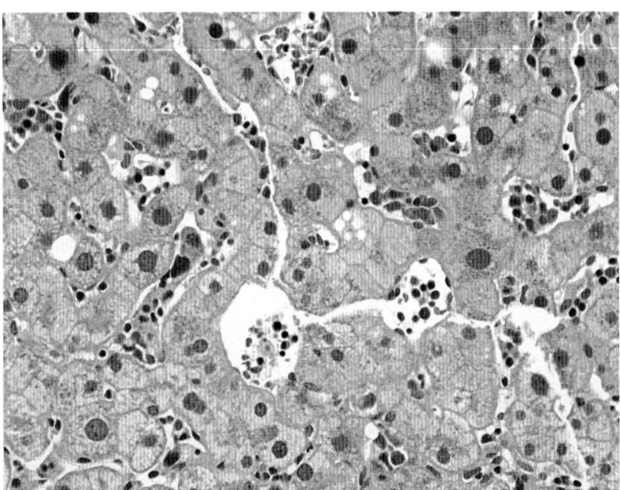

Figure 19.35 Extramedullary hematopoiesis. Small aggregates of hematopoietic cells, including megakaryocytes in sinusoids.

Hemophagocytic syndrome

Familial hemophagocytic lymphohistiocytosis is genetic based, but most cases of hemophagocytic syndrome are secondary or acquired. Familial hemophagocytic lymphohistiocytosis is a rare and usually fatal autosomal recessive disorder that is discussed in Chapter 30. Secondary hemophagocytic syndrome occurs after strong immunologic activation because of systemic infections, immunodysregulation, or malignancy. In these conditions, there can be abnormal activation of T lymphocytes and macrophages leading to severe clinical and hematologic abnormalities. Nearly all patients with hemophagocytic syndrome will have hepatomegaly, elevated liver enzymes, elevated lactate dehydrogenase, and elevated bilirubin levels. Abnormal coagulation tests are frequently seen because of hepatic dysfunction and/or disseminated intravascular coagulopathy.

Histologically, the hemophagocytic syndrome typically shows variably dilated sinusoids filled with numerous large histiocytes with hemophagocytosis (Fig. 19.36). Most cases have erythrophagocytosis only, although intracytoplasmic accumulation of pigment (either hemosiderin or bile) is also found. The portal tracts do not show hemophagocytosis and often contain nonspecific mild lymphocytic inflammation. Significant bile duct injury or bile ductular proliferation is usually absent. Other nonspecific findings can include focal hepatocyte spotty necrosis, mild macrovesicular steatosis, and lobular or portal granulomas.[105]

Thrombotic thrombocytopenic purpura

Thrombotic thrombocytopenic purpura is a rare clotting disorder characterized by clotting in the small blood vessels of different organ systems, resulting in a low platelet count. The disease can be caused by severe deficiency of ADAMTS13 activity because of autoantibodies against this protease. Secondary thrombotic thrombocytopenic purpura is associated with medication effect, bone marrow transplant, pregnancy, and paraneoplastic syndromes. Hyaline intravascular microthrombi may be found in the portal tracts (Fig. 19.37). The liver may also show mild patchy sinusoidal congestion with marked lobular disarray, scattered apoptosis, and marked hepatocyte nuclear pleomorphism. Although these findings are not specific, they are quite distinctive and can suggest the diagnosis.[106]

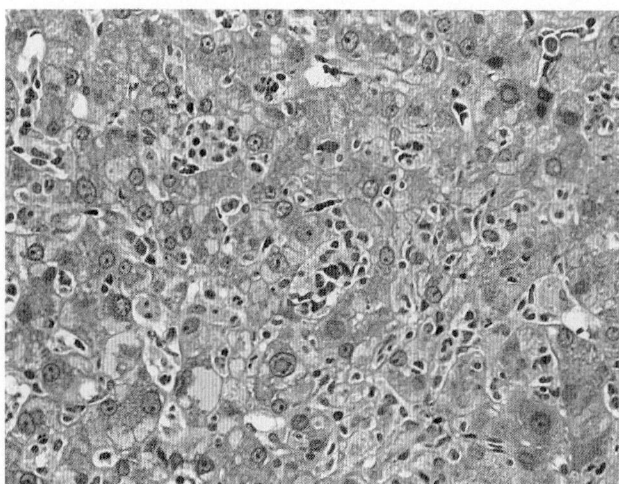

Figure 19.36 Hemophagocytic syndrome. Hepatic sinusoids packed with large activated histiocytes engulfing red blood cells and white blood cells.

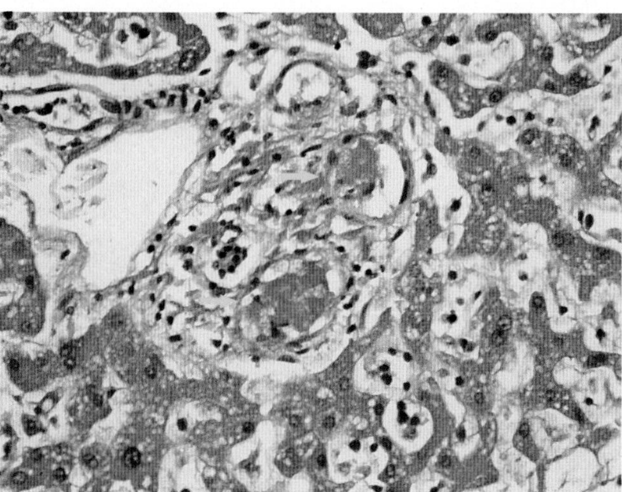

Figure 19.37 Thrombotic thrombocytopenic purpura. Intravascular microthrombi identified in portal vessels (*arrows*).

Sickle-cell disease

Sickle-cell disease is a group of hemoglobinopathies that results from single nucleotide mutations in the β-globin chain. The liver can be affected by the disease itself or by its treatment, such as multiple transfusions, which can increase the risk for viral hepatitis, iron overload, or gallstone formation. The term "sickle-cell hepatopathy" has been used to reflect the hepatic dysfunction in sickle-cell disease patients.[107] Acute elevations of serum ALT, AST, and alkaline phosphatase are seen in the setting of vaso-occlusive crises, whereas chronic liver enzymes elevations are usually because of coexisting hepatic pathology.

Mildly elevated bilirubin levels are almost universal in sickle-cell disease patients because of chronic hemolysis. The bilirubin levels can double during crises. Acute sickle hepatic crisis can occur in approximately 10% of patients with sickle-cell disease, which is caused by ischemia because of sinusoidal obstruction by diffuse red blood cell sickling and/or thrombi formation.[108] Patients usually present

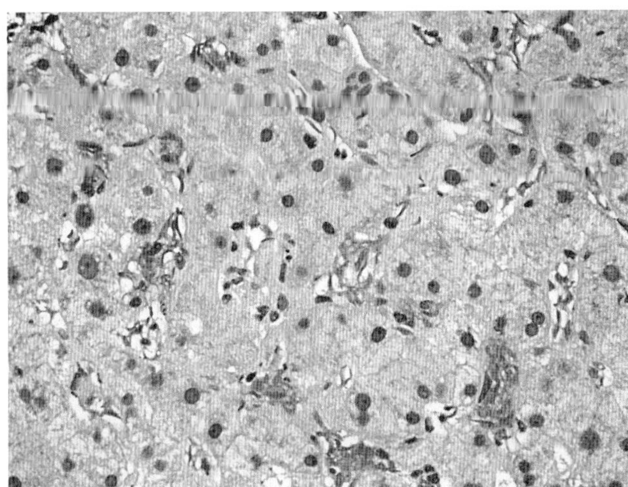

Figure 19.38 Sickle-cell disease involving liver. Extensive red blood cell sickling in sinusoids.

with acute right upper quadrant pain, tender hepatomegaly, low grade fevers, and jaundice. Hepatic sequestration crisis results from acute sequestration of large numbers of red blood cells in the liver and other organs, such as the spleen and lungs, which can lead to acute anemia, shock, and death.

In general, sickle-cell disease with acute hepatic disease is considered a contraindication for percutaneous liver biopsy. Serious hemorrhage and even death can occur in about one-third of sickle-cell disease patients who underwent percutaneous liver biopsy during acute sickle-cell disease.[109] When biopsied or at autopsy, the main histologic features in sickle-cell disease are diffuse sinusoidal dilatation with widespread red blood cell sickling, Kupffer cell hyperplasia, erythrophagocytosis, and hemosiderosis (Fig. 19.38). Crescent-shaped red blood cells are easily identified in the sinusoids and the Kupffer cells. An autopsy study showed that Kupffer cell erythrophagocytosis and sinusoidal distension by red blood cell sickling were universally present, whereas iron deposition, focal hepatocyte necrosis, extra medullary hematopoiesis, portal fibrosis, and nodular regenerative hyperplasia were also observed in some cases.[110] Of note, cirrhosis can develop in approximately 20% of patients with sickle-cell disease as a consequence of recurrent vascular obstruction, necrosis, and repair. Coexisting liver pathology, such as iron overload or chronic viral hepatitis, can also contribute to liver fibrosis.

Sickle-cell trait is the heterozygous form of sickle-cell disease and only rarely develops clinical manifestations of liver disease. Because of its high incidence (1 in 12 in African Americans), mild intrasinusoidal sickling with sinusoidal dilatation in perivenular areas can occasionally encountered in liver biopsy performed for other reasons. This incidental finding can be easily overlooked because of its subtle and nonspecific appearance.

19.11 LIVER CHANGES ADJACENT TO MASS-FORMING LESIONS

The nonneoplastic liver parenchyma adjacent to either primary or metastatic liver tumors exhibits a wide spectrum changes that result from mass effect, vascular or biliary obstruction by the tumor, or treatment-related changes.

Peritumoral changes

Mass-forming lesions can cause obstruction of the bile ducts or blood vessels, leading to biliary tract or vascular outflow changes, respectively. With biliary obstruction, the portal tracts show edema, ductular reactions, and nonspecific inflammation. The lobules can show cholestasis, and the zone 1 hepatocytes can show cholate stasis (Fig. 19.39). Ductopenia can be observed in some cases. With vascular obstruction, the lobular parenchyma can show marked sinusoidal dilation, hepatic plate atrophy, Kupffer cell hyperplasia, and mild nonspecific inflammation. As a more specific finding, the hepatocytes surrounding metastatic neuroendocrine tumors that produce insulin can show marked steatosis, a pattern that leads to a distinctive ring-like appearance on imaging.

Recognizing these peritumoral changes in liver biopsy is important when the biopsy is targeted toward a mass but contains no tumor. In many of these cases, the biopsy missed the tumor and sampled the peritumoral changes in the background liver. Re-biopsy is typically necessary in this situation in order to provide a diagnosis.

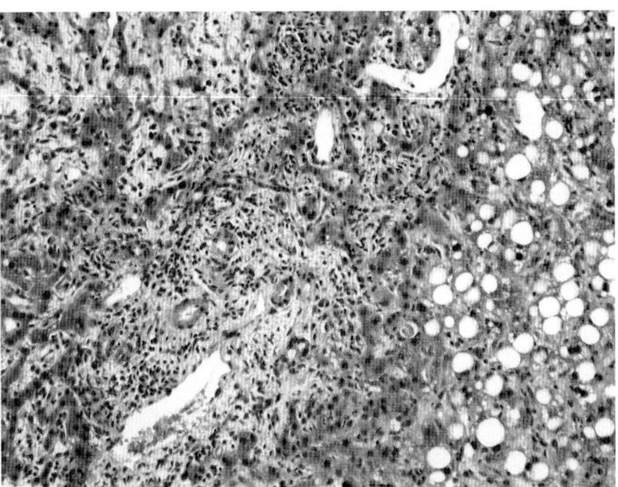

Figure 19.39 Liver changes in mass-forming lesions. Peritumoral effect, characterized by edema, nonspecific inflammation, bile ductular proliferation, and marked sinusoidal dilation with Kupffer cell hyperplasia.

Chemotherapy- and radiation-related changes

Nearly all chemotherapy agents can cause either direct or indirect hepatotoxicity. The clinical presentation can range from asymptomatic biochemical abnormalities to acute liver failure. The distinction between chemotherapy-related hepatotoxicity and other causes of liver injury can be difficult clinically. Other common causes of liver injury in this setting include tumor progression, coexisting liver disease, and adverse effects of other drugs. The clinical course often can help diagnose chemotherapy-related hepatotoxicity,[111] and biopsies may not be necessary. For example, in patients who lack a history of prior liver disease, chemotherapy-related hepatotoxicity is suggested when clinical symptoms or elevated liver enzymes develop after starting chemotherapy and improve after discontinuation of chemotherapy agents.

Although liver biopsy has limited value in this setting, the liver in chemotherapy-related hepatotoxicity can present with several basic patterns: (1) hepatocellular injury manifesting as a hepatitis with spotty liver necrosis; (2) cholestasis; (3) fatty liver disease; or (4) vascular injury with varying patterns, including zone 3 hepatocyte necrosis, sinusoidal obstructive syndrome/veno-occlusive disease, nodular regenerative hyperplasia, or peliosis.[112]

Radiation induces liver injury in 6% to 66% of patients, with injury usually manifesting 4 to 8 weeks after radiation exposure.[113] Patients can present with ascites, hepatomegaly, and abnormal liver enzyme tests. Most patients will recover completely in a few months, whereas some of them may develop chronic liver disease with liver fibrosis and liver failure. The main pathologic finding is sinusoidal obstructive syndrome, because radiation can cause endothelial damage and thrombi formation, leading to venous occlusion and sinusoidal congestion. Some cases develop advanced fibrosis, often with dense pericellular fibrosis.

Tumor ablation by either chemoembolization or radioembolization is an important nonsurgical approach for treating liver tumors. Treatment efficacy ranges from complete response to minimal response. The adjacent liver parenchyma can also be injured if embolization beads reach the non-tumor liver. These embolic beads can lead to foci of ischemic necrosis. In other cases, the liver parenchyma can show nonspecific reactive changes (Fig. 19.40). Macrovesicular steatosis, nodular regenerative hyperplasia, and veno-occlusive disease can also be observed. Ischemic cholangitis and bile duct necrosis can also occur after embolization.[114]

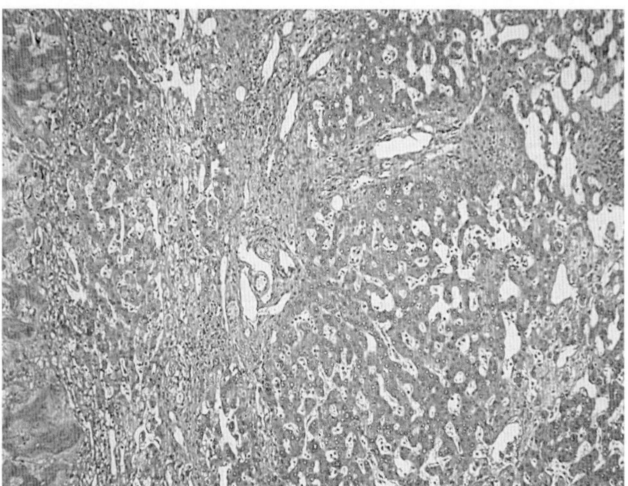

Figure 19.40 Liver changes after tumor ablation. Nonspecific inflammation, sinusoidal dilation with liver architectural disarray, and fibrosis. Note the necrotic tumor at the left.

19.12 LIVER IN PREGNANCY

Hepatic dysfunction occurs in 3% to 5% of pregnancies, and most cases are pregnancy-related. Preexisting liver diseases, such as autoimmune hepatitis or chronic viral hepatitis, may worsen during pregnancy. Liver diseases unique to pregnancy are the focus of this section (Table 19.3).

Liver in normal pregnancy

During a normal pregnancy, the serum levels of AST, ALT, and bilirubin are normal. Serum GGT activity is usually lower in the second and third trimesters. Alkaline phosphatase levels progressively rise in the last part of pregnancy. However, the elevated alkaline phosphatase is mainly from the placenta and bone formation, rather than being hepatic in origin.[115] Therefore, elevated alkaline phosphatase levels in pregnancy are not a good indicator of a biliary disease. On the other hand, any increase in serum transaminases, GGT levels, or bilirubin levels in pregnancy should be considered pathological, and further evaluation is warranted. The liver in normal pregnancies is normal or shows minimal nonspecific changes by light microscopy. Ultrastructurally, the hepatocytes can show nonspecific proliferation of smooth endoplasmic reticulum and enlarged mitochondria.[116]

Acute fatty liver of pregnancy

Definition

Acute fatty liver of pregnancy is a rare life-threatening complication unique to human pregnancies,

Table 19.3 Liver Diseases in Pregnancy

Disease	Trimester	Frequency (of Pregnancies)	Clinical Features	Liver Histology
Acute fatty liver of pregnancy	Third	1/10,000–20,000	Nausea, vomiting, abdominal pain, anorexia, and progressive jaundice; liver failure	Diffuse microvesicular steotosis
Hyperemesis gravidarum	First	1–20/1,000	Severe nausea and vomiting; dehydration; elevated liver enzymes, alanine transaminase (ALT) > aspartate transaminase (AST)	Normal histology or bland cholestasis
Intrahepatic cholestasis of pregnancy	Second or third	1%–6%, strong geographic variation	Pruritis with no rash; elevated bilirubin and/or ALT levels	Marked bland hepatocanalicular cholestasis with bile plugs
Preeclampsia/ eclampasia	Third	2%–8%	Hypertension with either proteinuria or end-organ dysfunction or both; ±HELLP syndrome; severe cases with liver infarction, hemorrahge, hematomas, and liver rupture	Periportal intrasinusoidal fibrin deposition with liver cell necrosis and hemorrahge; microvesicular steatosis

characterized by microvesicular fatty change of the hepatocytes and acute liver failure.

Clinical features

Acute fatty liver of pregnancy is rare, with a frequency of approximately 1/10,000 to 20,000 deliveries. The frequency is higher in women who are underweight or who have a history of multiple gestations. Acute fatty liver of pregnancy typically occurs in the last trimester and is always present before delivery, although it is not always clinically evident prior to delivery. Patients present with nausea, vomiting, abdominal pain, anorexia, and progressive jaundice. Signs of preeclampsia are present in about half of cases and can be severe. The medical course can also be complicated by portal hypertension, ascites, pancreatitis, or infection.

The exact etiology of acute fatty liver of pregnancy remains unknown but has been associated with inherited defects in mitochondrial β-oxidation of fatty acids, such as long-chain 3-hydroxyacyl CoA dehydrogenase deficiency (LCHAD).[117] In addition, defects in short- and medium-chain acyl-CoA dehydrogenase activity in infants have also been associated with acute fatty liver of pregnancy.[118]

Laboratory findings

Women with acute fatty liver of pregnancy have elevated liver enzymes and bilirubin levels. The serum transaminase levels usually range from modest values to 500 IU/L. Patients often have an elevated white blood cell count as well. A low platelet count is common and can be associated with other signs of disseminated intravascular coagulation. Severely affected patients also have elevations in serum ammonia, prolongation of prothrombin time, lactic acidosis, and hypoglycemia, and all of which are caused by hepatic insufficiency.

Imaging

Imaging by ultrasound or CT can demonstrate diffuse low-density signals in the liver, but detection of fatty changes in the liver with current imaging techniques is limited.[119] Ascites can also be present.

Gross findings

The liver is typically smaller and weighs less than normal because of liver cell loss. The cut surface usually shows a pale yellow color because of fatty infiltrate.

Microscopic findings

The diagnosis of acute fatty liver of pregnancy is often confirmed by liver biopsy. The key histological finding is diffuse microvesicular steatosis, predominantly involving zone 3 and zone 2 areas, with relative sparing of a rim of periportal hepatocytes (Fig. 19.41).[120,121] In the early phase of the disease, the hepatocytes can be markedly swollen, in which case the microvesicular steatosis is overlooked.[121] Occasional foci of intermediate and large droplet steatosis can also be found. Mild to moderate hepatocanalicular

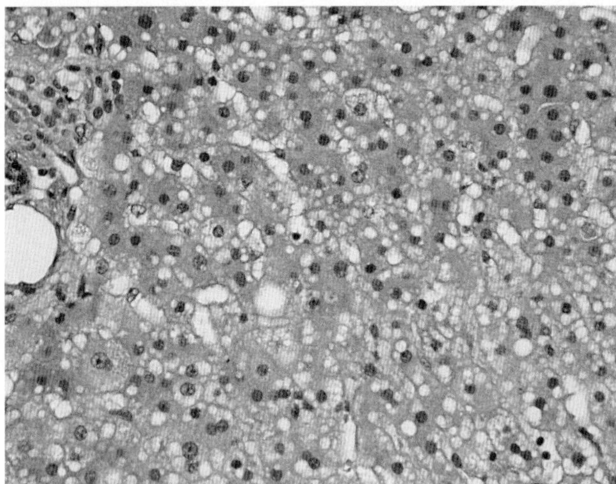

Figure 19.41 Acute fatty liver of pregnancy. Diffuse microvesicular steatosis with sparing of some periportal hepatocytes at the left.

cholestasis is present in most cases. Portal and lobular inflammation is usually mild. However, significant lymphoplasmacytic infiltrates mimicking viral hepatitis have been observed in some cases, although it is still uncertain if some of these cases actually represent coexisting liver insults.[122] Significant loss of hepatic parenchyma is seen in most cases because of necrosis and liver cell atrophy. Extramedullary hematopoiesis and giant mitochondria are often present. Kupffer cells with lipofuscin and/or lipids are seen in most cases as well.[121] The histological changes usually rapidly resolve after delivery, with no risk of progressing to chronic liver disease or fibrosis.

Immunohistochemistry and special stains

Immunohistochemical stains are of limited utility in acute fatty liver of pregnancy. When frozen tissue is available, Oil red O stains can confirm the presence of diffuse microvesicular steatosis, but this stain requires experience to avoid over interpretation. In any case, the diagnosis is based primarily on the H&E findings.

Ultrastructural findings

Electron microscopy shows diffuse microvesicular steatosis. There are dilated rough endoplasmic reticulum and paracrystalline inclusions. Mitochondria show significant variation in size with numerous megamitochondria.

Molecular genetic findings

Because an inherited enzyme deficiency in β-oxidation is found in some affected women, molecular testing for LCHAD deficiency, at least for the most common G1528C mutation, is currently recommended for all women with acute fatty liver of pregnancy and their children.[123] Additional testing for other defects in fatty acid oxidation may be offered if this mutation is not detected. Mutations in the *HADHA* gene can predispose the baby to subsequent episodes of life-threatening metabolic crises and sudden infant death.

Differential diagnosis

The differential diagnosis includes fulminant viral hepatitis, drug- or toxin-induced liver injury, adult-onset Reye syndrome, and HELLP syndrome. In the proper clinical setting, the presence of diffuse microvesicular steatosis establishes the diagnosis of acute fatty liver of pregnancy.

Treatment and prognosis

The primary treatment is prompt delivery of the fetus after maternal stabilization, regardless of gestational age. Most patients recover and do not progress to chronic liver disease. Liver transplant may occasionally be needed for those with irreversible liver failure despite delivery and aggressive supportive care. The maternal mortality is about 4% to 8%, and perinatal mortality rate is 120/1,000 births.[124] Of note, acute fatty liver of pregnancy can recur in subsequent pregnancies, and women with a history of acute fatty liver of pregnancy should be monitored closely during their pregnancies.

Hyperemesis gravidarum

Hyperemesis gravidarum occurs in 1 to 20 patients/1,000 pregnancies, generally in the first trimester. Hyperemesis gravidarum is characterized by severe nausea and vomiting that often leads to hospitalization because of dehydration. Up to half of patients can have abnormal liver enzymes, usually with ALT levels greater than AST levels. ALT levels may rise up to 200 IU/L but are generally less than 300 IU/L. However, if ALT levels are greater than 10 times the upper limit of normal or if there is jaundice, other causes of hepatitis should be carefully excluded. Enzyme levels return to normal when the vomiting resolves.[125] A liver biopsy is usually unnecessary, but if performed, typically snows either normal histology or bland cholestasis.[126]

Intrahepatic cholestasis of pregnancy

Intrahepatic cholestasis of pregnancy is the most common pregnancy-related liver disease. Approximately 1% to 6% of pregnancies in the United States are affected by this condition.[127] Interestingly, there is significant geographic variation in incidence. For

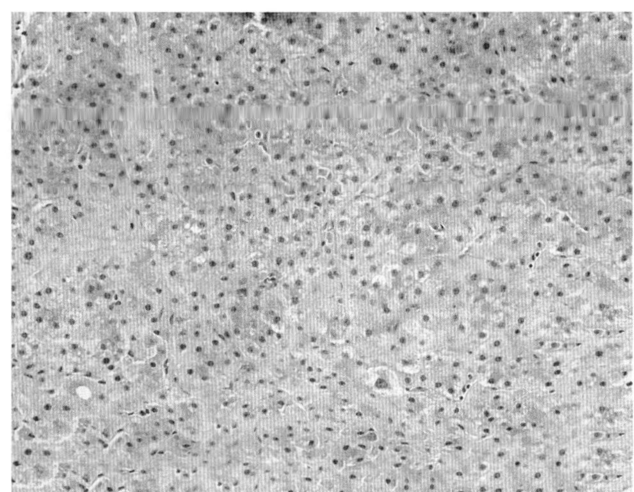

Figure 19.42 Intrahepatic cholestasis of pregnancy, characterized by marked bland hepatocanalicular cholestasis.

example, a subpopulation in Chile, the Araucanos Indians, have an incidence of 28%.[128] The etiology of intrahepatic cholestasis of pregnancy is still unclear but is believed to be multifactorial with environmental, hormonal, and genetic contributions. Multiple gestations, a family history of cholestatic syndrome when using oral contraceptives, and advanced maternal age, all increase the risk for intrahepatic cholestasis of pregnancy. Also at risk are women with mutations in genes that code for proteins involved in bile acid secretion and in bile acid detoxification and genes, such as *ABCB4*, *ABCB11*, *ATP8B1*, and *FXR*.[129,130] These same genes also play key roles in familial intrahepatic cholestasis.

Most affected women present in the second or third trimester with itching but without a rash. The pruritus characteristically starts on the soles of the feet and the palms of the hands and progresses to the trunk and face. The pruritus usually worsens at night. Laboratory tests show elevated bilirubin and/or ALT levels.

A liver biopsy is not required to make the diagnosis of intrahepatic cholestasis of pregnancy. Generally, intrahepatic cholestasis of pregnancy can be diagnosed in a pregnant woman beyond 25 weeks of gestation when there is pruritus without a rash, no known liver disease, and elevation of bilirubin and/or ALT levels. If liver biopsy is performed, it typically shows marked bland hepatocanalicular cholestasis. No evidence of bile duct injury or bile duct obstruction is seen (Fig. 19.42). Inflammation is usually absent or minimal.[131]

Intrahepatic cholestasis of pregnancy increases the risk for preterm delivery and also increases the risk for stillbirth. Ursodeoxycholic acid is the main medication for intrahepatic cholestasis of pregnancy and can reduce both pruritus and bilirubin levels. Delivery is recommended in the 38th week when fetal lung maturity has been established. Intrahepatic cholestasis of pregnancy can recur in subsequent pregnancies. If the postpartum bilirubin or ALT levels are persistently elevated, further evaluations are necessary to rule out an underlying genetic disorder or other chronic live diseases, such as chronic hepatitis C, gallstones, and primary biliary cirrhosis.[132]

Preeclampsia/eclampsia and HELLP syndrome

Preeclampsia is defined as new onset hypertension with either proteinuria or end-organ dysfunction, or both, after 20 weeks of gestation in a previously normotensive woman. It affects approximately 2% to 8% of all pregnancies worldwide.[133] When the liver is involved, women present with abdominal pain, nausea, vomiting, jaundice, and abnormal liver enzymes. Eclampsia is a more severe form of preeclampsia that is characterized by new onset of grand mal seizure activity and/or unexplained coma during pregnancy or postpartum.

The cause of preeclampsia remains unknown, but the disease is likely multifactorial and related to abnormal placentation, environmental factors, immunological factors, and pre-or coexisting maternal pathology. Risk factors include nulliparity, diabetes, a family history or prior history of preeclampsia, antiphospholipid antibody syndrome, hypertension, obesity, multiple gestation, and advanced maternal age (>35).[134] Approximately 10% to 20% of patients with severe preeclampsia or eclampsia can develop the HELLP syndrome, which is composed of hemolysis (H), elevated liver enzymes (EL), and low platelets (LP).[135] HELLP syndrome is associated with increased maternal and fetal morbidity and mortality. About one-third of cases of the HELLP syndrome can present postpartum.

The liver biopsy findings are generally mild and nonspecific in preeclampsia.[136] However, in some cases, particularly in severe and fatal cases, the liver biopsy shows periportal intrasinusoidal fibrin deposition, with liver cell necrosis and hemorrhage (Fig. 19.43).[137–139] Microvesicular steatosis can be seen, and a possible connection between preeclampsia and acute fatty liver of pregnancy has been proposed but is still unproven.[140] The vascular changes seen in other organs in severe preeclampsia can also occur in the arteries and arterioles of the liver, characterized by hyalinization of vessel walls and vessel thrombosis (Fig. 19.44). In severe cases, liver infarction, intrahepatic hemorrhage, or subcapsular hemorrhage with hematoma formation can occur and lead to spontaneous rupture of the liver.[141]

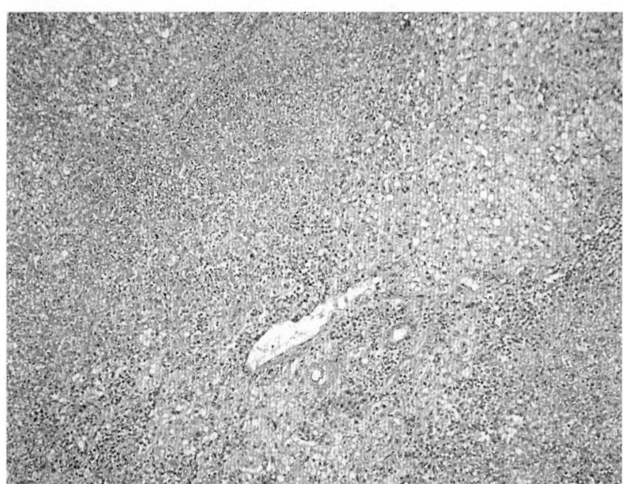

Figure 19.43 Liver in eclampsia with HELLP syndrome. Diffuse necrosis and hemorrhage with mild portal inflammation and steatosis in viable hepatocytes.

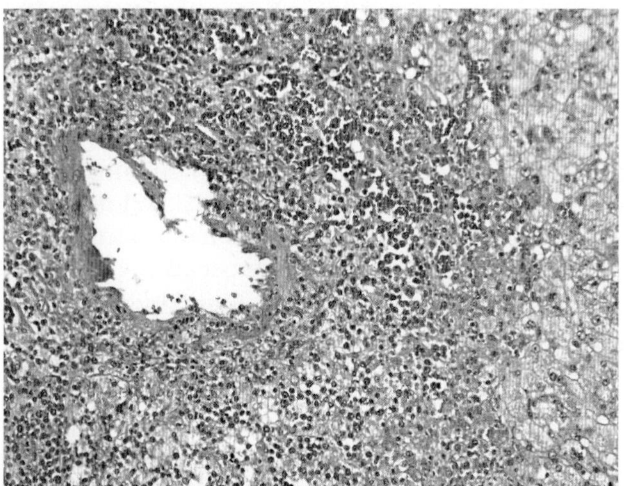

Figure 19.44 Liver in eclampsia with HELLP syndrome. Periportal fibrin deposition, portal lymphoplasmacytic infiltrate, and vascular damage.

The only cure for these conditions is delivery. Urgent delivery should be considered if gestation is >34 weeks or if there is fetal distress or signs of severe maternal bleeding. Signs and symptoms can completely disappear after delivery. Unfortunately, preeclampsia and eclampsia are still a leading cause of maternal and fetal morbidity and mortality and are estimated to be responsible for approximately 14% of maternal deaths per year.

REFERENCES

1. Lacaille F, Gupte G, Colomb V, et al. Intestinal failure-associated liver disease: a position paper of the ESPGHAN Working Group of Intestinal Failure and Intestinal Transplantation. *J Pediatr Gastroenterol Nutr*. 2015;60(2):272–283.
2. Peden VH, Witzleben CL, Skelton MA. Total parenteral nutrition. *J Pediatr*. 1971;78(1):180–181.
3. Chung C, Buchman AL. Postoperative jaundice and total parenteral nutrition-associated hepatic dysfunction. *Clin Liver Dis*. 2002;6(4):1067–1084.
4. Javid PJ, Malone FR, Dick AA, et al. A contemporary analysis of parenteral nutrition-associated liver disease in surgical infants. *J Pediatr Surg*. 2011;46(10):1913–1917.
5. Kaufman SS, Gondolesi GE, Fishbein TM. Parenteral nutrition associated liver disease. *Semin Neonatol*. 2003;8(5):375–381.
6. Beale EF, Nelson RM, Bucciarelli RL, et al. Intrahepatic cholestasis associated with parenteral nutrition in premature infants. *Pediatrics*. 1979;64(3):342–347.
7. Beath SV, Davies P, Papadopoulou A, et al. Parenteral nutrition-related cholestasis in postsurgical neonates: multivariate analysis of risk factors. *J Pediatr Surg*. 1996;31(4):604–606.
8. Lindor KD, Fleming CR, Abrams A, et al. Liver function values in adults receiving total parenteral nutrition. *JAMA*. 1979;241(22):2398–2400.
9. Fleming CR. Hepatobiliary complications in adults receiving nutrition support. *Dig Dis*. 1994;12(4):191–198.
10. Carter BA, Shulman RJ. Mechanisms of disease: update on the molecular etiology and fundamentals of parenteral nutrition associated cholestasis. *Nat Clin Pract Gastroenterol Hepatol*. 2007;4(5):277–287.
11. Buchman AL, Moukarzel A, Jenden DJ, et al. Low plasma free choline is prevalent in patients receiving long term parenteral nutrition and is associated with hepatic aminotransferase abnormalities. *Clin Nutr*. 1993;12(1):33–37.
12. Naini BV, Lassman CR. Total parenteral nutrition therapy and liver injury: a histopathologic study with clinical correlation. *Hum Pathol*. 2012;43(6):826–833.
13. Bowyer BA, Fleming CR, Ludwig J, et al. Does long-term home parenteral nutrition in adult patients cause chronic liver disease? *JPEN J Parenter Enteral Nutr*. 1985;9(1):11–17.
14. Javid PJ, Collier S, Richardson D, et al. The role of enteral nutrition in the reversal of parenteral nutrition-associated liver dysfunction in infants. *J Pediatr Surg*. 2005;40(6):1015–1018.
15. Willis TC, Carter BA, Rogers SP, et al. High rates of mortality and morbidity occur in infants with parenteral nutrition-associated cholestasis. *JPEN J Parenter Enteral Nutr*. 2010;34(1):32–37.
16. Kaufman SS, Pehlivanova M, Fennelly EM, et al. Predicting liver failure in parenteral nutrition-dependent short bowel syndrome of infancy. *J Pediatr*. 2010;156(4):580–585 e1.

17. Mauriac P. Gros ventre, hepatomegalie, troubles de las croissance chez les enfants diabetiques traits depuis plusieurs annes par l'insuline. *Gax Hebd Med Bordeaux*. 1930;26:8.
18. Torbenson M, Chen YY, Brunt E, et al. Glycogenic hepatopathy: an underrecognized hepatic complication of diabetes mellitus. *Am J Surg Pathol*. 2006;30(4):508–513.
19. Munns CF, McCrossin RB, Thomsett MJ, et al. Hepatic glycogenosis: reversible hepatomegaly in type 1 diabetes. *J Paediatr Child Health*. 2000;36(5):449–452.
20. Mukewar S, Sharma A, Lackore K, et al. Clinical, biochemical and histopathogical profile of subjects with glycogenic hepatopathy and comparison with type 1 diabetes patients unpublished data.
21. Wisell J, Boitnott J, Haas M, et al. Glycogen pseudoground glass change in hepatocytes. *Am J Surg Pathol*. 2006;30(9):1085–1090.
22. Iancu TC, Shiloh H, Dembo L. Hepatomegaly following short-term high-dose steroid therapy. *J Pediatr Gastroenterol Nutr*. 1986;5(1):41–46.
23. Tsujimoto T, Takano M, Nishiofuku M, et al. Rapid onset of glycogen storage hepatomegaly in a type-2 diabetic patient after a massive dose of long-acting insulin and large doses of glucose. *Intern Med*. 2006;45(7):469–473.
24. Chatila R, West AB. Hepatomegaly and abnormal liver tests due to glycogenosis in adults with diabetes. *Medicine*. 1996;75(6):327–333.
25. Umpaichitra V. Unusual glycogenic hepatopathy causing abnormal liver enzymes in a morbidly obese adolescent with well-controlled type 2 diabetes: resolved after A1c was normalized by metformin. *Clin Obes*. 2016;6(4):281–284.
26. Komuta M, Harada M, Ueno T, et al. Unusual accumulation of glycogen in liver parenchymal cells in a patient with anorexia nervosa. *Intern Med*. 1998;37(8):678–682.
27. Resnick JM, Zador I, Fish DL. Dumping syndrome, a cause of acquired glycogenic hepatopathy. *Pediatr Dev Pathol*. 2011;14(4):318–321.
28. Olsson R, Wesslau C, William-Olsson T, et al. Elevated aminotransferases and alkaline phosphatases in unstable diabetes mellitus without ketoacidosis or hypoglycemia. *J Clin Gastroenterol*. 1989;11(5):541–545.
29. Ludwig J, Viggiano TR, McGill DB, et al. Nonalcoholic steatohepatitis: Mayo clinic experiences with a hitherto unnamed disease. *Mayo Clin Proc*. 1980;55(7):434–438.
30. Nagore N, Scheuer PJ. The pathology of diabetic hepatitis. *J Pathol*. 1988;156(2):155–160.
31. Tolman KG, Fonseca V, Dalpiaz A, et al. Spectrum of liver disease in type 2 diabetes and management of patients with diabetes and liver disease. *Diabetes Care*. 2007;30(3):734–743.
32. Harrison SA, Brunt EM, Goodman ZD, et al. Diabetic hepatosclerosis: diabetic microangiopathy of the liver. *Arch Pathol Lab Med*. 2006;130(1):27–32.
33. Chen G, Brunt EM. Diabetic hepatosclerosis: a 10-year autopsy series. *Liver Int*. 2009;29(7):1044–1050.
34. Balakrishnan M, Garcia-Tsao G, Deng Y, et al. Hepatic arteriolosclerosis: a small-vessel complication of diabetes and hypertension. *Am J Surg Pathol*. 2015;39(7):1000–1009.
35. Biscoveanu M, Hasinski S. Abnormal results of liver function tests in patients with Graves' disease. *Endocr Pract*. 2000;6(5):367–369.
36. Barnes SC, Wicking JM, Johnston JD. Graves' disease presenting with cholestatic jaundice. *Ann Clin Biochem*. 1999;36 (Pt 5):677–679.
37. Khemichian S, Fong TL. Hepatic dysfunction in hyperthyroidism. *Gastroenterol Hepatol*. 2011;7(5):337–339.
38. Sola J, Pardo-Mindan FJ, Zozaya J, et al. Liver changes in patients with hyperthyroidism. *Liver*. 1991;11(4):193–197.
39. Boelaert K, Newby PR, Simmonds MJ, et al. Prevalence and relative risk of other autoimmune diseases in subjects with autoimmune thyroid disease. *Am J Med*. 2010;123(2):183 e1–9.
40. Tajiri J, Shimada T, Naomi S, et al. Hepatic dysfunction in primary hypothyroidism. *Endocrinol Jpn*. 1984;31(1):83–91.
41. Pagadala MR, Zein CO, Dasarathy S, et al. Prevalence of hypothyroidism in nonalcoholic fatty liver disease. *Dig Dis Sci*. 2012;57(2):528–534.
42. Torbenson M, Hart J, Westerhoff M, et al. Neonatal giant cell hepatitis: histological and etiological findings. *Am J Surg Pathol*. 2010;34(10):1498–1503.
43. Adams LA, Feldstein A, Lindor KD, et al. Nonalcoholic fatty liver disease among patients with hypothalamic and pituitary dysfunction. *Hepatology*. 2004;39(4):909–914.
44. Nishizawa H, Iguchi G, Murawaki A, et al. Nonalcoholic fatty liver disease in adult hypopituitary patients with GH deficiency and the impact of GH replacement therapy. *Eur J Endocrinol*. 2012;167(1):67–74.
45. Mendes FD, Levy C, Enders FB, et al. Abnormal hepatic biochemistries in patients with inflammatory bowel disease. *Am J Gastroenterol*. 2007;102(2):344–350.
46. Bargiggia S, Maconi G, Elli M, et al. Sonographic prevalence of liver steatosis and biliary tract stones in patients with inflammatory bowel disease: study of 511 subjects at a single center. *J Clin Gastroenterol*. 2003;36(5):417–420.
47. Riegler G, D'Inca R, Sturniolo GC, et al. Hepatobiliary alterations in patients with inflammatory bowel disease: a multicenter study.

Caprilli & Gruppo Italiano Studio Colon-Retto. *Scand J Gastroenterol*. 1998;33(1):93–98.
48. Callen JP, Soderstrom RM. Granulomatous hepatitis associated with salicylazosulfapyridine therapy. *South Med J*. 1978;71(9):1159–1160.
49. Balistreri WF. Hepatobiliary complications of inflammatory bowel disease: overview of the issues. *Inflamm Bowel Dis*. 1998;4(3):220–224.
50. Hagander B, Berg NO, Brandt L, et al. Hepatic injury in adult coeliac disease. *Lancet*. 1977;2(8032):270–272.
51. Sainsbury A, Sanders DS, Ford AC. Meta-analysis: coeliac disease and hypertransaminasaemia. *Aliment Pharmacol Ther*. 2011;34(1):33–40.
52. Bardella MT, Vecchi M, Conte D, et al. Chronic unexplained hypertransaminasemia may be caused by occult celiac disease. *Hepatology*. 1999;29(3):654–657.
53. Duggan JM, Duggan AE. Systematic review: the liver in coeliac disease. *Aliment Pharmacol Ther*. 2005;21(5):515–518.
54. da Rosa Utiyama SR, da Silva Kotze LM, Nisihara RM, et al. Spectrum of autoantibodies in celiac patients and relatives. *Dig Dis Sci*. 2001;46(12):2624–2630.
55. Volta U. Pathogenesis and clinical significance of liver injury in celiac disease. *Clin Rev Allergy Immunol*. 2009;36(1):62–70.
56. Mounajjed T, Oxentenko A, Shmidt E, et al. The liver in celiac disease: clinical manifestations, histologic features, and response to gluten-free diet in 30 patients. *Am J Clin Pathol*. 2011;136(1):128–137.
57. Reilly NR, Lebwohl B, Hultcrantz R, et al. Increased risk of non-alcoholic fatty liver disease after diagnosis of celiac disease. *J Hepatol*. 2015;62(6):1405–1411.
58. Riestra S, Dominguez F, Rodrigo L. Nodular regenerative hyperplasia of the liver in a patient with celiac disease. *J Clin Gastroenterol*. 2001;33(4):323–326.
59. Biecker E, Trebicka J, Fischer HP, et al. Portal hypertension and nodular regenerative hyperplasia in a patient with celiac disease. *Z Gastroenterol*. 2006;44(5):395–398.
60. Kendall MJ, Cockel R, Becker J, et al. Raised serum alkaline phosphatase in rheumatoid disease. An index of liver dysfunction? *Ann Rheum Dis*. 1970;29(5):537–540.
61. Fernandes L, Sullivan S, McFarlane IG, et al. Studies on the frequency and pathogenesis of liver involvement in rheumatoid arthritis. *Ann Rheum Dis*. 1979;38(6):501–506.
62. Thompson PW, Houghton BJ, Clifford C, et al. The source and significance of raised serum enzymes in rheumatoid arthritis. *Q J Med*. 1990;76(280):869–879.
63. Siede WH, Seiffert UB, Merle S, et al. Alkaline phosphatase isoenzymes in rheumatic diseases. *Clin Biochem*. 1989;22(2):121–124.
64. Lefkovits AM, Farrow IJ. The liver in rheumatoid arthritis. *Ann Rheum Dis*. 1955;14(2):162–169.
65. Ruderman EM, Crawford JM, Maier A, et al. Histologic liver abnormalities in an autopsy series of patients with rheumatoid arthritis. *Br J Rheumatol*. 1997;36(2):210–213.
66. Blendis LM, Lovell D, Barnes CG, et al. Oesophageal variceal bleeding in Felty's syndrome associated with nodular regenerative hyperplasia. *Ann Rheum Dis*. 1978;37(2):183–186.
67. Reynolds WJ, Wanless IR. Nodular regenerative hyperplasia of the liver in a patient with rheumatoid vasculitis: a morphometric study suggesting a role for hepatic arteritis in the pathogenesis. *J Rheumatol*. 1984;11(6):838–842.
68. Landas SK, Mitros FA, Furst DE, et al. Lipogranulomas and gold in the liver in rheumatoid arthritis. *Am J Surg Pathol*. 1992;16(2):171–174.
69. Smits JG, Kooijman CD. Rheumatoid nodules in liver. *Histopathology*. 1986;10(11):1211–1213.
70. van Hoek B. The spectrum of liver disease in systemic lupus erythematosus. *Neth J Med*. 1996;48(6):244–253.
71. Bessone F, Poles N, Roma MG. Challenge of liver disease in systemic lupus erythematosus: clues for diagnosis and hints for pathogenesis. *World J Hepatol*. 2014;6(6):394–409.
72. Carmona-Fernandes D, Santos MJ, Canhao H, et al. Anti-ribosomal P protein IgG autoantibodies in patients with systemic lupus erythematosus: diagnostic performance and clinical profile. *BMC Med*. 2013;11:98.
73. Zheng RH, Wang JH, Wang SB, et al. Clinical and immunopathological features of patients with lupus hepatitis. *Chin Med J*. 2013;126(2):260–266.
74. Chowdhary VR, Crowson CS, Poterucha JJ, et al. Liver involvement in systemic lupus erythematosus: case review of 40 patients. *J Rheumatol*. 2008;35(11):2159–2164.
75. Kaw R, Gota C, Bennett A, et al. Lupus-related hepatitis: complication of lupus or autoimmune association? Case report and review of the literature. *Dig Dis Sci*. 2006;51(4):813–818.
76. Agmon-Levin N, Shapira Y, Selmi C, et al. A comprehensive evaluation of serum autoantibodies in primary biliary cirrhosis. *J Autoimmun*. 2010;34(1):55–58.
77. Takahashi A, Abe K, Saito R, et al. Liver dysfunction in patients with systemic lupus erythematosus. *Intern Med*. 2013;52(13):1461–1465.
78. Morla RM, Ramos-Casals M, Garcia-Carrasco M, et al. Nodular regenerative hyperplasia of the liver and antiphospholipid antibodies: report of two cases and review of the literature. *Lupus*. 1999;8(2):160–163.

79. Zhang L, Smyrk TC. Autoimmune pancreatitis and IgG4-related systemic diseases. *Int J Clin Exp Pathol.* 2010;3(5):491–504.
80. Stone JH, Zen Y, Deshpande V. IgG4-related disease. *N Engl J Med.* 2012;366(6):539–551.
81. Zen Y, Fujii T, Sato Y, et al. Pathological classification of hepatic inflammatory pseudotumor with respect to IgG4-related disease. *Mod Pathol.* 2007;20(8):884–894.
82. Umemura T, Zen Y, Hamano H, et al. Immunoglobin G4-hepatopathy: association of immunoglobin G4-bearing plasma cells in liver with autoimmune pancreatitis. *Hepatology.* 2007;46(2):463–471.
83. Ghazale A, Chari ST, Zhang L, et al. Immunoglobulin G4-associated cholangitis: clinical profile and response to therapy. *Gastroenterology.* 2008;134(3):706–715.
84. Graham RP, Smyrk TC, Chari ST, et al. Isolated IgG4-related sclerosing cholangitis: a report of 9 cases. *Hum Pathol.* 2014;45(8):1722–1729.
85. Zhang L, Lewis JT, Abraham SC, et al. IgG4+ plasma cell infiltrates in liver explants with primary sclerosing cholangitis. *Am J Surg Pathol.* 2010;34(1):88–94.
86. Deshpande V, Sainani NI, Chung RT, et al. IgG4-associated cholangitis: a comparative histological and immunophenotypic study with primary sclerosing cholangitis on liver biopsy material. *Mod Pathol.* 2009;22(10):1287–1295.
87. Bauer M, Press AT, Trauner M. The liver in sepsis: patterns of response and injury. *Curr Opin Crit Care.* 2013;19(2):123–127.
88. Koskinas J, Gomatos IP, Tiniakos DG, et al. Liver histology in ICU patients dying from sepsis: a clinico-pathological study. *World J Gastroenterol.* 2008;14(9):1389–1393.
89. Iwata T, Hoshii Y, Kawano H, et al. Hepatic amyloidosis in Japan: histological and morphometric analysis based on amyloid proteins. *Hum Pathol.* 1995;26(10):1148–1153.
90. Buck FS, Koss MN. Hepatic amyloidosis: morphologic differences between systemic AL and AA types. *Hum Pathol.* 1991;22(9):904–907.
91. Park MA, Mueller PS, Kyle RA, et al. Primary (AL) hepatic amyloidosis: clinical features and natural history in 98 patients. *Medicine.* 2003;82(5):291–298.
92. Chopra S, Rubinow A, Koff RS, et al. Hepatic amyloidosis. A histopathologic analysis of primary (AL) and secondary (AA) forms. *Am J Pathol.* 1984;115(2):186–193.
93. Looi LM, Sumithran E. Morphologic differences in the pattern of liver infiltration between systemic AL and AA amyloidosis. *Hum Pathol.* 1988;19(6):732–735.
94. Chandan VS, Shah SS, Lam-Himlin DM, et al. Globular hepatic amyloid is highly sensitive and specific for LECT2 amyloidosis. *Am J Surg Pathol.* 2015;39(4):558–564.
95. Vrana JA, Gamez JD, Madden BJ, et al. Classification of amyloidosis by laser microdissection and mass spectrometry-based proteomic analysis in clinical biopsy specimens. *Blood.* 2009;114(24):4957–4959.
96. Sethi S, Vrana JA, Theis JD, et al. Laser microdissection and mass spectrometry-based proteomics aids the diagnosis and typing of renal amyloidosis. *Kidney Int.* 2012;82(2):226–234.
97. Herlenius G, Wilczek HE, Larsson M, et al. Ten years of international experience with liver transplantation for familial amyloidotic polyneuropathy: results from the Familial Amyloidotic Polyneuropathy World Transplant Registry. *Transplantation.* 2004;77(1):64–71.
98. Grois N, Potschger U, Prosch H, et al. Risk factors for diabetes insipidus in langerhans cell histiocytosis. *Pediatr Blood Cancer.* 2006;46(2):228–233.
99. Abdallah M, Genereau T, Donadieu J, et al. Langerhans' cell histiocytosis of the liver in adults. *Clin Res Hepatol Gastroenterol.* 2011;35(6–7):475–481.
100. Kaplan KJ, Goodman ZD, Ishak KG. Liver involvement in Langerhans' cell histiocytosis: a study of nine cases. *Mod Pathol.* 1999;12(4):370–378.
101. Mican JM, Di Bisceglie AM, Fong TL, et al. Hepatic involvement in mastocytosis: clinicopathologic correlations in 41 cases. *Hepatology.* 1995;22 (4 Pt 1):1163–1170.
102. Baron TH, Koehler RE, Rodgers WH, et al. Mast cell cholangiopathy: another cause of sclerosing cholangitis. *Gastroenterology.* 1995;109(5):1677–1681.
103. Sotlar K, Horny HP, Simonitsch I, et al. CD25 indicates the neoplastic phenotype of mast cells: a novel immunohistochemical marker for the diagnosis of systemic mastocytosis (SM) in routinely processed bone marrow biopsy specimens. *Am J Surg Pathol.* 2004;28(10):1319–1325.
104. Lemos LB, Baliga M, Benghuzzi HA, et al. Nodular hematopoiesis of the liver diagnosed by fine-needle aspiration cytology. *Diagn Cytopathol.* 1997;16(1):51–54.
105. de Kerguenec C, Hillaire S, Molinie V, et al. Hepatic manifestations of hemophagocytic syndrome: a study of 30 cases. *Am J Gastroenterol.* 2001;96(3):852–857.
106. Tasaki T, Yamada S, Nabeshima A, et al. An autopsy case of myocardial infarction due to idiopathic thrombotic thrombocytopenic purpura. *Diagn Pathol.* 2015;10:52.
107. Banerjee S, Owen C, Chopra S. Sickle cell hepatopathy. *Hepatology.* 2001;33(5):1021–1028.
108. Schubert TT. Hepatobiliary system in sickle cell disease. *Gastroenterology.* 1986;90(6):2013–2021.

109. Zakaria N, Knisely A, Portmann B, et al. Acute sickle cell hepatopathy represents a potential contraindication for percutaneous liver biopsy. *Blood*. 2003;101(1):101–103.
110. Bauer TW, Moore GW, Hutchins GM. The liver in sickle cell disease. A clinicopathologic study of 70 patients. *Am J Med*. 1980;69(6):833–837.
111. King PD, Perry MC. Hepatotoxicity of chemotherapy. *Oncologist*. 2001;6(2):162–176.
112. Ishak KG, Zimmerman HJ. Morphologic spectrum of drug-induced hepatic disease. *Gastroenterol Clin North Am*. 1995;24(4):759–786.
113. da Silveira EB, Jeffers L, Schiff ER. Diagnostic laparoscopy in radiation-induced liver disease. *Gastrointest Endosc*. 2002;55(3):432–434.
114. Makuuchi M, Sukigara M, Mori T, et al. Bile duct necrosis: complication of transcatheter hepatic arterial embolization. *Radiology*. 1985;156(2):331–334.
115. Bacq Y, Zarka O, Brechot JF, et al. Liver function tests in normal pregnancy: a prospective study of 103 pregnant women and 103 matched controls. *Hepatology*. 1996;23(5):1030–1034.
116. Perez V, Gorodisch S, Casavilla F, et al. Ultrastructure of human liver at the end of normal pregnancy. *Am J Obstet Gynecol*. 1971;110(3):428–431.
117. Treem WR, Rinaldo P, Hale DE, et al. Acute fatty liver of pregnancy and long-chain 3-hydroxyacyl-coenzyme A dehydrogenase deficiency. *Hepatology*. 1994;19(2):339–345.
118. Browning MF, Levy HL, Wilkins-Haug LE, et al. Fetal fatty acid oxidation defects and maternal liver disease in pregnancy. *Obstet Gynecol*. 2006;107(1):115–120.
119. Castro MA, Ouzounian JG, Colletti PM, et al. Radiologic studies in acute fatty liver of pregnancy. A review of the literature and 19 new cases. *J Reprod Med*. 1996;41(11):839–843.
120. Pockros PJ, Peters RL, Reynolds TB. Idiopathic fatty liver of pregnancy: findings in ten cases. *Medicine*. 1984;63(1):1–11.
121. Rolfes DB, Ishak KG. Acute fatty liver of pregnancy: a clinicopathologic study of 35 cases. *Hepatology*. 1985;5(6):1149–1158.
122. Riely CA, Latham PS, Romero R, et al. Acute fatty liver of pregnancy. A reassessment based on observations in nine patients. *Ann Intern Med*. 1987;106(5):703–706.
123. Ibdah JA. Acute fatty liver of pregnancy: an update on pathogenesis and clinical implications. *World J Gastroenterol*. 2006;12(46):7397–7404.
124. Nelson DB, Yost NP, Cunningham FG. Acute fatty liver of pregnancy: clinical outcomes and expected duration of recovery. *Am J Obstet Gynecol*. 2013;209(5):456 e1–7.
125. Conchillo JM, Pijnenborg JM, Peeters P, et al. Liver enzyme elevation induced by hyperemesis gravidarum: aetiology, diagnosis and treatment. *Neth J Med*. 2002;60(9):374–378.
126. Hay JE. Liver disease in pregnancy. *Hepatology*. 2008;47(3):1067–1076.
127. Joshi D, James A, Quaglia A, et al. Liver disease in pregnancy. *Lancet*. 2010;375(9714):594–605.
128. Reyes H, Gonzalez MC, Ribalta J, et al. Prevalence of intrahepatic cholestasis of pregnancy in Chile. *Ann Intern Med*. 1978;88(4):487–493.
129. van der Woerd WL, van Mil SW, Stapelbroek JM, et al. Familial cholestasis: progressive familial intrahepatic cholestasis, benign recurrent intrahepatic cholestasis and intrahepatic cholestasis of pregnancy. *Best Pract Res Clin Gastroenterol*. 2010;24(5):541–553.
130. Van Mil SW, Milona A, Dixon PH, et al. Functional variants of the central bile acid sensor FXR identified in intrahepatic cholestasis of pregnancy. *Gastroenterology*. 2007;133(2):507–516.
131. Mullally BA, Hansen WF. Intrahepatic cholestasis of pregnancy: review of the literature. *Obstet Gynecol Surv*. 2002;57(1):47–52.
132. Ropponen A, Sund R, Riikonen S, et al. Intrahepatic cholestasis of pregnancy as an indicator of liver and biliary diseases: a population-based study. *Hepatology*. 2006;43(4):723–728.
133. Al-Jameil N, Aziz Khan F, Fareed Khan M, et al. A brief overview of preeclampsia. *J Clin Med Res*. 2014;6(1):1–7.
134. Arulkumaran N, Lightstone L. Severe pre-eclampsia and hypertensive crises. *Best Pract Res Clin Obstet Gynaecol*. 2013;27(6):877–884.
135. Steegers EA, von Dadelszen P, Duvekot JJ, et al. Pre-eclampsia. *Lancet*. 2010;376(9741):631–644.
136. Antia FP, Bharadwaj TP, Watsa MC, et al. Liver in normal pregnancy, pre-eclampsia, and eclampsia. *Lancet*. 1958;2(7050):776–778.
137. Arias F, Mancilla-Jimenez R. Hepatic fibrinogen deposits in pre-eclampsia. Immunofluorescent evidence. *N Engl J Med*. 1976;295(11):578–582.
138. Rolfes DB, Ishak KG. Liver disease in toxemia of pregnancy. *Am J Gastroenterol*. 1986;81(12):1138–1144.
139. Tsokos M, Longauer F, Kardosova V, et al. Maternal death in pregnancy from HELLP syndrome. A report of three medico-legal autopsy cases with special reference to distinctive histopathological alterations. *Int J Legal Med*. 2002;116(1):50–53.
140. Dani R, Mendes GS, Medeiros Jde L, et al. Study of the liver changes occurring in preeclampsia and their possible pathogenetic connection with acute fatty liver of pregnancy. *Am J Gastroenterol*. 1996;91(2):292–294.
141. Sheikh RA, Yasmeen S, Pauly MP, et al. Spontaneous intrahepatic hemorrhage and hepatic rupture in the HELLP syndrome: four cases and a review. *J Clin Gastroenterol*. 1999;28(4):323–328.

20 Transplantation pathology

Roger K. Moreira, MD and Douglas A. Simonetto, MD

20.1 OVERVIEW

Chronic liver disease is a major cause of morbidity and mortality worldwide. In the United States alone, nearly 40,000 patients progress to liver failure and death annually. Liver transplantation is currently the standard treatment for various forms of severe liver disease, including acute liver failure or end-stage liver disease due to any etiology, as well as selected metabolic and neoplastic conditions.

Clinical findings

Chronic liver diseases are often silent until cirrhosis with clinical decompensation ensues. Events that define decompensation include ascites, hepatic encephalopathy, variceal bleeding, and nonobstructive jaundice, which are often triggered by precipitating factors such as bacterial infections, portal vein thrombosis, surgery, or hepatocellular carcinoma. Acute liver failure, on the other hand, is characterized by jaundice, coagulopathy, and the development of hepatic encephalopathy within 8 weeks of the onset of symptoms. Subacute liver failure has a similar presentation, except hepatic encephalopathy develops later, between 8 and 24 weeks of the onset of jaundice.

For both decompensated cirrhosis and acute/subacute liver failure, liver transplantation represents a lifesaving treatment. Unfortunately, however, liver allografts remain a scarce resource and, despite great improvements in the organ allocation system, approximately 2,500 to 3,000 patients are removed from the waiting list every year in the United States due to death or poor overall clinical status (Organ Procurement and Transplantation Network [OPTN] data, 2008 to 2015).

The organ transplant system in the United States is currently managed by a nonprofit organization—the United Network for Organ Sharing (UNOS). In 2002, the UNOS adopted the model of end-stage liver disease (MELD) score as the organ allocation system. The MELD score is an objective, laboratory-based measurement which has been validated in predicting 3-month waiting list mortality.[1] For children 12 years of age and under, the pediatric end-stage liver disease (PELD) score replaces MELD. In addition, some conditions are listed for liver transplant as UNOS status 1A, which takes priority over the MELD allocation score: acute liver failure, primary nonfunction of transplanted livers, hepatic artery thrombosis, and Wilson disease. The benefit of transplantation should be weighed against posttransplant morbidity

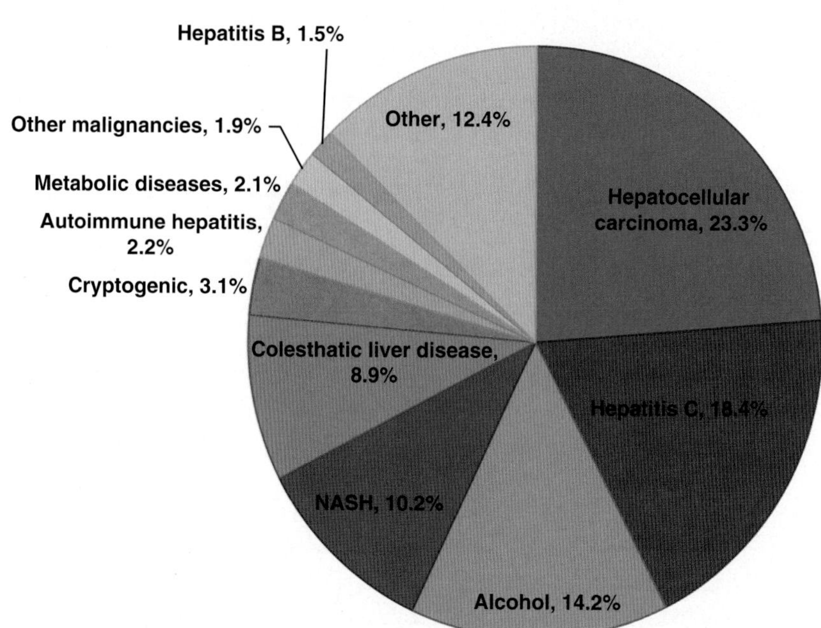

Figure 20.1 Etiology of liver disease in patients undergoing liver transplantation in the United States From UNOS database [2015]; 7,127 transplanted patients.

and mortality, being reserved for patients with considerable decline in their quality of life and/or high mortality without transplant.

Etiology

According to the UNOS database, 7,127 liver transplants were performed in the United States in 2015 and hepatocellular carcinoma was the most common indication for liver transplantation (often in the setting of cirrhosis due to various etiologies), followed by hepatitis C–related cirrhosis, alcoholic liver disease, and nonalcoholic fatty liver disease (Fig. 20.1). Acute liver failure accounts for less than 10% of all transplants performed in the United States annually, with acetaminophen overdose being responsible for almost half of these cases.

20.2 EVALUATION OF DONOR LIVER BIOPSY

Liver biopsy is an important adjunct tool in the evaluation of potential allografts. Its main role is to confirm the quality/viability of the donor organ and exclude features that would either contraindicate transplantation or increase the likelihood of various adverse short and long-term outcomes. As a result of organ shortage, increasing utilization of allografts from suboptimal donors has occurred in recent years, leading to a higher proportion of donor livers requiring pretransplantation frozen section evaluation. The so-called "extended donor criteria" includes several established risk factors for posttransplantation organ dysfunction and failure, such as old age (>60 years), hypernatremia (>155 mEq/L), macrovesicular steatosis >40%, cold ischemia time >12 hours, partial liver allografts, and donation after cardiac death (DCD) donors.[2] Suboptimal livers also include allografts from donors with prolonged hemodynamic instability, use of vasopressors, chronic viral hepatitis (B or C), as well as the presence of mass lesions or significant fibrosis. Although most risk factors are defined clinically, the main role of pathologists in the pretransplantation frozen section evaluation is to assess steatosis and exclude any miscellaneous findings (significant inflammation, necrosis, granulomatous processes, fibrosis, neoplasms, etc.) which may not have been detected on clinical evaluation.

In order to avoid diagnostic errors, the liver sample being submitted for frozen section by the transplant surgeon must be obtained and handled properly. Although a single biopsy is generally adequate (either needle core or wedge biopsy), additional samples should be obtained if the appearance of the liver is grossly heterogeneous. A large-core biopsy (i.e., away from the liver capsule) is preferred if there is concern for fibrosis, because subcapsular wedges can show nonspecific subcapsular fibrosis that is suboptimal for staging purposes.

The fresh tissue should ideally be carefully wrapped in a paper towel or gauze soaked in preservation solution and transported to the pathology lab immediately. Prolonged exposure to normal saline can cause significant histologic artifact, characterized by cellular discohesiveness and pyknosis-like chances of hepatocytes, mimicking necrosis (Fig. 20.2). Dry absorbent materials and sample compression can result in tissue dehydration and absorption of fat, potentially resulting in significant histologic changes and underestimation of steatosis. Tissue freezing itself frequently causes small cytoplasmic vacuoles in hepatocytes that are essentially indistinguishable from microvesicular steatosis on hematoxylin and eosin (H&E)–stained sections. Oil red O or other fat stains may aid in this distinction, but require experience for proper interpretation.

The importance of donor steatosis as a risk factor in the setting of liver transplantation is well established and consistently observed in several clinical and experimental studies.[3–6] Macrovesicular steatosis, defined histologically as one or a few large fat droplets that displace the hepatocyte nucleus to the periphery of the cell, represents the main finding in this context and has been associated with various adverse outcomes during the early transplantation period, including primary graft dysfunction and nonfunction, as well as prolonged intensive care unit and hospital stay.[7–9] This is thought to be related in part to the

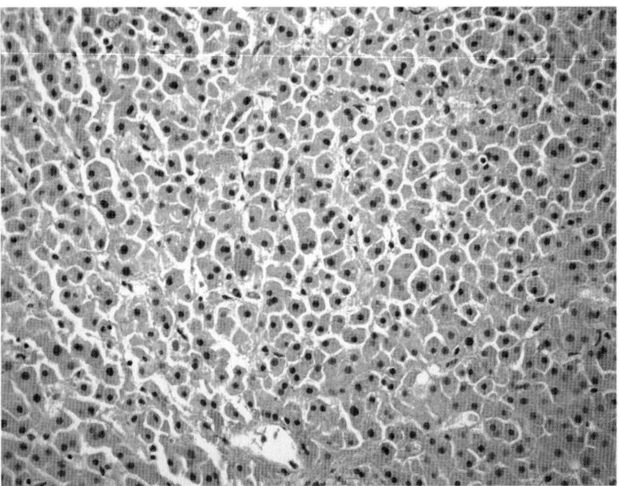

Figure 20.2 Saline preservation artifact. Hepatocytes appear discohesive, with glassy cytoplasm and piknotic-appearing nuclei, resembling early necrosis.

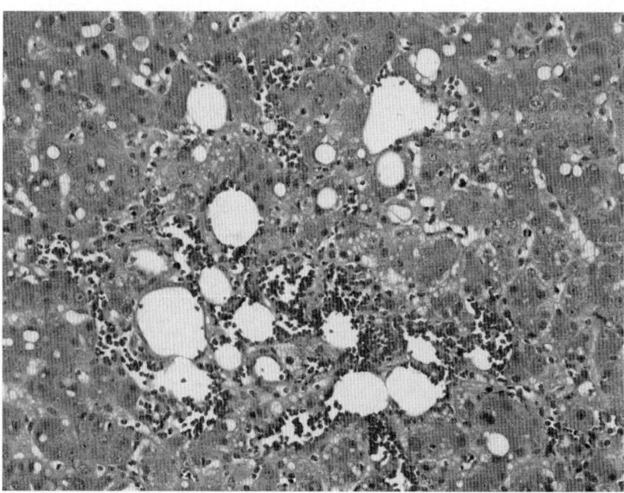

Figure 20.3 Lipopeliosis. Large coalescent fat globules extruded from hepatocytes are seen within congested sinusoids.

displacement of fat droplets from the cytoplasm of hepatocytes into sinusoids (because of mechanical factors and/or ischemia), leading to sinusoidal obstruction, lipid peroxidation and formation of free radicals upon reperfusion, and endothelial injury.[7] Examination of failed allografts owing to primary nonfunction and early posttransplant biopsies of steatotic allografts often show large, coalescent fat droplets within hepatic sinusoids—referred to as lipopeliosis (Fig. 20.3)—which illustrates one of the primary pathogenic mechanisms in this scenario.

Some confusion exists with regard to the nomenclature for the types of steatosis, making interpretation of the literature and communication of pathological findings quite challenging in certain situations. For example, the term *microvesicular steatosis* is often inappropriately used in the literature to refer to small-droplet steatosis, which virtually always coexist with typical large-droplet steatosis (as seen in nonalcoholic fatty liver disease, for example). In contrast, true microvesicular steatosis is characterized by very small lipid droplets which impart a "bubbly" appearance to the hepatocyte cytoplasm and that are often difficult to recognize on H&E stains (Fig. 20.4). Both small- and large-droplet fat are currently considered part of the spectrum of macrovesicular steatosis. Microvesicular steatosis is typically seen in specific clinical contexts that includes Reye syndrome, acute fatty liver of pregnancy, and toxicity by certain medications, and is thought to be related to mitochondrial toxicity. Unfortunately, in the context of liver transplantation, we must keep in mind that the terms *microvesicular steatosis* and *small-droplet steatosis* have been used interchangeably by some authors. See Chapter 16 for further discussion.

Although the specific method of interpretation differs slightly among pathologists, macrovesicular steatosis should be evaluated quantitatively (as a percentage). Macrovesicular steatosis is estimated as the percentage area of the hepatic lobules occupied by large-droplet steatosis (Fig. 20.5). Although no specific guidelines exist, livers with 30% large-droplet steatosis or less are considered adequate, without significant increased risk of adverse outcome, whereas allografts showing >60% are generally considered inadequate and, therefore, are not used for transplantation. Allografts with moderate (30% to 60%) large-droplet steatosis may or may not be utilized, depending on local

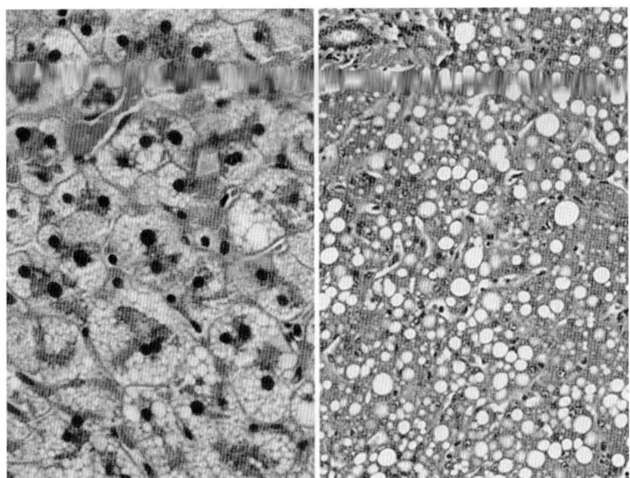

Figure 20.4 Microvesicular steatosis versus small-droplet steatosis. The left side of the panel shows true microvesicular steatosis, with very small fat droplets that impart a "bubbly" appearance to the cytoplasm. In contrast, small-droplet steatosis (seen on the right side of the panel in conjunction with large-droplet steatosis) is characterized by larger droplets than microvesicular steatosis, with greater variation in droplet size.

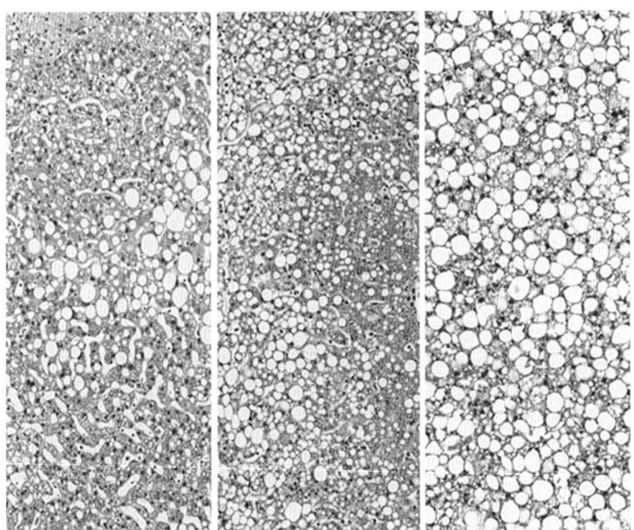

Figure 20.5 Semi-quantitative assessment of steatosis. Mild (5% to 33%), moderate (33% to 66%), and severe (>66%) steatosis are illustrated in the left, middle, and right parts of the panel, respectively.

preferences and additional risk factors related to both donor and recipient. Finally, digital/computerized tools are available to assist in this interpretation but yield values that are significantly different (approximately half) compared to visual (i.e., "eyeball") estimates by pathologists.[10] Therefore, validation of values yielded by digital analysis and correlation with outcomes is necessary before this technique is applied during liver allograft procurement.

20.3 THE LIVER TRANSPLANTATION PROCEDURE

Basic understanding of different surgical procedures utilized in liver transplantation is useful for pathologists, because certain posttransplant complications are associated with specific techniques. Orthotopic liver transplantation represents the most common procedure. A whole cadaveric liver is utilized to replace the diseased liver in its original location within the abdominal cavity. In orthotopic liver transplants, an end-to-end anastomosis is performed between donor and recipient vena cava, hepatic veins, hepatic arteries, and portal veins, whereas the bile duct anastomosis may be duct-to-duct or donor duct to recipient Roux-en-Y jejunostomy. Donor cholecystectomy is also routinely performed. Several technically more complex variations of the liver transplant procedure exist which require either surgical reconstruction of vascular structures, which is associated with increased risk of hepatic artery thrombosis, or surgical manipulation of the liver itself (e.g., "split" liver, reduced-size liver, and right or left lobe living donor procedure), which result in increased risk for both vascular and biliary complications.

20.4 TIMING OF POSTTRANSPLANT COMPLICATIONS

One of the most fundamental pieces of clinical information to take into account when assessing a liver transplant biopsy is the posttransplant time, because different categories of complications are strongly associated with specific posttransplant periods (Table 20.1). Although some variability and exceptions are recognized for most entities, posttransplant complications can broadly be classified into early (first week), delayed (second week to 3 to 6 months), and late (after 3 to 6 months). This classification is useful in narrowing our differential diagnosis and should be used routinely, in conjunction with other clinical data. Comparison with the donor (postperfusion) biopsy, if available, can also be helpful, excluding the possibility of preexisting (i.e., donor) and periprocedure changes, particularly when evaluating biopsies in the first few weeks posttransplantation.

20.5 PRESERVATION/REPERFUSION INJURY

Definition

Also known as *harvesting injury*, *ischemia/reperfusion injury*, and *functional cholestasis*, this diagnosis refers to a constellation of functional and histologic

Table 20.1	Timing of Posttransplantation Complications
Time zero (postperfusion)	Steatosis (most common) Chronic hepatitis, fibrosis (HCV+ donors, extended donor criteria) Centrilobular necrosis (due to preservation injury or premortem ischemic injury) Iron deposition
First week	Preservation/reperfusion injury Acute cellular rejection Humoral rejection
Second week to few (3–6) months	Vascular complications CMV and other infections Biliary strictures Acute cellular rejection Early-onset chronic rejection
Few (3–6) months and later	Recurrent viral hepatitis Recurrent autoimmune diseases (PBC, PSC, AIH, typically after a few years) De novo disease Chronic rejection PTLD

Abbreviations: HCV, hepatitis C virus; CMV, cytomegalovirus; PBC, primary biliary cirrhosis; PSC, primary sclerosing cholangitis; AIH, autoimmune hepatitis; PTLD, posttransplantation lymphoproliferative disease.

abnormalities related to harvesting, preservation, and reperfusion of allografts.

Clinical findings

Clinically, the terms *primary graft dysfunction, initial poor function*, and *primary nonfunction* are utilized to describe liver function abnormalities in the early posttransplantation period that are thought to at least in part be related to preservation/reperfusion injury. The liver dysfunction ranges from slightly delayed function and mild transaminase and bilirubin elevations to early allograft failure. Preservation/reperfusion injury represents a diagnosis of exclusion; therefore, vascular thrombosis, drug-induced injury, infections, and other causes of early graft dysfunction need to be reasonably excluded.

Etiology and pathogenesis

The pathogenesis of preservation/reperfusion injury is primarily related to damage of different cell types in the liver during warm ischemia, cold ischemia, and reperfusion. Warm ischemia refers to the period during which the liver is subjected to suboptimal perfusion at body temperature (before or during organ harvesting). During this phase, injury predominantly affects the hepatocytes, particularly if warm ischemia lasts more than 120 minutes.[11–13] Warm ischemia is particularly problematic in liver donation after cardiac death, because no blood flow to the liver occurs for a variable period of time before organ procurement. Cold ischemia refers to the period in which the allograft is perfused with preservation solution and kept in ice. This period is thought to primarily cause endothelial injury[14] and should ideally be less than 12 hours, because longer cold ischemia periods have been associated with early adverse graft outcomes.[15,16] Finally, during the reperfusion period, in which the allograft is reimplanted and perfused with blood at body temperature, there is further damage to both hepatocytes and endothelial cells, much of which is related to the release of reactive oxygen species and various inflammatory mediators from activated Kupffer cells.[17]

Histologic findings

Histologically, the most characteristic preservation/reperfusion injury–related changes are centrilobular hepatocyte swelling (Fig. 20.6) with associated hepatocanalicular cholestatasis. Scattered acidophil bodies and neutrophilic infiltration are also commonly seen. With more prominent injury, various degrees of parenchymal necrosis develop, sometimes associated with a ductular reaction. If significant steatosis is present, preservation/reperfusion injury–related hepatocyte injury can cause extrusion of fat droplets into sinusoids (i.e., "lipopeliosis") (Fig. 20.3). Some degree of microvesicular steatosis is also thought to develop during organ ischemia, presumably owing to

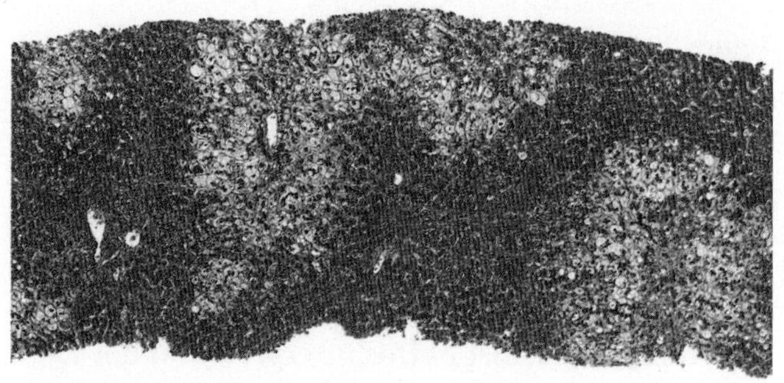

Figure 20.6 Preservation/reperfusion injury. Prominent zone 3 hepatocyte swelling. Zone 3 cholestasis was also present in this case (not shown).

mitochondrial dysfunction and abnormal fatty acid metabolism. Preservation/reperfusion injury–related histologic changes can persist for up to several weeks after transplantation in severe cases.

Differential diagnosis

The differential diagnosis for preservation/reperfusion injury primarily includes other forms of liver injury, which occur in the early posttransplantation period. Early biliary obstruction, hepatic artery thrombosis, drug-induced liver injury, and humoral rejection represent the main entities to be excluded. Although ductular reaction can be seen in preservation/reperfusion injury, portal/periductal edema, and portal/ductal neutrophilic infiltrate are usually absent. Endoscopic retrograde cholangiopancreatography (ERCP) or magnetic resonance retrograde cholangiopancreatography (MRCP) are often performed in the early transplantation period and provide useful information to evaluate bile duct obstruction or stricture. Arterial thrombosis can also closely mimic preservation/reperfusion injury, because changes are often centrilobular (swelling and necrosis) and a ductular reaction can be present (often associated with true biliary obstructive findings when there also is ischemic bile duct injury). Correlation with Doppler studies is essential to exclude this possibility. There also can be significant histologic overlap between preservation/reperfusion injury and humoral rejection. The presence of fibrin thrombi (in sinusoids, portal veins, and/or central veins), although rarely found, suggests humoral rejection. A C4d immunostain and correlation with donor-specific antibodies can also be helpful.

20.6 SMALL-FOR-SIZE SYNDROME

Definition

Portal hyperperfusion/small-for-size syndrome is an uncommon, pathologically difficult to recognize complication that occurs most commonly in allograft livers that are less than 30% of the ideal recipient liver volume or less than 0.8% of the recipient body weight.[18]

Clinical findings

The typical clinical scenario in portal hyperperfusion/small-for-size syndrome is unexplained cholestasis, coagulopathy, and ascites in the early posttransplant period, most commonly occurring in the setting of reduced-size or living donor allografts. The clinical features are not specific for this entity, mimicking several other posttransplant complications, but liver transplant surgeons are often aware of this possibility, being alerted when there is splanchnic congestion and portal hypertension upon revascularization of the allograft.

Etiology and pathogenesis

Portal hyperperfusion/small-for-size syndrome is thought to be related primarily to portal hyperperfusion, which leads to decreased levels of adenosine (a vasodilator) from the hepatic circulation (i.e., "adenosine washout"), which in turn causes hepatic artery vasoconstriction, with subsequent low arterial flow, thrombosis, and ischemic cholangitis.

Histologic findings

The histologic changes in portal hyperperfusion/small-for-size syndrome are rather subtle and nonspecific and a high degree of suspicion is required for this diagnosis. In early phases (starting minutes after transplantation), there is denudation of the endothelium of portal veins and sinusoids as well as hemorrhage into portal connective tissue. Subsequently, there is regeneration of the endothelium, reactive endothelial cells, subendothelial edema, and, eventually, fibrointimal hyperplasia, luminal obliteration, and recanalization. Nodular regenerative hyperplasia is also seen, presumably owing to vascular flow abnormalities. The hepatic lobules show a constellation of nonspecific abnormalities, including centrilobular cholestasis, microvesicular steatosis, parenchymal atrophy, and necrosis. In severe cases, ischemic cholangitis may be seen.[18]

Differential diagnosis

Portal hyperperfusion/small-for-size syndrome is essentially a diagnosis of exclusion. The possibility of arterial thrombosis/stricture, sepsis, biliary obstruction, ischemic cholangitis unrelated to portal hyperperfusion/small-for-size syndrome, and preservation injury should be carefully excluded. Vascular studies and ERCP/MRCP are helpful in excluding mechanical and/or anastomotic complications. Arteriography has been reported to show segmental narrowing, poor peripheral filling, and even reversal of flow in cases of portal hyperperfusion/small-for-size syndrome.[18]

Prognosis

The prognosis of portal hyperperfusion/small-for-size syndrome will depend on the severity of the disease. Some cases are effectively treated by decreasing portal venous flow using octreotide, splenic artery ligation, or mesocaval shunts.

20.7 ANTIBODY-MEDIATED REJECTION

Definition

Also known as *humoral* or *hyperacute* rejection, antibody-mediated rejection represents a form of graft injury/dysfunction, which occurs in the early posttransplantation period (hours to initial weeks) owing to preformed recipient antibodies or antidonor antibodies developed after transplantation. There is increasing evidence that antibody-mediated rejection also plays a role in complications occurring later, including acute cellular rejection and chronic rejection.[19]

Clinical findings

The typical pattern of hyperacute rejection (as described for other solid organs) may occur in unconditioned ABO-incompatible livers, but is very rarely seen in practice. This pattern of injury presents intraoperatively as uneven perfusion of the liver after vascular anastomosis, associated with swelling and dusky discoloration of the liver, and subsequent development of decreased bile production, coagulopathy and other signs of very early organ failure. A relatively more common scenario in liver transplantation is a slightly more protracted (acute) course, with varying degrees of liver dysfunction in the initial hours to several days posttransplant. This occurs in patients with positive donor-specific antibodies—often mimicking the presentation of acute cellular rejection. The liver dysfunction ranges from mild (delayed graft function) to complete loss of graft function with resulting patient death or need for retransplantation.[20,21]

Etiology and pathogenesis

Liver allografts are significantly less susceptible to antibody-mediated injury compared to other solid organ allografts. Nonetheless, antibody-mediated rejection seems to play an important role in a minority of cases of early liver allograft dysfunction, and there is mounting evidence that a humoral/antibody-mediated component also exists in cases of T-cell–mediated cellular rejection.[19,22] Endothelial cells are the main target of the antibody-mediated injury, with various antibodies binding to antigens expressed in hepatic endothelial cells (sinusoids and hepatic vessels), with resulting endothelial cell injury, inflammatory cell adhesion, thrombosis, and hemorrhage.[23] Antilymphocyte antibodies and, in rare cases, antiendothelial antibodies have been implicated in the pathogenesis of antibody-mediated rejection.

Histologic findings

The histologic findings in antibody-mediated rejection largely reflect its pathogenesis. In its early stages (first week posttransplantation), antibody-mediated rejection can very closely mimic preservation/reperfusion injury, with centrilobular hepatocyte injury and hepatocanalicular cholestasis, whereas the portal tract findings can be minimal to absent. As the process becomes more established (typically weeks 2 to 4 posttransplant), portal findings resembling biliary obstruction also become apparent, including portal edema, neutrophilic infiltrates, and ductular reaction (Fig. 20.7), often accompanied by a cholestatic pattern of liver enzyme elevations.[19,24] These "biliary-type" features in antibody-mediated rejection are thought to be owing to immune-mediated injury of the peribiliary vascular plexus, leading to biliary injury without obstruction. Central vein inflammation (usually neutrophilic and/or eosinophilic, rather than lymphocytic, as in acute cellular rejection) can also be seen in some cases. In a recent interinstitutional study by O'Leary et al.,[25] the histologic features most predictive of antibody-mediated rejection were portal eosinophilia, portal vein endothelial hypertrophy, and eosinophilic central venulitis. The overall histologic picture in antibody-mediated rejection, therefore, is not specific, and can mimic other early posttransplant complications. A high index of suspicion is needed for this diagnosis and the recognition of compatible morphologic findings should trigger further testing to exclude this possibility, including testing for donor-specific antibodoes and C4d immunostaining (see further discussion in "Special stains and immunostains").

Special stains and immunostains

Widely regarded as a reliable maker of antibody-mediated rejection in renal and cardiac allografts,[26,27] the precise significance of the various patterns of C4d staining by immunohistochemistry in liver allografts is not

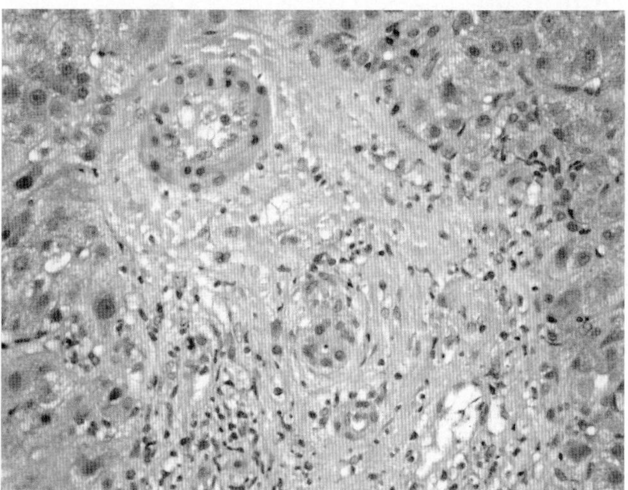

Figure 20.7 Antibody-mediated rejection. Portal tract with edema and ductular reaction, mimicking biliary tract obstruction.

as well established. In our liver pathology service, we only occasionally use this stain. Nonetheless, this technique has gained acceptance in recent years in the context of compatible histology and laboratory testing and should be used as an adjunct tool in cases showing features resembling either preservation/reperfusion injury or biliary-type features when there is no supporting clinical evidence or risk factors for these processes. C4d is deposited along the endothelial lining of hepatic vessels, being strongest in portal veins, venules, peribiliary plexus, and portal "stroma" (likely representing either C4d deposition within portal microvessels or complement spillage form injured vessels), then with progressively weaker staining within the lobular sinusoids (strongest in the periportal areas and weaker toward the central vein), in keeping with the direction of the blood supply to the liver (Fig. 20.8).[22,28,29] A "positive" interpretation for C4d immunostaining is typically reserved for cases showing expression in >50% of portal tracts. This approach represents the main criteria in most studies and is often accompanied by variable staining of portal vein endothelium and sinusoids.[30–32] The Banff Working Group has recently proposed a scoring system for C4d immunohistochemistry interpretation in liver allografts which is as follows: 0, no C4d deposition in portal microvasculature; 1, minimal (<10% of portal tracts) C4d deposition in >50% of the circumference of portal microvascular endothelia (portal veins and capillaries); 2, focal (10-50% of portal tracts) C4d deposition in >50% of the circumference of portal microvasculature endothelia; and 3, Diffuse (>50% of portal tracts) C4d deposition in >50% of the circumference of portal microvascular endothelia, often with extension into inlet venules or periportal sinusoids. It is worth emphasizing that variable staining (most often weak, but sometimes strong) can be seen in a wide range of liver diseases,[33] and C4d should only be considered a helpful adjunct study to be used in the presence of compatible/suspicious histologic changes and in correlation with recipient donor-specific antibody assays.

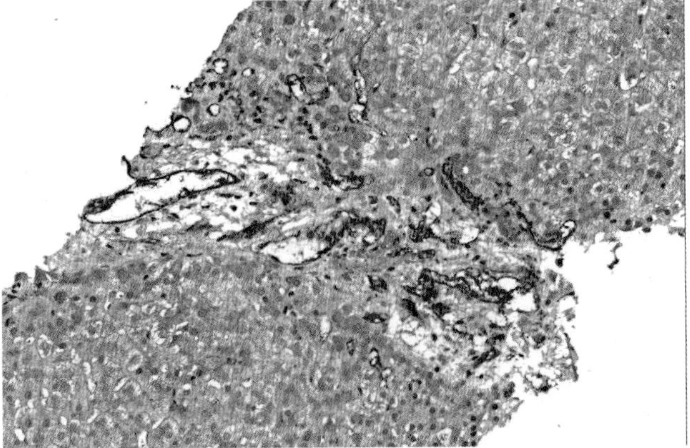

Figure 20.8 C4d immunostain. Strong staining of portal vein endothelium, portal capillaries, and some staining of portal stromal cells in this example of antibody-mediated rejection.

Differential diagnosis

Being essentially a complication of the early post-transplantation period, the differential diagnosis of antibody-mediated rejection mostly includes other processes that typically occur during this same time frame. The two primary differential diagnoses of antibody-mediated rejection are preservation/reperfusion injury and biliary obstruction. As discussed above, early changes of antibody-mediated rejection can closely mimic preservation/reperfusion injury, including changes of centrilobular hepatocyte swelling and cholestasis. Although some degree of ductular reaction can be seen in preservation/reperfusion injury, other biliary obstruction–type features such as portal edema and neutrophilic infiltrate (which can be seen in antibody-mediated rejection) are typically absent. Correlation with high-risk clinical features for preservation injury can also be helpful. The differential diagnosis with early biliary obstruction cannot be made reliably based on histologic features alone and the latter is best excluded clinically by ERCP/MRCP. Hepatic artery thrombosis should also be considered in the differential diagnosis, because it often presents with centrilobular-predominant findings (hepatocyte swelling or necrosis), sometimes with associated cholestasis and nonspecific portal changes. Correlation with Doppler studies is essential to exclude this possibility.

Prognosis

The prognosis of antibody-mediated rejection is difficult to establish because of various factors related to diagnostic criteria and definition of cases. Bona fide cases of antibody-mediated rejection can cause a wide range of graft injury, from subclinical to rapid early graft loss. The recognition and appropriate diagnosis of this entity is important in practice owing to the availability of potentially useful therapeutic interventions, including plasmapheresis, intravenous immunoglobulin (IVIG), splenectomy,[34] anti-CD-20 agents (e.g., rituximab), and lymphocyte depleting agents (e.g., bortezomib).[35]

20.8 ACUTE CELLULAR REJECTION

Definition

Acute cellular rejection is defined by a host immune response to foreign (donor) antigens present in the allograft. Acute cellular rejection is mainly driven by cytotoxic T lymphocytes. The liver shows characteristic histologic patterns of injury, which can result in allograft damage and dysfunction.

Clinical findings

In spite of significant improvements in immunosuppressive therapy and lower rates of acute cellular rejection after the introduction of current immunosuppressive agents, rejection remains an important cause of liver allograft dysfunction and graft loss.[36–38] Compared to other solid organ allografts, however, the liver is significantly more resistant to the deleterious effects of cellular rejection, with most episodes being either subclinical (i.e., seen in protocol biopsies without laboratory evidence of liver dysfunction) or mild, without associated long-term organ damage following treatment.[39,40]

Clinical factors associated with an increased risk for acute cellular rejection include older allograft donor age (≥30 years), prolonged cold ischemic time (≥15 hours), "healthy" recipients (young age, low Child–Pugh score, normal creatinine, etc.), HLA-DR mismatch, and baseline autoimmune conditions (autoimmune hepatitis, primary biliary cirrhosis, primary sclerosing cholangitis, etc.). Lower rates of rejection have been associated with pretransplant alcoholic liver disease.[41–46]

Mild acute cellular rejection is often clinically asymptomatic, typically presenting with isolated mild elevations of the liver enzymes. In moderate to severe rejection, fever, enlargement and tenderness of the allograft, and decreased bile output may be noted, along with leukocytosis and eosinophilia in some cases. Although allograft rejection characteristically presents with a predominantly "cholestatic" pattern of liver enzyme elevations (i.e., predominant elevation of bilirubin, alkaline phosphatase, and γ-glutamyl transpeptidase, with relatively minor elevation of transaminases), nonselective enzyme elevation is also rather common. Clinical and laboratory findings overall lack both sensitivity and specificity for the diagnosis of acute cellular rejection and histopathologic examination of a biopsy sample is required to confirm the diagnosis.[47] In practice, most cases of acute cellular rejection occur early in the posttransplantation period, most commonly in the first month. Late rejection (3–6 months posttransplantation or later) is less frequent and generally associated with suboptimal immunosuppression.

Etiology and pathogenesis

Although complex and still not entirely understood, the basic pathogenesis of acute cellular rejection is related to the recognition of alloantigens by antigen-presenting cells, with subsequent cytotoxic T-lymphocyte activation and cell-mediated injury to the allograft, primarily targeting interlobular bile ducts and hepatic microvasculature.

Histologic findings

Histopathologic examination represents the gold standard for the diagnosis of acute cellular rejection and is based on a triad of features which include: (1) portal inflammation, (2) lymphocytic cholangitis/bile duct injury, and (3) endotheliitis (Table 20.2). At least two of the components of this triad must be present for the diagnosis of acute cellular rejection according to the widely adopted Banff criteria for liver allograft rejection (Table 20.3).[47] Although the composition and intensity of portal inflammation varies significantly from case to case, depending on various factors (mainly posttransplantation period, as discussed below), typical "rejection-type" infiltrates are characterized by a mixture of lymphocytes that often display an "activated" or "blast-like" morphology—with slightly larger nuclei and with more cytoplasm. Scattered eosinophils (which tend to be more prominent in patients treated with steroid-sparing or lymphocyte-depleting immunosuppressive regimens), neutrophils, macrophages, and plasma cells can also be seen (Fig. 20.9). Interface activity is absent in mild cases but is seen in moderate and severe acute cellular rejection (Fig. 20.10).

Recognition of interlobular bile duct inflammation and injury is critical in the diagnosis of acute cellular rejection. In its early/mild form, there is lymphocytic infiltration through the epithelial basement membrane and lymphocytes are seen among bile duct epithelial cells (Fig. 20.11). Morphologic evidence of bile duct

Table 20.2 Banff Grading Criteria for Acute Cellular Rejection (Global Assessment)

Grade	Criteria
Indeterminate (nondiagnostic)	Portal inflammatory infiltrate that fails to meet the criteria for the diagnosis of acute rejection
Mild	Rejection infiltrate in a minority of the triads, which is generally mild and confined to the portal spaces
Moderate	Rejection infiltrate expanding most or all portal tracts
Severe	As above, with spillover of inflammatory cells into the periportal areas, with moderate to severe perivenular inflammation that extends into the hepatic parenchyma and is associated with perivenular liver cell necrosis

Adapted from Demetris AJ, Adeyi O, Bellamy COC, et al. Liver biopsy interpretation for causes of late liver allograft dysfunction. *Hepatology*. 2006;44(2):489–501, with permission from American Association for the Study of Liver Diseases. doi:10.1002/hep.21280.

Table 20.3	Banff Grading Criteria for Acute Cellular Rejection (Rejection Activity Index, RAI)
	Criteria
Portal inflammation	
1	Mostly lymphocytic inflammation involving, but not noticeably expanding, a minority of the triads
2	Expansion of most or all of the portal tracts by a mixed inflammatory infiltrate containing lymphocytes with occasional blasts, neutrophils, and eosinophils
3	Marked expansion of most or all of the triads by a mixed infiltrate containing numerous blasts and eosinophils, with inflammatory spillover into the periportal parenchyma
Bile duct inflammation/damage	
1	A minority of the ducts are cuffed and infiltrated by inflammatory cells and show only mild reactive changes such as increased nuclear/cytoplasmic ratio of the epithelial cells
2	Most or all of the ducts infiltrated by inflammatory cells. More than an occasional duct shows degenerative changes such as nuclear pleomorphism, disordered polarity and cytoplasmic vacuolization of the epithelium
3	As above for 2, with most or all of the ducts showing degenerative changes or focal lumenal disruption
Venous endothelial inflammation (endotheliitis)	
1	Subendothelial lymphocytic infiltration involving some, but not a majority of the portal and/or hepatic venules
2	Subendotheilal infiltration involving most or all of the portal and/or hepatic venules
3	As above for 2, with moderate or severe perivenular inflammation that extends into the perivenular parenchyma and is associated with perivenular hepatocyte necrosis

Adapted from Demetris AJ, Adeyi O, Bellamy COC, et al. Liver biopsy interpretation for causes of late liver allograft dysfunction. *Hepatology*. 2006;44(2):489–501, with permission from American Association for the Study of Liver Diseases. doi:10.1002/hep.21280.

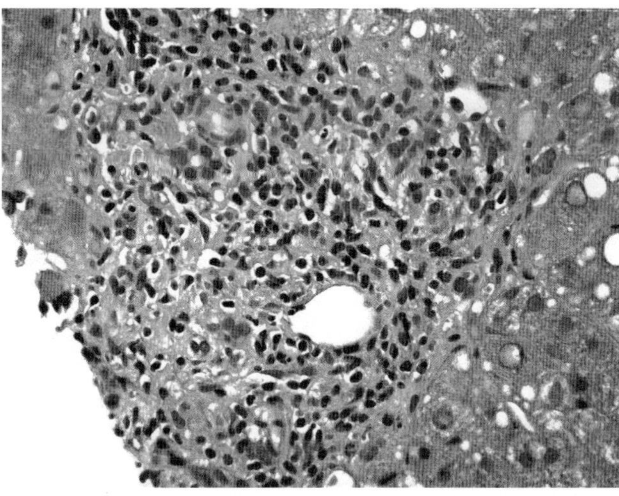

Figure 20.9 Acute cellular rejection, inflammation. Mixed portal inflammation with relatively large, "activated" lymphocytes and eosinophils.

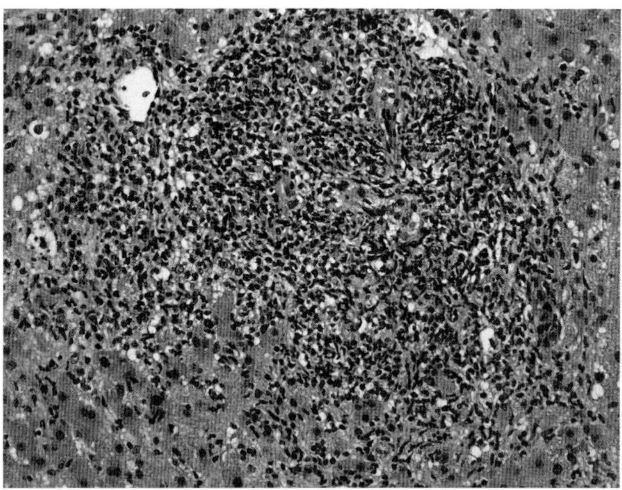

Figure 20.10 Acute cellular rejection, interface activity. A case of moderate to severe rejection showing interface activity.

epithelial injury subsequently appears in the form of nuclear enlargement, nuclear overlapping, occasional mitotic figures, and cytoplasmic vacuolization (Fig. 20.12). In severe cases, luminal obliteration occurs and the small bile ducts may be difficult to recognize within the inflammatory infiltrate (in which case a keratin immunostain may help). With persistent or recurring bile duct injury, nuclear pleomorphism, hyperchromasia, dyspolarity, cytoplasmic eosinophilia, and atrophic appearance of ducts (collectively referred to as *bile duct senescence*) can be seen and are generally thought to represent features of early chronic rejection.[47,48] In cases with significant bile duct injury and destruction, hepatocanalicular cholestasis can be present (see "Differential diagnosis" below for further discussion).

Finally, endotheliitis—the third component of the acute cellular rejection triad—is characterized

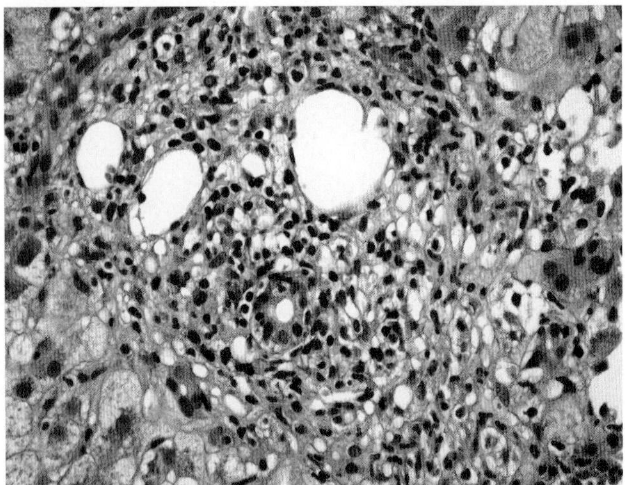

Figure 20.11 Acute cellular rejection, bile duct injury. Mild bile duct injury with subtle epithelial changes and focal lymphocytic infiltration.

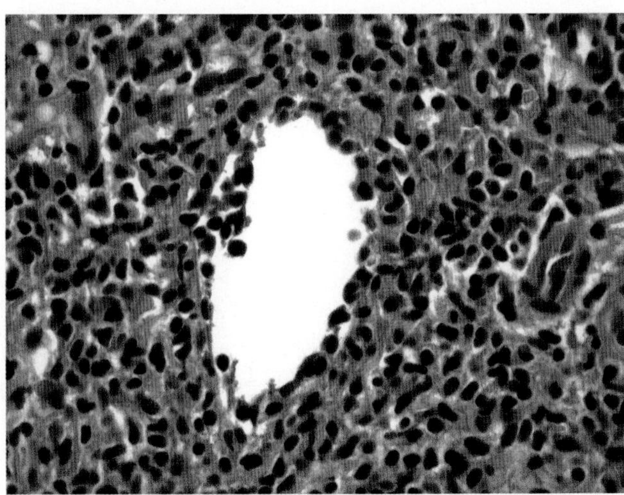

Figure 20.13 Acute cellular rejection, portal vein endotheliitis.

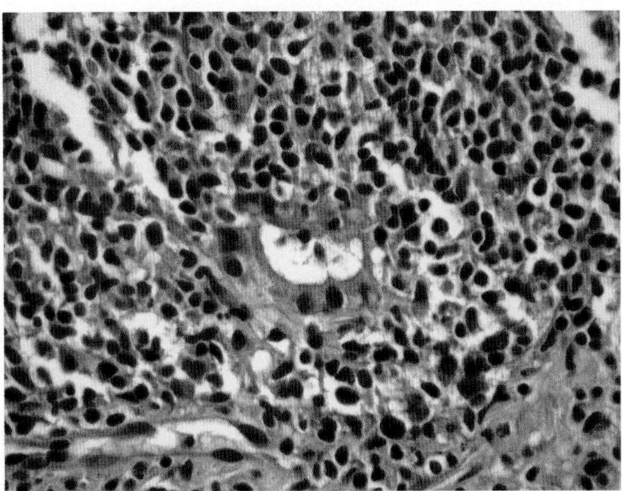

Figure 20.12 Acute cellular rejection, bile duct injury. More significant bile duct injury is seen in this case, which shows prominent epithelial injury and partial bile duct destruction.

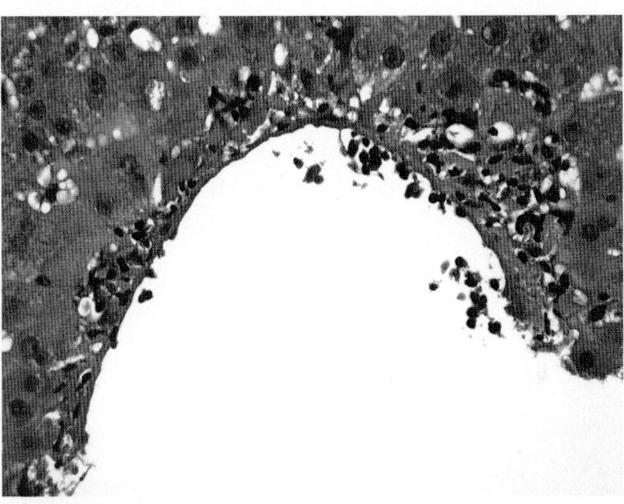

Figure 20.14 Acute cellular rejection, central vein endotheliitis.

by lymphocytic inflammation targeting the vascular endothelium of portal veins, central veins or, less commonly, hepatic arteries. Endotheliitis is histologically characterized by lymphocyte attachment to endothelial cells, generally associated with endothelial injury/reactive changes, or by the presence of subendothelial lymphocytes (subendotheliitis) causing detachment, or "lifting," of endothelial cells from the vascular basement membrane (Fig. 20.13). Portal vein branches are the most commonly affected structures, whereas central vein endotheliitis (often accompanied by centrilobular inflammation and injury—i.e., central perivenulitis) is more common in moderate to severe rejection or in late-occurring rejection (Fig. 20.14). Inflammatory or necrotizing arteritis is identified in rare instances of severe rejection, typically involving larger arteries near the hepatic hilum (therefore, not usually present in biopsy samples).[47,49–51]

In the most common form of acute cellular rejection, occurring in the initial 1 to 3 months posttransplantation, the histologic findings tend to be "typical," as described above, with lymphocytic portal inflammatory infiltrates, portal vein endotheliitis, and readily recognizable bile duct injury, with interface activity and central vein endothelialitis/central perivenulitis developing as rejection progresses toward the moderate to severe end of the spectrum. The diagnosis of acute cellular rejection during this period is usually obvious. In the late posttransplantation period (3 to 6 months or later), however, variant histologic patterns of rejection become more prevalent and may cause diagnostic difficulties[52] (described in detail below).

Finally, moderate to excellent interobserver agreement has been reported[11] for the various histologic criteria of acute cellular rejection: portal inflammation (κ= 0.86 to 0.88), subendothelial inflammation (κ = 0.39 to 0.63), and bile duct damage (κ = 0.42 to 0.49). The interobserver reproducibility for the overall diagnosis of acute cellular rejection in this study was good (κ = 0.50 to 0.62 in 2 separate interpretations), whereas the intraobserver reproducibility was good to excellent among five participating pathologists (κ = 0.53 to 0.89).

Histologic variants

Several variant histologic patterns are recognized in liver allografts and are thought to represent forms of alloimmune attack to the liver (i.e., rejection), all occurring predominantly in the late posttransplantation period.

Plasma cell–rich hepatitis

This term refers to a chronic hepatitis with markedly increased plasma cells, typically with prominent interface and lobular activity, resembling autoimmune hepatitis in native livers (Fig. 20.15). When occurring in patients with underlying autoimmune liver diseases (autoimmune hepatitis, primary biliary cirrhosis, primary sclerosing cholangitis, etc.) in their native livers, this is often considered to represent either recurrent or de novo autoimmune/alloimmune hepatitis. One study also identified an IgG4-rich subpopulation within cases of plasma cell hepatitis, which was associated with more aggressive histology and high rates of response to increased immunosuppression.[53]

The nomenclature (*[illegible]*[54] and *posttransplant plasma cell hepatitis*[55]) and the precise etiology in patients with concurrent recurrent hepatitis C has been a subject of debate. The prevailing evidence is that this pattern represents an alloimmune/rejection phenomenon, rather than a variant pattern of recurrent hepatitis C, as evidenced by an increased frequency of antinuclear antibodies and other autoantibodies, association with subtherapeutic levels of immunosuppression, and a trend toward a more favorable prognosis in response to increased immunosuppression. This pattern has been associated with progressive disease and poor prognosis.[54,55]

At Mayo clinic, our general approach in these posttransplant plasma cell–rich cases is to use the term *plasma cell hepatitis*, followed by grading and staging, favoring this pattern to represent an alloimmune phenomenon/rejection variant, noting that this pattern can sometimes be associated with an aggressive course.

Isolated central perivenulitis

Central perivenulitis is a term recognized by the Banff Working Party, which refers to centrilobular changes that include central vein endotheliitis, perivenular inflammation, and perivenular hepatocyte injury/dropout (Fig. 20.16). In allografts, central venulitis is most often associated with portal-based acute cellular rejection and commonly seen in the context of moderate to severe rejection. However, central perivenulitis occasionally can be seen as an isolated finding, with portal tracts that are either normal or

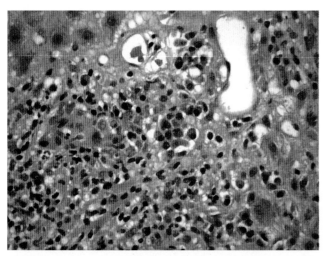

Figure 20.15 Acute cellular rejection, plasma cell–rich variant. Clusters of plasma cells are seen within this portal tract. Also notice the significant amount of bile duct injury and occasional eosinophils.

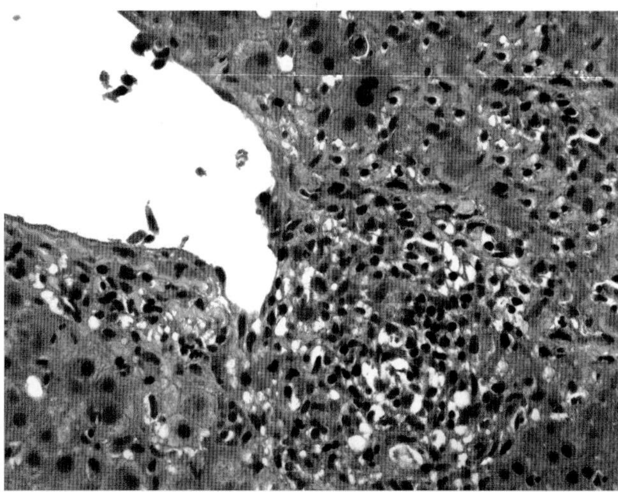

Figure 20.16 Acute cellular rejection, central perivenulitis. Prominent inflammation and hepatocyte dropout are seen adjacent to a central vein.

show only mild nonspecific inflammation. This entity is called isolated central perivenulitis and is generally thought to be a low-grade smoldering rejection, one that can often be treated with optimization of immunosuppressants.

One study identified this pattern of injury in 28% of liver transplant patients with long-term follow-up.[56] It was seen primarily in the late posttransplantation period, with many patients having histories of previous episodes of central perivenulitis in the early posttransplant period (usually with portal-based features of acute cellular rejection). Clinically, this pattern is most often associated with mild liver enzyme abnormalities. When untreated, a small minority of patients develop complications included zone 3 fibrosis, ductopenia, and de novo autoimmune/alloimmune hepatitis.

Chronic hepatitis pattern

When presenting in the late posttransplantation period, acute cellular rejection–related features are often more difficult to recognize, as bile duct injury, "activated" lymphocytes, and endotheliitis, can be sparse and some features can be absent. Thus the biopsy has to be carefully searched for features of acute cellular rejection and other causes of chronic hepatitis (such as recurrent disease, chronic hepatitis E, drug effect, etc.) have to be carefully excluded. When no cause is identified and no definite features or rejection are seen, the pattern of injury is called *idiopathic posttransplantation hepatitis* (Fig. 20.17). A significant proportion of allografts evolving to cirrhosis without a clear etiology persistently show this histologic pattern.[57–62] Chronic hepatitis E virus in particular should be carefully excluded, because

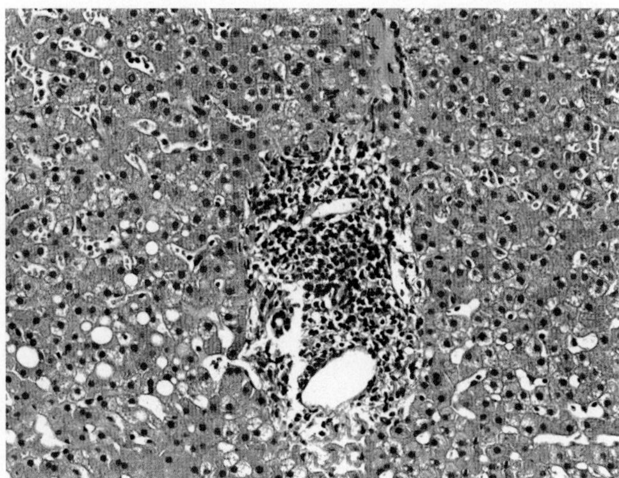

Figure 20.17 Idiopathic posttransplant hepatitis. Chronic portal inflammation without diagnostic features of acute cellular rejection.

chronic hepatitis E is a treatable cause of allograft dysfunction and failure[63,64] (see detailed discussion in the "Viral hepatitis" in Chapter 8).

Grading of acute cellular rejection

The grading system proposed by the Banff group[47,48]—an international consensus document devised by a panel of transplant pathologists, clinicians, and surgeons in 1997—remains the preferred method of grading rejection in transplant centers around the world. An important concept to keep in mind is that this system was designed exclusively as a grading tool. Therefore, the scoring system associated with this method cannot be used to assess a sample for the diagnosis of rejection per se—only to grade it once the diagnosis has independently been established.

The Banff system endorses two forms of rejection assessment: the "global assessment," whereby acute cellular rejection is classified as mild, moderate, or severe (or grade I–III), according to a specified set of criteria, and the "rejection activity index" (RAI), in which all three components of acute cellular rejection (portal inflammation, bile duct injury, and endothelialitis) are evaluated separately and ascribed a score from 0 to 3, with the overall rejection activity index being the sum of all three individual scores. This method has been validated by a number of subsequent studies, which have shown the Banff schema to be an accurate, reproducible, and clinically useful method for grading acute cellular rejection[40,65,66] (Tables 20.2 and 20.3).

One of the difficulties in grading rejection relates to the presence of histologic variants. Isolated central perivenulitis, for example, cannot be adequately graded by standard acute cellular rejection Banff criteria. According to the Banff group recommendations for interpretation of late liver allograft dysfuction,[67] these cases should be interpreted as minimal/indeterminate for rejection when perivenular inflammation involves a minority of central veins with patchy perivenular hepatocyte loss, mild rejection when the changes involve the majority of central veins, moderate rejection when there is at least focal confluent perivenular hepatocyte dropout, but without bridging necrosis, and severe rejection when confluent central-to-central necrosis is present (Table 20.4).

Differential diagnosis

The differential diagnosis for acute cellular rejection will depend on the posttransplant period and the specific histologic pattern. For "typical" cases of early acute cellular rejection, drug reactions are one of the closest mimics, because drug reactions can be associated with bile duct inflammation/duct injury and increased eosinophils. Endotheliitis, however,

Table 20.4 Grading of Late Rejection with Isolated Central Perivenulitis Pattern

Grade	Criteria
Minimal/ indeterminate	Perivenular inflammation involving a minority of terminal hepatic veins with patchy perivenular hepatocyte loss without confluent perinenular necrosis
Mild	As above, but involving a majority of terminal hepatic veins
Moderate	As above, with at least focal confluent perivenular hepatocyte dropout and mild moderate inflammation, but without bridging necrosis
Severe	As above, with confluent perivenular hepatocyte dropout and inflammation involving a majority of hepatic venules with central-to-central bridging necrosis

Adapted from Demetris AJ, Adeyi O, Bellamy COC, et al. Liver biopsy interpretation for causes of late liver allograft dysfunction. *Hepatology*. 2006;44(2):489–501, with permission from American Association for the Study of Liver Diseases. doi:10.1002/hep.21280.

represents a more specific rejection feature and is very helpful in this distinction. Drug reactions are also commonly associated with more pronounced lobular inflammation and sometimes with granulomas, both relatively uncommon in acute cellular rejection, particularly in the mild end of the spectrum. Hepatocanalicular cholestasis is also common in drug-related injury but only seen in moderate to severe rejection, typically with pronounced bile duct injury. Cholestasis that is out of proportion to the degree of bile duct injury, therefore, represents a useful feature to favor drug effect. Biliary obstruction may occasionally mimic rejection. However, biliary obstruction is typically associated with neutrophilic (rather than lymphocytic) cholangitis, significant ductular reaction, and portal edema—none of which is typical for rejection. The degree of portal infiltrate is also generally more pronounced in rejection. Again, endotheliitis, when present, favors rejection.

In the late posttransplantation period, atypical histologic features of rejection become more common (Table 20.5) and raise additional considerations in the differential diagnosis. Cases showing a plasma cell–rich chronic hepatitis morphology (discussed above) can closely mimic alloimmune or de novo autoimmune hepatitis, but this distinction cannot be accurately made on histologic grounds alone and a final diagnosis requires correlation with clinical, serological, and histological findings. Differentiating this pattern from that of recurrent hepatitis C, on the other hand, is

Table 20.5 Histologic Features of Early and Late Acute Cellular Rejection (ACR)

	Early ACR	Late ACR
Posttransplant period	Initial 1–3 months	3 months or later
Portal inflammation	Mixed, often containing activated (blast-like) lymphocytes and increased eosinophils	Often predominantly lymphocytic, resembling a chronic hepatitis
Bile duct injury	Variable, but often prominent in moderate and severe ACR	None or mild
Portal endothelialitis	Variable, but often prominent in moderate and severe ACR	None or mild
Interface hepatitis	Minimal or none, except for severe ACR	Often present, even in mild cases, resembling chronic hepatitis
Central perivenulitis	Moderate to severe rejection only; typically accompanied by ACR findings in portal tracts	Common; often not associated with diagnostic findings of ACR in portal tracts (i.e., isolated central perivenulitis)

Adapted from Moreira RK. Recurrent hepatitis C and acute allograft rejection: clinicopathologic features with emphasis on the differential diagnosis between these entities. *Adv Anat Pathol*. 2011;18(5): 393–405. doi:10.1097/PAP.0b013e31822a5a10.

very important for management purposes (increased immunosuppression for rejection and decreased immunosuppression, with or without antiviral therapy, for recurrent hepatitis C). Even in nontransplanted individuals with chronic hepatitis C, there can be some rejection-like features, including bile duct injury and endothelialitis.[68] However, these features in chronic hepatitis C are focal and mild and not the predominant pattern of injury. Thus, in most cases the distinction between recurrent hepatitis C and rejection is readily made (for details, see section on recurrent diseases).

Prognosis and treatment

Most cases of acute cellular rejection are mild (often subclinical, as seen in protocol biopsies), with no significant long-term adverse effect on graft outcome, when they are managed successfully with either optimization of immunosuppression alone or in conjunction with steroid therapy.[39,40] Currently, acute cellular rejection only uncommonly progresses to graft failure.[69] However, a large recent retrospective study showed that the long-term graft survival of patients with late acute cellular rejection (>90 days posttransplantation) is significantly worse compared with patients with early acute cellular rejection only.[70] Severe rejection and variant rejection patterns such as plasma cell hepatitis are more often associated with adverse graft outcomes. Finally, a minority of cases of acute cellular rejection are steroid resistant and management options for these patients include T-cell–depleting agents, thymoglobulin, mycophenolate mofetil, anti-IL-2, and OKT3.

20.9 CHRONIC (DUCTOPENIC) REJECTION

Definition

Chronic rejection is a form of immune-mediated liver allograft injury characterized by bile duct loss (ductopenia) and/or obliterative (foam cell) arteriopathy of medium- and large-sized vessels, often evolving to graft loss. Because most cases are diagnosed on liver biopsies (in which foam cell arteriopathy is rarely seen), the term *chronic ductopenic rejection* or *posttransplant vanishing bile duct syndrome* has been used.

Clinical findings

Chronic rejection historically accounted for up to 20% of all cases of allograft failure,[71,72] but the current incidence has substantially decreased (to as low as 3% of failed allografts), likely owing to improvements in immunosuppression therapy, monitoring, and early histologic recognition.[69] Chronic rejection is usually asymptomatic and most patients present with increasing liver enzymes showing a cholestatic pattern. Chronic rejection can eventually lead to jaundice as the disease progresses, typically in the setting of previous episodes of severe or steroid-resistant acute cellular rejection. The diagnosis of chronic rejection requires a liver biopsy that shows the presence of typical histologic features and the exclusion of other forms of biliary tract disease, particularly biliary obstruction. Other clinical risk factors for the development of chronic rejection include donor age >40, recipient age <30, and underlying primary biliary cirrhosis or autoimmune hepatitis.

Histologic findings

The histologic hallmarks of chronic rejection in liver allografts are: (1) bile duct loss (ductopenia) and/or

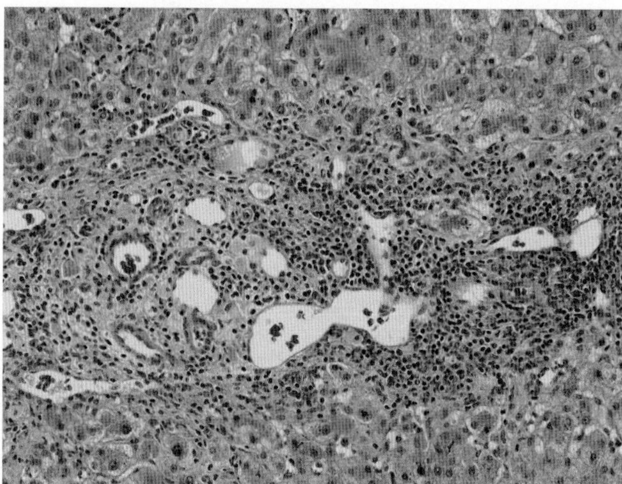

Figure 20.18 Ductopenia. No interlobular bile ducts are seen within this mildly inflamed portal tract. Notice the presence of several hepatic artery branch profiles, which should normally be accompanied by a similar-sized bile duct. Most portal tract lacked a bile duct in this case.

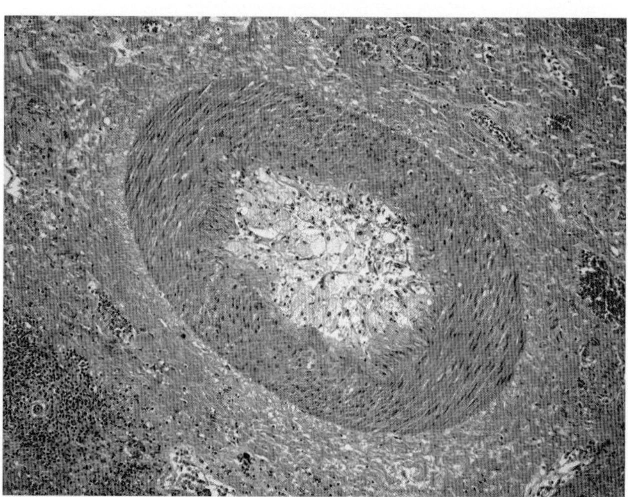

Figure 20.19 Foam cell arteriopathy. A medium-size arterial vessel close to the hepatic hilum showing prominent subintimal foamy macrophages in this failed allograft with chronic rejection.

(2) foam cell arteriopathy, along with several other less specific findings that are thought to be secondary to these two basic abnormalities. Of these two, ductopenia represents the main finding in the vast majority of chronic rejection cases (Fig. 20.18), because foam cell arteriopathy is relatively less common and primarily seen in medium- to large-sized arterial vessels that are not typically sampled in biopsies (Fig. 20.19).

Early in the course of the chronic rejection, a constellation of reactive bile duct epithelial changes can be seen, including marked nuclear pleomorphism, hyperchromasia, epithelial dyspolarity, cytoplasmic eosinophilia, epithelial flattening, and atrophic

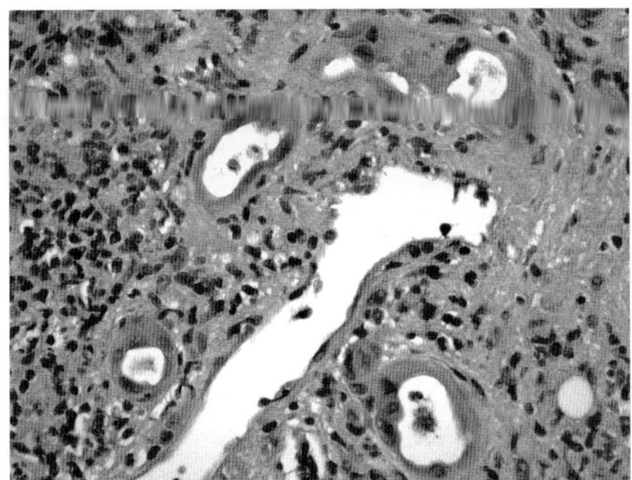

Figure 20.20 Early chronic rejection. The bile ducts in this example show pronounced epithelial dysmorphic changes, including marked nuclear enlargement, irregularity, overlapping, as well as flattening of the epithelium.

appearance of ducts (collectively referred to as *bile duct senescence*), without obvious bile duct loss (Fig. 20.20). Early chronic rejection, if untreated, can progress to ductopenic rejection.

Ductopenia is typically defined as the absence of bile ducts in >50% of portal tracts. The "50% rule" was developed in part from early morphometric studies of large tissue sections (autopsy and wedge biopsies), mostly from patients with Alagille syndrome[73] and primary biliary cirrhosis.[74] The same 50% rule is used with needle biopsies, but its application has several practical difficulties, including a significant proportion of incomplete and/or tangentially sectioned portal tracts, dense inflammatory infiltrates obscuring the visualization of bile ducts, and sometimes a very small number of portal tracts.[75] If a sufficient number of complete portal tracts are present within the sample, the absence of bile ducts in most portal tracts indicates ductopenia. In needle core biopsy samples, which typically have approximately 10 to 15 portal tracts per sample,[75,76] a useful method of assessing bile duct loss is to identify branches of the hepatic artery. These small arteries run side by side with similar-sized interlobular bile ducts within the portal tracts and both structures should normally be identified in close proximity on histologic sections (bile duct–hepatic artery parallelism). Cytokeratin 7 or 19 imunostains are also very useful for evaluating bile duct loss.

Foam cell arteriopathy (or "vascular chronic rejection") represents the most specific chronic rejection–related finding, but is most commonly recognized during examination of failed allografts, because this change typically involves large- and medium-sized arteries near the hepatic hilum. Foam cell arteriopathy is characterized by infiltration of foamy macrophages in the subintimal space and, less commonly, within deeper layers of the vascular wall. Some degree of [illegible] vascular inflammation and fibromuscular hyperplasia can also be seen. In cases of chronic vascular rejection, there may be a paucity of arterial profiles in the small, peripheral portal tracts—a finding that can occasionally be recognized on biopsy samples.

When the entire liver is carefully examined, ductopenic rejection and vascular rejection coexist in the majority (approximately 75%) of cases. In fact, it is possible that the bile duct injury/loss in chronic rejection is at least partially caused by ischemic changes that result from foam cell arteriopathy. However, there are well-documented cases in the literature in which purely ductopenic or purely vascular chronic rejection are seen.[77]

There are several relatively nonspecific, secondary changes found in the setting of chronic rejection, including hepato-canalicular cholestasis (which, as in many other diseases, is usually more pronounced in centrilobular regions), and centrilobular hepatocyte drop out (presumably caused by chronic ischemia), with subsequent development of centrilobular fibrosis. Secondary Kupffer cell hyperplasia often accompanies the cholestasis. Most cases of chronic ductopenic rejection show no significant ductular reaction, in spite of the severe cholestasis.

Differential diagnosis

The differential diagnosis of chronic rejection mainly includes other forms of cholestatic and/or ductopenic disorders. Chronic biliary obstruction is probably the most common entity in the differential diagnosis. Although biliary obstruction typically occurs earlier in the posttransplantation period than chronic rejection, biliary obstruction can also occur as a late complication. Histologically, biliary obstruction is associated with portal edema early in its course and significant ductular reaction later on, in contrast with ductopenic rejection, in which neither of these features should be present. It should be noted, however, that chronic biliary obstruction, particularly when associated with hepatic artery thrombosis/ischemia, can also lead to bile duct loss. Drug reaction should also be considered in the differential. Although significant cholestasis and bile duct changes can be seen in drug-related injury, bile duct loss is less common. Prominent portal or lobular inflammation or granulomas also favor drug reaction. Finally, recurrent ductopenic disorders such as primary biliary cirrhosis and primary sclerosing cholangitis can also mimic chronic rejection. Both recurrent primary biliary cirrhosis and primary sclerosing cholangitis typically show other changes of their respective diseases and not ductopenia in isolation.

Prognosis

Chronic rejection carries a high risk of evolution to graft failure and need for retransplantation, especially in cases with well-established ductopenia. Allograft salvage is possible in some cases with early intervention and optimization of immunosuppression.

20.10 HEPATIC ARTERY THROMBOSIS

Clinical findings

Hepatic artery thrombosis represents the most common vascular complication after liver transplantation, with an incidence of approximately 2% to 6% in adult orthotopic liver transplants.[78–80] Higher rates are seen in the pediatric population, with partial allografts (including living donor transplants), in the setting of hypercoagulable states, and in cases in which complex arterial reconstructions were performed. Hepatic artery thrombosis is a medically serious complication and routine surveillance with duplex ultrasound early in the posttransplant period is standard of care. Although often clinically silent early in the posttransplantation period, hepatic artery thrombosis can present clinically with fever, abdominal pain, and liver enzyme abnormalities. Transaminases can be markedly elevated in cases with significant parenchymal necrosis. A cholestatic pattern can develop, sometimes with clinical cholangitis or liver abscesses, in cases of ischemic bile duct injury.[81] Severe cases can present as acute or fulminant liver failure.

Histologic findings

The histologic findings of hepatic artery thrombosis are variable and often difficult to interpret on needle biopsy specimens owing to the highly heterogeneous/patchy nature of the parenchymal involvement by ischemic changes, especially at the peripheral areas of the liver. When present, changes in needle biopsies reflect either direct ischemic injury—which ranges from centrilobular hepatocyte swelling or centrilobular coagulative necrosis to complete parenchymal necrosis (Fig. 20.21)—or secondary features reflecting ischemic bile duct injury to the large hilar bile ducts, which in turn leads to biliary obstructive changes (portal edema, mixed inflammation, ductular reaction, hepatocanalicular cholestasis, etc.). With chronic, lower-grade vascular obstruction, the centrilobular areas may show atrophic changes and there may be an associated component of nodular regenerative hyperplasia. Chronic ischemia can also cause biliary epithelial senescence (characterized by dysmorphic/dysplasia-like epithelial changes), similar to those seen in early chronic rejection. As a very early injury pattern, hepatic artery thrombosis can present histologically as spotty necrosis (often combined with increased hepatocyte mitotic figures[82]), mimicking a hepatitic pattern. Therefore, any noninflammatory or pauci-inflammatory centrilobular injury, particularly early in the posttransplant period, with or without associated biliary obstructive changes, should raise suspicion for hepatic artery thrombosis. Although needle biopsy findings can strongly suggest ischemic-type injury, the final diagnosis requires correlation with vascular imaging studies.

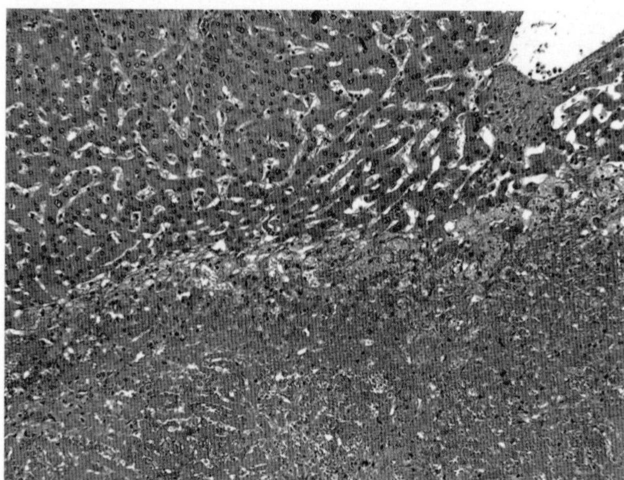

Figure 20.21 Hepatic artery thrombosis, parenchymal necrosis. Noninflammatory coagulative-type necrosis is seen in a well-demarkated area (**bottom** half of the image).

Upon examination of failed allografts, thrombi of varying ages and degrees of organization can be identified within the hepatic artery, most often around the vascular anastomotic site, sometimes with myointimal hyperplasia. The hilar bile ducts commonly show extensive ischemic injury, often with rupture, bile extravasation, and a histiocytic reaction (Fig. 20.22). Bile casts (sometimes associated clinically with biliary cast syndrome[83]) can also be seen in patients with hepatic artery thrombosis, presumably reflecting ischemic cholangiopathy (Fig. 20.23). Macroscopically, the liver parenchyma can also show patchy, well-defined areas of necrosis, sometimes in a distinctly wedge-shaped distribution (Fig. 20.24).

Differential diagnosis

Although the changes of hepatic artery thrombosis are relatively straightforward on failed allograft examination, the differential diagnosis on needle biopsies is broad, reflecting the various patterns of injury that can be seen with hepatic artery thrombosis. The association of hepatic artery thrombosis with biliary complications and hepatic artery abnormalities is strong enough that any biopsy showing

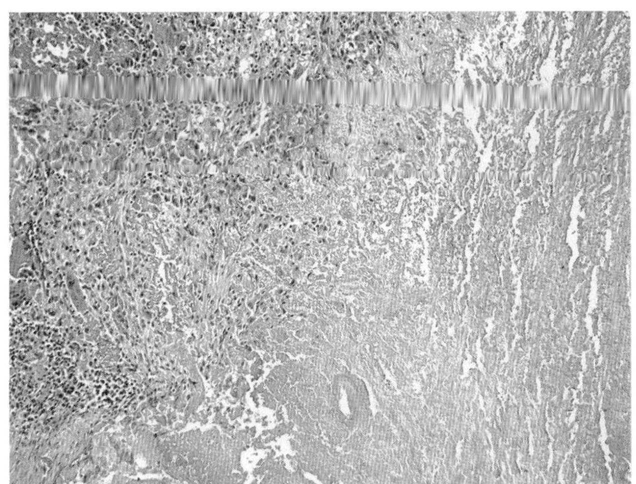

Figure 20.22 Hepatic artery thrombosis, bile duct necrosis. Bile extravazation with histiocytic reaction is seen in this case due to ischemia-related bile duct necrosis.

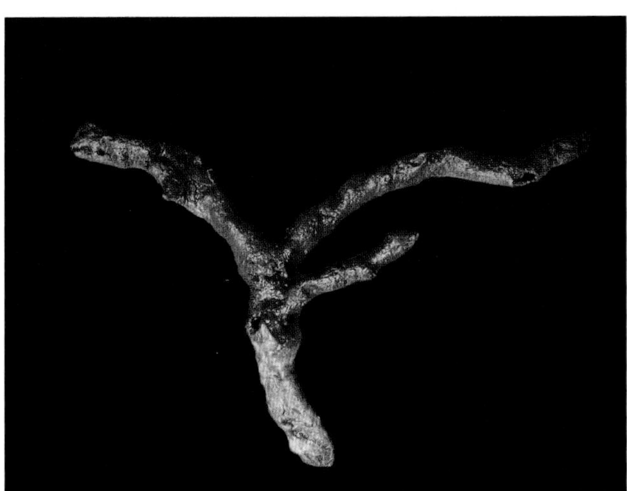

Figure 20.23 Biliary cast.

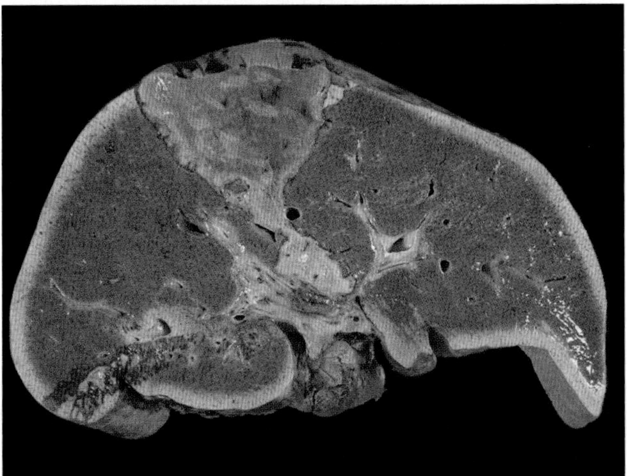

Figure 20.24 Hepatic artery thrombosis, gross. A failed allograft showing a large, well-delineated wedge-shaped area of ischemic necrosis due to hepatic artery thrombosis.

biliary obstructive features during the posttransplant period should prompt evaluation of hepatic artery patency. Centrilobular injury and necrosis can be seen in different settings, including rejection (both acute and chronic) and medication-induced injury. However, "bland" (noninflammatory/pauci-inflammatory) centrilobular necrosis, although not entirely specific, suggests ischemic injury.

Later, centrilobular injury due to chronic rejection also enters the differential diagnosis. Chronic rejection is more common than hepatic artery thrombosis in cases with a history of severe or refractory acute cellular rejection. Portal vein thrombosis, although significantly less common than hepatic artery thrombosis, should also be considered in the differential diagnosis, because portal vein thrombosis can be associated with variable (sometimes massive) hepatocellular coagulative necrosis, particularly in the early posttransplantation period, similar to that seen with hepatic artery thrombosis. However, in contrast to hepatic artery thrombosis, the necrosis that results from portal vein thrombosis can be predominantly periportal or mid-zonal.

Prognosis

The prognosis of hepatic artery thrombosis is variable, depending on disease severity, associated complications, posttransplantation period, and therapy. Overall, the mortality rate is approximately one third and over half of patients require retranplantation[81].

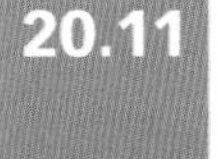

20.11 PORTAL VEIN THROMBOSIS AND VENOUS OUTFLOW IMPAIRMENT

Clinical findings

Transplant-related causes of portal vein thrombosis and venous outflow abnormalities are significantly less common than hepatic artery complications. Portal vein thrombosis occurs in less than 2% of all allografts, mostly in the early posttransplant period, but there is a higher incidence in reduced-sized livers, living donor transplants, pediatric recipients, and in the setting of pretransplant portal vein thrombosis. Because most of the blood flow to the liver is supplied by the portal vein and no significant collateral circulation is present shortly after transplantation, complete portal vein thrombosis can be associated with widespread parenchymal necrosis as well as clinical evidence of liver failure and severe portal hypertension.[84]

Various forms of venous outflow impairment are also seen in the posttransplant setting and can result from any pathologic process that interferes with normal blood drainage from the liver into the hepatic venous outflow tract. The major causes are divided into three groups of diseases:

1. Cardiovascular abnormalities, including congestive heart failure, right-sided heart failure, constrictive pericarditis, and obstructive processes of the vena cava.
2. Hepatic vein abnormalities (usually thrombosis, i.e., Budd–Chiari syndrome).
3. Diseases of the hepatic venules and sinusoids, that is, veno-occlusive disease/sinusoidal obstruction syndrome.

The clinical manifestations of venous outflow impairment depend on the etiology and the disease severity. Venous outflow impairment owing to heart failure typically presents with ascites, edema, and abdominal pain from liver congestion and enlargement, which often parallels the severity of cardiac dysfunction.

As in native livers, Budd–Chiari syndrome is typically seen in the setting of hypercoagulable states, including coagulation factor deficiencies, myelodysplastic syndromes, malignancies, use of oral contraceptives, and the antiphospholipid syndrome. Transplant-related risk factors for hepatic vein abnormalities include anastomotic problems, donor-recipient venous-size mismatch, and the "piggyback" anastomotic technique. The Budd–Chiari syndrome most commonly has a subacute presentation in liver transplant patients, with clinical signs and symptoms of liver congestion and portal hypertension. Acute/fulminant and "chronic" forms are also described but are less common.

Finally, veno-occlusive disease/sinusoidal obstruction syndrome—a disease of the hepatic sinusoidal endothelium—is most commonly seen in the setting of bone marrow transplantation, high-dose chemotherapy (especially cyclophosphamide and busulfan) and, occasionally, after ingestion of certain pyrrolizidine alkaloids in herbal medications (Jamaican bush tea). These injuries can have an acute, subacute, or chronic presentation. The clinical findings include varying degrees of hepatic congestion, portal hypertension, and liver dysfunction. In the post liver transplant setting, veno-occlusive disease/sinusoidal obstruction syndrome has also been associated with azathioprine and episodes of acute cellular rejection.[85,86]

Histologic findings

In portal vein thrombosis, the severity of the histologic changes will depend on the extent of the thrombosis, the location within the portal system, and the timing posttransplantation. The histologic findings will range from mild nonspecific hepatocyte swelling to massive ischemic-type necrosis. Unlike cirrhotic livers, which have extensive collateral circulation, the typical case of portal vein thrombosis in the setting of liver transplantation occurs early, during a period when the allograft has either no or very limited collateral circulation. In this setting, the liver allograft is highly susceptible to ischemia because of decreased portal venous flow. In long-standing/chronic portal vein thrombosis, nodular regenerative hyperplasia often develops.

In veno-occlusive disease/sinusoidal obstruction syndrome, the changes are identical to those seen in native livers (also see Chapter 21), with sinusoidal dilatation and congestion in zones 3 of the lobule (or zones 2 and 3 in more severe cases), as well as centrilobular sinusoidal fibrosis and hepatic plate atrophy within congested areas. In the acute phase, centrilobular congestion and hemorrhage can be seen, with red blood cell infiltration into the space of Disse. When severe, this can occasionally result in replacing the portions of the hepatic plates with red blood cells as a result of hepatocyte necrosis and hemorrhage into the space of Disse (referred to as *red blood cell–trabecular lesion*). Chronic cases can show marked centrilobular atrophy, dense zone 3 fibrosis, and nodular regenerative hyperplasia (with portal tracts at the center of regenerating periportal areas, in a "reverse lobulation" pattern). Changes related to the patient's primary diseases (such as amyloidosis, hemochromatosis, or sarcoidosis in cardiac disease) can also be present.

Differential diagnosis

In practice, nonspecific centrilobular sinusoidal dilatation (which could be due to biopsy-related artifacts, unrelated/extra-hepatic disease,[87] or normal variations) can sometimes be challenging to distinguish from true venous outflow impairment. In general, sinusoidal dilatation/congestion that is mild and not associated with sinusoidal fibrosis is usually nonspecific, whereas the presence of hepatocyte atrophy or sinusoidal fibrosis in the congested areas typically indicates true veno-occlusive disease/sinusoidal obstruction syndrome.

20.12 BILIARY COMPLICATIONS

Clinical findings

Biliary complications remain one of the most common problems in liver transplant patients. Among these, biliary strictures are one of the most significant, often requiring a liver biopsy as part of its workup. Biliary strictures occur in 5% to 15% of liver transplant patients (higher incidence in partial liver/living donor transplants). Biliary strictures most commonly represent a late complication, typically diagnosed between 6 and 12 months posttransplantation.[88,89] Biliary strictures present clinically with jaundice, fever, abdominal pain (when symptomatic), and a cholestatic pattern of abnormal liver tests. The diagnosis can often be made on imaging, where the most common finding is bile duct dilation proximal to the site of stricture.

Etiology and pathogenesis

Biliary strictures are generally divided into anastomotic and nonanastomotic strictures. Anastomotic strictures, as the name implies, involve the anastomosis site and are generally thought to be related to inadequate local healing owing to technical aspects of the surgery, local tissue ischemia, and/or bile leaks. Nonanastomotic strictures, on the other hand, are located in areas away from the anastomosis, can be localized, or can present as "diffuse" stricturing of the biliary system. Nonanastomotic strictures are mostly related to ischemic injury.[88] In fact, up to 50% of patients with nonanastomotic biliary strictures have been shown to have hepatic artery thrombosis.[90] In a minority of patients, the so-called biliary cast syndrome develops, which is characterized by casts of inspissated bile material of varying sizes obstructing the biliary tree (Fig. 20.23). This complication is typically associated with biliary strictures, but has also been linked to episodes of acute cellular rejection, biliary infections, and ischemia[91].

Histologic findings

The histologic features of biliary obstruction in allografts are essentially identical to those seen in native livers (please refer to Chapters 6 and 13). Early/acute changes include portal edema, mixed portal inflammation, and a ductular reaction. Later on, mild centrilobular hepatocanalicular cholestasis can develop. With long-standing obstruction, portal fibrosis can be seen and some cases can develop periductal onion-skin fibrosis and mild ductopenia. With prolonged cholestasis, cholate stasis is also seen, with periportal hepatocyte swelling/feathery degeneration, Mallory hyaline, and copper/copper-binding protein deposition in periportal hepatocytes.

Special stains and immunostains

There are two stains that are very useful in the setting of biliary obstruction: copper stains and CK7, although copper deposition is not found in the acute setting. Many stains are helpful in highlighting copper pigment (or copper-binding protein), including rhodanine, Victoria blue, and orcein stains. Copper deposition can be very focal, especially in early or mild biliary tract obstruction, and a useful practical strategy is to search within the hepatic plates immediately adjacent to portal tracts and to focus on the largest available portal tracts, because copper/copper-binding protein tends to be deposited preferentially in these locations initially. Although copper deposition is not specific for chronic biliary tract disease (also seen in Wilson disease and in relatively small amount as a nonspecific finding in advanced fibrosis/cirrhosis of any etiology), it is very helpful as an adjunct finding when other features suggestive of biliary tract disease are present, especially in a noncirrhotic liver.[92] Chronic cholestatic liver disease of any sort, including biliary obstruction, also leads to expression of CK7 in the periportal hepatocytes (intermediate hepatocytes). CK7 will also highlight the ductular proliferation in obstructive disease.

Differential diagnosis

Very early biliary tract obstruction is often the most difficult to diagnose, because the findings in the liver can be mild and patchy and the typical findings of large duct obstruction might not be seen on needle biopsy. Drug-induced injury and infections can also show some overlapping features with obstructive disease, but they both typically show more significant portal and lobular inflammation, which are not prominent features in biliary obstruction. Although histiocytic infiltrate around areas of bile infarcts can be present, granulomas are not part of the spectrum of biliary obstruction but can be seen in some drug reactions and certain infections.

Recurrent primary biliary cirrhosis or primary sclerosing cholangitis can mimic obstruction, though recurrent disease typically does not enter the differential diagnosis until several years after transplantation. The diagnosis of recurrent disease is discussed later but requires correlation with clinical and imaging findings. Primary biliary cirrhosis typically shows more pronounced portal chronic inflammation and the presence of lymphocytic cholangitis and/or florid bile duct lesions. Primary sclerosing cholangitis can be more difficult to distinguish from biliary obstruction because of other causes. The time course (early after transplantation suggests causes other than primary sclerosing cholangitis) and the location of the strictures (anastomic versus nonanastomatic) can help guide histological interpretation.

Fibrosing cholestatic hepatitis, which can be seen in the setting of hepatitis B or C, can also mimic biliary obstruction. The presence of marked lobular changes, including hepatocellular swelling and disarray, along with very high viral loads, favors fibrosing cholestatic hepatitis (see Chapter 8 for further information). In contrast, portal edema, ductular cholestasis, bile infarcts, as well as copper deposition and aberrant CK7 staining in periportal hepatocytes favor biliary obstruction.[93] Finally, cases showing histological biliary obstructive findings early in the posttransplantation period but without clinical/imaging evidence of obstruction should be evaluated for humoral rejection with C4d immunostain and, clinically, with donor-specific antibody panel.

20.13 OPPORTUNISTIC INFECTIONS

Cytomegalovirus

Clinical findings

Cytomegalovirus (CMV) is only rarely associated with liver infection and organ dysfunction in immunocompetent hosts but is among the most common opportunistic infections in liver transplant patients, with most cases presenting in the early posttransplantation period, between 4 and 12 weeks.

Etiology and pathogenesis

CMV is a DNA virus within the Herpesviridae family. Although a normal immune system is highly effective in preventing widespread infection by CMV, the high degree of immunosuppression seen with liver transplantation may lead to local or disseminated viral infection and organ damage. Latent viruses are thought to reside within granulocytes, monocytes, and endothelial cells, with sinusoidal endothelial cell infection representing an early step in the pathogenesis of liver allograft infection.[94,95] Both reactivation of latent disease and primary infection occurs after transplantation. Primary infection (highest risk in the donor-positive/recipient-negative scenario) is associated with a greater risk of significant disease and organ dysfunction compared to reactivation,[95–98] presumably owing to the partial protection conferred by previous immune activation.

Histologic findings

A high index of suspicion is required to recognize CMV infection histologically in liver allograft specimens, because the findings are frequently focal and often require the aid of immunostains for the diagnosis. In mild cases, localized areas of lobular injury can show a few injured/necrotic hepatocytes surrounded by neutrophils (referred to as a *microabscess*) or by clusters of histiocytes ("microgranuloma"). Within these foci, occasional enlarged cells sometimes show diagnostic CMV-type inclusions. CMV inclusions consist of large, somewhat irregular, glassy intranuclear eosinophilic inclusions surrounded by a clear halo, often accompanied by round cytoplasmic inclusions of varying sizes (Fig. 20.25). In early infection, viral inclusions are often inconspicuous or absent. With more severe infection, inclusions can be found in endothelial cells, stromal cells, hepatocytes, and biliary epithelium. Severe infections also show significant portal and lobular inflammation, predominantly lymphocytic, with abundant spotty necrosis and Kupffer cell hyperplasia.

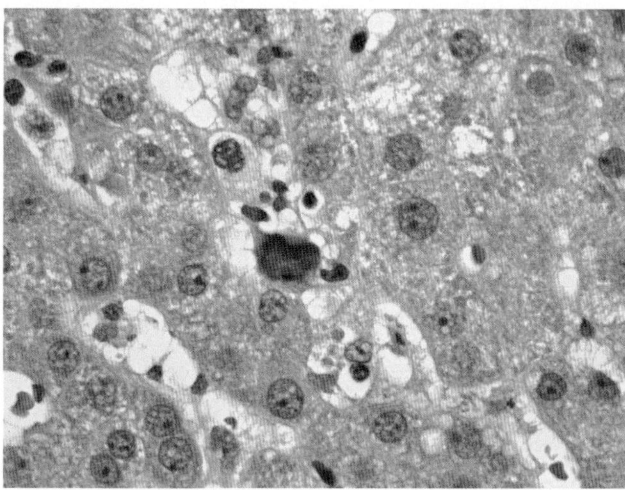

Figure 20.25 Cytomegalovirus. An typical CMV-type nuclear inclusion is seen in the center of the image.

It is important to recognize, however, that severe, widespread graft disease is rare in modern posttransplantation care, where there is close monitoring for CMV infection and use of prophylactic therapy in high-risk patients. Thus, the histologic diagnosis often relies on recognizing occasional infected cells. In cases where there is either clinical concern for CMV infection or suspicious histological findings, but no diagnostic inclusions, it is our practice to obtain additional H&E levels as well as CMV immunostain.

Special stains and immunostains

The typical case in modern practice contains few or no diagnostic cytomegalic cells on H&E, so ancillary techniques have an important role in the diagnosis of CMV infection. Immunohistochemistry is the most common method and recognizes the early or immediate early CMV nuclear protein, depending on the specific antibody used. In situ hybridization has also been studied but does not appear to have significant advantages over the widely available immunohistochemical antibodies.[99,100]

Occasionally, an obviously abnormal (cytomegalic) cell is seen on immunostain, which was not present on routine stains (i.e., a focus that appeared on the deeper tissue section used for immunostaining), representing a diagnostic finding for CMV disease. The presence of small (noncytomegalic) cells showing positivity for CMV on immunostains, in the absence of at least suspicious findings on H&E, on the other hand, is currently of unknown significance and could represent staining artifact or true CMV antigens within circulating cells. Clinical treatment decisions in these cases will depend on correlation with quantitative CMV levels in the blood as well as other clinical and biochemical findings (e.g., is there unexplained organ dysfunction?). As a diagnostic pitfall, plasma cells can sometimes show artifactual staining.

Differential diagnosis

Although typical inclusions are pathognomonic of CMV infection, the cytologic changes in practice are often equivocal. Reactive stromal and epithelial changes, particularly in the setting of significant inflammation, necrosis, or treatment effect (radiation, chemotherapy, etc.) can mimic viral cytopathic effect. True viral inclusions, including herpes simplex virus (HSV) and, to a lesser extent, adenovirus can also resemble CMV. The differential diagnosis can usually be resolved with the aid of immunostains. Other than viral inclusions, microabscesses represent the main histologic surrogate marker for the presence of CMV. Although all of these cases deserve further workup with CMV immunostains, the majority (approximately 80%) will be associated with other causes, including unrelated infections (bacteria, fungi, non-CMV viruses), graft ischemia, biliary obstruction, sepsis, or no identifiable etiology.[101]

Prognosis and treatment

CMV infection has been associated with an increased risk for hepatic artery thrombosis[102–104] and biliary complicatons[105] after liver transplantation, presumably owing to vascular endothelial infection and injury. CMV infection has also been implicated as a risk factor for chronic rejection[106,107] and increased severity of recurrent hepatitis C,[108] but these associations remain controvertial.[109,110] Prevention of CMV disease is recommended for high-risk liver transplant recipients (CMV mismatch). Preventive strategies include antiviral prophylaxis, with ganciclovir or valganciclovir, or preemptive therapy, which entails frequent posttransplant CMV testing and initiation of treatment if the virus is detected.[111] Treatment options for active CMV disease include ganciclovir, valganciclovir, foscarnet, and cidofovir. Intravenous ganciclovir and oral valganciclovir are similarly effective against posttransplant CMV infection[112] and are currently the drugs of choice.

Herpes simplex virus

Etiology, pathogenesis, and clinical findings

HSV hepatitis can be caused by either HSV type I or HSV type II and can represent reactivation, reinfection, or primary infection. Compared to immunocompetent individuals, HSV infection in transplant recipients has a more severe course with a higher rate of visceral or disseminated disease. Liver involvement (i.e., HSV hepatitis), although fairly uncommon, is often associated with massive/fulminant liver failure, leading to death or liver failure in the majority of cases. Most patients are immunosuppressed and approximately one third of cases occur in the setting of solid organ or bone marrow transplantation. Liver enzymes typically show a hepatitic pattern, with marked transaminase elevations, commonly associated with signs of acute/fulminant liver failure, including coagulopathy and encephalopathy. Mucocutaneous herpetic rashes are found in less than half of cases and can be either localized or disseminated. The majority of cases reported in literature were clinically unsuspected before tissue confirmation (either on autopsy or biopsy).[113,114] The diagnosis of HSV can be established by polymerase chain reaction assays from tissue sampling or blood, which has replaced tissue culture and direct fluorescent antibody as the preferred diagnostic test.[115] Serology testing is not useful for diagnosis. In the setting of solid organ transplantation, HSV tends to occur in the early posttransplant period (day 5 to 46).[114]

Histologic findings

The most typical histologic presentation of HSV hepatitis is characterized by relatively well-demarcated ("punched out") areas of necrosis that vary from small necrotic foci involving a few hepatocytes, often surrounded by macrophages and neutrophils, to massive areas of panlobular necrosis. HSV cytopathic effect generally involves hepatocytes adjacent to necrotic areas and is characterized by either a distinct nuclear inclusion surrounded by a halo (Cowdry type A) or, most commonly, by a diffuse glassy nuclear appearance, with margination of the chromatin toward the edge of the nucleus (Cowdry type B). Syncytial transformation and multinucleation of affected hepatocytes is also common and molding of juxtaposed infected nuclei may be present in some cases. The "3 Ms" of HSV cytopathic effect is a useful mnemonic and stands for margination, multinucleation, and molding (Fig. 20.26).

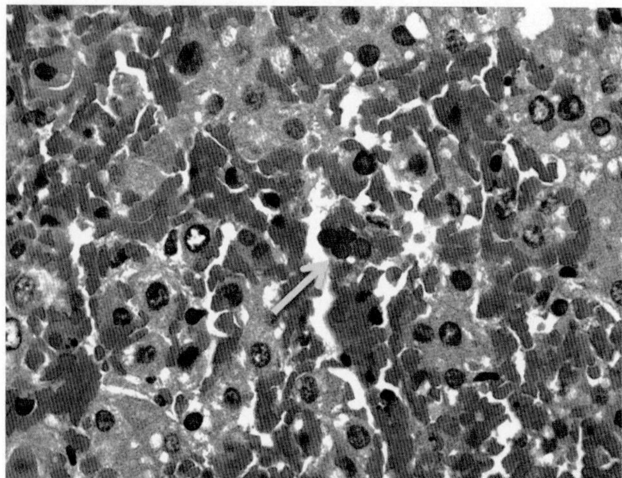

Figure 20.26 Herpes simplex virus hepatitis. HSV cytopathic effect (*arrow*), characterized by multinucleation, chromatin margination, and nuclear molding.

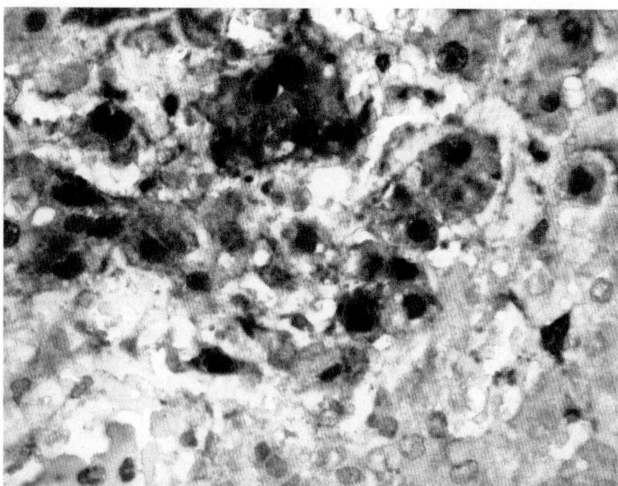

Figure 20.27 Herpes simplex virus immunohistochemistry.

Special stains and immunostains

Specific antibodies directed to HSV 1 and HSV 2 (and combined HSV1/2) by immunohistochemistry are very helpful and, if available, should be used to confirm the H&E findings (Fig. 20.27).

Differential diagnosis

Typical cases generally pose little diagnostic difficulty. In many cases, however, areas of cytopathic effect may be sparse and can be obscured by necrotic debris. Hepatocytes undergoing necrosis or apoptosis will commonly show some degree of nuclear "smudging," which is a common pitfall. CMV nuclear inclusions can mimic HSV cytopathic effect but are often associated with cytoplasmic inclusions, which are not seen in HSV infection. Adenovirus is also in the differential, because it may cause "geographic" areas of liver parenchymal necrosis and similar nuclear inclusions. Neither CMV nor adenovirus infection, however, shows hepatocyte multinucleation, which represents a somewhat specific HSV-related change, albeit not present in many cases. Varicella–Zoster virus hepatitis is very rare but shares most of the histologic changes with HSV and cannot be reliably distinguished from the latter without the aid of immunohistochemistry.

Prognosis and treatment

Although sampling can represent a problem given the patchy/geographic nature of the infection, the degree of liver involvement on biopsies seems to have prognostic implications. In one study, all patients with "diffuse disease" (presumably necrosis) died, whereas nearly half of the patients with "focal disease" survived.[114] Disseminated, visceral, or extensive cutaneous or mucosal HSV infection is treated with intravenous acyclovir.[116] Foscarnet can be used for acyclovir-resistance HSV infection.[117]

Epstein–Barr virus and posttransplantation lymphoproliferative disorder

Definition

Epstein–Barr virus (EBV) infection in the liver transplantation setting may be seen in two forms: (1) mononucleosis-like hepatitis, similar to native livers and (2) in association with a lymphoproliferative disorder. Posttransplantation lymphoproliferative disorder (PTLD) is a relatively common posttransplant complication, with an incidence of 10% in solid organ transplant recipients.[118] PTLD is subclassified into four histopathological categories according to World Health Organization (WHO) guidelines: early, polymorphic, monomorphic, and classical Hodgkin lymphoma (CHL)–type PTLD (see also Chapter 30).

Etiology, pathogenesis, and clinical findings

EBV is an enveloped, double-stranded DNA virus that, like HSV, can infect liver allografts by primary infection, reactivation, or reinfection, largely related to the degree of immunosuppression. Significant risk factors for PTLD in liver transplant recipients include EBV-negative status pretransplant, use of high-dose steroids, and use of OKT3 for treatment of rejection.[119] PTLD in the setting of liver transplantation typically occurs within the first year posttransplant and preferentially involves the liver allograft itself.[120,121] Patients can present with fever, lymphadenopathy, weight loss, nausea, abdominal pain or splenomegaly.[122]

Jaundice may be present, but hepatic failure due to PTLD is rare.

Histologic findings

EBV hepatitis in allografts shows similar features to those seen in native livers and is characterized by a primarily lobular infiltrate of mostly mature-appearing lymphocytes, with occasional atypical lymphocytes, often in a "lined-up" or "beaded" configuration within the hepatic sinusoids (Figs. 20.28 and 20.29). This is usually accompanied by some degree of hepatocellular disarray, scattered acidophilic bodies, sometimes with hepato-canalicular cholestasis. A mild degree of lymphocytic portal inflammation, occasionally with mild bile duct injury, is also part of the histologic picture.

Cases of PTLD are classified as "early," polymorphic, and monomorphic. Early lesions show a mononucleosis-like infiltrate of small lymphocytes and plasma cells with a small number of immunoblasts, which are frequently EBV-positive. Recognition of early PTLD requires a high level of suspicion from the pathologist. In polymorphic PTLD, there is a heterogeneous proliferation of small to intermediate-sized lymphocytes, plasma cells, and more immunoblasts than in early lesions. Again, these lesions are often EBV-positive. In monomorphic PTLD, there is a more uniform population of transformed/neoplastic lymphoid cells, with variable EBV expression. Monomorphic PTLD is further categorized according to the same WHO classification used in immunocompetent patients for B-cell and T/NK-cell neoplasms. Finally, Hodgkin lymphoma-type PTLD can also rarely occur.

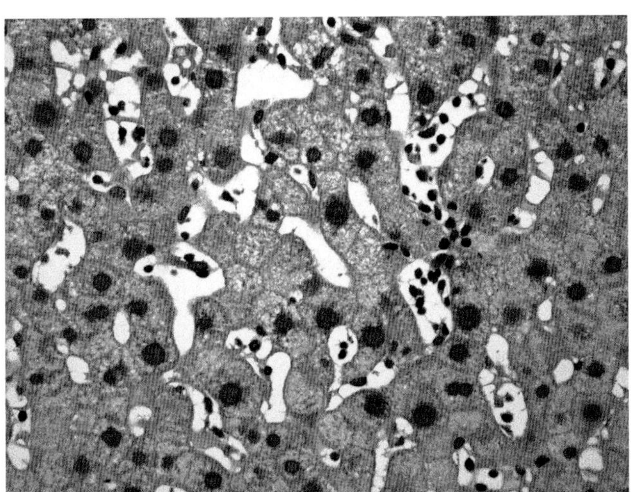

Figure 20.28 Epstein–Barr virus hepatitis. Sinusoidal lymphocytosis.

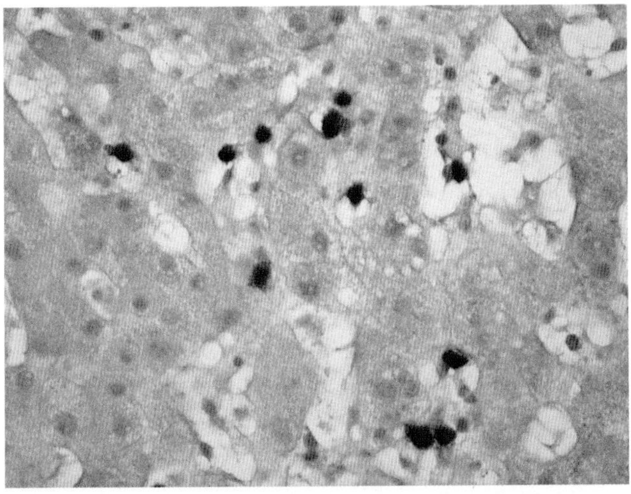

Figure 20.29 Epstein–Barr virus in situ hybridization.

Special stains and immunostains

In situ hybridization is the most commonly used ancillary method for EBV detection (immunohistochemistry for EBV-LMP-1 is not as sensitive) (Fig. 20.29).

Differential diagnosis

Given the high frequency of various inflammatory, unrelated infectious processes affecting liver allografts, and the very low overall incidence of EBV/PTLD, the diagnosis of PTLD is often overlooked. Early PTLD, in particular, is difficult to recognize and may mimic various common processes including rejection, recurrent viral hepatitis (especially hepatitis C), and other inflammatory diseases. Polymorphic PTLD is generally more striking histologically but can still be confused with various nonneoplastic inflammatory processes, especially acute rejection (in which somewhat enlarged/atypical blast-like lymphocytes may be present). Acute rejection tends to be associated with decreased/subtherapeutic levels of immunosuppression, whereas PTLD often occurs in the setting of high levels of immunosuppression. The monomorphic variant of PTLD shows features analogous to specific types of lymphomas in native livers, often forms mass lesions, and tends to cause less diagnostic difficulties.

Prognosis and therapy

The 5-year-survival after the diagnosis of PTLD ranges between 20% and 40%, but depends on the type of PTLD and the specific population, with the prognosis being worse in monomorphic PTLD and generally more favorable in children. Reduction of immunosuppression can lead to regression of PTLD within a few weeks, in particular early lesions and polymorphic lymphomas.[123] Rituximab may be used in patients with CD20-positive PTLD, leading to remission in a significant proportion of cases.[124] Antracycline-based chemotherapy is the preferred therapy for patients with high-grade lymphoma or treatment failure.[125]

20.14 BACTERIAL AND MYCOBACTERIAL INFECTIONS

Bacterial infections

Bacterial infections, whether involving the allograft primarily or as part of a systemic infection, represent the leading cause of infectious complications in liver transplant patients.[126] However, bacterial pathogens are only rarely diagnosed on tissue sections. Rather, tissue samples most commonly provide secondary evidence of a suppurative process or other patterns that are associated with bacterial infections. Sepsis, for instance, particularly from Gram-negative bacteria, is a frequent cause of cholestatic liver disease and typically presents histologically as various combinations of hepatocanalicular cholestasis with a mild ductular reaction, sometimes mimicking an obstructive process. The presence of ductular cholestasis (bile plugs within proliferating ductules in areas of ductular reaction) is not sensitive or specific but can also be seen in this setting (referred to as *cholangitis lenta*) (Fig. 20.30). Neutrophilic exudates within interlobular bile ducts may be seen in ascending cholangitis (Fig. 20.31), usually in the setting of biliary obstruction and bile stasis, which can rapidly lead to bacterial proliferation. Sepsis-related cholestasis and true biliary obstruction often coexist in these settings. Complicated cases of ascending cholangitis, as well as bacterial "seeding" from the bowel or systemic infections, can lead to bacterial abscesses in the liver.

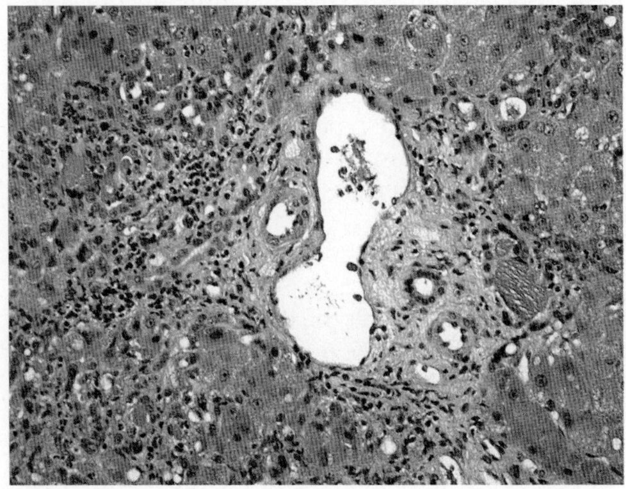

Figure 20.30 Ductular cholestasis. A portal tract showing large bile plugs within ductules in this case of sepsis-related cholestasis.

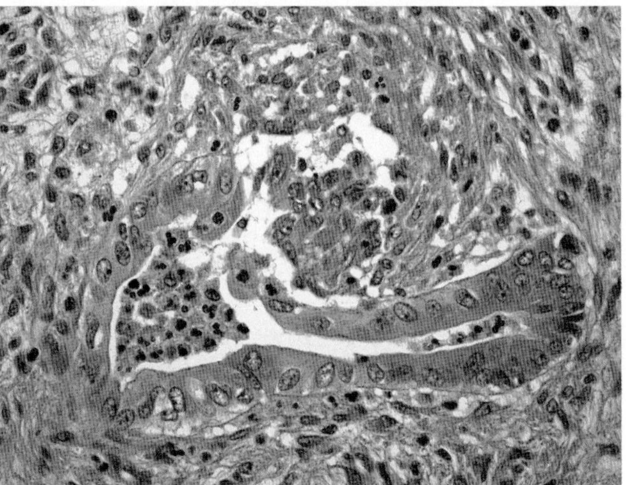

Figure 20.31 Acute cholangitis. A bile duct with intraluminal clusters of neutrophils and focal epithelial disruption in a case of ascending cholangitis due to large duct obstruction.

Liver transplant patients, as with all solid organ transplant recipients, are at markedly increased risk for tuberculosis compared to immunocompetent individuals, with an estimated 18-fold increase in the prevalence of active infection and 4-fold increase in disease-related mortality[127] compared to the general population.[128] Most cases represent reactivation of latent infection and typically occur in the first year posttransplantation. Donor-derived infection has also been reported, but accounts for less than 5% of cases.[129] Nontuberculous mycobacteria (most commonly *Mycobacterium abscessus* and *Mycobacterium avium* complex) can also involve liver allografts, generally as part of a systemic infection, but these are rare infections.

Histologically, cases of *M. tuberculosis* infection of liver allografts, as in other organs, present as granulomatous inflammation. Granulomas in allografts should always be further worked up for infectious processes (with Gomori methenamine silver [GMS] and acid-fast bacillus [AFB] stains at a minimum) given the greatly increased risk of infections in the setting of immunosuppression. Necrotizing granulomas should always raise strong suspicious for an infectious etiology, particularly mycobacterial. Because of immunosuppression, mycobacteria-related granulomas in liver allografts may be somewhat poorly formed and may not undergo necrosis. Tissue polymerase chain reaction can be very helpful in AFB stain-negative cases because of its higher sensitivity.

Fungal infections

Clinical findings

Fungal infections of the allograft are typically seen as part of multiorgan infections. The three most common invasive fungal infections in liver transplantation are *Candida* (accounting for the majority of cases; *albicans* being the most frequent, followed by *glabrata*, and *tropicalis*), *Aspergillus*, and *Cryptococcus*. Mucormycosis infection is occasionally seen in endemic areas, as are histoplasma and coccidiomycosis. The clinical presentation is generally rather nonspecific (fatigue, malaise, fever, leukocytosis), but significant liver dysfunction may be seen in cases of allograft involvement.[130–133]

Histologic findings

Although only rarely seen within the allograft itself, invasive fungal infections involving the liver can present histologically as an abscess, geographic areas of necrosis, or with necrotic bile ducts or thrombosed hepatic vessels (Fig. 20.32).[134–136] In general, the diagnosis of fungal infections in liver allografts requires a high index of suspicion and routine use of fungal stains (e.g., GMS and periodic acid–Schiff) in cases showing unexplained necrosis, histiocytic/giant cell reaction, or granulomas. *Candida* sp., the most commonly identified fungal organism in liver allograft samples, is characterized by budding yeast and pseudohyphae. *Aspergillus* organisms are seen as septate hyphae branching at 45° angles and can form abscess-like areas of necrosis with a capsule of fibrosis and histiocytic/giant cell reaction or can present as more widely infiltrating organisms (Fig. 20.33). In *Cryptococcus* infection, small round yeasts with narrow-based buds are present, ranging in size from 2 to 20 μm, usually seen within necrotic or granulomatous areas (Fig. 20.34). Although the morphologic findings of fungal organisms can be very helpful in suggesting a specific organism, definite fungal speciation requires correlation with cultures and/or molecular studies.

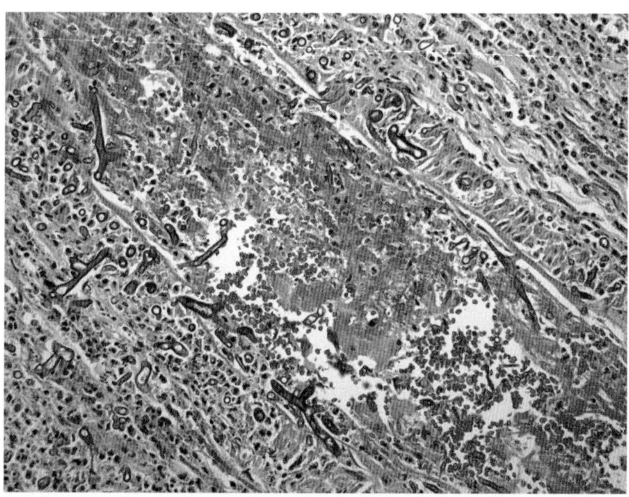

Figure 20.32 Fungal infection. An autopsy case showing invasive Mucormycosis. Organisms are seen invading a large blood vessel at the level of the hepatic hilum.

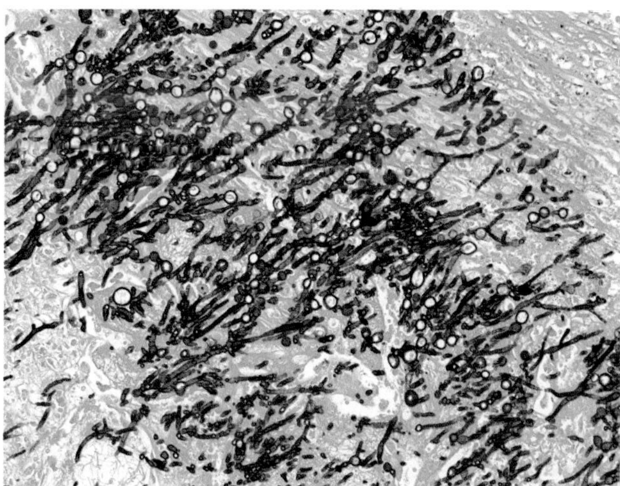

Figure 20.33 Fungal infection. Invasive Aspergillosis (Gomori methenamine silver stain) showing septated hyphae branching at 45° angles.

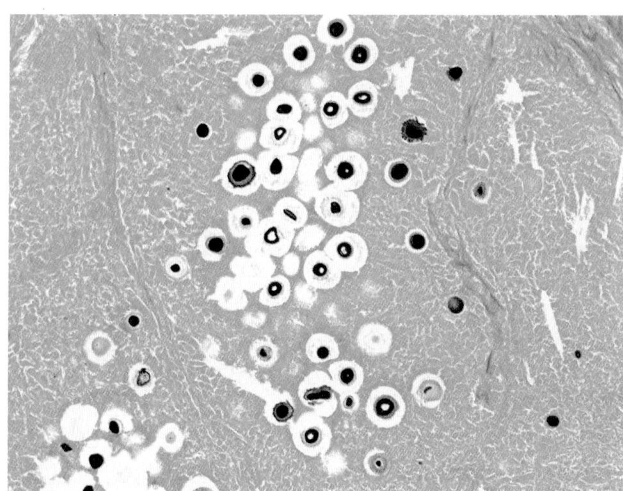

Figure 20.34 Fungal infection. Cryptococcus (Gomori methenamine silver stain).

20.15 HEPATITIS E VIRUS

Hepatitis E is typically associated with sporadic or epidemic cases of acute hepatitis in the general population. However, hepatitis E virus has been recognized since 2008 as a cause of both acute and chronic hepatitis in solid organ transplant patients (including liver transplant recipients).[137] In liver transplant patients, the documented cases of hepatitis E infection are because of genotype 3. The infections have a high propensity for becoming chronic and have been associated with accelerated fibrosis progression.[63] Hepatitis E viral infection in the setting of liver transplantation should be suspected in cases of unexplained chronic hepatitis. The biopsy findings tend to be mild and nonspecific, showing mild portal and lobular inflammation, occasionally with mild cholestasis. The management of chronic hepatitis E infection after transplantation includes reduction of immunosuppression and the use of pegylated-interferon and/or ribavirin.[138] Please refer to Chapter 8 for further discussion.

20.16 RECURRENT DISEASES

Hepatitis B

Clinical findings

Hepatitis B recurrence after liver transplantation has become uncommon with the advent of effective oral antiviral agents. Combined therapy with hepatitis B immune globulin (HBIg) and oral antivirals posttransplantation reduces the risk of recurrence to only 4% in the first 5 years after transplantation,[139] in contrast to a recurrence risk of 50% or higher without prophylaxis. Recipients of hepatitis B core antibody-positive and surface antibody-negative liver are also at risk of reactivation and require prophylaxis. Hepatitis B virus recurrence after liver transplant is usually a result of noncompliance with antiviral prophylaxis or the development of drug resistance. Other risk factors include detectable hepatitis B virus DNA levels pretransplant, HBeAg positivity, and HIV coinfection. Recurrence of infection is characterized by the reappearance of hepatitis B surface antigen and detectable levels of hepatitis B virus DNA in the serum. This is usually associated with biochemical evidence of hepatitis (elevated liver enzymes).

Etiology and pathogenesis

Hepatitis B is thought to reinfect the allograft through persistence in peripheral blood mononuclear cells as well as in various extrahepatic sites. Injury to the allograft occurs through two mechanisms: (1) immune attack that targets infected hepatocytes, triggered by CD8+ T cells through HLA class I recognition, leading to the typical acute or chronic hepatitis pattern seen in recurrent hepatitis B; and (2) a direct cytopathic effect when there is uncontrolled viral proliferation and markedly increased viral load in the setting of high-level immunosuppression. This second pattern is associated with variant patterns of hepatitis B infection (cholestatic forms) described below.

Histologic findings

The histologic findings in recurrent hepatitis B will vary according to the phase of infection. In the initial 1 to 2 months posttransplantation, the histological findings can be minimal and nonspecific findings, but HBc antigen immunohistochemistry can show focal nuclear or cytoplasmic positivity.[140] Thereafter, an "acute hepatitis" pattern is often seen, with varying degrees of spotty necrosis, Kupffer cell hyperplasia, hepatocellular disarray, and lobular inflammation. This "acute hepatitis" pattern transitions into a "chronic hepatitis" histologic pattern, with more pronounced portal inflammation, portal lymphoid aggregates, and varying degrees of fibrosis. Ground glass hepatocytes may not be seen for many months after reestablishment of hepatitis B reinfection (Fig. 20.35) and even then are present in only a subset of cases.

Variant histologic patterns of hepatitis B infection are seen in allografts and are generally thought to be due to direct viral cytopathic effect from uncontrolled viral replication because of immunosuppression. As described with other forms of immunosuppression (nonliver solid organ transplant, bone marrow transplantation, and cancer chemotherapy), fibrosing cholestatic hepatitis is characterized by a combination of marked hepatocellular swelling and disarray, hepatocanalicular cholestasis, and ductular reaction, typically with very little inflammation. This hepatitis B variant usually occurs early posttransplantation (within the first few months) and often leads to progressive fibrosis and organ failure if not successfully treated. There is usually widespread nuclear expression of HBc and variable HBs antigens by immunohistochemistry in these cases. Some cases of fibrosing cholestatic hepatitis also show prominent steatosis (including small-droplet steatosis) and have been

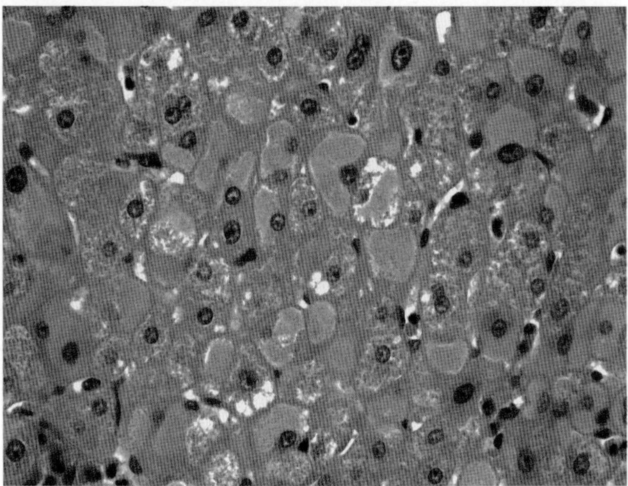

Figure 20.35 Recurrent hepatitis B. Numerous ground glass inclusions within hepatocytes are shown.

referred to as *steatoviral hepatitis.*[141] In the current era of highly effective antiviral treatment for hepatitis B, reinfection is unusual in most centers and fibrosing cholestatic hepatitis is now vanishingly rare.

Special stains and immunostains

HBs and HBc immunostains are extremely useful tools for confirming hepatitis B infection in allografts. It must be kept in mind, however, that both HBs and HBc are often absent in early phases of reinfection. Hepatocytes can also develop ground glass inclusions as a result of a drug effect, so all cases with ground glass–type inclusions should be stained for HBs by immunohistochemistry. Special stains such as Victoria blue and orcein also highlight ground glass inclusions but are not as specific as immunohistochemistry.

Differential diagnosis

The acute phase of reinfection is rather nonspecific histologically and can mimic various processes, including drug toxicity, other forms of viral hepatitis (hepatitis C), as well as nonhepatotropic viruses (CMVs, adenovirus, EBV, etc.). As the infection enters its chronic phase, ground glass hepatocytes represent the most specific finding. Ground glass hepatocytes can be seen late in infection (usually after several years) in a subset of cases. However, similar changes are seen in various conditions and can be virtually indistinguishable from hepatitis B–related ground glass cells on routine stains. In the posttransplant setting, polypharmacotherapy has been implicated in abnormal glycogen intracytoplasmic material causing striking pseudo ground glass change (Fig. 20.36).[142–144]

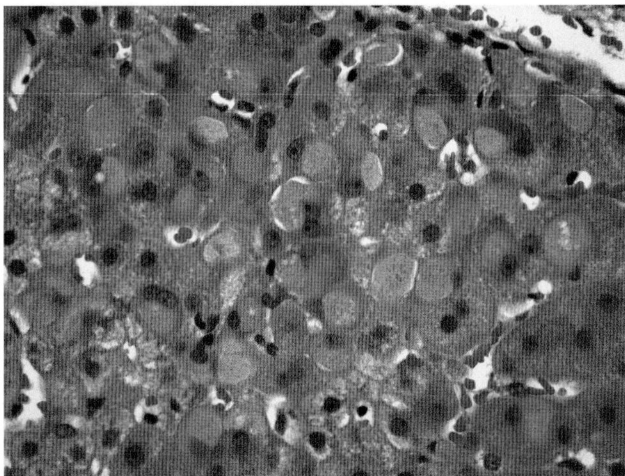

Figure 20.36 Pseudoground glass cells. Numerous cytoplasmic glassy inclusions are shown in this case of presumed medication-related injury (polypharmacotherapy), mimicking the appearance of hepatitis B–related ground glass inclusions.

Prognosis and treatment

The goal of hepatitis B treatment in end-stage liver disease is to achieve sustained virological suppression. New oral nucleosides and nucleotide analogues (tenofovir and entecavir) are currently the most effective inhibitors of hepatitis B replication and have the lowest rates of drug resistance. Other drugs used for prophylaxis or treatment of hepatitis B include lamivudine, adefovir and telbivudine. The use of combined prophylaxis with oral antiviral agents and intramuscular or intravenous hepatitis B immune globulin (HBIg) is recommended for all patients transplanted for hepatitis B. With this approach, the HBV recurrence rate has declined to 0% to 10% at 1 to 2 years after transplantation.[145,146] Treatment for recurrent disease depends on prior regimens used and it should include drugs with lower resistance rates, such as entecavir or tenofovir.

Hepatitis C

Clinical findings

Hepatitis C recurrence is essentially universal in patients with detectable hepatitis C virus RNA at the time of liver transplantation. Biochemical evidence of recurrent hepatitis (abnormal liver enzymes) is usually present 4 to 12 weeks postoperatively in most patients, who usually remain asymptomatic and typically evolve to a chronic hepatitis. Fibrosing cholestatic hepatitis, an uncommon and severe form of recurrent hepatitis C, usually presents later with a cholestatic pattern of enzyme elevation. Fibrosing cholestatic hepatitis is often associated with high-level immunosuppression, often in the setting of rejection treatment.[147]

Etiology and pathogenesis

Allograft infection by circulating viruses in hepatitis C–positive patients is thought to occur immediately after revascularization of the implanted liver.[36,148,149] A brief period of relatively low levels of viremia occurs during the "anhepatic" phase and immediately after implantation—during which hepatitis C infects allograft hepatocytes. Hepatitis C virus RNA levels then rapidly increase back to pretransplantation levels within approximately 72 hours[150] and shortly thereafter reach a steady state viral load that is typically 10 to 20 times higher than in the pretransplantation period.[151–153] This "acute hepatitis" phase essentially always progresses to a chronic hepatitis and, unlike native livers, spontaneous viral clearance has not been documented in the posttransplantation setting.[154]

Recurrent hepatitis C typically shows significantly faster disease progression than hepatitis C infection of native livers, with 10% to 30% of patients developing cirrhosis after 5 years and over 40% having cirrhosis after 10 years.[154–159] Fibrosis progression of 0.3 to 0.6 stages/year (using a 4-tiered system) is reported in the posttransplantation setting, compared with 0.1 to 0.2 stages/year in the nontransplant setting,[160–165] corresponding to an average time from transplantation to cirrhosis of approximately 9.5 years, compared with an average of 30 years from infection to cirrhosis in native livers.[154] Although numerous host and graft factors are involved, posttransplant immunosuppression largely accounts for the profound differences between hepatitis C infection in native liver compared to recurrent disease in the allograft. Heavy immunosuppression, primarily needed to treat rejection, can also lead to a particularly aggressive form of recurrent hepatitis C—fibrosing cholestatic hepatitis—which is associated with markedly faster fibrosis progression, frequently resulting in allograft failure. In these cases, the typical TH-1 immune response (mainly interleukin-2, interferon-γ, and tumor necrosis factor-α) to hepatitis C in both native livers and allografts is replaced by a TH-2 response (mainly interleukin-4 and interleukin-10) in fibrosing cholestatic hepatitis. The heavy immunosuppression in these patients leads to uncontrolled viral proliferation and extremely high intrahepatic viral loads.[166,167]

Histologic findings

The first histopathological manifestations in recurrent hepatitis C occur as early as the second week posttransplantation, but more typically appear between 1 and 3 months.[150,168] Initially, there are scattered acidophil bodies, mild lobular disarray, mild lobular inflammation, and Kupffer cell hyperplasia (Fig. 20.37). Portal tract abnormalities during this phase are absent or minimal, and there is no cholestasis. Prominent lobular inflammation with confluent or bridging necrosis, or predominantly centrilobular injury are not typical of recurrent hepatitis C infection and should raise suspicion for alternative diagnoses, including rejection, drug toxicity and, and in the late posttransplantation period, alloimmune hepatitis.

Within a few months (typically 3 to 6), more pronounced portal tract chronic inflammation develops, often with loose lymphoid aggregates, and variable—usually mild interface activity[154] (Fig. 20.38). The main differences between typical cases of recurrent hepatitis C in allografts and hepatitis C infection in native livers[52] are shown in Table 20.6.

The portal lymphoid aggregates in recurrent hepatitis C are formed predominantly of CD20+ B-lymphocytes, with a surrounding population of CD4+ T-helper cells, CD8+ cytotoxic T-cells, and scattered CD25+ regulatory T-cells. Prominent germinal centers are occasionally

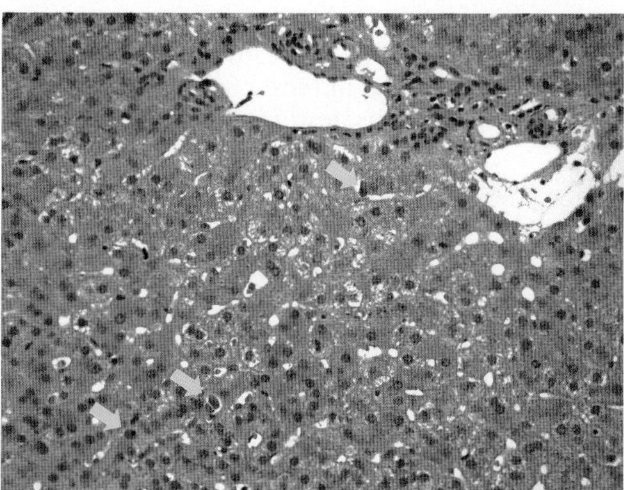

Figure 20.37 Recurrent hepatitis C. Early disease showing a mild acute hepatitis pattern with scattered acidophilic bodies (*arrows*).

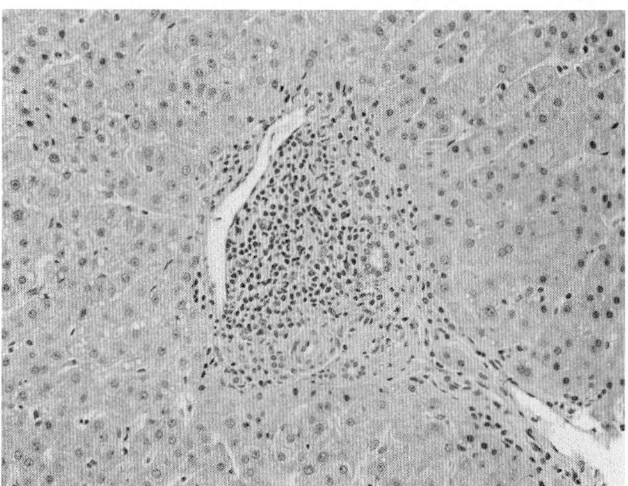

Figure 20.38 Recurrent hepatitis C. Established disease several months posttransplantation, with a mildly active chronic hepatitis pattern.

seen in recurrent hepatitis C but they are less common than in native livers. The lymphocytes within areas of interface hepatitis are predominantly CD4+ helper T-cells, whereas lymphocytes in the hepatic lobules are CD8+ suppressor/cytotoxic T-cells. A network of CD21+/CD35+ follicular dendritic cells is also present in lymphoid aggregates.[169] Scattered polytypic plasma cells are also commonly present in recurrent hepatitis C but should represent a small minority of cells within the inflammatory infiltrate and clusters of plasma cells should be absent. Eosinophils, likewise, are present in most cases in small numbers. Portal macrophages and sinusoidal Kupffer cells are both typically present in various amounts, reflecting the grade of inflammation and local injury.

Table 20.6 Histologic Features of Hepatitic C Infection in Native Livers versus Allografts

	Native livers	Allografts
Portal inflammation	Predominantly mature lymphocytes; lymphoid aggregates common, may have germinal centers	Lymphoid aggregates less prominent; germinal centers uncommon.
Ductular reaction	Uncommon, mild when present	May be more prominent when cholestatic
Lobular activity	Generally mild; severe inflammation distinctly uncommon	Generally mild, but moderate to severe inflammation may occur
Fibrosis progression	Average of 0.1–0.2 stages/year (four-tiered system) and 30 years from infection to cirrhosis	Average of 0.3–0.6 stages/year (four-tiered system) and 9.5 years from reinfection to cirrhosis

Adapted from Moreira RK. Recurrent hepatitis C and acute allograft rejection: clinicopathologic features with emphasis on the differential diagnosis between these entities. *Adv Anat Pathol*. 2011;18(5): 393–405. doi:10.1097/PAP.0b013e31822a5a10.

The lobular inflammation in recurrent hepatitis C is most commonly in the mild range but higher degrees of lobular activity than those typically seen in native livers can occur in the posttransplant setting.[155,170,171] A relatively mild degree of macrovesicular steatosis can also be seen with recurrent hepatitis C. Steatosis tends to be more common and prominent in hepatitis C genotype 3 infection, which is thought to cause steatosis through direct viral effect on hepatocyte lipid metabolism.[172] Additional unusual features that have been attributed to recurrent hepatitis C in the posttransplant setting include granulomatous inflammation,[173] but other causes need to be carefully excluded.

Bile duct injury can occur in hepatitis C[174] but is usually mild, nondestructive, present in a minority of portal tracts, and seen principally with moderate or greater portal lymphocyotic inflammation (Fig. 20.39). Similarly, scattered eosinophils are common in chronic hepatitis C (approximately 30% to 40% of cases)[68,175] and do not distinguish between rejection and recurrent hepatitis C. Finally, focal mild endothelialitis is well documented in a significant proportion of hepatitis C-infected livers.[68,176] Like bile duct injury, endothelialitis tends to be more common in cases showing higher inflammatory activity.

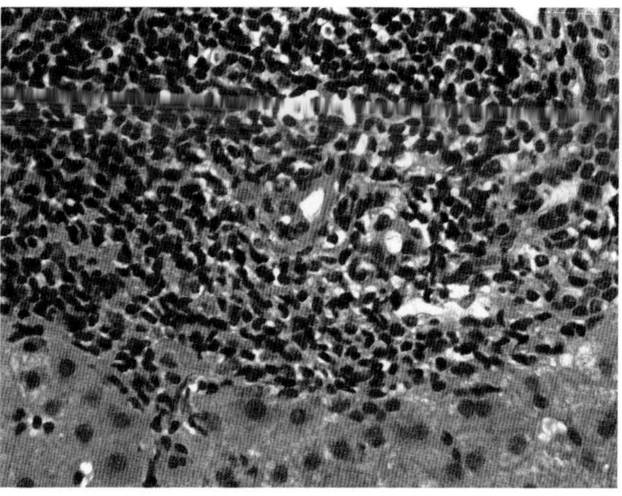

Figure 20.39 Recurrent hepatitis C. Bile duct injury within a densely inflamed portal tract.

Fibrosing cholestatic hepatitis

First described as a severe cholestatic disease affecting immunosuppressed patients with hepatitis B, fibrosing cholestatic hepatitis is now well described in the context of hepatitis C when there is heavy immunosuppression from several causes.[177–179] In recent years, most cases of fibrosing cholestatic hepatitis are associated with hepatitis C, because of the large number of hepatitis C–infected patients undergoing liver transplantation. Histologically, fibrosing cholestatic hepatitis C is characterized by the presence of many features that are typical of recurrent hepatitis C, including a similar degree of necroinflammation (as opposed to hepatitis B–related fibrosing cholestatic hepatitis that tends to be pauci-inflammatory). In addition, however, several features that are not part of the spectrum of typical recurrent hepatitis C are characteristic of fibrosing cholestatic hepatitis C (Figs. 20.40 and 20.41). Hepatocanalicular cholestasis, described as the earliest feature of fibrosing cholestatic hepatitis,[180] is present in most cases and is often pronounced. This is usually associated with a marked ductular reaction (mimicking a severe biliary obstructive process), marked hepatocyte swelling with lobular disarray (which can be centrilobular but is often diffuse), and periportal sinusoidal fibrosis. Biliary tract disease should be excluded in all cases before making a diagnosis of fibrosing cholestatic hepatitis. In most, cases there is also a history of heavy immunosuppression and viral loads are typically significantly above their posttransplant baseline.

Rather than representing a separate entity, fibrosing cholestatic hepatitis C represents the most severe end of the histologic spectrum of recurrent hepatitis C. In a recent study, the four fibrosing cholestatic hepatitis C–related findings mentioned above (cholestasis,

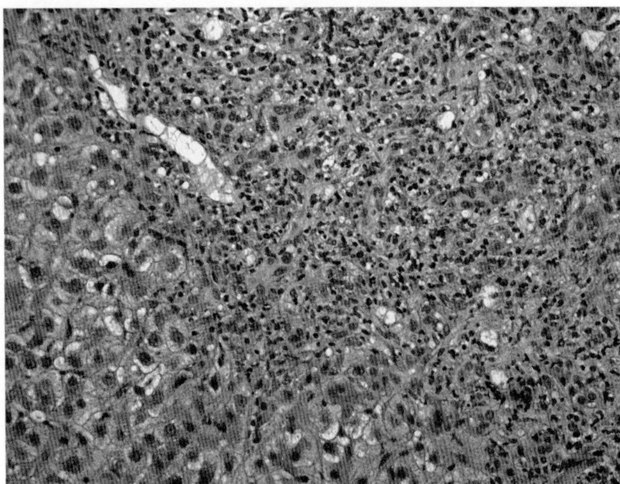

Figure 20.40 Recurrent hepatitis C, fibrosing cholestatic variant. Prominent ductular reaction and significant hepatocyte swelling are characteristic. Cholestasis was also present (not shown).

Table 20.7 Histologic Features Associated with Fibrosing Cholestatic Hepatitis (FCH) and the Hepatitis Aggressiveness Score (HAS)

Histologic features
1 Prominent ductular reaction, at least focally expanding portal tracts, mimicking biliary obstruction. 2 Prominent hepatocyte swelling, present in the majority of the sample, with lobular disarray. 3 Cholestasis of any degree. 4 Periportal sinusoidal fibrosis.
Final scoring
1 0 of 4 features: HAS 1 (nonaggressive hepatitis C). 2 1–2 of 4 features: HAS 2 (aggressive hepatitis C). 3 3–4 of 4 features: HAS 3 (fibrosing cholestatic hepatitis C).

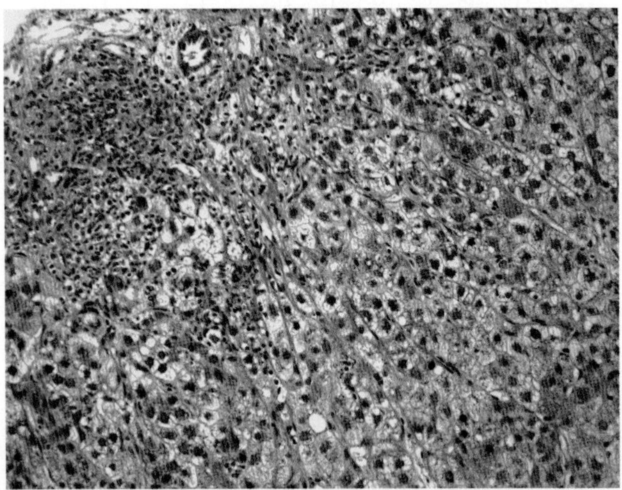

Figure 20.41 Recurrent hepatitis C, fibrosing cholestatic variant. Marked sinusoidal fibrosis.

marked ductular reaction, marked hepatocyte swelling, and sinusoidal fibrosis) were analyzed in the postliver transplant setting and the number of fibrosing cholestatic hepatitis–related features was highly predictive of overall patient survival, graft survival, and fibrosis progression. In fact, patients formed three groups: (1) typical hepatitis (none of the findings present), (2) aggressive hepatitis (1 to 2 features), and (3) fibrosing cholestatic hepatitis (3 to 4 features), with clearly distinct prognosis (Table 20.7).[181]

Therefore, the features of recurrent hepatitis C are generally similar to those seen in native livers, with a few particularities: (1) the "acute hepatitis" phase is rarely seen/biopsied in native livers but commonly seen on histologic samples in the early posttransplant setting; (2) transplant patients are at risk for fibrosing cholestatic hepatitis; (3) fibrosis progression is significantly faster (see additional details in Table 20.7).

Differential diagnosis

The histologic features of early recurrent hepatitis C are rather nonspecific (mild lobular inflammation and acidophilic bodies) and often raise additional diagnostic considerations, including drug-related injury and graft ischemia. This differential requires clinical correlation. Histologically, changes of recurrent hepatitis C are usually absent in the first 3 weeks to a month. Therefore, biopsy findings seen early after transplantation—particularly in the initial 2 weeks—are typically not hepatitis C–related. In later biopsies, especially those a year or more after transplantation, the histological findings are that of typical chronic hepatitis C. Although there are some share histological features with acute cellular rejection (bile duct injury, endothelialitis), these findings are focal and rare in recurrent hepatitis C and the distinction can usually be made without much trouble. However, some cases may pose significant diagnostic challenges. In practice, two facts must be kept in mind in this scenario: (1) hepatitis C–related changes are virtually always present after several weeks to a few months posttransplantation and the question is whether superimposed rejection is present and is of sufficient magnitude to warrant increased immunosuppression; (2) with established hepatitis C virus reinfection, acute cellular rejection–related features should be clearly evident and a diagnosis should not be based on equivocal findings of focal minimal duct injury or endothelialitis. This approach minimizes the

Table 20.8 Useful Histologic Features in the Differential Diagnosis between Recurrent Hepatitis C Virus and Acute Cellular Rejection

	Recurrent hepatitis C	Acute cellular rejection
Posttransplant period	2–3 months or later	Usually within initial 1–2 months, unless subtherapeutic levels of immunosuppression
Portal inflammation	Mature lymphocytes; few eosinophils typically present; lymphoid aggregates sometimes seen (germinal centers rare)	Inflammation often mixed, containing "activated" lymphocytes and eosinophils; lymphoid aggregates uncommon
Bile duct injury	Usually none; mild and in a minority of portal tracts when present	Variable, but often prominent in early ACR; should be more than focal and minimal in the setting of HCV infection
Endothelialitis	Usually none; mild and present in a minority of portal tracts and/or central veins when present	Variable, but often prominent in early ACR; should be more than focal and minimal in the setting of HCV infection
Ductular reaction	Commonly present; may be prominent	Uncommon
Interface activity	Common	Usually not a prominent feature in early ACR; may be more evident in late ACR
Lobular activity	Common, typically without zonal predilection	None or minimal, except in severe cases; when present, tends to involve centrilobular regions
Central perivenulitis	Uncommon	Present in moderate to severe early ACR and in late ACR; also present in plasma cell hepatitis
Histologic variants	Fibrosing cholestatic hepatitis	Isolated central perivenulitis Posttransplantation plasma cell hepatitis Idiopathic posttransplantation chronic hepatitis

Adapted from Moreira RK. Recurrent hepatitis C and acute allograft rejection: clinicopathologic features with emphasis on the differential diagnosis between these entities. *Adv Anat Pathol*. 2011;18(5):393–405. doi:10.1097/PAP.0b013e31822a5a10.

deleterious effect of increased immunosuppression in the recurrent hepatitis C population.[52,182] A summary of useful histologic features in the differential diagnosis between recurrent hepatitis C and acute cellular rejection[52] is provided in Table 20.8.

Plasma cell–rich hepatitis (also referred to as *posttransplantation plasma cell hepatitis*), can occasionally be seen in allograft liver biopsies of patients who also have recurrent hepatitis C. Overall, evidence suggests that this pattern is not hepatitis C–related, but instead is a rejection/alloimmune process. Plasma cell–rich hepatitis is associated with an increased frequency of antinuclear antibodies and other autoantibodies, a tendency to occur in patients with subtherapeutic levels of immunosuppressive medications, and a trend toward a favorable response to increased immunosuppression.

Finally, fibrosing cholestatic hepatitis can cause diagnostic challenges with bile duct obstruction. Several obstructive features, however, including portal edema, acute cholangitis, bile infarcts, periductal fibrosis, periportal copper deposition (on copper stains), and abnormal CK7 expression in periportal hepatocytes (by immunohistochemistry) are significantly more common in biliary obstruction, whereas hepatocyte injury, lobular disarray, and sinusoidal fibrosis favor fibrosing cholestatic hepatits.[93] Also, biliary obstruction should be clinically excluded before making a diagnosis of fibrosing cholestatic hepatitis.

Prognosis and treatment

Antiviral therapy remains the only therapeutic intervention capable of halting allograft fibrosis after liver transplant for hepatitis C. Management of liver transplant recipients with hepatitis C is rapidly evolving in the era of direct-acting antiviral agents.[183] Up until 2011, the standard treatment for hepatitis C recurrence involved 48 weeks of PEG-interferon and ribavirin. This regimen resulted in only a 30% sustained virological response rate[184] and was associated with significant side effects, including an increased risk of bacterial infections, cytopenias, and allograft rejection. In contrast, recent studies with direct-acting antiviral regimens have demonstrated greater than 90% sustained viral response rates with fewer side effects.[184,185] These regimens include a combination of a nucleotide analog inhibitor of NS5B polymerase (sofosbuvir) and a NS5A replication complex inhibitor (ledispavir or daclastavir) with or without ribavirin for 12 to 24 weeks. In the interferon era, treatment for hepatitis C recurrence was deferred until allograft fibrosis was detected (typically bridging fibrosis or higher). This strategy is being reevaluated, because earlier treatment with newer antiviral regimens seems to be safe and effective in the posttransplant setting, although the high costs of treatment remain a consideration.

Primary biliary cirrhosis

Primary biliary cirrhosis recurs in approximately one-third of cases after liver transplantation (reported numbers varying from 10% to 50%),[186–188] typically in the late posttransplant period (average of 3 to 5 years posttransplant).[189] The diagnosis of recurrent primary biliary cirrhosis can be challenging. As opposed to primary biliary cirrhosis in native livers, antimitochondrial antibody is not a reliable marker of disease recurrence, because antibody levels often remains elevated after transplantation.[190] Therefore, the diagnosis of recurrent primary biliary cirrhosis relies heavily on histologic findings. The histologic features of recurrent primary biliary cirrhosis are identical to those seen in native livers (see Chapter 13), with chronic inflammation that is essentially restricted to the portal tracts and is associated with lymphocytic cholangitis, bile duct epithelial injury, and, in typical cases, with granulomatous inflammation attacking bile ducts (i.e., florid bile duct lesion). Acute cellular rejection represents the main differential diagnosis in cases presenting with lymphocytic cholangitis alone. Primary biliary cirrhosis is favored in the presence of cholate stasis, ductular reaction, and periportal copper deposition. The diagnosis is usually straightforward when typical florid bile duct lesions are present. Granulomatous drug reactions occasionally cause florid bile duct lesion-like changes, but the background chronic inflammation and the chronic cholestatic changes seen in primary biliary cirrhosis are usually absent. Ursodeoxycholic acid is the standard treatment for recurrent primary biliary cirrhosis. Although ursodeoxycholic acid can lead to biochemical improvement, its use has not been shown to affect patient or graft survival.[191] Fortunately, the impact of primary biliary cirrhosis recurrence on long-term survival is only modest.

Primary sclerosing cholangitis

Primary sclerosing cholangitis, similarly to primary biliary cirrhosis, recurs in approximately one-third of patients, most commonly several years posttransplantation (median time to recurrence of approximately 3 to 5 years, but as early as 1 year),[192,193] and its pathologic features are essentially the same as in native livers (see Chapter 13). The diagnosis of recurrent primary sclerosing cholangitis relies not only on cholangiography and histology, but also on the exclusion of alternative etiologies.

The main differential diagnosis of recurrent primary sclerosing cholangitis, from a histologic perspective, is with biliary obstruction due to other etiologies. Typical periductal (onion skinning) fibrosis and fibro-obliterative lesions are only occasionally seen in biopsy samples and, even when present, are not diagnostic of primary sclerosing cholangitis, because some cases of chronic biliary obstruction of any etiology can also show similar changes. Therefore, the differential diagnosis between recurrent primary sclerosing cholangitis and other forms of biliary obstruction ultimately relies on histological, clinical, and imaging findings. Chronic rejection and recurrent primary sclerosing cholangitis (with small duct involvement and ductopenia) may also be difficult to distinguish based on histology alone. Chronic rejection, contrary to primary sclerosing cholangitis, typically lacks significant ductular reactions or portal-based fibrosis and often shows centrilobular hepatocyte cholestasis and swelling.

Although multiple risk factors for primary sclerosing cholangitis recurrence have been proposed, consistency among studies is lacking.[192,194] Active ulcerative colitis at the time of transplant seems to increase the risk for recurrence and total colectomy before or at the time of transplant may confer protection against primary sclerosing cholangitis recurrence.[193] Recurrent primary sclerosing cholangitis significantly reduces long-term graft and patient survival posttransplant.[195] Unfortunately, treatment options for recurrent disease are limited. Ursodeoxycholic acid can lead to biochemical improvement but its impact on survival has yet to be demonstrated.

Alloimmune/de novo autoimmune hepatitis

Similarly to both primary biliary cirrhosis and primary sclerosing cholangitis, autoimmune hepatitis recurs in up to a third of cases, usually several years (3 to 5 years on average) posttransplantation. The histologic features of alloimmune hepatitis, likewise, are comparable to those seen in the native liver, consisting of variable degrees of chronic portal inflammation, interface activity, and lobular inflammation. Untreated disease can show moderate to severe activity and high numbers of plasma cells. The degree of lobular injury, as in native livers, varies considerably, from mild to severe with confluent necrosis. Cases in the moderate to severe end of the spectrum can have associated cholestasis. Hepatocyte rosettes are also present, reflecting hepatocyte regeneration and/or cholestasis. Although a chronic hepatitis with increased plasma cells is highly suggestive of an alloimmune process, the final diagnosis requires exclusion of viral hepatitis, drug reaction, as well as correlation with autoantibodies and IgG levels, using similar parameters to those used in native livers.

Fatty liver disease and steatohepatitis

The reported frequency of recurrent alcoholic liver disease varies significantly, largely owing to the lack of standardization for the definition of recidivism. Likewise, the rate of recurrence in nonalcoholic fatty liver disease is difficult to estimate, because a large proportion of cases of "cryptogenic cirrhosis" are thought to be related to nonalcoholic fatty liver disease. Moreover, nonalcoholic fatty liver disease often coexists with other etiologies, such as viral hepatitis, but may not be identified before transplantation. In patients with known nonalcoholic fatty liver disease, the frequency of recurrent disease increases with the length of follow-up, with reported rates ranging from 30% to 100%.[196] Progression to steatohepatitis and advanced allograft fibrosis is less common, with reported rate of 10% at 10 years posttransplant. Although the overall survival is similar to that of patients undergoing transplantation for other indications, nonalcoholic fatty liver disease patients are at higher risk for cardiovascular-related death.[197] The histologic criteria for the diagnosis of steatosis and steatohepatitis are the same as in native livers.

20.17 MISCELLANEOUS FINDINGS IN LIVER TRANSPLANTATION

Several miscellaneous histologic changes are occasionally seen in liver allografts, including mild nonspecific portal and lobular inflammation, wall thickening and hyalinization of hepatic artery branches, portal venopathy, nodular regenerative hyperplasia, and sinusoidal fibrosis.[163,198–201] Although the usual differential diagnosis applies to these findings, their etiology commonly remains uncertain in spite of careful clinical correlation. Pseudoground glass inclusions in hepatocytes is also a finding that is more commonly seen in transplanted or otherwise immunosuppressed individuals, closely mimicking the appearance of hepatitis B–related ground glass cells (Fig. 20.37). Pseudoground glass change has been found to be because of abnormal glycogen accumulation within the cytoplasm of hepatocytes and typically occurs in the setting of multimedication therapy (no specific agent has been implicated to date).[142,143]

20.18 IMMUNOSUPPRESSIVE DRUGS

Posttransplant immunosuppression is required to prevent allograft rejection. Modern immunosuppressive regimens are based on the initial use of a combination of agents, followed by reduction in dosing and number of drugs.

Calcineurin inhibitors

Calcineurin is a calcium-dependent phosphatase important in T-cell activation and proliferation. The development of the first calcineurin inhibitor, cyclosporine, led to significant improvements in long-term allograft and patient survival. Tacrolimus was subsequently developed and became the calcineurin inhibitor of choice in 90% of liver transplant recipients.[202]

Antimetabolites

These agents act by blocking the synthesis of purine nucleotides, essential for DNA synthesis, thereby disrupting cellular division. Mycophenolate mofetil specifically blocks lymphocyte replication, affecting both cellular immunity and antibody production.[203] Mycophenolate mofetil is part of the standard maintenance immunosuppression, being used in over 75% of liver transplant recipients. Azathioprine, a prodrug of 6-mercaptopurine, is one of the oldest immunosuppressants used in transplant, but has largely been replaced by mycophenolate mofetil.[204]

Corticosteroid

Corticosteroids have numerous effects on the immune system. They produce a rapid decline in circulating T and B cells, while also impairing the function of various phagocytic cells. Corticosteroids are typically started as high-dose intravenous methylprednisolone posttransplant, followed by a prednisolone taper. They are also used in the setting of rejection.

Mammalian target of rapamycin inhibitors

Inhibition of the mammalian target of rapamycin (mTOR) pathway prevents cell cycle transition from G1 to S phase, thereby limiting proliferation and activation of lymphocytes. The mTOR inhibitors sirolimus and everolimus are commonly used posttransplant as calcineurin inhibitor-sparing agents, in patients experiencing renal dysfunction or neurotoxicity. Moreover, in contrast to calcineurin inhibitor, mTOR inhibitors have antineoplastic activity and may be preferred for patients transplanted for hepatocellular carcinoma.[205]

REFERENCES

1. Kamath P, Wiesner RH, Malinchoc M, et al. A model to predict survival in patients with end-stage liver disease. *Hepatology*. 2001;33(2):464–470. doi:10.1053/jhep.2001.22172.
2. Alkofer B, Samstein B, Guarrera JV, et al. Extended-donor criteria liver allografts. 2006;1(212):221–233. doi:10.1055/s-2006-947292.
3. Spitzer AL, Lao OB, Dick AAS, et al. The biopsied donor liver: incorporating macrosteatosis into high-risk donor assessment. *Liver Transplant*. 2010;16(7):874–884. doi:10.1002/lt.22085.
4. McCormack L, Petrowsky H, Jochum W, et al. Use of severely steatotic grafts in liver transplantation: a matched case-control study. *Ann Surg*. 2007;246(6):940-6-8. doi:10.1097/SLA.0b013e31815c2a3f.
5. Imber CJ, Peter SDS, Handa A, et al. Hepatic steatosis and its relationship to transplantation. *Liver Transplant*. 2002;8(5):415–423. doi:10.1053/jlts.2002.32275.
6. McCormack L, Dutkowski P, El-Badry AM, et al. Liver transplantation using fatty livers: Always feasible? *J Hepatol*. 2011;54(5):1055–1062. doi:10.1016/j.jhep.2010.11.004.
7. Todo S, Demetris AJ, Makowka L, et al. Primary nonfunction of hepatic allografts with preexisting fatty infiltration. *Transplantation*. 1989;47(5):903–905. http://www.pubmedcentral.nih.gov/articlerender.fcgi?artid=2967252&tool=pmcentrez&rendertype=abstract. Accessed May 30, 2016.
8. Ploeg RJ, D'Alessandro AM, Knechtle SJ, et al. Risk factors for primary dysfunction after liver transplantation--a multivariate analysis. *Transplantation*. 1993;55(4):807–813. http://www.ncbi.nlm.nih.gov/pubmed/8475556. Accessed May 30, 2016.
9. Canelo R, Braun F, Sattler B, et al. Is a fatty liver dangerous for transplantation? *Transplant Proc*. 31(1–2):414–415. http://www.ncbi.nlm.nih.gov/pubmed/10083167. Accessed May 30, 2016.
10. Marsman H, Matsushita T, Dierkhising R, et al. Assessment of donor liver steatosis: pathologist or automated software? *Hum Pathol*. 2004;35(4):430–435. http://www.ncbi.nlm.nih.gov/pubmed/15116323. Accessed May 30, 2016.
11. Takada Y, Taniguchi H, Fukunaga K, et al. Prolonged hepatic warm ischemia in non-heart-beating donors: protective effects of FK506 and a platelet activating factor antagonist in porcine liver transplantation. *Surgery*. 1998;123(6):692–698. http://www.ncbi.nlm.nih.gov/pubmed/9626320. Accessed May 30, 2016.
12. Kootstra G, Kievit J, Nederstigt A. Organ donors: heartbeating and non-heartbeating. *World J Surg*. 2002;26(2):181–184. doi:10.1007/s00268-001-0205-2.
13. Teoh NC, Farrell GC. Hepatic ischemia reperfusion injury: pathogenic mechanisms and basis for hepatoprotection. *J Gastroenterol Hepatol*. 2003;18(8):891–902. http://www.ncbi.nlm.nih.gov/pubmed/12859717. Accessed May 5, 2016.
14. Kakizoe S, Yanaga K, Starzl TE, et al. Evaluation of protocol before transplantation and after reperfusion biopsies from human orthotopic liver allografts: considerations of preservation and early immunological injury. *Hepatology*. 1990;11(6):932–941. http://www.pubmedcentral.nih.gov/articlerender.fcgi?artid=3022473&tool=pmcentrez&rendertype=abstract. Accessed May 30, 2016.
15. Busuttil RW, Tanaka K. The utility of marginal donors in liver transplantation. *Liver Transpl*. 2003;9(7):651–663. doi:10.1053/jlts.2003.50105.
16. Feng S, Goodrich NP, Bragg-Gresham JL, et al. Characteristics associated with liver graft failure: the concept of a donor risk index. *Am J Transplant*. 2006;6(4):783--790. doi:10.1111/j.1600-6143.2006.01242.x.
17. Bilzer M, Gerbes AL. Preservation injury of the liver: mechanisms and novel therapeutic strategies. *J Hepatol*. 2000;32(3):508–515. http://www.ncbi.nlm.nih.gov/pubmed/10735623. Accessed May 30, 2016.
18. Demetris AJ, Kelly DM, Eghtesad B, et al. Pathophysiologic observations and histopathologic recognition of the portal hyperperfusion or small-for-size syndrome. *Am J Surg Pathol*. 2006;30(8):986–993. http://www.ncbi.nlm.nih.gov/pubmed/16861970. Accessed May 30, 2016.
19. Musat AI, Agni RM, Wai PY, et al. The significance of donor-specific HLA antibodies in rejection and ductopenia development in ABO compatible liver transplantation. *Am J Transplant*. 2011;11(3):500–510. doi:10.1111/j.1600-6143.2010.03414.x.
20. Hübscher SG. Antibody-mediated rejection in the liver allograft. *Curr Opin Organ Transplant*. 2012;17(3):1. doi:10.1097/MOT.0b013e328353584c.
21. O'Leary JG, Shiller SM, Bellamy C, et al. Acute liver allograft antibody-mediated rejection: an inter-institutional study of significant histopathological features. *Liver Transplant*. 2014;20(10):1244–1255. doi:10.1002/lt.23948.
22. Lunz J, Ruppert KM, Cajaiba MM, et al. Re-examination of the lymphocytotoxic crossmatch in liver transplantation: can C4d stains help in monitoring? *Am J Transplant*. 2012;12(1):171–182. doi:10.1111/j.1600-6143.2011.03786.x.

23. Demetris AJ, Murase N, Nakamura K, et al. Immunopathology of antibodies as effectors of orthotopic liver allograft rejection. *Semin Liver Dis.* 1992;12(1):51–59. doi:10.1055/s-2007-1007376.
24. Kozlowski T, Rubinas T, Nickeleit V, et al. Liver allograft antibody-mediated rejection with demonstration of sinusoidal C4d staining and circulating donor-specific antibodies. *Liver Transpl.* 2011;17(4):357–368. doi:10.1002/lt.22233.
25. O'Leary JG, Shiller SM, Bellamy C, et al. Acute liver allograft antibody-mediated rejection: an inter-institutional study of significant histopathological features. *Liver Transplant.* 2014;20(10):1244–1255. doi:10.1002/lt.23948.
26. Takemoto SK, Zeevi A, Feng S, et al. National conference to assess antibody-mediated rejection in solid organ transplantation. *Am J Transplant.* 2004;4(7):1033–1041. doi:10.1111/j.1600-6143.2004.00500.x.
27. Colvin RB. Antibody-mediated renal allograft rejection: diagnosis and pathogenesis. *J Am Soc Nephrol.* 2007;18(4):1046–1056. doi:10.1681/ASN.2007010073.
28. Krukemeyer MG, Moeller J, Morawietz L, et al. Description of B lymphocytes and plasma cells, complement, and chemokines/receptors in acute liver allograft rejection. *Transplantation.* 2004;78(1):65–70. http://www.ncbi.nlm.nih.gov/pubmed/15257040. Accessed May 30, 2016.
29. Bellamy COC. Complement C4d immunohistochemistry in the assessment of liver allograft biopsy samples: applications and pitfalls. *Liver Transpl.* 2011;17(7):747–750. doi:10.1002/lt.22323.
30. Salah A, Fujimoto M, Yoshizawa A, et al. Application of complement component 4d immunohistochemistry to ABO-compatible and ABO-incompatible liver transplantation. *Liver Transpl.* 2014;20(2):200-209. doi:10.1002/lt.23789.
31. Haga H, Egawa H, Fujimoto Y, et al. Acute humoral rejection and C4d immunostaining in ABO blood type-incompatible liver transplantation. *Liver Transpl.* 2006;12(3):457–464. doi:10.1002/lt.20652.
32. Sakashita H, Haga H, Ashihara E, et al. Significance of C4d staining in ABO-identical/compatible liver transplantation. *Mod Pathol.* 2007;20(6):676–684. doi:10.1038/modpathol.3800784.
33. Ali S, Ormsby A, Shah V, et al. Significance of complement split product C4d in ABO-compatible liver allograft: diagnosing utility in acute antibody mediated rejection. *Transpl Immunol.* 2012;26(1):62–69. doi:10.1016/j.trim.2011.08.005.
34. Hanto DW, Fecteau AH, Alonso MH, et al. ABO-incompatible liver transplantation with no immunological graft losses using total plasma exchange, splenectomy, and quadruple immunosuppression: evidence for accommodation. *Liver Transpl.* 2003;9(1):22–30. doi:10.1053/jlts.2003.50011.
35. Paterno F, Shiller M, Tillery G, et al. Bortezomib for acute antibody-mediated rejection in liver transplantation. *Am J Transplant.* 2012;12(9):2526–2531. doi:10.1111/j.1600-6143.2012.04126.x.
36. Bartlett AS, Ramadas R, Furness S, et al. The natural history of acute histologic rejection without biochemical graft dysfunction in orthotopic liver transplantation: a systematic review. *Liver Transpl.* 2002;8(12):1147–1153. doi:10.1053/jlts.2002.36240.
37. Tippner C, Nashan B, Hoshino K, et al. Clinical and subclinical acute rejection early after liver transplantation: contributing factors and relevance for the long-term course. *Transplantation.* 2001;72(6):1122–1128. http://www.ncbi.nlm.nih.gov/pubmed/11579311. Accessed May 30, 2016.
38. Therapondos G, Hayes PC. Is this the end for protocol early posttransplant liver biopsies? *Liver Transpl.* 2002;8(12):1154–1155. doi:10.1053/jlts.2002.36731.
39. Górnicka B, Ziarkiewicz-Wróblewska B, Bogdan´ska M, et al. Pathomorphological features of acute rejection in patients after orthotopic liver transplantation: own experience. *Transplant Proc.* 2006;38(1):221–225. doi:10.1016/j.transproceed.2006.01.002.
40. Demetris AJ, Ruppert K, Dvorchik I, et al. Real-time monitoring of acute liver-allograft rejection using the Banff schema. *Transplantation.* 2002;74(9):1290–1296. doi:10.1097/01.TP.0000034517.01022.4E.
41. Neuberger J. Incidence, timing, and risk factors for acute and chronic rejection. *Liver Transpl Surg.* 1999;5(4 suppl 1):S30–S36. doi:10.1053/JTLS005s00030.
42. Berlakovich GA, Rockenschaub S, Taucher S, et al. Underlying disease as a predictor for rejection after liver transplantation. *Arch Surg.* 1998;133(2):167–172. http://www.ncbi.nlm.nih.gov/pubmed/9484729. Accessed May 30, 2016.
43. Seiler CA, Dufour JF, Renner EL, et al. Primary liver disease as a determinant for acute rejection after liver transplantation. *Langenbeck's Arch Surg/Dtsch Gesellschaft für Chir.* 1999;384(3):259–263. http://www.ncbi.nlm.nih.gov/pubmed/10437614. Accessed May 30, 2016.
44. Farges O, Saliba F, Farhamant H, et al. Incidence of rejection and infection after liver transplantation as a function of the primary disease: possible influence of alcohol and polyclonal immunoglobulins. *Hepatology.* 1996;23(2):240–248. doi:10.1053/jhep.1996.v23.pm0008591847.

45. Wiesner RH, Demetris AJ, Belle SH, et al. Acute hepatic allograft rejection: incidence, risk factors, and impact on outcome. *Hepatology*. 1998;28(3):638–645. doi:10.1002/hep.510280306.
46. Neuberger J, Adams DH. What is the significance of acute liver allograft rejection? *J Hepatol*. 1998;29(1):143–150. http://www.ncbi.nlm.nih.gov/pubmed/9696504. Accessed May 30, 2016.
47. Of D, Rejection A. Banff schema for grading liver allograft rejection: an international consensus document. *Hepatology*. 1997;25(3):658–663. doi:10.1002/hep.510250328.
48. Demetris A, Adams D, Bellamy C, et al. Update of the International Banff Schema for Liver Allograft Rejection: working recommendations for the histopathologic staging and reporting of chronic rejection. An International Panel. *Hepatology*. 2000;31(3):792–799. doi:10.1002/hep.510310337.
49. Demetris AJ, Qian SG, Sun H, et al. Liver allograft rejection: an overview of morphologic findings. *Am J Surg Pathol*. 1990;14 suppl 1:49–63. http://www.ncbi.nlm.nih.gov/pubmed/2183642. Accessed May 30, 2016.
50. Snover DC, Freese DK, Sharp HL, et al. Liver allograft rejection. An analysis of the use of biopsy in determining outcome of rejection. *Am J Surg Pathol*. 1987;11(1):1–10. http://www.ncbi.nlm.nih.gov/pubmed/3538917. Accessed May 30, 2016.
51. Demetris AJ, Belle SH, Hart J, et al. Intraobserver and interobserver variation in the histopathological assessment of liver allograft rejection. The Liver Transplantation Database (LTD) Investigators. *Hepatology*. 1991;14(5):751–755. http://www.ncbi.nlm.nih.gov/pubmed/1937381. Accessed May 30, 2016.
52. Moreira RK. Recurrent hepatitis C and acute allograft rejection: clinicopathologic features with emphasis on the differential diagnosis between these entities. *Adv Anat Pathol*. 2011;18(5):393–405. doi:10.1097/PAP.0b013e31822a5a10.
53. Castillo-Rama M, Sebagh M, Sasatomi E, et al. "Plasma cell hepatitis" in liver allografts: Identification and characterization of an IgG4-rich cohort. *Am J Transplant*. 2013;13(11):2966–2977. doi:10.1111/ajt.12413.
54. Khettry U, Huang W-Y, Simpson MA, et al. Patterns of recurrent hepatitis C after liver transplantation in a recent cohort of patients. *Hum Pathol*. 2007;38(3):443–452. doi:10.1016/j.humpath.2006.08.028.
55. Fiel MI, Agarwal K, Stanca C, et al. Posttransplant plasma cell hepatitis (de novo autoimmune hepatitis) is a variant of rejection and may lead to a negative outcome in patients with hepatitis C virus. *Liver Transpl*. 2008;14(6):861–871. doi:10.1002/lt.21447.
56. Krasinskas AM, Demetris AJ, Poterucha JJ, et al. The prevalence and natural history of untreated isolated central perivenulitis in adult allograft livers. *Liver Transpl*. 2008;14(5):625–632. doi:10.1002/lt.21404.
57. Neil DA, Hübscher SG. Current views on rejection pathology in liver transplantation. *Transpl Int*. 2010;23(10):971–983. doi:10.1111/j.1432-2277.2010.01143.x.
58. Gao Z. Seeking beyond rejection: an update on the differential diagnosis and a practical approach to liver allograft biopsy interpretation. *Adv Anat Pathol*. 2009;16(2):97–117. doi:10.1097/PAP.0b013e31819946aa.
59. Shaikh OS, Demetris AJ. Idiopathic posttransplantation hepatitis? *Liver Transpl*. 2007;13(7):943–946. doi:10.1002/lt.21202.
60. Syn W-K, Nightingale P, Gunson B, et al. Natural history of unexplained chronic hepatitis after liver transplantation. *Liver Transpl*. 2007;13(7):984–989. doi:10.1002/lt.21108.
61. Seyam M, Neuberger JM, Gunson BK, et al. Cirrhosis after orthotopic liver transplantation in the absence of primary disease recurrence. *Liver Transpl*. 2007;13(7):966–974. doi:10.1002/lt.21060.
62. Evans HM, Kelly DA, McKiernan PJ, et al. Progressive histological damage in liver allografts following pediatric liver transplantation. *Hepatology*. 2006;43(5):1109–1117. doi:10.1002/hep.21152.
63. Unzueta A, Rakela J. Hepatitis E infection in liver transplant Hepatitis E infection in liver transplant recipients . *Liver Transpl*. 2014;20(1):15–24. doi:10.1002/lt.23764.
64. Sue PK, Pisanic N, Heaney CD, et al. Hepatitis E virus infection among solid organ transplant recipients at a North American transplant center. *Open forum Infect Dis*. 2016;3(1):ofw006. doi:10.1093/ofid/ofw006.
65. Blakolmer K, Jain A, Ruppert K, et al. Chronic liver allograft rejection in a population treated primarily with tacrolimus as baseline immunosuppression: long-term follow-up and evaluation of features for histopathological staging. *Transplantation*. 2000;69(11):2330–2336. http://www.pubmedcentral.nih.gov/articlerender.fcgi?artid=2967190&tool=pmcentrez&rendertype=abstract. Accessed May 30, 2016.
66. Ormonde DG, de Boer WB, Kierath A, et al. Banff schema for grading liver allograft rejection: utility in clinical practice. *Liver Transpl Surg*. 1999;5(4):261–268. doi:10.1002/lt.500050418.
67. Demetris AJ, Adeyi O, Bellamy COC, et al. Liver biopsy interpretation for causes of late liver allograft dysfunction. *Hepatology*. 2006;44(2):489–501. doi:10.1002/hep.21280.
68. Souza P, Prihoda TJ, Hoyumpa AM, et al. Morphologic features resembling transplant rejection in core biopsies of native livers from patients with Hepatitis C. *Hum Pathol*. 2009;40(1):92–97. doi:10.1016/j.humpath.2008.06.020.

69. Matinlauri IH, Nurminen MM, Höckerstedt KA, et al. Changes in liver graft rejections over time. *Transplant Proc*. 2006;38(8):2663–2666. doi:10.1016/j.transproceed.2006.07.031.
70. Thurairajah PH, Carbone M, Bridgestock H, et al. Late acute liver allograft rejection; a study of its natural history and graft survival in the current era. *Transplantation*. 2013;95(7):955–959. doi:10.1097/TP.0b013e3182845f6c.
71. Pruthi J, Medkiff KA, Esrason KT, et al. Analysis of causes of death in liver transplant recipients who survived more than 3 years. *Liver Transpl*. 2001;7(9):811–815. doi:10.1053/jlts.2001.27084.
72. Kashyap R, Jain A, Reyes J, et al. Causes of retransplantation after primary liver transplantation in 4000 consecutive patients: 2 to 19 years follow-up. *Transplant Proc*. 33(1–2):1486–1487. http://www.pubmedcentral.nih.gov/articlerender.fcgi?artid=2987633&tool=pmcentrez&rendertype=abstract. Accessed May 30, 2016.
73. Alagille D, Odièvre M, Gautier M, et al. Hepatic ductular hypoplasia associated with characteristic facies, vertebral malformations, retarded physical, mental, and sexual development, and cardiac murmur. *J Pediatr*. 1975;86(1):63–71. http://www.ncbi.nlm.nih.gov/pubmed/803282. Accessed June 7, 2016.
74. Nakanuma Y, Ohta G. Histometric and serial section observations of the intrahepatic bile ducts in primary biliary cirrhosis. *Gastroenterology*. 1979;76(6):1326–1332. http://www.ncbi.nlm.nih.gov/pubmed/437429. Accessed June 7, 2016.
75. Moreira RK, Chopp W, Washington MK. The concept of hepatic artery-bile duct parallelism in the diagnosis of ductopenia in liver biopsy samples. *Am J Surg Pathol*. 2011;35(3):392–403. doi:10.1097/PAS.0b013e3182082ef6.
76. Crawford AR, Lin XZ, Crawford JM. The normal adult human liver biopsy: a quantitative reference standard. *Hepatology*. 1998;28(2):323–331. doi:10.1002/hep.510280206.
77. Deligeorgi-Politi H, White DGD, Calne RY. Chronic rejection of liver transplants revisited. *Transpl Int*. 1994;7(6):442–447. doi:10.1111/j.1432-2277.1994.tb01265.x.
78. Bhattacharjya S, Gunson BK, Mirza DF, et al. Delayed hepatic artery thrombosis in adult orthotopic liver transplantation-a 12-year experience. *Transplantation*. 2001;71(11):1592–1596. http://www.ncbi.nlm.nih.gov/pubmed/11435970. Accessed June 8, 2016.
79. Oh CK, Pelletier SJ, Sawyer RG, et al. Uni- and multi-variate analysis of risk factors for early and late hepatic artery thrombosis after liver transplantation. *Transplantation*. 2001;71(6):767–772. http://www.ncbi.nlm.nih.gov/pubmed/11330540. Accessed June 8, 2016.
80. Stange BJ, Glanemann M, Nuessler NC, et al. Hepatic artery thrombosis after adult liver transplantation. *Liver Transpl*. 2003;9(6):612–620. doi:10.1053/jlts.2003.50090.
81. Heaton ND. Hepatic artery thrombosis: conservative management or retransplantation? *Liver Transplant*. 2013;19(S2):S14–S16. doi:10.1002/lt.23739.
82. Liu T-C, Nguyen TT, Torbenson MS. Concurrent increase in mitosis and apoptosis: a histological pattern of hepatic arterial flow abnormalities in post-transplant liver biopsies. *Mod Pathol*. 2012;25(12):1594–1598. doi:10.1038/modpathol.2012.116.
83. Voigtländer T, Negm AA, Strassburg CP, et al. Biliary cast syndrome post-liver transplantation: risk factors and outcome. *Liver Int*. 2013;33(8):1287–1292. doi:10.1111/liv.12181.
84. Ponziani FR, Zocco MA, Campanale C, et al. Portal vein thrombosis: insight into physiopathology, diagnosis, and treatment. *World J Gastroenterol*. 2010;16(2):143–155. http://www.ncbi.nlm.nih.gov/pubmed/20066733. Accessed June 11, 2016.
85. Mion F, Cloix P, Boillot O, et al. Veno-occlusive disease after liver transplantation. Association of acute cellular rejection and toxicity of azathioprine. *Gastroentérol Clin Biol*. 1993;17(11):863–867. http://www.ncbi.nlm.nih.gov/pubmed/8143956. Accessed June 11, 2016.
86. Marín-Gómez LM, Álamo-Martínez JM, Suárez-Artacho G, et al. Is the sinusoidal obstructive syndrome post-liver transplantation a pathologic entity with a multifactorial etiology? *Rev española enfermedades Dig organo Of la Soc Española Patol Dig*. 2015;107(4):235–238. http://www.ncbi.nlm.nih.gov/pubmed/25824926. Accessed June 11, 2016.
87. Kakar S, Kamath PS, Burgart LJ. Sinusoidal dilatation and congestion in liver biopsy: is it always due to venous outflow impairment? *Arch Pathol Lab Med*. 2004;128(8):901–904. doi:10.1043/1543-2165(2004)1282.0.CO;2.
88. Kochhar G, Parungao JM, Hanouneh IA, et al. Biliary complications following liver transplantation. *World J Gastroenterol*. 2013;19(19):2841–2846. doi:10.3748/wjg.v19.i19.2841.
89. Sharma S, Gurakar A, Jabbour N. Biliary strictures following liver transplantation: past, present and preventive strategies. *Liver Transpl*. 2008;14(6):759–769. doi:10.1002/lt.21509.
90. Koneru B, Sterling MJ, Bahramipour PF. Bile duct strictures after liver transplantation: a changing landscape of the Achilles' heel. *Liver Transpl*. 2006;12(5):702–704. doi:10.1002/lt.20753.
91. Paik WH, Lee SH, Ryu JK, et al. Long-term clinical outcomes of biliary cast syndrome in liver transplant recipients. *Liver Transplant*. 2013;19(3):275–282. doi:10.1002/lt.23589.

92. Mounajjed T, Oxentenko AS, Qureshi H, et al. Revisiting the topic of histochemically detectable copper in various liver diseases with special focus on venous outflow impairment. *Am J Clin Pathol.* 2013;139(1):79–86. doi:10.1309/AJCPDZR4OHDQNG3L.
93. Salomao M, Verna EC, Lefkowitch JH, et al. Histopathologic distinction between fibrosing cholestatic hepatitis C and biliary obstruction. *Am J Surg Pathol.* 2013;37(12):1837–1844. doi:10.1097/PAS.0b013e31829b626c.
94. Toorkey CB, Carrigan DR. Immunohistochemical detection of an immediate early antigen of human cytomegalovirus in normal tissues. *J Infect Dis.* 1989;160(5):741–751. http://www.ncbi.nlm.nih.gov/pubmed/2553823. Accessed June 18, 2016.
95. Theise ND, Conn M, Thung SN. Localization of cytomegalovirus antigens in liver allografts over time. *Hum Pathol.* 1993;24(1):103–108. http://www.ncbi.nlm.nih.gov/pubmed/8380273. Accessed June 18, 2016.
96. Bronsther O, Makowka L, Jaffe R, et al. Occurrence of cytomegalovirus hepatitis in liver transplant patients. *J Med Virol.* 1988;24(4):423–434. http://www.ncbi.nlm.nih.gov/pubmed/2835433. Accessed June 18, 2016.
97. Snover DC, Hutton S, Balfour HH, et al. Cytomegalovirus infection of the liver in transplant recipients. *J Clin Gastroenterol.* 1987;9(6):659–665. http://www.ncbi.nlm.nih.gov/pubmed/2832467. Accessed June 18, 2016.
98. Wiesner RH, Marin E, Porayko MK, et al. Advances in the diagnosis, treatment, and prevention of cytomegalovirus infections after liver transplantation. *Gastroenterol Clin North Am.* 1993;22(2):351–366. http://www.ncbi.nlm.nih.gov/pubmed/8389735. Accessed June 18, 2016.
99. Colina F, Jucá NT, Moreno E, et al. Histological diagnosis of cytomegalovirus hepatitis in liver allografts. *J Clin Pathol.* 1995;48(4):351–357. http://www.ncbi.nlm.nih.gov/pubmed/7615856. Accessed June 19, 2016.
100. Espy MJ, Paya CV, Holley KE, et al. Diagnosis of cytomegalovirus hepatitis by histopathology and in situ hybridization in liver transplantation. *Diagn Microbiol Infect Dis.* 14(4):293–296. http://www.ncbi.nlm.nih.gov/pubmed/1716192. Accessed June 19, 2016.
101. Lamps LW, Pinson CW, Raiford DS, et al. The significance of microabscesses in liver transplant biopsies: a clinicopathological study. *Hepatology.* 1998;28(6):1532–1537. doi:10.1002/hep.510280613.
102. Vivarelli M, Cucchetti A, La Barba G, et al. Ischemic arterial complications after liver transplantation in the adult: multivariate analysis of risk factors. *Arch Surg.* 2004;139(10):1069–1074. doi:10.1001/archsurg.139.10.1069.
103. Gunsar F, Rolando N, Pastacaldi S, et al. Late hepatic artery thrombosis after orthotopic liver transplantation. *Liver Transpl.* 2003;9(6):605–611. doi:10.1053/jlts.2003.50057.
104. Pastacaldi S, Teixeira R, Montalto P, et al. Hepatic artery thrombosis after orthotopic liver transplantation: a review of nonsurgical causes. *Liver Transpl.* 2001;7(2):75–81. doi:10.1053/jlts.2001.22040.
105. Halme L, Hockerstedt K, Lautenschlager I. Cytomegalovirus infection and development of biliary complications after liver transplantation. *Transplantation.* 2003;75(11):1853–1858. doi:10.1097/01.TP.0000064620.08328.E5.
106. Lautenschlager I, Höckerstedt K, Jalanko H, et al. Persistent cytomegalovirus in liver allografts with chronic rejection. *Hepatology.* 1997;25(1):190–194. doi:10.1053/jhep.1997.v25.pm0008985289.
107. O'Grady JG, Alexander GJ, Sutherland S, et al. Cytomegalovirus infection and donor/recipient HLA antigens: interdependent co-factors in pathogenesis of vanishing bile-duct syndrome after liver transplantation. *Lancet (London, England).* 1988;2(8606):302–305. http://www.ncbi.nlm.nih.gov/pubmed/2899720. Accessed June 19, 2016.
108. Bosch W, Heckman MG, Pungpapong S, et al. Association of cytomegalovirus infection and disease with recurrent hepatitis C after liver transplantation. *Transplantation.* 2012;93(7):723–728. doi:10.1097/TP.0b013e3182472876.
109. Paya CV, Wiesner RH, Hermans PE, et al. Lack of association between cytomegalovirus infection, HLA matching and the vanishing bile duct syndrome after liver transplantation. *Hepatology.* 1992;16(1):66–70. http://www.ncbi.nlm.nih.gov/pubmed/1319956. Accessed June 19, 2016.
110. Teixeira R, Pastacaldi S, Davies S, et al. The influence of cytomegalovirus viraemia on the outcome of recurrent hepatitis C after liver transplantation. *Transplantation.* 2000;70(10):1454–1458. http://www.ncbi.nlm.nih.gov/pubmed/11118089. Accessed June 19, 2016.
111. Bodro M, Sabé N, Lladó L, et al. Prophylaxis versus preemptive therapy for cytomegalovirus disease in high-risk liver transplant recipients. *Liver Transpl.* 2012;18(9):1093–1099. doi:10.1002/lt.23460.
112. Asberg A, Humar A, Jardine AG, et al. Long-term outcomes of CMV disease treatment with valganciclovir versus IV ganciclovir in solid organ transplant recipients. *Am J Transplant.* 2009;9(5):1205–1213. doi:10.1111/j.1600-6143.2009.02617.x.
113. Norvell JP, Blei AT, Jovanovic BD, et al. Herpes simplex virus hepatitis: an analysis of the published

literature and institutional cases. *Liver Transpl.* 2007;13(10):1428–1434. doi:10.1002/lt.21250.

114. Kusne S, Schwartz M, Breinig MK, et al. Herpes simplex virus hepatitis after solid organ transplantation in adults. *J Infect Dis.* 1991;163(5):1001–1007. http://www.ncbi.nlm.nih.gov/pubmed/1850439. Accessed June 25, 2016.
115. Wald A, Huang M-L, Carrell D, et al. Polymerase chain reaction for detection of herpes simplex virus (HSV) DNA on mucosal surfaces: comparison with HSV isolation in cell culture. *J Infect Dis.* 2003;188(9):1345–1351. doi:10.1086/379043.
116. Basse G, Mengelle C, Kamar N, et al. Disseminated herpes simplex type-2 (HSV-2) infection after solid-organ transplantation. *Infection.* 2008;36(1):62–64. doi:10.1007/s15010-007-6366-7.
117. Safrin S, Crumpacker C, Chatis P, et al. A controlled trial comparing foscarnet with vidarabine for acyclovir-resistant mucocutaneous herpes simplex in the acquired immunodeficiency syndrome. The AIDS Clinical Trials Group. *N Engl J Med.* 1991;325(8):551–555. doi:10.1056/NEJM199108223250805.
118. Burns DM, Crawford DH. Epstein–Barr virus-specific cytotoxic T-lymphocytes for adoptive immunotherapy of post-transplant lymphoproliferative disease. *Blood Rev.* 2004;18(3):193–209. doi:10.1016/j.blre.2003.12.002.
119. Kremers WK, Devarbhavi HC, Wiesner RH, et al. Post-transplant lymphoproliferative disorders following liver transplantation: incidence, risk factors and survival. *Am J Transplant.* 2006;6(5 Pt 1):1017–1024. doi:10.1111/j.1600-6143.2006.01294.x.
120. Opelz G, Döhler B. Lymphomas after solid organ transplantation: a collaborative transplant study report. *Am J Transplant.* 2004;4(2):222–230. http://www.ncbi.nlm.nih.gov/pubmed/14974943. Accessed July 10, 2016.
121. Izadi M, Taheri S. Features, predictors and prognosis of lymphoproliferative disorders post-liver transplantation regarding disease presentation time: report from the PTLD.Int. survey. *Ann Transplant.* 16(1):39–47. http://www.ncbi.nlm.nih.gov/pubmed/21436773. Accessed July 10, 2016.
122. Kamdar KY, Rooney CM, Heslop HE. Posttransplant lymphoproliferative disease following liver transplantation. *Curr Opin Organ Transplant.* 2011;16(3):274–280. doi:10.1097/MOT.0b013e3283465715.
123. Tsai DE, Nearey M, Hardy CL, et al. Use of EBV PCR for the diagnosis and monitoring of post-transplant lymphoproliferative disorder in adult solid organ transplant patients. *Am J Transplant.* 2002;2(10):946–954. http://www.ncbi.nlm.nih.gov/pubmed/12482147. Accessed July 10, 2016.
124. Blaes AH, Peterson BA, Bartlett N, et al. Rituximab therapy is effective for posttransplant lymphoproliferative disorders after solid organ transplantation: results of a phase II trial. *Cancer.* 2005;104(8):1661–1667. doi:10.1002/cncr.21391.
125. Parker A, Bowles K, Bradley JA, et al. Management of post-transplant lymphoproliferative disorder in adult solid organ transplant recipients—BCSH and BTS Guidelines. *Br J Haematol.* 2010;149(5):693–705. doi:10.1111/j.1365-2141.2010.08160.x.
126. Hernandez MDP, Martin P, Simkins J. Infectious complications after liver transplantation. *Gastroenterol Hepatol (N Y).* 2015;11(11):741–753. http://www.ncbi.nlm.nih.gov/pubmed/27134589. Accessed June 26, 2016.
127. Aguado JM, Herrero JA, Gavaldá J, et al. Clinical presentation and outcome of tuberculosis in kidney, liver, and heart transplant recipients in Spain. Spanish Transplantation Infection Study Group, GESITRA. *Transplantation.* 1997;63(9):1278–1286. http://www.ncbi.nlm.nih.gov/pubmed/9158022. Accessed June 26, 2016.
128. Holty J-EC, Gould MK, Meinke L, et al. Tuberculosis in liver transplant recipients: a systematic review and meta-analysis of individual patient data. *Liver Transpl.* 2009;15(8):894–906. doi:10.1002/lt.21709.
129. Subramanian AK, Morris MI, AST Infectious Diseases Community of Practice. Mycobacterium tuberculosis infections in solid organ transplantation. *Am J Transplant.* 2013;13 suppl 4:68–76. doi:10.1111/ajt.12100.
130. Liu X, Ling Z, Li L, et al. Invasive fungal infections in liver transplantation. *Int J Infect Dis.* 2011;15(5):e298–e304. doi:10.1016/j.ijid.2011.01.005.
131. Saliba F, Delvart V, Ichaï P, et al. Fungal infections after liver transplantation: outcomes and risk factors revisited in the MELD era. *Clin Transplant.* 27(4):E454–E461. doi:10.1111/ctr.12129.
132. Ok Atılgan A, Özdemir BH, Kırnap M, et al. Invasive fungal infections in liver transplant recipients. *Exp Clin Transplant.* 2014;12 suppl 1:110–116. http://www.ncbi.nlm.nih.gov/pubmed/24635806. Accessed June 12, 2016.
133. Sganga G, Bianco G, Frongillo F, et al. Fungal infections after liver transplantation: incidence and outcome. *Transplant Proc.* 2014;46(7):2314–2318. doi:10.1016/j.transproceed.2014.07.056.
134. Said A, Safdar N, Lucey MR, et al. Infected bilomas in liver transplant recipients, incidence, risk factors and implications for prevention. *Am J Transplant.* 2004;4(4):574–582. doi:10.1111/j.1600-6143.2004.00374.x.
135. Marcó del Pont J, De Cicco L, Gallo G, et al. Hepatic arterial thrombosis due to Mucor species in a child following orthotopic liver transplantation. *Transpl*

Infect Dis. 2000;2(1):33–35. http://www.ncbi.nlm.nih.gov/pubmed/11429008. Accessed June 12, 2016.

136. Lowell JA, Coopersmith CM, Shenoy S, et al. Unusual presentations of nonmycotic hepatic artery pseudoaneurysms after liver transplantation. *Liver Transpl Surg*. 1999;5(3):200–203. doi:10.1002/lt.500050306.

137. Kamar N, Selves J, Mansuy J-M, et al. Hepatitis E virus and chronic hepatitis in organ-transplant recipients. *N Engl J Med*. 2008;358(8):811–817. doi:10.1056/NEJMoa0706992.

138. Kamar N, Garrouste C, Haagsma EB, et al. Factors associated with chronic hepatitis in patients with hepatitis E virus infection who have received solid organ transplants. *Gastroenterology*. 2011;140(5):1481–1489. doi:10.1053/j.gastro.2011.02.050.

139. Gane EJ, Angus PW, Strasser S, et al. Lamivudine plus low-dose hepatitis B immunoglobulin to prevent recurrent hepatitis b following liver transplantation. *Gastroenterology*. 2007;132(3):931–937. doi:10.1053/j.gastro.2007.01.005.

140. Demetris AJ, Todo S, Van Thiel DH, et al. Evolution of hepatitis B virus liver disease after hepatic replacement. Practical and theoretical considerations. *Am J Pathol*. 1990;137(3):667–676. http://www.ncbi.nlm.nih.gov/pubmed/2399936. Accessed June 26, 2016.

141. Phillips MJ, Cameron R, Flowers MA, et al. Post-transplant recurrent hepatitis B viral liver disease. Viral-burden, steatoviral, and fibroviral hepatitis B. *Am J Pathol*. 1992;140(6):1295–1308. http://www.ncbi.nlm.nih.gov/pubmed/1376555. Accessed June 26, 2016.

142. Lefkowitch JH, Lobritto SJ, Brown RS, et al. Ground-glass, polyglucosan-like hepatocellular inclusions: A "new" diagnostic entity. *Gastroenterology*. 2006;131(3):713-718. doi:10.1053/j.gastro.2006.07.006.

143. Wisell J, Boitnott J, Haas M, et al. Glycogen pseudoground glass change in hepatocytes. *Am J Surg Pathol*. 2006;30(9):1085–1090. doi:10.1097/01.pas.0000208896.92988.fc.

144. Bejarano PA, Garcia MT, Rodriguez MM, et al. Liver glycogen bodies: ground-glass hepatocytes in transplanted patients. *Virchows Arch*. 2006;449(5):539–545. doi:10.1007/s00428-006-0286-2.

145. Katz LH, Paul M, Guy DG, et al. Prevention of recurrent hepatitis B virus infection after liver transplantation: hepatitis B immunoglobulin, antiviral drugs, or both? Systematic review and meta-analysis. *Transpl Infect Dis*. 2010;12(4):292–308. doi:10.1111/j.1399-3062.2009.00470.x.

146. Idilman R, Akyildiz M, Keskin O, et al. The long-term efficacy of combining nucleos(t)ide analog and low-dose hepatitis B immunoglobulin on post-transplant hepatitis B virus recurrence. *Clin Transplant*. July 2016. doi:10.1111/ctr.12804.

147. Verna EC, Abdelmessih R, Salomao MA, et al. Cholestatic hepatitis C following liver transplantation: an outcome-based histological definition, clinical predictors, and prognosis. *Liver Transpl*. 2013;19(1):78–88. doi:10.1002/lt.23559.

148. Ramírez S, Pérez-Del-Pulgar S, Forns X. Virology and pathogenesis of hepatitis C virus recurrence. *Liver Transpl*. 2008;14 suppl 2:S27–S35. doi:10.1002/lt.21644.

149. McCaughan GW, Shackel NA, Bertolino P, et al. Molecular and cellular aspects of hepatitis C virus reinfection after liver transplantation: how the early phase impacts on outcomes. *Transplantation*. 2009;87(8):1105–1111. doi:10.1097/TP.0b013e31819dfa83.

150. Garcia-Retortillo M, Forns X, Feliu A, et al. Hepatitis C virus kinetics during and immediately after liver transplantation. *Hepatology*. 2002;35(3):680–687. doi:10.1053/jhep.2002.31773.

151. Berenguer M. Natural history of recurrent hepatitis C. *Liver Transplant*. 2002;8(10):S14–S18. doi:10.1053/jlts.2002.35781.

152. Brown RS. Hepatitis C and liver transplantation. *Nature*. 2005;436(7053):973–978. doi:10.1038/nature04083.

153. Sreekumar R, Gonzalez-Koch A, Maor-Kendler Y, et al. Early identification of recipients with progressive histologic recurrence of hepatitis C after liver transplantation. *Hepatology*. 2000;32(5):1125–1130. doi:10.1053/jhep.2000.19340.

154. Gane EJ. The natural history of recurrent hepatitis C and what influences this. 2008;14(10):36–44. doi:10.1002/lt.

155. Gane EJ, Portmann BC, Naoumov NV, et al. Long-term outcome of hepatitis C infection after liver transplantation. *N Engl J Med*. 1996;334(13):815–820. doi:10.1056/NEJM199603283341302.

156. Mattman A, Huntsman D, Lockitch G, et al. Re: Brunt et. al.--Histological evaluation of iron in liver biopsies: relationship to HFE mutations. *Am J Gastroenterol*. 2001;96(3):926. doi:10.1111/j.1572-0241.2001.03653.x.

157. Pelletier SJ, Iezzoni JC, Crabtree TD, et al. Prediction of liver allograft fibrosis after transplantation for hepatitis C virus: persistent elevation of serum transaminase levels versus necroinflammatory activity. *Liver Transplant*. 2000;6(1):44–53. doi:10.1002/lt.500060111.

158. Neumann UP, Berg T, Bahra M, et al. Fibrosis progression after liver transplantation in patients with recurrent hepatitis C. *J Hepatol*. 2004;41(5):830–836. doi:10.1016/j.jhep.2004.06.029.

159. Yilmaz N, Shiffman ML, Stravitz RT, et al. A prospective evaluation of fibrosis progression in patients with recurrent hepatitis C virus following liver transplantation. *Liver Transpl*. 2007;13(7):975–983. doi:10.1002/lt.21117.
160. Firpi RJ, Abdelmalek MF, Soldevila-Pico C, et al. One-year protocol liver biopsy can stratify fibrosis progression in liver transplant recipients with recurrent hepatitis C infection. *Liver Transpl*. 2004;10(10):1240–1247. doi:10.1002/lt.20238.
161. Berenguer M, Ferrell L, Watson J, et al. HCV-related fibrosis progression following liver transplantation: increase in recent years. *J Hepatol*. 2000;32(4):673–684. doi:10.1016/S0168-8278(00)80231-7.
162. Wali M, Harrison RF, Gow PJ, et al. Advancing donor liver age and rapid fibrosis progression following transplantation for hepatitis C. *Gut*. 2002;51(2):248–252. http://www.ncbi.nlm.nih.gov/pubmed/12117889. Accessed July 2, 2016.
163. Sebagh M, Rifai K, Féray C, et al. All liver recipients benefit from the protocol 10-year liver biopsies. *Hepatology*. 2003;37(6):1293–1301. doi:10.1053/jhep.2003.50231.
164. Belli LS, Burroughs AK, Burra P, et al. Liver transplantation for HCV cirrhosis: improved survival in recent years and increased severity of recurrent disease in female recipients: results of a long term retrospective study. *Liver Transpl*. 2007;13(5):733–740. doi:10.1002/lt.21093.
165. Baiocchi L, Angelico M, Petrolati A, et al. Correlation between liver fibrosis and inflammation in patients transplanted for HCV liver disease. *Am J Transplant*. 2008;8(3):673–678. doi:10.1111/j.1600-6143.2007.02107.x.
166. Zekry A, Bishop GA, Bowen DG, et al. Intrahepatic cytokine profiles associated with posttransplantation hepatitis C virus-related liver injury. *Liver Transpl*. 2002;8(3):292–301. doi:10.1053/jlts.2002.31655.
167. McCaughan GW, Bowen DG. Pathogenesis of cholestatic hepatitis C. *J Hepatol*. 2011;54(2):392–394. doi:10.1016/j.jhep.2010.09.010.
168. Demetris AJ. Evolution of hepatitis C virus in liver allografts. *Liver Transpl*. 2009;15 suppl 2:S35–S41. doi:10.1002/lt.21890.
169. Mosnier J-FF, Degott C, Marcellin P, et al. The intraportal lymphoid nodule and its environment in chronic active hepatitis C: an immunohistochemical study. *Hepatology*. 1993;17(3):366–371. doi:10.1002/hep.1840170304.
170. Guido M, Fagiuoli S, Tessari G, et al. Histology predicts cirrhotic evolution of post transplant hepatitis C. *Gut*. 2002;50(5):697–700. http://www.ncbi.nlm.nih.gov/pubmed/11950819. Accessed July 3, 2016.
171. Saxena R, Crawford JM, Navarro VJ, et al. Utilization of acidophil bodies in the diagnosis of recurrent hepatitis C infection after orthotopic liver transplantation. *Mod Pathol*. 2002;15(9):897–903. doi:10.1038/modpathol.3880626.
172. Negro F, Sanyal AJ. Hepatitis C virus, steatosis and lipid abnormalities: clinical and pathogenic data. *Liver Int*. 2009;29 suppl 2:26–37. doi:10.1111/j.1478-3231.2008.01950.x.
173. Vakiani E, Hunt KK, Mazziotta RM, et al. Hepatitis C-associated granulomas after liver transplantation: morphologic spectrum and clinical implications. *Am J Clin Pathol*. 2007;127(1):128–134. doi:10.1309/NN03WMD8V0GK6HFW.
174. Poulsen H, Christoffersen P. Abnormal bile duct epithelium in liver biopsies with histological signs of viral hepatitis. *Acta Pathol Microbiol Scand*. 1969;76(3):383–390. http://www.ncbi.nlm.nih.gov/pubmed/5823358. Accessed July 3, 2016.
175. Tarantino G, Cabibi D, Cammà C, et al. Liver eosinophilic infiltrate is a significant finding in patients with chronic hepatitis C. *J Viral Hepat*. 2008;15(7):523–530. doi:10.1111/j.1365-2893.2008.00976.x.
176. Steatohepatitis N, Yeh MM, Larson AM, et al. Endotheliitis in chronic viral hepatitis A comparison with acute cellular rejection and. 2006;30(6):727–733.
177. Teresa Izquierdo M, Almenar L, Zorio E, et al. Hepatitis colestásica fibrosante relacionada con el virus de la hepatitis C tras el trasplante cardíaco. *Med Clin (Barc)*. 2007;129(3):117–118. doi:10.1157/13107371.
178. Zylberberg H, Carnot F, Mamzer MF, et al. Hepatitis C virus-related fibrosing cholestatic hepatitis after renal transplantation. *Transplantation*. 1997;63(1):158–160. http://www.ncbi.nlm.nih.gov/pubmed/9000679. Accessed July 3, 2016.
179. Rosenberg PM, Farrell JJ, Abraczinskas DR, et al. Rapidly progressive fibrosing cholestatic hepatitis--hepatitis C virus in HIV coinfection. *Am J Gastroenterol*. 2002;97(2):478–483. doi:10.1111/j.1572-0241.2002.05459.x.
180. Dixon LR, Crawford JM. Early histologic changes in fibrosing cholestatic hepatitis C. 2007;13(2):219–226. doi:10.1002/lt.
181. Moreira RK, Salomao M, Verna EC, et al. The Hepatitis Aggressiveness Score (HAS): a novel classification system for post-liver transplantation recurrent hepatitis C. *Am J Surg Pathol*. 2013;37(1):104–113. doi:10.1097/PAS.0b013e31826a92ac.
182. Demetris AJ, Eghtesad B, Marcos A, et al. Recurrent hepatitis C in liver allografts: prospective assessment of diagnostic accuracy, identification of pitfalls, and observations about pathogenesis. *Am J Surg Pathol*.

2004;28(5):658–669. http://www.ncbi.nlm.nih.gov/pubmed/15105656. Accessed July 9, 2016.
183. Majumdar A, Kitson MT, Roberts SK. Systematic review: current concepts and challenges for the direct-acting antiviral era in hepatitis C cirrhosis. *Aliment Pharmacol Ther*. 2016;43(12):1276–1292. doi:10.1111/apt.13633.
184. Berenguer M. Systematic review of the treatment of established recurrent hepatitis C with pegylated interferon in combination with ribavirin. *J Hepatol*. 2008;49(2):274–287. doi:10.1016/j.jhep.2008.05.002.
185. Poordad F, Schiff ER, Vierling JM, et al. Daclatasvir with sofosbuvir and ribavirin for hepatitis C virus infection with advanced cirrhosis or post-liver transplantation recurrence. *Hepatology*. 2016;63(5):1493–1505. doi:10.1002/hep.28446.
186. Guy JE, Qian P, Lowell JA, et al. Recurrent primary biliary cirrhosis: peritransplant factors and ursodeoxycholic acid treatment post-liver transplant. *Liver Transpl*. 2005;11(10):1252–1257. doi:10.1002/lt.20511.
187. Neuberger J, Gunson B, Hubscher S, et al. Immunosuppression affects the rate of recurrent primary biliary cirrhosis after liver transplantation. *Liver Transpl*. 2004;10(4):488–491. doi:10.1002/lt.20123.
188. Sanchez EQ, Levy MF, Goldstein RM, et al. The changing clinical presentation of recurrent primary biliary cirrhosis after liver transplantation. *Transplantation*. 2003;76(11):1583–1588. doi:10.1097/01.TP.0000090867.83666.F7.
189. Silveira MG, Talwalkar JA, Lindor KD, et al. Recurrent primary biliary cirrhosis after liver transplantation. *Am J Transplant*. 2010;10(4):720–726. doi:10.1111/j.1600-6143.2010.03038.x.
190. Hashimoto E, Shimada M, Noguchi S, et al. Disease recurrence after living liver transplantation for primary biliary cirrhosis: a clinical and histological follow-up study. *Liver Transplant*. 2001;7(7):588–595. doi:10.1053/jlts.2001.25357.
191. Charatcharoenwitthaya P, Pimentel S, Talwalkar JA, et al. Long-term survival and impact of ursodeoxycholic acid treatment for recurrent primary biliary cirrhosis after liver transplantation. *Liver Transpl*. 2007;13(9):1236–1245. doi:10.1002/lt.21124.
192. Alexander J, Lord JD, Yeh MM, et al. Risk factors for recurrence of primary sclerosing cholangitis after liver transplantation. *Liver Transpl*. 2008;14(2):245–251. doi:10.1002/lt.21394.
193. Alabraba E, Nightingale P, Gunson B, et al. A re-evaluation of the risk factors for the recurrence of primary sclerosing cholangitis in liver allografts. *Liver Transpl*. 2009;15(3):330–340. doi:10.1002/lt.21679.
194. Cholongitas E, Shusang V, Papatheodoridis GV, et al. Risk factors for recurrence of primary sclerosing cholangitis after liver transplantation. *Liver Transpl*. 2008;14(2):138–143. doi:10.1002/lt.21260.
195. Hildebrand T, Pannicke N, Dechene A, et al. Biliary strictures and recurrence after liver transplantation for primary sclerosing cholangitis: a retrospective multicenter analysis. *Liver Transpl*. 2016;22(1):42–52. doi:10.1002/lt.24350.
196. Patel YA, Berg CL, Moylan CA. Nonalcoholic fatty liver disease: key considerations before and after liver transplantation. *Dig Dis Sci*. 2016;61(5):1406–1416. doi:10.1007/s10620-016-4035-3.
197. Yalamanchili K, Saadeh S, Klintmalm GB, et al. Nonalcoholic fatty liver disease after liver transplantation for cryptogenic cirrhosis or nonalcoholic fatty liver disease. *Liver Transpl*. 2010;16(4):431–439. doi:10.1002/lt.22004.
198. Pappo O, Ramos H, Starzl TE, et al. Structural integrity and identification of causes of liver allograft dysfunction occurring more than 5 years after transplantation. *Am J Surg Pathol*. 1995;19(2):192–206. http://www.ncbi.nlm.nih.gov/pubmed/7832279. Accessed July 15, 2016.
199. Gane E, Portmann B, Saxena R, et al. Nodular regenerative hyperplasia of the liver graft after liver transplantation. *Hepatology*. 1994;20(1 Pt 1):88–94. http://www.ncbi.nlm.nih.gov/pubmed/8020909. Accessed July 15, 2016.
200. Rosenthal P, Emond JC, Heyman MB, et al. Pathological changes in yearly protocol liver biopsy specimens from healthy pediatric liver recipients. *Liver Transpl Surg*. 1997;3(6):559–562. http://www.ncbi.nlm.nih.gov/pubmed/9404953. Accessed July 15, 2016.
201. Slapak GI, Saxena R, Portmann B, et al. Graft and systemic disease in long-term survivors of liver transplantation. *Hepatology*. 1997;25(1):195–202. doi:10.1002/hep.510250136.
202. Wiesner RH, Fung JJ. Present state of immunosuppressive therapy in liver transplant recipients. *Liver Transpl*. 2011;17 suppl 3:S1–S9. doi:10.1002/lt.22410.
203. Mele TS, Halloran PF. The use of mycophenolate mofetil in transplant recipients. *Immunopharmacology*. 2000;47(2):215–245. doi:10.1016/S0162-3109(00)00190-9.
204. Dumortier J, Guillaud O, Pittau G, et al. Introduction of mycophenolate mofetil in maintenance liver transplant recipients: what can we expect? Results of a 10-year experience. *Transplant Proc*. 2010;42(7):2602–2606. doi:10.1016/j.transproceed.2010.05.170.
205. Menon KV, Hakeem AR, Heaton ND. Meta-analysis: recurrence and survival following the use of sirolimus in liver transplantation for hepatocellular carcinoma. *Aliment Pharmacol Ther*. 2013;37(4):411–419. doi:10.1111/apt.12185.

21 Vascular disorders

Lizhi Zhang, MD

21.1 INTRODUCTION

The liver has a dual blood supply. The portal vein provides approximately two-thirds of blood flow to the liver, with blood that is rich in nutrients. The hepatic artery supplies the rest of the blood, with blood that is oxygen rich. The hepatic veins drain the venous blood into the inferior vena cava and then back to the right side of the heart. A variety of abnormalities can occur at any level of blood inflow to the liver or blood outflow of the liver. These abnormalities can be either extrahepatic or intrahepatic and can lead to ischemia, portal hypertension, liver fibrosis and cirrhosis, or liver architectural alterations.

21.2 CONGENITAL ABNORMALITIES AND VASCULAR MALFORMATIONS

Normal variants

Variations in the anatomy of the portal vein and the hepatic artery are common. For example, variants in the branching pattern of intrahepatic portal veins are observed in approximately 20% of the population. The most common of these variant patterns include trifurcation of the main portal vein, or a right posterior segmental branch arising from the main portal vein, or a right anterior segmental branch arising from the left portal vein.[1] Variations in the classic branching of the hepatic artery are seen in 40% to 45% of people, with the most common patterns being a right hepatic artery arising from the superior mesentery artery or a left hepatic artery arising from the left gastric artery. Interestingly, an abnormal origin of the hepatic artery is frequently associated with biliary atresia.[2] Knowing these variants is particularly important for liver transplant surgeons because ligation of these branches may lead to liver necrosis, bile duct injury, or allograft failure.

Arteriovenous malformation

Arteriovenous malformations are congenitally abnormal direct connections between arteries and veins, which are usually localized to one lobe of the liver. Neonates with hepatic arteriovenous malformations can present clinically with congestive heart failure, anemia, hepatomegaly, and portal hypertension. Syndromic forms of vascular malformations, such as hereditary hemorrhagic telangiectasia, can also have arteriovenous malformations that manifest in late childhood with congestive heart failure and portal hypertension. Hepatic arteriovenous malformations are typically diagnosed by imaging or angiography and are rarely biopsied. In some cases, they may be resected.

Microscopically, arteriovenous malformations are characterized by large vessels with thick fibromuscular walls (Fig. 21.1). The center of the lesion can show infarction, hemorrhage, and calcification, whereas the peripheral of the lesion typically shows a marked fibrovascular proliferation (Fig. 21.2). Of note, infantile hemangioma has some overlapping clinical and radiologic features with arteriovenous malformations.[3,4] However, they are biologically and histologically distinct lesions. GLUT-1 immunostain can also help distinguish these two entities because the endothelial cells are positive for GLUT-1 in infantile hemangiomas but are negative in arteriovenous malformations.[5]

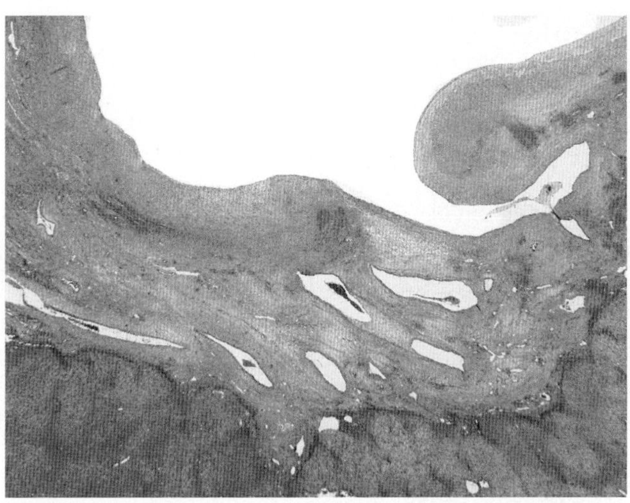

Figure 21.1 Hepatic arteriovenous malformation. The lesion is composed of large vessels with thick fibromuscular walls.

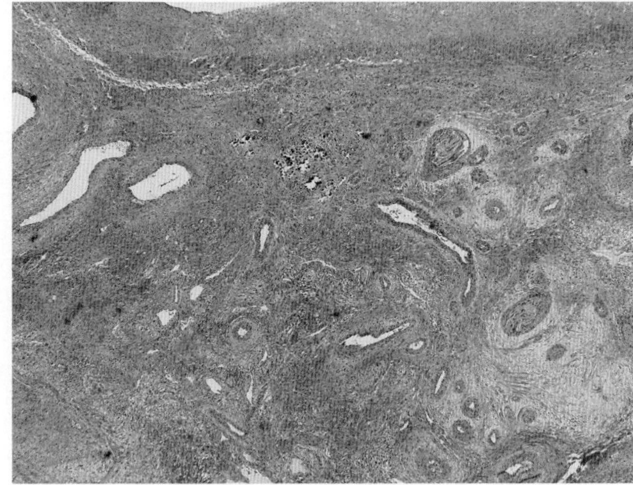

Figure 21.2 Hepatic arteriovenous malformation. There is a fibrovascular proliferation with calcification at the periphery.

Arterioportal fistula

Although most arterioportal fistulas are acquired because of cirrhosis, other rare causes include hepatic neoplasms, trauma, and rare cases of congenital arterioportal fistulas. Most patients with congenital arterioportal fistulas become symptomatic within the first year of life owing to portal hypertension, but the age of presentations varies. Arterioportal fistulas can also be associated with biliary atresia or hereditary hemorrhagic telangiectasia, although no other disease is seen in most cases.[6] Doppler ultrasound is the most useful method for making the diagnosis, which typically shows enlargement of the hepatic artery and dilatation of the segment of the portal vein, where the fistula is located. If left untreated, the liver may develop portal fibrosis and hepatoportal sclerosis.

Extrahepatic portosystemic shunt (Abernethy malformation)

Extrahepatic portosystemic shunt, also known as Abernethy malformation, is a rare congenital malformation in which portal blood is diverted away from the liver and drains into systemic veins. It has been classified into two subgroups. In type 1, there is congenital absence of the portal vein, and the portal blood is completely diverted into the inferior vena cava. This subgroup is further subdivided into type 1a, in which the splenic and superior mesenteric veins drain separately into the systemic veins, and type 1b, in which the splenic and superior mesenteric veins join to form a common trunk before draining into the inferior vena cava. In the type 2 Abernethy malformation, the portal vein is present and there is partial portal blood flow to the liver, but some of the portal flow is diverted into the inferior vena cava through a side-to-side extrahepatic communication.[7]

The clinical presentation of Abernethy malformation varies significantly. Some cases may be entirely asymptomatic or only have mild elevations of liver enzymes and bilirubin levels, whereas other cases may have serious complications, such as pulmonary hypertension, hepatopulmonary syndrome, hyperammonemia, or hepatic encephalopathy.[8] Abernethy malformation is occasionally diagnosed in adulthood. Abernethy malformations are also associated with the development of focal nodular hyperplasia, hepatic adenomas, and hepatocellular carcinoma.[9,10] Cross-sectional imaging can readily identify the portosystemic shunt and the absent vessels.

Microscopically, the liver parenchyma changes in Abernethy malformation are characterized by the absence or paucity of portal vein branches in the small portal tracts, and hypoplastic veins or fibrotic remnants in medium-sized portal tracts. The hepatic arteries are large and thickened, crowding the portal tracts with a disordered tangle of vessels (Figs. 21.3 and 21.4). Bile duct changes are generally absent to mild, but there can be a mild bile ductular proliferation and focal periductal fibrosis. Prominent, dilated lymphatic channels at the periphery of portal tracts are described in some cases. The lobules often show mild sinusoidal dilation, small lobular arterioles, and nodular regenerative hyperplasia. Nodular regenerating hyperplasia, when present, can be highlighted by a reticulin stain. Trichrome stains usually show mild portal fibrosis, fibrotic remnants of portal veins, and hypoplastic portal vein branches with narrow lumens and thickened muscle bundles.[10]

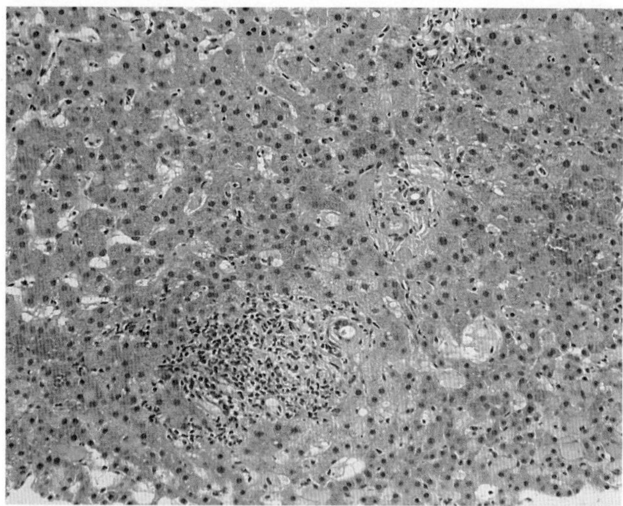

Figure 21.3 Abernethy malformation. The biopsy shows portal tracts without portal vein branches.

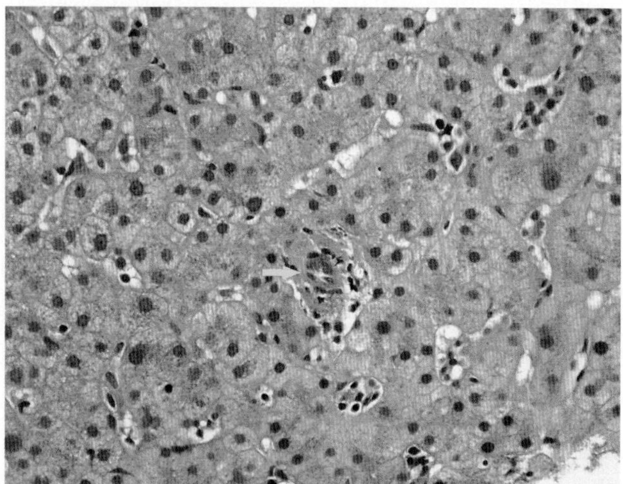

Figure 21.4 Abernethy malformation. An isolated capillary is seen in the lobule (arrow).

Abernethy malformations can occasionally be encountered in liver resections for hepatocellular carcinoma arising in noncirrhotic livers.[10]

Intrahepatic portosystemic shunt

Congenital intrahepatic portosystemic shunts are abnormal intrahepatic connections between branches of the portal veins and the hepatic veins. This condition can be complicated by congestive heart failure, portal hypertension, portosystemic encephalopathy, and cirrhosis. In the most common form, there is a connection between the right portal vein and the inferior vena cava through a single large shunting vessel. Congenital intrahepatic portosystemic shunts can also present with a localized communication or multiple communications between peripheral portal veins and hepatic veins.[11] A persistent ductus venosus is also considered to be a type of portosystemic shunt. The diagnosis is usually made with Doppler ultrasound, which demonstrates the vascular nature of the shunt and the amount of blood being shunted. As a result of the abnormal blood flow, the liver can develop nodular regenerative hyperplasia and/or focal nodular hyperplasia.[12] There are also acquired forms of intrahepatic portosystemic shunts that are associated with cirrhosis, hepatocellular carcinoma, or traumatic injuries to the liver.

Hepatic vascular disorders associated with other congenital syndromes

VACTERL association

VACTERL association (also known as VATER association) is a nonrandom association of birth defects in the vertebrae, anus and rectum, heart, trachea, esophagus, radius, and kidney. The etiology is unknown. The liver can also be involved, presenting as unexplained abnormal liver enzyme elevations or portal hypertension. Focal nodular hyperplasias and lymphatic cysts have also been described.[13,14] The microscopic features are similar to those in Abernethy malformations, including absent or atrophic portal veins associated with increased numbers and prominence of hepatic arterioles in the portal tracts.

Turner syndrome

Turner syndrome is one of the most common chromosomal abnormalities and results from a missing X chromosome in females. There is a wide range of signs and symptoms, and some affected individuals may have less obvious or less severe physical findings. The classic phenotype of Turner syndrome is short stature, broad chest, webbed neck, low set ears, and gonadal dysgenesis. Abnormal liver tests are frequent in patients with the Turner syndrome, and most of them present with steatosis and steatohepatitis due to being overweight. Biliary disease has also been reported, including a wide range of findings such as biliary atresia, sclerosing cholangitis, and paucity of bile ducts.[15] Liver architectural changes can also develop, such as nodular regenerative hyperplasia or focal nodular hyperplasia, which are associated with vascular changes, including obliterative portal venopathy, or with congenital vascular disorders such as hypoplasia or agenesis of the portal venous system.[15,16] Cirrhosis may develop in some affected individuals, but it is often unclear if the cirrhosis is due to the fatty liver disease or the vascular abnormalities, or both.[15]

Hereditary hemorrhagic telangiectasia

Hereditary hemorrhagic telangiectasia, also known as Osler–Weber–Rendu syndrome, is an autosomal dominant genetic disorder leading to abnormal blood vessel formation in the skin, mucous membranes, and various organs including the liver. There are five genetic types of hereditary hemorrhagic telangiectasia. Mutations have been identified in three specific genes (*ENG*, *ALK1*, and *SMAD4*), whereas the other two types of hereditary hemorrhagic telangiectasia have to date been linked only to loss of DNA on a particular locus. The subtype associated with *ALK1* mutations is most likely to have liver disease.

Hereditary hemorrhagic telangiectasia is manifested by telangiectasia (small vessel malformations) and arteriovenous malformations (large vessel malformations). Liver involvement is common in hereditary hemorrhagic telangiectasia, but the majority of individuals are asymptomatic. Overall, 10% of individuals can present with clinical findings that result from portal hypertension, biliary disease, or high-output heart failure.[17] Hepatic arteriovenous malformations can be seen in 50% to 75% of individuals, whereas telangiectasias are less commonly seen.[18] Livers are generally not biopsied in cases of known hereditary hemorrhagic telangiectasia because of the risk of bleeding. However, some cases undergo liver biopsy because imaging studies show lesions in individuals without a known diagnosis of hereditary hemorrhagic telangiectasia. Histologically, arteriovenous malformations are characterized by large caliber vessels with abnormal thick fibromuscular walls and direct shunts between portal arterioles and veins. These shunts can lead to focal nodular hyperplasias, which are the most common mass lesions found in patients with hereditary hemorrhagic telangiectasia. Histologically, the focal nodular hyperplasias are similar to those in the sporadic setting.[19]

Other vascular lesions are telangiectasias. These lesions can be focal microscopic collections of dilated inter-anastomosing vessels in the portal tracts, with sinusoidal dilation at the periphery (Fig. 21.5). In other cases, the telangiectasias can be large and mass forming. Mass-forming lesions are characterized by interanastomosing vascular channels that in some areas can show direct connections to the portal veins (Fig. 21.6). The lesion is composed of thin-walled vascular channels that are lined by bland endothelium with a very low or absent proliferative rate. The channels can dissect into the hepatic parenchyma, leaving intact portal tracts and hepatic lobules. The hepatic lobules can also show sinusoidal dilation and mild hyperplasia but do not show well-defined regenerative nodules. Focal hemorrhage with fibrosis and hemosiderin-laden macrophages are often seen within larger telangiectasias. Hepatocellular carcinomas have also been reported.[20]

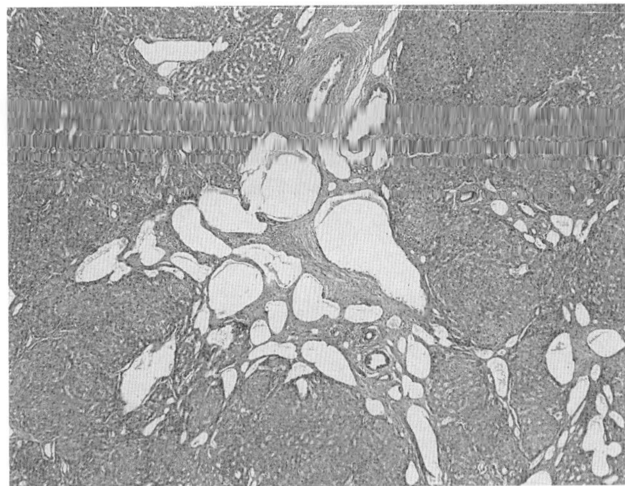

Figure 21.5 Liver involvement in hereditary hemorrhagic telangiectasia (HHT). Arteriovenous malformation in HHT characterized by dilated vessels with thick fibromuscular walls and direct shunts between portal arterioles and veins.

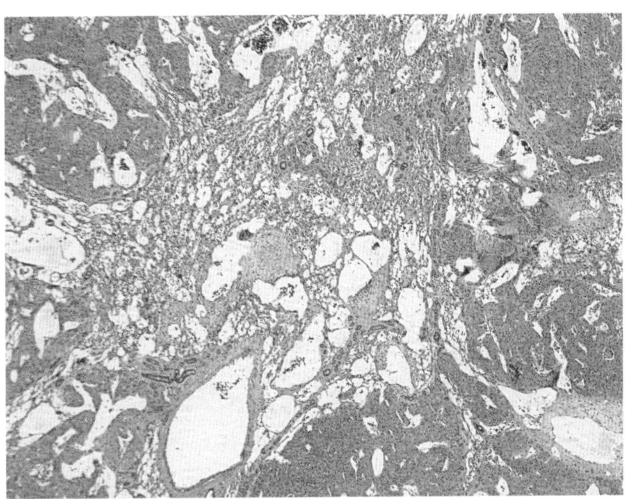

Figure 21.6 Mass-forming telangiectasia in hereditary hemorrhagic telangiectasia. The lesion is characterized by interanastomosing vessels connected directly with the portal veins.

Hereditary hemorrhagic telangiectasia is usually managed conservatively, but liver transplantation is used in cases with cardiac failure, liver failure, massive biliary necrosis, or severe portal hypertension. Vascular abnormalities and lesions, such as arteriovenous malformations, intrahepatic shunts, hemangioma, hemorrhagic foci, ischemic liver and biliary necrosis, and peliosis, are universally identified in the explants (Fig. 21.7). The explanted livers show a range of findings, but commonly include nodular regenerative hyperplasia (in noncirrhotic livers), focal nodular hyperplasia, arteriovenous malformations, and telangiectasias. Advanced fibrosis or cirrhosis is seen up to one-third of patients.[21]

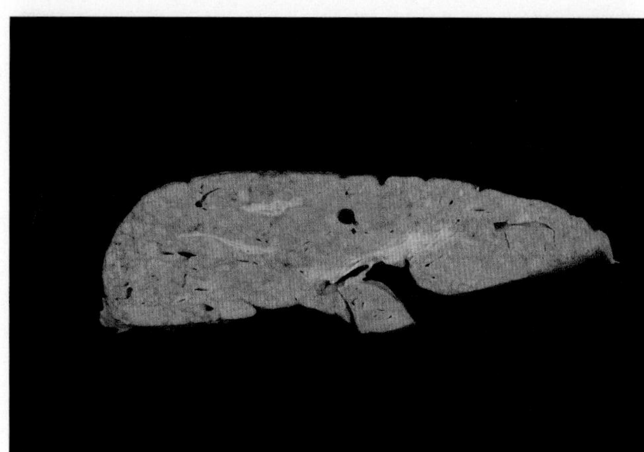

Figure 21.7 A liver explant of hereditary hemorrhagic telangiectasia shows patchy red telangiectasias.

21.3 PORTAL VEIN DISORDERS

Portal vein thrombosis

Definition

Portal vein thrombosis is an obstruction or narrowing of the hepatic portal vein by a thrombus, leading to portal hypertension and a reduction in the blood supply to the liver.

Clinical features

Portal vein thrombosis is a relatively rare disorder with an overall incidence of 0.05% to 0.5%, but the reported incidence in people with cirrhosis varies from 0.6% to 16%.[22] In the acute phase, patients may be asymptomatic or have nonspecific features such as fever or abdominal pain. In chronic cases, symptoms and signs related to portal hypertension can develop. In fact, approximately 5% to 10% of all cases of portal hypertension are due to portal vein thrombosis.

The clinical presentations also vary with different underlying causes of liver disease, which can be either inherited or acquired. In children and neonates, intra-abdominal infection is the leading cause of portal vein thrombosis, with the remaining cases due to congenital anomalies of the portal venous system, or due to neonatal sepsis with umbilical catheter placement. In adults, cirrhosis and neoplasms are the main causes. Individuals with coagulopathy are at particularly high risk of thrombosis. Of note, 8% to 15% of portal vein thrombosis cases are idiopathic.[23]

Laboratory findings

In patients with portal vein thrombosis, the liver enzymes are generally normal or only mildly elevated, unless there is coexistence of an underlying liver disease or cirrhosis. Coagulation tests are often abnormal because of the inherited coagulation disorders and/or underlying hepatic insufficiency.

Imaging

Ultrasound can quickly establish the diagnosis of portal vein thrombosis by revealing the presence of solid, hyperechoic material in a distended portal vein or its tributaries and the presence of collateral vessels. Doppler imaging can confirm the absence of flow in part or all of the vessel lumen. Endoscopic ultrasound is even more sensitive and specific and can detect small and nonoccluding thrombi. Computed tomography (CT) scan demonstrates hyperattenuating material in the portal vein lumen and the absence of enhancement after contrast injection.

Gross findings

The liver can be diffusely atrophic if the main portal vein trunk is blocked. Liver parenchyma remodeling occurs after partial recanalization of the vein, or with compensatory hyperflow from the hepatic artery. This parenchymal remodeling can lead to generalized nodular regenerative hyperplasia or focal nodular hyperplasia.

Acute thrombosis of small hepatic veins can lead to pseudoinfarctions, also known as Zahn infarcts, characterized by a focal area of congestion associated with hepatocellular atrophy but no necrosis.

Liver explants with portal vein thrombosis usually show underlying cirrhosis because of concurrent chronic liver diseases, such as chronic viral hepatitis or fatty liver disease. Organized thrombi or webs can be identified in the portal vein branches (Fig. 21.8).

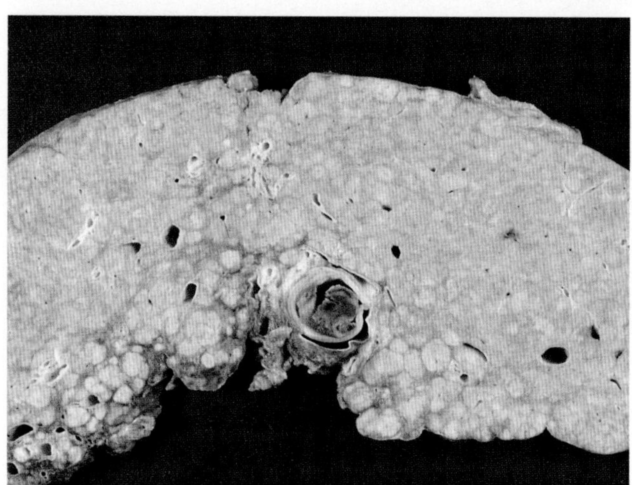

Figure 21.8 Portal vein thrombosis. A large thrombus was identified in liver explant.

Microscopic findings

Changes in the portal veins include organizing and recanalized thrombi, eccentric intimal fibrosis of the vein wall, luminal webs, and in long standing cases, partial or complete absence of the veins, being replaced by fibrotic scars (Fig. 21.9). The morphologic changes within the hepatic lobules are mild and often subtle. Typical features of nodular regenerative hyperplasia may be present. In many cases, the main finding is hepatoportal sclerosis, characterized by atrophy or complete absence of the smaller branches of the portal veins. Other portal tracts can show an increased number of small caliber portal veins or dilated portal vein branches "herniating" into the surrounding parenchyma with an "ectopic" appearance (Fig. 21.10). However, the changes of hepatoportal sclerosis are subtle and can be easily overlooked because the biopsies can appear "almost normal" on first examination. One important clue can be a clinical diagnosis of portal hypertension, but no significant fibrosis present in the biopsy.

Portal biliopathy, also known as pseudosclerosing cholangitis, is a term that describes biliary abnormalities secondary to portal hypertension.[24] Most cases of portal biliopathy result from extrahepatic portal vein thrombosis,[25] resulting in external compression of the bile ducts by large collaterals, leading to ischemia and strictures with subsequent episodes of infection. The portal tracts may show changes compatible with large bile duct obstruction.

Molecular genetic findings

Molecular genetic testing is not used to diagnose portal vein thrombosis but is important after a diagnosis is made in order to rule out inherited coagulation disorders such as Factor V Leiden mutation, protein C deficiency, or prothrombin mutations.

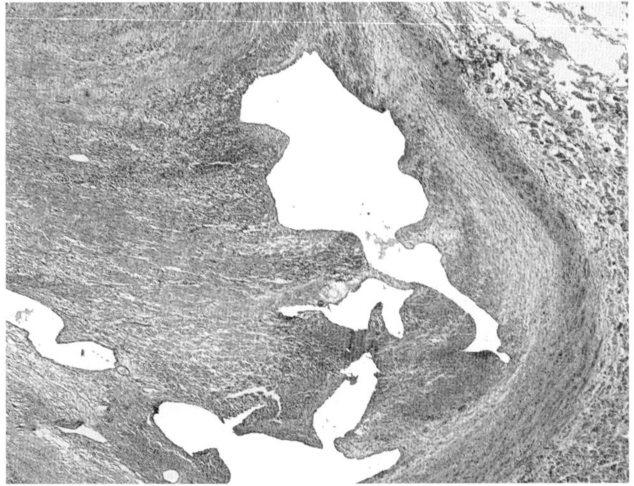

Figure 21.9 Portal vein thrombosis. Microscopic findings of an organizing portal vein thrombus with recanalization.

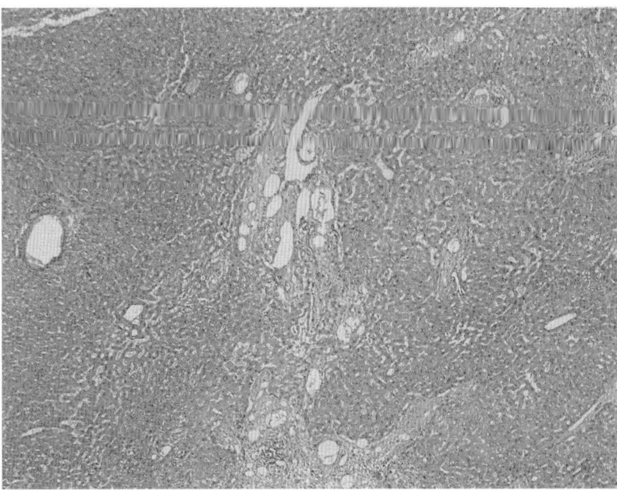

Figure 21.10 Portal vein thrombosis. Parenchyma changes are characterized by nodular appearance with atrophy and absent of the portal veins in the small portal tracts. Also seen are dilated portal vein branches that "herniate" into the surrounding parenchyma.

Differential diagnosis

The clinical diagnosis of portal vein thrombosis is usually established by imaging studies. The main histologic differential diagnosis includes other causes of hepatoportal sclerosis and/or noncirrhotic portal hypertension (Table 21.1).

Prognosis and treatment

The prognosis of portal vein thrombosis depends on the underlying liver disease and any systemic disease. In noncirrhotic and nonneoplastic patients, the prognosis of portal vein thrombosis is generally good. The overall mortality has been reported to be less than 10% in this setting, but rises to 25% in patients with malignancy or cirrhosis.[26] Although spontaneous resolution of portal vein thrombosis has been reported,[27] this is very rare and all cases are treated clinically, with the goal of treatment to correct underlying risk factors, prevent thrombosis extension, achieve portal vein patency, and manage complications related to portal hypertension. Portal vein thrombosis used to be considered a contraindication for liver transplant, but with the advent of new surgical techniques, a subset of patients can undergo liver transplant and achieve long-term survival.[28]

Table 21.1 Histopathologic features of common causes of noncirrhotic portal hypertension due to vascular disorders[a]

	PVT	HPS	SOS	BCS	CH	NRH
Venous inflow or outflow obstruction	Thrombosis in large portal veins and may extend into medium to small intrahepatic branches	Phlebosclerosis in portal tracts may coexist with PVT	Obliteration of the small central vein branches and terminal venules	Thrombotic or nonthrombotic obstruction at any level from intrahepatic veins to inferior vena cava	Right heart failure	Can be associated with any cause of hepatic blood flow alterations
OPV	Present	Present	Usually absent	May present if complicated with PVT	Absent	Not common
Aberrant or dilated portal veins in portal tracts	Present	Present	Absent	May present if complicated with PVT	Absent	Absent
Perivenular congestion	Absent	Absent	Marked	Marked	Marked	Absent
Sinusoidal dilatation	Mild	Mild	Variable	Marked	Marked	Absent to mild
Perivenular liver cell atrophy	Mild	Mild	Mild to marked	Mild to marked	Mild to marked	Mild to marked
Liver parenchyma loss	Absent	Absent	Marked in severe cases	Marked in severe cases	Marked in severe cases	Absent
RBC extravasation	Absent	Absent	Not common	Present	Present	Absent
Perisinusoidal fibrosis	Absent or mild	Absent or mild	Significant	Significant	Significant	Absent or mild
Portal fibrosis	Absent or mild	Absent or mild	Absent or mild	Absent or mild	Absent or mild	Absent or mild
Periportal fibrosis	Absent or mild	Absent or mild	Absent or mild	Absent or mild	Absent or mild	Absent
Progression to cirrhosis	Yes	No	Rarely	Yes	Yes	No
NRH-like architectural changes	May present	May present	May present	Absent	Absent	Present
Bile duct changes	Sclerosing cholangitis	No or mild bile ductular proliferation	No or mild bile ductular proliferation	No or mild bile ductular proliferation	No or mild bile ductular proliferation	No

[a] There are many overlapped histological features among these entities. Correlation with clinical and radiologic information is necessary to determine the etiology and level of blood flow blockage.

Abbreviations: PVT, portal vein thrombosis; HPS, hepatoportal sclerosis; SOS, sinusoidal obstruction syndrome; BCS, Budd–Chiari syndrome; CH, congestive hepatopathy; NRH, nodular regenerative hyperplasia; OPV, obliterative portal venopathy; RBC, red blood cell.

Hepatoportal sclerosis

Definition

Hepatoportal sclerosis is a rare disorder characterized by sclerosis of the intrahepatic portal veins leading to noncirrhotic portal hypertension.

Clinical features

Hepatoportal sclerosis is the main histologic finding of idiopathic noncirrhotic portal hypertension.[29] It can occur in both pediatric populations and in adults. The etiology of hepatoportal sclerosis is idiopathic in many cases, but it can be associated with a variety of conditions including chronic or recurrent infections, hematologic disorders, exposures to drugs or toxins, immunologic disorders, genetic disorders, and hypercoagulability. Clinical manifestations are characterized by portal hypertension, but liver failure with ascites and/or encephalopathy is rare. Portal vein thrombosis is common during the course of the disease.

Laboratory findings

Liver enzymes are usually normal or just mildly elevated. Anemia, leukopenia, and thrombocytopenia are common because of hypersplenism.

Imaging

Imaging studies can reveal diffuse nodularity of the liver, mimicking cirrhosis. Portal vein thrombosis and ascites can be present in some patients.

Gross findings

The liver explants can appear normal, show mild atrophy, or demonstrate a nodular parenchymal pattern. In many cases, organizing thrombi can be identified in large portal vein branches.

Microscopic findings

The diagnosis of hepatoportal sclerosis relies on identifying characteristic histopathologic features in liver biopsy specimens. A history of portal hypertension but no fibrosis on liver biopsy is an important clue to look carefully for this diagnosis. The primary findings are obliterative portal venopathy associated with liver parenchyma remodeling.[29,30] The classical changes of obliterative portal venopathy include luminal narrowing and obliteration of the small portal vein branches. Other findings include the complete absence, atrophy, or fibrous scarring of portal veins (Figs. 21.11, 21.12, and 21.13). The atrophic portal veins

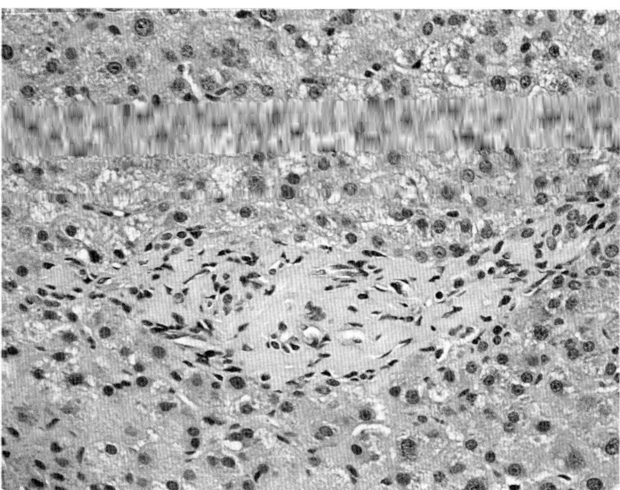

Figure 21.11 Hepatoportal sclerosis. Obliterative portal venopathy.

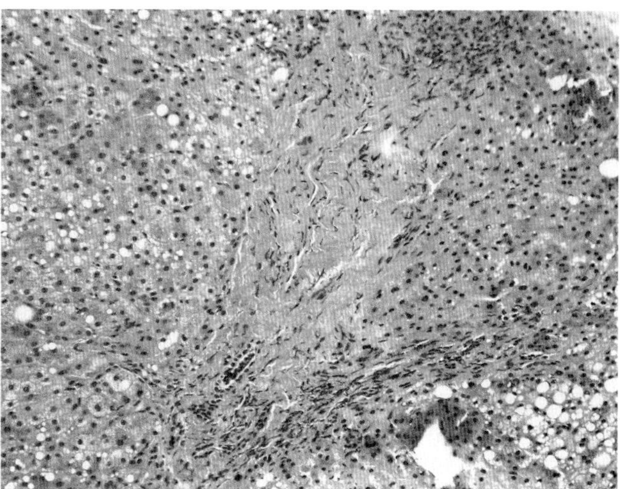

Figure 21.12 Hepatoportal sclerosis. An atrophic portal vein with dense fibrosis in a large portal tract.

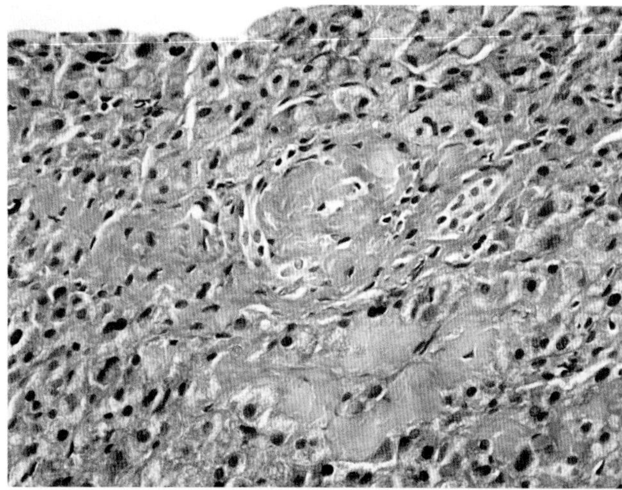

Figure 21.13 Hepatoportal sclerosis. Remnants of a portal vein are seen as a fibrotic scar in a portal tract (Trichrome stain).

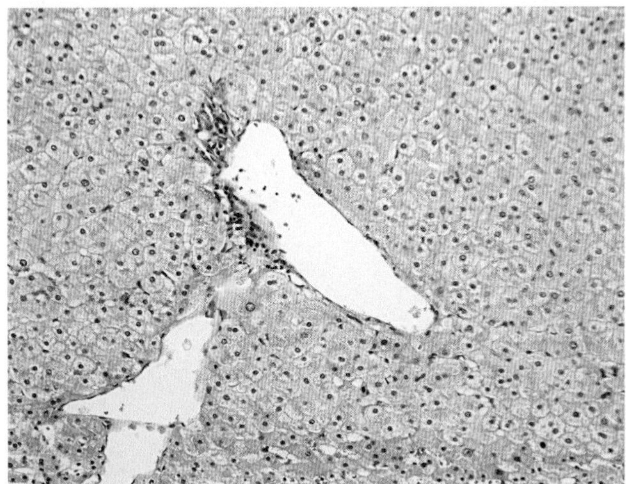

Figure 21.14 Hepatoportal sclerosis. Dilated portal veins "herniating" into the surrounding liver parenchyma.

are much smaller in caliber, often being similar in size to that of the hepatic arterioles or bile ducts. There can be increased numbers of small caliber portal veins as well. Some portal tracts may contain prominent dilated portal vein branches "herniating" into the surrounding liver parenchyma (Fig. 21.14). The lobular parenchyma can be unremarkable or nodular regenerative hyperplasia.[30] Partial nodular transformation in perihilar areas has also been observed, but this diagnosis needs to be correlated with gross or imaging findings.[31]

Fibrosis is usually absent or mild. Trichrome stains can demonstrate mild portal fibrosis, but advanced fibrosis is absent. The lobules can also show perisinusoidal fibrosis,[32,33] but this finding is not specific and overall tends to occur more frequently with other etiologies such as chronic venous outflow impairment or sinusoidal obstruction syndrome.

Immunohistochemistry and special stains

Trichrome stains can show portal sclerosis and fibrotic remnants of portal veins in portal tracts. Some cases may have incomplete septal fibrosis, characterized by delicate "incomplete" septal fibrosis giving a nodular appearance of liver parenchyma. Reticulin stains can highlight the changes of nodular regenerative hyperplasia.

Differential diagnosis

Hepatoportal sclerosis can be idiopathic or associated with a wide range of congenital and acquired conditions, such as Abernethy malformation or portal vein thrombosis.[34] Therefore, after the pathologic findings of hepatoportal sclerosis are identified on liver biopsy, clinical workup for specific disorders causing noncirrhotic portal hypertension is necessary (Table 21.1).

Prognosis and treatment

The management of hepatoportal sclerosis is to control portal hypertension-related complications. Liver transplantation is reserved for those individuals with severe portal hypertension or liver failure. The outcome of liver transplantation is generally good and portal hypertension tends not to recur.[35]

21.4 HEPATIC ARTERY DISEASES

Hepatic artery thrombosis

Hepatic artery thrombosis is a major cause of graft loss and mortality after liver transplantation (Fig. 21.15).[36] It occurs more frequently in the pediatric population because of the smaller caliber of the vessels and greater fluctuations in the concentration of coagulation factors. Early onset hepatic artery thrombosis can be clinically severe and histologically can show ischemic hepatitis and biliary ischemic injury. Of note, about a third of cases of hepatic artery thrombosis can be asymptomatic.

Depending on the size and degree of thrombosis, the histologic findings can be subtle with increased lobular spotty necrosis, increased hepatocyte mitoses, and variable degrees of cholestasis (Fig. 21.16). In more severe cases, there can be bland zone 3 hepatocyte necrosis or panacinar cell necrosis. In some cases, the ischemic injury can lead to bile duct necrosis, strictures, and cholangiectases in the perihilar extrahepatic bile ducts and the large intrahepatic bile ducts.[37] In these cases, peripheral liver biopsies show changes that resemble biliary obstruction, with portal edema, cholangitis, and bile ductular reaction.

In nontransplant cases, hepatic artery thrombosis can develop due to a variety of causes such as hypercoagulability disorders, severe arteriosclerosis,

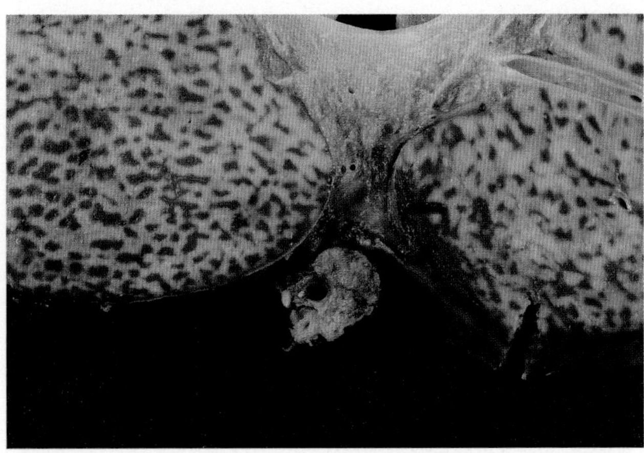

Figure 21.15 Hepatic artery thrombosis. A thrombus identified in portal artery in the liver explant.

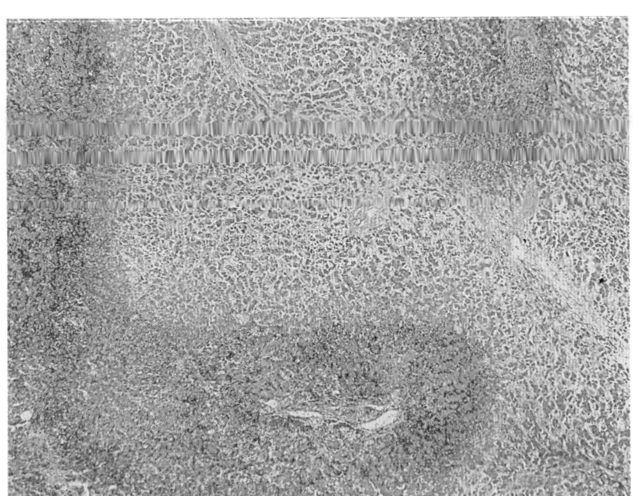

Figure 21.16 Hepatic artery thrombosis. Bland ischemic necrosis predominantly involving zones 3 and 2 regions.

vasculitis, hepatic artery aneurysm, or iatrogenic (ligation during surgery or therapeutic embolization). Individuals may be asymptomatic because of the dual blood supply of the liver, but a subset of patients may develop ischemic hepatitis with jaundice and elevated liver aminotransferase levels. Liver infarcts are more likely to occur when artery thrombosis is also associated with compromised portal vein blood flow.[38] Liver infarcts are characterized by panacinar parenchymal necrosis with little or no inflammation. In some cases, the panacinar necrosis will contain residual portal tracts surrounded by a thin rim of viable liver cells. Of note, liver infarction can form a mass lesion that mimics a neoplasm.[39]

Hepatic artery aneurysm

Hepatic artery aneurysm is uncommon but can be caused by arteriosclerosis, infections, trauma, and vasculitis. Most aneurysms are located in the extrahepatic artery. Ruptured aneurysms may lead to death, with bleeding into the common bile duct (hemobilia), abdominal cavity, or adjacent hollow viscera.[40] The diagnosis is established by imaging studies.

21.5 HEPATIC SINUSOID DISORDERS

Overview

The hepatic sinusoids are lined with highly fenestrated endothelial cells and contain numerous Kupffer cells. The sinusoidal spaces and the cellular components of the sinusoids are typically not prominent on hematoxylin and eosin (H&E) under normal conditions. However, in certain disorders, the sinusoids can show significant architectural changes or accumulation of abnormal cells or deposits. Sinusoidal obstructive syndrome, also known as veno-occlusive disease, is believed to be caused by direct injury of the endothelial cells of the sinusoids and/or central veins, and will be discussed in detail later.

Mild Kupffer cell hyperplasia is a common finding in liver injuries because of all kinds of causes. Significant intrasinusoidal neutrophils are frequently seen in liver biopsy specimens taken during abdominal surgeries, a finding referred to as "surgical hepatitis" (Fig. 21.17). This phenomenon is probably due to hypoxia or mechanical effects and is not a true hepatitic process. The sinusoidal neutrophils are found in zone 3, surrounding the central veins.

Sinusoidal lymphocytosis is commonly seen in acute and chronic hepatitis. The so-called "beaded" pattern of lymphocytosis, where lymphocytes are found as linear cords of cells in the sinusoids, resembling four to five beads on a string, has been associated with Epstein–Barr virus (EBV) hepatitis (Fig. 21.18). Although distinctive, this pattern is neither sensitive nor specific

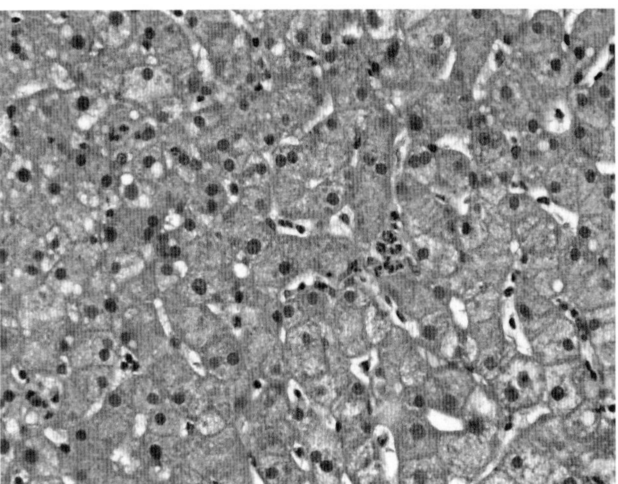

Figure 21.17 Surgical hepatitis. Abundant sinusoidal neutrophils are seen.

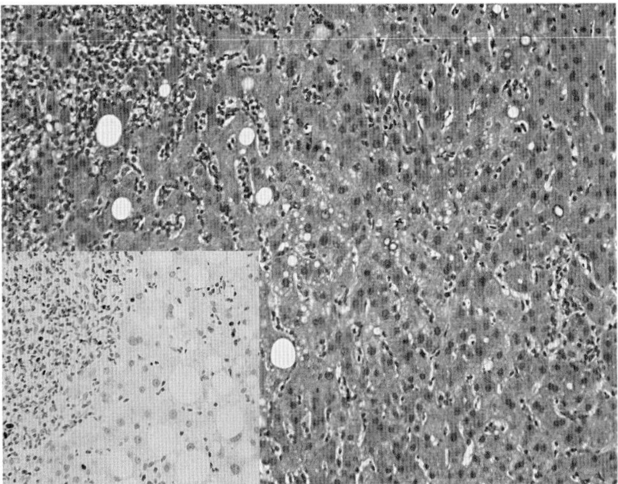

Figure 21.18 EBV hepatitis. Sinusoidal lymphocytes in a beaded pattern (inset, EBV in situ hybridization).

for EBV hepatitis. Other abnormal cellular or non-cellular accumulations in the sinusoids are discussed elsewhere in this book, including metastatic tumor cell infiltrates, Ito cell hyperplasia (or Hypervitaminosis A), sickle-cell disease, hemophagocytic syndrome (Fig. 21.19), storage diseases such as Nimann–Pick disease or Guanche, amyloidosis, and fibrin thrombi in disseminated intravascular coagulation. Other examples of sinusoidal disease include pseudopeliotic steatosis (also known as lipopeliosis), which results from ischemic injury after liver transplantation, with death of zone 3 hepatocytes containing fat. The released fat accumulates near the hepatic venules, some of which can enter the damaged sinusoids in the areas of necrosis (Fig. 21.20).

The most common abnormality of the sinusoids seen on liver biopsy is sinusoidal dilation. Of note, mild sinusoidal dilation is a fairly common and nonspecific finding in liver biopsy specimens (Fig. 21.21). In addition, diffuse and homogenous sinusoidal dilation is a well-known artifact in autopsy liver specimens owing to shrinking artifact (Fig. 21.22). Sinusoidal dilation is more likely to be clinically significant when it is associated with congestion, liver plate atrophy, perisinusoidal fibrosis, or liver cell dropout.

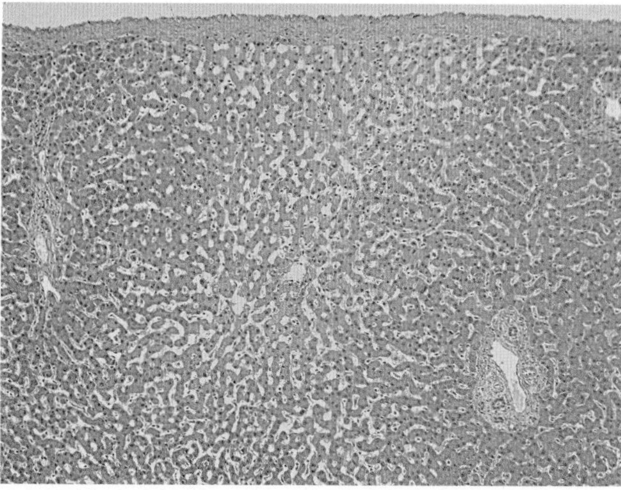

Figure 21.21 Nonspecific sinusoidal dilation. Nonspecific sinusoidal dilation in wedge liver biopsy specimen.

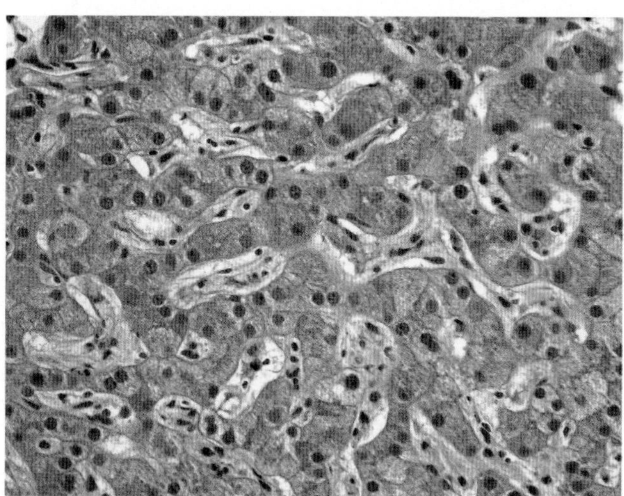

Figure 21.19 Hemophagocytosis. Activated macrophages engulfing red blood cells are seen in the sinusoids.

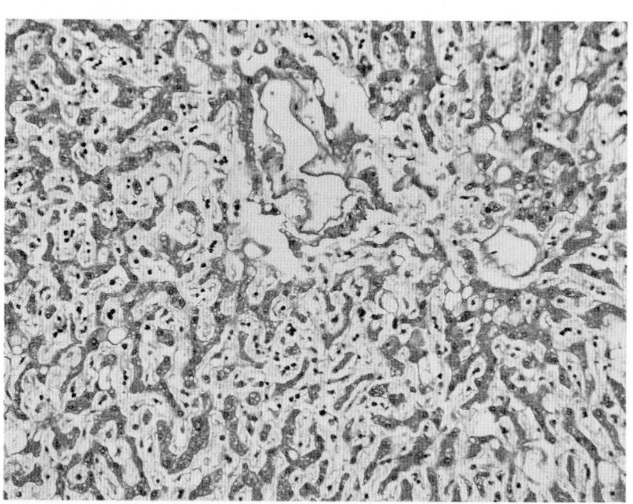

Figure 21.22 Artifactual diffuse sinusoidal dilation. Diffuse sinusoidal dilation in autopsy liver specimen.

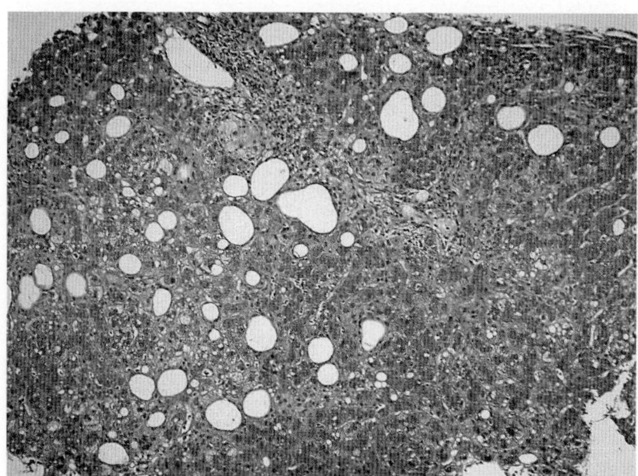

Figure 21.20 Lipopeliosis. Accumulation of large lipid droplets in the sinusoids.

Sinusoidal obstruction syndrome (or veno-occlusive disease)

Definition

Hepatic sinusoidal obstruction syndrome is also known as veno-occlusive disease. This condition is caused by inflammatory or toxic damage of sinusoidal and/or central vein endothelial cells, leading to occlusion of terminal hepatic venules and hepatic sinusoids.

Clinical features

Sinusoidal obstruction syndrome most often occurs after hematopoietic stem cell transplantation, with reported incidences ranging from approximately 5% to 60%.[41] In the nontransplantation setting, potential causes include chemotherapeutic agents such as oxalipatin, gemtuzumab, ozogamicin, etoposide, etc., and immunosuppressive agents including azathioprine and methotrexate. Other causes include total body or hepatic radiation therapy and alkaloid toxins in herbal teas or remedies.

Most patients initially present with unexplained weight gain because of fluid and sodium retention and ascites. Patients quickly develop firm and painful hepatomegaly and jaundice. Approximately half of patients will also have the hepatorenal syndrome, leading to renal insufficiency requiring hemodialysis. Severe cases may advance to multiorgan failure, hepatic encephalopathy, and death. Two different sets of criteria have been described for the clinical diagnosis of sinusoidal obstruction syndrome after hematopoietic stem cell transplantation: the revised Seattle criteria[42] and the Baltimore criteria.[43] Both sets of criteria are based on using clinical findings such as jaundice, weight gain, hepatomegaly, and ascites, after excluding other possible etiologies. However, neither approach has proven to be a reliable tool for either recognizing or excluding the diagnosis of sinusoidal obstruction syndrome. Liver biopsy is still considered the most accurate method to confirm a diagnosis of the sinusoidal obstruction syndrome.[44]

Laboratory findings

Patients with the sinusoidal obstruction syndrome usually present with elevated liver transaminases, alkaline phosphatase levels, and bilirubin levels. The hyperbilirubinemia usually develops after the weight gain and hepatomegaly and ranges from 12 to 18 mg/dL. In severe cases, liver synthetic function may be affected, leading to coagulopathy. Thrombocytopenia with refractoriness to platelet transfusion is common. About half of cases have abnormal renal function tests due to hepatorenal syndrome.

Imaging

Ultrasound with Doppler examination may identify hepatomegaly, ascites, an abnormal portal vein waveform, reversal of flow in the portal vein, and marked thickening of the gallbladder wall, but none of these findings are diagnostic for sinusoidal obstruction syndrome.

Gross findings

The liver is generally enlarged with congestion. Necrotic and hemorrhagic foci can be seen.

Microscopic findings

The key morphologic changes of this disorder are obliteration of the small central vein branches. Probably owing to sampling, this change is found in about 50% to 75% of liver biopsy cases with sinusoidal obstruction syndrome. The endothelial damage leads to subintimal edema and fibrin deposition (Figs. 21.23 and 21.24). The

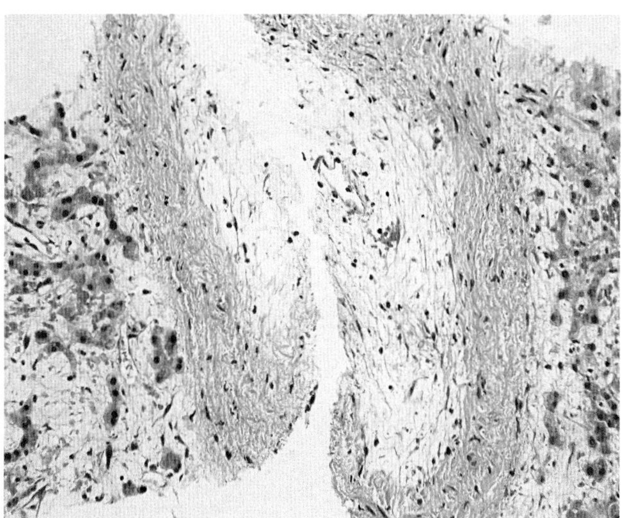

Figure 21.23 Hepatic sinusoidal obstruction syndrome. Early changes include subintimal edema and fibrin deposition in the central veins.

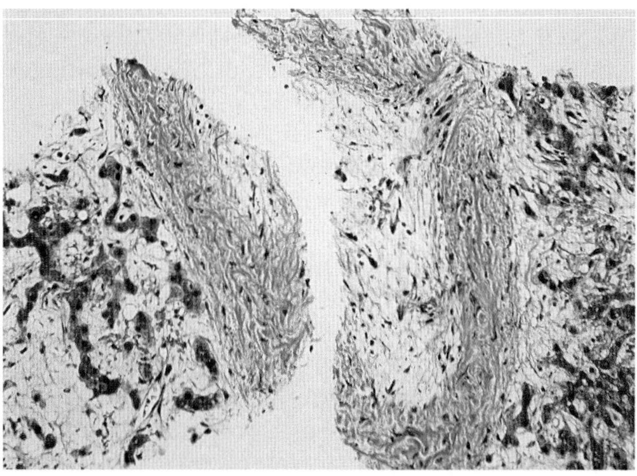

Figure 21.24 Hepatic sinusoidal obstruction syndrome. A trichrome stain of the same lesion from Figure 21.23.

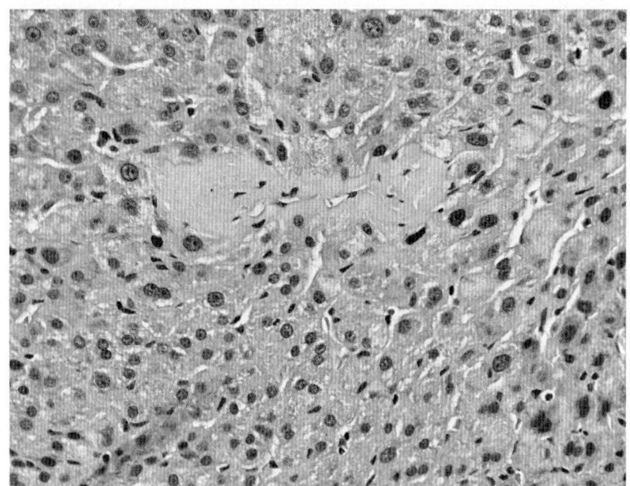

Figure 21.25 Hepatic sinusoidal obstruction syndrome. Venous occlusive changes by collagen depositions.

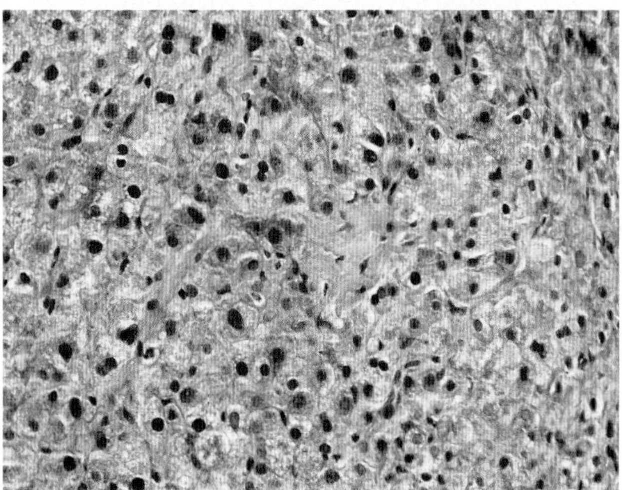

Figure 21.26 Hepatic sinusoidal obstruction syndrome. A trichrome stain of the same lesion from Figure 21.25.

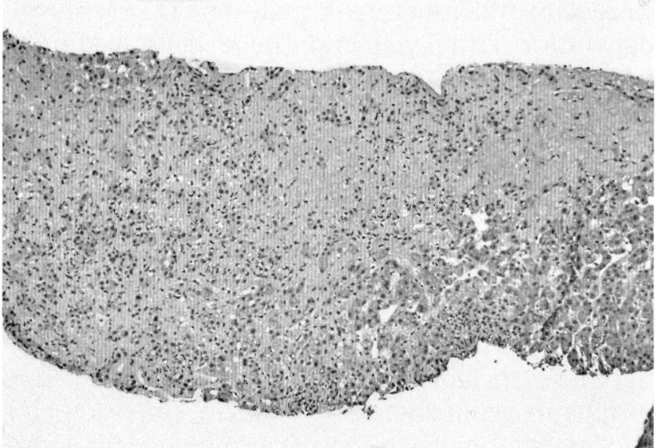

Figure 21.27 Hepatic sinusoidal obstruction syndrome. Bridging congestion with parenchymal loss is seen.

vein lumens are narrowed or obliterated by concentric or eccentric loose collagen deposition. Trichrome and elastic stains can be helpful in identify the damaged central veins (Figs. 21.25 and 21.26).[45–47] Thrombi are usually not recognized.

Other changes in the lobules tend to have a zone 3 distribution, including variable sinusoidal dilation with congestion, liver cell dropout, and liver plate atrophy. In severe cases, there can be zone 3 bridging necrosis, congestion, and larger areas of parenchymal loss (Fig. 21.27). Inflammation is usually absent or may be present as mild portal lymphocytic infiltrates with occasional acidophil bodies. Kupffer cell hyperplasia with increased iron accumulation can be seen in long-standing cases. Overall, the severity of the morphologic findings tends to correlate with the clinical severity of the disease.[47]

In mild cases, the liver can also develop nodular regenerative hyperplasia. In more severe cases, the liver can develop fibrosis. The fibrosis usually has a perivenular pattern but in severe cases, bridging fibrosis and eventually cirrhosis can develop. The cirrhosis is of the "congestive" type because of relatively sparing of the portal tracts. The regenerative nodules contain intact portal tracts with dilated portal veins in the center.

Immunohistochemistry and special stains

Reticulin stains can highlight architectural changes of the liver parenchyma, such as nodular regenerative hyperplasia or liver plate atrophy. Trichrome stains can reveal fibrous obliteration of central vein branches. Elastic stains can be used to highlight residual vascular structures.

Differential diagnosis

Clinically, other complications after hematopoietic stem cell transplantation can resemble sinusoidal obstruction syndrome, including acute graft-versus-host disease, hepatic infection, or drug toxicity. Liver biopsies are useful because they show very different morphologic changes from sinusoidal obstruction syndrome.

As noted previously, mild nonspecific sinusoidal dilation is a common finding. However, these cases will lack congestion, liver plate atrophy, and/or fibrosis. Budd–Chiari syndrome is also in the histologic differential (Table 21.1). The Budd–Chiari syndrome results from thrombosis of the largest branches of the intrahepatic central veins and/or extrahepatic veins. On peripheral needle biopsy, the Budd–Chiari syndrome tends show more striking zone 3 congestion and/or necrosis than is seen in the sinusoidal obstruction syndrome. In addition, the typical fibrotic obliterative changes in central veins and small venules in the sinusoidal obstruction syndrome are usually not present in the Budd–Chiari syndrome, or when present, are a minor component of the overall histologic findings. However, there can be histologic overlap, and correlation with imaging findings is important to rule out the Budd–Chiari syndrome.[48] Finally, fibrous obliteration of small hepatic veins is not specific for the sinusoidal obstruction syndrome, also being found as a secondary change in alcoholic liver disease and cirrhosis.[49,50]

Prognosis and treatment

Sinusoidal obstruction syndrome is a potentially fatal disorder. The mortality rate of severe sinusoidal obstruction syndrome after hematopoietic stem cell transplant is about 80%.[41] Careful management of risk factors can reduce the incidence and/or severity of the sinusoidal obstruction syndrome. Defibrotide has been shown promising results for the prevention and treatment of the sinusoidal obstruction syndrome. This drug has protective effects on the small vessel endothelium cells through its antithrombotic, anti-ischemic, and anti-inflammatory activities.[51,52] The usage of heparin and ursodeoxycholic acid for prevention of sinusoidal obstruction syndrome is still controversial. Liver transplantation may be required for very severe sinusoidal obstruction syndrome.

Peliosis hepatis

Definition

Peliosis hepatis is a rare vascular disorder characterized by randomly distributed areas of sinusoidal dilation and multiple blood-filled cavities throughout the liver. Similar changes can also occur in spleen, lymph nodes, or other organs.

Clinical features

The microscopic form of peliosis hepatis is characterized by small cysts and sinusoidal dilation and is usually asymptomatic. However, patients with the macroscopic form develop large cysts occupying significant portions of the liver and can develop abdominal pain, jaundice, hepatomegaly, portal hypertension, liver failure, or intrahepatic or peritoneal hemorrhage due to cyst rupture.[53]

The etiology of peliosis hepatis is not fully understood. A variety of conditions have been associated with peliosis hepatis, including chronic wasting diseases (particularly untreated tuberculosis and malignant tumors), multiple drugs such as estrogenic and androgenic steroids, renal transplantation, hairy cell leukemia, and HIV infection. Bacillary peliosis hepatis is an important form of peliosis hepatis that is caused by infection from *Bartonella henselae* or less frequently by *Bartonella quintana*.[54]

Laboratory findings

Mild elevations in liver enzymes are common in peliosis hepatis. In contrast, alkaline phosphates levels can be markedly elevated in cases of bacillary peliosis hepatis.

Imaging

The imaging features of peliosis hepatis vary with the type of the disease, the size and extent of the lesions, and the presence of thrombi or hemorrhage. The microscopic form tends to have no specific features on imaging, whereas the large vascular lesions in the macroscopic form can be visualized by various imaging techniques.

Gross findings

The liver surface may have small purplish areas. On cut surface, randomly distributed blood-filled cavities are present throughout the liver, ranging from a few millimeters to a few centimeters. Large intrahepatic hemorrhagic or infarct areas may also be present.

Microscopic findings

Liver biopsy is usually not performed for a suspected peliotic lesions because of the risk of bleeding. Liver involvement with peliosis hepatis can be disuse or focal. There are two morphologic patterns described in the literatures.[55] The parenchymal type is characterized by irregular blood-filled cavities with no endothelial lining. The cavities are connected to dilated sinusoids (Fig. 21.28). Patchy parenchymal loss is often present in the adjacent liver parenchyma. The phlebitic type, on the other hand, is composed of irregular cavities lined by either endothelial cells or fibrous tissue. The cavities tend to be distributed in centrilobular areas and communicate with the sinusoids and central veins. Thrombosis and organization may be observed at the edges of cavities. However, classification based on the presence or absence of an endothelial lining may not be biologically meaningful because blood cavities with no endothelial lining can quickly become endothelialized (Fig. 21.29). The noninvolved liver is usually unremarkable with no cirrhosis, significant inflammation, or changes of sinusoidal obstructive syndrome or venous outflow impairment.

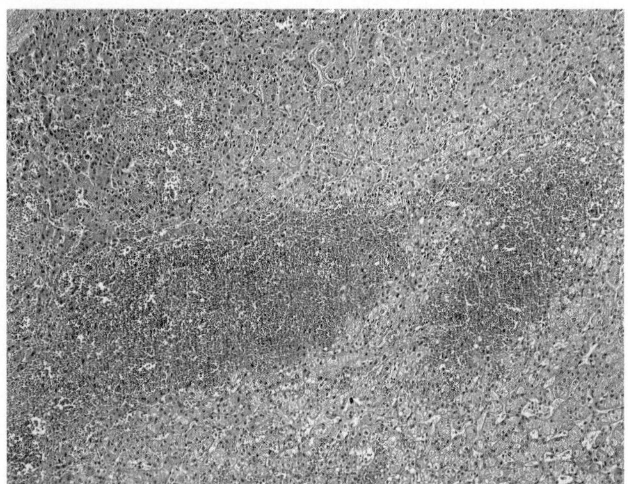

Figure 21.28 Peliosis hepatis, parenchymal type. Irregular blood-filled cavities are seen, with no endothelial lining.

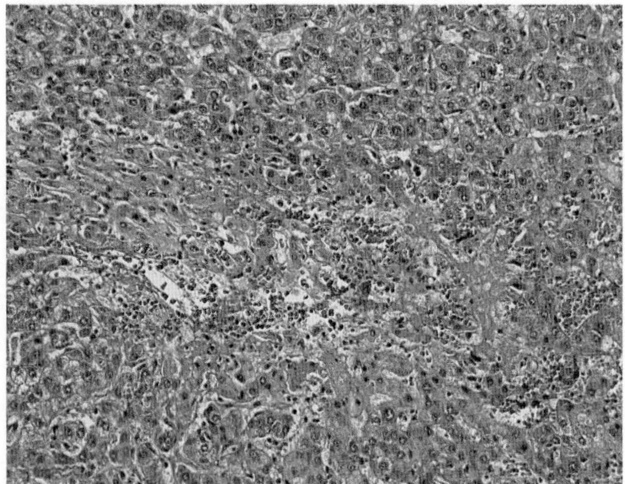

Figure 21.29 Peliosis hepatis, phlebitis type. Re-endothelialization and fibrosis of a blood-filled cavity.

Immunohistochemistry and special stains

Warthin–Starry stains are useful to evaluate for *Bartonella* infection.

Differential diagnosis

Dilated sinusoids due to other causes can resemble peliosis hepatis microscopically, including liver congestion secondary to heart failure, Budd–Chiari syndrome, or sinusoidal obstructive syndrome. However, the sinusoidal dilatation in these disorders has a centrilobular pattern and not the random distribution seen in peliosis hepatis. Hepatocellular adenomas, especially the inflammatory subtype, can show sinusoidal dilatation and blood pools, but these features are usually focal, and other diagnostic features of a hepatocellular neoplasm are readily identified. Low-grade angiosarcomas can also have areas of peliotic change, with hemorrhage mimicking the blood-filled cavities of peliosis hepatis. In these cases, the atypical hyperchromatic cells lining the dilated sinusoids and blood pools will lead to the correct diagnosis of angiosarcoma.

Prognosis and treatment

There is no specific treatment of peliosis hepatis. Early detection and discontinuation of the causative agent or treatment of the underlying condition may result in regression of the hepatic lesions, such as antibiotics in bacillary peliosis hepatis. Rare patients with severe liver failure from peliosis hepatis benefit from liver transplantation.

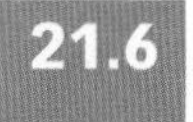

21.6 HEPATIC VEIN AND VENOUS OUTFLOW DISORDERS

Overview

Blood leaves the liver by draining through the right, left, and middle hepatic veins into the inferior vena cava and back to the right heart. Hepatic venous outflow impairment is divided into three categories according to the level of venous obstruction. Hepatic sinusoidal obstructive syndrome represents obstruction at the level of the sinusoids and terminal venules that are usually smaller than 300 μm. Budd–Chiari syndrome is due to the obstruction at any level from the intrahepatic hepatic veins to the inferior vena cava. Congestive hepatopathy results from passive congestion due to heart failure. These three conditions have many overlapping clinical and histopathologic features (Table 21.1).

The generic term “venous outflow impairment” may be used when interpreting liver biopsy specimens. The final diagnosis requires correlation with clinical and radiologic findings to determine the site of venous obstruction. The major histopathologic features of chronic venous outflow impairment are found in zone 3, including perivenular congestion and sinusoidal dilatation, hepatocyte atrophy, and hepatocyte necrosis (Figs. 21.30 and 21.31). Acute cases may also have extravasation of red blood cells into the space of Disse (Fig. 21.32). Chronic changes include perivenular sinusoidal fibrosis and centrizonal scarring (Figs. 21.33 and 21.34). Some cases will progress to cirrhosis without treatment.

In addition, the perivenular fibrosis and centrizonal scar can contain aberrant arterioles, metaplastic ductules, CK7 positive intermediate hepatocytes, and loss of the normal perivenular glutamine synthetase staining pattern. The combination of these features can make the centrizonal scars resemble portal tracts (Fig. 21.35).[56] In these cases, the liver biopsy findings can be misinterpreted as chronic biliary disease with

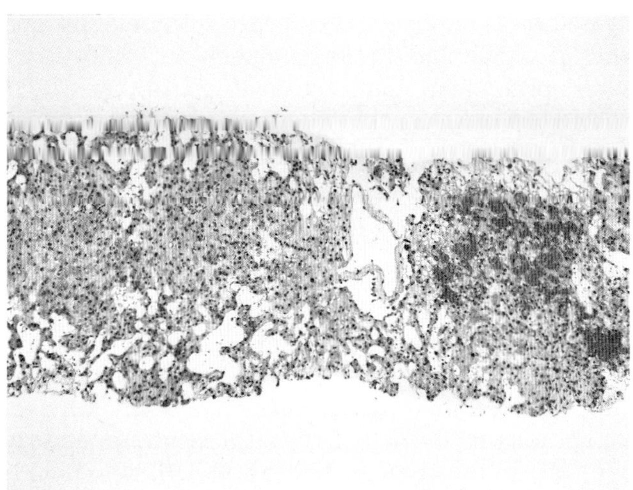

Figure 21.30 Chronic venous outflow impairment. Marked zone 3 changes including congestion, sinusoidal dilation, liver plate atrophy, and focal liver parenchymal loss.

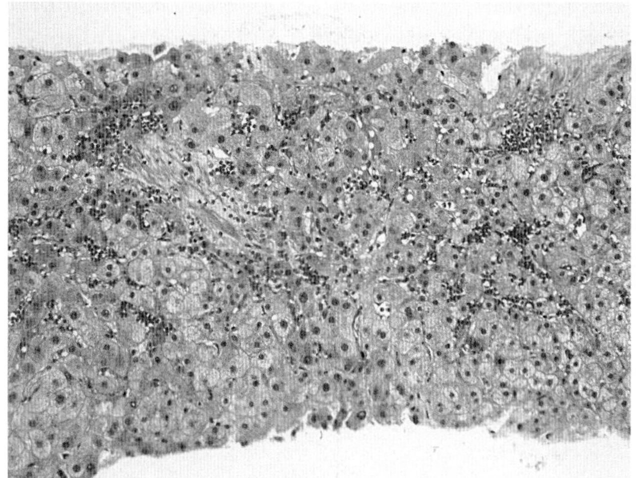

Figure 21.31 Chronic venous outflow impairment. Subtle zone 3 changes include mild congestion, sinusoidal dilation, and liver plate atrophy.

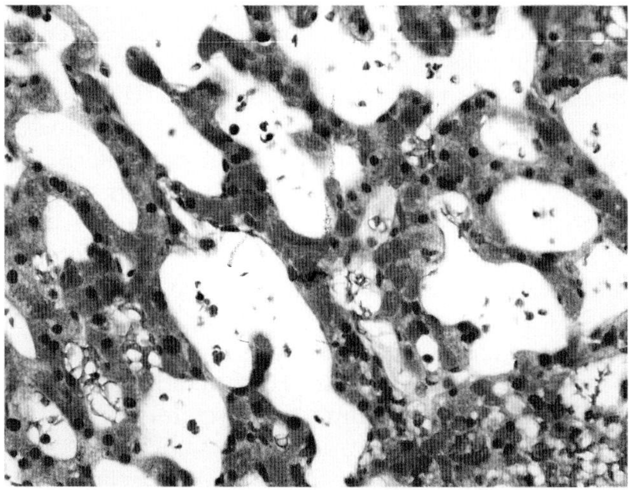

Figure 21.32 Chronic venous outflow impairment. Red blood cell extravasation into spaces of Disse (Trichrome stain).

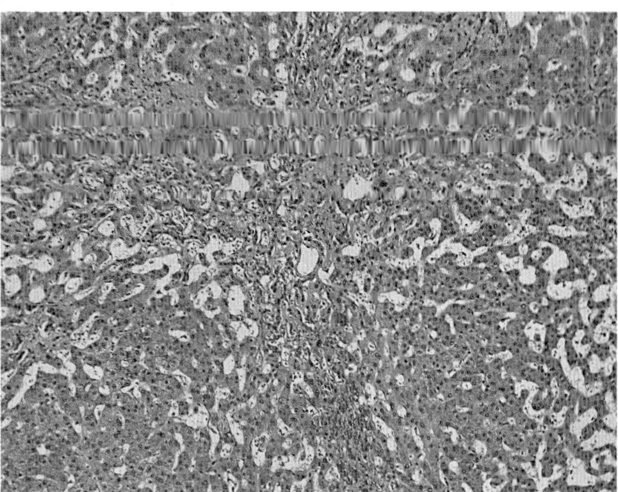

Figure 21.33 Chronic venous outflow impairment. Veno-to-venous congestion of fibrosis.

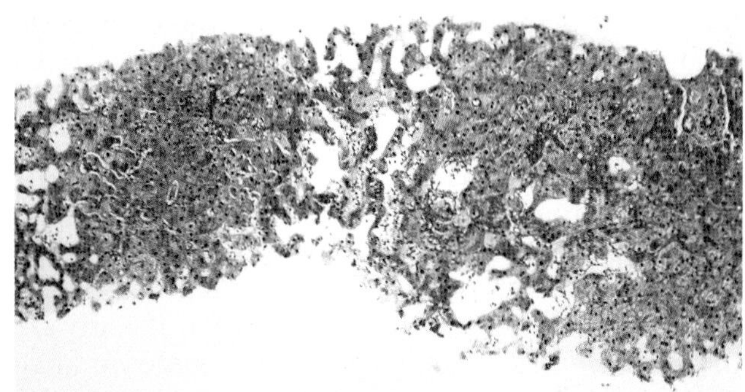

Figure 21.34 Chronic venous outflow impairment. Perivenular and sinusoidal fibrosis (Trichrome stain).

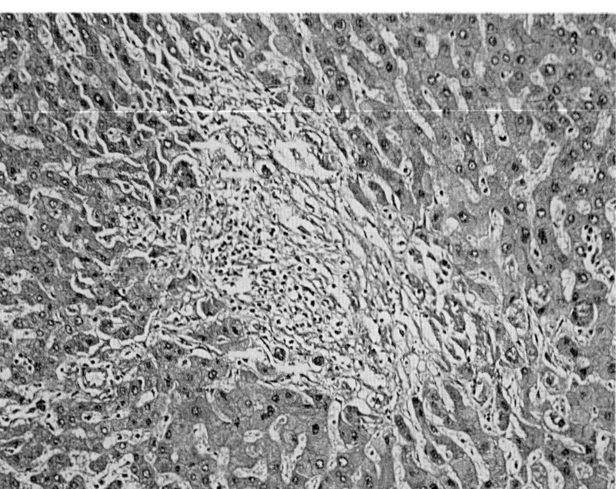

Figure 21.35 Chronic venous outflow impairment. A central scar in chronic venous outflow impairment mimics a portal tract by the presence of small vessels and bile ductular metaplasia (arrows).

loss of bile ducts because of the above-mentioned abnormal changes, especially when individuals with venous outflow impairment also have cholestatic liver tests.[57]

Budd–Chiari syndrome

Definition

Budd–Chiari syndrome is defined as thrombotic or nonthrombotic hepatic venous outflow obstruction at any level from the intrahepatic hepatic veins to the junction of the inferior vena cava with the right atrium.

Clinical features

Budd–Chiari syndrome can be classified as primary or secondary according to the cause, with no underlying etiologies identified in about 20% of cases. Primary Budd–Chiari syndrome is caused by intravascular thrombosis, whereas secondary Budd–Chiari syndrome is due to compression or invasion of the hepatic veins and/or the inferior vena cava by an outside lesion such as tumor or infection.[58] Blockage at the level of the hepatic veins is more common in western countries, primarily affecting women in their third or fourth decade of life. In contrast, blockage at the level of the inferior vena cava or combined blockage of the inferior vena cava and hepatic veins are more common in Asia, with a slight predominance of men.[59] At least 75% of patients with Budd–Chiari syndrome have hypercoagulable states due to either hereditary or acquired coagulative disorders, such as protein C deficiency, protein S deficiency, Factor V Leiden mutation, antiphospholipid syndrome, myeloproliferative disorders, pregnancy, malignancy, or use of oral contraceptives, etc.[60]

Budd–Chiari syndrome has a wide spectrum of clinical presentations, which depend on the location, extent, and rapidity of the obstructive process, as well as any underlying diseases. The clinical presentation has been classified into five categories based on the disease duration and severity[61]: (1) approximately 5% to 20% Budd–Chiari syndrome patients are asymptomatic. The disease is usually incidentally found during working up for abnormal liver function tests; (2) acute or fulminant liver failure, while uncommon, is caused by rapid and complete blockage of all hepatic veins. The patients rapidly develop hepatic encephalopathy with jaundice, markedly elevated transaminases, renal failure, and coagulopathy; (3) acute Budd–Chiari syndrome develops over the course of weeks with severe right upper quadrant pain, hepatomegaly, ascites and liver necrosis; (4) the subacute form has an insidious onset, and a disease course that develops over several months, with no symptoms or minimal ascites, hepatosplenomegaly, and mild jaundice; and (5) approximately 60% of patients with Budd–Chiari syndrome develop cirrhosis, which is referred to as the chronic form, and these patients first present with complications of cirrhosis.

Laboratory findings

The liver function tests may be slightly abnormal in patients with asymptomatic or subacute Budd–Chiari syndrome. In patients with acute liver failure or acute Budd–Chiari syndrome, the liver enzymes and bilirubin levels are markedly elevated. The transaminases can be over 600 IU/L, and the alkaline phosphatase is typically in the range of 300 to 400 IU/L.

Imaging

Imaging studies play a key role in diagnosing the Budd–Chiari syndrome. Doppler ultrasonography is the primary method, with a sensitivity and specificity of nearly 85%. Ultrasound shows obliteration of hepatic veins, thrombosis or stenosis, spiderweb vessels, or large collateral vessels. CT or magnetic resonance imaging (MRI) can be performed to confirm the diagnosis and assess liver parenchymal disease, but they are not as sensitive or specific as Doppler ultrasonography. Hepatic venography is the gold standard for diagnosing Budd–Chiari syndrome and can also demonstrate which vessels are involved, directing subsequent treatment. However, venography is not essential for most cases, which are diagnosed using noninvasive methods.

Gross findings

The macroscopic changes in the Budd–Chiari syndrome depend on the duration and pattern of venous blockage. In the acute phase, the liver is congested with patchy necrosis and hemorrhage. Later, regenerative nodules can develop (Fig. 21.36). Thrombi can be identified in hepatic vein branches. The hepatic portion of the inferior vena cava can show fibrotic thickening and narrowing, or a thin valve-like membrane. The portions of the liver with patent hepatic veins show hypertrophy, especially the caudate lobe, where venous outflow can drain directly into inferior vena cava. In the chronic cases, the liver is cirrhotic with a mixed micro- and macronodular pattern of cirrhosis. Large regenerative nodules may mimic focal nodular hyperplasia. Hepatic adenoma and hepatocellular carcinoma can also develop,[62,63] so all nodules should be adequately sampled. Scarred areas of parenchyma are also found, especially after large area of necrosis or infarction in the setting of coexisting portal vein thrombosis.[64]

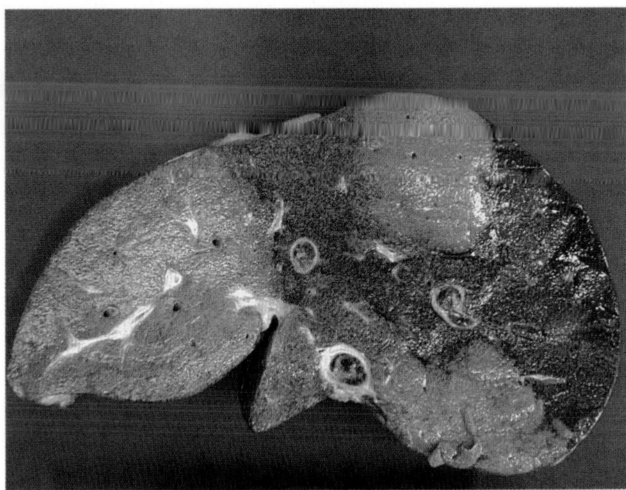

Figure 21.36 Budd–Chiari syndrome. There are thrombi in hepatic veins and large areas of hemorrhage and parenchymal collapse.

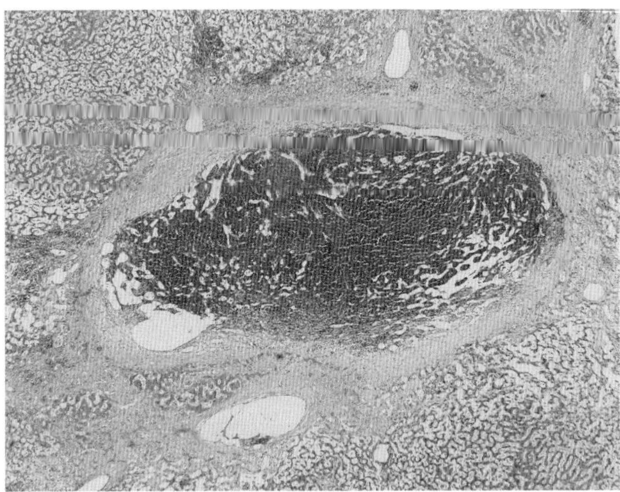

Figure 21.37 Budd–Chiari syndrome. An organizing thrombus in a small hepatic vein branch with diffuse sinusoidal dilation and liver plate atrophy.

Microscopic findings

Microscopically, the main features are those of chronic venous outflow impairment (Fig. 21.37). Hepatic vein thrombi are typically not identified in peripheral liver biopsies, except for thrombi originating in the smaller sized intrahepatic veins, or with propagation of the thrombi leading to extension from outside the liver into the hepatic veins. The zone 3 sinusoids are congested and dilated. The liver plates and hepatocytes are often atrophic and there can be hepatocyte dropout. With acute obstruction, red blood cells can migrate into the space of Disse. The extravasation of red blood cells is usually focal and often difficult to confidently identify. This finding may be easier to recognize on trichrome stains because the spaces of Disse become more apparent.

In the acute phase, variable degrees of perivenular liver necrosis and hemorrhage are also present. No significant inflammation is present in either the portal tracts or the lobular parenchyma. However, the portal tracts can show a mild bile ductular proliferation. There is no bile duct loss. In chronic disease, perivenular and perisinusoidal fibrosis is common, along with liver plate atrophy and liver cell dropout. Incomplete septa fibrosis can form, linking hepatic veins and leading to the venocentric pattern of cirrhosis, with the portal tracts showing little or no fibrosis (Fig. 21.38); however, if both hepatic veins and portal veins are blocked, venoportal cirrhosis can develop.[65] The scarred central veins can also sometimes show an ingrowth of bile ducts, making the liver architecture challenging to recognize. CK7 immunohistochemistry can show intermediate hepatocytes in zone 3. Obliterative portal venopathy is observed in some cases, because 25% of cases with Budd–Chiari syndrome have coexisting portal vein thrombosis.

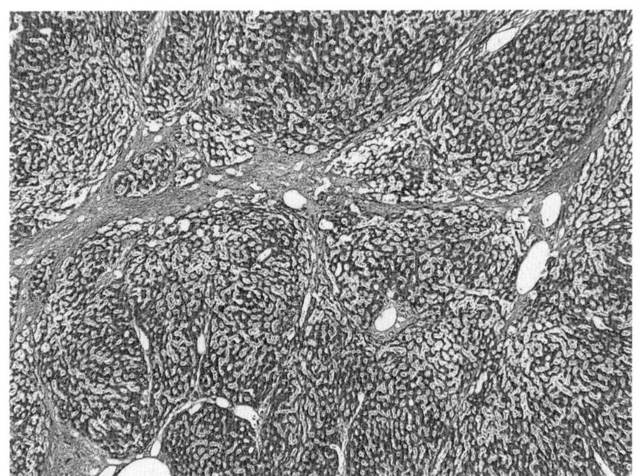

Figure 21.38 Budd–Chiari syndrome. Bridging fibrosis is seen (Trichrome stain).

Liver biopsies may appear normal if the tissue is taken away from the affected areas. For this reason, at least two biopsies from different lobes are recommended when evaluating for the Budd–Chiari syndrome. Although liver biopsy is not absolutely necessary for diagnosing Budd–Chiari syndrome, transjugular liver biopsy is often obtained during venography to assist clinicians in management decisions. For example, surgical shunts may be indicated if there is necrosis or liver transplantation when there is cirrhosis.

Immunohistochemistry and special stains

Trichrome stains are important for evaluating fibrosis.

Molecular genetic findings

Molecular genetic tests are not used to diagnose Budd–Chiari syndrome but are important to evaluate for coagulation deficiencies.

Differential diagnosis

Chronic venous outflow impairment due to congestive hepatopathy from heart failure has the similar histologic changes and histology alone cannot determine the level and cause of venous outflow blockage. Sinusoidal obstructive syndrome can also have some similar findings, but tends to have only mild sinusoidal dilatation and congestion. Fibrotic obliteration of the terminal hepatic venules, with no or mild sinusoidal dilatation, is typical of sinusoidal obstructive syndrome and rarely seen on liver biopsies in Budd–Chiari syndrome.

Prognosis and treatment

Survival depends on the duration and severity of the disease as well as treatment response and the underlying causes. More than two-thirds of patients survive over 5 years. A prognostic model using the presence of encephalopathy, ascites, prothrombin time, and bilirubin levels has been proposed, which classifies patients into good, intermediate, and poor prognostic groups. These groups have 5-year survival rates of 89%, 74%, and 42%, respectively.[66]

The management of Budd–Chiari syndrome focuses on restoring venous outflow by thrombolytic therapy or invasive procedures, such as percutaneous angioplasty, transjugular intrahepatic portosystemic shunts, or other shunt surgery. Medical treatment focuses on controlling ascites, preventing extension of the thrombosis, preserving liver function, and correcting underlying causes when possible. Liver transplantation is used for individuals with cirrhosis, fulminant liver failure, or biochemical evidence of decompensated liver function.

Congestive hepatopathy

Congestive hepatopathy results from hepatic venous outflow impairment due to any of the causes of right heart failure, including constrictive pericarditis, tricuspid regurgitation, mitral stenosis, cor pulmonale, or cardiomyopathies. The liver injury is caused by both passive hepatic congestion and coexisting reduced cardiac output. Most patients with congestive hepatopathy are asymptomatic, and liver disease is incidentally detected because of mildly abnormal liver enzymes. Mild jaundice is also common at clinical presentation. Some patients can have tender hepatomegaly, ascites, and jugular venous distention. Rare cases with congestive hepatopathy present with acute or fulminant liver failure or even death, but this severe form is mainly caused by shock or ischemic liver injury due to poor cardiac output, rather than passive congestion.[67]

Patients can be mistakenly diagnosed clinically as having a cholestatic or biliary disorder because laboratory tests usually show mildly elevated bilirubin and alkaline phosphatase levels.[57] Liver transaminase levels are mildly elevated in about one-third of patients, with the degree of elevation correlating with the extent of zone 3 necrosis seen on liver biopsy. Patients with hypotension or reduced cardiac output and extensive hepatic necrosis can present with strikingly high transaminase levels that can mimic acute viral hepatitis.

Grossly, the liver in congestive hepatopathy typically shows a "nutmeg" pattern (Fig. 21.39) because of the contrast between the congested and/or hemorrhagic zone 3 areas (red color) and the surrounding normal or fatty liver areas (yellow color). In long-standing cases, the liver can develop fibrosis and progress to cardiac cirrhosis.

The microscopic features of congestive hepatopathy are similar to the changes seen in Budd–Chiari syndrome, including zone 3 sinusoidal dilatation with congestion, atrophy of liver plates, hepatocyte dropout or necrosis, and variable degrees of perivenular and/or sinusoidal fibrosis (Fig. 21.40). In severe cases, lobular changes can extend into zone 2 or 1, resulting in larger areas of parenchymal loss (Fig. 21.41). Advanced fibrosis shows a venocentric bridging pattern and eventually leads to cardiac cirrhosis (Fig. 21.42). Some authors have suggested that congestive hepatopathy should

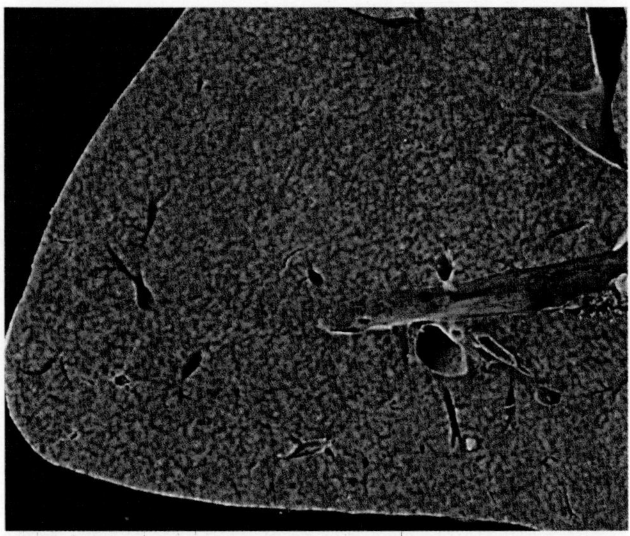

Figure 21.39 Congestive hepatopathy. "Nutmeg" appearance of liver on cut surface.

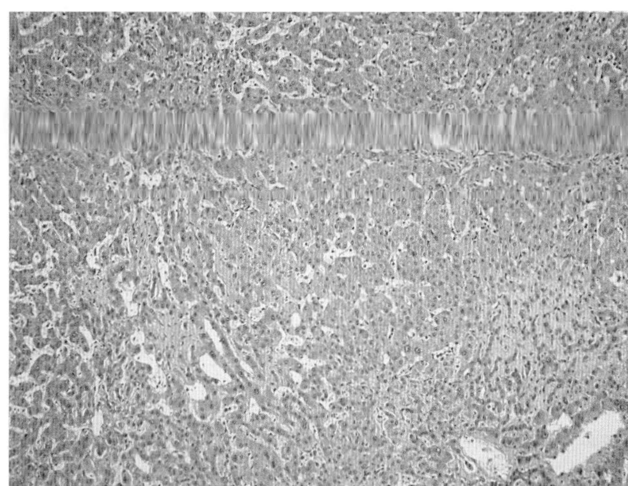

Figure 21.40 Congestive hepatopathy. Zone 3 changes including mild congestion, sinusoidal dilation, liver plate atrophy, and perisinusoidal fibrosis.

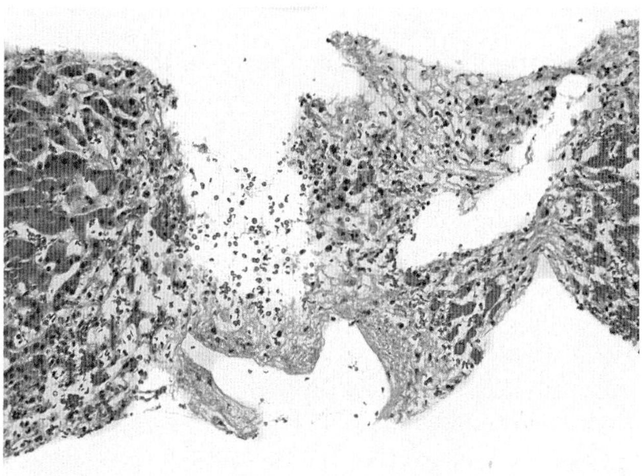

Figure 21.41 Congestive hepatopathy. Perivenular parenchymal loss is seen in a case of long-standing congestive hepatopathy.

be considered as the underlying cause of cirrhosis if the cirrhotic liver shows a venocentric fibrosis pattern, where regenerative nodules have spared portal tracts in the center, sometimes accompanied by marked sinusoidal dilatation. However, histology alone cannot distinguish congestive hepatopathy from Budd–Chiari syndrome, and correlation with imaging findings and clinical information is required.

The primary treatment of congestive hepatopathy focuses on managing the underlying cardiac or pulmonary disease. Early liver changes may resolve and fibrosis progression can be halted if the cardiac function is restored. Most individuals with congestive hepatopathy die of cardiac causes. Overall, the fibrosis stage of the liver correlates with the severity of heart disease, which is measured by hemodynamic

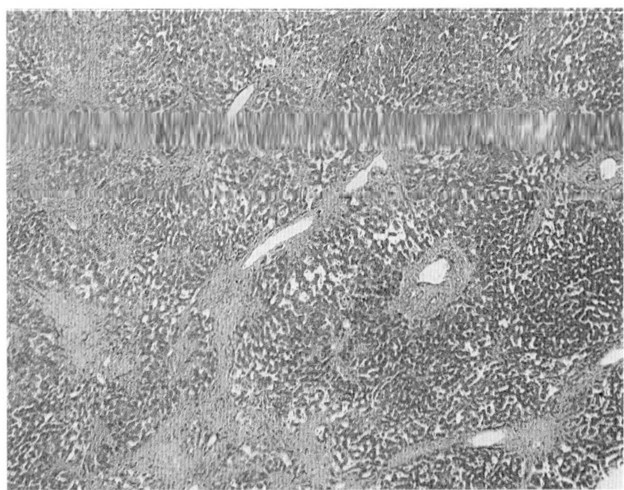

Figure 21.42 Congestive hepatopathy. Cardiac cirrhosis (Trichrome stain).

and echocardiographic parameters.[68] If patients with congestive hepatopathy develop cirrhosis, the risk of cardiac surgery and heart transplantation is significantly increased. Liver biopsy is a part of preoperative evaluation, especially when patients present with abnormal liver function tests or ascites. The presence of cirrhosis may exclude the possibility of heart transplantation, although combined heart–liver transplantations have been attempted. Patients with bridging fibrosis on liver biopsy may still undergo heart transplantation successfully.[69]

21.7 ARCHITECTURAL CHANGES AND TUMOR-LIKE LESIONS ASSOCIATED WITH VASCULAR DISORDERS

Nodular regenerative hyperplasia

Definition

Nodular regenerative hyperplasia is defined as diffuse small nodular transformation of the liver parenchyma with no or minimal fibrosis. Nodular regenerative hyperplasia can lead to noncirrhotic portal hypertension.

Clinical features

Nodular regenerative hyperplasia is a rare disorder of the liver with a reported incidence at autopsy of about 2%,[30] but it counts for approximately 20% of cases of noncirrhotic portal hypertension.[70,71] The majority of patients diagnosed with nodular regenerative hyperplasia are between 25 and 60 years old, but rare cases in children and even fetuses have been reported.[72] In early disease, individuals with nodular regenerative hyperplasia may be asymptomatic or have only mild nonspecific symptoms, such as fatigue, weight loss, upper abdominal pain, or mild elevation of liver enzymes. Disease progression is usually slow, but approximately 50% of patients with nodular regenerative hyperplasia at some point develop overt clinical portal hypertension.[73]

Although the pathogenesis is not fully understood, nodular regenerative hyperplasia is generally believed to represent an adaptive regenerative process of the liver, where the hepatocytes are responding to liver blood flow alterations at the level of microvasculature, either due to mechanical obstruction or vascular injury. The hepatocytes in the hypoperfused area undergo atrophy and apoptosis, whereas the hepatocytes in areas with maintained blood flow or hyperperfusion become hypertrophic. The alternating areas of atrophy and hypertrophy lead to diffuse nodular transformation of the liver. Oblitertive portal venopathy has been observed in many cases of nodular regenerative hyperplasia.[30,71] Medication-induced endothelium damage of the small hepatic veins has also been widely reported to lead to nodular regenerative hyperplasia, including immune modulators such as thiopurines for inflammatory bowel disease,[74] didanosine for HIV treatment,[75] and chemotherapy agents such as busulphan, thioguanine, cyclophosphamide, or oxaliplatin.[76]

Most cases of nodular regenerative hyperplasia are associated with an underlying disease, but some cases are idiopathic. The most common underlying causes include autoimmune disease such as systemic lupus erythematosus, scleroderma, rheumatoid arthritis, celiac disease, or sarcoidosis; inflammatory disease such as inflammatory bowel disease or HIV infection; malignant tumors including lymphoma; transplantation; hematologic disorders such as myeloproliferative diseases and congenital thrombophilias; pulmonary fibrosis or pulmonary hypertension.

Laboratory findings

Serum transaminase levels are usually normal or only minimally elevated, whereas alkaline phosphatase levels are disproportionately elevated. Elevated bilirubin levels are rare. Thrombocytopenia may occur in some cases early in the course of disease.

Imaging

Imaging studies usually show mild hepatomegaly and a diffusely heterogeneous hepatic parenchyma. However, these findings have poor sensitivity and specificity for detecting nodular regenerative hyperplasia. Ultrasound usually cannot detect nodular regenerative hyperplasia because of the smaller size and isoechogenicity of the nodules. CT or MRI scans can show isodense or hypodense small nodules, which appear different than focal nodular hyperplasia or hepatic adenomas.

Gross findings

Nodular regenerative hyperplasia is characterized by diffuse fine nodularity of the liver on cut surface and granularity of the capsular surface, often closely mimicking cirrhosis (Fig. 21.43). The nodules may be distinctly paler compared to the surrounding liver tissue. The nodules are small and usually measure 1 to 3 mm in diameter. However, the nodules may coalesce into larger nodules or pseudotumors in rare cases.[77]

Microscopic findings

Microscopically, the small regenerative nodules have two zones. The central zone consists of hypertrophied hepatocytes often forming double-celled liver plates. The sinusoids are compressed, and the terminal central veins can also be compressed and difficult to see on H&E. The surrounding peripheral zone of hepatocytes is usually in zone 3 and is characterized by thinner liver plates composed of smaller, atrophic hepatocytes. The sinusoids at the peripheral areas can be compressed or mildly dilated. These alternating areas of atrophic and hypertrophic hepatocytes lead to a vague nodularity of the liver parenchyma, often best appreciated at low power (Figs. 21.44 and 21.45).

Nodular regenerative hyperplasia can be associated with portal vein abnormalities, such as thrombosis. In these cases, the portal veins can show atrophy, fibrosis, or obliterative portal venopathy. Portal inflammation

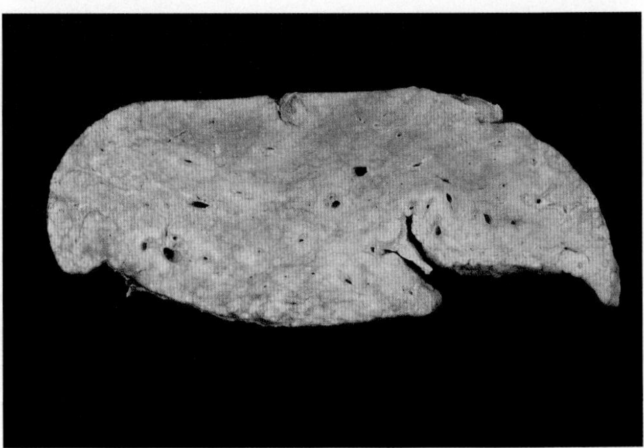

Figure 21.43 Nodular regenerative hyperplasia. Diffuse nodular formation is seen grossly.

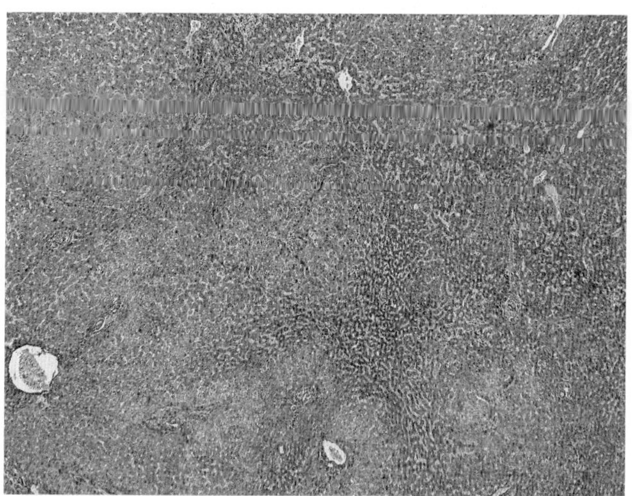

Figure 21.44 Nodular regenerative hyperplasia. Alternative hypertrophic and atrophic zones give the liver a nodular appearance.

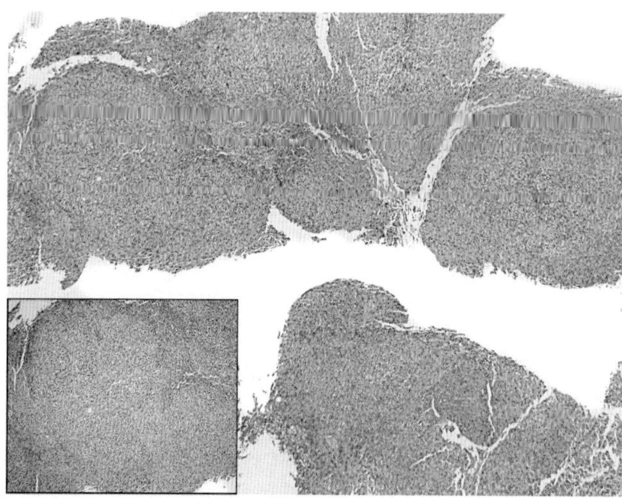

Figure 21.46 Nodular regenerative hyperplasia. A subtle nodular appearance is seen on liver needle biopsy (inset showing a nodule with atrophy at the periphery).

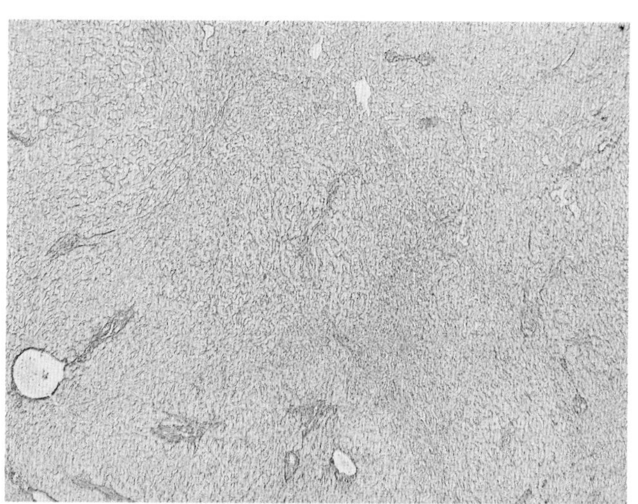

Figure 21.45 Nodular regenerative hyperplasia. A reticulin stain on the same case in Figure 44.

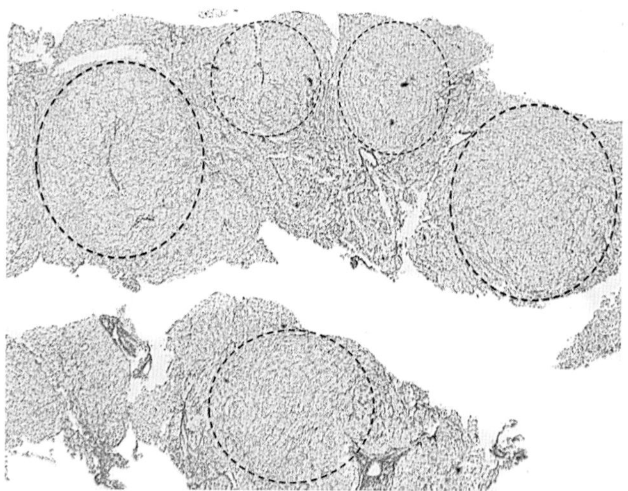

Figure 21.47 Nodular regenerative hyperplasia. A reticulin stain on the same case in Figure 21.46 (circles outlining the nodularity).

and bile ductular proliferation are absent. The lobules show no significant inflammation or fatty change. In some cases, the liver biopsy may appear almost normal, but a nodular appearance without obvious fibrosis is revealed after careful examination, often being best demonstrated by a reticulin stain (Figs. 21.46 and 21.47). Although the initial diagnostic criteria of nodular regenerative hyperplasia included focal incomplete septal fibrosis surrounding the nodules,[30] more recent definitions require no or very mild fibrosis. When present, there can be mild perisinusoidal or portal fibrosis.

Even though the diagnostic criteria of nodular regenerative hyperplasia have been well described, recognizing nodular regenerative hyperplasia in liver biopsy is often challenging, even for experienced liver pathologists. The interobserver agreement of diagnosing nodular regenerative hyperplasia among pathologists is still poor.[78] However, this applies to cases on the more subtle end of the spectrum. Well-developed cases of nodular regenerative hyperplasia are readily identifiable. Other factors that can limit recognition of this entity include small-sized biopsies.[79] The diagnosis of nodular regenerative hyperplasia is also very challenging to make in the setting of coexisting liver diseases, such as fatty liver disease, chronic biliary disease, or hepatitis. In these setting, the findings of nodular regenerative hyperplasia should be well developed prior to making such a diagnosis, in order to avoid overdiagnosis.

Immunohistochemistry and special stains

The reticulin stain is an important tool in recognizing nodular regenerative hyperplasia, highlighting the alternating areas of thickened liver plates and atrophic liver plates. The trichrome stain should show no fibrosis or very mild perisinusoidal or portal fibrosis. The presence of dense perisinusoidal fibrosis or more than mild portal fibrosis essentially rules out nodular regenerative hyperplasia as the primary diagnosis.

Differential diagnosis

The differential diagnosis for nodular regenerative hyperplasia includes other nodular lesions of the liver and other causes of idiopathic noncirrhotic portal hypertension (Table 21.1). Chronic venous outflow impairment also demonstrates significant zone 3 changes, but the sinusoidal dilatation with congestion and the dense perivenular and perisinusoidal fibrosis are inconsistent with nodular regenerative hyperplasia. Finally, some biopsies may have paler cytoplasmic staining of the zone 3 hepatocytes (glycogen accumulation), often in the setting of the metabolic syndrome and insulin resistance, which may give a vague nodular appearance to the liver parenchyma at low power, but the liver plates do not exhibit a hypertrophic and hypotrophic pattern.

Prognosis and treatment

Nodular regenerative hyperplasia is a slowly progressive disease, and the prognosis is related to the severity of the underlying diseases and the complications of portal hypertension. Therefore, timely recognition of nodular regenerative hyperplasia and elimination of the underlying causes are the primary treatment.

Focal nodular hyperplasia

Focal nodular hyperplasia is a common non-neoplastic nodular lesion of liver caused by hyperplastic/regenerative response to a localized hyperperfusion, one that develops as a result of arterial blood shunting through anomalous arteries, which are often identified in the center of the lesion (Fig. 21.48).[80] Focal nodular hyperplasia may occasionally receive blood flow support from portal veins if thromboses develop in the anomalous arteries.[81] Focal nodular hyperplasia can be seen in a wide variety of hepatic vascular disorders, including Abernathy syndrome, focal vascular shunts, and chronic venous outflow impairment.[10,12,82–84] The clinical and histopathologic features of focal nodular hyperplasia are discussed in Chapter 27.

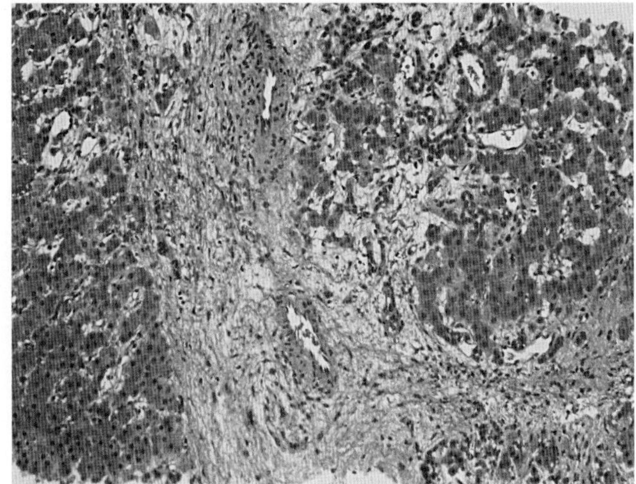

Figure 21.48 Focal nodular hyperplasia. Aberrant thickened-wall vessels in a focal nodular hyperplasia.

Segmental atrophy of liver

Segmental atrophy of liver is a pseudotumor caused by vascular injury leading to sequential pathologic changes, starting with parenchymal collapse, followed by an elastosis stage, and eventually a fibrotic stage.[85,86] Patients present with right upper quadrant abdominal pain or mass lesions that can be incidental findings identified at the time of surgery for other reasons, or by imaging.

Grossly, most lesions are subcapsular, firm, and have a whitish discoloration. The average size of mass is 5.2 cm, and they can be up to 10 cm. Microscopically, a sequential pattern has been described.[85] The earliest changes are parenchymal collapse with scattered islands of residual hepatocytes. Mild chronic inflammation and brisk bile duct proliferation are frequently seen. Elastosis within this stage is mild and focal (Fig. 21.49). The second stage of the lesion shows an increased amount of elastosis, with elastosis comprising 10% to 80% of the lesion (Fig. 21.50), whereas bile ductular proliferation and chronic inflammation are less prominent. The third stage is characterized by nodular elastosis. The lesions are almost entirely composed of distinctive well-delineated nodules of elastotic fibers, with scattered small islands of admixed residual hepatocytes and portal tracts (Fig. 21.51). The lesion in the final stage is composed mostly of dense fibrosis with occasional small islands of hepatocytes (Fig. 21.52).

Abnormal blood vessels can be found in all cases, which can show a mixture of thickened arterioles and venules with thromboses, fibrosis, and recanalization (Figs. 21.52 and 21.53). These vascular changes imply ischemic injury as the etiology, leading to atrophy of the liver segment with subsequent development of elastosis and fibrosis. The amphophilic extracellular

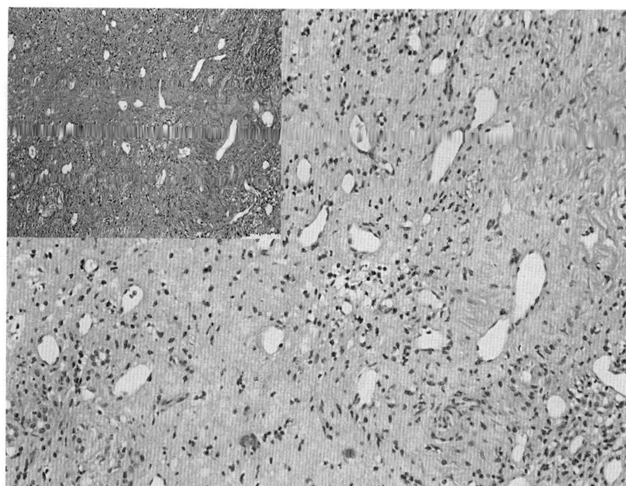

Figure 21.49 Segmental atrophy of liver. Parenchymal collapse with mild chronic inflammation, bile duct proliferation, and mild elastosis (inset, elastin stain) at the first stage.

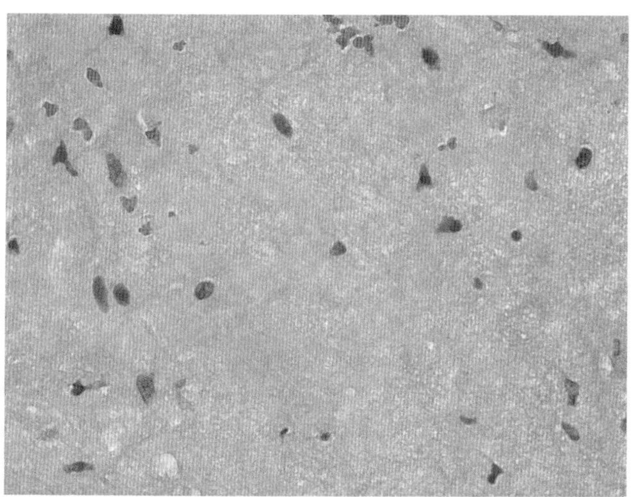

Figure 21.50 Segmental atrophy of liver. Elastosis is prominent.

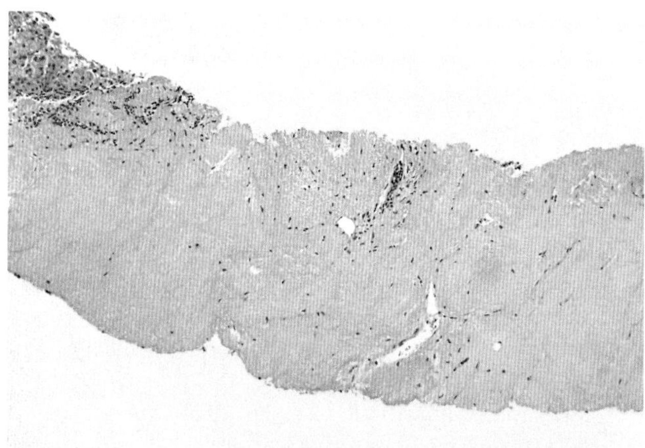

Figure 21.51 Segmental atrophy of liver. Distinctive nodular elastosis with scattered residual hepatocytes.

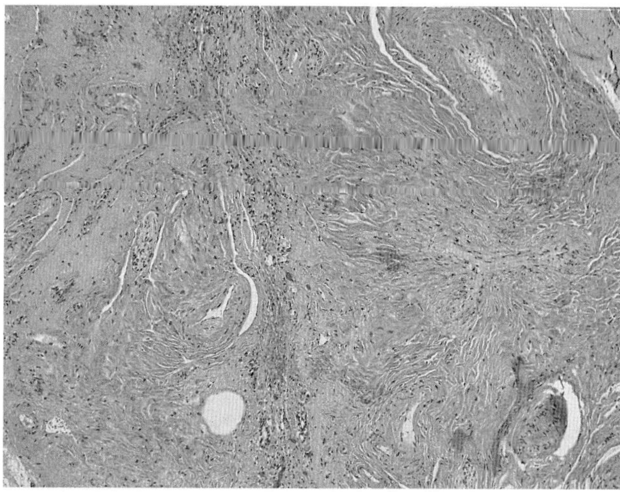

Figure 21.52 Segmental atrophy of liver. Dense fibrosis is seen in an end stage lesion. Note the abnormal vessels in the lesion.

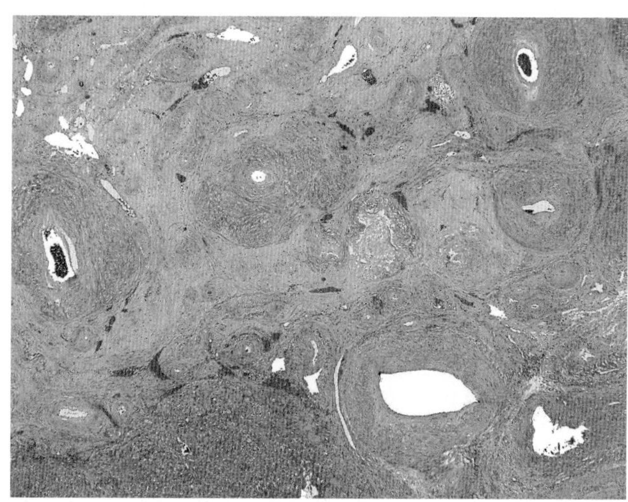

Figure 21.53 Segmental atrophy of liver. Abnormal vessels in different forms.

matrix of nodular elastosis should be distinguished from amyloidosis or myxoid stroma in epithelioid hemangioendothelioma. In addition, many cases also develop secondary simple biliary cysts, which result from bile duct obstruction (Fig. 21.54).

Partial nodular transformation

Partial nodular transformation is a rare condition characterized by nodular formation in the liver hilum, without significant liver fibrosis. This pattern of injury can result in portal hypertension.[31] The term partial nodular transformation was used to differentiate this injury pattern from nodular regenerative hyperplasia (diffuse nodular transformation, usually with smaller nodules) and focal nodular hyperplasia (discrete mass-forming lesions). Partial

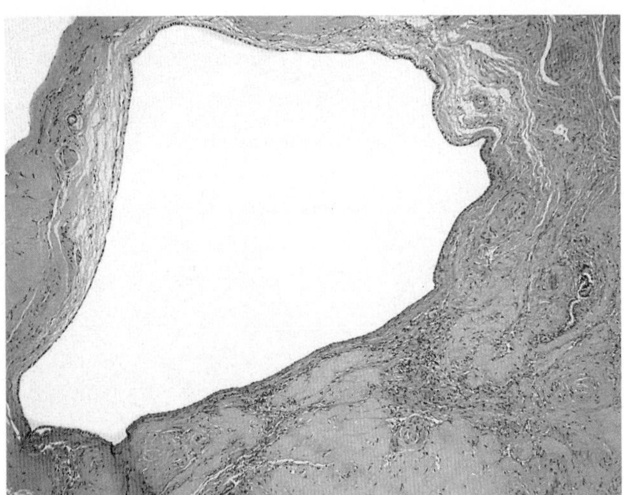

Figure 21.54 Segmental atrophy of liver. Formation of biliary simple cyst.

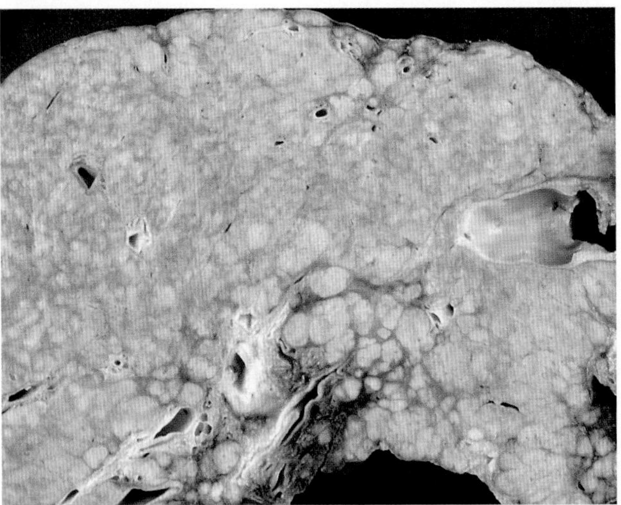

Figure 21.55 Partial nodular transformation. Coalescent nodular formation in the liver hilum.

nodular transformation results from the remodeling of liver parenchyma in the hilum after portal vein thrombosis.[87] Grossly, partial nodular transformation is composed of numerous coalescent nodules in the liver hilum (Fig. 21.55). The peripheral liver may be normal, atrophic, or have a nodular regenerative hyperplasia-like appearance. Microscopically, the nodules are composed of hyperplastic liver cells, but there are no fibrotic septa or rim surrounding the nodules (Fig. 21.56). Obliterative portal venopathy may be seen in the lesion or adjacent area.

Hepatocellular neoplasm with hepatic vascular disorders

Hepatocellular neoplasms can also develop in the setting of chronic vascular disorders of the liver.[88] For example,

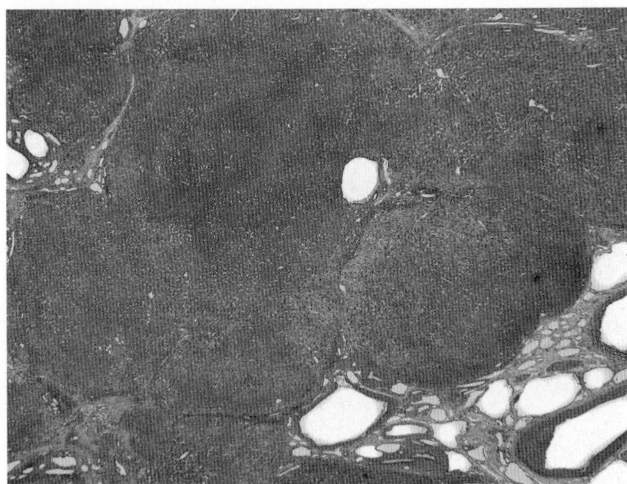

Figure 21.56 Partial nodular transformation. Nodular appearance of perihilar liver parenchyma with no significant fibrosis.

hepatocellular adenomas can occur in the setting of Budd–Chiari syndrome.[89] Hepatocellular carcinomas can also develop in different chronic vascular disorders, even without hepatic fibrosis or cirrhosis.[63,88,90] The morphology of those lesions is the same as hepatocellular adenomas and carcinomas arising in other diseases.

REFERENCES

1. Fraser-Hill MA, Atri M, Bret PM, et al. Intrahepatic portal venous system: variations demonstrated with duplex and color Doppler US. *Radiology*. 1990;177(2):523–526.
2. Carmi R, Magee CA, Neill CA, et al. Extrahepatic biliary atresia and associated anomalies: etiologic heterogeneity suggested by distinctive patterns of associations. *Am J Med Genet*. 1993;45(6):683–693.
3. Boon LM, Burrows PE, Paltiel HJ, et al. Hepatic vascular anomalies in infancy: a twenty-seven-year experience. *J Pediatr*. 1996;129(3):346–354.
4. Prokurat A, Kluge P, Chrupek M, et al. Hemangioma of the liver in children: proliferating vascular tumor or congenital vascular malformation? *Med Pediatr Oncol*. 2002;39(5):524–529.
5. Mo JQ, Dimashkieh HH, Bove KE. GLUT1 endothelial reactivity distinguishes hepatic infantile hemangioma from congenital hepatic vascular malformation with associated capillary proliferation. *Hum Pathol*. 2004;35(2):200–209.
6. Lane MJ, Jeffrey RB Jr, Katz DS. Spontaneous intrahepatic vascular shunts. *AJR Am J Roentgenol*. 2000;174(1):125–131.
7. Morgan G, Superina R. Congenital absence of the portal vein: two cases and a proposed classification system for portasystemic vascular anomalies. *J Pediatr Surg*. 1994;29(9):1239–1241.

8. De Gaetano AM, Gui B, Macis G, et al. Congenital absence of the portal vein associated with focal nodular hyperplasia in the liver in an adult woman: imaging and review of the literature. *Abdom Imaging*. 2004;29(4):455–459.
9. Kobayashi N, Niwa T, Kirikoshi H, et al. Clinical classification of congenital extrahepatic portosystemic shunts. *Hepatol Res*. 2010;40(6):585–593.
10. Lisovsky M, Konstas AA, Misdraji J. Congenital extrahepatic portosystemic shunts (Abernethy malformation): a histopathologic evaluation. *Am J Surg Pathol*. 2011;35(9):1381–1390.
11. Park JH, Cha SH, Han JK, et al. Intrahepatic portosystemic venous shunt. *AJR Am J Roentgenol*. 1990;155(3):527–528.
12. Lee SA, Lee YS, Lee KS, et al. Congenital intrahepatic portosystemic venous shunt and liver mass in a child patient: successful endovascular treatment with an amplatzer vascular plug (AVP). *Korean J Radiol*. 2010;11(5):583–586.
13. Chawla A, Kahn E, Becker J, et al. Focal nodular hyperplasia of the liver and hypercholesterolemia in a child with VACTERL syndrome. *J Pediatr Gastroenterol Nutr*. 1993;17(4):434–437.
14. Distefano G, Rodono A, Smilari P, et al. The VACTERL association: a report of a clinical case with hepatic cystic lymphangiectasis. *Pediatr Med Chir*. 1998;20(3):223–226.
15. Roulot D, Degott C, Chazouilleres O, et al. Vascular involvement of the liver in Turner's syndrome. *Hepatology*. 2004;39(1):239–247.
16. Noe JA, Pittman HC, Burton EM. Congenital absence of the portal vein in a child with Turner syndrome. *Pediatr Radiol*. 2006;36(6):566–568.
17. Garcia-Tsao G, Korzenik JR, Young L, et al. Liver disease in patients with hereditary hemorrhagic telangiectasia. *N Engl J Med*. 2000;343(13):931–936.
18. Scardapane A, Ficco M, Sabba C, et al. Hepatic nodular regenerative lesions in patients with hereditary haemorrhagic telangiectasia: computed tomography and magnetic resonance findings. *Radiol Med*. 2013;118(1):1–13.
19. Brenard R, Chapaux X, Deltenre P, et al. Large spectrum of liver vascular lesions including high prevalence of focal nodular hyperplasia in patients with hereditary haemorrhagic telangiectasia: the Belgian Registry based on 30 patients. *Eur J Gastroenterol Hepatol*. 2010;22(10):1253–1259.
20. Mavrakis A, Demetris A, Ochoa ER, et al. Hereditary hemorrhagic telangiectasia of the liver complicated by ischemic bile duct necrosis and sepsis: case report and review of the literature. *Dig Dis Sci*. 2010;55(7):2113–2117.
21. Lerut J, Orlando G, Adam R, et al. Liver transplantation for hereditary hemorrhagic telangiectasia: report of the European liver transplant registry. *Ann Surg*. 2006;244(6):854–862; discussion 62–64.
22. Chawla Y, Duseja A, Dhiman RK. Review article: the modern management of portal vein thrombosis. *Aliment Pharmacol Ther*. 2009;30(9):881–894
23. Ogren M, Bergqvist D, Bjorck M, et al. Portal vein thrombosis: prevalence, patient characteristics and lifetime risk: a population study based on 23,796 consecutive autopsies. *World J Gastroenterol*. 2006;12(13):2115–2119.
24. Chandra R, Kapoor D, Tharakan A, et al. Portal biliopathy. *J Gastroenterol Hepatol*. 2001;16(10):1086–1092.
25. Khuroo MS, Yattoo GN, Zargar SA, et al. Biliary abnormalities associated with extrahepatic portal venous obstruction. *Hepatology*. 1993;17(5):807–813.
26. Sogaard KK, Astrup LB, Vilstrup H, et al. Portal vein thrombosis; risk factors, clinical presentation and treatment. *BMC Gastroenterol*. 2007;7:34.
27. Sheen CL, Lamparelli H, Milne A, et al. Clinical features, diagnosis and outcome of acute portal vein thrombosis. *QJM*. 2000;93(8):531–534.
28. Ramos AP, Reigada CP, Ataide EC, et al. Portal vein thrombosis and liver transplantation: long term. *Transplant Proc*. 2010;42(2):498–501.
29. Schouten JN, Garcia-Pagan JC, Valla DC, et al. Idiopathic noncirrhotic portal hypertension. *Hepatology*. 2011;54(3):1071–1081.
30. Wanless IR. Micronodular transformation (nodular regenerative hyperplasia) of the liver: a report of 64 cases among 2,500 autopsies and a new classification of benign hepatocellular nodules. *Hepatology*. 1990;11(5):787–797.
31. Sherlock S, Feldman CA, Moran B, et al. Partial nodular transformation of the liver with portal hypertension. *Am J Med*. 1966;40(2):195–203.
32. Sciot R, Staessen D, Van Damme B, et al. Incomplete septal cirrhosis: histopathological aspects. *Histopathology*. 1988;13(6):593–603.
33. Bernard PH, Le Bail B, Cransac M, et al. Progression from idiopathic portal hypertension to incomplete septal cirrhosis with liver failure requiring liver transplantation. *J Hepatol*. 1995;22(4):495–499.
34. Ohbu M, Okudaira M, Watanabe K, et al. Histopathological study of intrahepatic aberrant vessels in cases of noncirrhotic portal hypertension. *Hepatology*. 1994;20(2):302–308.
35. Dumortier J, Bizollon T, Scoazec JY, et al. Orthotopic liver transplantation for idiopathic portal hypertension: indications and outcome. *Scand J Gastroenterol*. 2001;36(4):417–422.
36. Silva MA, Jambulingam PS, Gunson BK, et al. Hepatic artery thrombosis following orthotopic

liver transplantation: a 10-year experience from a single centre in the United Kingdom. *Liver Transpl.* 2006;12(1):146–151.
37. Ludwig J, Batts KP, MacCarty RL. Ischemic cholangitis in hepatic allografts. *Mayo Clin Proc.* 1992;67(6):519–526.
38. Francque S, Condat B, Asselah T, et al. Multifactorial aetiology of hepatic infarction: a case report with literature review. *Eur J Gastroenterol Hepatol.* 2004;16(4):411–415.
39. Mendes B, Oderich, GS, Macedo TA, et al. Ischemic liver lesions mimicking neoplasm in a patient with severe chronic mesenteric ischemia. *J Vasc Surg Cases.* 2015;1:4.
40. Psathakis D, Muller G, Noah M, et al. Present management of hepatic artery aneurysms. Symptomatic left hepatic artery aneurysm; right hepatic artery aneurysm with erosion into the gallbladder and simultaneous colocholecystic fistula--a report of two unusual cases and the current state of etiology, diagnosis, histology and treatment. *Vasa.* 1992;21(2):210–215.
41. Coppell JA, Richardson PG, Soiffer R, et al. Hepatic veno-occlusive disease following stem cell transplantation: incidence, clinical course, and outcome. *Biol Blood Marrow Transplant.* 2010;16(2):157–168.
42. McDonald GB, Hinds MS, Fisher LD, et al. Veno-occlusive disease of the liver and multiorgan failure after bone marrow transplantation: a cohort study of 355 patients. *Ann Intern Med.* 1993;118(4):255–267.
43. Jones RJ, Lee KS, Beschorner WE, et al. Venoocclusive disease of the liver following bone marrow transplantation. *Transplantation.* 1987;44(6):778–783.
44. Carreras E, Granena A, Navasa M, et al. On the reliability of clinical criteria for the diagnosis of hepatic veno-occlusive disease. *Ann Hematol.* 1993;66(2):77–80.
45. Fajardo LF, Colby TV. Pathogenesis of veno-occlusive liver disease after radiation. *Arch Pathol Lab Med.* 1980;104(11):584–588.
46. Weitz H, Gokel JM, Loeschke K, et al. Veno-occlusive disease of the liver in patients receiving immunosuppressive therapy. *Virchows Arch A Pathol Anat Histol.* 1982;395(3):245–256.
47. Shulman HM, Fisher LB, Schoch HG, et al. Veno-occlusive disease of the liver after marrow transplantation: histological correlates of clinical signs and symptoms. *Hepatology.* 1994;19(5):1171–1181.
48. Saint-Marc Girardin MF, Zafrani ES, Prigent A, et al. Unilobar small hepatic vein obstruction: possible role of progestogen given as oral contraceptive. *Gastroenterology.* 1983;84(3):630–635.
49. Goodman ZD, Ishak KG. Occlusive venous lesions in alcoholic liver disease. A study of 200 cases. *Gastroenterology.* 1982;83(4):786–796.
50. Nakanuma Y, Ohta G, Doishita K. Quantitation and serial section observations of focal venocclusive lesions of hepatic veins in liver cirrhosis. *Virchows Arch A Pathol Anat Histopathol.* 1985;405(4):429–438.
51. Corbacioglu S, Cesaro S, Faraci M, et al. Defibrotide for prophylaxis of hepatic veno-occlusive disease in paediatric haemopoietic stem-cell transplantation: an open-label, phase 3, randomised controlled trial. *Lancet.* 2012;379(9823):1301–1309.
52. Richardson PG, Soiffer RJ, Antin JH, et al. Defibrotide for the treatment of severe hepatic veno-occlusive disease and multiorgan failure after stem cell transplantation: a multicenter, randomized, dose-finding trial. *Biol Blood Marrow Transplant.* 2010;16(7):1005–1017.
53. Wang SY, Ruggles S, Vade A, et al. Hepatic rupture caused by peliosis hepatis. *J Pediatr Surg.* 2001;36(9):1456–1459.
54. Relman DA, Falkow S, LeBoit PE, et al. The organism causing bacillary angiomatosis, peliosis hepatis, and fever and bacteremia in immunocompromised patients. *N Engl J Med.* 1991;324(21):1514.
55. Yanoff M, Rawson AJ. Peliosis hepatis. An anatomic study with demonstration of two varieties. *Arch Pathol.* 1964;77:159–165.
56. Krings G, Can B, Ferrell L. Aberrant centrizonal features in chronic hepatic venous outflow obstruction: centrilobular mimicry of portal-based disease. *Am J Surg Pathol.* 2014;38(2):205–214.
57. Kakar S, Batts KP, Poterucha JJ, et al. Histologic changes mimicking biliary disease in liver biopsies with venous outflow impairment. *Mod Pathol.* 2004;17(7):874–878.
58. Bogin V, Marcos A, Shaw-Stiffel T. Budd–Chiari syndrome: in evolution. *Eur J Gastroenterol Hepatol.* 2005;17(1):33–35.
59. Plessier A, Valla DC. Budd–Chiari syndrome. *Semin Liver Dis.* 2008;28(3):259–269.
60. Valla DC. Hepatic vein thrombosis (Budd–Chiari syndrome). *Semin Liver Dis.* 2002;22(1):5–14.
61. Hadengue A, Poliquin M, Vilgrain V, et al. The changing scene of hepatic vein thrombosis: recognition of asymptomatic cases. *Gastroenterology.* 1994;106(4):1042–1047.
62. Sempoux C, Paradis V, Komuta M, et al. Hepatocellular nodules expressing markers of hepatocellular adenomas in Budd–Chiari syndrome and other rare hepatic vascular disorders. *J Hepatol.* 2015;63(5):1173–1180.
63. Paul SB, Shalimar, Sreenivas V, et al. Incidence and risk factors of hepatocellular carcinoma in patients with hepatic venous outflow tract obstruction. *Aliment Pharmacol Ther.* 2015;41(10):961–971.

64. Cazals-Hatem D, Vilgrain V, Genin P, et al. Arterial and portal circulation and parenchymal changes in Budd–Chiari syndrome: a study in 17 explanted livers. *Hepatology*. 2003;37(3):510–519.
65. Tanaka M, Wanless IR. Pathology of the liver in Budd–Chiari syndrome: portal vein thrombosis and the histogenesis of veno-centric cirrhosis, veno-portal cirrhosis, and large regenerative nodules. *Hepatology*. 1998;27(2):488–496.
66. Darwish Murad S, Valla DC, de Groen PC, et al. Determinants of survival and the effect of portosystemic shunting in patients with Budd–Chiari syndrome. *Hepatology*. 2004;39(2):500–508.
67. Kisloff B, Schaffer G. Fulminant hepatic failure secondary to congestive heart failure. *Am J Dig Dis*. 1976;21(10):895–900.
68. Dai DF, Swanson PE, Krieger EV, et al. Congestive hepatic fibrosis score: a novel histologic assessment of clinical severity. *Mod Pathol*. 2014;27(12):1552–1558.
69. Louie CY, Pham MX, Daugherty TJ, et al. The liver in heart failure: a biopsy and explant series of the histopathologic and laboratory findings with a particular focus on pre-cardiac transplant evaluation. *Mod Pathol*. 2015;28(7):932–943.
70. Naber AH, Van Haelst U, Yap SH. Nodular regenerative hyperplasia of the liver: an important cause of portal hypertension in non-cirrhotic patients. *J Hepatol*. 1991;12(1):94–99.
71. Nakanuma Y, Hoso M, Sasaki M, et al. Histopathology of the liver in non-cirrhotic portal hypertension of unknown aetiology. *Histopathology*. 1996;28(3):195–204.
72. Hillaire S, Bonte E, Denninger MH, et al. Idiopathic non-cirrhotic intrahepatic portal hypertension in the West: a re-evaluation in 28 patients. *Gut*. 2002;51(2):275–280.
73. Ferlitsch A, Teml A, Reinisch W, et al. 6-thioguanine associated nodular regenerative hyperplasia in patients with inflammatory bowel disease may induce portal hypertension. *Am J Gastroenterol*. 2007;102(11):2495–2503.
74. Shastri S, Dubinsky MC, Fred Poordad F, et al. Early nodular hyperplasia of the liver occurring with inflammatory bowel diseases in association with thioguanine therapy. *Arch Pathol Lab Med*. 2004;128(1):49–53.
75. Vispo E, Moreno A, Maida I, et al. Noncirrhotic portal hypertension in HIV-infected patients: unique clinical and pathological findings. *Aids*. 2010;24(8):1171–1176.
76. Ryan P, Nanji S, Pollett A, et al. Chemotherapy-induced liver injury in metastatic colorectal cancer: semiquantitative histologic analysis of 334 resected liver specimens shows that vascular injury but not steatohepatitis is associated with preoperative chemotherapy. *Am J Surg Pathol*. 2010;34(6):784–791.
77. Dachman AH, Ros PR, Goodman ZD, et al. Nodular regenerative hyperplasia of the liver: clinical and radiologic observations. *AJR Am J Roentgenol*. 1987;148(4):717–722.
78. Jharap B, van Asseldonk DP, de Boer NK, et al. Diagnosing nodular regenerative hyperplasia of the liver is thwarted by low interobserver agreement. *PLoS One*. 2015;10(6):e0120299.
79. Rousselet MC, Michalak S, Dupre F, et al. Sources of variability in histological scoring of chronic viral hepatitis. *Hepatology*. 2005;41(2):257–264.
80. Fukukura Y, Nakashima O, Kusaba A, et al. Angioarchitecture and blood circulation in focal nodular hyperplasia of the liver. *J Hepatol*. 1998;29(3):470–475.
81. Nakanuma Y. Non-neoplastic nodular lesions in the liver. *Pathol Int*. 1995;45(10):703–714.
82. Ibarrola C, Castellano VM, Colina F. Focal hyperplastic hepatocellular nodules in hepatic venous outflow obstruction: a clinicopathological study of four patients and 24 nodules. *Histopathology*. 2004;44(2):172–179.
83. Bouyn CI, Leclere J, Raimondo G, et al. Hepatic focal nodular hyperplasia in children previously treated for a solid tumor. Incidence, risk factors, and outcome. *Cancer*. 2003;97(12):3107–3113.
84. Choi JY, Lee HC, Yim JH, et al. Focal nodular hyperplasia or focal nodular hyperplasia-like lesions of the liver: a special emphasis on diagnosis. *J Gastroenterol Hepatol*. 2011;26(6):1004–1009.
85. Singhi AD, Maklouf HR, Mehrotra AK, et al. Segmental atrophy of the liver: a distinctive pseudotumor of the liver with variable histologic appearances. *Am J Surg Pathol*. 2011;35(3):364–371.
86. Spolverato G, Anders R, Kamel I, et al. Segmental atrophy of the liver: an uncommon and often unrecognized pseudotumor. *Dig Dis Sci*. 2014;59(12):3122–3125.
87. Terayama N, Terada T, Hoso M, et al. Partial nodular transformation of the liver with portal vein thrombosis. A report of two autopsy cases. *J Clin Gastroenterol*. 1995;20(1):71–76.
88. Kobayashi S, Matsui O, Gabata T, et al. Radiological and histopathological manifestations of hepatocellular nodular lesions concomitant with various congenital and acquired hepatic hemodynamic abnormalities. *Jpn J Radiol*. 2009;27(2):53–68.
89. Sobhonslidsuk A, Jeffers LJ, Acosta RC, et al. Budd–Chiari-like presentation of hepatic adenoma. *J Gastroenterol Hepatol*. 2005;20(4):653–656.
90. Park H, Yoon JY, Park KH, et al. Hepatocellular carcinoma in Budd–Chiari syndrome: a single center experience with long-term follow-up in South Korea. *World J Gastroenterol*. 2012;18(16):1946–1952.

22 Cytopathology of the liver

Yajue Huang, MD, Andrea Jones, MD, Michael Rivera, MD

22.1 INTRODUCTION

Fine needle aspiration (FNA) is a commonly used approach to determine the nature of a liver mass.[1–3] The average sensitivity of FNA is about 85%, and the specificity has been reported to be as high as 100%.[1,4–10] It is important to understand the clinical history of the patient in order to make the best use of the FNA material. In situations where immediate on-site evaluation is being provided, the cytopathologist can play an important role in making sure that the biopsy material is optimally prepared. In many cases, cell block material may be required to perform immunostains or molecular studies. In addition, in cases where lymphoma may be suspected, needle rinses in RPMI can be performed for flow cytometry analysis. Moreover, in some cases, cytology and cell block material may be insufficient to determine if a hepatocytic tumor is benign or malignant. In such cases, it is prudent to suggest a core biopsy. In some cases, the clinician may opt to perform a core biopsy upfront, in which case touch imprints or smears can be prepared from the core.

Liver FNA biopsy can be performed by individual puncture, coaxial biopsy, or tandem needle biopsy.[2,11,12] Each method has its own unique advantages, and the preferred method may vary according to the operators comfort level and the clinical circumstances of the patient. For instance, in the tandem method, an additional reference needle is utilized in parallel to guide the biopsy needle. This allows multiple passes to be performed, limiting the need for repeated imaging between passes.

22.2 NORMAL CYTOLOGY

FNA of normal or reactive liver parenchyma is comprised mostly of bland appearing hepatocytes. Hepatocytes appear as cells showing abundant polygonal cytoplasm with one to two uniform appearing nuclei (Fig. 22.1). The cytoplasm of hepatocytes shows a granular appearance and may contain lipofuscin pigment.[13] Bile pigment may also be identified. The nuclei frequently possess an easily identifiable central nucleolus. The hepatocytes are frequently arranged as flat sheets, but scattered single cells may also be seen. Intrahepatic bile ducts can also be seen in benign FNA specimens, represented as small clusters or sheets of cells with indistinct cell borders and small round

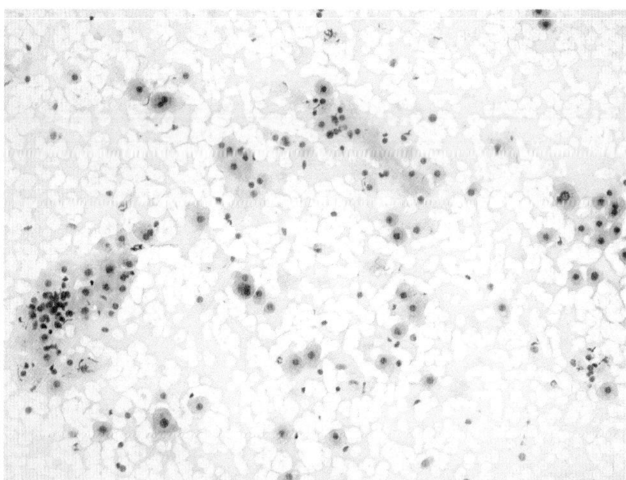

Figure 22.1 **Benign reactive hepatocytes.**

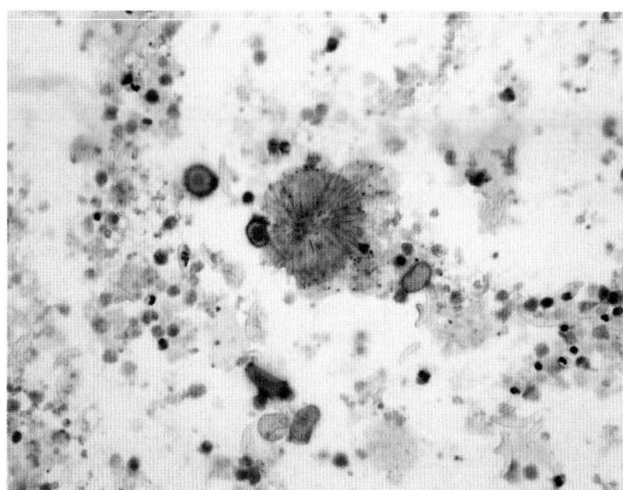

Figure 22.3 **Hooklets of *Echinococcus granulosus*.**

evenly spaced nuclei. Endothelial cells are usually inconspicuous; however, the elongated nuclei of endothelial cells can occasionally be seen along the edges of hepatocyte clusters. Prominent endothelial wrapping around hepatocyte clusters is usually not seen in benign liver samples. Kupffer cells can be seen in liver aspirates as single cells attached to hepatocytes. Kupffer cells contain round to oval nuclei with some of the nuclei showing reniform contours.

22.3 BENIGN LESIONS

Infections involving the liver can present as a mass lesion. An abscess is usually straight forward to identify because the smears are dominated by neutrophils and other inflammatory cells (Fig. 22.2). Clusters of epithelioid histiocytes, which may include multinucleated giant cells, indicate granulomatous inflammation. Although infection is a primary consideration when granulomas are seen, malignancies such as lymphoma, germ cell malignancy, and squamous cell carcinoma can also be associated with granulomatous inflammation. If a core biopsy or cell block is available, then special stains should be performed for microorganisms such as fungi, parasites, or mycobacterium. Parasites are difficult to detect on FNA but certain structures, such as the hooklets of *Echinococcus*, would be pathognomonic for parasitic infestation[14,15] (Fig. 22.3).

Focal nodular hyperplasia and hepatic adenoma are common hepatocytic tumors that are often biopsied. Both tumors show bland appearing hepatocytes that cytologically overlap greatly with the appearance of reactive changes, such as those seen in cirrhotic nodules. In focal nodular hyperplasia, fragments of stromal tissue and bile duct epithelium can also be seen.[16] Adenomas are typically comprised exclusively of hepatocytes; necrosis and hemorrhage can sometimes be seen in the background (Fig. 22.4).[4]

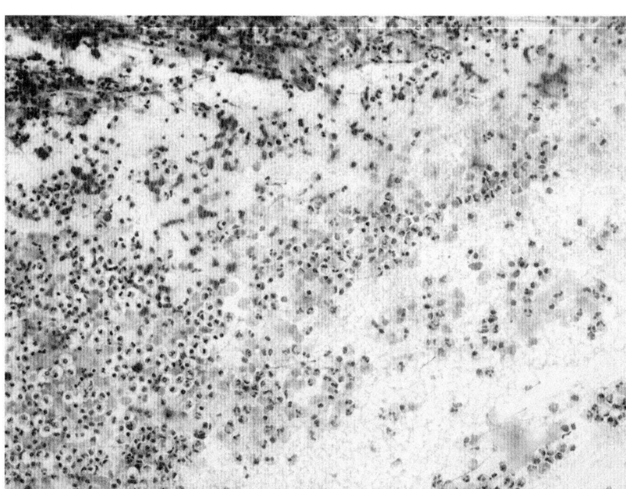

Figure 22.2 **Abundant neutrophils consistent with abscess.**

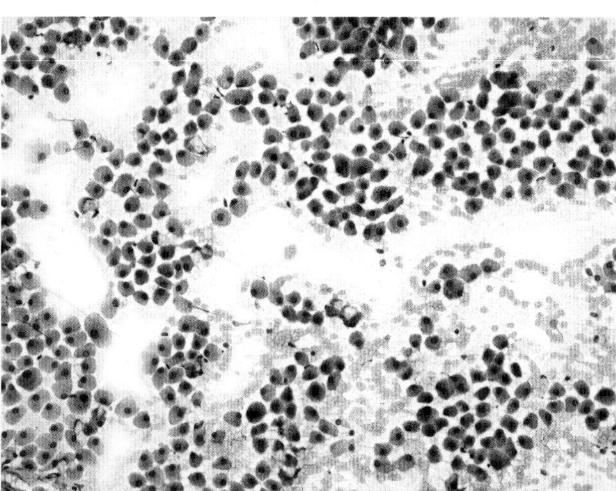

Figure 22.4 **Hepatic adenoma showing cellular smears comprised exclusively of bland hepatocytes.**

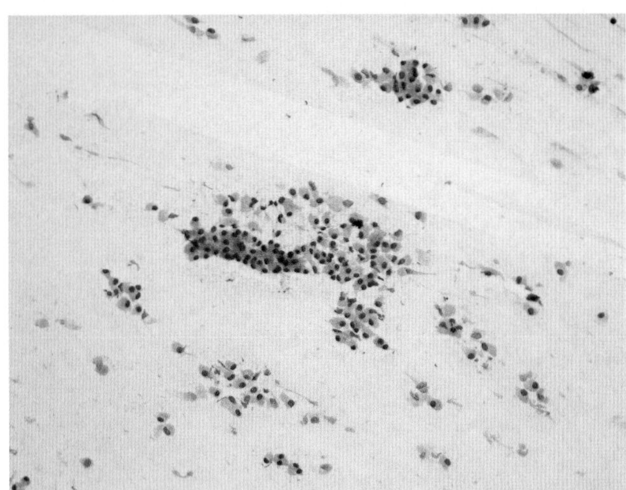

Figure 22.5 **Benign appearing glandular cells in bile duct adenoma.**

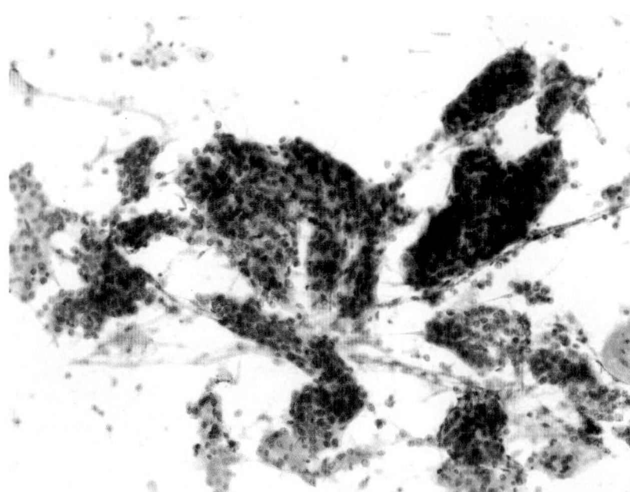

Figure 22.6 **Well-differentiated HCC showing thick irregular trabeculae.**

Bile duct adenomas and hamartomas are benign tumors of bile duct origin. Bile duct hamartoma and adenoma produce smears predominated by clusters of bland ductal cells with evenly spaced uniform nuclei (Fig. 22.5). The appearance of the clusters has been likened to that of a "honeycomb."

22.4 HEPATOCELLULAR CARCINOMA

Hepatocellular carcinoma usually occurs in the background of cirrhosis (~80%). Patients with hepatocellular carcinoma are typically older male individuals with a history of chronic liver disease. Although the cytopathologist should avoid biasing himself or herself with the clinical history alone, a diagnosis of hepatocellular carcinoma should be rendered with care when the clinical findings are not typical.

The gross appearance of smears from a hepatocellular carcinoma usually has a dispersed granular appearance in contrast to benign hepatocytic lesions which tend to produce smears with larger tissue fragments.[17]

Well-differentiated hepatocellular carcinoma can be difficult to diagnose on cytomorphology alone because the nuclei frequently do not look overtly malignant.[18,19] Cytologically, the low-power appearance of well-differentiated hepatocellular carcinoma usually consists of clusters of hepatocytes arranged as rounded nests and thickened trabeculae (Fig. 22.6). The trabaculae are usually three cells or more in thickness.

The clusters of tumor cells can be wrapped in endothelial cells (Fig. 22.7). Endothelial cell wrapping is relatively specific for hepatocellular carcinoma and is usually absent in nodules of cirrhosis.[19] However, benign hepatic lesions can also occasionally show endothelial cell wrapping. Therefore, endothelial cell wrapping of hepatocyte clusters should be interpreted in the context of the overall cytomorphology.[20] Thin-walled capillaries coursing through the tumor clusters, called "transgressing vessels," may also be present (Fig. 22.8). At times, the transgressing vessels show an arborizing pattern.[21]

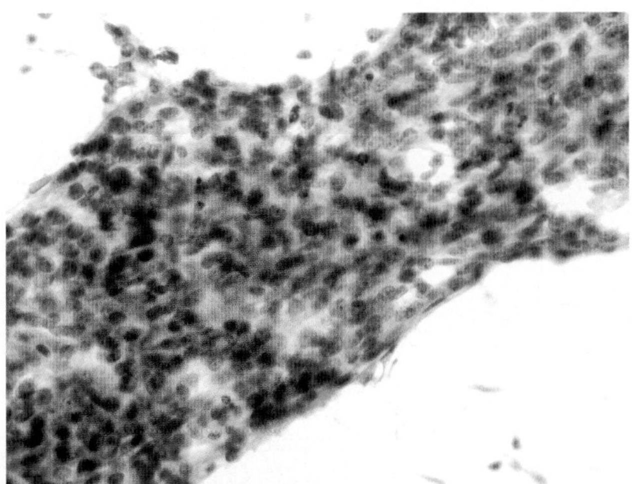

Figure 22.7 **Endothelial cell wrapping as seen by cells with elongated nuclei along lower border of cluster.**

Tumor clusters may be comprised of small hepatocytes with a high N/C ratio, as a consequence of a diminished amount of cytoplasm compared to normal hepatocytes. Large macronucleoli usually indicate malignancy. Moderately and poorly differentiated hepatocellular carcinoma tends to have granular appearing smears that result from the fragmentation of delicate cell membranes or from necrosis. As a result, numerous naked nuclei can be seen (Fig. 22.9). It has

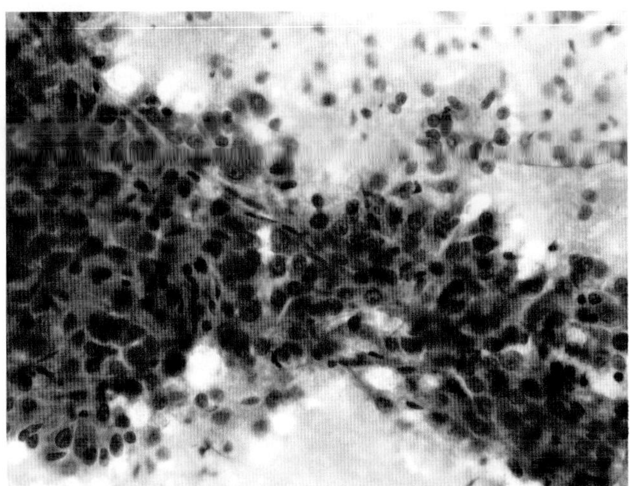

Figure 22.8 Transgressing vessel seen near center of tumor cluster.

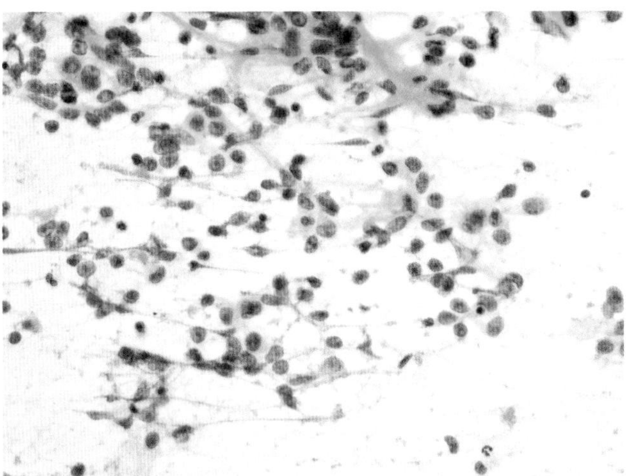

Figure 22.9 Naked nuclei in HCC.

been suggested that the presence of many naked nuclei will help distinguish hepatocellular carcinoma from other malignant tumors, but this not a completely specific feature.[22] In the case of moderately differentiated hepatocellular carcinoma, the cytology shows small intact clusters of cells having a similar degree of nuclear atypia, but having abundant polygonal cytoplasm. In addition, some cases of moderately differentiated hepatocellular carcinoma retain trabecular aggregates with endothelial wrapping, strongly supporting the diagnosis of hepatocellular carcinoma. Poorly differentiated hepatocellular carcinoma can be difficult to recognize because many of the typical features of hepatocellular carcinoma are absent (Fig. 22.10). Poorly differentiated hepatocellular carcinoma can resemble other carcinomas, including intrahepatic cholangiocarcinoma. It should be noted that combined tumors containing both adenocarcinoma and

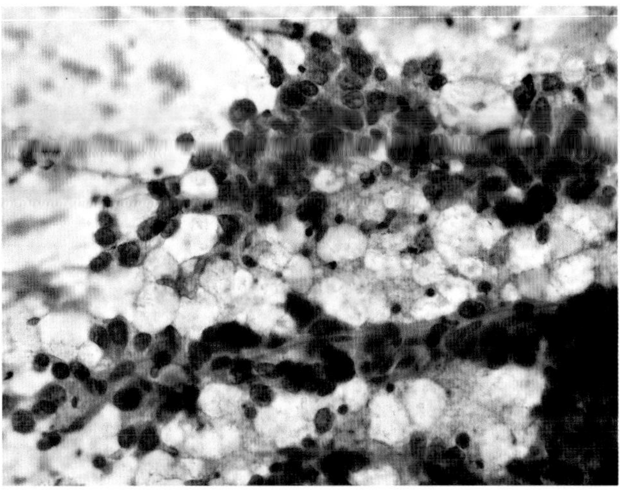

Figure 22.10 Poorly differentiated HCC.

hepatocellular carcinoma also exist. In cases of poorly differentiated hepatocellular carcinoma, acquisition of cell block material or a core biopsy is needed to perform immunohistochemical stains. Immunostains for markers of hepatic differentiation, such as HePar-1 and Arginase, as well as a battery of other stains to exclude various types of metastatic tumors, are usually needed.[23]

Several variants of hepatocellular carcinoma can be mistaken for other tumor types. Hepatocellular carcinomas with psuedoglands can be mistaken for adenocarcinoma. When numerous gland-like or acinar structures are present, the diagnosis of adenocarcinoma should be excluded. Large three-dimensional rounded aggregates may be a clue to the diagnosis of adenocarcinoma. Wrapping of endothelial cells around acinar or rounded clusters of cells usually indicates hepatocytic differentiation. Clear cell hepatocellular carcinoma, as the name indicates, is comprised primarily of cells with clear cytoplasm because of the accumulation of glycogen. The tumor cells may appear vacuolated. As a result, clear cell hepatocellular carcinoma can mimic metastatic adrenal cortical carcinoma or renal cell carcinoma (Fig. 22.11). It should also be noted that large tumors directly involving the liver and either the adrenal gland or kidney can have a complicated clinical-pathologic picture without a clear site of origin. Clues that assist in the diagnosis of hepatocellular carcinoma include the presence of bile, trabecular arrangements of tumor cells wrapped by endothelial cells, and Mallory bodies.[24] Immunostains for hepatocytic differentiation are of great use in this scenario, as are immunostains for renal cortical differentiation such as PAX-8.

Fibrolamellar carcinoma (FLC) has unique clinical and morphologic features. Smears prepared from FLC are comprised mostly of single cells containing large

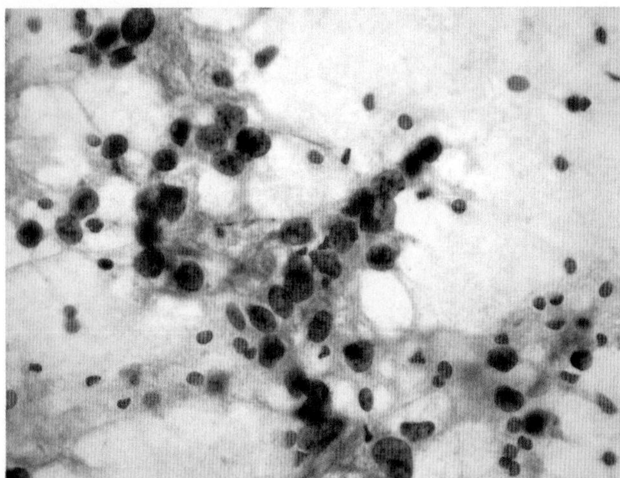
Figure 22.11 Clear cell HCC.

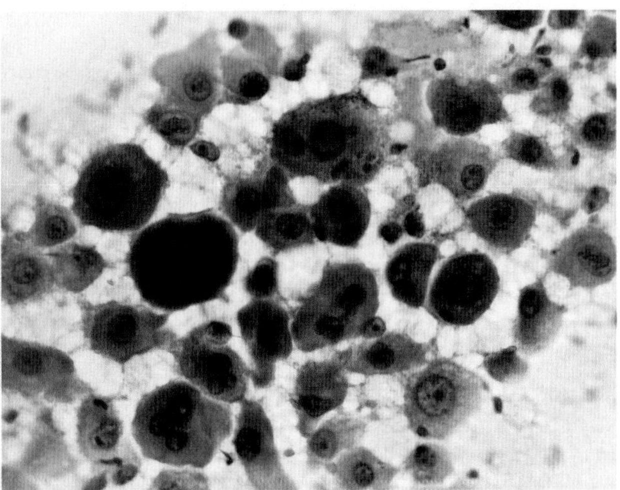
Figure 22.12 Fibrolammellar HCC showing single cells with abundant granular cytoplasm.

nuclei and prominent red nucleoli (Fig. 22.12). The tumor cells of FLC also contain abundant granular cytoplasm. Cytoplasmic pale bodies are also frequently seen. The abundance of cytoplasm may lead to the erroneous conclusion that the nuclei are not enlarged, because the N/C ratio may appear relatively normal. Trabecular aggregates and endothelial wrapping are not usually seen in cytology preparations of FLC.[25] Fragments of hyalinized stroma can also be identified, either in isolation or intimately admixed with tumor cells.

22.5 HEPATOBLASTOMA

Hepatoblastoma is a rare tumor of the liver that occurs in children, with 70% occurring before the age of 2. It is an embyronal neoplasm that derives from mutipotent cells. Hepatoblastoma has been reported in association with Prader–Wili and Beckwith–Wiederman syndrome. Hepatoblastoma can be classified as epithelial or mixed epithelial and mesenchymal types. Most cases occur as a single liver mass, however, up to 20% of cases show multiple masses. The epithelial types consist of embryonal or fetal appearing hepatocytic cells with oval to fusiform shapes containing large nuclei with prominent nucleoli. In cytology specimens, the cells are arranged as loose sheets, cords, and rosette-like structures (Fig. 22.13).[26] Pseudopapillary structures may also be observed. The small cell undifferentiated growth pattern is comprised of primitive appearing cells with sparse cytoplasm, imparting a small blue round cell appearance. When a mesenchymal component is present, spindled cells with dark nuclei and poorly defined cell borders can be seen. Osteoid may be seen, as can other forms mesenchymal differentiation such as skeletal muscle and cartilage. The differential diagnosis can include other primitive neoplasms such as metastatic neuroblastoma or Wilm tumor and rhabdomyosarcoma. Immunostains and molecular studies may be required to distinguish hepatoblastoma from other primitive appearing malignancies.

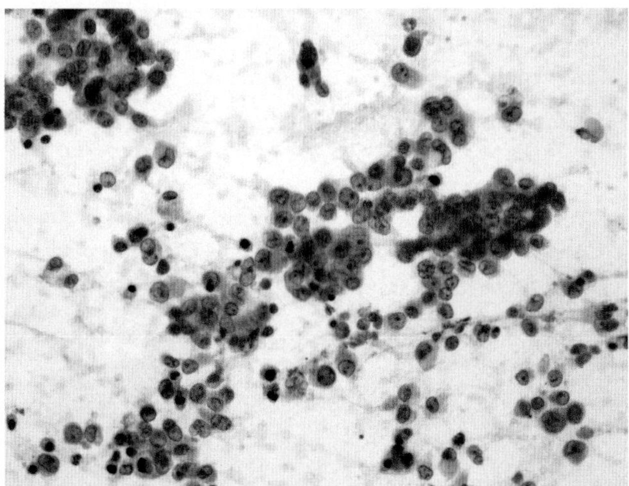
Figure 22.13 Hepatoblastoma showing primitive appearing cells with irregular nuclei.

22.6 NONHEPATOCYTIC EPITHELIAL TUMORS, PRIMARY AND METASTATIC

Almost all malignant tumor types have been reported to metastasize to the liver, and most malignant tumors involving the liver are of metastatic origin. The distinction between a primary malignant liver tumor and a metastasis is an essential, albeit sometimes difficult, task for cytopathology. Of course, in many cases, the diagnosis of metastatic disease can be strongly inferred clinically by the presence of numerous tumor nodules involving the liver on imaging. Most metastatic tumors to the liver are adenocarcinomas. The most common metastasis to the liver is from colorectal adenocarcinoma.[27] Metastatic adenocarcinomas have to be distinguished from primary cholangiocarcinoma.

Cholangiocarcinoma

Aspirates of intrahepatic (primary) cholangiocarcinoma produce smears comprised of three-dimensional clusters of tumor cells with all the hallmarks of adenocarcinoma (see later). They usually show significant nuclear pleomorphism and appear poorly differentiated. However, there are no specific cytomorphologic features to distinguish primary intrahepatic cholangiocarcinoma from adenocarcinomas of other sites. Immunostains are used to identify metastatic adenocarcinomas from other sites, such as pulmonary, mammary, or mullerian origin. Unfortunately, no specific immunohistochemical stains exist to confirm the diagnosis of intrahepatic cholangiocarcinoma. Instead, the diagnosis of intrahepatic chalngiocarcinoma rests on the exclusion of other possibilities by utilizing a combination of clinical, pathologic, and radiographic features.

Colorectal carcinoma

FNA specimens from colorectal carcinomas frequently show necrotic debris on the slides. The necrotic debris contains fragments of pyknotic nuclear debris that appears deeply basophilic on diff-quick stains and black/dark blue on pap-stained slides. Abundant neutrophils can also be present. Although necrosis is often a signal of malignancy, it should be kept in mind that an abscess cavity can produce a similar necrotic background associated with abundant neutrophils. Therefore, confirmation of malignancy rests on identifying the malignant epithelial cells. Adenocarcinomas typically produce three-dimensional clusters on smears.[9] The clusters found in metastatic colorectal adenocarcinoma can have a rounded appearance; however, branching imparting a trabecular appearance can also be seen. The clusters are usually tightly cohesive, but scattered single cells may be found in the background. The tumor cells usually contain cytoplasm with a delicate, lacy appearance. Cytoplasmic vacuoles may be seen, some containing mucin. When conspicuous, the presence of cytoplasmic vacuoles usually indicates glandular differentiation. Nuclear pleomorphism, coarse chromatin, and prominent central nucleoli are frequently observed. The histologic appearance of stratified nuclei imparting a "picket fence" arrangement can also be appreciated on cytology specimens, when the glands are oriented on edge (Fig. 22.14). This finding can also sometimes be appreciated at the edges of large rounded clusters of tumor cells as well. Although the aforementioned clues are helpful in identifying metastatic colorectal adenocarcinoma, no one cytomorphological feature is specific. Other adenocarcinomas, especially those showing enteric differentiation, can have a similar appearance, including cholangiocarcinoma (whether intrahepatic or extrahepatic in origin) or adenocarcinomas from sites other than the gastrointestinal tract. Positive staining for CDX-2 combined with a CK20 positive, CK7 negative cytokeratin profile can help support a colorectal origin in the appropriate clinical context.

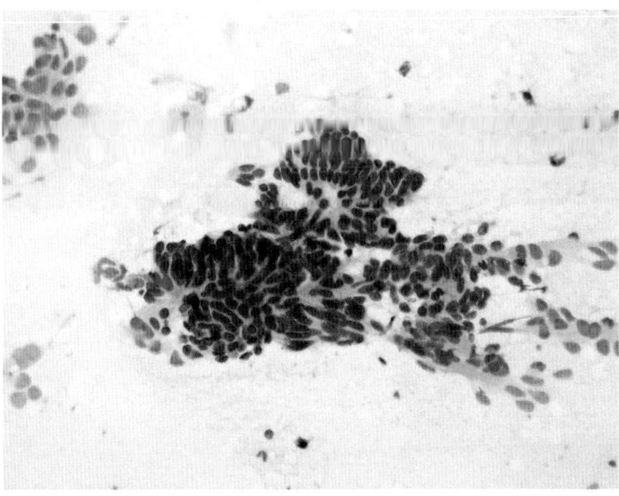

Figure 22.14 Picket fence arrangement of nuclei seen along the edge of the clusters from metastatic colorectal adenocarcinoma.

Prostate adenocarcinoma

Metastatic adenocarcinoma from the prostate frequently forms branched or acinar appearing clusters of tumor cells (Fig. 22.15). The nuclei are enlarged, but frequently show a uniform appearance with minimal pleomorphism. Large central nucleoli are a consistent feature. Higher grade prostate adenocarcinomas may not show acinar formations and may show significant nuclear pleomorphism. The uniformity of the nuclei in prostate adenocarcinoma may mimic the uniform appearance seen in well-differentiated neuroendocrine tumors. Immunostaining for PSA and prostatic acid phosphatase performed on cell block/core biopsy material are usually needed in this situation. Caution should be exercised not to interpret positive immunostains for chromogranin and synaptophysin as

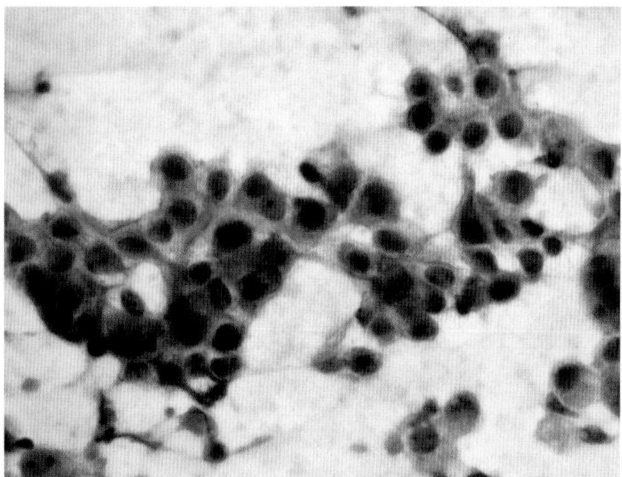

Figure 22.15 Metastatic prostate adenocarcinoma.

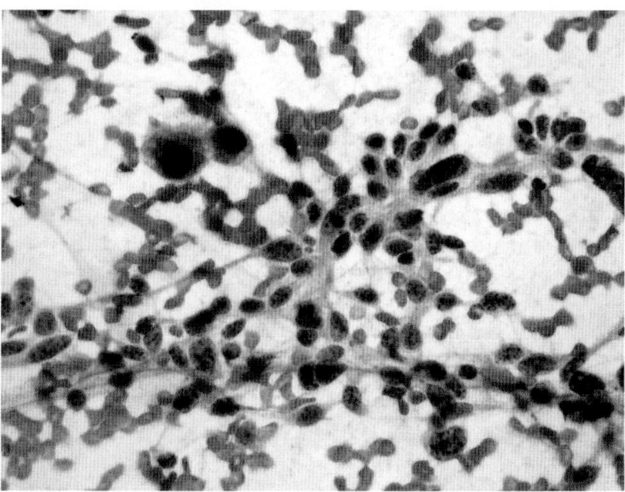

Figure 22.16 Metastatic well-differentiated neuroendocrine tumor with "salt and pepper" chromatin.

pathognomonic for the diagnosis of a neuroendocrine tumor in the setting of known metastatic prostate adenocarcinoma. Some prostate adenocarcinomas can show neuroendocrine differentiation, especially those tumors that become insensitive to androgen depravation therapy.

Neuroendocrine tumors

Well-differentiated neuroendocrine tumors involving the liver, whether primary or metastatic, have a unique appearance that usually reliably separates this group of tumors from other epithelial malignancies.[27] The smears of neuroendocrine tumors can produce clusters that appear acinar, trabecular, or branching, but usually have a flatter depth when compared with adenocarcinomas. Usually, the clusters are only loosely cohesive, with many single cells present in the background. Alternatively, the smears may be predominately single cells. The nuclei are enlarged, being two to three times the diameter of an erythrocyte; however, only mild nuclear pleomorphism is usually seen. Indeed, the monomorphic appearance of the nuclei can serve as a useful clue to identify neuroendocrine tumors.[18] The nuclei are frequently eccentrically placed in the tumor cells, imparting a plasmacytoid appearance. The chromatin has a finely granular look, which is commonly referred to as "salt and pepper" chromatin (Fig. 22.16).

High-grade neuroendocrine carcinomas can have either large or small cell morphology. Smears of small cell carcinomas are usually highly cellular with a background of necrosis. Sometimes, the necrotic background predominates with only a few viable tumor cells present. Small cell carcinoma can show the classic "oat cell" morphology, characterized by nuclei that are roughly two times the size of an average lymphocyte. The tumor cells of small cell carcinoma contain sparse cytoplasm and therefore have a very high nuclear to cytoplasmic ratio (Fig. 22.17). The nuclei are hyperchromatic in appearance, with finely granular chromatin. Nucleoli are either absent or inconspicuous. The nuclei are frequently degenerated, imparting a pyknotic appearance. Closely opposed nuclei creating a molded appearance can be identified.

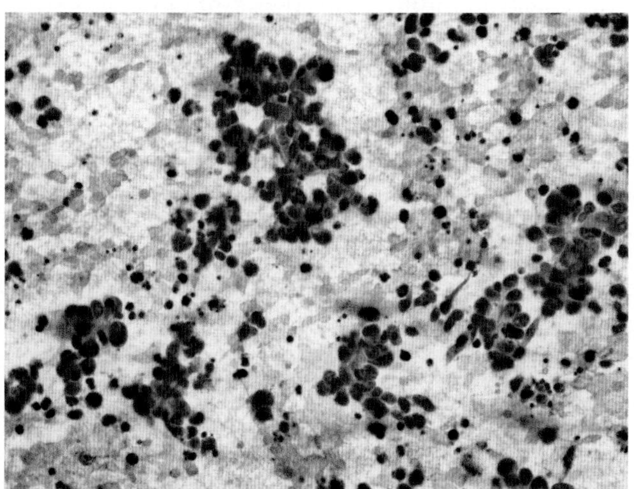

Figure 22.17 Metastatic small cell carcinoma.

The tumor cells of small cell carcinoma are delicate and are easily disrupted by the mechanical shearing forces that occur during smearing. The result is that the tumor cells frequently appear crushed. In addition, the nuclei can have a streaked appearance that is created as the nuclei are drawn out into elongated filaments or string-like structures. The appearance is somewhat similar to azzopardi artifact in histologic sections.

Variations in the appearance of small cell carcinoma may create diagnostic difficulties, such as spindled morphology or tumor cells with more abundant cytoplasm than usual. In addition, the appearance may overlap with other malignancies showing small round cell morphology, such as primitive neuroectodermal tumor or lymphoma. The presence of cytoplasmic fragments simulating lymphoglandular bodies can mimic the appearance of lymphoma. However, in the case of high-grade lymphoma, the chromatin is usually coarser, and multiple chromocenters are usually present. When performing rapid on-site assessment, it is usually a good idea to ask for a core biopsy or acquire material for a cell block preparation to perform immunostains for the confirmation of the diagnosis of small cell carcinoma.

Squamous cell carcinoma

Metastatic keratinizing (well or moderately differentiated) squamous cell carcinoma usually presents no major diagnostic difficulty because the dense cytoplasm of the cells and the presence of keratinization are usually a strong indication of squamous differentiation. Squamous differentiation is best demonstrated on Papanicolaou-stained slides by the appearance of dense cytoplasm with a hyaline or glassy appearance. In addition, the hue of the cells is either deeply cyanophilic or orangeophilic (Fig. 22.18). The cells of squamous cell carcinoma frequently show a wide array of shapes and sizes, including spindle- and tadpole-shaped cells. Significant nuclear pleomorphism is usually seen, with the nuclei usually appearing markedly hyperchromatic and frequently pyknotic. As the chromatin is densely staining, nucleoli are less readily observed compared to adenocarcinoma. However, it should be noted that mixed carcinomas such as adenosquamous carcinoma and combined small cell carcinoma exist. The presence of squamous differentiation does not negate the presence of other clues that may indicate a carcinoma with mixed differentiation. In the case of combined (mixed) small-cell carcinoma, this may result in significant treatment differences. Poorly differentiated squamous cell carcinoma can be difficult to distinguish from other poorly differentiated and high-grade carcinomas, such as poorly differentiated adenocarcinoma, and immunostains are often needed.

Adrenal cortical carcinoma

Metastatic adrenal cortical carcinoma can be challenging to differentiate from hepatocellular carcinoma in FNA specimens.[29] Most adrenal cortical carcinomas present with large adrenal masses.[30] Therefore, when examining FNAs from the liver, it is usually prudent to review the radiographic findings. If there are any additional mass lesions in adjacent organs, such as the kidney and adrenal gland, then careful consideration should be given to the possibility of a metastatic adrenal or renal tumor. Metastatic adrenal carcinoma usually produces cellular smears comprised of cells with abundant, finely granular cytoplasm (Fig. 22.19). Vacuolated cells or cells with a foamy appearance can be seen. Nuclear pleomorphism is common, and stripped naked nuclei may be seen. The tumor cells are usually arranged singly and in flattened clusters. The clusters may contain thin-walled blood vessels that can mimic transgressing vessels seen in hepatocellular carcinoma. Peripheral wrapping of endothelial cells can also be occasionally seen. Oncocytic adrenal carcinomas can be particularly challenging

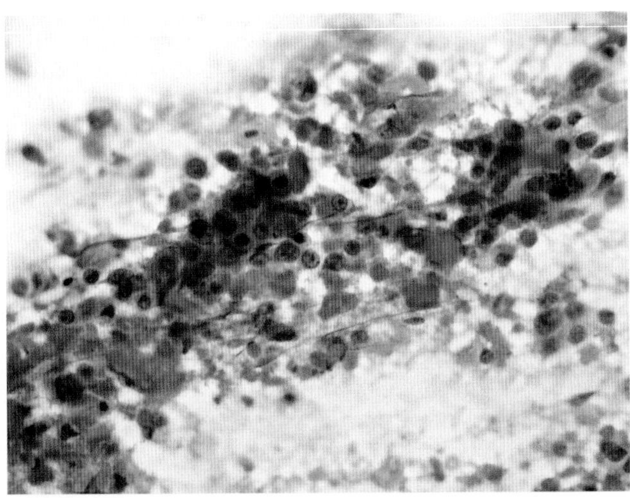

Figure 22.18 Metastatic squamous cell carcinoma.

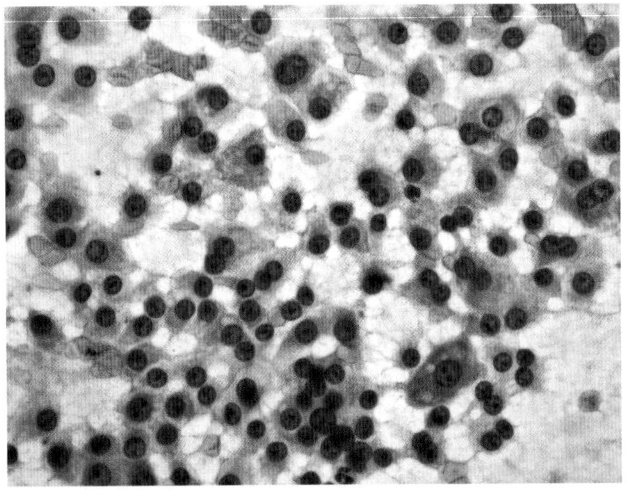

Figure 22.19 Metastatic adrenal cortical carcinoma.

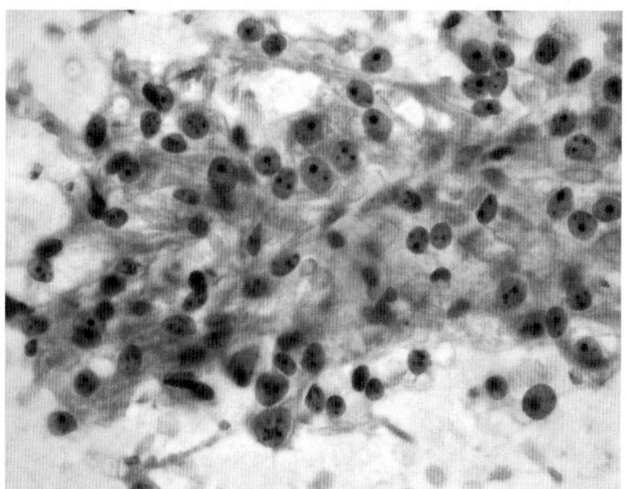

Figure 22.20 **Metastatic renal cell carcinoma.**

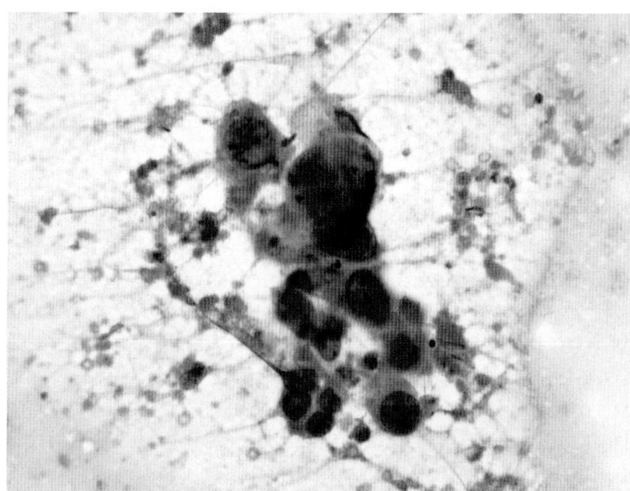

Figure 22.21 **Syncytiotropblast and cytotrophoblast cells of metastatic choriocarcinoma.**

to distinguish from hepatocellular carcinoma owing to their cytological similarity to hepatocytes. A cell block or core biopsy is usually necessary to perform immunostains such as melan-A, inhibin, and calretinin (along with markers of hepatocytic differentiation) to determine the nature of the lesion.

Renal cell carcinoma

The morphology of metastatic renal cell carcinoma varies depending on the subtype. The most common type, clear cell renal cell carcinoma, usually consists of cells with foamy, vacuolated, or granular cytoplasm[31] (Fig. 22.20). The tumor cells are arranged singly or in relatively flat sheets. The tumor cells contain nuclei with conspicuous central nucleoli, which become larger as the tumor becomes higher grade. The cytoplasm of tumor cells in high-grade clear cell renal cell carcinoma usually becomes densely granular and can be difficult to distinguish from hepatocellular carcinoma without using immunohistochemistry. Because clear cell renal cell carcinoma is a very vascular tumor, many erythrocytes are usually seen in the background. The tumor clusters frequently contain branching capillaries that resemble transgressing vessels of hepatocellular carcinoma. However, wrapping of tumor clusters by endothelial cells is uncommon in renal cell carcinoma.

Germ cell malignancies

Metastatic germ cell tumors show diverse morphologic and cytologic features, which can be a source of confusion diagnostically. Most patients with germ cell tumors are younger in age and many present in the second to third decade of life. In patients with extragonadal disease, a mean age of 19.9 years is reported.[32] Seminoma/dysgerminoma smears are highly cellular, showing mostly single cells with large nuclei, coarse chromatin, and a large nucleolus. Strands of cytoplasm containing, proteinaceous fluid, and glycogen form the characteristic reticular, or "tigroid," pattern in the background.

Yolk sac tumor shows cohesive groups of cells with traversing vessels. Papillary clusters may be seen. Hyaline basement membrane-like material may be closely associated with the tumor clusters, appearing green or blue in color on Papanicolaou stains.[32] The hepatoid variant of yolk sac tumor can be a source of diagnostic confusion with hepatocellular carcinoma on cytology specimens.[33] The polygonal appearance of the tumor cells and the presence of entrapped endothelial cells can resemble the appearance of hepatocellular carcinoma. In most cases, knowledge of the clinical history and imaging studies and can avert a mistaken diagnosis.

Metastatic embryonal carcinoma shows cohesive aggregates of tumor cells with marked nuclear pleomorphism. The appearance most frequently mimics nonhepatocytic tumors, such as adenocarcinoma. Rarely, metastatic choriocarcinoma can be seen, which produces bloody smears containing a combination of loose clusters and single cells with marked nuclear pleomorphism. Multinucleated cells representing syncytiotrophoblast cells can be seen (Fig. 22.21).

Lymphoid malignancies

The most common lymphoma to involve the liver is diffuse large B-cell lymphoma. However, almost all lymphoid malignancies have been reported to involve the liver, including plasma cell myeloma, Hodgkin lymphoma, hairy cell leukemia, and T-cell lymphoma.[34] In the case of high-grade lymphomas,

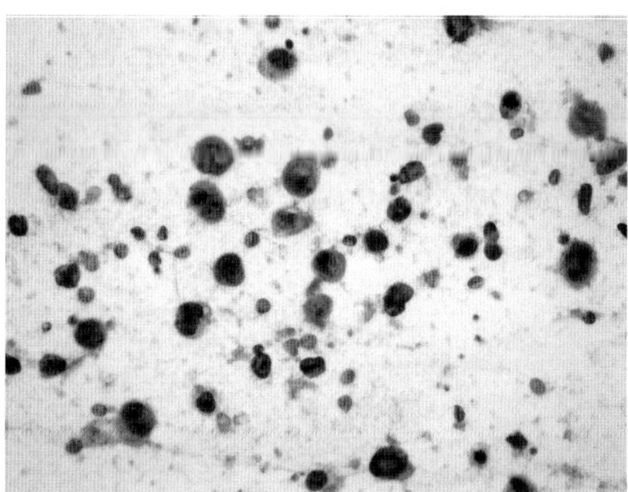

Figure 22.22 Diffuse large B-cell lymphoma. Note lymphoglandular bodies.

like diffuse large B-cell lymphoma, cellular smears are seen, comprised mostly of single cells. Clumps of cytoplasm are frequently present in the background, a finding termed lymphoglandular bodies (Fig. 22.22). The nuclei are enlarged, show coarse chromatin, and may contain multiple large nucleoli or chromocenters.

The plasma cells in multiple myeloma can mimic the appearance of a well-differentiated neuroendocrine tumor, given that the tumor cells can share a plasmacytoid appearance in both tumors (Fig. 22.23). However, the chromatin of plasma cells has a clumping pattern that resembles a "clock face" or "cartwheel" rather than the "salt and pepper" appearance typically seen in well-differentiated neuroendocrine tumors. Plasma cells usually show a perinuclear hof, resulting from the presence of a prominent golgi apparatus.

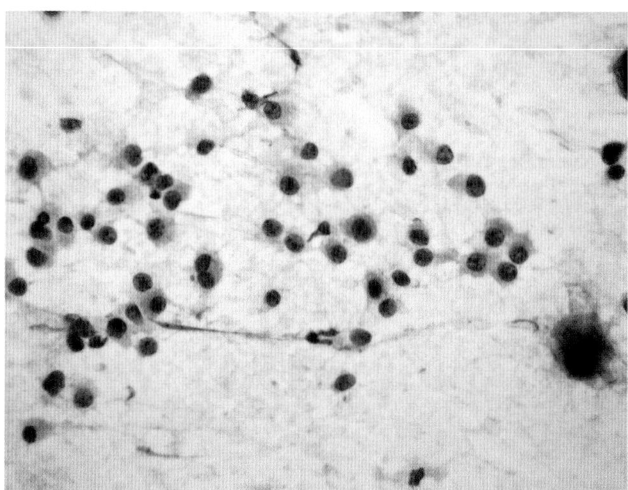

Figure 22.23 Plasma cell myeloma. Nuclei show "clock face chromatin."

When lymphoma or a plasma cell neoplasm is suspected during rapid on-site evaluation, it is prudent to save material for a cell block preparation or to request core biopsy material for immunohistochemical characterization. Submission of material for flow cytometry can also be of value, but will not be of assistance in cases of Hodgkin lymphoma. In addition, some high-grade lymphomas such as diffuse large B-cell lymphoma can produce nondiagnostic flow cytometry results, because high-grade lymphomas may be subject to disruption of cell membranes during specimen acquisition and processing.

Metastatic melanoma

When dealing with a poorly differentiated high-grade tumor, the possibility of metastatic melanoma should be considered. Many patients will have an established history of melanoma; however, the first presentation of melanoma may be its metastasis. Mucosal melanomas add additional difficulty because they may not be clinically evident at first presentation. Compounding the clinical difficulties in diagnosis, the cytomorphologic appearance of melanoma is among the most diverse seen among malignant tumors. Able to mimic almost any tumor, the cells can form clusters having the appearance of carcinoma, appear entirely spindled like a sarcoma, or even have a small cell appearance that can be confused with small-cell carcinoma or lymphoma.[35,36] When pigmentation is present, this finding is usually a strong clue to the diagnosis of melanoma. However, caution should be exercised to not mistake hemosiderin for melanin. Hemosiderin usually has a more "golden brown" appearance and is more retractile on Papanicolaou stain. Also, typical examples of melanoma usually consist of smears showing mostly single cells or poorly cohesive clusters. The tumor cells contain large nuclei and often contain conspicuous macronucleoli (Fig. 22.24). The nuclei are frequently eccentric, imparting a plasmacytoid appearance. Nuclear pseudoinclusions can also be seen. Binucleated cells with a symmetrical appearance can also be seen which has invoked the name D-MIN (double mirror image nuclei) cells.

Mesenchymal tumors

A plethora of mesenchymal tumors can occur in the liver, both primary and metastatic. The most common primary mesenchymal tumor occurring in the liver is hemangioma. As in other sites, hemangiomas of the liver produce bloody aspirates containing bland spindle cells arranged singly and as compact dense coils.[37] Epithelioid hemangiomas can mimic an epithelial tumor. However, a bloody background and admixture of spindle cells can suggest the vascular nature of the tumor.

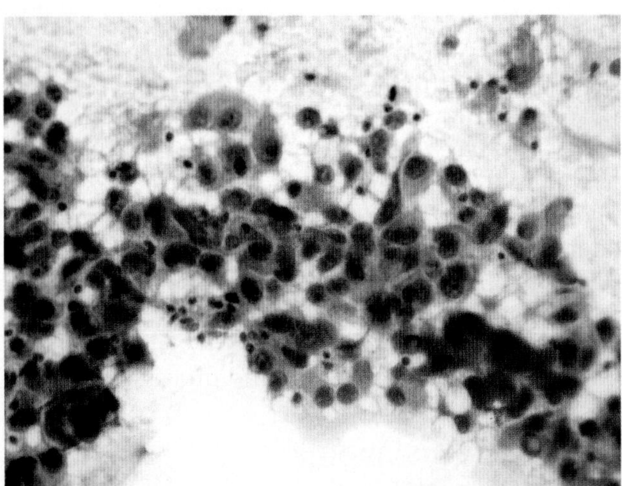

Figure 22.24 Metastatic melanoma showing melanin pigment.

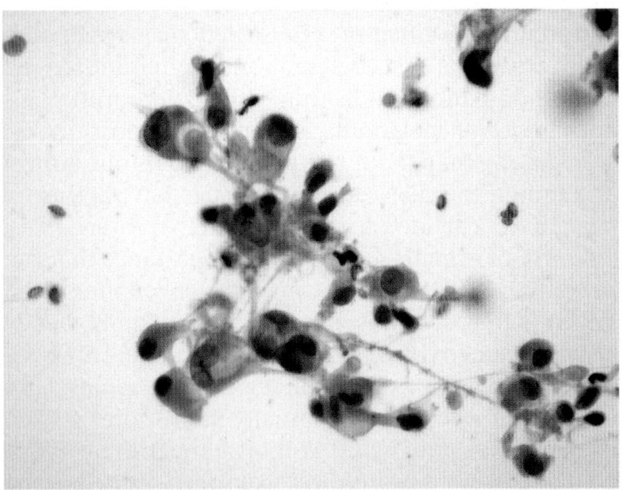

Figure 22.25 Epithelioid hemangioendothelioma. Note cell with intracytoplasmic lumen in upper left of image.

Epithelioid hemangioendothelioma shows smears that contain ovoid to polygonal cells with eccentric nuceli and finely granular chromatin. Binucleated cells can also be present. Cells containing cytoplasmic lumina (with erythrocytes) and intranuclear inclusions may be seen (Fig. 22.25).[38] A somewhat myxoid background can also be evident, a finding that is usually more prominent in diff-quick slides. If a cell block is available, the diagnosis can be confirmed by markers of endothelial differentiation.

Angiosarcoma frequently shows higher grade features that can mask the vascular character of the tumor. The aspirates can be bloody; however, necrosis is also a frequent feature. The tumor cells often contain hyperchromatic nuclei with coarse chromatin. A variable degree of nuclear pleomorphism can be seen. The nuclei may be oval to spindle shaped and hyperchromatic. The chromatin pattern varies from fine to coarse. Macronucleoli may be present. Tubular or rosette-like structures representing formations of vascular channels can be present and can be mistaken for glands.[39]

Angiomyolipomas are frequently identified by their characteristic imaging features because of the presence of adipose tissue. Angiomyolipomas show smears containing a mixture of elements. Fragments of mature adipose tissue are usually evidence for the diagnosis of angiomyolipoma.[40] Fragments of smooth muscle may also be seen. The smears may consist primarily of perivascular epithelioid cells, which form clusters of cells that can mimic both renal cell carcinoma and hepatocellular carcinoma. The cells contain clear to granular cytoplasm and rounded nuclei with small punctuate central nucleoli. These cells can be intimately associated with vessels, some of which appear to be thick walled (best seen on cell block or core biopsy material). Seeing the epithelioid cells in close association with thick-walled blood vessels, smooth muscle, or adipose tissue can help avoid the pitfall of mistaking the findings for an epithelial tumor.

Epithelioid angiomyolipomas can be mistaken for hepatocellular carcinoma, given the granularity of the tumor cells and the presence of large nuclei with prominent nucleoli (Fig. 22.26).[41] However, the cytoplasm in epithelioid angiomyolipomas is usually more abundant than seen in hepatocellular carcinoma. In addition, the cell cytoplasm frequently has a foamy histiocytic quality. Immunostains such as HMB-45 and Melan-A should be performed to help establish the diagnosis.

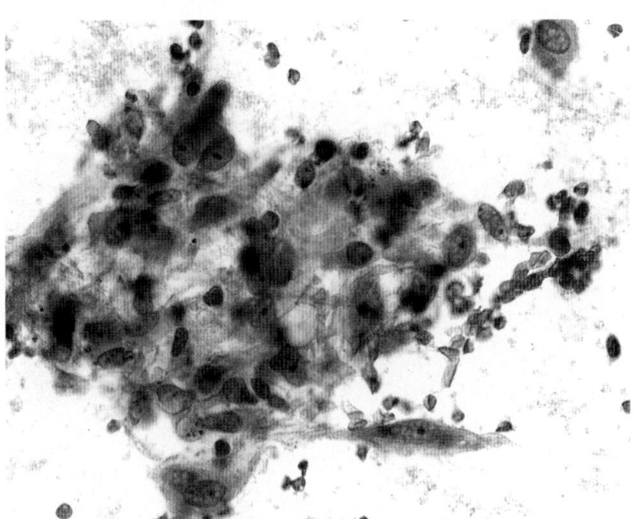

Figure 22.26 Epithelioid angiomyolipoma. Note the abundance of foamy to granular cytoplasm.

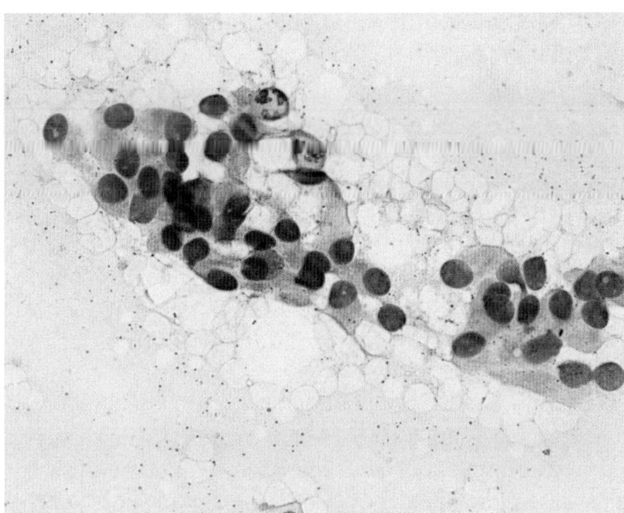

Figure 22.27 Metastatic epithelioid GIST.

Gastrointestinal stromal tumor (GIST) aspirates show loose clusters of spindle cells. Single cells are also present. The nuclei are oval and hyperchromatic with finely granular chromatin. Nucleoli are frequently absent or inconspicuous.[42] Epithelioid gastrointestinal stromal tumors produce smears that may resemble an epithelial tumor, including hepatocellular carcinoma, because the abundance of cytoplasm can mimic hepatocytes. In addition, epithelioid gastrointestinal stromal tumors show tumor cells with eccentric nuclei, mimicking a neuroendocrine tumor (Fig. 22.27). Immunostains for DOG-1 and C-KIT can establish the diagnosis of GIST.

REFERENCES

1. Kuo FY, Lin YM, Lin KJ, et al. Fine needle aspiration cytodiagnosis of liver tumors. *Acta Cytol.* 2004;48(2):142–148.
2. Nguyen P, Feng JC, Chang KJ. Endoscopic ultrasound (EUS) and EUS-guided fine-needle aspiration (FNA) of liver lesions. *Gastrointest Endosc.* 1999;50(3):357–361.
3. Hill KA, Nayar R, DeFrias DV. Cytohistologic correlation of cirrhosis and hepatocellular carcinoma. Pitfall in diagnosis? *Acta Cytol.* 2004;48(2):127–132.
4. Chhieng DC. Fine needle aspiration biopsy of liver – an update. *World J Surg Oncol.* 2004;2:5.
5. Walker AN, Feldman PS, Covell JL, et al. Fine needle aspiration under percutaneous transhepatic cholangiographic guidance. *Acta Cytol.* 1982;26(6):767–771.
6. Schwerk WB, Schmitz-Moormann P. Ultrasonically guided fine-needle biopsies in neoplastic liver disease: cytohistologic diagnoses and echo pattern of lesions. *Cancer.* 1981;48(6):1469–1477.
7. Samaratunga H, Wright G. Value of fine needle aspiration biopsy cytology in the diagnosis of discrete hepatic lesions suspicious for malignancy. *ANZ J Surg.* 1992;62(7):540–544.
8. Hertz G, Reddy VB, Green L, et al. Fine needle aspiration biopsy of the liver: a multicenter study of 602 radiologically guided FNA. *Diagn Cytopathol.* 2000;23(5):326–328.
9. Tao LC, Pearson FG, Delarue NC, et al. Percutaneous fine-needle aspiration biopsy. I. Its value to clinical practice. *Cancer.* 1980;45(6):1480–1485.
10. McGahan JP, Bishop J, Webb J, et al. Role of FNA and core biopsy of primary and metastatic liver disease. *Int J Hepatol.* 2013;2013:174103.
11. Dusenbery D, Ferris JV, Thaete FL, et al. Percutaneous ultrasound-guided needle biopsy of hepatic mass lesions using a cytohistologic approach. Comparison of two needle types. *Am J Clin Pathol.* 1995;104(5):583–587.
12. DeWitt J, LeBlanc J, McHenry L, et al. Endoscopic ultrasound-guided fine needle aspiration cytology of solid liver lesions: a large single-center experience. *Am J Gastroenterol.* 2003;98(9):1976–1981.
13. Das DK. Cytodiagnosis of hepatocellular carcinoma in fine-needle aspirates of the liver: its differentiation from reactive hepatocytes and metastatic adenocarcinoma. *Diagn Cytopathol.* 1999;21(6):370–377.
14. Saenz-Santamaria J, Moreno-Casado J, Nunez C. Role of fine-needle biopsy in the diagnosis of hydatid cyst. *Diagn Cytopathol.* 1995;13(3):229–232.
15. Saenz-Santamaria J, Catalina-Fernandez I, Fernandez de Mera JJ. Hydatid cyst in soft tissues mimicking malignant tumors. Diagnosis by fine needle aspiration cytology. *Acta Cytol.* 2003;47(3):337–340.
16. Ruschenburg I, Droese M. Fine needle aspiration cytology of focal nodular hyperplasia of the liver. *Acta Cytol.* 1989;33(6):857–860.
17. Yang GC, Yang GY, Tao LC. Distinguishing well-differentiated hepatocellular carcinoma from benign liver by the physical features of fine-needle aspirates. *Mod Pathol.* 2004;17(7):798–802.
18. Longchampt E, Patriarche C, Fabre M. Accuracy of cytology vs. microbiopsy for the diagnosis of well-differentiated hepatocellular carcinoma and macroregenerative nodule. Definition of standardized criteria from a study of 100 cases. *Acta Cytol.* 2000;44(4):515–523.
19. de Boer WB, Segal A, Frost FA, et al. Cytodiagnosis of well differentiated hepatocellular carcinoma: can indeterminate diagnoses be reduced? *Cancer.* 1999;87(5):270–277.
20. Yu GH, Gustafson KS, Pan ST, et al. Peripheral endothelial cells are not reliable in differentiating primary benign and malignant hepatocellular lesions in fine needle aspirates of the liver. *Cytopathology.* 2002;13(3):145–151.

21. Pitman MB. Fine needle aspiration biopsy of the liver. Principal diagnostic challenges. *Clin Lab Med.* 1998;18(3):483–506, vi.
22. Pedio G, Landolt U, Zöbeli L, et al. Fine needle aspiration of the liver. Significance of hepatocytic naked nuclei in the diagnosis of hepatocellular carcinoma. *Acta Cytol.* 1988;32(4):437–442.
23. Saleh HA, Aulicino M, Zaidi SY, et al. Discriminating hepatocellular carcinoma from metastatic carcinoma on fine-needle aspiration biopsy of the liver: the utility of immunocytochemical panel. *Diagn Cytopathol.* 2009;37(3):184–190.
24. Singh HK, Silverman JF, Geisinger KR. Fine-needle aspiration cytomorphology of clear-cell hepatocellular carcinoma. *Diagn Cytopathol.* 1997;17(4):306–310.
25. Perez-Guillermo M, Masgrau NA, García-Solano J, et al. Cytologic aspect of fibrolamellar hepatocellular carcinoma in fine-needle aspirates. *Diagn Cytopathol.* 1999;21(3):180–187.
26. Gupta RK, Naran S, Alansari AG. Fine needle aspiration cytodiagnosis in a case of hepatoblastoma. *Cytopathology.* 1994;5(2):114–117.
27. Soudah B, Masgrau NA, García-Solano J, et al. Overview and evaluation of the value of fine needle aspiration cytology in determining the histogenesis of liver nodules: 14 years of experience at Hannover Medical School. *Oncol Rep.* 2015;33(1):81–87.
28. Gupta RK, Naran S, Lallu S, et al. Fine needle aspiration diagnosis of neuroendocrine tumors in the liver. *Pathology.* 2000;32(1):16–20.
29. Serrano R, Rodríguez-Peralto JL, Santos-Briz A, et al. Fine needle aspiration cytology of metastatic hepatic adrenocortical carcinoma mimicking hepatocellular carcinoma: a case report. *Acta Cytol.* 2001;45(5):768–770.
30. Aubert S, Wacrenier A, Leroy X, et al. Weiss system revisited: a clinicopathologic and immunohistochemical study of 49 adrenocortical tumors. *Am J Surg Pathol.* 2002;26(12):1612–1619.
31. Lew M, Foo WC, Roh MH. Diagnosis of metastatic renal cell carcinoma on fine-needle aspiration cytology. *Arch Pathol Lab Med.* 2014;138(10):1278–1285.
32. Gupta R, Mathur SR, Arora VK, et al. Cytologic features of extragonadal germ cell tumors: a study of 88 cases with aspiration cytology. *Cancer.* 2008;114(6):504–511.
33. Ceyhan K, Utkan G, Dincol D, et al. Fine needle aspiration biopsy features with histologic correlation in mediastinal hepatoid yolk sac tumor presenting with sternum metastasis: a case report. *Acta Cytol.* 2007;51(4):610–615.
34. Swadley MJ, Deliu M, Mosunjac MB, et al. Primary and secondary hepatic lymphomas diagnosed by image-guided fine-needle aspiration: a retrospective study of clinical and cytomorphologic findings. *Am J Clin Pathol.* 2014;141(1):119–127.
35. Buehler D, Waknitz M, Rehrauer W, et al. Small cell variant of malignant melanoma masquerading as lymphoma on fine-needle aspiration cytology: a case report. *Diagn Cytopathol.* 2012;40(7):619–623.
36. Piao Y, Guo M, Gong Y. Diagnostic challenges of metastatic spindle cell melanoma on fine-needle aspiration specimens. *Cancer.* 2008;114(2):94–101.
37. Caturelli E, Rapaccini GL, Sabelli C, et al. Ultrasound-guided fine-needle aspiration biopsy in the diagnosis of hepatic hemangioma. *Liver.* 1986;6(6):326–330.
38. Campione S, Cozzolino I, Mainenti P, et al. Hepatic epithelioid hemangioendothelioma: pitfalls in the diagnosis on fine needle cytology and "small biopsy" and review of the literature. *Pathol Res Pract.* 2015;211(9):702–705.
39. Geller RL, Hookim K, Sullivan HC, et al. Cytologic features of angiosarcoma: a review of 26 cases diagnosed on FNA. *Cancer Cytopathol.* 2016;124(9):659–668.
40. Crapanzano JP. Fine-needle aspiration of renal angiomyolipoma: cytological findings and diagnostic pitfalls in a series of five cases. *Diagn Cytopathol.* 2005;32(1):53–57.
41. Xie L, Jessurun J, Manivel JC, et al. Hepatic epithelioid angiomyolipoma with trabecular growth pattern: a mimic of hepatocellular carcinoma on fine needle aspiration cytology. *Diagn Cytopathol.* 2012;40(7):639–650.
42. Padilla C, Saez A, Vidal A, et al. Fine-needle aspiration cytology diagnosis of metastatic gastrointestinal stromal tumor in the liver: a report of three cases. *Diagn Cytopathol.* 2002;27(5):298–302.

23 Molecular genetics of liver diseases

Rondell P. Graham, MBBS

23.1 INTRODUCTION

Molecular techniques are increasingly used in the characterization of diseases and specimens in clinical practice and research. These scientific advances have advanced the understanding of liver diseases. This chapter will provide an overview of the most commonly used molecular techniques for diagnostic and theranostic purposes. Thereafter, this chapter will review the clinically relevant molecular discoveries to date in common primary liver tumors. The liver is a common site for metastatic disease. As such, this chapter will also review molecular targets for a select group of metastases to the liver. Finally, the chapter will review the molecular defects in a collection of hereditary liver diseases, which may lead to early cirrhosis.

23.2 MOLECULAR TECHNIQUES

The most commonly employed modality for germline genetic testing is Sanger sequencing. This method works by dideoxy termination and allows for amplification and sequencing of part of a gene or an entire single gene at a time. This method has been the main workhouse in clinical laboratories for some time, but the advent of next-generation sequencing has changed this. Next-generation sequencing employs a massively parallel sequencing approach, allowing for the sequencing of several genes or the entire exome (DNA) or transcriptome (RNA) at a given time. Whole exome sequencing has been shown to be a cost-effective and powerful approach for germline molecular diagnostics in several studies and is now in routine use in large academic centers.[1–3] Smaller sequencing panels that evaluate genes known to be involved in specific disorders have also been created for more focused testing, as exemplified by a recent report on Wilson disease.[4]

Targeted genotyping assays are used for diseases that result from one or two mutations in a single gene, for example, in *HFE*-related hereditary hemochromatosis and α-1-antitrypsin deficiency. These targeted assays may be based on a number of different platforms, but they all operate on the same principles as sequencing. It is important to note that targeted assays will only detect the alteration(s) for which they were designed.

Other approaches are also being developed. As one example, mass spectrometry–based testing can identify the S and Z alleles of

SERPINA1 based on the affect these alleles have on the mass-to-charge ratio of the peptides of the SERPINA1 (α-1-antitrypsin) protein.[5] The main advantage of this assay is that it is significantly less expensive than targeted genotyping assays. However, it has the same limitations as other targeted assays for α-1-antitrypsin deficiency in that it cannot detect mutations for which it was not specifically designed.[5]

For somatic tumor testing, sequencing assays such as those described above play a very important role. Given the improved analytic and clinical sensitivity of next-generation sequencing and its reduced cost, whole exome or large gene panel sequencing assays are being utilized with increasing frequency.[6–10] Also, the characterization of an increasing number of tumors as translocation-associated tumors has led to the use of RNA sequencing clinically to support diagnoses.[11–14] Frozen tissue provides a better quality and quantity of nucleic acids for somatic testing than formalin-fixed paraffin-embedded tissue.[15–18] However, most pathology practices do not have the resources for routine collection of frozen tissue for clinical care. Fortunately, numerous studies have shown successful global transcriptome (RNA) and multigene DNA sequencing studies from formalin-fixed paraffin-embedded tissue.[6–9,19–25] Indeed, clinically validated assays for large gene panels from formalin-fixed paraffin-embedded tissue are commercially available and in use in clinical care. Despite this broad success, individual cases may not yield sufficient quantity or quality nucleic acids leading to noninformative test results.

The most commonly identified alterations from DNA sequencing are point mutations and small insertions and deletions. As mentioned above, RNA sequencing can detect translocation events which produce a novel fusion transcript, in addition to detecting sequence alterations. It is important to point out that RNA sequencing cannot directly detect translocations (i.e., genomic rearrangements) that lead to a promoter switch or a change in regulatory region/elements of a gene, but do not create a fusion transcript. Instead, these latter changes are best detected in clinical practice by fluorescent in situ hybridization (FISH). Mate pair sequencing and other methods can also be used for detecting such large structural changes, but these latter methods are not routinely used in clinical practice.

Several more targeted test methods are still very commonly used. Reverse transcriptase polymerase chain reaction (PCR) is widely used for the detection of specific fusion transcripts that characterize a variety of different tumor types. This technique includes extraction of total RNA from tissue followed by reverse transcription to cDNA. Primers for specific fusion event(s) are then used to amplify the fusion transcript, if it is present. Next, the results of the reaction are detected by any of a number of techniques. Classically, gel electrophoresis is used to detect the amplification products (Fig. 23.1).

PCR-based detection of nucleic acids of microorganisms in formalin-fixed paraffin-embedded tissue is being increasingly employed.[26] These assays use a variety of detection systems including Taqman or FRET probes, depending on whether or not melt curve analysis is desired.[26] As one example, the molecular detection of viral hepatitis E RNA has contributed to considerable improvement in the clinical care of immunocompromised solid organ transplant recipients.[27,28] Briefly, it has recently been recognized that viral hepatitis E can cause chronic liver disease in the immunosuppressed patient, manifesting with a nonspecific histologic picture of chronic hepatitis.[27–29] Chronic viral hepatitis E can lead to allograft loss, and serologic tests for hepatitis E are difficult to interpret. Detection of hepatitis E RNA can definitively make the diagnosis of chronic hepatitis E infection of the allograft, which can be cured with antiviral therapy.[30] This example illustrates the power of molecular techniques in clinical scenarios where serology and morphology do not allow for specific diagnosis of an infectious organism involving the liver.

FISH is another modality often used for molecular cytogenetic characterization of liver neoplasms. FISH can be used to detect translocations or to identify copy number abnormalities. For the former, different color probes are used that are specific to the genes or regions involved in the genomic change. The presence of the translocation gives rise to an altered signal pattern with probes being brought together (fusion

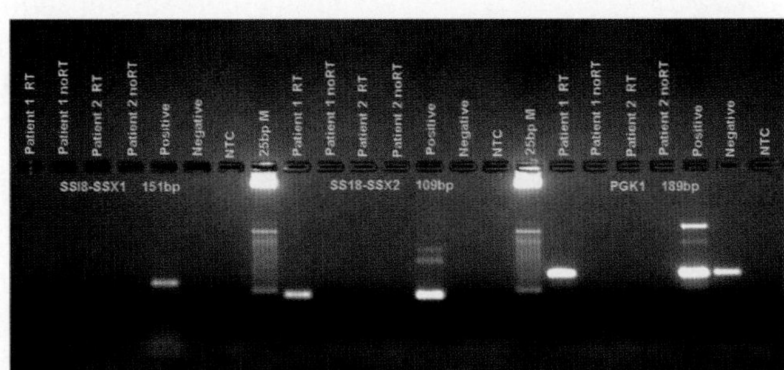

Figure 23.1 This is a representative gel image from RT-PCR for *SS18-SSX* fusion genes. The control gene *PGK1* **(right of image)** was amplified in patient 1. This indicates that the RNA from patient 1 is of sufficient quality for testing. The positive and negative controls also include good-quality RNA and the no tissue control (NTC) is negative excluding contamination. Only the positive control is amplified in the *SS18-SSX1* reaction as seen on the left of the gel image. Patient 1 is therefore negative for *SS18-SSX1*. In the *SS18-SSX2* reaction, patient 1 and the positive control are amplified. The controls react appropriately **(center of image)**. The detection of *SS18-SSX2* supports the diagnosis of synovial sarcoma in this illustrative example.

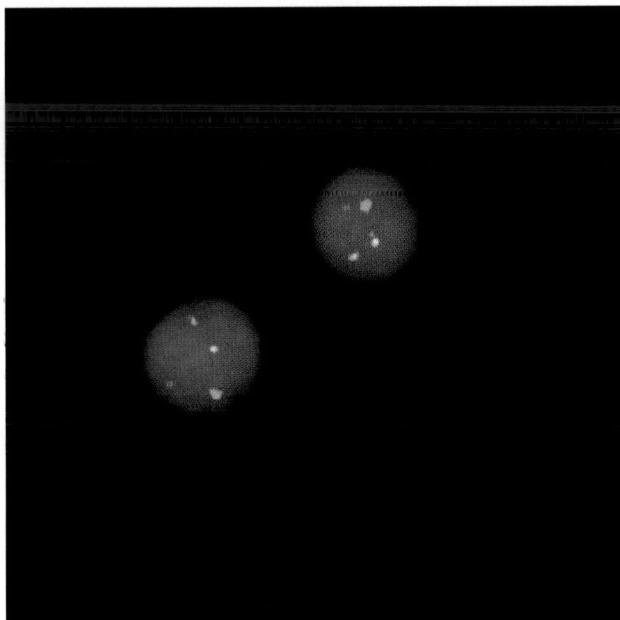

Figure 23.2 This is a representative interphase FISH image from a dual fusion FISH assay. A cell without the translocation event would harbor two separate red and two separate green signals. The observation of red and green signals coming together to form two yellow signals is indicative of a reciprocal translocation of the two genes.

probe set; Fig. 23.2) or probes being separated (break apart probe set; Fig. 23.3). For copy number changes different color probes to the gene/locus of interest and the centromere of the chromosome in question are used to enumerate the number of copies of the gene and the chromosome (Fig. 23.4). Multiple probes can

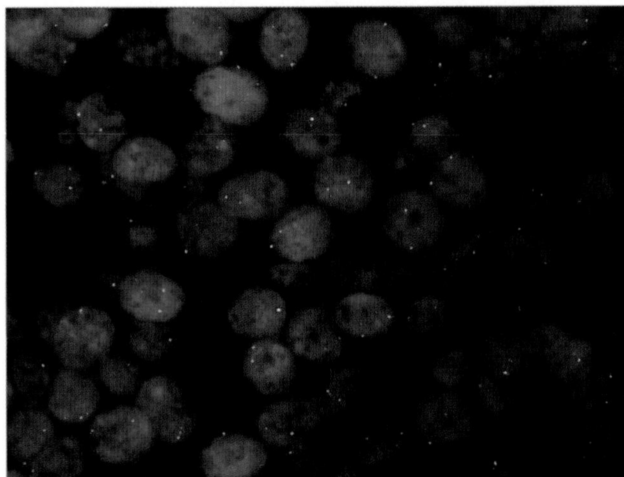

Figure 23.3 This is a representative interphase FISH image of a break apart FISH strategy. A normal cell should display two intact *yellow* signals. In this example, *red* and *green* signal are separated indicative of a rearrangement of the locus (i.e., the gene is involved in a translocation).

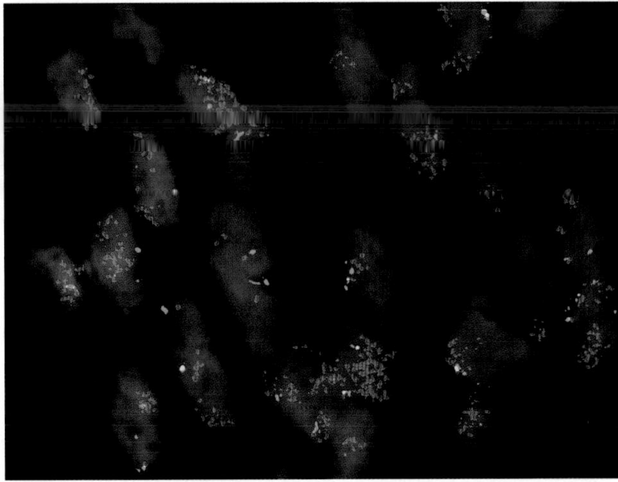

Figure 23.4 In this enumeration FISH strategy, there is a green probe for the centromere of the chromosome where the locus of interest is located. The *red* probe is to the locus of interest. In a normal cell the *green* and *red* signals should be in a 1:1 ratio. Typically, there would be two signals for each probe per cell. In this tumor, it is clear that there amplification at the locus is highlighted by the *red* probe with a marked gain in the number of copies at that locus relative to the *green* probe.

be combined to allow for simultaneous enumeration of several loci or chromosomes. This combination of multiple enumeration probes is used in the biliary FISH assay used to evaluate bile duct brushings for neoplasia, which will be discussed later in this chapter.

Array comparative genomic hybridization (array CGH) provides a pan-genomic view of the copy number state of a large number of genomic loci, the autosomes, and the X chromosome. The density of the array determines the resolution of the platform. A platform for formalin-fixed paraffin-embedded tissue is commercially available. Despite the potential of array CGH to simultaneously evaluate for a large number of copy number alterations, this technology is not currently in routine use for the evaluation of liver neoplasms.

23.3 TUMORS

Hepatocellular carcinoma

Hepatocellular carcinoma is the most common primary hepatic malignancy. Several large-scale exome and transcriptome sequencing studies have been reported in the literature, which have repeatedly yielded a pattern of low-frequency mutations for a number of genetic drivers.[31–34] The most common alterations are in *TP53*, *CTNNB1* (beta catenin gene), *CDKN2A*, and the promoter of *TERT*. *TERT* promoter mutations are present in approximately 50% of hepatocellular carcinoma, with *β-catenin* and *TP53* mutations in approximately 25% and 20% of hepatocellular carcinoma respectively.[31,32,34] *CDKN2A* mutations are present in approximately 10% of hepatocellular carcinoma. All other mutations are identified at a much lower frequency. The patterns of mutations present across large cohorts of hepatocellular carcinoma have been correlated to various etiologic agents.[33,35,36] One study revealed a correlation between alcohol and *β-catenin* mutations and viral hepatitis B and *TP53* mutations.[36] In another study, *TERT* promoter mutations were significantly correlated with Wnt pathway activation in nonviral hepatitis B cases.[34] Finally, *ARID2* mutations, which are uncommon in hepatocellular carcinoma overall (approximately 6%), were found to be enriched in individuals with underlying chronic viral hepatitis C.[33] Currently, none of these mutations represent targets for therapy and a role in routine diagnostics has not yet been shown.

Fibrolamellar carcinoma

Fibrolamellar carcinoma is currently classified as a variant of hepatocellular carcinoma. However, fibrolamellar carcinoma shows several distinctive features: (1) the tumors have a predilection for younger patients (>85% of patients are under 35 years at diagnosis)[37]; (2) the tumors arise in livers without chronic liver disease[38]; (3) the tumor shows characteristic histologic features (almost all fibrolamellar carcinomas look the same)[38]; (4) the neoplastic cells typically display coexpression of cytokeratin 7 and CD68[39]; and (5) the tumors have a recurrent fusion gene that is found in fibrolamellar carcinoma but not in conventional hepatocellular carcinoma.[40,41]

Almost all fibrolamellar carcinomas are characterized genetically by the recurrent *DNAJB1-PRKACA* fusion gene, owing to an intrachromosomal deletion at chromosome 19p13.[40] This fusion gene is the oncogenic driver of the fibrolamellar carcinomas.[40] Detection of this fusion transcript is specific for the diagnosis of fibrolamellar carcinoma in the context of primary hepatic neoplasms.[41] A commercially available FISH test to detect *PRKACA* rearrangement has been clinically validated and can also be used to confirm the diagnosis of fibrolamellar carcinoma. The FISH test displays a sensitivity of 99% and specificity of 100% in the context of primary hepatocellular neoplasms and is informative even when there are as few as 50 tumor nuclei available for analysis.[42] Very rare cases of fibrolamellar carcinoma are negative for the *DNAJB1-PRKACA* translocation and instead reveal *PRKAR1A* biallelic inactivation in the context of the Carney complex.[42] Biallelic inactivation of *PRKAR1A* provides an alternate means for activation of the Protein kinase A pathway, which appears to be a major driver of tumorigenesis in fibrolamellar carcinoma. No molecularly targeted treatment has yet been developed for fibrolamellar carcinoma.

Hepatocellular adenoma

Hepatocellular adenomas are molecularly heterogeneous tumors, reflecting dysregulation of a number of different pathways.[43] The epidemiology, morphology, and immunohistochemical stains used in the classification of these tumors are discussed in detail in Chapter 27. However, the salient molecular features will be described here. The first type of hepatocellular adenomas are the *HNF1-α* inactivated adenomas.[43–45] These are characterized by loss of LFABP expression and tumors can occur sporadically (most cases) or occur in patients bearing germline *HNF1-α* mutations. *HNF1-α* functions as a tumor suppressor, and both copies of the gene require inactivation for tumorigenesis. Germline *HNF1-α* mutations are also associated with maturity onset diabetes of the young type 3.

The second type of hepatocellular adenoma displays activation of the oncogene, *β-catenin*, which leads to dysregulated signaling of the Wnt pathway.[43–45] Activation of the Wnt signaling pathway may or may not be associated with *β-catenin* mutations. Mutations can be detected by sequencing, but tumors in clinical practice are most commonly assessed by *β-catenin* immunohistochemistry instead, where nuclear staining serves as a surrogate marker for mutations, albeit with an imperfect correlation. Strong and diffuse glutamine synthetase staining within the tumor also serves as broad marker for Wnt signaling activation, and can be seen with or without *β-catenin* mutations.

β-Catenin activation can also be seen in inflammatory adenomas (~10%). Activation of β-catenin is thought to increase the risk for malignant transformation.[43–45] As such, detection of β-catenin–activated hepatocellular adenoma on biopsy requires careful clinical follow-up, and many cases undergo surgical resection.

The third type of hepatocellular adenoma is called the inflammatory type and is characterized by activation of the JAK/STAT pathway.[43–45] Most commonly, this is because of an activating mutation in *IL6ST* (~65%), with some cases showing *STAT3* mutations instead. In still other cases, *GNAS* mutations underlie this type of adenoma. Postzygotic mosaic *GNAS* mutations are responsible for the McCune–Albright syndrome, and inflammatory adenomas have been described in patients with this syndrome. Cross talk between the cyclic AMP and JAK/STAT pathways is believed to explain the phenotype in this subgroup of adenomas.[46] In approximately 15% of type 3 hepatocellular adenomas, the genetic basis is unknown. As mentioned above, approximately 10% of otherwise typical type 3 adenomas can show *β-catenin* activation.[44,47]

The final group of hepatocellular adenomas does not have any unifying molecular features and remains molecularly unclassified.[44,47] Table 23.1 shows a summary of the molecular abnormalities in the various types of hepatocellular adenoma.

There are some parallels between the molecular abnormalities seen in hepatocellular carcinoma and hepatocellular adenoma. For example, *TERT* promoter mutations have been found in a subset of hepatocellular adenomas and in hepatocellular carcinomas.[34] Also, evidence of *HNF1-α* inactivation and *β-catenin* mutations have been found in subsets of both hepatocellular adenomas and hepatocellular carcinomas.[48] As such, detection of any of these molecular aberrations alone does not allow for distinction of hepatocellular adenoma from hepatocellular carcinoma. These similarities are not explained by hepatocellular adenomas preceding the development of hepatocellular carcinoma, as only a small subset of hepatocellular adenomas undergo malignant transformation, and most hepatocellular carcinomas do not arise from adenomas, even in noncirrhotic livers.[49,50] Instead, these findings illustrate that common pathways are dysregulated in hepatocellular neoplasms of various types.

Table 23.1 Genes Involved in Hepatocellular Adenoma Subtypes

Type of hepatocellular adenoma	Characteristic mutated genes	Mechanism	Immuno histochemical surrogate
1	*HNF1-α*	Loss of function	LFABP (loss of expression in tumors; retained expression in background liver)
2	*CTNNB1*	Activation	*β-catenin* (nuclear accumulation and/or glutamine synthetase (strong and diffuse staining)
3	*IL6ST, STAT3, GNAS*	Gain of function	CRP and serum amyloid A

Hepatoblastoma

Hepatoblastoma is the most common primary liver malignancy in children less than 2 years of age. The histology, embryology, and diagnosis of hepatoblastoma are presented in Chapter 25, and this section will focus on the main molecular finding in hepatoblastoma. Hepatoblastomas have been evaluated at genomic and RNA levels. Similar to the biology of hepatocellular adenomas and hepatocellular carcinomas, the oncogenesis of hepatoblastomas is driven by activation of the Wnt signaling pathway. In this regard, the most important consistent finding has been recurrent *β*-catenin mutations, found in almost all cases, with rare cases showing germline adenomatous polyposis coli (*APC*) mutations.[51,52] The latter mutations are responsible for familial *APC*, which is a known risk factor for hepatoblastomas. Beckwith–Weidemann syndrome is a risk factor for hepatoblastoma, but the molecular mechanisms[53] for this predisposition are unknown.

Cholangiocarcinoma

Cholangiocarcinomas are invasive adenocarcinomas with biliary differentiation and may be intrahepatic, (peri)hilar, or extrahepatic (distal) in location. Currently, molecular techniques are used for both therapeutic and diagnostic purposes in cholangiocarcinoma.

Molecular characterization of cholangiocarcinomas has yielded identification of several therapeutic targets in cholangiocarcinoma (Table 23.2).[25,54–64] Notably, these therapeutic targets display clustering that corresponds to the location of the tumor. Briefly, *FGFR2* fusions and *BRAF* mutations have been detected exclusively

Table 23.2 Common molecular abnormalities in cholangiocarcinoma

Molecular findings	Intrahepatic CCA (%)	Perihilar and extrahepatic CCA (%)
FGFR2 fusions	~20–25	0
ERBB2 amplification	0	~15–20
Somatic mutations		
BAP1	11	2
BRAF	5	0
IDH1/2	15	2
KRAS	19	19
TP53	16	26

in intrahepatic cholangiocarcinomas, whereas *ERBB2* (*HER2*) amplification is found in perihilar or distal cholangiocarcinomas.[61–63] *IDH1/2* point mutations are also enriched in intrahepatic tumors when compared to perihilar or distal cholangiocarcinoma.[55,56,65,66] Targeted inhibitors of each of these molecular alterations (*FGFR2* fusion, *ERRB2* amplification, and *BRAF* and *IDH* mutations) are available and are being tested in clinical trials.[55,57,64,67]

At the diagnostic level, there is significant clinical, radiologic, and morphologic overlap between benign and malignant extrahepatic biliary strictures. Consequently, biliary specimens from extrahepatic biliary strictures or filling defects may be assessed by molecular techniques. The most extensive clinical experience in this clinical situation has been with the use of FISH on biliary brushing specimens.[68–70] Early studies of FISH described significantly improved diagnostic sensitivity over routine cytology with a specificity of approximately 90%.[68,69] Nonetheless, the sensitivity was still approximately 50%. Therefore, investigators have developed an optimized FISH probe set, which has improved the diagnostic resolution of biliary FISH.[70] Interestingly, another group has reported that a next-generation sequencing assay focused on detecting mutations known to be seen in biliary carcinomas shows equivalent performance, but the clinical validation of that report is currently pending.[71]

Metastatic disease

The most common liver tumors encountered in clinical practice are metastases. Recent molecular advances have led to the identification of therapeutic targets for several types of metastatic tumors. It is useful for the practicing pathologist to be aware of the molecular targets assayed in common metastases in order to facilitate or guide appropriate test ordering. Table 23.3 provides an overview of the genes and mutations of clinical significance in a select group of tumors which commonly metastasize to the liver.

23.4 NONTUMOR DISEASES

Hereditary liver diseases

The category of hereditary liver diseases includes a group of genetic defects which impair liver metabolism and or function. Table 23.4 provides a summary of the frequency, pattern of inheritance, typical clinical

Table 23.3 Molecular targets for select metastases to the liver

Tumor type	Genes	Somatic alteration	Clinical significance	Genes associated with hereditary predisposition
Breast carcinoma	*ERBB2*[75]	*ERBB2* amplification	Predicts responsiveness to HER2 antibodies	*BRCA1, BRCA2, CDH1, PTEN, STK11, PALB2*[76]
Lung adenocarcinoma	*EGFR, ALK, RET, ROS1, BRAF, MET, KRAS*[77–82]	*EGFR* exon 18–21 mutations	*EGFR* exon 18–21 mutations predict responsiveness to anti-EGFR therapy.	*EGFR* T790M[83]
		EGFR T790M	*EGFR* T790M predicts resistance to anti-EGFR therapy.	
		ALK, RET and *ROS1* rearrangements	*ALK, RET* and *ROS1* rearrangements predict responsiveness to tyrosine kinase inhibitors.	
		BRAF V600E	*BRAF* V600E may predict response to BRAF inhibition.	
		MET amplification	*MET* amplification predicts resistance to EGFR inhibition.	
		KRAS mutations	*KRAS* mutations predict resistance to EGFR inhibition.	
Colorectal carcinoma	*KRAS, HRAS, NRAS, BRAF*[84–86]	*RAS* mutations	Predict resistance to anti-EGFR therapy	*APC*, MMR*, *MYH, NTHL1*[87]

(continued)

Table 23.3 Molecular targets for select metastases to the liver (*continued*)

Tumor type	Genes	Somatic alteration	Clinical significance	Genes associated with hereditary predisposition
Malignant melanoma	*BRAF, KIT, GNAQ, GNA11*[88–90]	*BRAF* V600 mutations	Predict responsiveness to BRAF inhibition	*CDKN2A, CDK4, TERT, MITF, BAP1*[91]
		KIT mutations	Predict responsiveness to tyrosine kinase inhibitors	
		GNAQ/GNA11 mutations	Detection of *GNAQ* or *GNA11* supports the diagnosis of a central nervous system melanoma primary	
Gastrointestinal stromal tumor	*KIT, PDGFRA, BRAF*[92–94]	*KIT* mutations	Predict responsiveness to tyrosine kinase inhibition	*KIT, PDGFRA, SDHB, SDHC, SDHD NF1*[95,96]
		PDFGRA mutations	Predict responsiveness to tyrosine kinase inhibition	
		BRAF V600E	Possibly predict resistance to imatinib therapy	

MMR*—mismatch repair genes: *MLH1*, *MSH2*, *MSH6*, and *PMS2*. Though not related to a molecular therapy, detection of microsatellite instability may predict responsiveness to immune checkpoint inhibition.

Table 23.4 A summary of hereditary diseases that may be occasionally or rarely encountered in practice but which may progress to cirrhosis

Disease	Gene	Frequency	Pattern of inheritance	Clinical presentation	Main diagnostic features
Hereditary hemochromatosis	*HFE*	1:250	AR	Often asymptomatic	Increased iron deposition in hepatocytes
Juvenile onset hemochromatosis	*HAMP, HFE2*	<1: 1,000,000	AR	Cardiomyopathy and hypogonadism	Serum transferrin saturation and serum ferritin are markedly elevated
Hemochromatosis type 3	*TFR2*	<1:1,000, 000	AR	Often asymptomatic	Low hepcidin. Increased hepatocyte iron.
α-1-antitrypsin deficiency	*SERPINA1*	1:2,000	AR	Emphysema. Variable liver manifestations	PAS-D positive periportal globules. Low serum A1AT
Wilson disease	*ATP7B*	1:30,000	AR	Variable liver manifestations which usually precede neurologic disease	Low serum ceruloplasmin, increased liver tissue copper, Kayser-Fleischer rings
Type 1 Tyrosinemia	*FAH*	1:100,000	AR	Ascites, jaundice	Increased plasma and urine succinylacetone
Hereditary fructose intolerance	*ALDOB*	1:20,000	AR	Diarrhea, hypoglycemia, failure to thrive, seizures	Abnormal fructose tolerance breath test. Gene sequencing

(continued)

Table 23.4 A summary of hereditary diseases that may be occasionally or rarely encountered in practice but which may progress to cirrhosis (*continued*)

Disease	Gene	Frequency	Pattern of inheritance	Clinical presentation	Main diagnostic features
Glycogen storage disease, type IV	*GBE1*	1:600,000	AR	Failure to thrive, hepatomegaly	Abnormal hepatic glycogen. Abnormal fibroblast, liver or muscle enzyme activity.
Cholesteryl ester storage disease	*LIPA*	1:40,000 (Germany) 1:300,000	AR	Hepatomegaly and cirrhosis	Hepatosplenomegaly with high cholesterol and low HDL. Low lysosomal acid lipase activity.
"Telomere disease"	*TERT, TERC*	NA	AD	Usual interstitial pneumonia (Idiopathic pulmonary fibrosis) and cirrhosis. Affected individuals or relatives may have bone marrow failure.	Usual interstitial pneumonia. Gene sequencing.

Abbreviation: NA, not available.

presentation, and main diagnostic features of a select group of hereditary liver diseases that have been well characterized at a molecular level and progress to cirrhosis.[72–74] Each of these diseases can be diagnosed by germline sequencing. In most instances, the disorders are inherited in an autosomal recessive manner, and two mutations need to be identified for diagnosis. In conditions with this pattern of inheritance, both parents need to be carriers for the disease (i.e., have an abnormal gene copy), but neither is affected by the disease. The notable exception is telomere disease which is inherited in an autosomal dominant manner. One abnormal gene copy (i.e., one abnormal allele) in diseases with autosomal dominant inheritance will produce the phenotype. Therefore, only a single parent will need to be affected in order for a child to manifest the disease. Diseases which are associated with biliary-type cirrhosis are not included but are discussed in Chapter 14.

REFERENCES

1. Posey JE, Rosenfeld JA, James RA, et al. Molecular diagnostic experience of whole-exome sequencing in adult patients. *Genet Med.* 2016;18(7):678–685.
2. Yang Y, Muzny DM, Reid JG, et al. Clinical whole-exome sequencing for the diagnosis of mendelian disorders. *N Engl J Med.* 2013;369(16):1502–1511.
3. Yang Y, Muzny DM, Xia F, et al. Molecular findings among patients referred for clinical whole-exome sequencing. *JAMA.* 2014;312(18):1870–1879.
4. Nemeth D, Arvai K, Horvath P, et al. Clinical use of next-generation sequencing in the diagnosis of Wilson's disease. *Gastroenterol Res Pract.* 2016;2016:4548039.
5. Chen Y, Snyder MR, Zhu Y, et al. Simultaneous phenotyping and quantification of alpha-1-antitrypsin by liquid chromatography-tandem mass spectrometry. *Clin Chem.* 2011;57(8):1161–1168.
6. Mody RJ, Wu YM, Lonigro RJ, et al. Integrative clinical sequencing in the management of refractory or relapsed cancer in youth. *JAMA.* 2015;314(9):913–925.
7. Young G, Wang K, He J, et al. Clinical next-generation sequencing successfully applied to fine-needle aspirations of pulmonary and pancreatic neoplasms. *Cancer Cytopathol.* 2013;121(12):688–694.
8. Cheng DT, Mitchell TN, Zehir A, et al. Memorial sloan kettering-integrated mutation profiling of actionable cancer targets (MSK-IMPACT): a hybridization capture-based next-generation sequencing clinical assay for solid tumor molecular oncology. *J Mol Diagn.* 2015;17(3):251–264.
9. Hagemann IS, Devarakonda S, Lockwood CM, et al. Clinical next-generation sequencing in patients with non-small cell lung cancer. *Cancer.* 2015;121(4):631–639.
10. Marino-Enriquez A. Advances in the molecular analysis of soft tissue tumors and clinical implications. *Surg Pathol Clin.* 2015;8(3):525–537.
11. Walther C, Hofvander J, Nilsson J, et al. Gene fusion detection in formalin-fixed paraffin-embedded

benign fibrous histiocytomas using fluorescence in situ hybridization and RNA sequencing. *Lab Invest*. 2015;95(9):1071–1076.
12. Cieslik M, Chugh R, Wu YM, et al. The use of exome capture RNA-seq for highly degraded RNA with application to clinical cancer sequencing. *Genome Res*. 2015;25(9):1372–1381.
13. Hofvander J, Tayebwa J, Nilsson J, et al. RNA sequencing of sarcomas with simple karyotypes: identification and enrichment of fusion transcripts. *Lab Invest*. 2015;95(6):603–609.
14. Byron SA, Van Keuren-Jensen KR, Engelthaler DM, et al. Translating RNA sequencing into clinical diagnostics: opportunities and challenges. *Nat Rev Genet*. 2016;17(5):257–271.
15. De Paoli-Iseppi R, Johansson PA, Menzies AM, et al. Comparison of whole-exome sequencing of matched fresh and formalin fixed paraffin embedded melanoma tumours: implications for clinical decision making. *Pathology*. 2016;48(3):261–266.
16. Oh E, Choi YL, Kwon MJ, et al. Comparison of accuracy of whole-exome sequencing with formalin-fixed paraffin-embedded and fresh frozen tissue samples. *PLoS One*. 2015;10(12):e0144162.
17. Srinivasan M, Sedmak D, Jewell S. Effect of fixatives and tissue processing on the content and integrity of nucleic acids. *Am J Pathol*. 2002;161(6):1961–1971.
18. Hedegaard J, Thorsen K, Lund MK, et al. Next-generation sequencing of RNA and DNA isolated from paired fresh-frozen and formalin-fixed paraffin-embedded samples of human cancer and normal tissue. *PLoS One*. 2014;9(5):e98187.
19. Ross JS, Wang K, Gay L, et al. Comprehensive genomic profiling of carcinoma of unknown primary site: new routes to targeted therapies. *JAMA Oncol*. 2015;1(1):40–49.
20. Froyen G, Broekmans A, Hillen F, et al. Validation and application of a custom-designed targeted next-generation sequencing panel for the diagnostic mutational profiling of solid tumors. *PLoS One*. 2016;11(4):e0154038.
21. Fisher KE, Zhang L, Wang J, et al. Clinical validation and implementation of a targeted next-generation sequencing assay to detect somatic variants in non-small cell lung, melanoma, and gastrointestinal malignancies. *J Mol Diagn*. 2016;18(2):299–315.
22. de Leng WW, Gadellaa-van Hooijdonk CG, Barendregt-Smouter FA, et al. Targeted next generation sequencing as a reliable diagnostic assay for the detection of somatic mutations in tumours using minimal dna amounts from formalin fixed paraffin embedded material. *PLoS One*. 2016;11(2):e0149405.
23. Van Allen EM, Wagle N, Stojanov P, et al. Whole-exome sequencing and clinical interpretation of formalin-fixed, paraffin-embedded tumor samples to guide precision cancer medicine. *Nat Med*. 2014;20(6):682–688.
24. Chau NG, Li YY, Jo VY, et al. Incorporation of next-generation sequencing into routine clinical care to direct treatment of head and neck squamous cell carcinoma. *Clin Cancer Res*. 2016;22(12):2939–2949.
25. Voss JS, Holtegaard LM, Kerr SE, et al. Molecular profiling of cholangiocarcinoma shows potential for targeted therapy treatment decisions. *Hum Pathol*. 2013;44(7):1216–1222.
26. Espy MJ, Uhl JR, Sloan LM, et al. Real-time PCR in clinical microbiology: applications for routine laboratory testing. *Clin Microbiol Rev*. 2006;19(1):165–256.
27. Galante A, Pischke S, Polywka S, et al. Relevance of chronic hepatitis E in liver transplant recipients: a real-life setting. *Transpl Infect Dis*. 2015;17(4):617–622.
28. Protzer U, Bohm F, Longerich T, et al. Molecular detection of hepatitis E virus (HEV) in liver biopsies after liver transplantation. *Mod Pathol*. 2015;28(4):523–532.
29. Haagsma EB, van den Berg AP, Porte RJ, et al. Chronic hepatitis E virus infection in liver transplant recipients. *Liver Transpl*. 2008;14(4):547–553.
30. Kamar N, Izopet J, Tripon S, et al. Ribavirin for chronic hepatitis E virus infection in transplant recipients. *N Engl J Med*. 2014;370(12):1111–1120.
31. Guichard C, Amaddeo G, Imbeaud S, et al. Integrated analysis of somatic mutations and focal copy-number changes identifies key genes and pathways in hepatocellular carcinoma. *Nat Genet*. 2012;44(6):694–698.
32. Cleary SP, Jeck WR, Zhao X, et al. Identification of driver genes in hepatocellular carcinoma by exome sequencing. *Hepatology*. 2013;58(5):1693–1702.
33. Li M, Zhao H, Zhang X, et al. Inactivating mutations of the chromatin remodeling gene ARID2 in hepatocellular carcinoma. *Nat Genet*. 2011;43(9):828–829.
34. Nault JC, Calderaro J, Di Tommaso L, et al. Telomerase reverse transcriptase promoter mutation is an early somatic genetic alteration in the transformation of premalignant nodules in hepatocellular carcinoma on cirrhosis. *Hepatology*. 2014;60(6):1983–1992.
35. Edamoto Y, Hara A, Biernat W, et al. Alterations of RB1, p53 and Wnt pathways in hepatocellular carcinomas associated with hepatitis C, hepatitis B and alcoholic liver cirrhosis. *Int J Cancer*. 2003;106(3):334–341.
36. Schulze K, Imbeaud S, Letouze E, et al. Exome sequencing of hepatocellular carcinomas identifies new mutational signatures and potential therapeutic targets. *Nat Genet*. 2015;47(5):505–511.

37. Ang CS, Kelley RK, Choti MA, et al. Clinicopathologic characteristics and survival outcomes of patients with fibrolamellar carcinoma: data from the fibrolamellar carcinoma consortium. *Gastrointest Cancer Res.* 2013;6(1):3–9.
38. Torbenson M. Fibrolamellar carcinoma: 2012 update. *Scientifica*. 2012;2012:743790.
39. Ross HM, Daniel HD, Vivekanandan P, et al. Fibrolamellar carcinomas are positive for CD68. *Mod Pathol.* 2011;24(3):390–395.
40. Honeyman JN, Simon EP, Robine N, et al. Detection of a recurrent DNAJB1-PRKACA chimeric transcript in fibrolamellar hepatocellular carcinoma. *Science*. 2014;343(6174):1010–1014.
41. Graham RP, Jin L, Knutson DL, et al. DNAJB1-PRKACA is specific for fibrolamellar carcinoma. *Mod Pathol.* 2015;28(6):822–829.
42. Graham RYM, Lam-Himlin D, Terracciano LM, et al. PRKACA fluorescent in situ hybridization reveals novel findings in fibrolamellar carcinoma. *Mod Pathol.* 2016;29:420A.
43. Zucman-Rossi J, Jeannot E, Nhieu JT, et al. Genotype-phenotype correlation in hepatocellular adenoma: new classification and relationship with HCC. *Hepatology*. 2006;43(3):515–524.
44. Nault JC, Zucman Rossi J. Molecular classification of hepatocellular adenomas. *Int J Hepatol.* 2013;2013:315947.
45. Bioulac-Sage P, Rebouissou S, Thomas C, et al. Hepatocellular adenoma subtype classification using molecular markers and immunohistochemistry. *Hepatology*. 2007;46(3):740–748.
46. Nault JC, Fabre M, Couchy G, et al. GNAS-activating mutations define a rare subgroup of inflammatory liver tumors characterized by STAT3 activation. *J Hepatol.* 2012;56(1):184–191.
47. Paradis V. Hepatocellular adenomas: WHO classification and immunohistochemical workup. *Surg Pathol Clin.* 2013;6(2):311–331.
48. Liu L, Shah SS, Naini BV, et al. Immunostains used to subtype hepatic adenomas do not distinguish hepatic adenomas from hepatocellular carcinomas. *Am J Surg Pathol.* 2016;40(8):1062-1069 .
49. Micchelli ST, Vivekanandan P, Boitnott JK, et al. Malignant transformation of hepatic adenomas. *Mod Pathol.* 2008;21(4):491–497.
50. Stoot JH, Coelen RJ, De Jong MC, et al. Malignant transformation of hepatocellular adenomas into hepatocellular carcinomas: a systematic review including more than 1600 adenoma cases. *HPB*. 2010;12(8):509–522.
51. Eichenmuller M, Trippel F, Kreuder M, et al. The genomic landscape of hepatoblastoma and their progenies with HCC-like features. *J Hepatol.* 2014;61(6):1312–1320.
52. Czauderna P, Lopez-Terrada D, Hiyama E, et al. Hepatoblastoma state of the art: pathology, genetics, risk stratification, and chemotherapy. *Curr Opin Pediatr*. 2014;26(1):19–28.
53. Herzog CE, Andrassy RJ, Eftekhari F. Childhood cancers: hepatoblastoma. *Oncologist*. 2000;5(6):445–453.
54. Andersen JB, Spee B, Blechacz BR, et al. Genomic and genetic characterization of cholangiocarcinoma identifies therapeutic targets for tyrosine kinase inhibitors. *Gastroenterology*. 2012;142(4):1021–1031 e15.
55. Borad MJ, Champion MD, Egan JB, et al. Integrated genomic characterization reveals novel, therapeutically relevant drug targets in FGFR and EGFR pathways in sporadic intrahepatic cholangiocarcinoma. *PLoS Genet.* 2014;10(2):e1004135.
56. Jiao Y, Pawlik TM, Anders RA, et al. Exome sequencing identifies frequent inactivating mutations in BAP1, ARID1A and PBRM1 in intrahepatic cholangiocarcinomas. *Nat Genet.* 2013;45(12):1470–1473.
57. Ross JS, Wang K, Gay L, et al. New routes to targeted therapy of intrahepatic cholangiocarcinomas revealed by next-generation sequencing. *Oncologist.* 2014;19(3):235–242.
58. Sia D, Tovar V, Moeini A, et al. Intrahepatic cholangiocarcinoma: pathogenesis and rationale for molecular therapies. *Oncogene*. 2013;32(41):4861–4870.
59. Simbolo M, Fassan M, Ruzzenente A, et al. Multigene mutational profiling of cholangiocarcinomas identifies actionable molecular subgroups. *Oncotarget*. 2014;5(9):2839–2852.
60. Wang P, Dong Q, Zhang C, et al. Mutations in isocitrate dehydrogenase 1 and 2 occur frequently in intrahepatic cholangiocarcinomas and share hypermethylation targets with glioblastomas. *Oncogene*. 2013;32(25):3091–3100.
61. Arai Y, Totoki Y, Hosoda F, et al. Fibroblast growth factor receptor 2 tyrosine kinase fusions define a unique molecular subtype of cholangiocarcinoma. *Hepatology*. 2014;59(4):1427–1434.
62. El Khatib M, Bozko P, Palagani V, et al. Activation of Notch signaling is required for cholangiocarcinoma progression and is enhanced by inactivation of p53 in vivo. *PLoS One*. 2013;8(10):e77433.
63. Graham RP, Barr Fritcher EG, Pestova E, et al. Fibroblast growth factor receptor 2 translocations in intrahepatic cholangiocarcinoma. *Hum Pathol.* 2014;45(8):1630–1638.
64. Borad MJ, Gores GJ, Roberts LR. Fibroblast growth factor receptor 2 fusions as a target for treating cholangiocarcinoma. *Curr Opin Gastroenterol.* 2015;31(3):264–268.

65. Kipp BR, Voss JS, Kerr SE, et al. Isocitrate dehydrogenase 1 and 2 mutations in cholangiocarcinoma. *Hum Pathol.* 2012;43(10):1552–1558.
66. Fujimoto A, Furuta M, Shiraishi Y, et al. Whole-genome mutational landscape of liver cancers displaying biliary phenotype reveals hepatitis impact and molecular diversity. *Nat Commun.* 2015;6:6120.
67. Rizvi S, Borad MJ, Patel T, et al. Cholangiocarcinoma: molecular pathways and therapeutic opportunities. *Semin Liver Dis.* 2014;34(4):456–464.
68. Fritcher EG, Kipp BR, Halling KC, et al. A multivariable model using advanced cytologic methods for the evaluation of indeterminate pancreatobiliary strictures. *Gastroenterology.* 2009;136(7):2180–2186.
69. Kipp BR, Barr Fritcher EG, Pettengill JE, et al. Improving the accuracy of pancreatobiliary tract cytology with fluorescence in situ hybridization: a molecular test with proven clinical success. *Cancer Cytopathol.* 2013;121(11):610–619.
70. Barr Fritcher EG, Voss JS, Brankley SM, et al. An optimized set of fluorescence in situ hybridization probes for detection of pancreatobiliary tract cancer in cytology brush samples. *Gastroenterology.* 2015;149(7):1813–1824 e1.
71. Dudley JC, Zheng Z, McDonald T, et al. Next-generation sequencing and fluorescence in situ hybridization have comparable performance characteristics in the analysis of pancreaticobiliary brushings for malignancy. *J Mol Diagn.* 2016;18(1):124–130.
72. Scorza M, Elce A, Zarrilli F, et al. Genetic diseases that predispose to early liver cirrhosis. *Int J Hepatol.* 2014;2014:713754.
73. Calado RT, Brudno J, Mehta P, et al. Constitutional telomerase mutations are genetic risk factors for cirrhosis. *Hepatology.* 2011;53(5):1600–1607.
74. Torbenson M. Iron in the liver: a review for surgical pathologists. *Adv Anat Pathol.* 2011;18(4):306–317.
75. Wolff AC, Hammond ME, Hicks DG, et al. Recommendations for human epidermal growth factor receptor 2 testing in breast cancer: American Society of Clinical Oncology/College of American Pathologists clinical practice guideline update. *J Clin Oncol.* 2013;31(31):3997–4013.
76. Kleibl Z, Kristensen VN. Women at high risk of breast cancer: molecular characteristics, clinical presentation and management. *Breast.* 2016;28:136–144.
77. Dacic S. Molecular genetic testing for lung adenocarcinomas: a practical approach to clinically relevant mutations and translocations. *J Clin Pathol.* 2013;66(10):870–874.
78. Drilon A, Wang L, Hasanovic A, et al. Response to Cabozantinib in patients with RET fusion-positive lung adenocarcinomas. *Cancer Discov.* 2013;3(6):630–635.
79. Engelman JA, Zejnullahu K, Mitsudomi T, et al. MET amplification leads to gefitinib resistance in lung cancer by activating ERBB3 signaling. *Science.* 2007;316(5827):1039–1043.
80. Kwak EL, Bang YJ, Camidge DR, et al. Anaplastic lymphoma kinase inhibition in non-small-cell lung cancer. *N Engl J Med.* 2010;363(18):1693–1703.
81. Lynch TJ, Bell DW, Sordella R, et al. Activating mutations in the epidermal growth factor receptor underlying responsiveness of non-small-cell lung cancer to gefitinib. *N Engl J Med.* 2004;350(21):2129–2139.
82. Roberts PJ, Stinchcombe TE. KRAS mutation: should we test for it, and does it matter? *J Clin Oncol.* 2013;31(8):1112–1121.
83. Gazdar A, Robinson L, Oliver D, et al. Hereditary lung cancer syndrome targets never smokers with germline EGFR gene T790M mutations. *J Thorac Oncol.* 2014;9(4):456–463.
84. Douillard JY, Oliner KS, Siena S, et al. Panitumumab-FOLFOX4 treatment and RAS mutations in colorectal cancer. *N Engl J Med.* 2013;369(11):1023–1034.
85. Karapetis CS, Khambata-Ford S, Jonker DJ, et al. K-ras mutations and benefit from cetuximab in advanced colorectal cancer. *N Engl J Med.* 2008;359(17):1757–1765.
86. De Roock W, Claes B, Bernasconi D, et al. Effects of KRAS, BRAF, NRAS, and PIK3CA mutations on the efficacy of cetuximab plus chemotherapy in chemotherapy-refractory metastatic colorectal cancer: a retrospective consortium analysis. *Lancet Oncol.* 2010;11(8):753–762.
87. Short E, Thomas LE, Hurley J, et al. Inherited predisposition to colorectal cancer: towards a more complete picture. *J Med Genet.* 2015;52(12):791–796.
88. Carvajal RD, Antonescu CR, Wolchok JD, et al. KIT as a therapeutic target in metastatic melanoma. *JAMA.* 2011;305(22):2327–2334.
89. Flaherty KT, Puzanov I, Kim KB, et al. Inhibition of mutated, activated BRAF in metastatic melanoma. *N Engl J Med.* 2010;363(9):809–819.
90. Van Raamsdonk CD, Griewank KG, Crosby MB, et al. Mutations in GNA11 in uveal melanoma. *N Engl J Med.* 2010;363(23):2191–2199.
91. Soura E, Eliades PJ, Shannon K, et al. Hereditary melanoma: update on syndromes and management: emerging melanoma cancer complexes and genetic counseling. *J Am Acad Dermatol.* 2016;74(3):411–420; quiz 21–22.
92. Agaram NP, Wong GC, Guo T, et al. Novel V600E BRAF mutations in imatinib-naive and imatinib-resistant gastrointestinal stromal tumors. *Genes Chromosomes Cancer.* 2008;47(10):853–859.

93. Rammohan A, Sathyanesan J, Rajendran K, et al. A gist of gastrointestinal stromal tumors: a review. *World J Gastrointest Oncol*. 2013;5(6):102–112.
94. Miranda C, Nucifora M, Molinari F, et al. KRAS and BRAF mutations predict primary resistance to imatinib in gastrointestinal stromal tumors. *Clin Cancer Res*. 2012;18(6):1769–1776.
95. Patil DT, Rubin BP. Genetics of gastrointestinal stromal tumors: a heterogeneous family of tumors? *Surg Pathol Clin*. 2015;8(3):515–524.
96. Burgoyne AM, Somaiah N, Sicklick JK. Gastrointestinal stromal tumors in the setting of multiple tumor syndromes. *Curr Opin Oncol*. 2014;26(4):408–414.

24

Imaging of liver tumors

Michael L. Wells, MD, Sudhakar K. Venkatesh, MD

Radiologic evaluation represents a critical component of liver tumor detection and characterization. After discovery of a liver mass, the radiologic findings will typically provide guidance for patient management. Management may include imaging follow-up, percutaneous biopsy, or surgical resection. Radiologic findings can safely diagnose benign lesions such as cysts or hemangiomas with sufficient confidence that further workup is unnecessary. However, for most complex cystic and solid liver masses the imaging findings are often not entirely specific, and a differential diagnosis of pathologic entities are provided. When a benign entity is favored, many patients will be given imaging follow-up to determine stability of the mass over time. In challenging cases, a mass discovered by imaging must ultimately be diagnosed by percutaneous biopsy or surgical resection. Radiologic–pathologic collaboration, with careful correlation between the initial imaging findings and the pathology findings, is often helpful to arrive at the correct diagnosis. Radiologic imaging is very helpful for describing the size, anatomic extent, and number of masses, which may not be entirely included within a biopsy or surgical specimen. Correlation with prior imaging is often necessary to ensure diagnostic concordance and can prevent errors in diagnosis by revealing inadequate sampling of a tumor or sampling of the wrong lesion.

The vast majority of liver mass evaluations entail cross-sectional imaging using ultrasound (US), computed tomography (CT), and magnetic resonance imaging (MRI). A basic understanding of the principles of operation and the terminology used to describe the images is helpful for each of these modalities. A brief introduction of these modalities is provided below. Liver mass evaluation is further supplemented with additional radiologic modalities including positron emission tomography (PET), scintigraphy using a variety of radiopharmaceuticals, and fluoroscopic angiography. Discussion of these modalities will be limited and provided in the context of individual pathologic liver entities.

24.1 IMAGING MODALITIES

Ultrasound

Ultrasound (US) is often the first-line test used to examine the liver because of its low cost, lack of ionizing radiation, and accessibility. US produces images by imparting sound waves into the tissues at a high frequency, typically between 3 and 7 MHz. Lower frequencies travel further into the tissues, allowing deeper tissues to be visualized, whereas the higher frequencies provide better spatial resolution and anatomic detail with more limited depth of penetration. As sound waves travel into the liver, they encounter tissues that transmit the sound waves at different speeds (e.g., transmission speed in liver is 1,570 m/s, in water is 1,489 m/s and within fat is 1,450 m/s). Interfaces between these tissues result in a change in transmission speed and the reflection of sound waves back to the transducer, where they are detected and used to form an image. The US images of a liver mass are described in terms of relative echogenicity, with areas of the mass that are brighter than the background liver referred to as *hyperechoic*, areas that are similar in brightness referred to as *isoechoic*, areas that are darker referred to as *hypoechoic*, and areas with an absence of any signal referred to as *anechoic*. It is important to note that the background liver can have abnormally increased echogenicity in the setting of steatosis or fibrosis, which can alter the US appearance of liver masses.

Doppler imaging is used to assess blood flow within the liver. As sound waves encounter moving elements within the blood, not only are the sound waves are reflected back to the transducer, but the movement of the object alters the frequency of the reflected waves. This phenomenon is analogous to the higher pitched sound of a train horn while it is moving toward you and lower pitch while it is moving away. Detecting this change in frequency allows calculation of the direction and velocity of the flowing blood. This property can be used to assess flowing blood within the vasculature and within liver tumors.

The strengths of US include its ability to assess the liver parenchyma, biliary tree, and vascular supply of the liver. In the evaluation of liver masses, US is primarily useful for mass detection and for its ability to differentiate between cystic and solid lesions. US is limited by its inability to penetrate bone or gas filled organs. Overlying ribs and gas-containing bowel or lung tissue occasionally results in regions of the liver that cannot be adequately visualized. The depth of sound wave penetration is also limited, which can lead to incomplete parenchymal evaluation. This is particularly a problem in obese patients, where there is increased thickness of subcutaneous fat, and in livers with poor penetration because of parenchymal disease such as steatosis or fibrosis. Of note, liver evaluation with US is highly operator dependent. Sonographers working in a low-volume practices may be prone to inadequate evaluation of the entire liver parenchyma, or not optimizing the scanner settings to demonstrate cystic components of a mass or internal blood flow.

Computed tomography

Computed tomography (CT) is commonly used to evaluate liver tumors because of its accessibility, reproducibility, and its relative simplicity to perform and interpret. CT produces images by generating high-energy photons (typically up to 140 keV), which are a transmitted through the patient and are received by a detector on the opposite side of the patient. The photon generator and detector are mounted on a gantry, which rotates around the patient in a helical pattern. Tissues of different composition attenuate photons to varying degrees. These differences in attenuation result in contrast, which is used to generate a CT image. Bright regions of a CT image are referred to as *high attenuation* or hyperdensity and dark regions as *low attenuation* or hypodensity. Attenuation of tissue substances on CT images are often measured in terms of Hounsfield units (HU). Hounsfield units are a measure of relative attenuation and calculated by the formula $HU = 1{,}000 \times (\mu - \mu_{water})/(\mu_{water} - \mu_{air})$, where μ is the linear attenuation coefficient. For reference, common HU include air = −1,000, fat = −100 to −50, water = 0, blood = 30 to 45, liver 40 to 60, and bone 700 to 3,000.

Iodine-containing contrast medium is routinely injected intravenously into the patient to increase contrast between tissues. Iodinated contrast injection provides information regarding the anatomic vascular supply, the rate of blood flow, and the volume of distribution within tissue. These characteristics are very useful for describing and categorizing liver masses. Increased attenuation of tissue in response to IV contrast uptake is referred to as *enhancement*. In the first few minutes following contrast injection, the relative amount of iodinated contrast changes rapidly within tissues of different composition. This change is typically assessed by scanning the patients multiple times to provide a dynamic evaluation.

The time at which a patient is scanned after injection is referred to as the *phase* of contrast enhancement. The most important phases of contrast enhancement for liver tumor characterization include the late arterial phase, the portal venous phase, and the delayed (or equilibrium) phase. The late arterial phase is the time at which the injected contrast bolus has opacified the hepatic arteries and has just begun to opacify the portal veins; this typically occurs 15 to 35 seconds after contrast injection. Imaging at time points earlier than this may fail to show enhancement in tumors with hepatic arterial vascular supply. The portal venous phase is defined as the time at which the contrast bolus has opacified the portal veins and has just begun to opacify the hepatic veins; this occurs roughly 60 seconds after injection. This is typically the time at which the hepatic parenchyma is maximally enhanced. The delayed or equilibrium phase includes imagings that are usually performed between 3 and 10 minutes after injection. Most iodinated IV contrast agents used for CT remain within the extracellular compartment of tissues. Over time, these contrast agents diffuse through the extracellular space to equilibrate between the extracellular intravascular and extravascular compartments. Fibrotic or sclerotic tissues remain enhanced in the delayed phases because of large extracellular spaces associated with fibrosis.

CT has several advantages, including its ability to scan rapidly and to provide a comprehensive assessment for metastatic disease. CT examinations are often performed for liver mass evaluation out of convenience, as the entire body can be quickly assessed for metastatic disease in a single setting. The ability to acquire an imaging data set within a few seconds is a major advantage for patients who cannot hold their breath or cannot breathe consistently, as is required for MRI. An inability to adequately suspend respiration can render an abdominal MRI nondiagnostic. CT is also able to acquire high spatial resolution, 3D image data sets that can be reformatted in any plane. These types of data sets are difficult to acquire at MRI and, with current technology, most MRI images are acquired with the intention of being viewed in a single plane.

Specific limitations of CT include inferior soft-tissue and IV contrast resolution when compared with MRI. The limited soft-tissue contrast can create difficulty differentiating a low-attenuation solid mass from a cystic mass or lipid-containing tissue. Similarly, high-attenuation tissue or calcification can occasionally be difficult to differentiate from iodine-containing contrast media. Despite these limitations, CT has a very high sensitivity for detection of small calcifications and gas, when compared with either MRI or US. The radiation exposure imposed by CT is another limitation, one that frequently restricts the number of phases obtained during an examination and the frequency of follow-up exams. However, in the presence of malignancy or in advanced patient age, the risk imposed to the patient because of radiation exposure at CT is probably negligible.

Magnetic resonance imaging

MRI provides the best discrimination between soft tissues of different types and is the modality of choice for both liver mass detection and liver mass characterization. MRI uses a strong static magnetic field, weak gradient magnetic fields, and radiofrequency transmission coils to alter the orientation of protons found within hydrogen atoms, which are the most abundant element in the human body. Protons are imaged by specifically changing gradient field strengths, applying energy through radiofrequency transmissions, and recording signal from the tissue at varying time points. The combinations of the steps required to produce images are referred to as *pulse sequences*.

In a strong static magnetic field, the axis of a proton's magnetic dipole will tend to align with that of the static magnetic field. The axis of a proton's dipole is not aligned exactly with that of the magnet but slightly off center and precesses (rotates) around it at a frequency proportional to the strength of the magnetic field. This precessional frequency is specific to particular protons and can be exploited by using an applied radiofrequency electromagnetic pulse at the same frequency to shift proton orientation away from that of the magnetic field. After protons have been shifted, they will relax (or reorient) with the direction of the static magnetic field.

There are two basic ways in which protons relax after being stimulated by a radiofrequency pulse: T1 (or longitudinal) relaxation and T2 (or transverse) relaxation. These two types of relaxation occur at different rates, which are affected by a proton's surrounding magnetic micro-environment or tissue type. Measuring differences in the T1 and T2 relaxation rates between different tissues creates contrast. This contrast in turn forms the basis for creating images at MRI. When reviewing MRI images, bright regions of the image are referred to as having *high signal* or *hyperintense* and dark regions as *low signal* or *hypointense*.

A typical liver imaging protocol includes a combination of pulse sequences designed to show contrast differences between T1 and T2 relaxation rates of different tissue and are referred to as *T1-weighted* and *T2-weighted* images. Images of each sequence are specifically used to reveal different anatomic features or abnormalities of tissue content, so characterization of a tumor using MRI requires review of several image sets.

A basic knowledge of typical tissue signal intensities on MRI images is necessary for image review. On T1-weighted images, water is low in signal and fat is high in signal. On T2-weighted images, both water and fat are high in signal. The weighting of an image can often be determined by looking at the signal of cerebrospinal fluid in the spinal canal. T2-weighted images are predominantly used to image water content of tissues. An extreme example of T2-weighted image is magnetic resonance cholangiography, in which the images are very heavily T2-weighted, such that the only structures clearly visible on the images are fluid-containing structures, such as the bile ducts and renal collecting system. It is important to know that both T1- and T2-weighted images are often altered by suppressing the signal from fat. This is accomplished by a variety of techniques and allows increased dynamic range of the images, increased conspicuity of liver parenchyma, and detection of fat-containing structures.

Specialized MRI techniques that are used to image the liver include in-phase and opposed-phase imaging and diffusion-weighted imaging. Protons within water precess at a slightly different frequency than those found in fat. When T1-weighted image acquisition is timed so that the magnetic dipoles of both water and fat are oriented in the same direction, the signal intensities from both tissue types are additive; this produces an in-phase image. When the timing of image acquisition is altered so that the dipoles of fat and water are oriented in opposite directions, the signal intensities cancel out and the overall signal intensity decreases, this produces an opposed-phase image.

These properties can be exploited to identify tissues that contain elements of both water and fat. When the signal from a voxel (a position in a 3 dimensional image) of an image of tissue originates from 50% water and 50% fat, the signal intensity of that voxel should be near zero on the out-of-phase image. Because of this, lesions that drop in signal intensity on the opposed-phase image, when compared to in-phase image, are likely to have fat.

Diffusion-weighted imaging basically measures the Brownian motion of water molecules. Tissues that are either very cellular or swollen tend to have restricted motion on diffusion-weighted imaging. Diffusion-weighted imaging is a technique in which specialized gradient magnetic fields are added to a T2-weighted image. These gradients fields are designed such that bound protons that are unable to move (their ability to diffuse is restricted) do not lose signal, whereas moving protons lose signal rapidly. The most common explanation for restricted diffusion in tissues is increased cellularity, in which a greater percentage of the imaged protons are within cells and their movement is physically restricted by cellular membranes. Another common reason for restricted diffusion includes abscess formation, in which the protons are extracellular but free diffusion is restricted by the highly viscous and proteinaceous environment. The resulting diffusion-weighted image shows areas of high signal, which could represent either an intrinsically T2 hyperintense tissue or a tissue with restricted diffusion. Multiple diffusion-weighted images are produced with increasing strengths of the gradient fields. The relative change in signal of each pixel over the series of images is used to calculate an apparent diffusion coefficient (ADC) map. The apparent diffusion coefficient map shows pixels on the diffusion-weighted image, with true restricted diffusion showing low-signal intensity, whereas regions of high-signal intensity that are seen on both diffusion-weighted image and the ADC map represent tissue with intrinsically high T2 signal (on the diffusion-weighted image these regions are referred to as *T2 shine through*) and/or unrestricted diffusion.

IV contrast-enhanced MRI imaging of the liver is typically performed with fat saturated T1-weighted sequences. IV gadolinium shortens the T1 relaxation time of tissues, resulting in higher signal intensity. Most gadolinium contrast agents are extracellular and have dynamic enhancement properties similar to those discussed previously for iodinated CT contrast agents. The phases of dynamic contrast enhancement that are routinely acquired at MRI are the same as those acquired at CT. MRI contrast agents, referred to as *hepatobiliary agents*, are also available. These agents are actively taken up into hepatocytes and excreted into the bile ducts. The most commonly used is disodium gadoxetate (Gd-EOB-DTPA; Eovist; Bayer Corporation, Pittsburgh, PA) and gadobenate dimeglumine (Gd-BOPTA; MultiHance; Bracco Diagnostics Inc, Princeton, NJ). These contrast agents are typically imaged in a dynamic fashion similar to extracellular agents. Additional images at delays of 20 to 120 minutes are referred to as the *hepatobiliary phase*. During the hepatobiliary phase, the normal liver is diffusely high signal and contrast agent increases the signal intensity of the biliary tree. These images have a high sensitivity for detection of liver masses that do not contain hepatocytes and thus do not retain the contrast agent.

MRI is considered the preferred modality for liver mass evaluation.[1] MRI pulse sequences are exquisitely sensitive to changes in normal liver parenchymal composition and are highly sensitive for detection of liver masses.[2–4] MRI is more sensitive than CT or US for detection of substances such as fat or iron.[3] Despite these advantages MRI does have limitations, including cost and patient contraindications to the MRI scanner. Many metallic implanted foreign bodies and pacemakers are not compatible with the strong magnetic fields and radiofrequency gradient pulses. Patient inability to cooperate can also result in a severely limited MRI exam. Acquisition of MRI images takes a relatively long time and patients who cannot hold their breath or cannot breathe at a consistent rate will result in images with substantial motion artifact. MRI is also limited by a number of image artifacts because of magnetic susceptibility of metallic foreign bodies, pulsation artifacts from vessels, and other artifacts when patients are large in size or have significant ascites. A detailed discussion of these artifacts is beyond the scope of this chapter, but it is important to recognize that these artifacts can impair the interpretation of images and occasionally simulate liver pathology.

24.2 RADIOLOGIC DESCRIPTION OF SPECIFIC LIVER MASSES

Simple hepatic cyst

Simple liver cysts are readily diagnosed on imaging. By US evaluation, the contents of a simple cyst should be anechoic (Fig. 24.1). The cyst walls should be thin or imperceptible. The lack of internal architecture to attenuate sound waves results in higher amplitude of echoes in the tissues directly posterior to the cyst, a phenomenon referred to as *posterior acoustic enhancement*. There should be no detectable Doppler vascular flow within a cyst. CT findings of a homogenously low-attenuation mass (0 to 20 HU) with sharp borders and no internal enhancement are consistent with a benign cyst.[5] MRI will show a cyst to be homogenously high signal on T2-weighted images; low signal on T1-weighted images with no detectable internal enhancement. A simple cyst will be high signal on both diffusion weighted imaging and apparent diffusion coefficient, reflecting its "T2 shine through" effect and the lack of true restricted diffusion. At hepatobiliary phase imaging, excretion of contrast material into the biliary tree will not demonstrate uptake into a simple cyst, because of lack of biliary communication.

The finding of a simple cyst in a subcapsular location of hepatic segment IV suggests that it is a ciliated foregut cyst.[6] The finding of numerous tiny (<15 mm) simple cysts within the liver is suggestive of biliary hamartomas (von Meyenburg Complexes).[6]

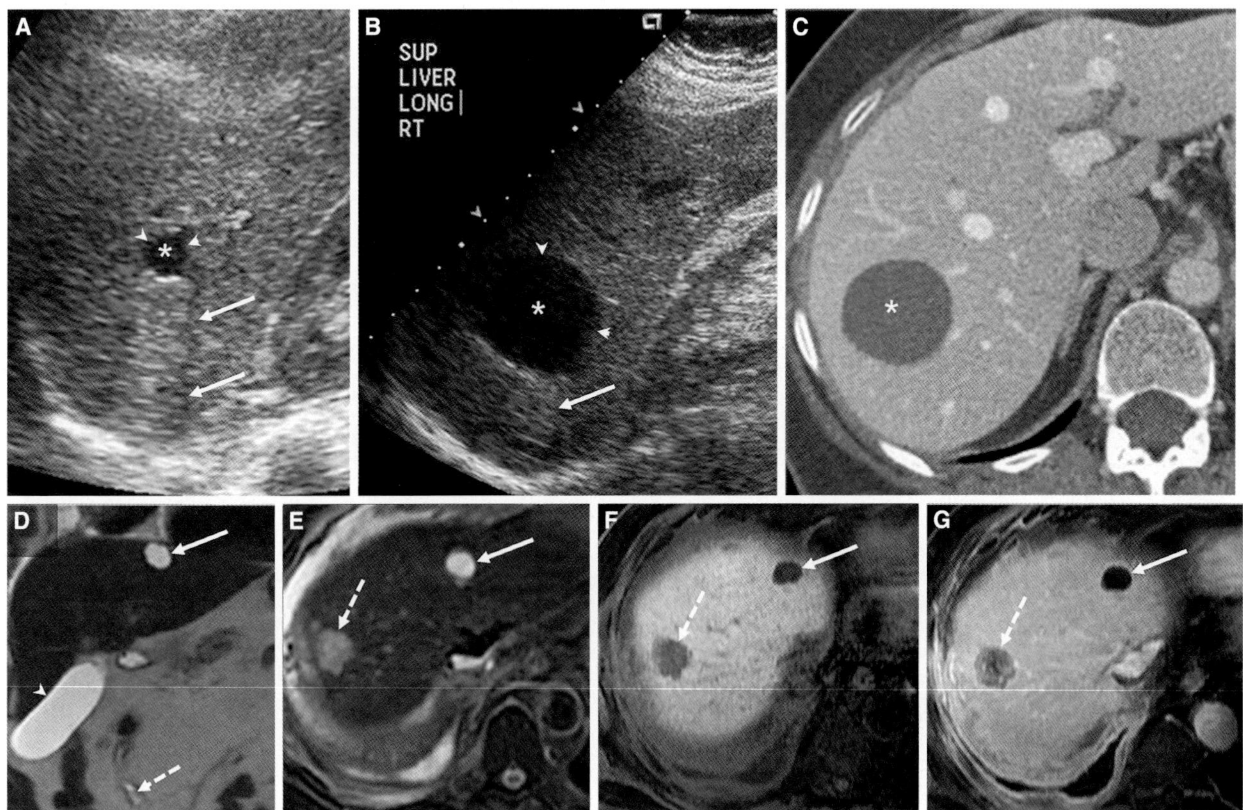

Figure 24.1 (A) Simple cyst demonstrated on US. Typical features include an anechoic cyst (*asterisk*) with thin or imperceptible walls (*arrowheads*) and posterior acoustic enhancement (*arrows*). **(B)** Grayscale US performed on the same patient 6 years later shows increased size of the mass, but similar imaging findings diagnostic of a benign cyst. **(C)** Axial image from a contrast-enhanced CT scan performed to evaluate the cyst shows CT features of a simple cyst (*asterisk*) including homogenous internal fluid (0–20 HU) attenuation, thin or imperceptible walls, and lack of enhancement. **(D)** Coronal T2-weighted MRI image showing a simple cyst (*arrow*) with very high T2 signal identical to that found in the gallbladder (*arrowhead*) and bowel lumen (*dashed arrow*). **(E)** Axial T2-weighted MRI image shows the same cyst (*arrow*) to be much higher in signal intensity when compared with a nearby adenocarcinoma metastasis (*dashed arrow*). **(F)** Axial fat-suppressed T1-weighted image shows the cyst (*arrow*) to be very low in signal intensity consistent with simple fluid. The cyst is much lower in signal when compared to the nearby metastasis (*dashed arrow*). **(G)** Axial fat-suppressed T1-weighted image with intravenous contrast enhancement in the portal venous phase shows no enhancement of the cyst (*arrow*), whereas the metastasis (*dashed arrow*) shows irregular peripheral increased signal because of accumulation of contrast.

Numerous larger hepatic cysts (typically several centimeters in size) can be seen with autosomal dominant polycystic liver and kidney disease. In this condition, the intraparenchymal liver cysts can be accompanied by numerous small peribiliary cysts and cysts within the kidneys. Cysts that have hemorrhage can result in increased echogenicity at US, increased attenuation at CT, and increased T1 signal at MRI. Cysts complicated by infection can have imaging findings identical to an abscess.

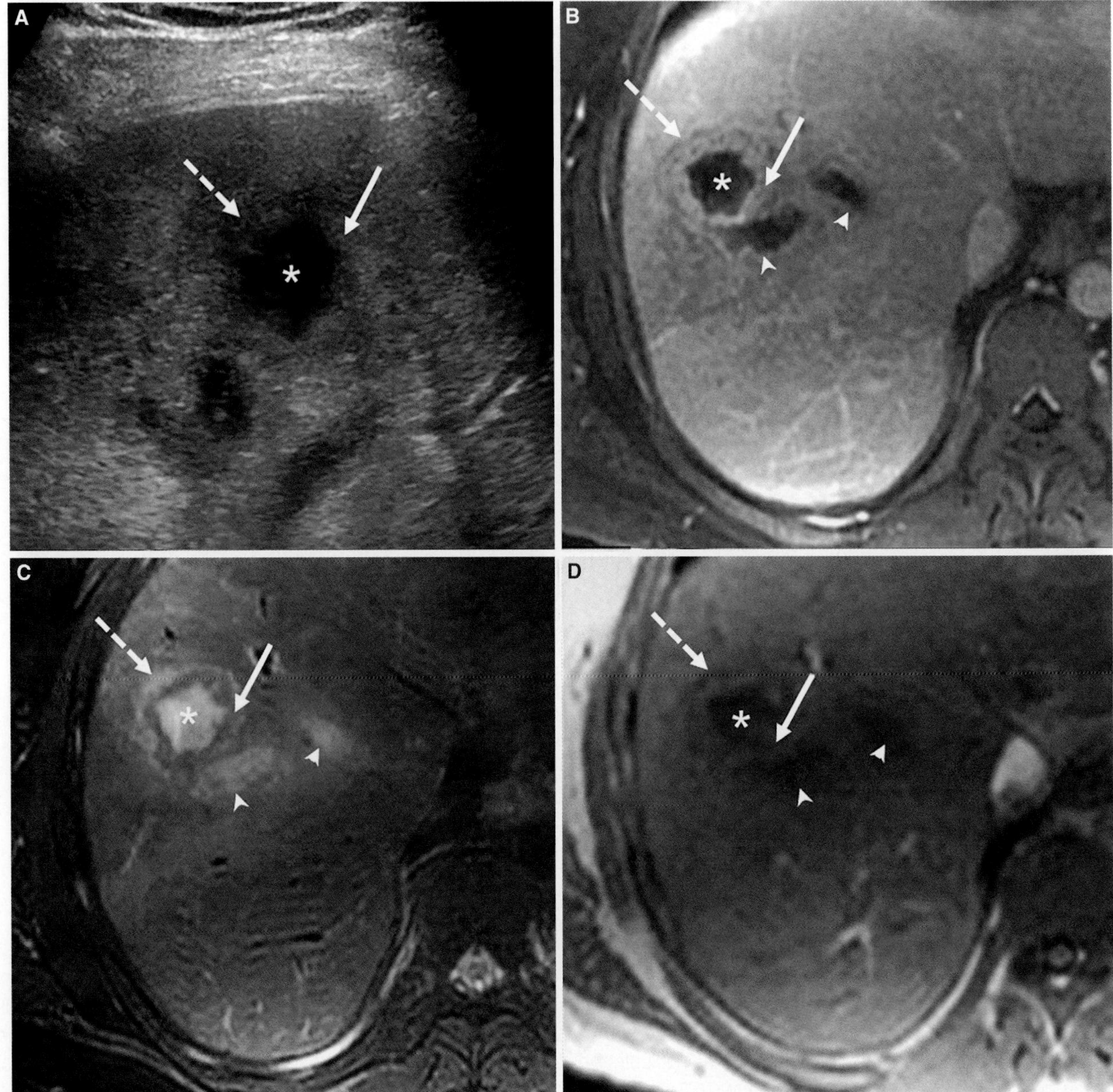

Figure 24.2 **(A)** Grayscale US image of a hepatic abscess. Abscess cavity (*asterisk*) is hypoechoic surrounded by an irregular wall (*arrow*). A thin low-echogenicity band surrounds the abscess cavity corresponding to edematous hepatic parenchyma (*dashed arrow*). **(B, C)** Axial fat-suppressed T1-weighted contrast-enhanced MRI image **(B)**, axial fat-suppressed T2-weighted MRI image **(C)**, and axial T1-weighted MRI image **(D)** show similar findings including a nonenhancing central cavity (*asterisk*) surrounded by an irregular enhancing abscess wall (*arrows*) and a band of low T1 and high T2 signal edema (*dashed arrows*). **(E, F)** Axial diffusion-weighted image **(D)** and apparent diffusion coefficient map **(E)** show high and low signal of the abscess cavity (*asterisk*) respectively indicated marked restricted diffusion. Structures incompletely included on these images (**B–F**, *arrowheads*) represent septic thrombophlebitis within the hepatic veins.

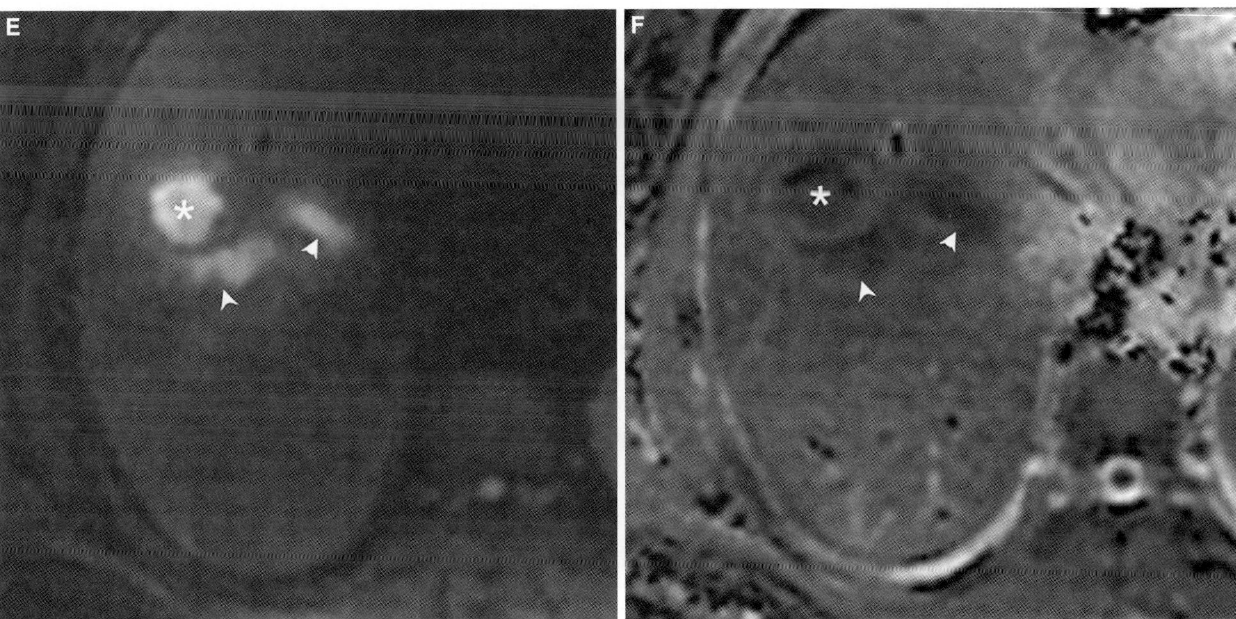

Figure 24.2 *(continued)*

Abscess

A pyogenic liver abscess can occasionally simulate a liver tumor at imaging. The lesions are often multiple and may be clustered in one region of the liver, becoming confluent over time. Pyogenic abscess because of *Klebsiella pneumoniae* are typically multiseptated or multi-loculated whereas an amebic (*Entamoeba histolytica*) liver abscess is unilocular and often single. At US, liver abscesses tend to have poorly defined borders because of adjacent inflammation (Fig. 24.2). The internal contents vary in appearance but they typically appear hyperechoic early and become hypoechoic over time, sometimes with the development of internal septations.[7] Despite internal echogenicity, abscesses show posterior acoustic enhancement, which is a clue to its internal fluid content. CT typically demonstrates a hypoattenuating mass with an irregular margin. Early in abscess formation, the lesion may enhance homogenously. After necrosis has occurred and fluid has accumulated, adjacent inflammation and hyperemia will result in rim enhancement and central avascularity. Inflammation can cause transient segmental perfusion abnormalities in the adjacent liver, which are characterized by geographic regions of arterial hyperenhancement, which fade to isoattenuation on delayed images. CT identification of internal gas in the absence of instrumentation or air introduction from the biliary tree is diagnostic of an abscess. On MRI, an abscess is T1 hypointense and T2 hyperintense.[8] Reactive edema within the adjacent hepatic parenchyma appears as a hazy T2 hyperintense halo. As with CT, rim enhancement and adjacent perfusion abnormalities may be present. An abscess typically results in significant restricted diffusion, which can be a helpful diagnostic finding.

Numerous tiny hepatic microabscesses (<2 cm) can be seen with conditions such as disseminated candidiasis and staphylococcus septicemia.[9] These cases may show similar findings in the spleen and lungs. The lesions appear as small hypoechoic or hypoattenuating nodules at US and CT respectively. At MRI, they appear similar to larger pyogenic abscesses in that they are T2 hyperintense and show restricted diffusion. The imaging differential diagnosis for these findings typically includes metastatic disease, sarcoidosis, and lymphoma.

Focal hepatic steatosis and focal fatty sparing

Hepatic steatosis shows a variety of patterns on imaging. The changes are most commonly diffuse, but can also appear segmental, perivascular, or focal. Focal steatosis can simulate a mass on both US and CT imaging (Fig. 24.3). MRI using in and opposed-phase imaging is very sensitive to the presence of fat and the diagnosis is often readily apparent.[10] On US, regions of hepatic steatosis are hyperechoic relative to normal parenchyma and at CT they are hypoattenuating compared to normal parenchyma. Conversely, a diffusely steatotic liver with a region of focal sparing can simulate a hypoechoic mass on US, and on CT can appear as a hyperattenuating or hyperenhancing mass. At imaging, regions of steatosis can show

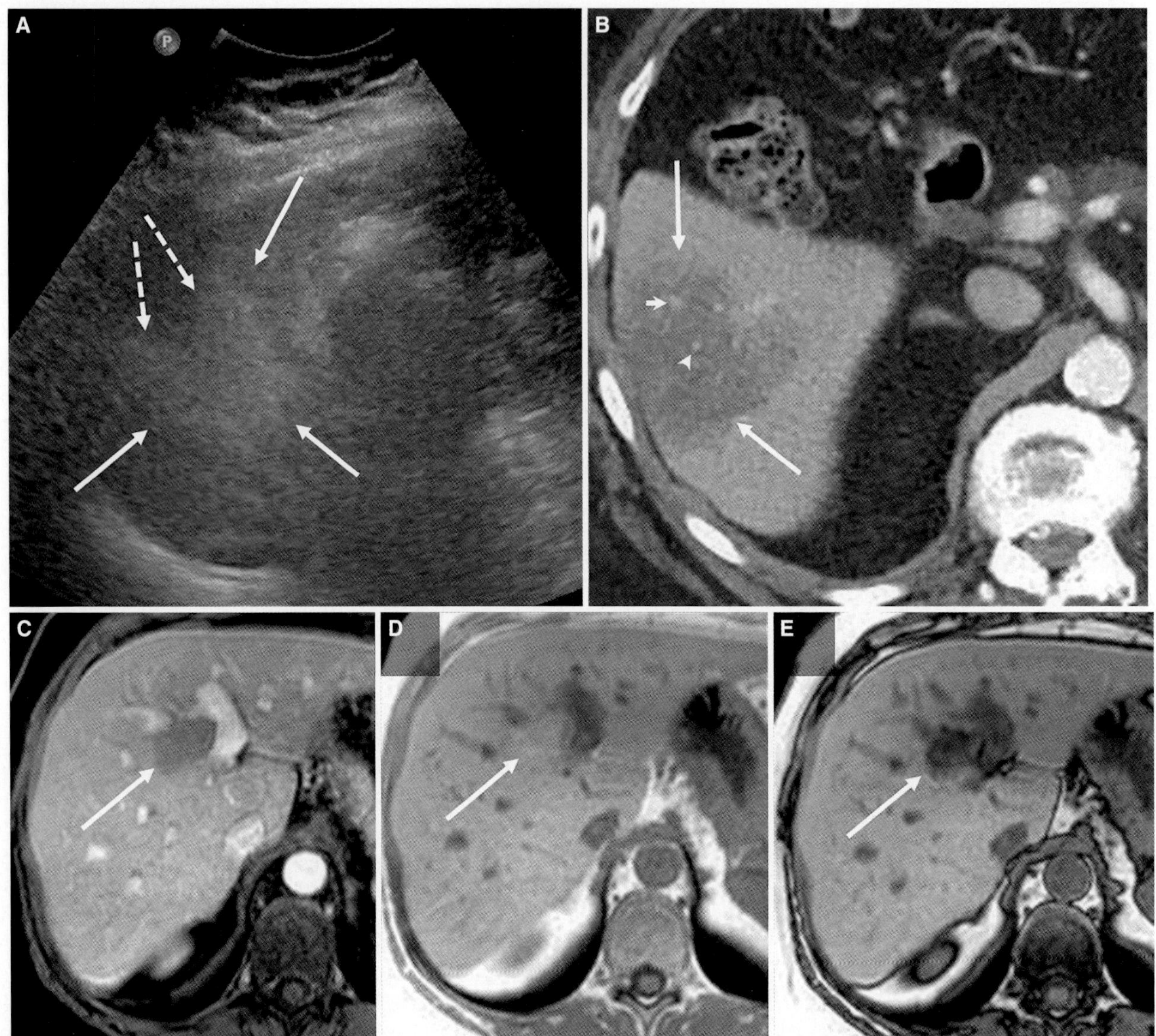

Figure 24.3 (A, B) Apparent hyperechoic mass in the right hepatic lobe discovered on US (**A**, *arrows*). The mass was further evaluated at CT and shown to be focal hepatic steatosis (**B**, *arrows*). Characteristic findings include geographic pattern of distribution, angulated margins (**A**, *dashed arrow*), and lack of mass effect with portal veins (**B**, *arrow heads*) coursing normally through the parenchyma. **(C–E)** Axial hepatobiliary agent contrast-enhanced MRI obtained at 20-minute delay shows an apparent mass within hepatic segment IV (**C**, *arrow*). The abnormality is barely visible on axial T1-weighted in-phase image (**D**, *arrow*). Significant loss of signal on axial T1-weighted out-of-phase image (**E**, *arrow*) shows the lesion to be composed of intracellular lipid. Not shown, the absence of a fat-containing mass was further proven in this case by lack of concerning findings on T2 and diffusion-weighted sequences.

focal nodular or segmental patterns that simulate a malignancy and should be considered in the differential diagnosis of focal lesions. Clues to the correct diagnosis include a lack of mass effect on adjacent liver borders, undisturbed course of bile ducts and/or blood vessels, geographic and/or linear borders, and typical location along the gallbladder fossa and falciform ligament. When biopsy of a suspected mass reveals normal liver parenchyma, careful review of the patient's imaging should be performed to exclude the possibility of a benign condition, such as focal steatosis, and to ensure the biopsy was performed at the proper location.

Cavernous hemangioma

Cavernous hemangiomas typically appear as well circumscribed, round or lobulated mass. On US, hemangiomas are typically homogenously hyperechoic with posterior acoustic enhancement (Fig. 24.4). The

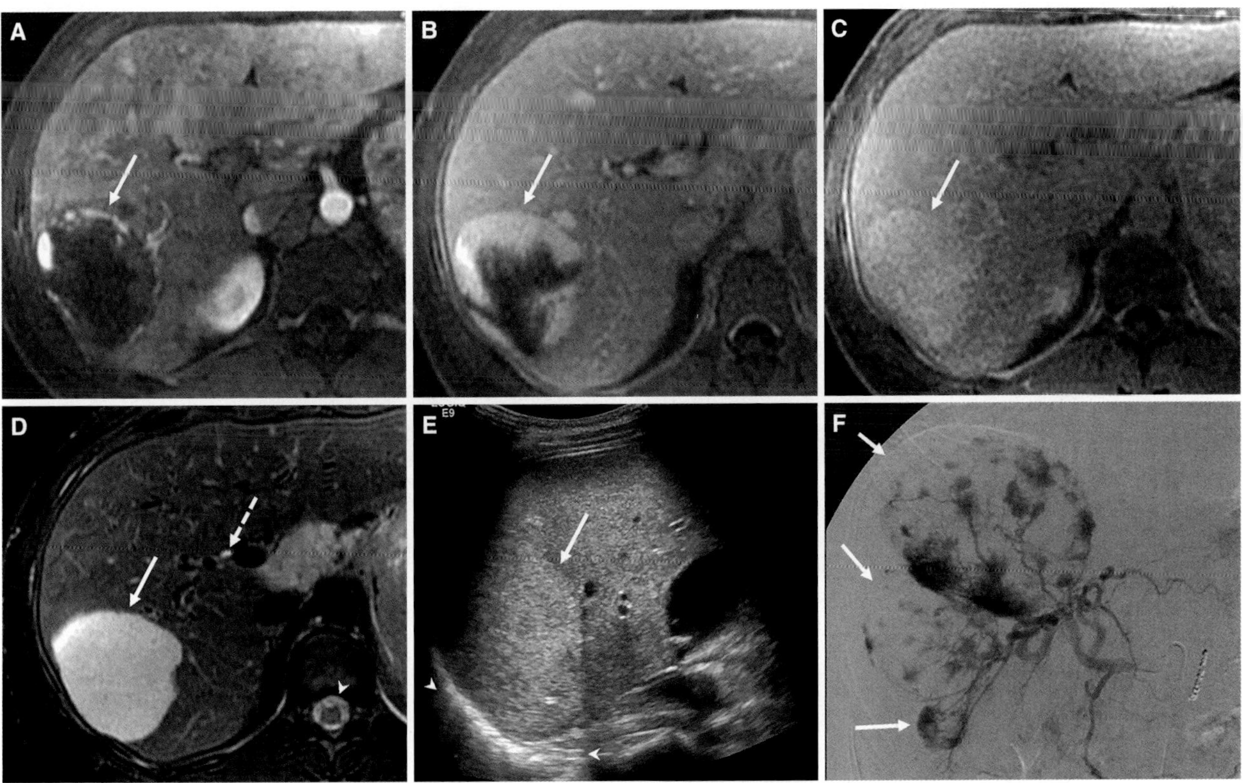

Figure 24.4 Typical hemangioma. **(A–C)** Axial T1-weighted contrast-enhanced MRI images in the late arterial **(A)**, portal venous **(B)**, and 15-minute delayed phase **(C)** show the classic peripheral, nodular, discontinuous enhancement with progressive centripetal central enhancement. Importantly, the hemangioma is isointense to the aortic blood pool on all images, retains contrast even when imaged at a long delay, and fills completely. **(D)** Axial T2-weighted fat-saturated MRI image shows the characteristic high T2 signal of a hemangioma, which is similar to free water in the biliary tree (*dashed arrow*) and spinal canal (*arrow head*). **(E)** Grayscale US image shows the typical well-circumscribed and homogenously hyperechoic appearance of a hemangioma. Note also the finding of posterior acoustic enhancement, which is often also seen with hemangiomas (*arrow head*). **(F)** Angiogram performed by injection of the common hepatic artery shows three separate hemangiomas with peripheral nodular contrast enhancement (each hemangioma is indicated by a separate arrow).

diffuse hyperechogenicity is thought to be caused by reflections from the walls of numerous internal blood filled channels. In 20% to 40% of hemangiomas, US shows a peripheral rim of hyperechogenicity and central hypoechogenicity, a less common but recognized pattern.[11] At CT, hemangiomas are typically homogenously hypoattenuating on precontrast images. Dynamic contrast enhancement on CT and MRI shows a characteristic pattern of peripheral discontinuous globular enhancement with progressive centripetal enhancement (moving toward the center) on subsequent phases.[5] Hemangiomas tend to fill in completely and retain contrast on delayed-phase images. On all phases, the appearance of the contrast within the hemangioma is similar to that of the aortic blood pool.[12] This characteristic enhancement pattern is considered highly specific for hemangiomas.[13] Small hemangiomas and atypical larger hemangiomas may "flash fill," in which the entire lesion enhances homogenously, but again the degree of the enhancement is similar to that of the aorta. MRI is very helpful in the diagnosis of hemangiomas by demonstrating high T2 signal, near that of simple fluid. Combining the findings of high T2 signal with characteristic enhancement pattern allows a confident diagnosis to be made in most cases.

Large hemangiomas (greater than 5 cm in size) are often referred to as *giant hemangiomas*. These tend to show atypical enhancement, with lack of complete central filling because of the presence of a central scar.[14,15] The central portion of the lesion, which does not enhance, is typically markedly hypoattenuating on CT, markedly T2 hyperintense, and T1 hypointense at MRI (Fig. 24.5). Larger lesions can also demonstrate inhomogeneous T2 signal intensity because of regions of thrombosis or fibrosis.[16] CT can occasionally demonstrate internal calcification within a giant hemangioma.[14] Hyalinized or sclerosed hemangiomas do not have the typical T2 signal characteristics or enhancement patterns of conventional hemangiomas

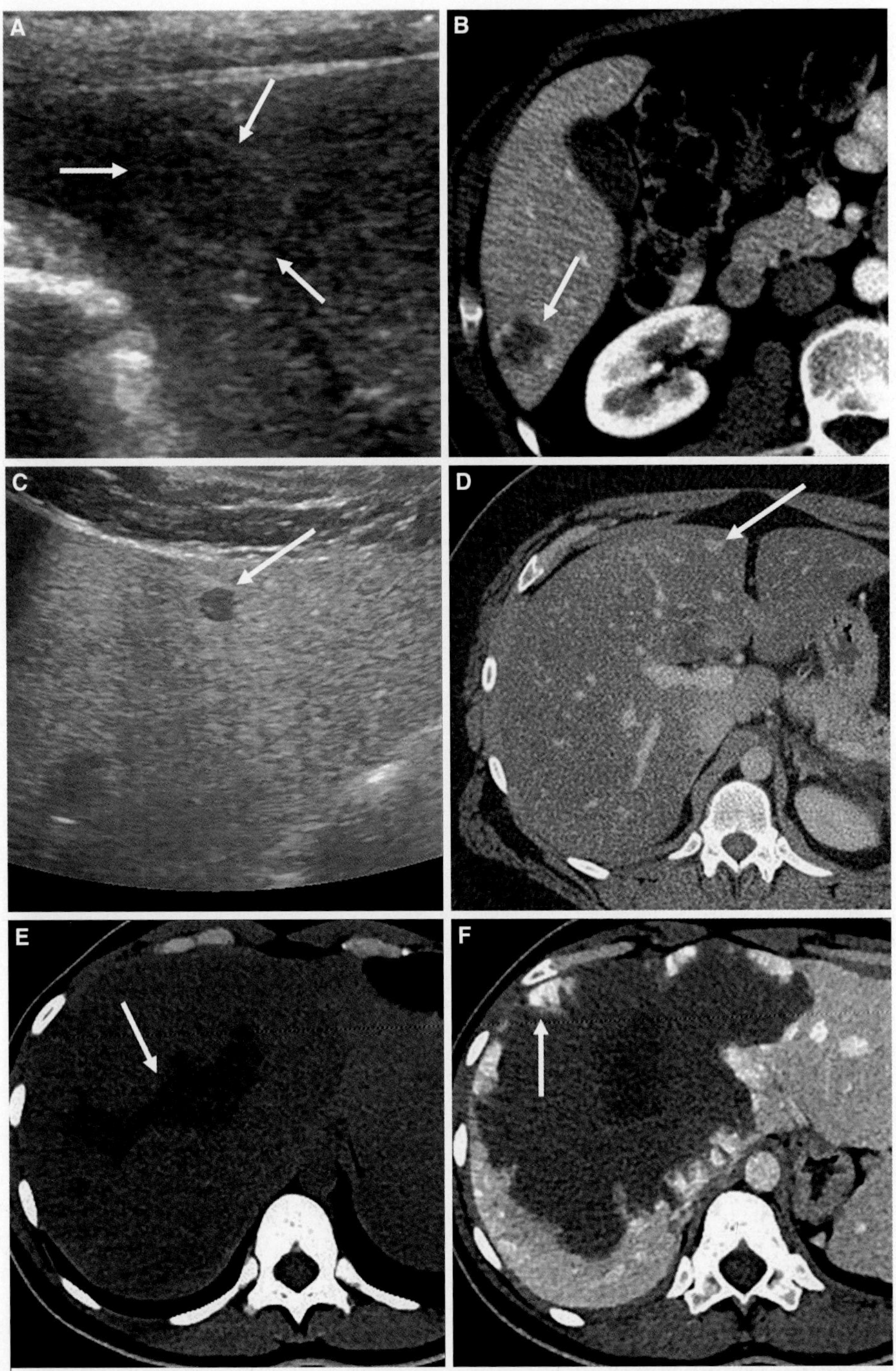

Figure 24.5 Atypical appearances of hemangioma. **(A, B)** Grayscale US image of a hepatic hemangioma showing a frequently seen atypical appearance in which the periphery of the lesion is hyperechoic (*arrows*) and central portion is isoechoic or hypoechoic. Corresponding portal venous phase axial CT scan image shows the characteristic peripheral globular enhancement pattern of the hemangioma (*arrow*, **B**). **(C, D)** Grayscale US image showing a hemangioma as a hypoechoic mass (**C**, *arrow*). The appearance is caused by a diffusely steatotic liver, which abnormally increases the echogenicity of the background parenchyma. Corresponding axial image from a CT scan performed in the portal venous phase shows the hemangioma (**D**, *arrow*) in an abnormally low attenuation liver. **(E–G)** Axial CT images in the precontrast **(E)**, portal venous **(F)**, and delayed phases **(G)** showing a giant hemangioma with a central scar (**E**, *arrow*) and typical peripheral progressive enhancement of a hemangioma (**F, G**, *arrows*). **(H)** Sulfur colloid scintigraphy of the giant hemangioma shows radiotracer uptake diffusely throughout the hemangioma (*arrows*) except for the central scar.

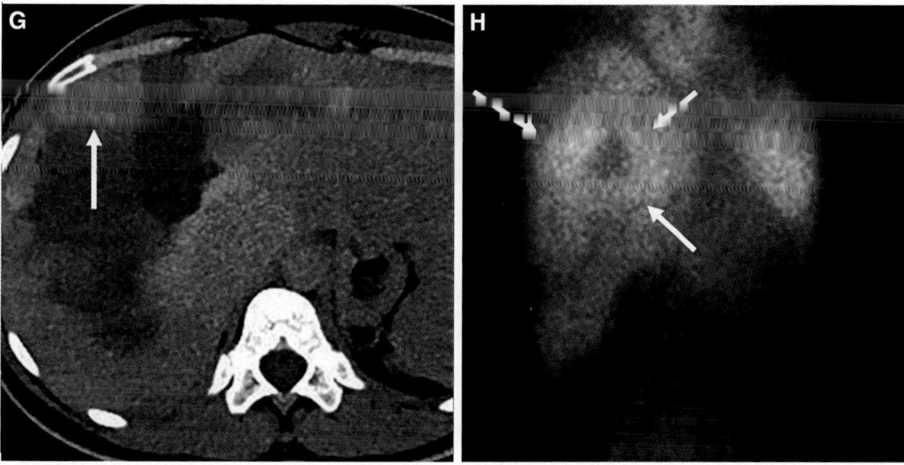

Figure 24.5 *(continued)*

and they are often difficult to adequately characterize on imaging.[17]

Radionucleotide imaging with technetium labeled red blood cells (Tc-RBC) is only rarely performed to confirm the diagnosis of cavernous hemangioma. In Tc-RBC studies, the typical scintigraphic findings include poor radiotracer uptake of the hemangioma relative to the adjacent liver on immediate images, and relatively increased tracer uptake on delayed images, which may be performed several hours after tracer injection.[18] In large hemangiomas, areas of poor delayed tracer uptake can be present. These areas correspond to the regions of scarring/thrombus better seen on cross-sectional imaging with CT or MRI.

Focal nodular hyperplasia

Focal nodular hyperplasia typically presents on imaging as a solitary well circumscribed mass. The US appearance of focal nodular hyperplasia is nonspecific and most commonly shows an isoechoic or slightly hypoechoic mass.[19] Doppler analysis can demonstrate a feeding artery entering the center of the mass, which branches into a stellate or "spoke-wheel" pattern (Fig. 24.6). On CT and MRI, focal nodular hyperplasia appears similar to the background parenchyma, being nearly isoattenuating at CT, and typically slightly T1 hypointense to isointense or slightly T2 hyperintense to isointense.

Because of their similar appearance to the liver parenchyma, focal nodular hyperplasia in some cases can remain undetected on imaging, which led to their name "stealth lesions." The lesions may have a characteristic central scar, reported to occur in 35% of lesions less than 3 cm and 65% of larger lesions.[20] When present, the central scar is considered to be a specific finding.[21] The central scar appears hypoattenuating on CT images and T2 hyperintense on MRI images. The characteristic dynamic contrast enhancement appearance of focal nodular hyperplasia at CT and MRI is a homogenously hyperenhancing mass on late arterial phase images, which fades to isointensity/isoattenuation at delayed-phase imaging.[20,22,23] The central scar enhances poorly on early phase imaging but characteristically shows delayed-phase enhancement.

Occasionally, enlarged feeding arteries are associated with the lesion. Focal nodular hyperplasia occasionally contains detectable fat at MRI, although this is considered unusual, and it often occurs most often in the setting of background hepatic steatosis.[24] Imaging with hepatobiliary agent is useful for making the diagnosis of focal nodular hyperplasia. This is particularly important when encountering an arterially hyperenhancing mass, where the differential diagnosis frequently includes hepatic adenoma, hepatocellular carcinoma, and fibrolamellar carcinoma (Table 24.1). Focal nodular hyperplasia tends to retain hepatobiliary agents to a similar degree or greater than the adjacent liver parenchyma, which is rarely found in the alternative lesions in the differential.[25]

Radionucleotide imaging of focal nodular hyperplasia with technetium sulfur colloid (Tc-SC) is rarely performed today, but was used in the past to help differentiate focal nodular hyperplasia from other lesions, such as hepatic adenoma or hepatocellular carcinoma. Tc-SC with particle sizes of 0.3 to 1.0 μm are taken up by Kupffer cells within the liver. Focal nodular hyperplasia typically contains Kupffer cells and will demonstrate Tc-SC activity greater than the background liver in 40%, similar in 30%, and less in 30%.[26] By comparison the majority of hepatic adenomas and hepatocellular carcinoma appear as a photopenic defect within the liver because they have less Kupffer cells than the background liver.

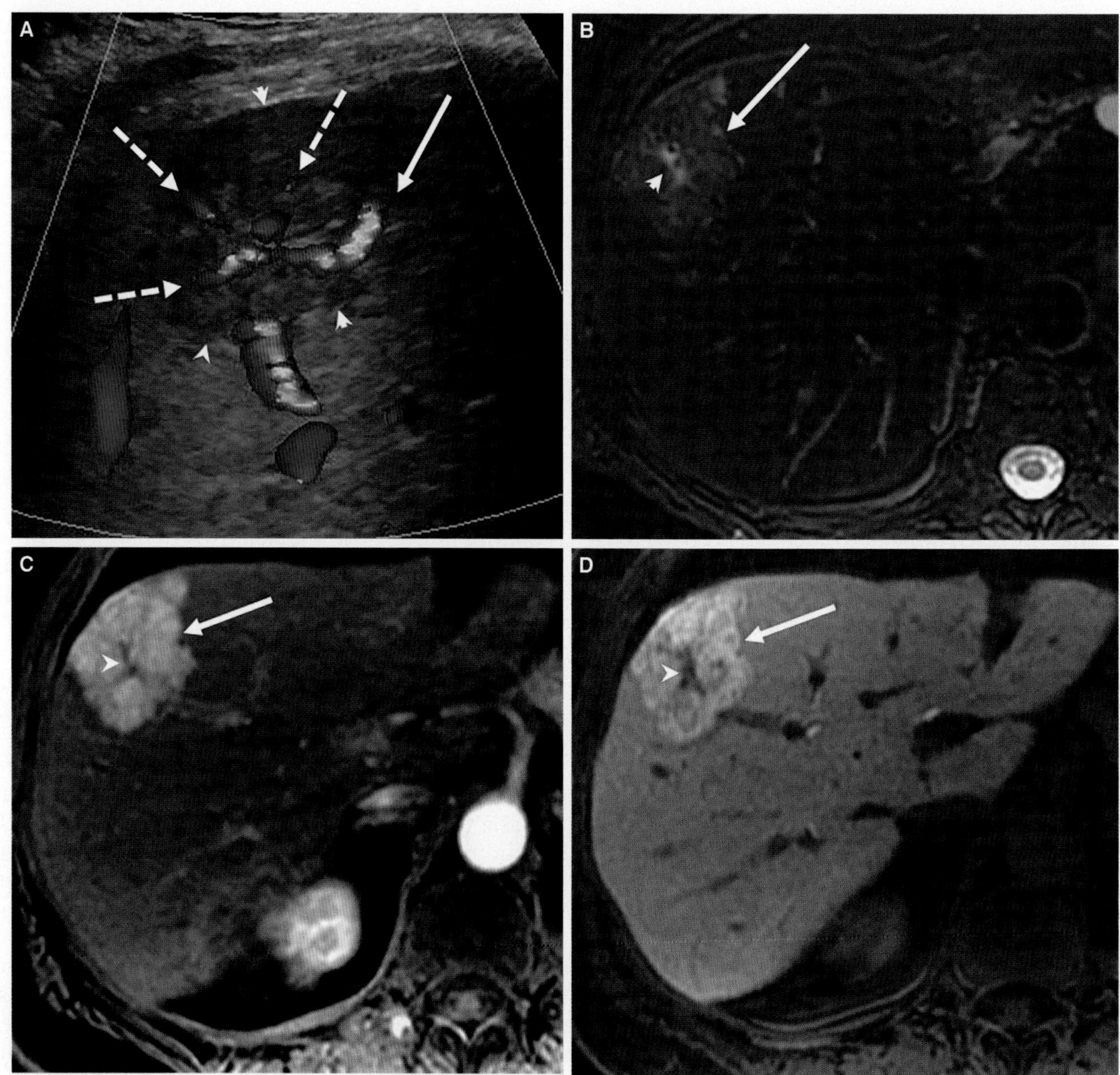

Figure 24.6 Focal nodular hyperplasia. **(A)** US image with Doppler flow overlay showing a hypoechoic mass (*arrowheads*). A feeding artery (*arrow*) is seen coursing into the center of the mass and smaller arteries are seen radiating from the center to the periphery of the mass (*dashed arrows*). This is the classic "spoke wheel" vascularity of an FNH. **(B)** Axial fat-suppressed T2-weighted MRI image shows the same mass (*arrow*) as T2 hyperintense to the remaining liver parenchyma with a centrally markedly T2 hyperintense central scar (*arrow head*). **(C, D)** Axial fat-suppressed T1-weighted images enhanced with hepatobiliary agent in the late arterial **(C)** and 20-minute delayed phases **(D)**. Late arterial phase image shows diffuse avid contrast enhancement (**C**, *arrow*) with a T1 hypointense central scar (**C**, *arrowhead*). 20-minute delayed phase shows retention of contrast agent (**D**, *arrow*) to a degree greater than the surrounding liver, which is typical of an FNH. The central scar does not retain hepatobiliary contrast agent (**D**, *arrowhead*).

Radionucleotide imaging with the hepatobiliary agent technetium iminodiacetic acid (Tc-IDA) analogs show uptake in normal hepatocytes and excretion into the biliary tree. When focal nodular hyeprlasia is imaged with these agents, rapid uptake and delayed clearance are seen in over 90% of patients.[18] By contrast, adenomas do not take up the agent, whereas hepatocellular carcinomas often show only some delayed retention, although this is absent in poorly differentiated tumors.

Table 24.1 Comparison of common hyperenhancing liver masses

Lesion	Imaging characteristics			
	Attenuation at CT	T1 Signal	T2 Signal	Enhancement
Hemangioma	Hypoattenuating	Hypointense	Marked Hyperintensity	Peripheral globular discontinuous enhancement with gradual complete central filling. Regions of contrast enhancement should appear similar to the aortic blood pool
Focal nodular hyperplasia	Isoattenuating with hypoattenuating central scar	Isointense to slightly hypointense	Isointense to slightly hyperintense	Diffuse late arterial hyperenhancement with fade to isoenhancement on delayed phases
Adenoma	Generally heterogeneously hypoattenuating with regions of hemorrhage appearing hyperattenuating and lipid-containing regions hypoattenuating	Generally heterogeneously hypointense with regions of hemorrhage appearing hyperintense and lipid-containing regions hyperintense (hypointense if fat saturation applied)	Hyperintense. Lipid rich lesions may appear hypointense on fat saturated sequences.	Heterogeneously hyperenhancing in the late arterial phase with fade to isoenhancement on delayed phases. Delayed-phase hypointensity (washout) may be present.
Regenerative nodule	Isoattenuating	Isointense	Isointense	Iso to slightly hypoenhancing
Dysplastic nodule	Isoattenuating or slightly hyperattenuating	Isointense to slightly hyperintense	Isointense	Iso to hyperenhancing in the late arterial phase with fade to isointensity on delayed phases
Hepatocellular carcinoma	Variable. Generally hypoattenuating but often heterogeneously isoattenuating or hyperattenuating because of the presence of iron, hemorrhage and lipid.	Generally hypointense with regions of hemorrhage appearing hyperintense and lipid-containing regions hyperintense (hypointense if fat saturation applied)	Moderately T2 hyperintense but variable depending on necrosis, hemorrhage, iron, lipid content.	Hyperenhancing in the late arterial phase with hypointensity on portal venous or delayed phases (washout). Enhancement is often heterogeneous.

Hepatic adenoma

Hepatic adenomas vary in their imaging appearance because of their varying cellular composition. Classically, hepatic adenomas are characterized as late arterial hyperenhancing masses, which are heterogeneous in appearance because of the presence of internal fat, necrosis, and hemorrhage. The heterogeneous appearance is considered a characteristic feature and heterogeneity increases with the size of the tumors.[27]

Portions of an adenoma-containing fat appear hyperechoic at US. Fat appears hypoattenuating on CT imaging and can be confused with regions of poor enhancement or necrosis. MRI is highly sensitive and accurate for correctly identifying regions of internal fat.

Adenomas have a tendency to hemorrhage. Hemorrhage varies in appearance based on its age. At US, hemorrhage can result in heterogeneously echogenic regions containing debris or it can appear hypoechoic.[28] On CT images, early hemorrhage appears hyperattenuating and decreases in attenuation with age of the hemorrhage. At MRI, hemorrhage is typically identified by its T1 hyperintensity. Hemorrhage can also be identified by a loss of signal on the in-phase images relative to out-of-phase images. Adenomas typically do not contain calcification, being found in only 10% of cases.[28]

The imaging findings of focal nodular hyperplasia and hepatocellular adenoma overlap, creating difficulty in arriving at a definitive imaging diagnosis. Imaging with hepatobiliary contrast agent can be helpful when identifying a mass in a healthy young patient, as the lack of retention in the delayed phase strongly supports a diagnosis of adenoma, as opposed to focal nodular hyperplasia.[29]

The vascularity in hepatic adenomas appears variable on both cross-sectional contrast-enhanced imaging and Doppler US. Adenomas are typically hyperenhancing in the late arterial phase of contrast enhancement and then fade to isointensity in the portal venous or delayed phases.[27] Occasionally, adenomas can remain hyperenhancing in the portal venous and delayed phases or show washout. At Doppler US, identification of venous waveforms can be observed within the mass.[30] This has been described as a useful finding to help differentiate hepatic adenoma from focal nodular hyperplasia, in which venous waveforms are absent. Conversely, the US finding of a central feeding artery with a stellate appearance that is typical of focal nodular hyperplasia is absent in hepatic adenomas. Studies of hepatic adenomas with CT and US images that are enhanced with an intravenous microbubble contrast agent have shown a centripetal pattern (moving toward the center) of enhancement. This is related to the presence of subcapsular feeding arteries and can be a useful discriminator of focal nodular hyperplasia, which shows a centrifugal (moving away from the center) or homogeneous pattern of enhancement.[31]

Patterns of imaging findings in hepatic adenomas have been associated with the known pathologic subtypes, such as inflammatory adenoma, HNF-1α inactivated adenoma, and β-catenin activated adenoma. The described patterns represent the typical imaging appearance of each subtype, but are not consistently present.[32] Inflammatory adenomas are characteristically T2 hyperintense, thought to be related to the presence of dilated sinusoids and inflammation (Fig. 24.7). A peripheral rim of increased T2 signal has been described and is referred to as the *Atoll sign*. This sign is considered a specific finding of inflammatory adenomas.[33] Enhancement within inflammatory adenomas is typically heterogeneous and these tumors can occasionally retain hepatobiliary contrast agent in a heterogeneous pattern.[34] The retention of hepatobiliary contrast agent in these adenomas can create confusion with focal nodular hyperplasia, but the presence of associated T2 hyperintensity will favor the diagnosis of adenoma. The degree of intratumoral fat is typically less in inflammatory adenomas than in HNF-1α mutated adenomas. The finding of diffuse steatosis and is considered to be a fairly specific finding of HNF-1α mutated adenomas (Fig. 24.7).[32,33] After contrast administration, this subtype of adenoma can also display hypointensity (washout) on portal venous and delayed phases, which may raise suspicion for hepatocellular carcinoma. β-catenin mutated adenomas are not associated with any specific imaging findings. However, the presence of a vague central scar characterized by T2 hyperintense lines that enhance in the portal phase has been reported in association with this adenoma subtype.[33]

Hepatocellular carcinoma

The imaging findings of hepatocellular carcinoma have been extensively described and hepatocellular carcinoma is the only primary liver cancer that can be diagnosed based on clinical, laboratory, and imaging findings alone, without histologic confirmation. Characteristic imaging features are seen at cross-sectional imaging that allows a highly specific imaging diagnosis to be made in patients at risk for hepatocellular carcinoma. These at risk patients include those with chronic viral hepatitis and patients with cirrhosis of any cause.[35] Periodic liver US is typically used to screen patients at risk for the development of hepatocellular carcinoma. With the development of screening programs, most hepatocellular carcinomas that are identified at imaging are small, measuring no more than a few centimeters in size. Although US is effective at identifying suspicious lesions, the imaging findings are not specific, and US is not reliable for differentiating hepatocellular carcinoma from dysplastic nodules or cirrhotic nodules. At US, hepatocellular carcinoma is typically a hypoechoic mass but may appear hyperechoic or heterogeneous, particularly if the mass contains internal fat or hemorrhage.[36] Most cases of suspected hepatocellular carcinoma identified at US will be further evaluated with CT or MRI.

CT and MRI studies of hepatocellular carcinoma identify characteristic abnormal blood flow patterns at dynamic imaging. Cirrhotic nodules have a predominantly portal venous blood supply, whereas hepatocellular carcinomas have a blood supply from the hepatic arteries.[37] Typical cirrhotic or regenerative nodules enhance in a similar pattern as the background liver.[38] For dysplastic nodules, the relative proportion of feeding arteries increases compared to the background cirrhotic nodules and the nodules become hyperenhancing relative to the adjacent parenchyma on late arterial phase images. A hyperenhancing mass that

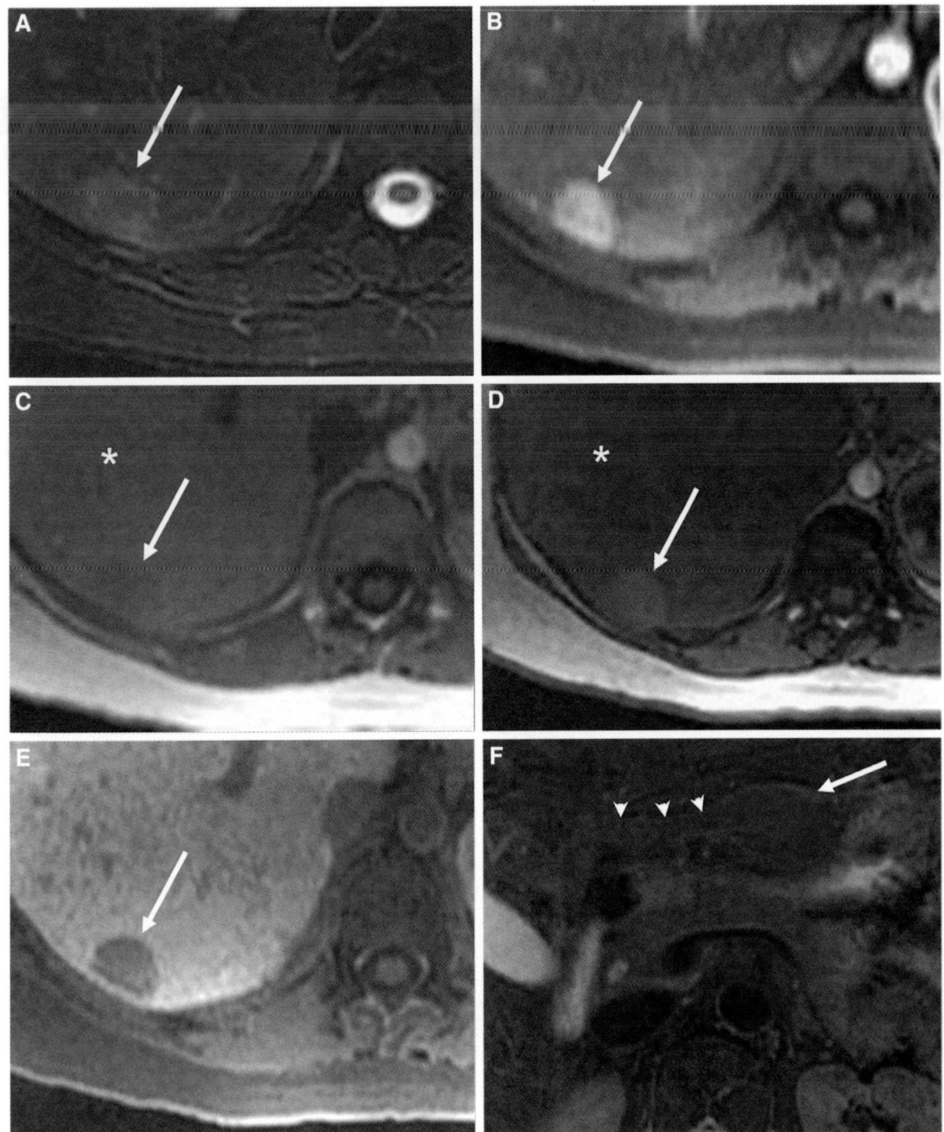

Figure 24.7 **(A–E)** Typical imaging findings of an inflammatory adenoma. **(A)** Axial fat-suppressed T2-weighted MRI imaging showing heterogeneous peripheral high T2 signal intensity (*arrow*). **(B)** Axial fat-suppressed T1-weighted imaging with contrast enhancement in the arterial phase showing heterogeneous hyperenhancement (*arrows*). **(C)** Axial T1-weighted in-phase **(C)** and opposed-phase **(D)** images. Despite the appearance, the signal intensity of the mass did not significantly change (*arrows*), however the background liver parenchyma is markedly steatotic (*asterisk*). **(E)** Axial fat-suppressed T1-weighted image enhanced with hepatobiliary contrast agent showing lack of uptake (*arrow*) on a 20-minute delayed image. **(F–J)** Typical imaging findings of an HNF-1a inactivated hepatic adenoma. **(F)** Axial fat-suppressed T2-weighted image showing a mass (*arrows*), which is isointense to the surrounding liver parenchyma (*arrowheads*). **(G, H)** Axial fat-suppressed T1-weighted images with IV contrast enhancement show the mass to be heterogeneously hyperenhancing in the late arterial phase (**G**, *arrows*) and hypoenhancing in the portal venous phase (**H**, *arrows*). (**I, J**) In-phase **(I)** and opposed-phase **(J)** images show significant and diffuse loss of signal on the out-of-phase images (**J**, *arrow*) consistent with lesional steatosis. Adenomas are often hyperintense on T2-weighted images, the fat suppression applied in image f helps to explain the isointensity seen in this case and the apparent washout seen on the portal venous phase image I.

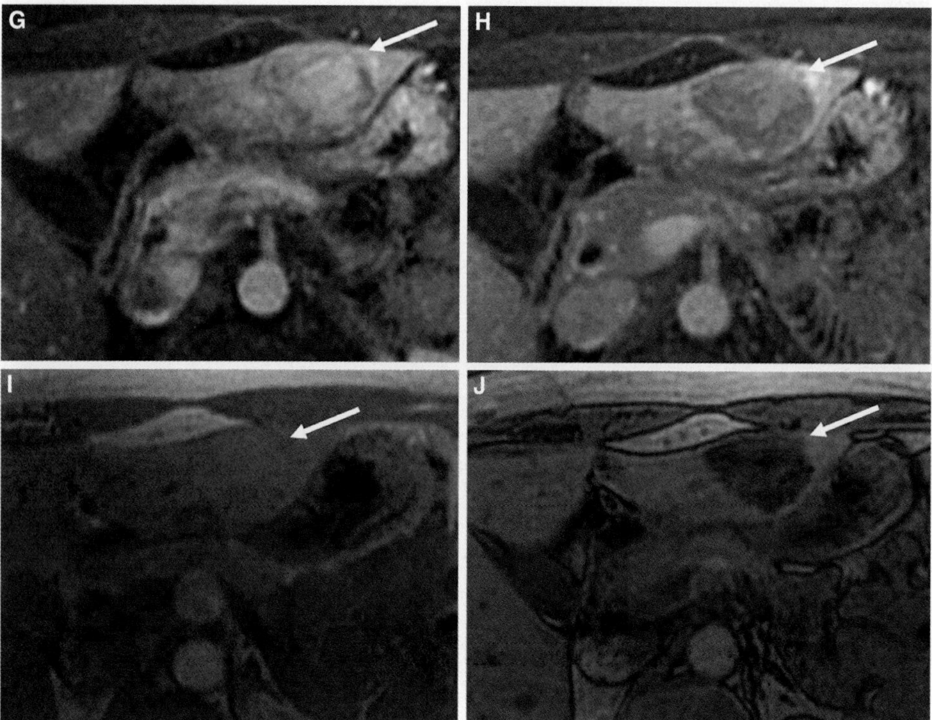

Figure 24.7 *(continued)*

fades to isoenhancement on portal or delayed-phase images is not specific and may represent a dysplastic nodule or early hepatocellular carcinoma. In larger hepatocellular carcinomas, the vascular supply becomes entirely arterial and late arterial hyperenhancing nodules become hypoattenuating or hypointense on portal venous and/or delayed imaging phases (Fig. 24.8). This imaging finding of hypoattenuation on CT (or hypointensity on MRI) is referred to as *washout* and is a feature highly specific for hepatocellular carcinoma.[39] A delayed enhancing pseudocapsule is another feature considered to be a major criterion for the diagnosis of hepatocellular carcinoma. A pseudocapsule is defined as a thin band of increased peripheral enhancement, which progressively increases in conspicuity on subsequent imaging phases. The capsule can also been seen on nonenhanced MRI images as a T1 hypointense and T2 hyperintense thin band, however, the nonenhanced appearance does not contribute to the imaging diagnosis.

Rapid growth of a mass is also considered a major criterion for the diagnosis of hepatocellular carcinoma. The growth rate of hepatocellular carcinoma has been shown to be highly variable,[40,41] but a growth of more than 50% diameter within 6 months suggests a diagnosis of carcinoma.

Hepatocellular carcinoma has a tendency to invade the hepatic and portal veins. This finding can be grossly visible on imaging and is a diagnostic finding of hepatocellular carcinoma in patients at risk (e.g., those with cirrhosis). Tumor invasion into the veins is referred to as *tumor thrombus* and must be distinguished from a bland thrombus, which is commonly found in the setting of cirrhosis. Imaging findings that support the diagnosis of a tumor thrombus include early enhancement of the portal veins, which is caused by arterial blood flow coursing through the tumor tissue in tumors with arterial to portal venous shunts. The moderate T2 signal intensity and restricted diffusion of a tumor thrombus typically appears similar to that of the intraparenchymal portion of the tumor. A finding that is often present and strongly suggests the presence of tumor thrombus is expansion of the vessel. An acute bland thrombus may cause mild transient expansion of a vein; however the expansion created by invading carcinoma is typically much greater in degree and easily identified.

The major criteria for the imaging diagnosis of hepatocellular carcinoma are the enhancement patterns seen at CT and MRI, significant interval tumor growth, and venous invasion. Many additional findings are considered important ancillary findings in judging the likelihood of carcinoma. These findings relate to the internal enhancement pattern or architecture of a nodule, hepatobiliary phase hypointensity, the presence of internal fat or hemorrhage, focal iron sparing, restricted diffusion, and T2 signal intensities. Patterns of internal enhancement that are concerning for hepatocellular carcinoma are referred to as *mosaic enhancement*. This term includes masses with a nodule-in-nodule appearance and compartmentalized or septated masses. A small focus of hepatocellular

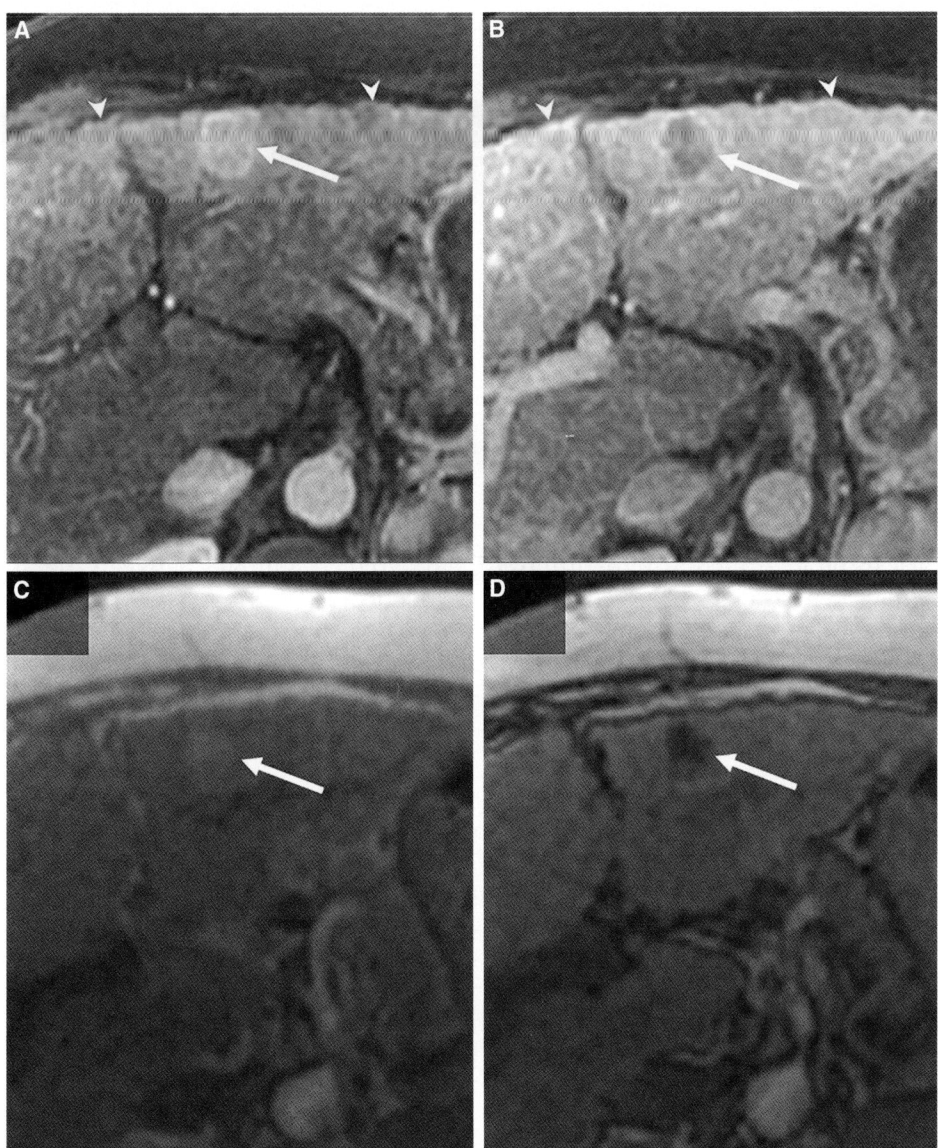

Figure 24.8 **(A, B)** Axial fat-suppressed contrast-enhanced images in the late arterial **(A)** and portal venous **(B)** phases show an arterial hyperenhancing nodule (**A**, *arrow*) with portal venous hypointensity or washout (**B**, *arrow*). This finding in the nodular cirrhotic liver (*arrowheads*) is highly specific for hepatocellular carcinoma. **(C, D)** Axial T1-weighted in-phase **(C)** and opposed-phase **(D)** images show loss of signal on opposed-phase images (*arrows*) indicating intravoxel lipid. The presence of detectable fat within a nodule of a cirrhotic liver is considered an ancillary finding of hepatocellular carcinoma and typically seen in well differentiated nodules.

carcinoma developing within a larger regenerative or dysplastic nodule is occasionally identified at imaging. The appearance of nodule-in-nodule architecture specifically refers to this pattern. This pattern can be seen as a small hyperenhancing focus within a larger nodule or as a T2 hyperintense focus within a T2 hypointense siderotic nodule.

The expression of organic anion transport protein (OATP) on hepatocyte membranes, which are necessary for the uptake of hepatobiliary agent into a hepatocyte, are lower in hepatocellular carcinoma compared to regenerative nodules.[42] This results in hypointensity of the mass at hepatobiliary phase imaging. As mentioned above, dysplastic nodules and early hepatocellular carcinoma initially loose portal flow prior to becoming arterially supplied and hypervascular. This phenomenon results in some hepatocellular carcinoma being arterially isoenhancing or hypoenhancing when imaged with extracellular contrast agents.[23] Imaging with hepatobiliary contrast agents is gaining popularity and has shown promise as a method for identifying these early tumors, which will not meet major criteria for imaging diagnosis.[43]

The abnormal fibrosis that is present in cirrhosis results in abnormal background liver signal at MRI. Areas of fibrosis contain a relatively greater amount of extracellular fluid, resulting in mild T1 hypointensity and T2 hyperintensity. This finding can create the appearance of T1 hyperintensity and T2 hypointensity in cirrhotic nodules. Dysplastic nodules can also contain variable amounts of substances such as protein, copper or iron. These substances can result in increased attenuation at CT. At MRI, these substances can result in decreased T2 signal and either increased (protein, copper) or decreased (iron) T1 signal.[38] Moderately increased T2 signal is an uncommon finding in benign lesions and suggests hepatocellular carcinoma.[37] Hepatocellular carcinomas often have less iron accumulation than the background cirrhotic liver. These nodules with less iron content than the background liver can be identified as hyperintense on T2-weighted images or by a lack of signal loss on T1-weighted in-phase images, when compared with opposed-phase images.

Intracellular fat is found in a subset of cases of early hepatocellular carcinoma and less commonly in dysplastic nodules (Fig. 24.8).[44] The identification of internal fat may cause difficulty at imaging, as an arterially enhancing and fat-containing hepatocellular carcinoma has an appearance that can simulate an adenoma. Additional difficulty is encountered at imaging as hepatocellular carcinomas may originate within preexisting hepatic adenomas.

Sporadic hepatocellular carcinomas (those without risk factors such as underlying liver cirrhosis) often present as a large, heterogeneous hepatic tumors (Fig. 24.9). The imaging findings of large hepatocellular carcinomas differ from the small masses typically discovered in hepatocellular carcinoma screening programs. The larger masses are generally heterogeneous and have an irregular central scar. The central scar is different from that associated with focal nodular hyperplasia, in that it tends to be low in MRI signal on both T1- and T2-weighted sequences and it lacks delayed enhancement. Large hepatocellular carcinomas often have evidence of prior hemorrhage. Importantly, sporadic hepatocellular carcinoma often present with hemorrhage, which can occasionally extend into the peritoneal cavity.

Fibrolamellar carcinoma

Fibrolamellar carcinoma typically presents as large lobulated mass in the setting of a normal liver. The characteristic imaging feature of fibrolamellar carcinoma is the large central scar (present in 65% to 70% of cases) and radiating septa (Fig. 24.10).[45] The finding of a large mass with central scar in a healthy young person may lead to misdiagnosis on imaging as focal nodular hyperplasia. Central scars are also commonly seen in giant hemangiomas and large hepatocellular carcinomas. In fibrolamellar carcinoma, the central scar typically shows low attenuation and is low in signal on both T1- and T2-weighted sequences.[45,46] The central scar may show delayed enhancement, which can also result in confusion with focal nodular hyperplasia.[45]

The cellular portion of fibrolamellar carcinoma is hypointense on T1-weighted images and iso to slightly hyperintense on T2-weighted images. The enhancement pattern of fibrolamellar carcinoma is heterogeneous late arterial phase hyperenhancement followed by iso or hypoenhancement in the portal venous and delayed phases. On delayed-phase images, the heterogeneous appearance becomes progressively more homogenous as extracellular contrast material equilibrates between the fibrous and cellular portions of the mass.[47] Fibrolamellar carcinoma commonly contains areas of calcification which can involve the central scar, a finding that is unusual in focal nodular hyperplasia.[48] Fibrolamellar carcinoma does not retain hepatobiliary contrast agents, which represents another useful differentiator from focal nodular hyperplasia. Fibrolamellar carcinomas do not contain fat on imaging studies even though fat is not uncommon histologically.[45]

Intrahepatic cholangiocarcinoma

Radiologically, intrahepatic cholangiocarcinoma is divided into three categories based on the location and appearance: intrahepatic mass forming, periductal infiltrating, and intraductal.[49] Intrahepatic mass forming cholangiocarcinoma typically forms a large, lobulated mass which is hypoattenuating at CT (Fig. 24.11). Areas of necrosis and calcification may be present.[47] At MRI, the mass is T1 hypointense and T2 hyperintense. Dynamic contrast enhancement findings reflect the underlying histologic patterns of increased peripheral cellularity with a central predominance of fibrous tissue. After contrast administration the cellular periphery of the mass demonstrates irregular peripheral enhancement in the arterial and portal phases. This is followed by characteristic slow central accumulation of contrast as the extracellular contrast material diffuses into the expanded extracellular space of the fibrous regions. At long delays of 5 to 15 minutes after contrast administration, the fibrous regions of the tumor can become hyperenhancing relative to the adjacent liver parenchyma.[50] At US the periphery of the mass often appears hypoechoic with increased echogenicity centrally. These dynamic enhancement and US findings are not specific for cholangiocarcinoma and are commonly seen with metastatic disease.

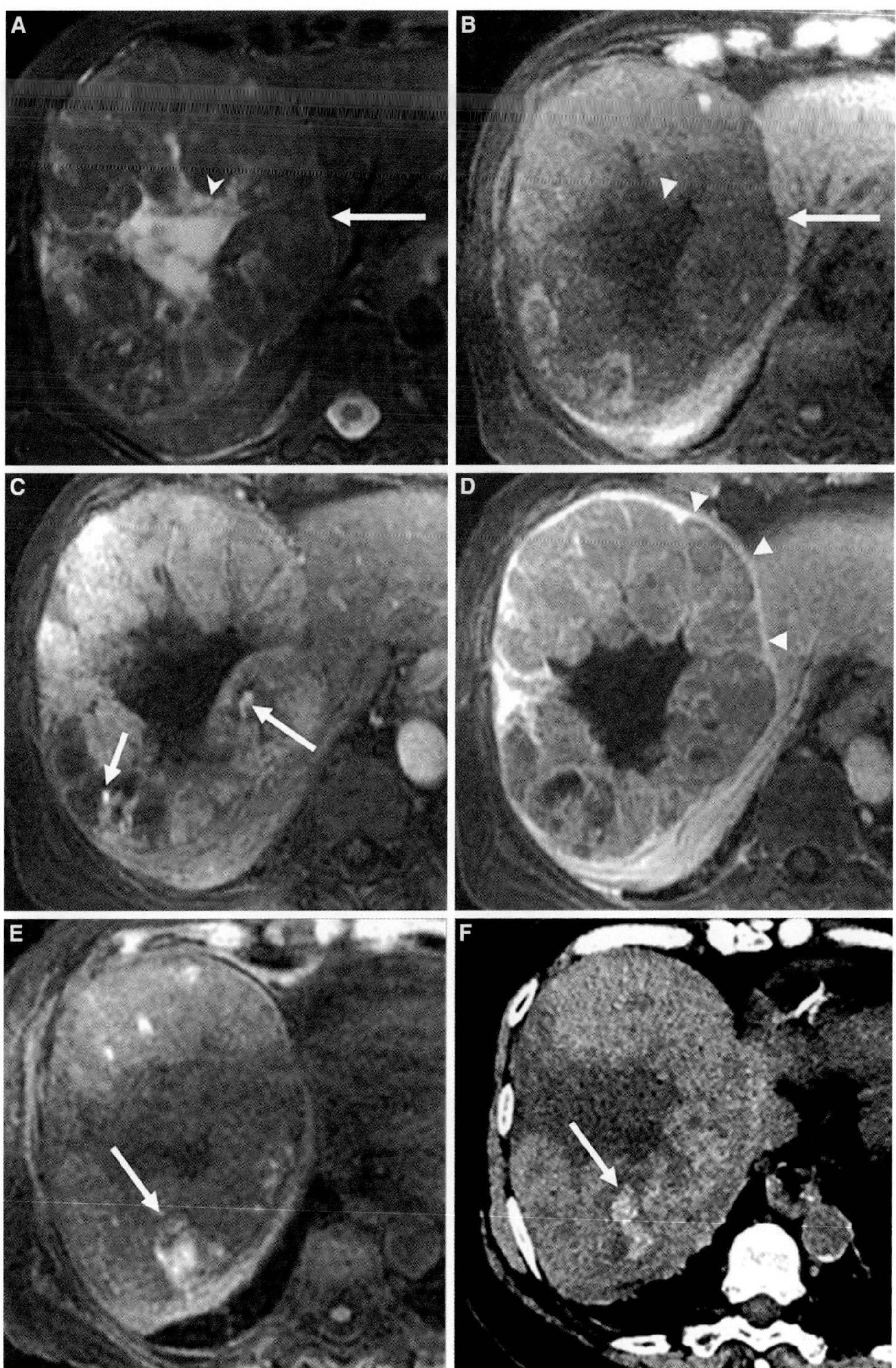

Figure 24.9 Well differentiated hepatocellular carcinoma. Large hepatocellular carcinoma presenting in a patient without cirrhosis. **(A)** T2-weighted MRI image shows a large mass with signal intensity slightly greater than that of the background liver (*arrows*). The mass has formed a central scar, which is atypical of a classic HCC in that it is T2 hyperintense (*arrow head*) **(B)** T1-weighted MRI image shows the mass to be predominantly hypointense to liver parenchyma (*arrow*). The central scar is markedly T1 hypointense. **(C)** Late arterial phase MRI image shows the mass to be hyperenhancing. Several abnormal and aneurysmal vessels can be seen (*arrows*). **(D)** Delayed-phase MRI image showing hypointensity (washout) of the tumor tissue relative to liver. A well defined enhancing pseudocapsule extends around the mass (*arrow heads*). **(E, F)** T1-weighted precontrast MRI image **(E)** showing hyperintense blood products from recent hemorrhage (*arrow*). A CT scan without IV contrast performed a few weeks earlier shows the blood products in the same region to be hyperattenuating (*arrow*). CT image also shows the central scar to be low attenuation.

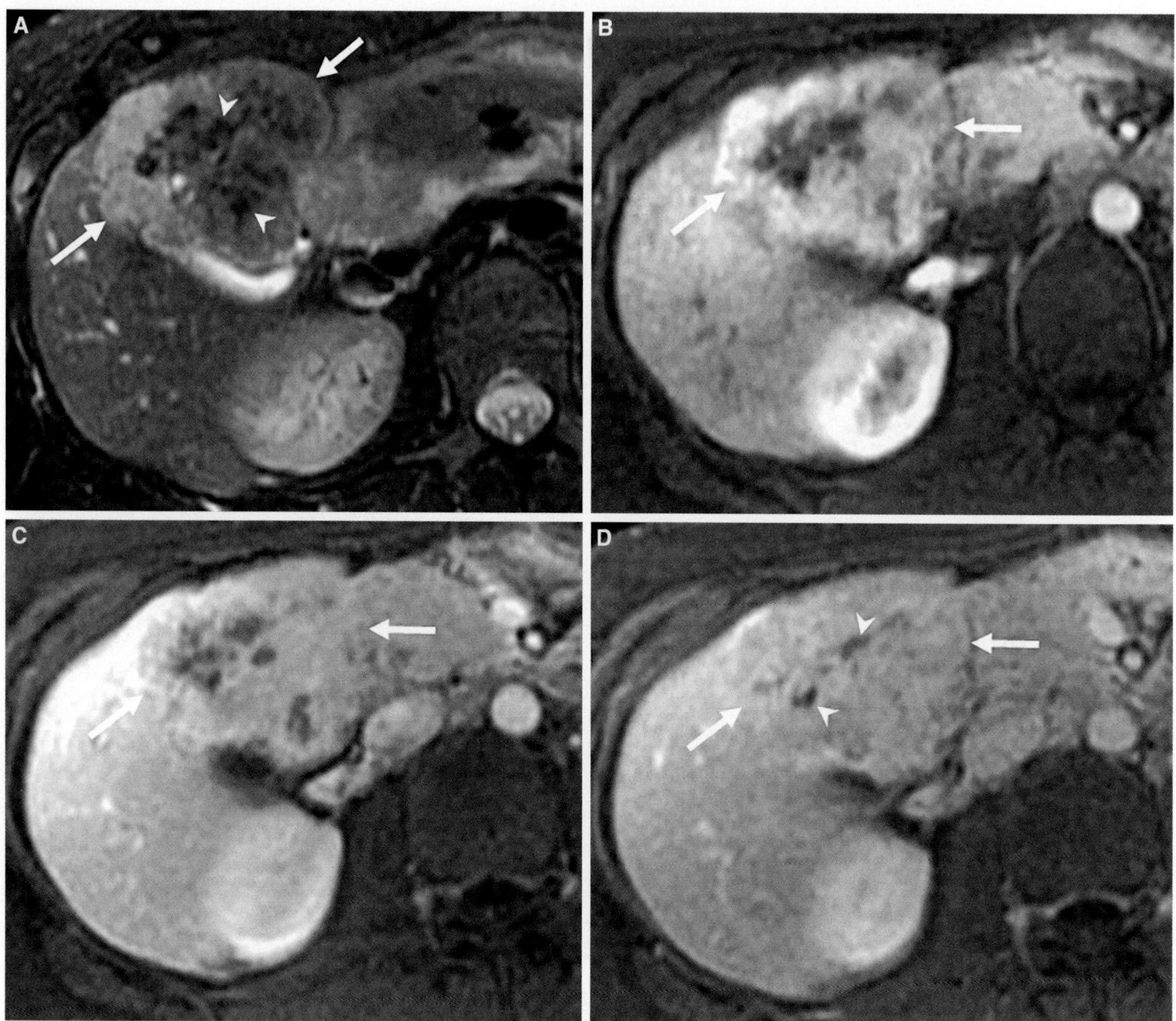

Figure 24.10 Fibrolamellar carcinoma. **(A)** Axial fat-suppressed T2-weighted image demonstrates a T2 hyperintense lobulated mass (*arrows*) with an irregularly shaped, T2 hypointense central scar (*arrowheads*). **(B–D)** Axial fat-suppressed T1-weighted IV contrast-enhanced images in the late arterial **(B)**, portal venous **(C)**, and delayed phases **(D)**. The mass (*arrows*) is shown to be peripherally hyperenhancing with T1 hypointense central scar and incomplete gradual central enhancement. The majority of the mass fades to isointensity on the delayed phase, however portions of central scar do not enhance (**D**, *arrowheads*).

Several associated findings can be seen that support an imaging diagnosis of cholangiocarcinoma. A major finding is the frequent tendency of cholangiocarcinoma to cause severe biliary obstruction. The obstruction often occurs in association with obstruction of the portal vein and is associated with atrophy of the affected portion of the liver parenchyma.[51] This result in compensatory hypertrophy of the surrounding liver, a characteristic finding referred to as *atrophy-hypertrophy* complex. Retraction of the overlying liver capsule and vascular encasement without formation of tumor thrombus are additional characteristic findings.[49] Cholangiocarcinoma does not retain hepatobiliary contrast agent, similar to hepatocellular carcinoma.

Small, mass-forming cholangiocarcinomas are occasionally hyperenhancing in the arterial phase and may simulate a small hepatocellular carcinoma.[52] These small tumors can be misdiagnosed as hepatocellular carcinoma on imaging studies. This problem can lead to inappropriate management including liver transplant.[53] Another pitfall is the potential for the hyperenhancing periphery of a mass forming cholangiocarcinoma to washout in the portal venous or delayed phase. This finding also has the potential for a misdiagnosis of hepatocellular carcinoma. Identifying the combination of peripheral hyperenhancement and delayed central enhancement along with other helpful findings, such as marked restricted diffusion,

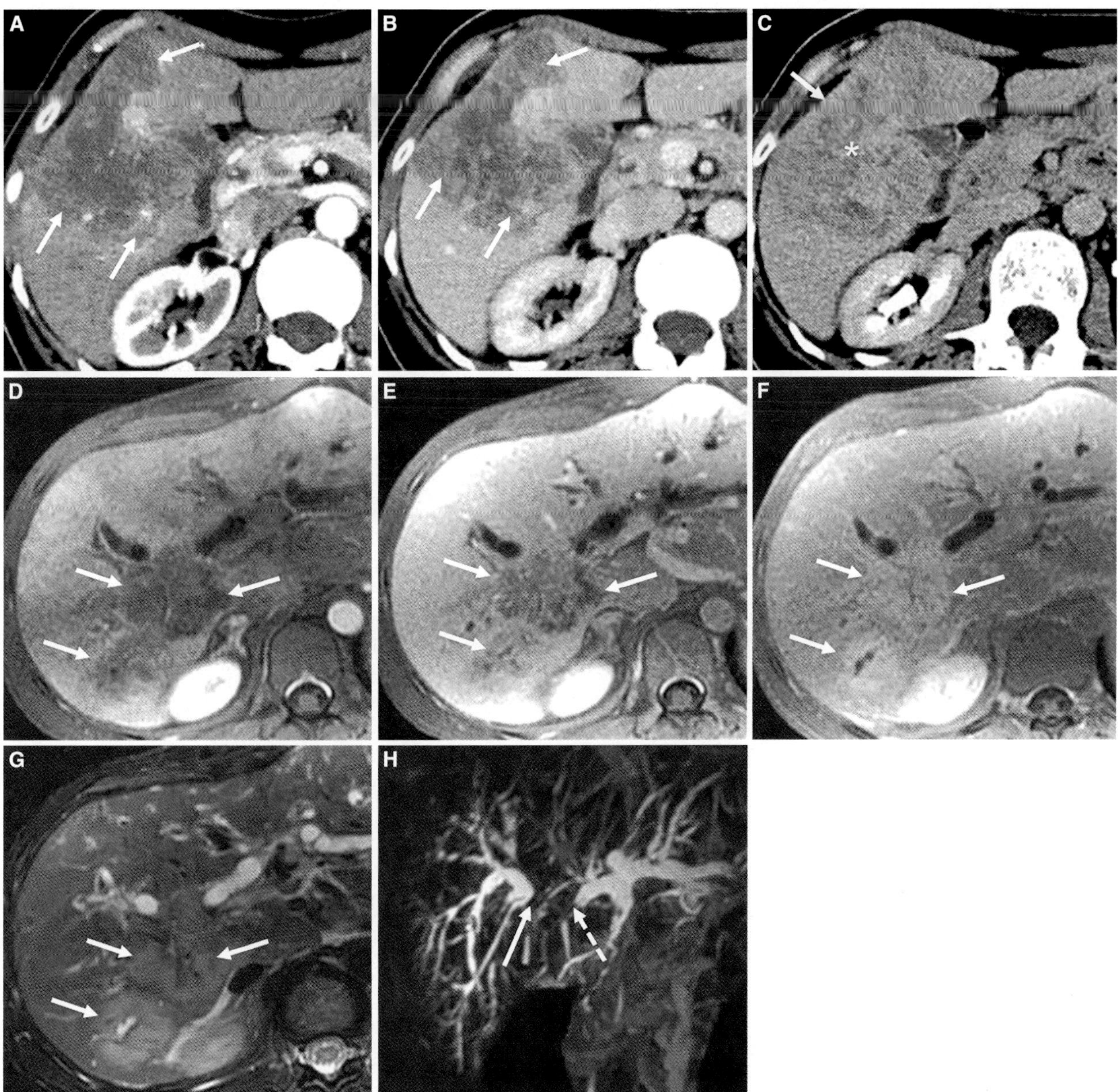

Figure 24.11 (A–C) Axial contrast-enhanced CT images in the late arterial **(A)**, portal venous **(B)** and 10-minute delayed **(C)** phases show the typical appearance of an intrahepatic mass forming cholangiocarcinoma. Mass demonstrates irregular continuous peripheral enhancement (**A, B**, *arrows*) with gradual central accumulation of contrast material over time **(C)**. Notice the characteristic retraction of the overlying liver margin (**C**, *arrow*). **(D–F)** Axial fat-suppressed T1-weighted images with contrast enhancement in the late arterial **(D)**, portal venous **(E)**, and 5-minute delay **(F)** phases. Images show a hypoenhancing mixed mass-forming and periductal infiltrating mass growing primarily within the posterior hepatic sector (**D, E**, *arrows*). In the delayed phase the mass has accumulated contrast and become hyperintense to the adjacent parenchyma (**F**, *arrows*). (**G**) Axial fat-suppressed T2-weighted image showing the tumor to be T2 hyperintense (*arrows*). **(H)** Image taken from a 3D rendering of a heavily T2-weighted magnetic resonance cholangiopancreatography sequence shows abrupt obstruction of the right (*arrow*) and left (*dashed arrow*) hepatic bile ducts with marked upstream dilation caused by involvement by the central part of the mass.

may help prevent misdiagnosis as hepatocellular carcinoma.[54] A small cholangiocarcinoma with peripheral enhancement may occasionally be misdiagnosed as a benign hemangioma on CT and MRI scans. This imaging misdiagnosis of a hemangioma can be avoided by correctly recognizing the continuous rim of enhancement, which is typically less intense than that of the aortic blood pool. Unless there are central regions of necrosis, the high T2 signal that is typical of hemangiomas will be also absent in cholangiocarcinomas when evaluated with MRI.

Periductal infiltrating cholangiocarcinoma is a rare form of intrahepatic cholangiocarcinoma that does not form a well-defined mass.[49] The malignant cells extend along the biliary tree. At imaging, these tumors are suggested by identifying a narrowed or obstructed bile duct with associated peribiliary soft-tissue thickening and enhancement (Fig. 24.12). At MRI, abnormally high peribiliary T2 signal may also be seen. This type of growth is most commonly seen in tumors located at the hepatic hilum.[49]

Papillary intraductal cholangiocarcinoma manifests as one or more enhancing masses within the biliary tree.[47] The mass can be associated with significant biliary dilation or obstruction. Some intraductal cholangiocarcinomas are associated with significant

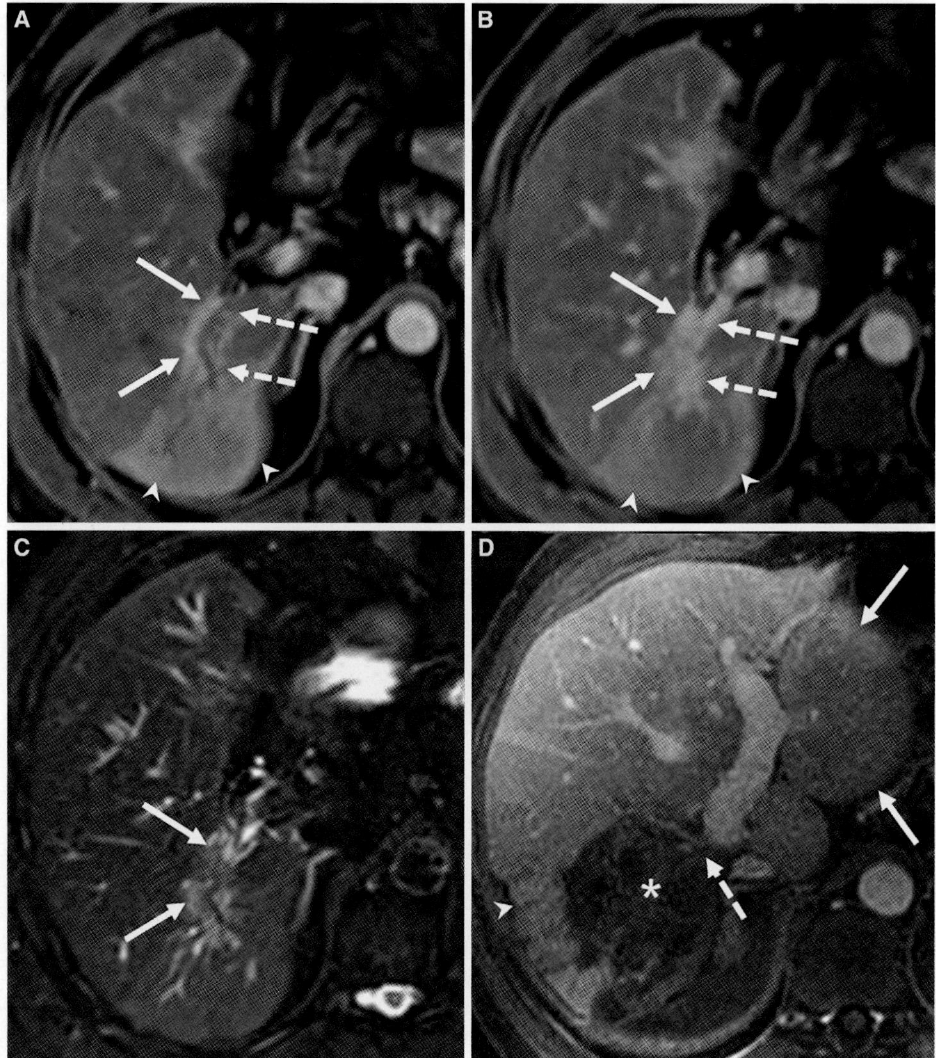

Figure 24.12 **(A, B)** Axial fat-suppressed T1-weighted images with IV contrast enhancement in the late arterial **(A)** and portal venous phases **(B)**. Abnormal enhancement is seen extending along the bile duct draining the posterior hepatic sector (**A, B**, *arrows*), directly adjacent to the portal vein. There is an associated transient perfusion irregularity of the adjacent liver parechyma (**A, B**, *arrowheads*). **(C)** Axial fat-suppressed T2-weighted image shows abnormal T2 hyperintensity associated with the tumor (*arrows*). **(D)** Axial fat-suppressed T1-weighted image with IV contrast enhancement in the portal venous phase obtained 1 year later shows marked enlargement of the mass (*asterisk*) with occlusion of the right portal triad (*dashed arrow*). Also notice the atrophy of the right posterior hepatic parenchyma (*arrow heads*) and compensatory hypertrophy of the left lobe (*arrows*, only partially shown).

mucin production, resulting in dilation of the adjacent biliary tree, including the downstream duct.

Mucinous cystic neoplasms

Biliary mucinous cystic neoplasms present as a large unilocular or multilocular cystic mass (Fig. 24.13). Mucinous cystic neoplasms are typically suggested on imaging when encountering a cystic lesion several centimeters in size in a middle-aged female, which represents the typical demographics for this tumor. At US, CT, and MRI the typical findings include a thick fibrous capsule, internal septations and mural nodules.[55] The internal fluid content generally appears similar to simple fluid, but these tumors can contain complex internal contents, which may be echogenic, high in attenuation, or high in T1 signal. Complex internal fluid, may be the result of prior hemorrhage.[56] Calcifications along the walls and septa may be present. The masses can prolapse into the biliary tree.[56] The presence of mural nodules and papillary growths favors the diagnosis of adenocarcinoma arising in the a mucinous cystic neoplasm, but can be seen in both entities.[55] The possibility of malignancy within a mucinous cystic neoplasm cannot be excluded by imaging and histologic diagnosis is necessary.

Epithelioid hemangioendothelioma

Epithelioid hemangioendotheliomas tend to present as multiple peripherally distributed masses at imaging, which tend to coalesce as they grow (Fig. 24.14).[57] At US, the masses are typically hypoechoic without detectable Doppler flow.[58] At CT, the masses show low attenuation and calcifications are found in up to 20% of cases.[59] T2-weighted MRI images show a typical

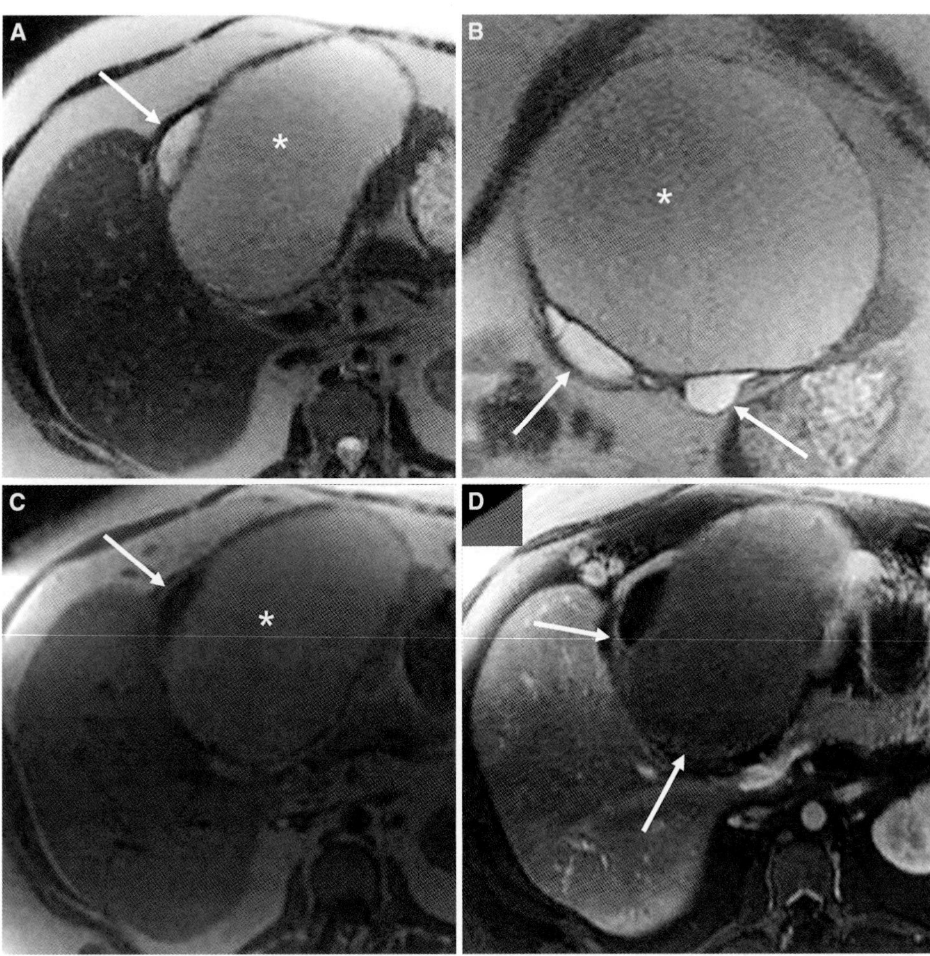

Figure 24.13 Biliary cystadenoma. Axial **(A)** and coronal **(B)** T2-weighted MRI images show a large cystic mass (*asterisk*) arising from the liver with loculated components of higher T2 signal intensity (*arrows*) located along its periphery. **(C)** Axial T1-weighted image shows most of the fluid within the mass to have high T1 signal (*asterisk*) consistent with proteinaceous or hemorrhagic contents. Fluid within the loculated components (*arrow*) along the periphery show low T1 signal indicating simple fluid. **(D)** Axial fat-suppressed T1-weighted image with IV contrast in the portal venous phase shows minimal enhancement along the periphery of the mass (*arrows*) with no internal enhancing component.

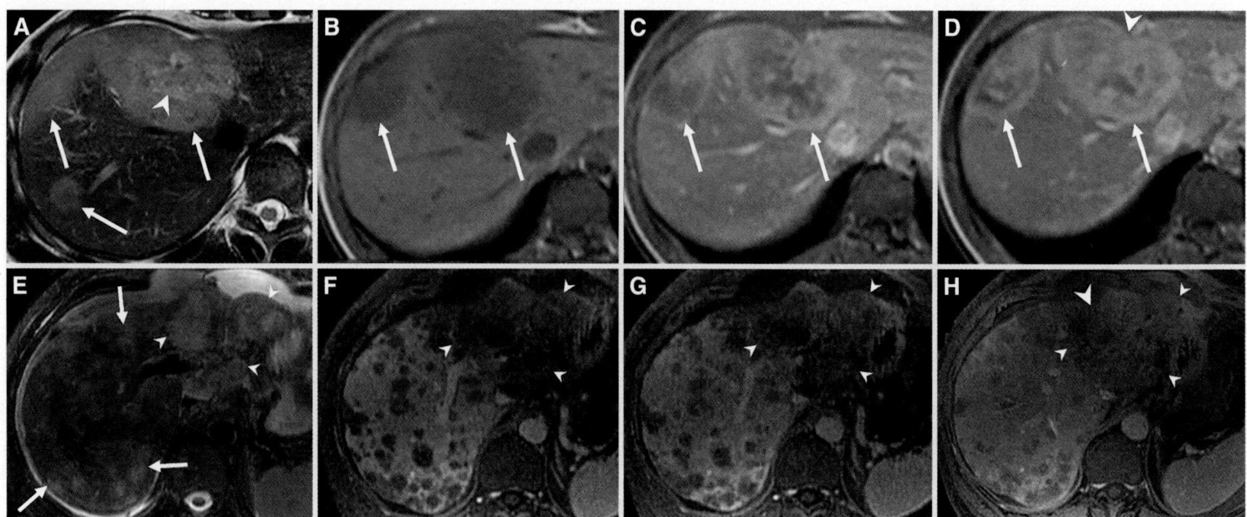

Figure 24.14 (A–D) Axial fat-suppressed T2-weighted image shows multiple (*arrows*) masses of epithelioid hemangioendothelioma as a T2 hyperintense with central region of slightly higher T2 signal (*arrowhead*). Axial fat-suppressed T1-weighted images without **(B)** and with IV contrast in the portal venous **(C)** and delayed **(D)** phases show peripheral hyperenhancement with gradual central accumulation of contrast material. **(E–H)** Another patient with epithelioid hemangioendothelioma. Axial T2-weighted images showing innumerable T2 hyperintense masses (*arrows*), which have formed a conglomerate mass in the left liver (*arrowheads*). Axial fat-suppressed T1-weighted images with IV contrast enhancement in the portal venous **(F)**, 3-minute delay **(G)**, and 5-minute delay **(H)** show the individual (*arrows*) and conglomerate (*arrowheads*) to slowly accumulate contrast in a centripetal pattern. Capsular retraction is present associated with both cases (**D** and **H**, *arrowheads*).

"target" sign of alternating high and low intensity rings. Dynamic contrast enhancement at CT and MRI shows rim-like enhancement with occasionally a thin hypoenhancing outer rim.[58] Delayed central enhancement of the masses can be seen in the presence of central fibrosis. Findings considered to be helpful in the diagnoses of these tumors include coalescence of multiple masses over time and retraction of the liver capsule adjacent to superficial masses. Epithelioid hemangioendothelioma can lead to compression of adjacent structures, however gross invasion of portal or hepatic veins is not a typical finding.[58] Imaging findings of epithelioid hemangioendothelioma can be suggestive but are not diagnostic. The imaging differential diagnosis often includes cholangiocarcinoma, metastatic carcinoma, angiosarcoma, and multifocal hepatocellular carcinoma. For this reason, histologic confirmation is necessary.

Angiosarcoma

Angiosarcoma often presents as a multifocal mass, but occasionally may present as a single or infiltrating lesion.[60,61] Lesions tend to be large at initial imaging and frequently present with intrahepatic or intraperitoneal hemorrhage. Angiosarcoma is hypoattenuating on CT. MRI demonstrates heterogeneous high T2 and low T1 signal. If hemorrhage is present, portions of the mass may appear hyperattenuating at CT or high in T1 signal at MRI. Lesions are vascular and display irregular peripheral early enhancement with a progressive centripetal pattern (moving toward the center) of contrast accumulation on delayed images. Angiosarcoma has previously been described as having a similar appearance to typical hemangiomas, but multiphase imaging is generally able to effectively exclude hemangioma from the differential diagnosis.[61] Heterogeneous T2 signal, an irregular pattern of peripheral enhancement, regions of early central enhancement, and varying intensity of contrast material attenuation or signal intensity with respect to the blood pool all help to differentiate these lesions from benign hemangiomas.[60]

Cystic regions containing blood products and debris may be present.[47,61] Findings of compartmentalization within the tumor with septum-like regions showing low T2 signal or rounded areas of low T2 signal may be present.[62] An additional helpful imaging that can support the diagnosis of angiosarcoma is the detection of simultaneous splenic lesions or splenic metastases, which are uncommon with other tumors but can be found in relatively high frequency in angiosarcoma.[62]

Lymphoma

Primary lymphomas of the liver most commonly manifest as a single solitary lesion (60% of cases), but can present as multiple lesions or as diffusely

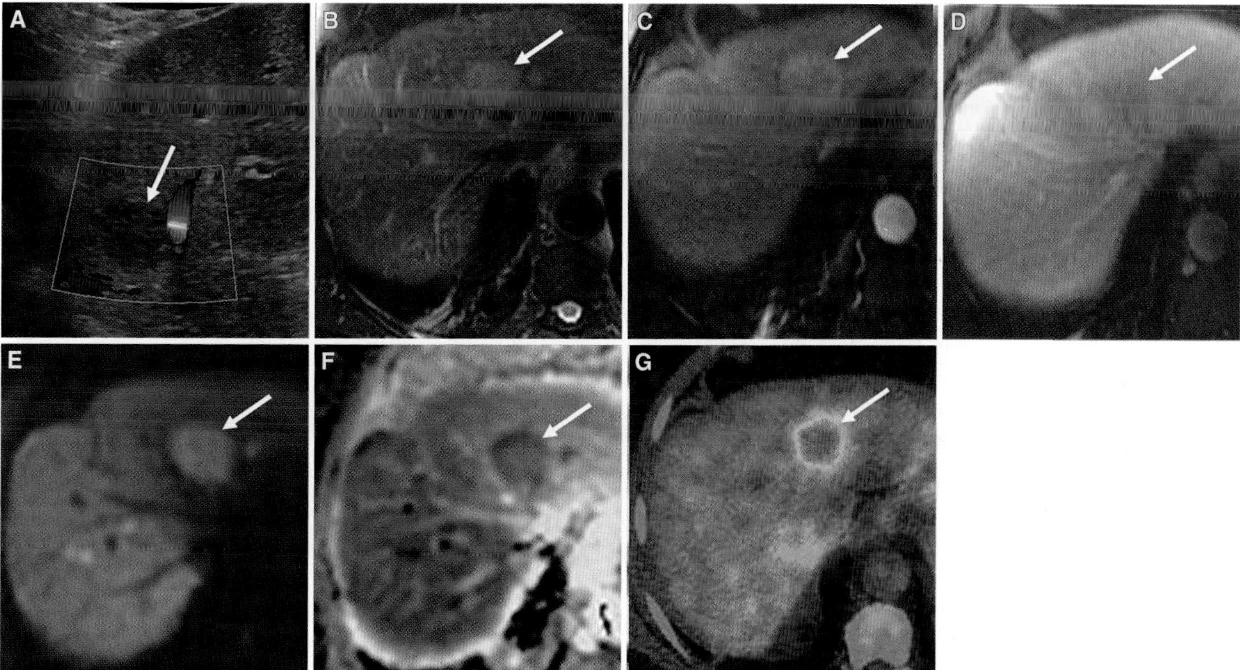

Figure 24.15 Patient with diffuse large B-cell lymphoma secondarily involving the liver. **(A)** Grayscale US with Doppler overlay shows a hypoechoic mass (*arrow*) in the liver dome without detectable vascular flow. **(B)** Axial fat-suppressed T2-weighted MRI image shows a mildly T2 hyperintense mass (*arrow*) in the hepatic dome. **(C, D)** Axial fat-suppressed T1-weighted images with IV contrast enhancement in the late arterial **(C)** and portal venous phase **(D)** show the mass to be arterially hyperenhancing (**C**, *arrow*) with washout on the portal venous phase (**D**, *arrow*). Findings are atypical for lymphoma, which often enhances similar to or less than the background liver. **(E, F)** Diffusion-weighted **(E)** and apparent diffusion coefficient **(F)** maps show high and low signal intensity (*arrows*), respectively, indicating marked restricted diffusion. **(G)** Positron emission tomography showing the mass to be markedly hypermetabolic (*arrow*), which is a typical finding of hepatic lymphoma.

infiltrating disease (Fig. 24.15).[63] Secondary lymphomatous involvement of the liver most commonly presents as multiple lesions or diffuse infiltration (90% of cases), as opposed to a solitary mass. Extrahepatic involvement of the spleen and abdominal lymph nodes are commonly seen in secondary lymphomas.

At US, mass forming lymphomas are characteristically hypoechoic and may be anechoic. This finding is because of the tightly packed homogenous tumor cells, which do not create surfaces for internal reflection, in contrast to that seen in other liver tumors. The absence of posterior acoustic enhancement can be a clue that the lesion is solid and not cystic.[63] Similarly, at CT the mass typically shows homogenously soft-tissue attenuation and at MRI is T2 hyperintense and T1 hypointense. Lymphoma may also show a target appearance similar to a metastasis or a central scar.[64] Calcification is rare. Lymphoma is typically hypoenhancing on all phases at CT and MRI. Identification of enhancing vessels passing through the lesion can be helpful for recognizing the infiltrating growth pattern of lymphoma and arriving at the correct diagnosis.[64] The dense cellularity of lymphoma creates high signal on diffusion-weighted imaging, which is considered a sensitive sequence for detection of this tumor.[65]

Diffuse infiltrative involvement of the liver is common with secondary lymphoma.[64] This pattern of infiltration may be difficult or impossible to detect on anatomic imaging, in which the only imaging finding may be hepatomegaly. In the case of segmental or incomplete infiltration, findings of mild T2 hyperintensity and restricted diffusion can be identified.

Metastases

Liver metastases have variable imaging appearances depending on the tumor type and size of the lesion (Fig. 24.16). The imaging findings reflect the typical structure of a metastasis, which is often composed of malignant cellular tissue surrounding a region of central necrosis. A few lesions such as melanoma or breast carcinoma are notable for producing infiltrative metastases that can present with segmental or diffuse enlargement of the liver (Fig. 24.16).

At US, metastases are typically round and hypoechoic or have a "targetoid" pattern of peripheral hyperechogenicity and central hypoechogenicity. At CT,

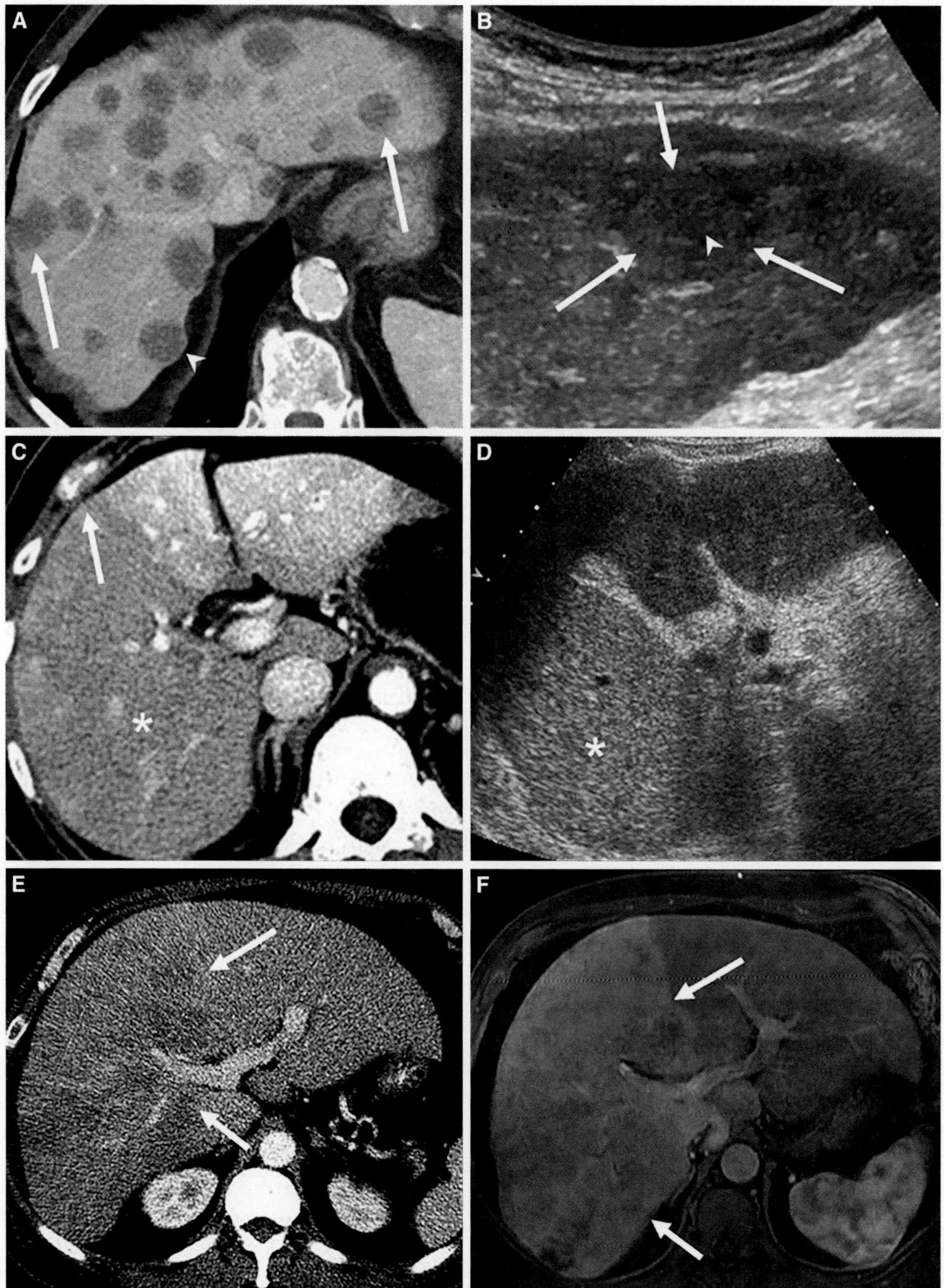

Figure 24.16 (A) Axial CT with IV contrast enhancement in the portal venous phase demonstrates the typical appearance of metastases with multiple low attenuation masses scattered within the liver (*arrows*), some of which distort the normal parenchymal architecture (*arrowhead*). **(B)** Grayscale US from the same patient showing a typical hypoechoic mass (*arrow*) with a central region of lower echogenicity (*arrowhead*) giving a "targetoid" appearance. **(C)** Axial CT with IV contrast enhancement in the portal venous phase shows diffuse low attenuation of the right hepatic lobe (*asterisk*) initially thought to be because of steatosis, however, note the slightly expanded border of the liver (*arrow*) indicating abnormal mass effect from an underlying malignancy. **(D)** Subsequent US in the same patient shows increased echogenicity of the right lobe (*asterisk*) also thought to be because of steatosis. Subsequent biopsy performed for rising liver enzymes and history of breast carcinoma confirmed infiltrating metastatic adenocarcinoma consistent with breast primary. **(E)** Axial CT with IV contrast enhancement in the portal venous phase from a different patient again demonstrates heterogeneous low attenuation of the right liver (*arrows*). **(F, G)** Axial fat-suppressed T1-weighted MRI images with IV contrast enhancement in the late arterial **(H)** and delayed **(G)** phases shows heterogeneous arterial hyperenhancement throughout the right lobe (**H**, *arrows*), which fades to near isointensity on the delayed phase. **(I)** Axial diffusion-weighted image clearly delineates the high signal intensity extent of the tumor. The tumor was subsequently biopsied and found to be metastatic melanoma.

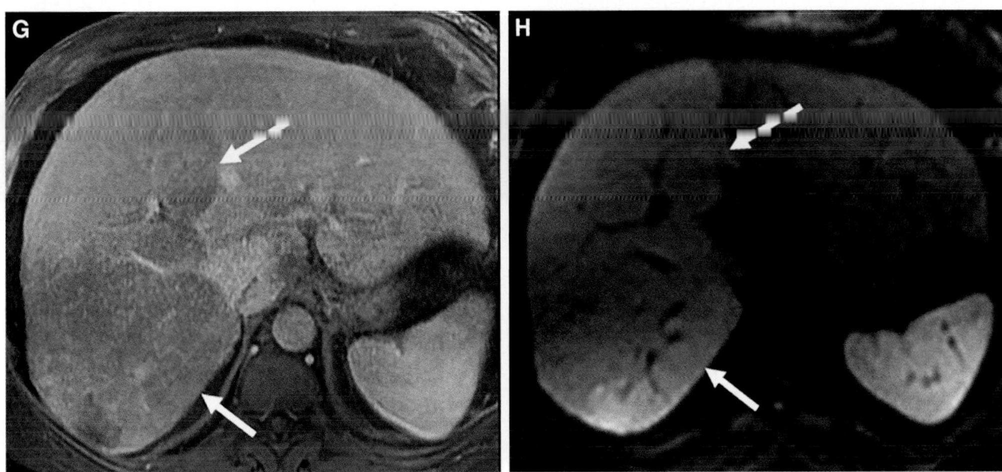

Figure 24.16 *(continued)*

most metastases appear hypoattenuating. At MRI they appear T2 hyperintense and T1 hypointense. Notable exceptions to this pattern are metastases that have internal hemorrhage or rare metastases that contain internal lipid. Regions of hemorrhage appear hypo to hyperechoic at US, depending on the age of the hemorrhage, and are generally hyperattenuating at CT and have high T1 signal at MRI. Regions of tissue containing lipid appear hyperechoic at US, have low attenuation at CT, and lose signal on opposed-phase imaging at MRI.

Neuroendocrine tumors synthesizing compounds such as vasoactive intestinal polypeptide or insulin may produce perilesional steatosis. Melanin within melanoma metastases may appear T1 hyperintense.

The CT and MRI enhancement characteristics also vary, but most metastases are hyperenhancing with a "targetoid" pattern of peripheral ring enhancement and variable central accumulation of contrast material on delayed phases.[66] Hyperenhancing metastases are seen with vascular rich metastases from melanoma, kidney, thyroid, and neuroendocrine origin.[66] The cellular portions of a metastasis may washout in the delayed phase.[67] This is considered characteristic for metastasis and is more commonly seen with vascular rich metastases.[66,67] Hepatic metastases typically do not retain hepatobiliary contrast agent.

Metastases are often imaged with FDG-PET/CT. This modality is well established for tumors such as colorectal carcinoma, in which it has shown a high sensitivity for detecting hepatic metastasis and occult extrahepatic metastases.[68] Metastases typically demonstrate increased activity compared to the adjacent parenchyma. Occasionally, false positives can include inflammatory lesions such as abscesses or rarely hepatic adenomas.[69] Benign primary tumors such as hemangioma, focal nodular hyperplasia, and hepatic adenoma typically show activity at a level that is similar to or less than the background liver.[70]

24.3 TUMORS TYPICALLY FOUND IN PEDIATRIC POPULATION

Hepatoblastoma

Hepatoblastoma typically presents as a single large, well circumscribed mass (Fig. 24.17).[71] The masses tend to be hyperechoic at US, hypoattenuating at CT, and T1 hypointense and T2 hyperintense at MRI. The purely epithelial hepatoblastomas are associated with a homogenous appearance, whereas the mixed epithelial-mesenchymal variant tends to have a heterogeneous appearance.[72] The masses frequently contain hemorrhage and calcification.[72] The calcification tends to be coarse or dense, in comparison to the fine granular calcification of infantile hemangioma.[71] Calcification also suggests a component of osteoid formation.[71] Fibrotic septa may be seen, which are hypoechoic at US and hypointense on T1- and T2-weighted MRI images. The masses are hypervascular but tend to enhance less than the surrounding liver.[71] Vessels running within the fibrous septa can create a "spoke-wheel" appearance at fluoroscopic angiography.[47] The hepatoblastomas can invade into the hepatic and portal veins, similar to hepatocellular carcinoma. The imaging features are not specific and histologic confirmation is needed

Infantile hemangioma

Infantile hemangiomas may present as a large vascular mass, multifocal masses, or diffuse lesions that result in massive hepatomegaly.[49] The masses are well

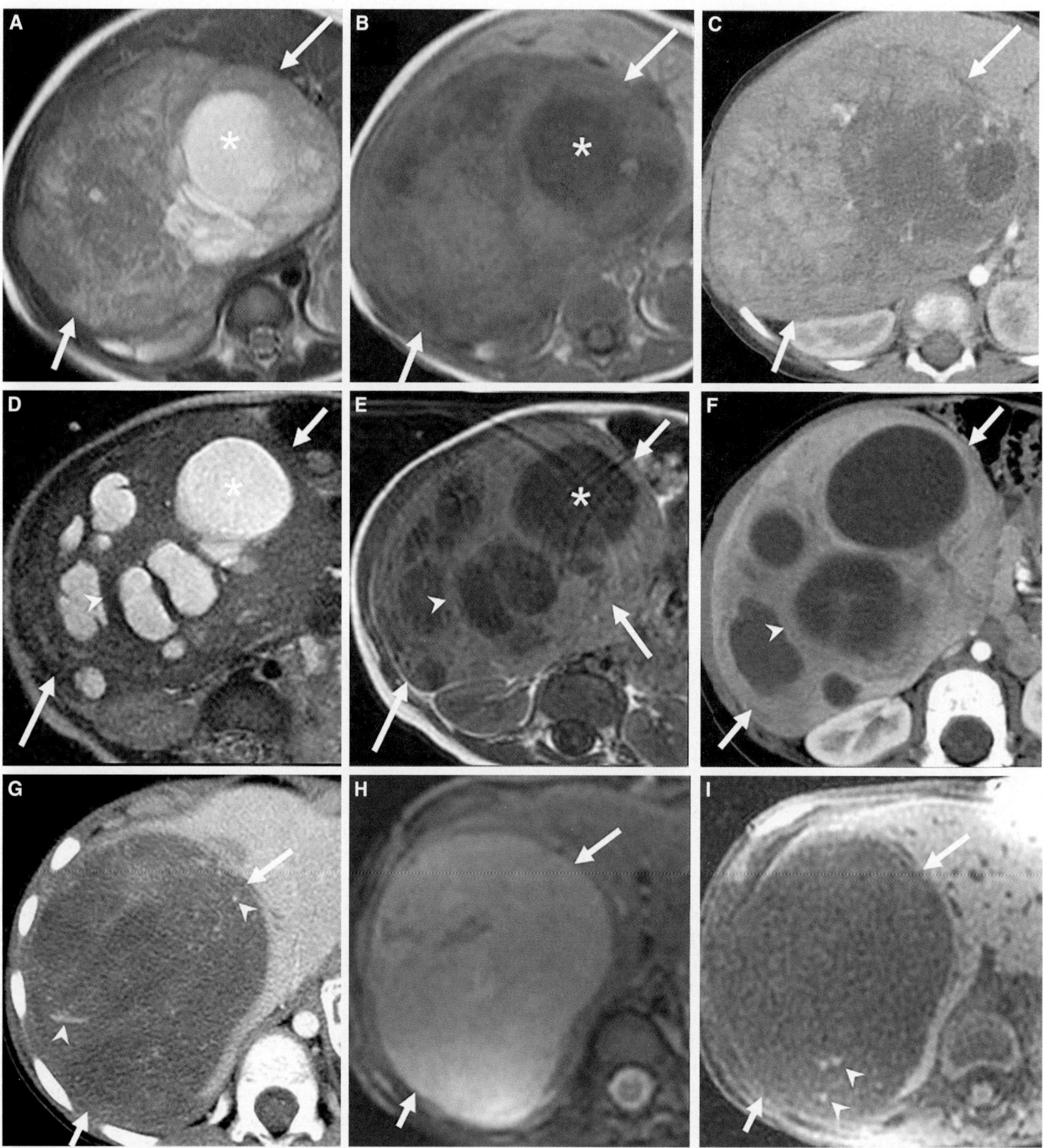

Figure 24.17 Liver tumors typically found in children. **(A–C)** Hepatoblastoma in a 1-year-old boy. Axial T2-weighted **(A)**, T1-weighted **(B)** MRI images show a predominantly solid tumor (*arrows*) with heterogeneous high T2 signal, low T1 signal and complex cystic regions (*asterisk*). **(C)** Axial CT with IV contrast enhancement in the late arterial phase shows heterogeneous enhancement of the solid portions of tumor (*arrows*). **(D–F)** Mesenchymal hamartoma in a 1 year old boy. Axial T2-weighted **(D)**, T1-weighted **(E)** MRI images show a mass (*arrows*) with multiple cystic regions (*asterisk*) with thick fibrous septa (*arrowheads*) low in T1 and T2 signal. **(F)** Axial CT with IV contrast enhancement in the portal venous phase shows low level enhancement within the mass (*arrows*) and its fibrous septa (*arrowhead*); **(G–L)** Embryonal sarcoma in a 7 year old boy. **(G)** Axial CT with IV contrast enhancement in the late arterial phase shows a complex cystic appearing mass (*arrows*) containing small enhancing vessels (*arrowheads*). **(H, I)** Axial fat-suppressed T2-weighted **(H)** and T1-weighted **(I)** MRI images show the tumor (*arrows*) to have heterogeneous high T2 and low T1 signal. Focal hemorrhage within the mass is high signal on T1-weighted images (**I**, *arrowheads*). **(J–L)** Axial fat-suppressed T1-weighted MRI images with IV contrast enhancement in the late arterial **(J)**, portal venous **(K)** and delayed phases **(L)** show slow heterogeneous contrast accumulation within the mass (*arrows*) typical of a mass with solid myxoid composition.

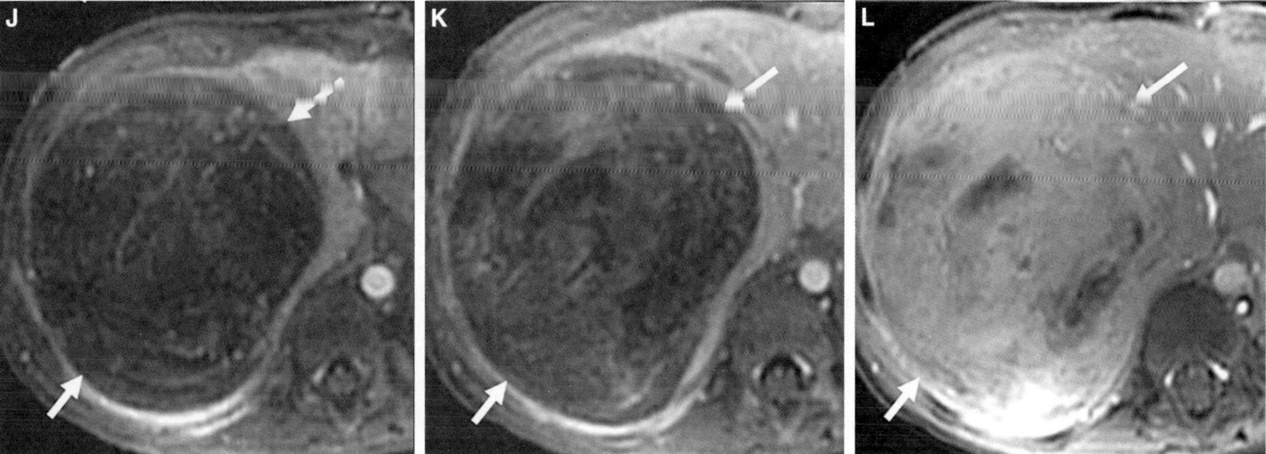

Figure 24.17 *(continued)*

circumscribed at imaging. At US the masses appear solid with mixed echogenicity, most commonly hypoechoic.[49] US may show internal vascularity with large vessels and arteriovenous shunting.[73] At CT, the masses are hypoattenuating and may show regions of heterogeneity when hemorrhage is present. Calcifications can be seen in a third to half of tumors, typically within the larger tumors.[73,74] MRI demonstrates T1 hypointensity and characteristic marked T2 hyperintensity. High flow vessels within the tumor may show a "flow void" or focal loss of signal along the path of flowing blood on MRI images. The masses enhance in a centripetal pattern (moving toward the center) and can demonstrate peripheral nodular enhancement similar to a hemangioma.[47] When masses are multifocal, the enhancement tends to be homogenous with complete filling in the delayed phase. Large, solitary masses tend to have internal hemorrhage, necrosis, and fibrosis resulting in an irregular pattern of enhancement with frequent incomplete central filling.[73,74] Enlarged hepatic arteries and veins may be present and represent a secondary indication of high vascular flow of the tumor.[49]

Mesenchymal hamartoma

At imaging, mesenchymal hamartoma most commonly presents as a large septated cystic mass, but may also be mixed cystic/solid or a solid mass.[47,75] The cystic regions within the tumor demonstrate typical imaging findings of an anechoic lesion at US, fluid attenuation at CT, and low T1 and high T2 signal at MRI (Fig. 24.17). Occasionally, internal debris or fluid/fluid levels can be found within the cystic portions.[75] The cystic regions are often separated by thick septa. If a mass is predominantly composed of solid stromal components, the tissue tends to be hyperechoic at US, hypoattenuating at CT, and hypointense on T1-weighted MRI. Solid fibrous components of the mass are usually hypointense on T2-weighted images.[72] Imaging findings of hemorrhage and calcification are characteristically absent.[47,49] These masses are hypovascular and can show mild enhancement of fibrous septa and mild heterogeneous enhancement of solid stromal components.

Embryonal sarcoma

Embryonal sarcomas typically present as large well circumscribed solid masses.[60] Myxoid components of the mass may give the appearance of a septated cystic mass at CT and MRI because of its fluid attenuation, low T1 signal, and very high T2 signal (Fig. 24.17).[76] US is effective at demonstrating the solid nature of the mass, despite the cystic appearance at CT and unenhanced MRI. The mass typically appears heterogeneously hyperechoic at US. IV contrast-enhanced imaging is also effective at excluding a cystic mass. Delayed-phase imaging shows irregular peripheral enhancement with progressive, heterogeneous accumulation of contrast within the myxoid tissue, a finding that would not be seen with a cystic mass. Internal septations tend to be relatively high signal on CT and low signal on both T1- and T2-weighted MRI. Septations, solid nodular components, and the periphery of the mass tend to show low-level enhancement. Regions of high T1 signal and low T2 signal may be present because of intratumoral hemorrhage.[47,60] Internal calcification is a rare finding.

24.4 SUMMARY

Radiologic imaging is an important part of the evaluation and management of liver tumors. The diagnosis of certain benign lesions like cysts, hemangiomas, abscesses, and focal nodular hyperplasia are possible when characteristic imaging findings and supportive clinical history are present. Confirmatory diagnosis of hepatocellular carcinoma is possible with dynamic CT or MRI in the right clinical setting. Metastases are often diagnosed when the primary tumor is known and there are no other features to suggest another diagnosis. Many tumors have overlapping imaging features necessitating histologic confirmation. In such situations, radiologic pathologic correlation is beneficial for biopsy guidance and verifying features detected at histology.

REFERENCES

1. Fowler KJ, Brown JJ, Narra VR. Magnetic resonance imaging of focal liver lesions: approach to imaging diagnosis. *Hepatology*. 2011;54(6):2227–2237.
2. Blyth S, Blakeborough A, Peterson M, et al. Sensitivity of magnetic resonance imaging in the detection of colorectal liver metastases. *Ann R Coll Surg Engl*. 2008;90(1):25–28.
3. Albiin N. MRI of focal liver lesions. *Curr Med Imaging Rev*. 2012;8(2):107–116.
4. Hammerstingl R, Huppertz A, Breuer J, et al. Diagnostic efficacy of gadoxetic acid (Primovist)-enhanced MRI and spiral CT for a therapeutic strategy: comparison with intraoperative and histopathologic findings in focal liver lesions. *Eur Radiol*. 2008;18(3):457–467.
5. Berland LL, Silverman SG, Gore RM, et al. Managing incidental findings on abdominal CT: white paper of the ACR incidental findings committee. *J Am Coll Radiol*. 2010;7(10):754–773.
6. Borhani AA, Wiant A, Heller MT. Cystic hepatic lesions: a review and an algorithmic approach. *AJR Am J Roentgenol*. 2014;203(6):1192–1204.
7. Newlin N, Silver TM, Stuck KJ, et al. Ultrasonic features of pyogenic liver abscesses. *Radiology*. 1981;139(1):155–159.
8. Balci NC, Sirvanci M. MR imaging of infective liver lesions. *Magn Reson Imaging Clin N Am*. 2002;10(1):121–135, vii.
9. Mortele KJ, Segatto E, Ros PR. The infected liver: radiologic-pathologic correlation. *Radiographics*. 2004;24(4):937–955.
10. Dao TH, Mathieu D, Thu NT, et al. Value of MR imaging in evaluating focal fatty infiltration of the liver: preliminary study. *Radiographics*. 1991;11(6):1003–1012.
11. Kim KW, Kim TK, Han JK, et al. Hepatic hemangiomas: spectrum of US appearances on gray-scale, power Doppler, and contrast-enhanced US. *Korean J Radiol*. 2000;1(4):191–197.
12. Quinn SF, Benjamin GG. Hepatic cavernous hemangiomas: simple diagnostic sign with dynamic bolus CT. *Radiology*. 1992;182(2):545–548.
13. Leslie DF, Johnson CD, Johnson CM, et al. Distinction between cavernous hemangiomas of the liver and hepatic metastases on CT: value of contrast enhancement patterns. *AJR Am J Roentgenol*. 1995;164(3):625–629.
14. Prasanna PM, Fredericks SE, Winn SS, et al. Best cases from the AFIP: giant cavernous hemangioma. *Radiographics*. 2010;30(4):1139–1144.
15. Coumbaras M, Wendum D, Monnier-Cholley L, et al. CT and MR imaging features of pathologically proven atypical giant hemangiomas of the liver. *AJR Am J Roentgenol*. 2002;179(6):1457–1463.
16. Ros PR, Lubbers PR, Olmsted WW, et al. Hemangioma of the liver: heterogeneous appearance on T2-weighted images. *AJR Am J Roentgenol*. 1987;149(6):1167–1170.
17. Doyle DJ, Khalili K, Guindi M, et al. Imaging features of sclerosed hemangioma. *AJR Am J Roentgenol*. 2007;189(1):67–72.
18. Ziessman HA, O'Malley JP, Thrall JH. *Nuclear medicine: the requisites in radiology*. 3rd ed. Philadelphia, PA: Mosby Elsevier; 2006.
19. Venturi A, Piscaglia F, Vidili G, et al. Diagnosis and management of hepatic focal nodular hyperplasia. *J Ultrasound*. 2007;10(3):116–127.
20. Brancatelli G, Federle MP, Grazioli L, et al. Focal nodular hyperplasia: CT findings with emphasis on multiphasic helical CT in 78 patients. *Radiology*. 2001;219(1):61–68.
21. Mortele KJ, Praet M, Van Vlierberghe H, et al. CT and MR imaging findings in focal nodular hyperplasia of the liver: radiologic-pathologic correlation. *AJR Am J Roentgenol*. 2000;175(3):687–692.
22. Choi BY, Nguyen MH. The diagnosis and management of benign hepatic tumors. *J Clin Gastroenterol*. 2005;39(5):401–412.
23. Choi CS, Freeny PC. Triphasic helical CT of hepatic focal nodular hyperplasia: incidence of atypical findings. *AJR Am J Roentgenol*. 1998;170(2):391–395.
24. Ronot M, Paradis V, Duran R, et al. MR findings of steatotic focal nodular hyperplasia and comparison with other fatty tumours. *Eur Radiol*. 2013;23(4):914–923.
25. Zech CJ, Grazioli L, Breuer J, et al. Diagnostic performance and description of morphological features of focal nodular hyperplasia in Gd-EOB-DTPA-enhanced liver magnetic resonance imaging: results of a multicenter trial. *Invest Radiol*. 2008;43(7):504–511.
26. Mettler FA, Guiberteau MJ. *Essentials of nuclear medicine imaging*. 5th ed. Philadelphia, PA: Saunders/Elsevier; 2006.

27. Hussain SM, van den Bos IC, Dwarkasing RS, et al. Hepatocellular adenoma: findings at state-of-the-art magnetic resonance imaging, ultrasound, computed tomography and pathologic analysis. *Eur Radiol.* 2006;16(9):1873–1886.
28. Grazioli L, Federle MP, Brancatelli G, et al. Hepatic adenomas: imaging and pathologic findings. *Radiographics*. 2001;21(4):877–892; discussion 92–94.
29. Grazioli L, Bondioni MP, Haradome H, et al. Hepatocellular adenoma and focal nodular hyperplasia: value of gadoxetic acid-enhanced MR imaging in differential diagnosis. *Radiology*. 2012;262(2):520–529.
30. Bartolozzi C, Lencioni R, Paolicchi A, et al. Differentiation of hepatocellular adenoma and focal nodular hyperplasia of the liver: comparison of power Doppler imaging and conventional color Doppler sonography. *Eur Radiol.* 1997;7(9):1410–1415.
31. Kim TK, Jang HJ, Burns PN, et al. Focal nodular hyperplasia and hepatic adenoma: differentiation with low-mechanical-index contrast-enhanced sonography. *AJR Am J Roentgenol.* 2008;190(1):58–66.
32. Grazioli L, Olivetti L, Mazza G, et al. MR imaging of hepatocellular adenomas and differential diagnosis dilemma. *Int J Hepatol.* 2013;2013:374170.
33. van Aalten SM, Thomeer MG, Terkivatan T, et al. Hepatocellular adenomas: correlation of MR imaging findings with pathologic subtype classification. *Radiology*. 2011;261(1):172–181.
34. Agarwal S, Fuentes-Orrego JM, Arnason T, et al. Inflammatory hepatocellular adenomas can mimic focal nodular hyperplasia on gadoxetic acid-enhanced MRI. *AJR Am J Roentgenol.* 2014;203(4):W408–414.
35. Bruix J, Sherman M. Management of hepatocellular carcinoma: an update. *Hepatology*. 2011;53(3):1020–1022.
36. McEvoy SH, McCarthy CJ, Lavelle LP, et al. Hepatocellular carcinoma: illustrated guide to systematic radiologic diagnosis and staging according to guidelines of the American Association for the Study of Liver Diseases. *Radiographics*. 2013;33(6):1653–1668.
37. Willatt JM, Hussain HK, Adusumilli S, et al. MR Imaging of hepatocellular carcinoma in the cirrhotic liver: challenges and controversies. *Radiology*. 2008;247(2):311–330.
38. Choi JY, Lee JM, Sirlin CB. CT and MR imaging diagnosis and staging of hepatocellular carcinoma: part I. Development, growth, and spread: key pathologic and imaging aspects. *Radiology*. 2014;272(3):635–654.
39. Marrero JA, Hussain HK, Nghiem HV, et al. Improving the prediction of hepatocellular carcinoma in cirrhotic patients with an arterially-enhancing liver mass. *Liver Transpl.* 2005;11(3):281–289.
40. Furlan A, Marin D, Agnello F, et al. Hepatocellular carcinoma presenting at contrast-enhanced multi-detector-row computed tomography or gadolinium-enhanced magnetic resonance imaging as a small (</=2 cm), indeterminate nodule: growth rate and optimal interval time for imaging follow-up. *J Comput Assist Tomogr.* 2012;36(1):20–25.
41. Barbara L, Benzi G, Gaiani S, et al. Natural history of small untreated hepatocellular carcinoma in cirrhosis: a multivariate analysis of prognostic factors of tumor growth rate and patient survival. *Hepatology*. 1992;16(1):132–137.
42. Golfieri R, Grazioli L, Orlando E, et al. Which is the best MRI marker of malignancy for atypical cirrhotic nodules: hypointensity in hepatobiliary phase alone or combined with other features? Classification after Gd-EOB-DTPA administration. *J Magn Reson Imaging.* 2012;36(3):648–657.
43. Kogita S, Imai Y, Okada M, et al. Gd-EOB-DTPA-enhanced magnetic resonance images of hepatocellular carcinoma: correlation with histological grading and portal blood flow. *Eur Radiol.* 2010;20(10):2405–2413.
44. Rimola J, Forner A, Tremosini S, et al. Non-invasive diagnosis of hepatocellular carcinoma </= 2 cm in cirrhosis. Diagnostic accuracy assessing fat, capsule and signal intensity at dynamic MRI. *J Hepatol.* 2012;56(6):1317–1323.
45. Ganeshan D, Szklaruk J, Kundra V, et al. Imaging features of fibrolamellar hepatocellular carcinoma. *AJR Am J Roentgenol.* 2014;202(3):544–552.
46. Mattison GR, Glazer GM, Quint LE, et al. MR imaging of hepatic focal nodular hyperplasia: characterization and distinction from primary malignant hepatic tumors. *AJR Am J Roentgenol.* 1987;148(4):711–715.
47. Gore RM, Levine MS. *Textbook of gastrointestinal radiology*. 4th ed.
48. Brandt DJ, Johnson CD, Stephens DH, et al. Imaging of fibrolamellar hepatocellular carcinoma. *AJR Am J Roentgenol.* 1988;151(2):295–299.
49. Chung YE, Kim MJ, Park YN, et al. Varying appearances of cholangiocarcinoma: radiologic-pathologic correlation. *Radiographics*. 2009;29(3):683–700.
50. Valls C, Guma A, Puig I, et al. Intrahepatic peripheral cholangiocarcinoma: CT evaluation. *Abdom Imaging*. 2000;25(5):490–496.
51. Hann LE, Getrajdman GI, Brown KT, et al. Hepatic lobar atrophy: association with ipsilateral

portal vein obstruction. *AJR Am J Roentgenol.* 1996;167(4):1017–1021.

52. Huang B, Wu L, Lu XY, et al. Small intrahepatic cholangiocarcinoma and hepatocellular carcinoma in cirrhotic livers may share similar enhancement patterns at multiphase dynamic MR imaging. *Radiology.* 2016:151205.
53. Sapisochin G, Fidelman N, Roberts JP, et al. Mixed hepatocellular cholangiocarcinoma and intrahepatic cholangiocarcinoma in patients undergoing transplantation for hepatocellular carcinoma. *Liver Transpl.* 2011;17(8):934–942.
54. Potretzke TA, Tan BR, Doyle MB, et al. Imaging features of biphenotypic primary liver carcinoma (hepatocholangiocarcinoma) and the potential to mimic hepatocellular carcinoma: LI-RADS analysis of CT and MRI features in 81 cases. *AJR Am J Roentgenol.* 2016:1–7.
55. Mortele KJ, Ros PR. Cystic focal liver lesions in the adult: differential CT and MR imaging features. *Radiographics.* 2001;21(4):895–910.
56. Kawashima A, Fishman EK, Hruban RH, et al. Biliary cystadenoma with intratumoral bleeding: radiologic-pathologic correlation. *J Comput Assist Tomogr.* 1991;15(6):1035–1038.
57. Azzam RI, Alshak NS, Pham HP. AIRP best cases in radiologic-pathologic correlation: hepatic epithelioid hemangioendothelioma. *Radiographics.* 2012;32(3):789–794.
58. Earnest Ft, Johnson CD. Case 96: hepatic epithelioid hemangioendothelioma. *Radiology.* 2006;240(1):295–298.
59. Makhlouf HR, Ishak KG, Goodman ZD. Epithelioid hemangioendothelioma of the liver: a clinicopathologic study of 137 cases. *Cancer.* 1999;85(3):562–582.
60. Yu RS, Chen Y, Jiang B, et al. Primary hepatic sarcomas: CT findings. *Eur Radiol.* 2008;18(10):2196–2205.
61. Peterson MS, Baron RL, Rankin SC. Hepatic angiosarcoma: findings on multiphasic contrast-enhanced helical CT do not mimic hepatic hemangioma. *AJR Am J Roentgenol.* 2000;175(1):165–170.
62. Koyama T, Fletcher JG, Johnson CD, et al. Primary hepatic angiosarcoma: findings at CT and MR imaging. *Radiology.* 2002;222(3):667–673.
63. Tomasian A, Sandrasegaran K, Elsayes KM, et al. Hematologic malignancies of the liver: spectrum of disease. *Radiographics.* 2015;35(1):71–86.
64. Rajesh S, Bansal K, Sureka B, et al. The imaging conundrum of hepatic lymphoma revisited. *Insights Imaging.* 2015;6(6):679–692.
65. van Ufford HM, Kwee TC, Beek FJ, et al. Newly diagnosed lymphoma: initial results with whole-body T1-weighted, STIR, and diffusion-weighted MRI compared with 18F-FDG PET/CT. *AJR Am J Roentgenol.* 2011;196(3):662–669.
66. Danet IM, Semelka RC, Leonardou P, et al. Spectrum of MRI appearances of untreated metastases of the liver. *AJR Am J Roentgenol.* 2003;181(3):809–817.
67. Mahfouz AE, Hamm B, Wolf KJ. Peripheral washout: a sign of malignancy on dynamic gadolinium-enhanced MR images of focal liver lesions. *Radiology.* 1994;190(1):49–52.
68. Sacks A, Peller PJ, Surasi DS, et al. Value of PET/CT in the management of liver metastases, part 1. *AJR Am J Roentgenol.* 2011;197(2):W256–259.
69. Tan GJ, Berlangieri SU, Lee ST, et al. FDG PET/CT in the liver: lesions mimicking malignancies. *Abdom Imaging.* 2014;39(1):187–195.
70. Sacks A, Peller PJ, Surasi DS, et al. Value of PET/CT in the management of primary hepatobiliary tumors, part 2. *AJR Am J Roentgenol.* 2011;197(2):W260–265.
71. Dachman AH, Pakter RL, Ros PR, et al. Hepatoblastoma: radiologic-pathologic correlation in 50 cases. *Radiology.* 1987;164(1):15–19.
72. Chung EM, Lattin GE, Jr, Cube R, et al. From the archives of the AFIP: Pediatric liver masses: radiologic-pathologic correlation. Part 2. Malignant tumors. *Radiographics.* 2011;31(2):483–507.
73. Kassarjian A, Zurakowski D, Dubois J, et al. Infantile hepatic hemangiomas: clinical and imaging findings and their correlation with therapy. *AJR Am J Roentgenol.* 2004;182(3):785–795.
74. Roos JE, Pfiffner R, Stallmach T, et al. Infantile hemangioendothelioma. *Radiographics.* 2003;23(6):1649–1655.
75. Kim SH, Kim WS, Cheon JE, et al. Radiological spectrum of hepatic mesenchymal hamartoma in children. *Korean J Radiol.* 2007;8(6):498–505.
76. Crider MH, Hoggard E, Manivel JC. Undifferentiated (embryonal) sarcoma of the liver. *Radiographics.* 2009;29(6):1665–1668.

25 Pediatric liver tumors

Saba Yasir, MBBS

25.1 HEPATOBLASTOMA

Definition

Hepatoblastomas are malignant epithelial neoplasms that are primary to the liver and show a range of hepatocellular differentiation, recapitulating various stages of hepatic development. The tumor is composed of various combinations of epithelial and sometimes mesenchymal components.

Clinical features

Hepatoblastomas are the most common liver tumors in infants and children. Overall, 90% of cases are diagnosed before the age of 5 years.[1] There is a modest male predominance with about a male to female ratio of 2:1.[1] Clinical findings at presentation are nonspecific but can include a palpable abdominal mass, abdominal pain, weight loss, and jaundice.[2] A variety of paraneoplastic findings have also been reported, and the most common are anemia and thrombocytosis. Rarely, hepatoblastomas produce human chorionic gonadotropin and lead to virilization and precocious puberty.[3] Patients do not have underlying chronic liver disease. Hepatoblastomas rarely have been reported in adults, though many of these cases are somewhat suspect, not being sufficiently well documented to rule out other potential mimics.

The etiology of hepatoblastomas is unknown, but there is a strong association with prematurity and low birth weight, especially <1,500 g. Hepatoblastomas are also associated with several clinical syndromes including familial adenomatosis polyposis[4] and the Beckwith–Wiedemann syndrome.[5]

A marked elevation in serum α fetoprotein (AFP) is noted in >90% of cases and is an important tool in the diagnostic workup. However, elevated serum AFP levels are not specific to hepatoblastoma because they can be seen in other benign and malignant liver tumors, including mesenchymal hamartomas[6] and hepatocellular carcinomas. Also of note, a small subset of hepatoblastomas (2% to 4%) has normal or mildly elevated serum AFP levels (<100 ng/mL).[7] This group of tumors has a worse prognosis, in most cases because of an association with the more aggressive small cell undifferentiated morphology.

Gross findings

Hepatoblastomas are well-circumscribed and usually solitary lesions (Fig. 25.1), but they can be multifocal. The background liver is noncirrhotic, but there can be a rim of inflamed and fibrotic background liver at the tumor–nontumor interface. The cut surface of the tumor has a variegated appearance, reflecting the different components of the tumor. The epithelial components tend to be tan brown in color, whereas the mesenchymal areas tend to be more grey-white in color. Areas of necrosis, hemorrhage, and cystic degeneration can be encountered, especially in cases with neoadjuvant therapy. Adequate tumor sampling is critical for proper tumor evaluation, allowing the identification of the various epithelial and mesenchymal components. Per standardized protocol, at least one section per centimeter of tumor diameter should be submitted.[8]

Histologic subtypes

Hepatoblastomas display a wide variety of histologic patterns, including various combinations of epithelial as well as mixed epithelial and mesenchymal components. By definition, an epithelial component is needed for the diagnosis. Most hepatoblastomas (70%) are purely epithelial, while the remaining cases have both epithelial and mesenchymal components. Hepatoblastomas are currently subclassified into the following subtypes[8]:

1. Hepatoblastoma, pure fetal with low mitotic activity (≤2 mitoses/10 high-power fields)
2. Hepatoblastoma, pure fetal, mitotically active (>2 mitoses/10 high-power fields)
3. Hepatoblastoma, epithelial type, pleomorphic fetal
4. Hepatoblastoma, epithelial type, embryonal
5. Hepatoblastoma, epithelial type, macrotrabecular
6. Hepatoblastoma, epithelial type, small cell undifferentiated
7. Hepatoblastoma, epithelial type, cholangioblastic

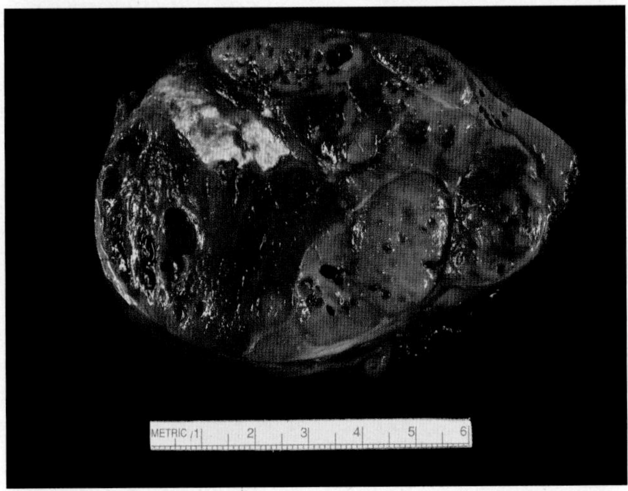

Figure 25.1 Hepatoblastoma gross features. The cut surface has variegated appearance; periphery of the tumor is tan brown, while central areas are greyish. Areas of necrosis and hemorrhage are also seen.

8. Hepatoblastoma, mixed epithelial type (combination of any or all of the above components)
9. Hepatoblastoma, mixed epithelial and mesenchymal components
   a. Without teratoid features
   b. With teratoid features

The fetal pattern is the most common type of epithelium, being found in 80% to 90% of cases, either alone or in combination with other types of epithelium. Overall, about one-third of hepatoblastomas are composed solely of fetal type epithelium. In contrast, the embryonal pattern is present in 30% of cases, where it is almost always admixed with fetal type epithelium. The other epithelial types are seen in 5% of cases or less and are also typically admixed with other epithelial subtypes.

Small cell undifferentiated

The small cell undifferentiated subtype is composed of discohesive sheets, nests, and clusters of small cells that resemble the cells of neuroblastoma or other small round blue cell tumors. Sometimes, the clusters of cells are embedded in a myxoid matrix. This subtype typically lacks well-defined acini, trabeculae, or rosette/pseudogland formation. The cells demonstrate very high nuclear–cytoplasmic ratios, scant cytoplasm, relatively fine nuclear chromatin, and inconspicuous nucleoli (Fig. 25.2). This subtype frequently displays numerous mitotic figures. Immunostains for INI-1 should also be performed because loss of INI-1 has been reported in some cases with small cell undifferentiated histology.[9] Small cell undifferentiated hepatoblastomas usually have normal or mildly elevated serum AFP levels.[9]

This subgroup of hepatoblastomas has a more aggressive behavior and worse survival.[9] Per current Children's Oncology Group (COG) protocol, specimens with any percentage of small cell undifferentiated histology may require more extensive therapy, and the presence and percent of tumor (estimated to nearest 10%) with small cell undifferentiated morphology should be included in the pathology report.

Embryonal pattern

The embryonal pattern has small basophilic epithelial cells with angulated nuclei and relatively high nuclear–cytoplasmic ratios. The tumor cells mostly show a solid growth pattern but also have scattered areas of rosettes or pseudogland formation (Fig. 25.3). The embryonal pattern is only rarely seen in isolation, in most cases being found with the fetal pattern. This makes the fetal pattern easier to see because the basophilic embryonal cells are juxtaposed to more eosinophilic fetal cells (Fig. 25.4). Extramedullary hematopoiesis can be present (Fig. 25.5). The tumor cells of the embryonal pattern can sometimes resemble the tumor cells in the small cell undifferentiated pattern. However, the tumor cells in the embryonal pattern have a more basophilic appearance at low power, slightly bigger nuclei, and have more cytoplasm.

Fetal pattern

The fetal pattern is the most common histologic pattern in hepatoblastomas. The fetal type epithelium is more mature appearing than the tumor cells of the small cell undifferentiated or the embryonal patterns. The fetal growth pattern shows bland-appearing

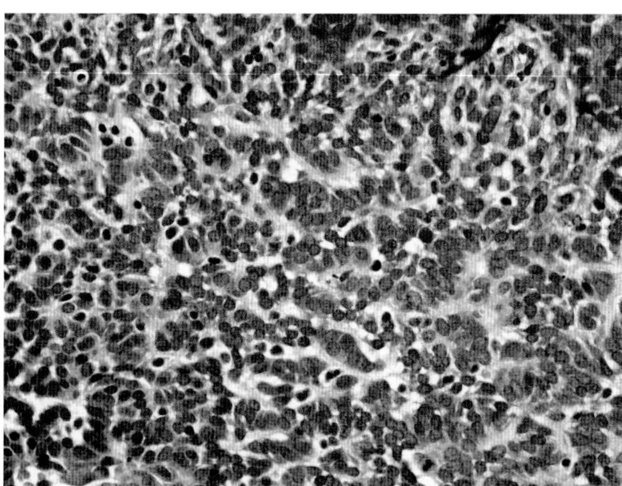

Figure 25.2 Small cell undifferentiated component. The cells have scant cytoplasm, high nuclear–cytoplasmic ratio, and fine nuclear chromatin.

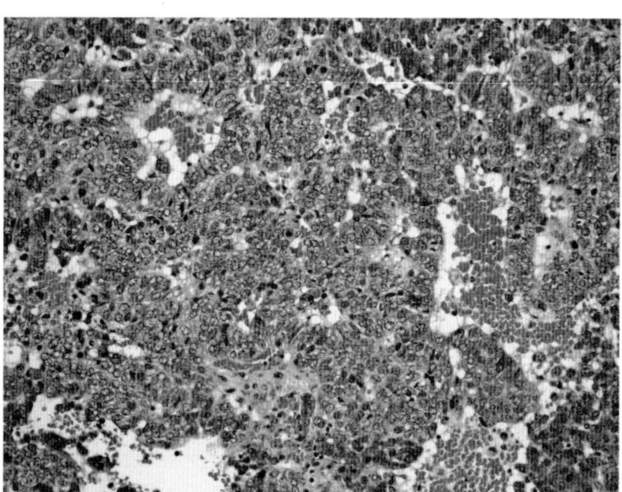

Figure 25.3 Embryonal pattern. Rosettes or pseudogland formation is noted. The cells have basophilic appearance with relatively high nuclear–cytoplasmic ratio.

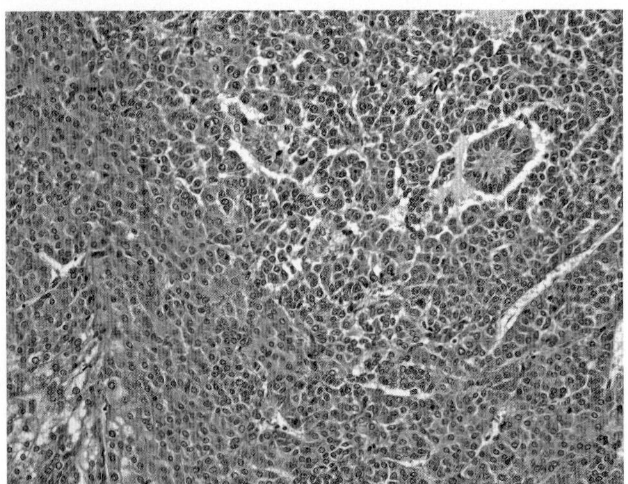

Figure 25.4 Embryonal pattern with fetal pattern. A basophilic appearing embryonal component (upper right) is juxtaposed to eosinophilic fetal component.

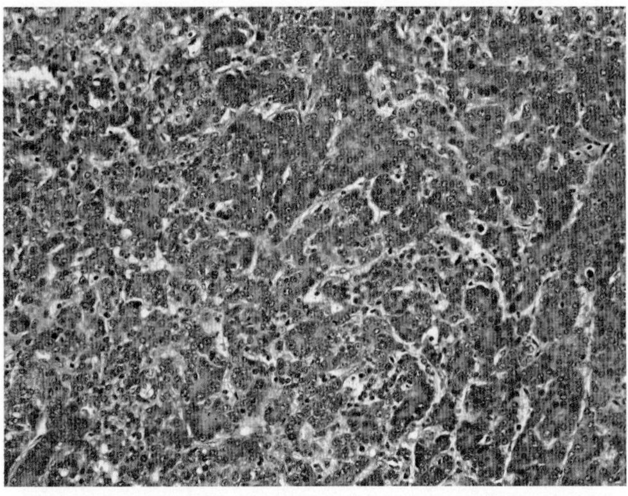

Figure 25.6 Fetal component. The more mature appearing tumor cells grow as thin trabeculae (2–3 cells thick) and have eosinophilic cytoplasm.

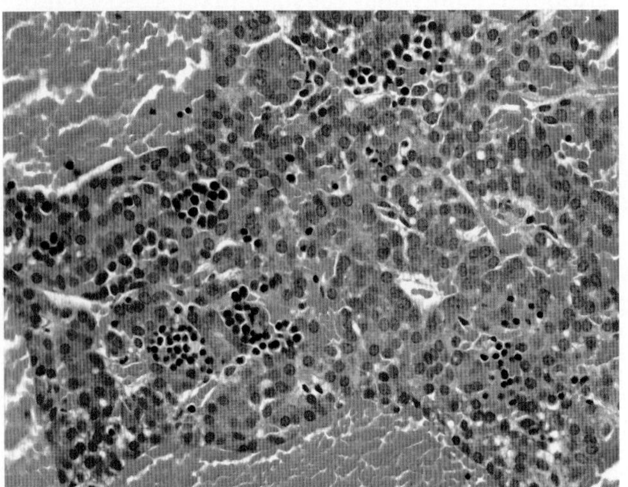

Figure 25.5 Extramedullary hematopoiesis. Immature hematopoietic elements seen in hepatoblastoma.

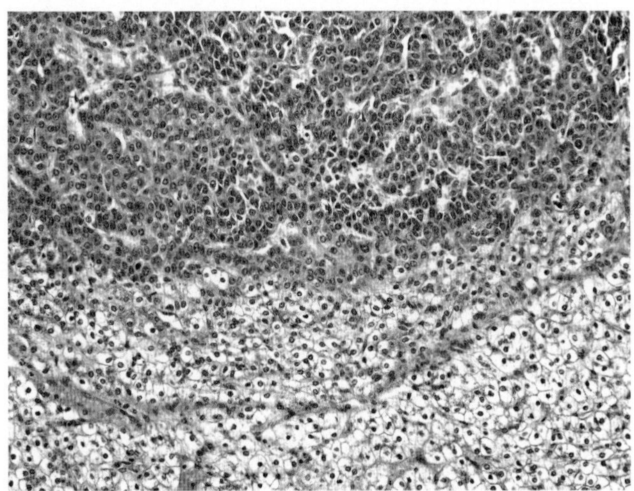

Figure 25.7 Fetal component. Alternating light (clear cells) and dark zones are seen.

tumor cells with moderate amounts of eosinophilic cytoplasm. The cells have recognizable hepatocyte differentiation (Fig. 25.6). In some areas, the tumor cells will show clear cell change because of glycogen accumulation. The tumor cells grow as solid sheets or thin trabeculae (2 to 3 cells thick) and can show a "light and dark pattern" because of patchy glycogen accumulation (Fig. 25.7). These alternating light and dark zones can be further highlighted by periodic acid–Schiff (PAS) stains, but are not specific for hepatoblastoma.

Hepatoblastomas that are composed entirely of tumor cells showing a fetal morphology are further divided into those with low mitotic activity (previously called well-differentiated fetal hepatoblastomas), and mitotically active hepatoblastomas (previously called "crowded fetal hepatoblastoma"), using a cutoff of less than or equal to 2 mitoses per 10 high-power fields (40×). The pure fetal hepatoblastoma with low mitotic activity has a favorable prognosis. Complete surgical resection with negative margins is curative, and no adjuvant chemotherapy is required. Pure fetal hepatoblastoma, mitotically active, has more than 2 mitoses per 10 high power fields (40×) (Fig. 25.8) and has less favorable prognosis.

Pleomorphic pattern

The pleomorphic pattern is uncommon. It is not a primitive appearing growth pattern, but instead demonstrates definite hepatocellular differentiation that can resemble adult type hepatocellular carcinomas. The tumor cells in the pleomorphic pattern show

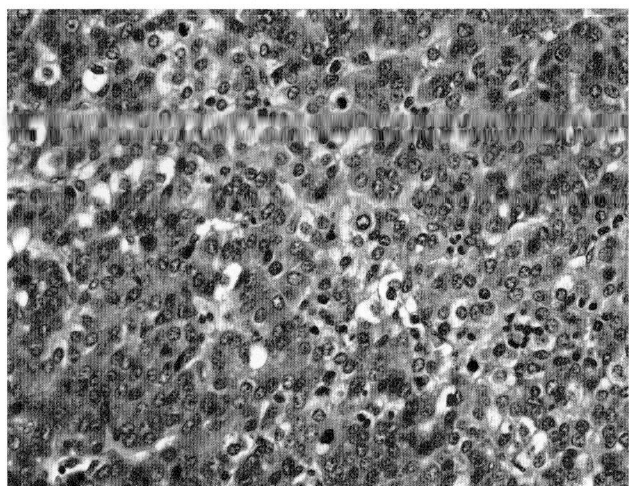

Figure 25.8 Fetal component, mitotically active. Four mitotic figures are seen (40×).

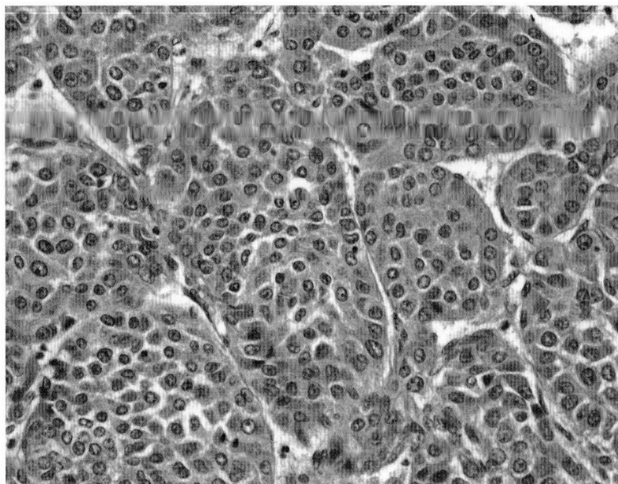

Figure 25.10 Macrotrabecular pattern. The tumor is growing in thick trabeculae.

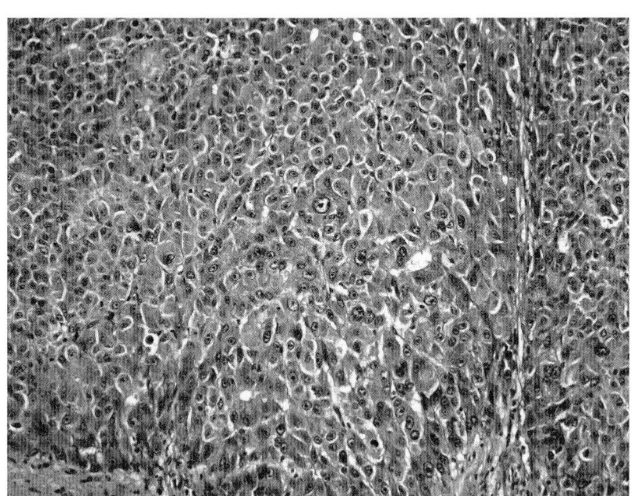

Figure 25.9 Pleomorphic pattern. The cells have moderate degree of nuclear pleomorphism with prominent nucleoli.

more striking nuclear atypia than the fetal growth pattern. There is moderate nuclear pleomorphism with coarse, basophilic chromatin, and prominent nucleoli (Fig. 25.9).

Macrotrabecular pattern

The macrotrabecular pattern is rare, being found in <5% of cases. The individual tumor cells usually have a fetal morphology. This subtype is defined by its distinctive growth pattern, characterized by very thick, broad trabeculae (>10 cells thick, Fig. 25.10). This pattern of thick trabeculae can be nicely highlighted by a CD34 immunostain. The macrotrabecular pattern is almost always seen admixed with other patterns.

Cholangioblastic pattern

The cholangioblastic pattern is very rare, but can be more evident in treated cases. The tumor shows scattered small duct-like structures, usually in a loose mesenchymal background. Sometimes, the findings can resemble a benign reactive ductular proliferation. In most cases, there is sufficient cytological atypia to confidently recognize the cells as neoplastic. The location of the duct-like structures can be another useful clue: tumor–nontumor interface versus deeper in the tumor (Fig. 25.11), the latter location making a benign ductular proliferation unlikely. Immunohistochemistry for β-catenin can be helpful, as strong diffuse nuclear β-catenin expression indicates malignant process.

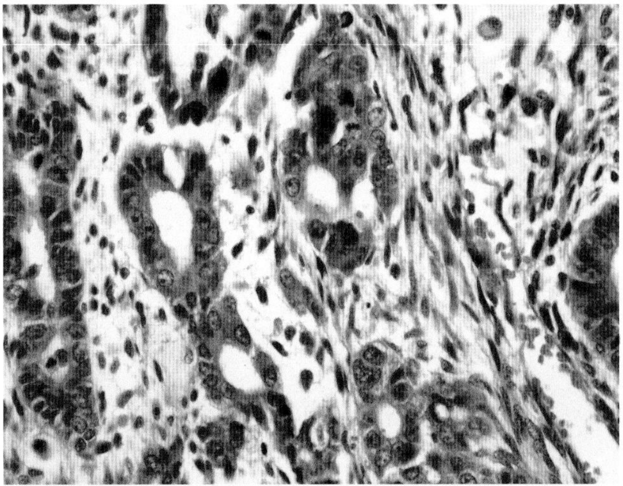

Figure 25.11 Cholangioblastic pattern. Malignant gland-like structures are seen.

Mesenchymal component

About 20% to 40% of hepatoblastomas have a mesenchymal component. The mesenchymal components show various morphologies, but are mostly a mixture of undifferentiated spindle cells and osteoid formation (Fig. 25.12). Rarely, teratoid components are found, which include endodermal derivatives (squamous, glandular, mucinous epithelium, etc.) and neuroectodermal derivatives such as neuroglial elements or melanin-containing cells (Fig. 25.13).

Immunohistochemical and molecular findings

Hepar-1 and Arginase are typically positive in fetal and embryonal patterns, but negative in the small cell undifferentiated pattern. β-Catenin is normally expressed as membranous staining in benign hepatocytes and bile ducts. Two abnormal patterns of β-catenin expression are found in hepatoblastomas: nuclear staining (Fig. 25.14) or diffuse cytoplasmic staining. Abnormal nuclear expression is best seen in the embryonal pattern. The fetal pattern can show only focal or patchy β-catenin nuclear staining. Glypican-3 can be positive in any of the patterns. INI-1 immunostain should be performed on hepatoblastomas with a small cell undifferentiated morphology because loss of INI-1 expression can be seen in a subset of cases.[9] Cases with INI-1 loss typically require more aggressive chemotherapy.

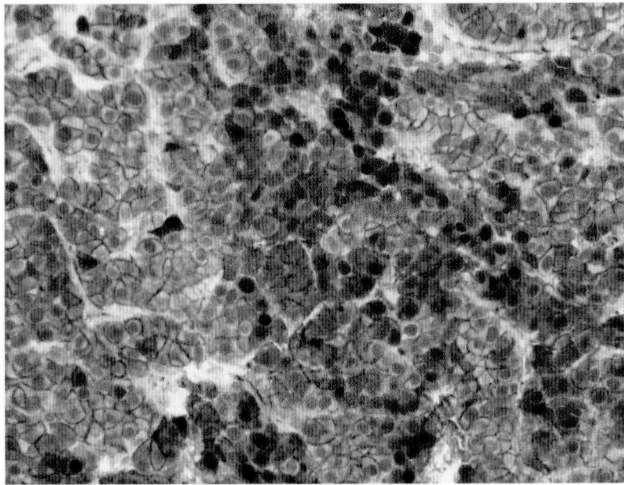

Figure 25.14 β-Catenin immunostain. Nuclear β-catenin expression is noted.

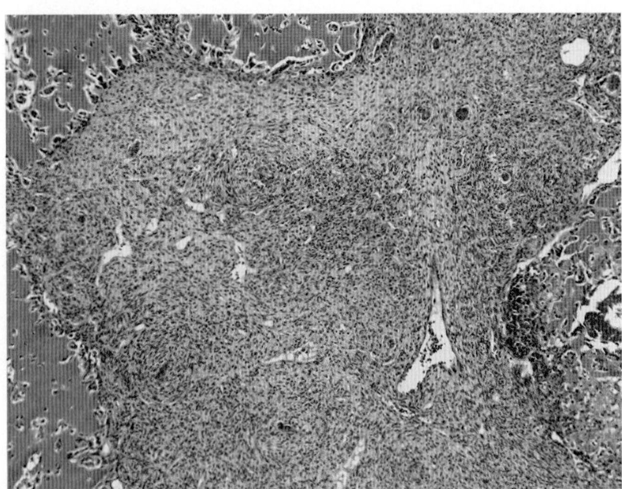

Figure 25.12 Mesenchymal component. Undifferentiated spindle cell areas are seen as well as an osteoid component.

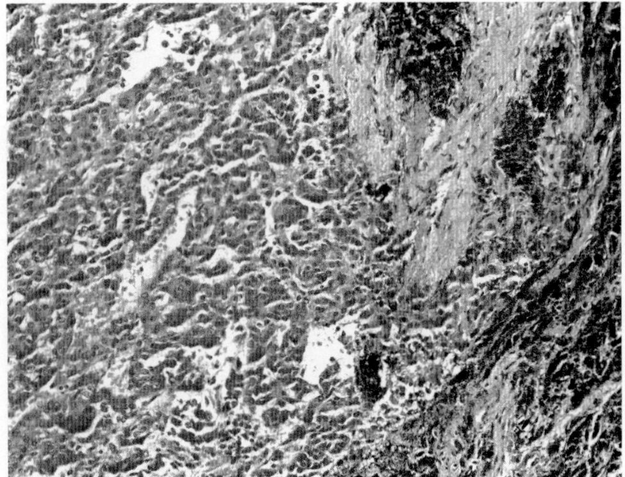

Figure 25.13 Melanin. This hepatoblastoma had aggregates of melanin producing cells (right side of image) scattered throughout the tumor.

The main molecular finding in hepatoblastomas is mutations involving exon 3 of the *CTNNB1* gene (β-catenin). The majority of mutations are deletions and these lead to nuclear accumulation of β-catenin protein and aberrant activation of the Wnt signaling pathway. Neither the genetic changes nor nuclear accumulation of β-catenin is specific for hepatoblastoma, being found in other tumors of the liver including conventional hepatocellular carcinoma.

Differential diagnosis

The differential diagnosis depends on the histologic pattern or combination of patterns seen in any particular case. In cases with fetal or pleomorphic patterns, the main differential diagnosis is conventional hepatocellular carcinoma. The presence of other histologic components of hepatoblastoma, including mesenchymal pattern, helps establish the diagnosis of hepatoblastoma. Underlying liver disease strongly favors hepatocellular carcinoma. In

Table 25.1 Staging of hepatoblastoma, Children's Oncology Group (COG)

Stage 1	Complete resection, margins grossly and microscopically negative for tumor
Stage 2	Microscopic residual tumor present 1. Microscopic residual tumor present at hepatic resection margin 2. Microscopic residual tumor present at extrahepatic resection margin 3. Intraoperative tumor spill
Stage 3	Gross residual tumor present 1. Macroscopic tumor visible at resection margin(s) 2. Lymph node metastasis present
Stage 4	Metastatic disease present 1. Primary tumor completely resected 2. Primary tumor not completely resected

addition, correlation with clinical findings (including age of the patient, serum AFP levels) is helpful. Hepatoblastoma typically arises in children under age 5. High serum AFP levels are not helpful because they are seen in both hepatocellular carcinoma and hepatoblastomas. However, normal or mildly elevated AFP in any tumor with obvious hepatocellular differentiation argues strongly against the possibility of hepatoblastoma. Immunohistochemical stains, including β-catenin do not reliably differentiate these two entities.

Small cell undifferentiated hepatoblastomas can mimic other small round blue cell tumors. Identifying other components (embryonal, fetal) will establish a diagnosis of hepatoblastoma. A panel of immunostains can be performed if needed to exclude entities like Ewing sarcoma (positive for CD99), lymphoma (positive for lymphoid markers), and Wilm tumor (WT-1, keratins).

Staging

Two staging systems are currently used for hepatoblastomas: the first is the COG system and the second is the PRETEXT (pretreatment extent of disease) staging system. The COG system is a post-surgical staging system adopted by the American Children Oncology Group that recommends surgical resection as the initial treatment (Table 25.1). The PRETEXT system is a preoperative or pretreatment staging system and is based on pretreatment imaging findings to determine the size, site, and extent of disease. This system is helpful to determine risk stratification, monitor response to chemotherapy, and predicts surgical respectability. In this system, the liver is divided into four segments, and each segment is evaluated for involvement by the tumor. This system has four categories (PRETEXT I, II, III, and IV) depending on the number of segments involved by the tumor (Fig. 25.15).

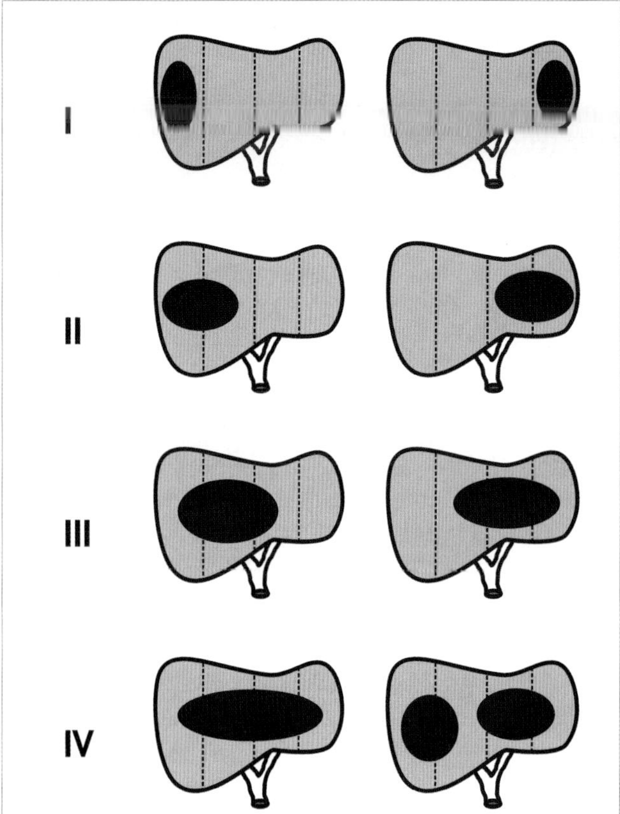

Figure 25.15 PRETEXT staging. The liver is divided into four sections with boundaries being the right and middle hepatic veins and the umbilical fissure. Stage 1 disease is defined by three contiguous disease-free sections of the liver; Stage 2 by two contiguous disease-free sections of the liver; Stage 3 by one disease-free sections of the liver; Stage 4 disease involving all sections of the liver. When hepatoblastomas are multifocal, additional combinations are possible but are not illustrated for Stages II and III.

Metastasis and recurrence

Approximately 20% of hepatoblastomas are metastatic at the time of initial diagnosis.[10] The lungs are the most common site of metastases.[11] Hepatoblastomas developing in utero may metastasize to the placenta.[12] The recurrence rate of hepatoblastomas after complete remission is about 10%.[13] The median time to relapse after initial diagnosis is about 12 months. The major risk factors for recurrence of hepatoblastoma are as follows: PRETEXT IV, metastases at presentation, older age at diagnosis, low AFP level, the presence of vascular involvement, and the presence of a small cell undifferentiated component.[14] The most common sites of recurrence are liver, lungs, peritoneum, and brain.[14]

Prognosis and treatment

Surgical resection and chemotherapy (pre- or post-surgery) are the main therapeutic modalities for hepatoblastoma. There are several treatment protocols designed by major study groups that use a combination of surgery and/or chemotherapy. In clinical trials designed by International Childhood Liver Tumor Strategy Group (SIOPEL), all hepatoblastomas are treated with neoadjuvant chemotherapy followed by surgical resection. In contrast to this approach, American COG recommends surgical resection of hepatoblastoma as the initial treatment.

The current survival rate is about 80%. The most important negative prognostic factors are advanced PRETEXT stage, older age at the time of diagnosis, AFP levels (very high or very low), the presence of metastases, small cell undifferentiated histology,[15] unresectable vessel involvement, positive surgical margins, or tumor rupture.[16,17] In contrast, children with pure fetal hepatoblastoma with low mitotic activity can be treated with complete surgical resection and have excellent long-term outcomes without additional chemotherapy.[18]

25.2 MALIGNANT RHABDOID TUMOR

Definition

Malignant rhabdoid tumors are extremely rare and aggressive neoplasms. These tumors display characteristic rhabdoid cytology, loss of nuclear INI-1 expression, and mutations/deletions in the *SMARCB1/INI-1* gene on chromosome 22. They have no hepatic differentiation even when primary to the liver.

Clinical features

Malignant rhabdoid tumors are rare, but can be primary to the liver. In the largest studies to date, the median age of presentation was 8 months and mean age was 2 years.[19] There is modest male predominance. Patients present with nonspecific findings that can include palpable abdominal masses, hepatomegaly, fever, anorexia, vomiting, and lethargy. Common laboratory findings include anemia, thrombocytopenia, and elevated liver enzyme levels. Serum AFP levels are normal or minimally activated. Spontaneous tumor rupture occurs in up to 20% of cases.[20] Sixty percent of patients have metastatic disease at the time of presentation.[19]

Gross findings

The tumors are typically very large and frequently involve multiple lobes of the liver. Tumors have variegated lobulated cut surfaces, with areas of hemorrhage, necrosis, calcifications, and sometimes large areas of cystic degeneration.

Histologic findings

Malignant rhabdoid tumors are epithelioid malignant neoplasms with predominantly solid and thick trabecular growth patterns, but there can be spindled or pseudoacinar morphology. The neoplastic cells are large, round to polygonal, and discohesive with abundant dense eosinophilic cytoplasm (Fig. 25.16). They have round vesicular nuclei that are eccentrically located in the cell cytoplasm, along with prominent nucleoli. In a subset of cases, the cytoplasm contains distinctive round hyaline filamentous perinuclear inclusions that push the nucleus to the edge of the cell. Extensive areas of necrosis are common and can elicit a reactive lymphohistiocytic infiltrate and myxoid stromal changes.

Immunohistochemical findings

The most important stain is INI-1, which is a very sensitive and specific marker for the diagnosis of malignant rhabdoid tumor. The loss of nuclear INI-1 expression by immunohistochemical stain results from mutations/deletions in the *SMARCB1/INI-1*. Markers of epithelial differentiation are frequently positive. The majority

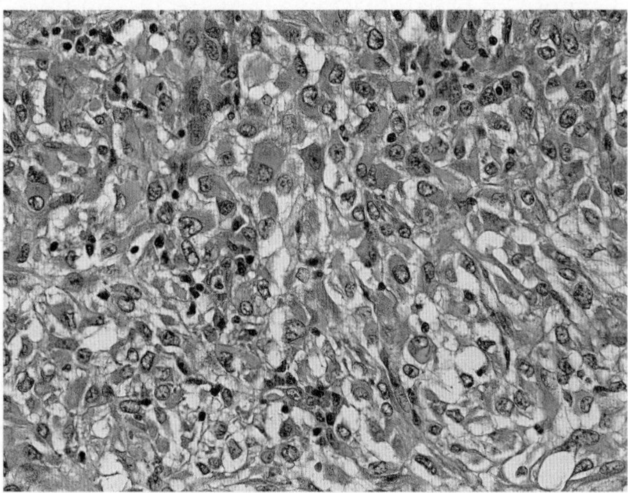

Figure 25.16 Malignant rhabdoid tumor. The tumor cells are round and have abundant dense eosinophilic cytoplasm with eccentrically located vesicular nuclei.

of tumors are positive for pancytokeratin (AE1/AE3, OSCAR), CK8 (low molecular weight keratin), and epithelial membrane antigen (EMA) . The extent of keratin expression varies from focal or patchy to diffuse staining. Vimentin can show strong paranuclear expression. Of note, these tumors do not express markers of skeletal muscle differentiation such as myogenin or myo-D1. Glypican-3 is positive in two-third of cases,[21,22] but more specific markers of hepatic differentiation are negative, including HePar1 and Arginase. Other markers such as S-100, NSE, synaptophysin, SMA, CD34, and CD99 can show variable nonspecific immunostaining.

Molecular and other special techniques

The vast majority of malignant rhabdoid tumors are characterized by loss of function mutations affecting the *SMARCB1/INI-1* gene on chromosome 22. Approximately 15% to 20% of all rhabdoid tumors have an underlying germ line *SMARCB1* mutation, and other members of the patient's family are at risk for developing malignancies.[23]

Differential diagnosis

A subset of small cell undifferentiated hepatoblastomas has been reported to show loss of nuclear INI-1 expression, similar to malignant rhabdoid tumors, posing a classification challenge. Adequate sampling is critical in making the appropriate diagnosis. Typical rhabdoid morphology favors malignant rhabdoid tumors. The identification of other fetal or embryonal patterns indicates a hepatoblastoma. Markers of hepatic differentiation (hepar-1 and Arginase) are helpful when positive, but are not informative when negative because both small cell undifferentiated hepatoblastomas and malignant rhabdoid tumors are negative. Glypican-3 staining is also noninformative, as it can be positive or negative in both tumors.

Depending on the morphology, other differential considerations can include tumors with "small round blue cell" morphology, such as lymphoma, Ewing sarcoma/primitive neuroectodermal tumors, and rhabdomyosarcomas. A diagnostic workup in a particular case can include stains to evaluate for these possibilities, including CD45/CD20 (lymphoma), CD99/FLI-1 (Ewing sarcoma/primitive neuroectodermal tumors), myogenin/Myo-D1 (rhabdomyosarcomas), and INI-1.

Prognosis and treatment

Malignant rhabdoid tumors have an aggressive clinical course with a poor prognosis. The overall median survival is 1.5 months, with a range of 2 days to 18 months.[24] Complete surgical resection is performed when possible, followed by chemotherapy. The most commonly used chemotherapeutic agents are doxorubicin, vincristine, etoposide, cisplatin, carboplatin, ifosfamide, and cyclophosphamide.[19,24] The most common metastatic sites are the lungs (65% of cases), lymph nodes (35%), and the central nervous system (10%).[24]

25.3 CALCIFYING NESTED STROMAL-EPITHELIAL TUMOR

Definition

Calcifying nested stromal-epithelial tumors are extremely rare primary liver neoplasms that are characterized by nests of epithelial cells associated with a desmoplastic stromal component. The tumors often show ossification and calcification.

Clinical features

In one large series, the age at presentation ranged from 2 to 33 years with a median age of 20 years.[25] Most cases occur in female patients. The tumor is an incidental finding in the majority of patients.[25,26] Calcifying nested stromal-epithelial tumors can mimic other neoplasms on imaging, for example, resembling calcified hemangiomas.[25] Several case series have reported an association with a paraneoplastic Cushing syndrome,[25,26] In addition, there are cases of calcifying nested stromal-epithelial tumors associated with Wilm tumor[26] and with the Beckwith–Wiedemann syndrome.[27] There are no specific serum markers for calcifying nested stromal-epithelial tumors, but adrenocorticotropic hormone levels are elevated in some individuals. Serum AFP levels are not elevated.

Gross findings

Tumors are well circumscribed and most occur as isolated nodules, ranging in size from 4 to 30 cm.[26] The tumors usually have a multilobulated, pale, yellow appearance on cut surface, sometimes with cystic and calcified areas.

Microscopic findings

Calcifying nested stromal-epithelial tumors are composed of well-demarcated nests of bland-appearing epithelial cells with a surrounding cuff of desmoplastic stroma (Fig. 25.17). The epithelial component shows round to elongated cells with relatively mild cytological atypia (Fig. 25.18). The cells are rather nondescript, with no clear line of differentiation on hematoxylin and eosin. They do not particularly look like hepatocytes and there is no gland formation or trabecular architecture.

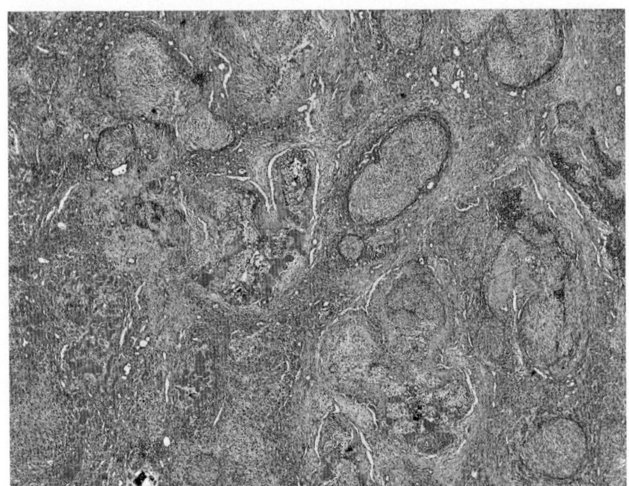

Figure 25.17 Calcifying nested stromal-epithelial tumor. Well-demarcated epithelial nests with desmoplastic stroma.

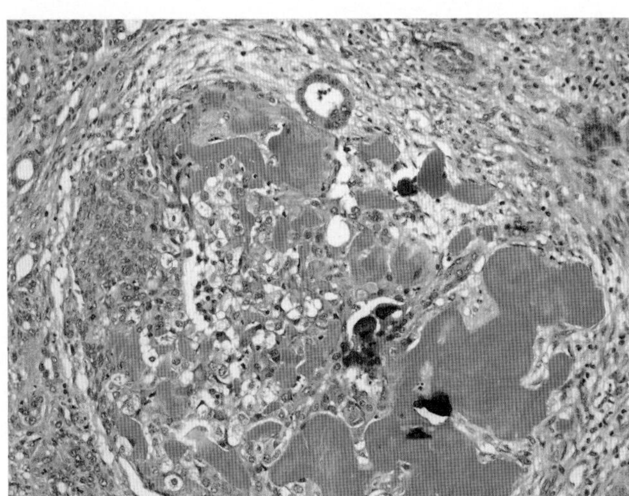

Figure 25.19 Calcifying nested stromal-epithelial tumor. Osteoid formation with calcifications.

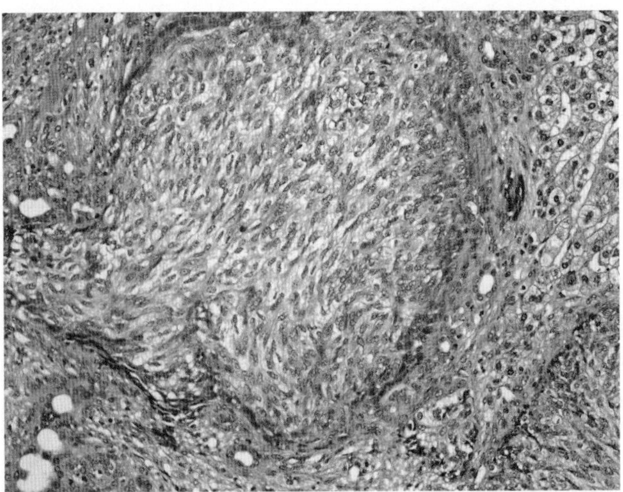

Figure 25.18 Calcifying nested stromal-epithelial tumor. The epithelial cells are round to elongated with clear cytoplasm.

The mitotic activity ranges from 1 to 5/per 10 high-power fields.[25] The reactive stromal component has a variegated appearance with densely fibrous and collagenized stroma in the center of the lesion, whereas the stroma is more loose and myxoid at the periphery of the lesion. Areas of osteoid formation and calcification (Fig. 25.19), often psammomatous, are noted and can be focal or extensive. Additional histologic features include osteoid-like material, necrosis, and cystic degeneration. At the edges, the tumor infiltrates into the surrounding hepatic parenchyma. Rarely, vascular invasion can be seen.[25]

Immunohistochemical findings

The epithelial component is positive for keratins, including AE1/AE3, CAM5.2, CK7, CK8, and CK19. The epithelial cells show nuclear positivity for β-catenin on immunostain.[28] The tumor cells are also positive for vimentin, NSE, and WT1. Markers of hepatic differentiation, including hapar-1, Arginase, and Albumin in situ hybridization are negative.[25,26] Synaptophysin, chromogranin, ER, AFP, and S-100 immunostains are negative.

Prognosis and treatment

The treatment is complete surgical resection when possible. The overall prognosis is favorable after complete resection. However, a few cases have reported recurrences, lymph node metastases, lung metastases, and even death.[29–31] Factors associated with recurrence include large tumor size, vascular invasion, necrosis, and elevated mitotic activity.[25]

25.4 PEDIATRIC HEPATOCELLULAR CARCINOMA

Hepatocellular carcinoma is rare in the pediatric population and accounts for <1% of all hepatocellular carcinoma cases.[32] Pediatric hepatocellular carcinoma can be *de novo*, with no underlying liver disease, or can arise in the setting of chronic liver disease, with or without cirrhosis.[32,33] The most common underlying chronic liver diseases include biliary atresia, chronic hepatitis B infection, bile acid synthesis/transport defects such as MDR3 deficiency, glycogen storage disease, and hereditary tyrosinemia.[34–37]

The morphologic features and immunohistochemical profile of hepatocellular carcinoma in children are essentially the same as observed in adult hepatocellular carcinoma. In one study,[38] the vast majority of pediatric cases were conventional hepatocellular carcinomas (74.7%), followed by fibrolamellar carcinoma (24.1%) and clear cell hepatocellular carcinoma (1.2%).

The main differential diagnosis is the fetal type hepatoblastoma. Clinical findings can be helpful, including the age of the patient and serum AFP levels. Serum AFP levels can be elevated in either hepatoblastoma or hepatocellular carcinoma. Normal or borderline elevation of serum AFP levels in a tumor with obvious hepatocellular differentiation strongly favors hepatocellular carcinoma. Patients with hepatoblastoma usually present with very high serum AFP levels, with the exception of those with predominately small cell undifferentiated morphology, which is unlikely to be confused with conventional hepatocellular carcinoma. Primary hepatic malignant tumors in children <3 years of age are mostly hepatoblastomas. Primary hepatic malignant tumors in children >5 years of age are almost all hepatocellular carcinomas. The finding of background liver disease or cirrhosis is a very helpful feature that strongly favors hepatocellular carcinoma.

25.5 PEDIATRIC HEPATOCELLULAR ADENOMAS

Hepatocellular adenoma is a benign primary hepatic neoplasm. Hepatocellular adenomas are extremely rare in childhood. One large series of pediatric tumors reported only 22 hepatocellular adenomas in a period of 12 years.[39] Most pediatric hepatocellular adenomas are diagnosed in late childhood (mean age of presentation is 14 years). In contrast to adult hepatocellular adenomas, which are more common in women, there is no sex predilection in pediatric hepatocellular adenomas. Pediatric hepatocellular adenomas are more frequently associated with predisposing factors such as glycogen storage diseases Type I, Type III, and less commonly Type VI.[40–42] Other factors associated with pediatric hepatocellular adenomas are anabolic androgenic steroid treatments, congenital or surgical portosystemic shunt,[43] germline mutations of the *HNF1*-α gene, and familial adenomatosis polyposis.[44] Rarely, hepatocellular adenomas arise without known predisposing factors. The morphologic characteristics and subclassification approach for pediatric hepatocellular adenomas are the same as that for adult tumors.

25.6 PEDIATRIC FOCAL NODULAR HYPERPLASIA

Focal nodular hyperplasia is nonneoplastic benign proliferation of mature hepatocytes secondary to vascular abnormalities. Focal nodular hyperplasia is very rare in the pediatric population. There have been about 200 cases reported in literature as case reports and small case series.[39,45,46] Focal nodular hyperplasia has been reported in all age groups, including prenatal and neonatal cases, though most of these cases were classified as telangiectatic focal nodular hyperplasia and it is not clear if some would be now classified as inflammatory type hepatocellular adenomas.[47,48] Some common predisposing factors are biliary atresia, chemotherapy, and radiotherapy in patients with known malignancies, and portal vascular flow impairments in congenital and surgical portosystemic shunts. Focal nodular hyperplasia can be multifocal, especially when arising in a setting of prior chemotherapy.[45] Focal nodular hyperplasia is more frequently symptomatic in children than it is in adults. Symptoms include abdominal pain and rarely weight loss and weakness. The morphologic findings and immunostain results are the same in pediatric cases as they are in adult cases.

25.7 INFANTILE HEMANGIOMA

Definition

Infantile hemangioma is a benign vascular neoplasm of the pediatric liver. This tumor was formerly known as infantile hemangioendothelioma.

Clinical features

Infantile hemangioma is the most common benign liver tumor and the second most common liver tumor (after hepatoblastoma) in the pediatric population.[49] The vast majority of cases are diagnosed in children <6 months of ages and almost all cases occur before the age of 3 years.[49,50] There is a slight female predominance (2:1) and an association with numerous congenital anomalies including Beckwith–Wiedemann syndrome, hemihypertrophy, meningomyelocele, and bilateral renal agenesis.[51] Sometimes, infantile hemangiomas present with hepatomegaly, congestive heart failure, thrombocytopenia, or hemoperitoneum.[51] A subset of cases (approximately 10%) has vascular lesions involving extrahepatic sites, including skin, lungs, gastrointestinal tract, and adrenal gland.

Gross findings

Infantile hemangiomas are usually well-demarcated and nonencapsulated. The tumor can be solitary or multifocal and range in size from <1.0 to 15 cm. The cut surface is usually soft, cystic, and hemorrhagic. Solid areas, calcification, and necrosis can be seen in larger lesions.

Histologic findings

Infantile hemangioma is characterized by a proliferation of small, dilated, capillary-like vascular channels. The vascular channels are lined by single layer of bland-appearing, flat endothelial cells with no or minimal cytological atypia (Fig. 25.20). There can be increased mitotic activity (up to 15 mitoses/10 high-power fields). The presence of increased mitosis alone does not indicate malignancy. The lesion is nonencapsulated, but often shows a layer of compressed fibrous tissue at the periphery. The lesion is typically well circumscribed grossly but demonstrates infiltration into surrounding liver parenchyma histologically, often leaving remnant entrapped bile ducts. This finding should not be interpreted as evidence for malignancy. Areas of calcifications, fibrosis, infarction, and cystic degeneration are common in large tumors. Large tumors can also demonstrate central areas of larger caliber and dilated vascular channels, similar to those seen in cavernous hemangiomas.

Infantile hemangiomas can show architecturally complex solid, papillary, and kaposiform-like growth as well as striking cytological atypia (Figs. 25.21 and 25.22). These areas are classified as foci of malignant transformation. Therefore, adequate tumor sampling in resection specimen is very important to identify focal malignant transformation. Although the data are limited, case reports and small series have demonstrated a low but clear risk for aggressive behavior in tumors with foci of malignant transformation. Although the clinical outcome in most cases is similar regardless of the presence or absence of foci of malignant transformation, almost all tumors with aggressive behavior have areas malignant transformation. Tumor recurrence is more common than metastases.

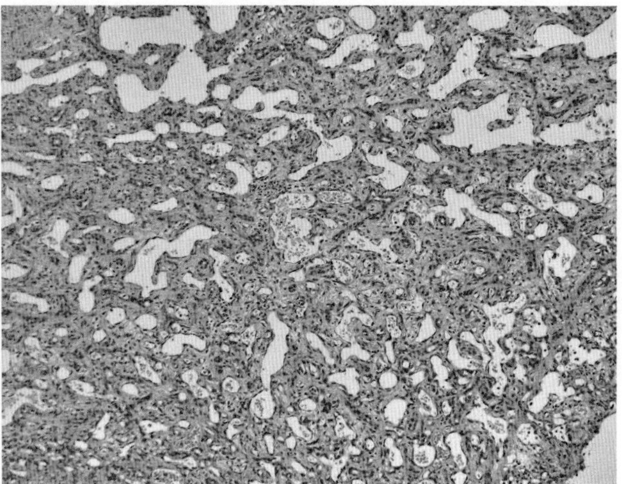

Figure 25.20 Infantile hemangioma. Vascular channels lined by single layer flat endothelial cells.

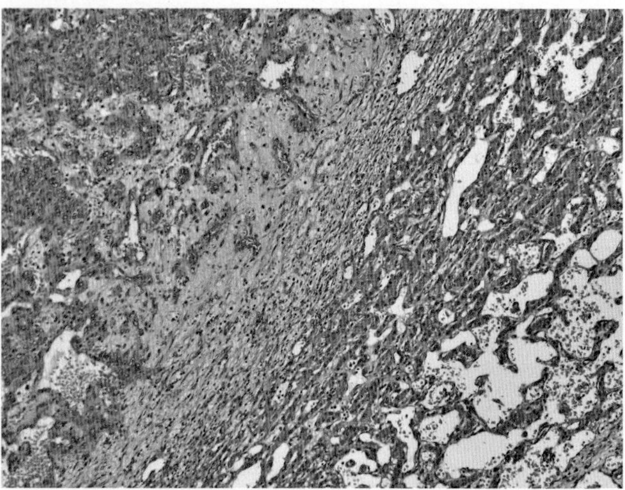

Figure 25.21 Infantile hemangioma with malignant transformation. This infantile hemangioma shows more complex solid growth, seen on the upper left of the image.

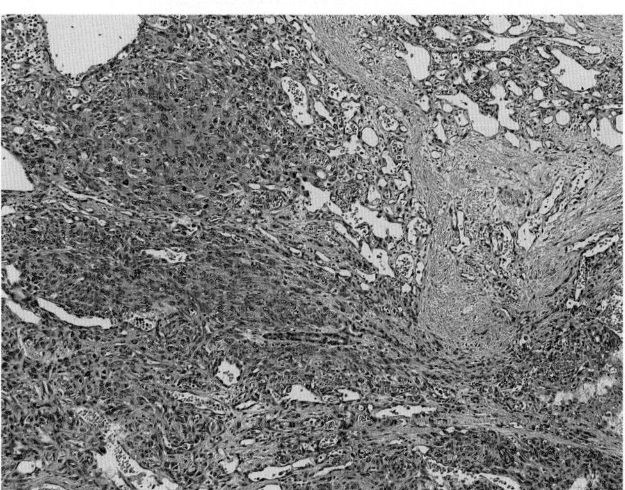

Figure 25.22 Infantile hemangioma with malignant transformation. Another example of a foci of malignant transformation.

Immunohistochemical findings

The tumor is positive for vascular markers including CD31, CD34, von Willebrand factor, ERG, and FLI1. Infantile hemangiomas are also positive for GLUT1.[52]

Differential diagnosis

The main differential diagnoses are hepatic vascular malformations and angiosarcomas.

Infantile hemangiomas and hepatic vascular malformations may have overlapping clinical features because children with hepatic vascular malformations can present with abdominal masses, cardiomegaly, anemia, and congestive heart failure. Imaging of hepatic vascular malformations typically shows a single large mass with extensive central hemorrhage, calcification, and large vascular shunts. Histologic evaluation reveals a mixture of abnormal thin walled and large tortuous blood vessels associated with reactive fibrovascular stroma and areas of hemorrhagic infarction. Hepatic vascular malformation can have some areas with prominent capillary proliferation, mimicking infantile hemangioma. GLUT-1 immunostains can be helpful because they are negative in vascular malformations but positive in infantile hemangiomas.[52] Angiosarcomas are very rare in children. Overall, angiosarcomas typically affect older children than infantile hemangiomas and are characterized by infiltrative growth, architectural complexity, unequivocal cytological atypia, and necrosis.

Prognosis and treatment

Some infantile hemangiomas regress spontaneously in months or years. Other cases are treated with corticosteroids or α interferons. Cases failing to respond to these modalities undergo surgical wedge resection or arterial embolization or rarely transplantation.

25.8 MESENCHYMAL HAMARTOMA

Definition

Mesenchymal hamartomas are benign neoplasms composed of various tissue types found in the normal liver, including loose mesenchymal tissue, bile ducts, and small islands or cords of hepatocytes. The hepatocytes and bile ducts are entrapped and not neoplastic.

Clinical findings

Mesenchymal hamartomas present before the age of 3 years in 85% of cases,[53] but can rarely first present in adult years.[54] Rare cases have been detected in utero by prenatal ultrasound. There is a slight male predominance. The presenting signs and symptoms are nonspecific, but often include painless but progressive abdominal distension. Of note, serum AFP levels are elevated in up 40% of cases,[55] which can lead to clinical concern for hepatoblastoma or hepatocellular carcinoma.

The etiology of mesenchymal hamartoma is uncertain, but multiple case reports have described an association with placental mesenchymal dysplasia,[56–58] the latter being a hydropic change in placental villi that resembles the findings in a partial mole, but has no chromosomal abnormalities. Mesenchymal hamartomas historically were thought to be developmental abnormalities, thus termed as hamartoma, but recent molecular findings have shown somatic chromosomal translocations involving chromosome 19, indicating the tumor is neoplastic. The translocation is not found in the entrapped bile ducts and hepatocytes.[59]

Gross findings

Mesenchymal hamartomas are single tumors in most cases (90%). Most tumors (75%) arise in the right lobe[53] and about 20% are pedunculated.[53] On gross examination, mesenchymal hamartomas are well-demarcated and usually unencapsulated tumors. The tumors are composed of solid and cystic spaces, with some tumors being predominately solid, while others are largely cystic. The cystic spaces lack communication with the bile ducts. They range in size from microscopic to very large, including reports of cystic spaces measuring 30 cm in diameter. The cystic spaces contain clear fluid or gelatinous material. Foci of necrosis or hemorrhage or foci of grossly distinct subnodules are generally not seen in typical mesenchymal hamartomas and should be carefully sampled to rule out malignant transformation.

Microscopic findings

Most tumors are composed primarily of loose mesenchyme tissue that is typically edematous and paucicellular, containing only scattered cytologically bland spindle cells (Fig. 25.23). The background matrix can be either myxoid or densely collagenized, the latter being more common in cases in older children or adults.[54] When the mesenchymal tissue is loose and edematous, variably sized cystic spaces are seen

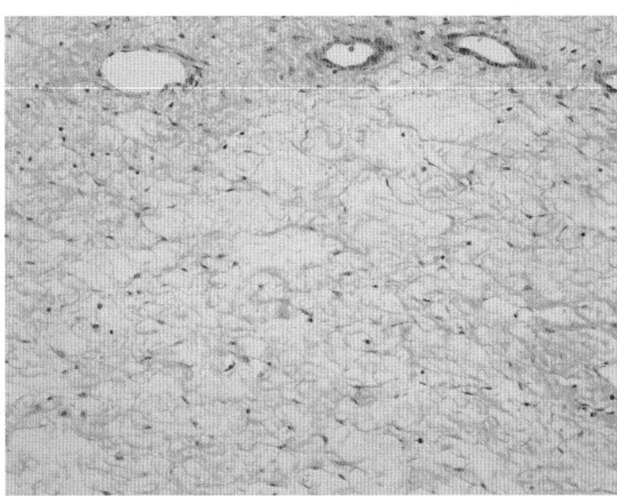

Figure 25.23 Mesenchymal hamartoma. The tumor is composed of cytologically bland spindle cells in a background of loose edematous connective tissue.

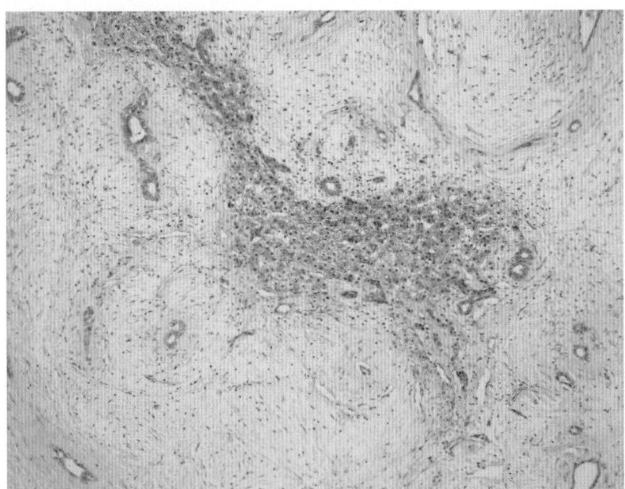

Figure 25.24 Mesenchymal hamartoma. A small island of benign hepatocytes is seen.

and represent a reactive/degenerative change. These spaces are not lined by epithelium, so are not true cysts. Extramedullary hematopoiesis is common in pediatric cases, less so in adult tumors.[54]

Clusters of hepatocytes can be found scattered within the mesenchymal background (Fig. 25.24). The hepatocytes are cytological bland and mature appearing, growing in small islands or cords. Somewhat disorganized clusters of bile ducts and blood vessels can also be found. In some cases, the biliary structures can resemble a ductal plate malformation. Small, simple biliary cysts can also develop. Rare cases have been reported with both mesenchymal hamartoma and infantile hemangioma components[60,61] or with prominent myoid differentiation within the mesenchymal hamartoma.[62]

Immunohistochemical findings

The mesenchymal cells are vimentin positive and show variable staining for smooth muscle actin and desmin.[63,64] The entrapped hepatocytes stain with HepPar and Arginase, as well as glypican-3.[65] In this setting, glypican-3 staining does not suggest malignancy. Also of note, the hepatic islands and bile ducts can sometimes be positive for AFP, but this also does not indicate malignancy. The bile duct epithelium shows a typical staining profile, being positive for CK7 and CK19.

Prognosis and treatment

Mesenchymal hamartomas are treated by surgical resection. The overall survival rate is approximately 90%. The tumors do not recur after resection, but rare cases can undergo malignant transformation to embryonal sarcoma, and the embryonal sarcoma component can recur and/or metastasize.

25.9 EMBRYONAL SARCOMA

Definition

Embryonal sarcomas are undifferentiated sarcomas seen most commonly in the pediatric population. In the literature, other terms used for this entity include "undifferentiated embryonal sarcoma" or "hepatic undifferentiated sarcoma."

Clinical findings

The median age at presentation is around 9 years,[66,67] but embryonal sarcomas can also present in adults. Although data are limited, the adult cases appear to have different underlying genetic changes than pediatric cases.[59] The male to female ratio is about equal.[67] The etiology for embryonal sarcoma is unknown, but a proportion of them develop from malignant transformation of mesenchymal hamartomas.[68] A large number of cases are misdiagnosed clinically and radiologically prior to resection or biopsy, being mistaken for hepatocellular carcinomas or hepatoblastomas.[69] Metastatic disease is found in 15% of individuals at presentation.[67]

Gross findings

Embryonal sarcomas have a median size of 14 cm,[67] but can range from a few centimeter to 25 plus centimeters. The tumors are soft, white-tan (Fig. 25.25), and often cystic, with cyst-like areas containing a thick myxoid material that can be brown from remote hemorrhage. The tumors can show partial or rarely complete capsules.[69]

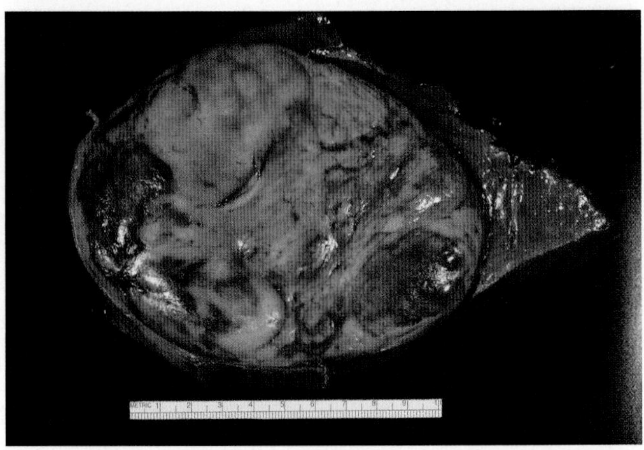

Figure 25.25 Embyronal sarcoma. The tumor is soft and white with areas of hemorrhage at the periphery.

Histological findings

Embryonal sarcomas are composed of undifferentiated spindled cells that are medium to large in size and show striking and diffuse cytological atypia (Fig. 25.26). Foci of giant cell transformation are common (Fig. 25.27). Hyaline globules can be found in some tumor cells and sometimes outside of tumor cells in the stroma, but are not necessary for the diagnosis and can be lacking. Also of note, hyaline globules are not specific for embryonal sarcoma, being found in a number of other sarcomas and carcinomas. The tumor cellularity in embryonal sarcoma varies and in some cases the malignant cells can be less prominent than the background stroma. The stroma can range from loose and myxoid tissue to more densely fibrotic tissue. Cystic degeneration is also common and in some cases can dominate the radiological and gross findings.[70,71]

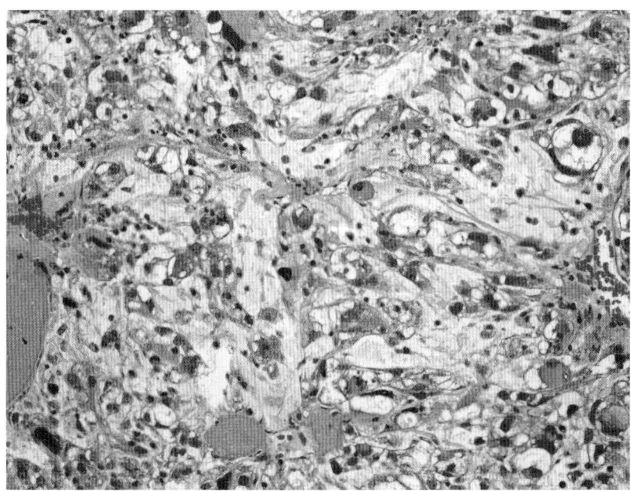

Figure 25.26 Undifferentiated embryonal sarcoma. The tumor shows diffuse striking anaplasia.

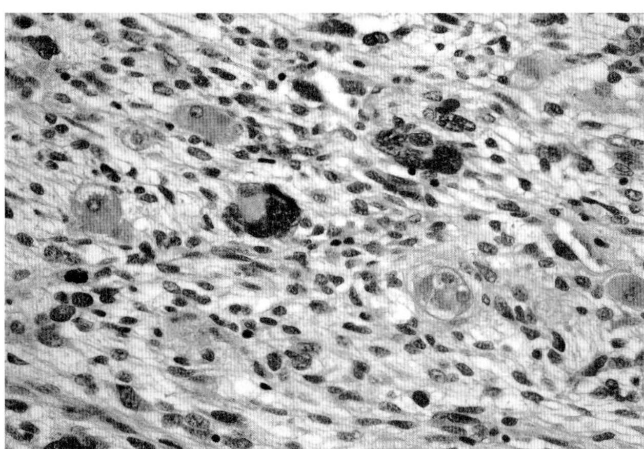

Figure 25.27 Undifferentiated embryonal sarcoma. Scattered tumor giant cells are seen.

Immunohistochemical findings

There is no distinct immunostain profile for embryonal sarcoma, and stains are not needed to make the diagnosis, but can be helpful to rule out other potential entities in the differential. Negative stains include myogenin,[66,72] myoglobin (focal positivity in rare cases), smooth muscle myosin, h-caldesmon, CD34 (focal positivity in rare cases), CD31, Alk-1, S-100 (focal positivity in rare cases), HMB45, KIT, Arginase, and HepPar1.[72,73]

There are many stains that can be positive, but none are diagnostic. Vimentin and CD68 are routinely positive in the malignant cells.[73,74] Desmin and smooth muscle actin stains are positive in 30% to 50% of cases, usually with a patchy staining pattern.[72,73,75] Membranous CD56 and CD10 staining has also been reported,[76] as has glypican-3.[65] Other stains that can be positive include α-1 antitrypsin, α-1 antichymotrypsin, BCL2, CD68, and P53.[69,72,73] A PAS-D stain can be used to highlight the globules because they are diastase resistant. As a potential diagnostic pitfall, embryonal sarcomas can be positive for a variety of different keratins including cytokeratin AE1/AE3 and Cam5.2.[72,73,76] In most cases, the keratin staining tends to be patchy. A perinuclear dot-like positivity for the keratins has also been reported.[76]

Differential diagnosis

In the pediatric population, biliary tract rhabdomyosarcoma is the primary consideration. Biliary tract rhabdomyosarcomas are positive for myogenin and MyoD1, while embryonal sarcomas are negative.[66] Metastatic sarcomas should be ruled out especially in the adult population.

Prognosis and treatment

Surgical resection when possible is the mainstay of treatment, typically supplemented with chemotherapy. The overall 5-year survival in the largest study to date, with 103 patients, was 86%.[67]

REFERENCES

1. Lack EE, Neave C, Vawter GF. Hepatoblastoma. A clinical and pathologic study of 54 cases. *Am J Surg Pathol*. 1982;6:693–705.
2. Darbari A, Sabin KM, Shapiro CN, et al. Epidemiology of primary hepatic malignancies in U.S. children. *Hepatology*. 2003;38:560–566.
3. Eren E, Demirkaya M, Cakir ED, et al. A rare cause of precocious puberty: hepatoblastoma. *J Clin Res Pediatr Endocrinol*. 2009;1:281–283.

4. Giardiello FM, Petersen GM, Brensinger JD, et al. Hepatoblastoma and APC gene mutation in familial adenomatous polyposis. *Gut*. 1996;39:867–869.
5. DeBaun MR, Tucker MA. Risk of cancer during the first four years of life in children from The Beckwith-Wiedemann Syndrome Registry. *J Pediatr*. 1998;132:398–400.
6. Unal E, Koksal Y, Akcoren Z, et al. Mesenchymal hamartoma of the liver mimicking hepatoblastoma. *J Pediatr Hematol Oncol*. 2008;30:458–460.
7. De Ioris M, Brugieres L, Zimmermann A, et al. Hepatoblastoma with a low serum alpha-fetoprotein level at diagnosis: the SIOPEL group experience. *Eur J Cancer*. 2008;44:545–550.
8. Lopez-Terrada D, Alaggio R, de Davila MT, et al. Towards an international pediatric liver tumor consensus classification: proceedings of the Los Angeles COG liver tumors symposium. *Mod Pathol*. 2014;27:472–491.
9. Trobaugh-Lotrario AD, Tomlinson GE, Finegold MJ, et al. Small cell undifferentiated variant of hepatoblastoma: adverse clinical and molecular features similar to rhabdoid tumors. *Pediatr Blood Cancer*. 2009;52:328–334.
10. Brown J, Perilongo G, Shafford E, et al. Pretreatment prognostic factors for children with hepatoblastoma--results from the International Society of Paediatric Oncology (SIOP) study SIOPEL 1. *Eur J Cancer*. 2000;36:1418–1425.
11. Feusner JH, Krailo MD, Haas JE, et al. Treatment of pulmonary metastases of initial stage I hepatoblastoma in childhood. Report from the Childrens Cancer Group. *Cancer*. 1993;71: 859–864.
12. Endo EG, Walton DS, Albert DM. Neonatal hepatoblastoma metastatic to the choroid and iris. *Arch Ophthalmol*. 1996;114:757–761.
13. Hishiki T, Matsunaga T, Sasaki F, et al. Outcome of hepatoblastomas treated using the Japanese Study Group for Pediatric Liver Tumor (JPLT) protocol-2: report from the JPLT. *Pediatr Surg Int*. 2011;27:1–8.
14. Semeraro M, Branchereau S, Maibach R, et al. Relapses in hepatoblastoma patients: clinical characteristics and outcome--experience of the International Childhood Liver Tumour Strategy Group (SIOPEL). *Eur J Cancer*. 2013;49:915–922.
15. Maibach R, Roebuck D, Brugieres L, et al. Prognostic stratification for children with hepatoblastoma: the SIOPEL experience. *Eur J Cancer*. 2012;48:1543–1549.
16. Fuchs J, Rydzynski J, Von Schweinitz D, et al. Pretreatment prognostic factors and treatment results in children with hepatoblastoma: a report from the German Cooperative Pediatric Liver Tumor Study HB 94. *Cancer*. 2002;95:172–182.
17. Meyers RL, Rowland JR, Krailo M, et al. Predictive power of pretreatment prognostic factors in children with hepatoblastoma: a report from the Children's Oncology Group. *Pediatr Blood Cancer*. 2009;53:1016–1022.
18. Malogolowkin MH, Katzenstein HM, Meyers RL, et al. Complete surgical resection is curative for children with hepatoblastoma with pure fetal histology: a report from the Children's Oncology Group. *J Clin Oncol*. 2011;29:3301–3306.
19. Trobaugh-Lotrario AD, Finegold MJ, Feusner JH. Rhabdoid tumors of the liver: rare, aggressive, and poorly responsive to standard cytotoxic chemotherapy. *Pediatr Blood Cancer*. 2011;57:423–428.
20. Kachanov D, Teleshova M, Kim E, et al. Malignant rhabdoid tumor of the liver presented with initial tumor rupture. *Cancer Genet*. 2014;207:412–414.
21. Chan ES, Pawel BR, Corao DA, et al. Immunohistochemical expression of glypican-3 in pediatric tumors: an analysis of 414 cases. *Pediatr Dev Pathol*. 2013;16:272–277.
22. Kohashi K, Nakatsura T, Kinoshita Y, et al. Glypican 3 expression in tumors with loss of SMARCB1/INI1 protein expression. *Hum Pathol*. 2013;44:526–533.
23. Eaton KW, Tooke LS, Wainwright LM, et al. Spectrum of SMARCB1/INI1 mutations in familial and sporadic rhabdoid tumors. *Pediatr Blood Cancer*. 2011;56:7–15.
24. Oita S, Terui K, Komatsu S, et al. Malignant rhabdoid tumor of the liver: a case report and literature review. *Pediatr Rep*. 2015;7:5578.
25. Makhlouf HR, Abdul-Al HM, Wang G, et al. Calcifying nested stromal-epithelial tumors of the liver: a clinicopathologic, immunohistochemical, and molecular genetic study of 9 cases with a long-term follow-up. *Am J Surg Pathol*. 2009;33:976–983.
26. Heerema-McKenney A, Leuschner I, Smith N, et al. Nested stromal epithelial tumor of the liver: six cases of a distinctive pediatric neoplasm with frequent calcifications and association with cushing syndrome. *Am J Surg Pathol*. 2005;29:10–20.
27. Malowany JI, Merritt NH, Chan NG, et al. Nested stromal epithelial tumor of the liver in Beckwith-Wiedemann syndrome. *Pediatr Dev Pathol*. 2013;16:312–317.
28. Assmann G, Kappler R, Zeindl-Eberhart E, et al. beta-Catenin mutations in 2 nested stromal epithelial tumors of the liver: a neoplasia with defective mesenchymal-epithelial transition. *Hum Pathol*. 2012;43:1815–1827.
29. Brodsky SV, Sandoval C, Sharma N, et al. Recurrent nested stromal epithelial tumor of the liver with extrahepatic metastasis: case report and review of literature. *Pediatr Dev Pathol*. 2008;11:469–473.
30. Hommann M, Kaemmerer D, Daffner W, et al. Nested stromal epithelial tumor of the liver: liver

transplantation and follow-up. *J Gastrointest Cancer*. 2011;42:292–295.

31. Heywood G, Burgart LJ, Nagorney DM. Ossifying malignant mixed epithelial and stromal tumor of the liver: a case report of a previously undescribed tumor. *Cancer*. 2002;94:1018-22.
32. Emre S, McKenna GJ. Liver tumors in children. *Pediatr Transplant*. 2004;8:632–638.
33. Czauderna P, Mackinlay G, Perilongo G, et al. Hepatocellular carcinoma in children: results of the first prospective study of the International Society of Pediatric Oncology group. *J Clin Oncol*. 2002;20:2798–2804.
34. Zhang XF, Liu XM, Wei T, et al. Clinical characteristics and outcome of hepatocellular carcinoma in children and adolescents. *Pediatr Surg Int*. 2013;29:763–770.
35. Vij M, Safwan M, Shanmugam NP, et al. Liver pathology in severe multidrug resistant 3 protein deficiency: a series of 10 pediatric cases. *Ann Diagn Pathol*. 2015;19(5):277–282.
36. van Ginkel WG, Gouw AS, van der Jagt EJ, et al. Hepatocellular carcinoma in tyrosinemia type 1 without clear increase of AFP. *Pediatrics*. 2015;135:e749–752.
37. Franco LM, Krishnamurthy V, Bali D, et al. Hepatocellular carcinoma in glycogen storage disease type Ia: a case series. *J Inherit Metab Dis*. 2005;28:153–162.
38. Lau CS, Mahendraraj K, Chamberlain RS. Hepatocellular carcinoma in the pediatric population: a population based clinical outcomes study involving 257 patients from the Surveillance, Epidemiology, and End Result (SEER) database (1973-2011). *HPB Surg*. 2015;2015:670728.
39. Kochin IN, Miloh TA, Arnon R, et al. Benign liver masses and lesions in children: 53 cases over 12 years. *Isr Med Assoc J*. 2011;13:542–547.
40. Labrune P, Trioche P, Duvaltier I, et al. Hepatocellular adenomas in glycogen storage disease type I and III: a series of 43 patients and review of the literature. *J Pediatr Gastroenterol Nutr*. 1997;24:276–279.
41. Alshak NS, Cocjin J, Podesta L, et al. Hepatocellular adenoma in glycogen storage disease type IV. *Arch Pathol Lab Med*. 1994;118:88–91.
42. Manzia TM, Angelico R, Toti L, et al. Glycogen storage disease type Ia and VI associated with hepatocellular carcinoma: two case reports. *Transplant Proc*. 2011;43:1181–1183.
43. Franchi-Abella S, Branchereau S, Lambert V, et al. Complications of congenital portosystemic shunts in children: therapeutic options and outcomes. *J Pediatr Gastroenterol Nutr*. 2010;51:322–330.
44. Bioulac-Sage P, Sempoux C, Possenti L, et al. Pathological diagnosis of hepatocellular cellular adenoma according to the clinical context. *Int J Hepatol*. 2013;2013:253261.
45. Bouyn CI, Leclere J, Raimondo G, et al. Hepatic focal nodular hyperplasia in children previously treated for a solid tumor. Incidence, risk factors, and outcome. *Cancer*. 2003;97:3107–3113.
46. Lautz T, Tantemsapya N, Dzakovic A, et al. Focal nodular hyperplasia in children: clinical features and current management practice. *J Pediatr Surg*. 2010;45:1797–1803.
47. Kang J, Choi HJ, Yu E, et al. A case report of fetal telangiectatic focal nodular hyperplasia. *Pediatr Dev Pathol*. 2007;10:416–417.
48. Okamura N, Nakadate H, Ishida K, et al. Telangiectatic focal nodular hyperplasia of the liver in the perinatal period: case report. *Pediatr Dev Pathol*. 2005;8:581–586.
49. Stocker JT. Hepatic tumors in children. *Clin Liver Dis*. 2001;5:259–281, viii–ix.
50. Sevinir B, Ozkan TB. Infantile hepatic hemangioendothelioma: clinical presentation and treatment. *Turk J Gastroenterol*. 2007;18:182–187.
51. Samuel M, Spitz L. Infantile hepatic hemangioendothelioma: the role of surgery. *J Pediatr Surg*. 1995;30:1425–1429.
52. Mo JQ, Dimashkieh HH, Bove KE. GLUT1 endothelial reactivity distinguishes hepatic infantile hemangioma from congenital hepatic vascular malformation with associated capillary proliferation. *Hum Pathol*. 2004;35:200–209.
53. Stringer MD, Alizai NK. Mesenchymal hamartoma of the liver: a systematic review. *J Pediatr Surg*. 2005;40:1681–1690.
54. Cook JR, Pfeifer JD, Dehner LP. Mesenchymal hamartoma of the liver in the adult: association with distinct clinical features and histological changes. *Hum Pathol*. 2002;33:893–898.
55. Chang HJ, Jin SY, Park C, et al. Mesenchymal hamartomas of the liver: comparison of clinicopathologic features between cystic and solid forms. *J Korean Med Sci*. 2006;21:63–68.
56. Francis B, Hallam L, Kecskes Z, et al. Placental mesenchymal dysplasia associated with hepatic mesenchymal hamartoma in the newborn. *Pediatr Dev Pathol*. 2007;10:50–54.
57. Mack-Detlefsen B, Boemers TM, Groneck P, et al. Multiple hepatic mesenchymal hamartomas in a premature associated with placental mesenchymal dysplasia. *J Pediatr Surg*. 2011;46:e23–25.
58. Harris K, Carreon CK, Vohra N, et al. Placental mesenchymal dysplasia with hepatic mesenchymal hamartoma: a case report and literature review. *Fetal Pediatr Pathol*. 2013;32:448–453.
59. Mathews J, Duncavage EJ, Pfeifer JD. Characterization of translocations in mesenchymal hamartoma and undifferentiated

embryonal sarcoma of the liver. *Exp Mol Pathol.* 2013;95:319–324.
60. Bejarano PA, Serrano MF, Casillas J, et al. Concurrent infantile hemangioendothelioma and mesenchymal hamartoma in a developmentally arrested liver of an infant requiring hepatic transplantation. *Pediatr Dev Pathol.* 2003;6:552–557.
61. Hsiao KH, Lin LH, Chen DF, et al. Hepatic mesenchymal hamartoma combined with infantile hepatic hemangioendothelioma in an infant. *J Formos Med Assoc.* 2007;106:S1–4.
62. Gornicka B, Ziarkiewicz-Wroblewska B, Wroblewski T, et al. Myoid hamartoma of the liver: a novel variant of hamartoma developing in the hilar region and imitating a malignant liver tumor. *Med Sci Monit.* 2004;10:CS23–CS26.
63. von Schweinitz D, Dammeier BG, Gluer S. Mesenchymal hamartoma of the liver: new insight into histogenesis. *J Pediatr Surg.* 1999;34:1269–1271.
64. Shintaku M, Watanabe K. Mesenchymal hamartoma of the liver: a proliferative lesion of possible hepatic stellate cell (Ito cell) origin. *Pathol Res Pract.* 2010;206:532–536.
65. Levy M, Trivedi A, Zhang J, et al. Expression of glypican-3 in undifferentiated embryonal sarcoma and mesenchymal hamartoma of the liver. *Hum Pathol.* 2012;43:695–701.
66. Nicol K, Savell V, Moore J, et al. Distinguishing undifferentiated embryonal sarcoma of the liver from biliary tract rhabdomyosarcoma: a Children's Oncology Group study. *Pediatr Dev Pathol.* 2007;10:89–97.
67. Shi Y, Rojas Y, Zhang W, et al. Characteristics and outcomes in children with undifferentiated embryonal sarcoma of the liver: a report from the National Cancer Database. *Pediatr Blood Cancer.* 2017;64(4):e26272.
68. Lauwers GY, Grant LD, Donnelly WH, et al. Hepatic undifferentiated (embryonal) sarcoma arising in a mesenchymal hamartoma. *Am J Surg Pathol.* 1997;21:1248–1254.
69. Li Y, Cai Q, Jia N, et al. Pre-operatively misdiagnosed undifferentiated embryonal sarcoma of the liver: analysis of 16 cases. *Ann Transl Med.* 2015;3:353.
70. Buetow PC, Buck JL, Pantongrag-Brown L, et al. Undifferentiated (embryonal) sarcoma of the liver: pathologic basis of imaging findings in 28 cases. *Radiology.* 1997;203:779–783.
71. Yoon JY, Lee JM, Kim do Y, et al. A case of embryonal sarcoma of the liver mimicking a hydatid cyst in an adult. *Gut Liver.* 2010;4:245–249.
72. Kiani B, Ferrell LD, Qualman S, et al. Immunohistochemical analysis of embryonal sarcoma of the liver. *Appl Immunohistochem Mol Morphol.* 2006;14:193–197.
73. Zheng JM, Tao X, Xu AM, et al. Primary and recurrent embryonal sarcoma of the liver: clinicopathological and immunohistochemical analysis. *Histopathology.* 2007;51:195–203.
74. Nishio J, Iwasaki H, Sakashita N, et al. Undifferentiated (embryonal) sarcoma of the liver in middle-aged adults: smooth muscle differentiation determined by immunohistochemistry and electron microscopy. *Hum Pathol.* 2003;34:246–252.
75. Lepreux S, Rebouissou S, Le Bail B, et al. Mutation of TP53 gene is involved in carcinogenesis of hepatic undifferentiated (embryonal) sarcoma of the adult, in contrast with Wnt or telomerase pathways: an immunohistochemical study of three cases with genomic relation in two cases. *J Hepatol.* 2005;42:424–429.
76. Perez-Gomez RM, Soria-Cespedes D, de Leon-Bojorge B, et al. Diffuse membranous immunoreactivity of CD56 and paranuclear dot-like staining pattern of cytokeratins AE1/3, CAM5.2, and OSCAR in undifferentiated (embryonal) sarcoma of the liver. *Appl Immunohistochem Mol Morphol.* 2010;18:195–198.

26 Benign and malignant mesenchymal tumors of the liver

Rondell P. Graham, MBBS, Andrew L. Folpe, MD

26.1 INTRODUCTION

Mesenchymal tumors of the liver can be challenging because they are not common in clinical practice. In this chapter, we will provide our general approach to the diagnosis of mesenchymal tumors of the liver. Then, we will delve into the characteristics of the most frequent primary neoplasms, describe how to distinguish them from mimics, and highlight ancillary tests which allow confirmation of specific diagnoses.

26.2 THE DIAGNOSTIC APPROACH

As in other anatomic sites, mesenchymal tumors of the liver are much less common than epithelial tumors. Therefore, it is prudent to exclude a nonmesenchymal tumor (e.g., carcinoma, melanoma, and lymphoma) before making the diagnosis of a mesenchymal tumor. The liver provides an added layer of challenge in that metastases significantly outnumber primary tumors. These considerations should be borne in mind when faced with a liver mass, particularly in a liver without cirrhosis. It is useful to note the patient's age and gender, an antecedent history of carcinoma, melanoma, or other tumors, and their primary site, histologic grade or type and the temporal relationship to the current liver mass(es). Where applicable, review of the slides from the original tumor may be helpful in confirming or excluding a metastasis. The presence of multiple liver masses favors metastasis, but there are many exceptions. Correlation with radiologic imaging may be of value, especially for small biopsies.

As always, a systematic approach to the histology is best. We recommend initial review of the liver mass to determine the growth pattern, circumscription and cellular composition of the tumor, and the presence or absence of a matrix. When immunostains are performed, they are often best done in panels, which not only support the primary diagnosis under consideration but also exclude other entities in the differential diagnosis. Table 26.1 presents an initial panel of immunostains which the authors find helpful in a number of common scenarios where mesenchymal tumors come in to consideration.

Table 26.1 Initial immunostain panels for select morphologic scenarios and the differential diagnoses for which they provide support

Morphologic scenario	Select differential diagnoses	Initial immunostain panel
Spindle cell neoplasm without specific features	Sarcomatoid carcinoma, malignant melanoma, GIST, smooth muscle tumor, myofibroblastic tumor	OSCAR cytokeratin, KIT, DOG1, S100, HMB45, SMA
Epithelioid neoplasm negative for cytokeratins	Malignant melanoma, GIST, rhabdomyosarcoma, angiosarcoma, histiocytic neoplasm	S100, HMB45, SOX10, KIT, ERG/FLI1, CD163, Desmin
Plasmacytoid neoplasm	Carcinoma, GIST, neuroendocrine tumor, acinar cell carcinoma, malignant melanoma, rhabdomyosarcoma, plasma cell neoplasm	OSCAR cytokeratin, trypsin, chromogranin, synaptophysin, S100, SOX10, Desmin, MUM1
Poorly differentiated neoplasm or small round blue cell tumor	High-grade carcinoma, malignant melanoma, hematopoietic neoplasm, rhabdomyosarcoma, high-grade sarcoma	OSCAR cytokeratin, AE1/AE3, S100, SOX10, Desmin, SMA, CD45 TLE1—screen for synovial sarcoma CD99—screen for Ewing sarcoma

26.3 VASCULAR TUMORS

Hepatic hemangioma

Definition

Hepatic hemangioma is a benign proliferation of vascular channels lined by endothelial cells in the liver.

Etiology

The etiology of hemangiomas is unknown, although usage of steroids, female sex hormones, and pregnancy have been postulated to be related to the growth of hepatic hemangiomas.[1–3]

Clinical features

Hepatic hemangioma is the most common primary mesenchymal tumor of the liver.[4] The reported incidence ranges from 0.4% to 7.4%.[4,5] It occurs more often in women with a female-to-male ratio of about 3:1.[6] Hemangiomas are often incidentally discovered on imaging, at surgery, or at autopsy.[7] Occasional cases of massive hemangiomas or thrombosed hemangiomas can be associated with abdominal discomfort and thrombocytopenia.[4] Hemangiomas arise sporadically as solitary masses in most cases, but there can be multiple hemangiomas in rare conditions such as Von Hippel–Lindau syndrome or systemic hemangiomatosis syndromes.[8,9]

Gross findings

Hepatic hemangiomas are usually solitary, but rarely can be multiple. The sizes can range from a few millimeters to up to 30 cm. Grossly, hemangiomas appear as red-brown or red-blueish, well-demarcated lesions with a spongy cut surface (Fig. 26.1). Some long-standing cases may contain white fibrotic areas.

Microscopic findings and histological types

Hepatic hemangiomas are uniformly well-circumscribed lesions and may be of three types. The first and most common type is cavernous hemangioma. Much less common hepatic hemangiomas include capillary hemangiomas and anastomosing hemangiomas.

Cavernous hemangiomas. Cavernous hemangiomas are characterized by widely dilated vascular channels with fibrous walls lined by a single layer of flattened inconspicuous endothelial cells devoid of cytological atypia (Fig. 26.2). They are sharply demarked from the surrounding liver parenchyma on gross examination but often have an "infiltrative growth" at their edges on histology.[10] Liver acini or portal tracts are absent within the lesion. Mitotic figures are absent. The lumens of vascular channels are usually filled with blood, but recently formed thrombi or organized thrombi are often seen as well. Some cavernous hemangiomas may undergo partial or complete sclerosis and thrombosis with calcification, and these lesions are known as sclerosed hemagiomas.

The term giant cavernous hemangioma is commonly used when tumors are >4 cm or 5 cm. The giant cavernous hemangiomas have similar histologic features to smaller cavernous hemangiomas. Some giant cavernous hemangiomas can have poorly defined

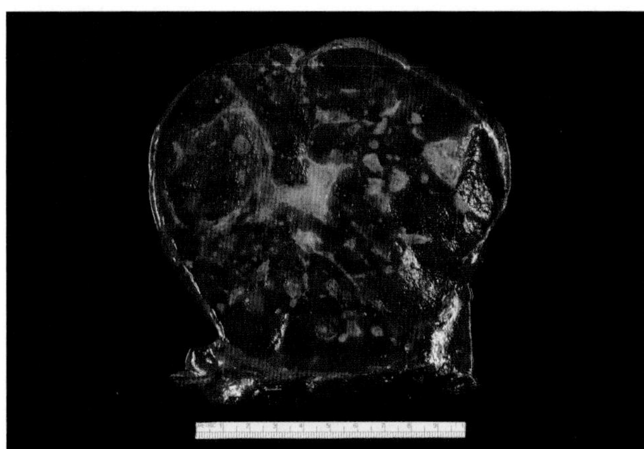

Figure 26.1 Cavernous hemangioma. The macroscopic appearance of a cavernous hemangioma. The mass displays a red-brown spongy appearance with tan branching septa corresponding to areas of sclerosis.

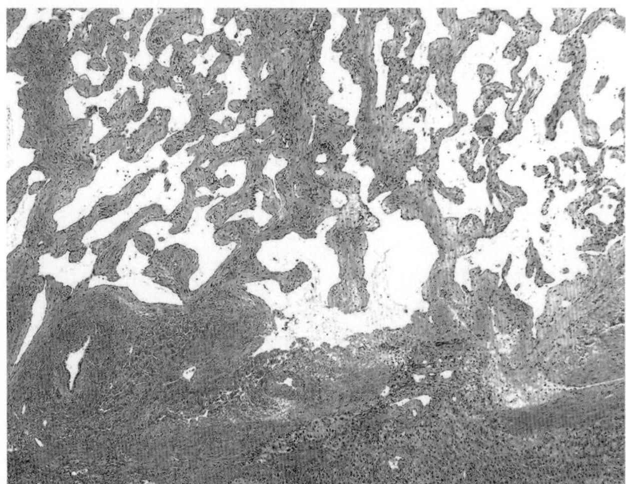

Figure 26.2 Cavernous hemangioma. This is a cavernous hemangioma composed of variably sized vascular spaces lined by attenuated endothelial cells.

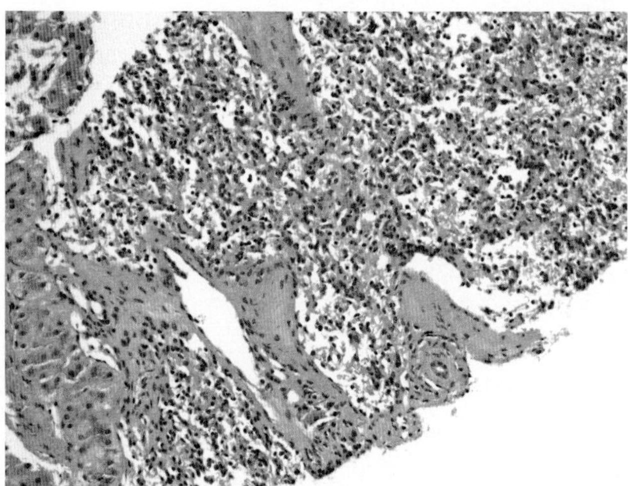

Figure 26.4 Anastomosing hemangioma. The tumor shows an interanastomosing proliferation of capillary-sized vessels. The neoplastic endothelial cells are characteristically devoid of hyperchromasia and significant nuclear atypia.

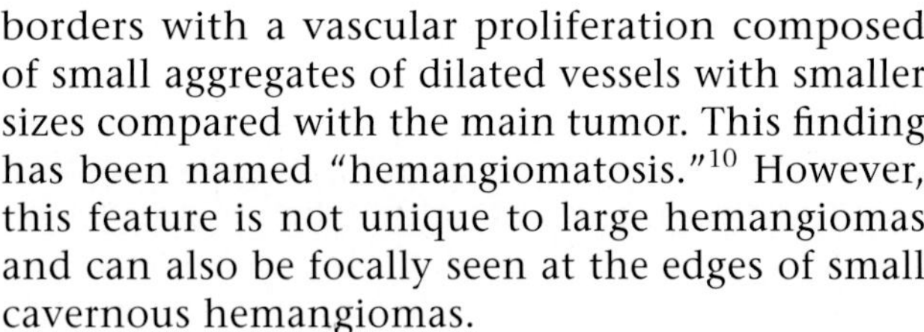

borders with a vascular proliferation composed of small aggregates of dilated vessels with smaller sizes compared with the main tumor. This finding has been named "hemangiomatosis."[10] However, this feature is not unique to large hemangiomas and can also be focally seen at the edges of small cavernous hemangiomas.

Capillary hemangioma. Capillary hemangioma is very rare in liver, with just a handful of case reports.[11] The morphology of hepatic capillary hemangioma is the same as those arising in the soft tissues. The lesion may have a fibrous capsule and consists of capillary-sized proliferating vessels arranged in a lobular configuration (Fig. 26.3). The endothelial cells are plump without atypia. Sometimes the plump cells may be confluent and obscure the vascular channels. Immunostains can be used to confirm the vascular nature of the tumor.

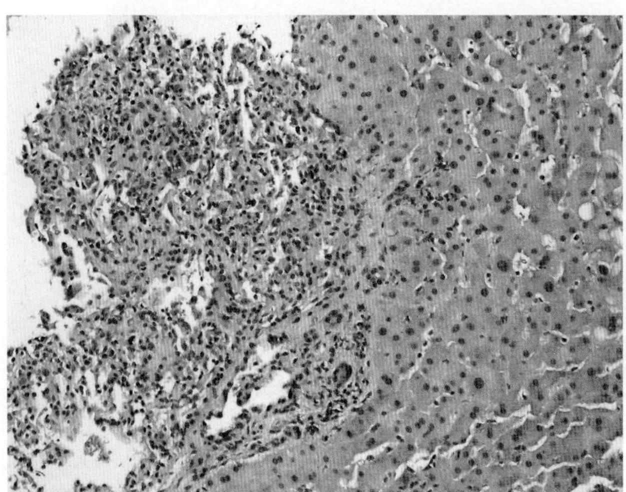

Figure 26.3 Capillary hemangioma.

Anastomosing hemangioma. Anastomosing hemangioma is a relatively rare and recently recognized variant of hepatic hemangioma, which is generally well circumscribed and is characterized by a nonlobular, interanastomosing, sinusoidal proliferation of capillary-sized vessels[12] (Fig. 26.4). The interanastomosing pattern may raise concern for well-differentiated angiosarcoma, but mitotic figures and multilayering of the neoplastic endothelial cells are absent. The endothelial cells of anastomosing hemangioma may be slightly prominent with a "hobnail" appearance, but lack nuclear hyperchromatism and irregularity. Some cases have intermixed features of conventional cavernous hemangioma. Other useful clues to the diagnosis of anastomosing hemangioma are small thrombi, mature adipose tissue, and extramedullary hematopoiesis.[12–14]

Immunohistochemical findings

Immunostains are not routinely used for diagnosing typical cases, but they may be helpful to confirm the endothelial phenotype of the lesional cells in small biopsy specimens or sclerosed hemangiomas. The endothelial cells lining hemangiomas are positive for all vascular markers, including CD31, CD34, von Willebrand factor, ERG, and FLI1.

Differential diagnosis

Hemangiomas are typically diagnosed without difficulty, except when there is extensive sclerosis of a cavernous hemangioma, mimicking a localized scar. In such cases, the presence of adjacent dilated blood vessels can be an important clue to the diagnosis of sclerotic hemangioma.

In the case of anastomosing hemangioma, distinction from angiosarcoma can be somewhat challenging on a needle biopsy due to the interconnecting vascular channels and the presence of "hobnail" endothelial cells, which can be seen in both tumors. In contrast to anastomosing hemangiomas, angiosarcomas are diffusely infiltrative, show irregularly shaped vascular lumina, multilayering of endothelial cells, mitoses, and cytological atypia. Necrosis may be seen in some angiosarcomas but is absent in anastomosing hemangioma.[12–14]

A recent study has identified a small subset of hepatic hemangiomas characterized by small vessel proliferation mimicking anastomosing hemangioma but showing some atypical features (Fig. 26.5), including subtle infiltration into hepatic sinusoids, mild cytological atypia, slightly higher Ki-67 index than cavernous hemagioma, and activating mutations in *GNAQ* and *PIK3CA*.

Prognosis and treatment

Hepatic hemangiomas are not associated with aggressive behavior or malignant transformation. Most hemangiomas are small and asymptomatic, and no treatment is required besides radiologic follow-up for 6 to 12 months after initial diagnosis. Long-term follow-up is usually not necessary unless there are risk factors, such as new onset abdominal pain and larger size (>10 cm). Surgical resection, enucleation, or minimally invasive therapies, such as arterial embolization and radiofrequency ablation, are reserved for those patients with large tumors (>10 cm) or significant symptoms.[16,17]

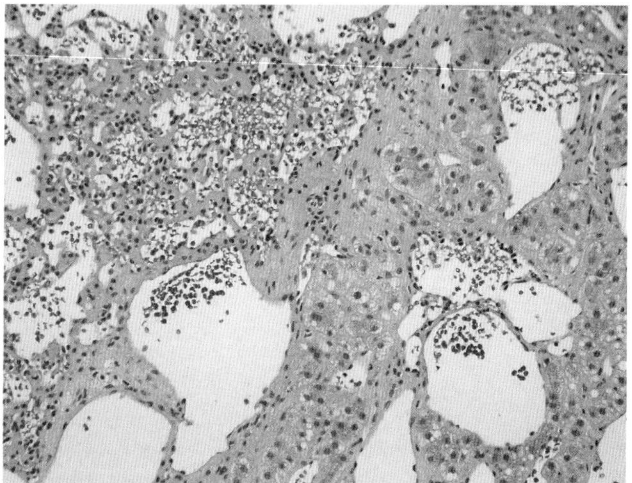

Figure 26.5 Atypical hemangioma. This lesion had some atypical features, with infiltration into hepatic sinusoids and a slightly increased Ki-67 proliferative rate.

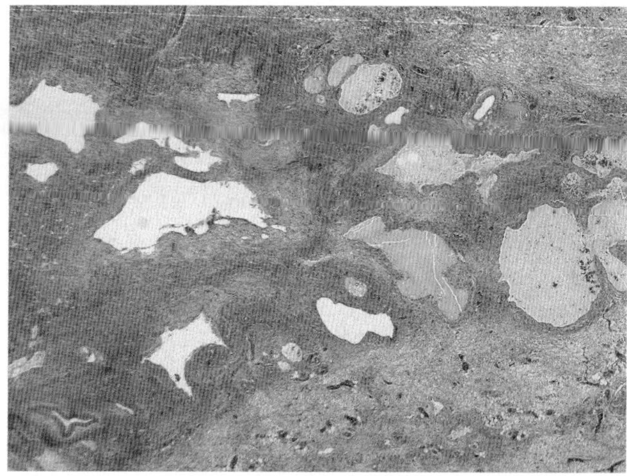

Figure 26.6 Lymphoangioma. Cystic spaces contain clear fluid and are lined by a single layer of flat endothelial cells.

Lymphangioma

Hepatic lymphangiomas are rare tumors, which are commonly associated with systemic lymphangiomatosis.[18,19] Grossly, the hepatic lymphangiomas typically present as multiple variable-sized cysts containing clear or chylous fluid. Single hepatic lymphangiomas are rare. Microscopically, the lesion is composed of variable-sized cystic spaces containing clear lymph fluid and lined by a single layer of flat endothelial cells (Fig. 26.6). The endothelial cells are bland and can have a papillary architecture in some cases. They are readily distinguished from cavernous hemangioma because of lack of red blood cells in the luminal space.

Kaposi sarcoma

Kaposi sarcoma is a low-grade malignant tumor that has a characteristic slit-like pattern of growth on histology. It is most commonly seen in AIDS patients and is uniformly associated with human herpes virus 8 (HHV-8) infection. Although Kaposi sarcoma most often affects skin and mucosal sites, liver involvement may occur in 34% of patients with Kaposi sarcoma.[20] There are four different forms of Kaposi sarcoma and all can involve liver: (1) the "classic" form typically affects elderly individuals (>60 years), mainly in the Eastern Europe and the Mediterranean region; (2) the "African endemic" form affects young adults of equatorial Africa and is characterized by localized nodular lesions; (3) the "epidemic" form occurs in patients with AIDS; and (4) the "iatrogenic" form is caused by immunosuppressive drugs administered after organ transplant and has aggressive behavior with a tendency to spread.

Microscopically, Kaposi sarcoma usually involves the portals tracts, but the tumor can infiltrate into the adjacent liver parenchyma. The lesion shows a characteristic slit-like pattern of proliferating vessels lined by spindle cells with large plump nuclei admixed with collagen fibers, extravasated red blood cells, and hemosiderin-laden macrophages. Mitotic figures are present but are low in number. Periodic acid–Schiff (PAS)-positive hyaline globules, which may represent destroyed red blood cells, are frequently found in neoplastic cells. The neoplastic cells are positive for endothelial markers including CD31, CD34, FLI-1, and ERG, but factor VIII immunostain is usually negative. In addition, lymphatic markers such as D2-40 and podoplanin are also positive. Almost all cases display strong nuclear staining of HHV-8, regardless of their subtypes.

Epithelioid hemangioendothelioma

Definition

Epithelioid hemangioendothelioma is a low-grade malignant vascular neoplasm, which is characterized by a distinctive myxoid or fibrous stroma and a more favorable clinical course than conventional angiosarcoma.

Etiology

Epithelioid hemangioendothelioma is caused by *WWTR1-CAMTA1* gene fusions in ~90% of cases.[21–23] An unusual vasoformative neoplasm containing the *YAP1-TFE3* fusion gene has been reported as a variant of epithelioid hemangioendothelioma, but more likely represents a distinct entity.[24]

Clinical features

Epithelioid hemangioendothelioma is often incidentally discovered, and lung or other metastases may be present at the time of diagnosis.[25,26] Some patients present with ascites and portal hypertension because of venous occlusion by tumor.[27,28] There is a slight female predominance, with a female-to-male ratio of 3:2. The mean age at diagnosis is 41.7 years (range: 3 to 86 years).[25,26]

Gross findings

Epithelioid hemangioendothelioma is characteristically multifocal and forms ill-defined bilobar tan nodules (Fig. 26.7). The nodule sizes may range from a few millimeters to several centimeters. Some tumor nodules may appear white and firm, often mimicking metastatic carcinoma. Calcifications may also be present.

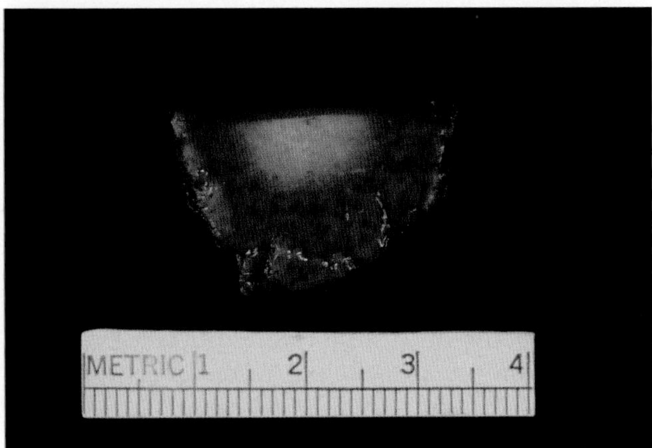

Figure 26.7 Epithelioid hemangioendothelioma. An ill-defined tan nodule of epithelioid hemangioendothelioma. Multiple nodules such as this are seen grossly in most cases.

Microscopic findings

Epithelioid hemangioendothelioma frequently encircles bile ducts and hepatocytes, and shows a propensity for portal vein and central vein invasion.[25,29] Histologically, epithelioid hemangioendothelioma is characterized by cords, chains, and single file arrays of small, bland endothelial cells growing in a distinctive myxoid to fibrous stroma[25,29,30] (Fig. 26.8). In the liver, the matrix in the center of the lesion often has

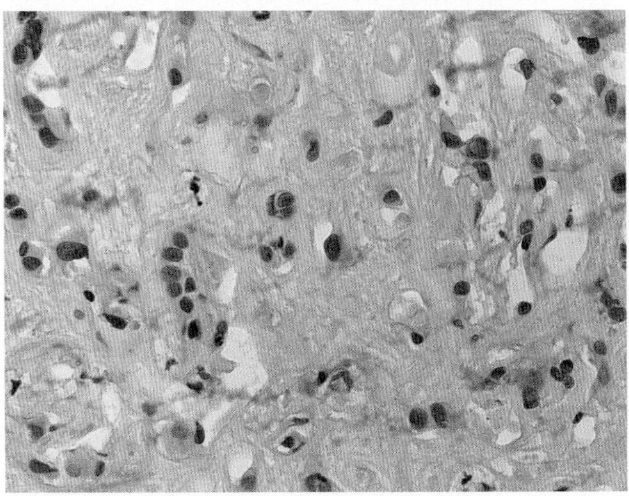

Figure 26.8 Epithelioid hemangioendothelioma. The tumor is defined by a distinctive myxoid matrix as shown in this example. The neoplastic cells form linear arrays and show intracytoplasmic "blisters."

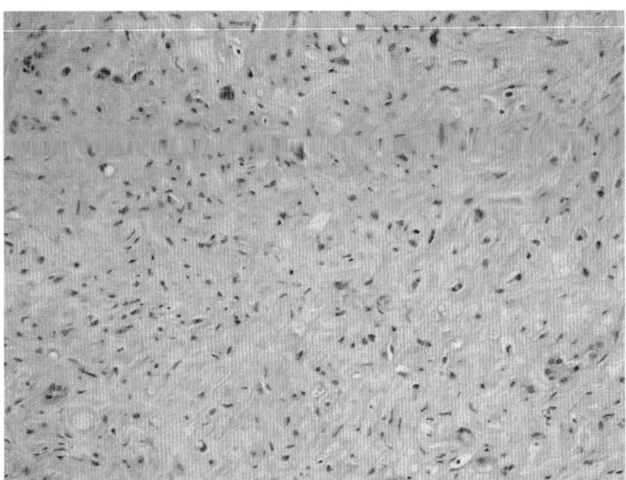

Figure 26.9 Epithelioid hemangioendothelioma. In the liver, tumors frequently show a "burnt out" center which is characterized by hyalinization of the stroma. Intracytoplasmic blister cells can be seen.

a "burnt out," fibrotic appearance (Fig. 26.9). At the peripheral of the lesion, the tumor cells tend to grow along hepatic sinusoids. Although the underlying hepatic acinar architecture is preserved, the liver cell plates become gradually atrophic, and eventually disappear and are replaced by tumor. Careful inspection shows scattered tumor cells with intracytoplasmic "blisters" or "vacuoles," containing red blood cells sometimes, representing primitive vascular lumen formation. In some cases, the neoplastic cells may be obscured by the accompanying inflammatory infiltrate.[29]

Immunohistochemical findings

The vascular markers CD31, CD34,[29] von Willebrand factor, ERG, and FLI1 are positive in the neoplastic cells and in this morphological context confirms the diagnosis (Fig. 26.10). Anomalous cytokeratin expression may be present, leading to confusion with adenocarcinoma, in particular cholangiocarcinoma.[30] Taking advantage of the identification of the genetic driver of epithelioid hemangioendothelioma, nuclear expression of carboxyl-terminus CAMTA1 can be used to support the diagnosis of epithelioid hemangioendothelioma.[31,32]

Molecular and special techniques

Approximately 90% of cases of epithelioid hemangioendothelioma are characterized by the recurrent fusion gene *WWTR1-CAMTA1* which is the genetic driver of the tumor. Detection of this fusion transcript by RT-PCR confirms the diagnosis of epithelioid hemangioendothelioma.[21,23]

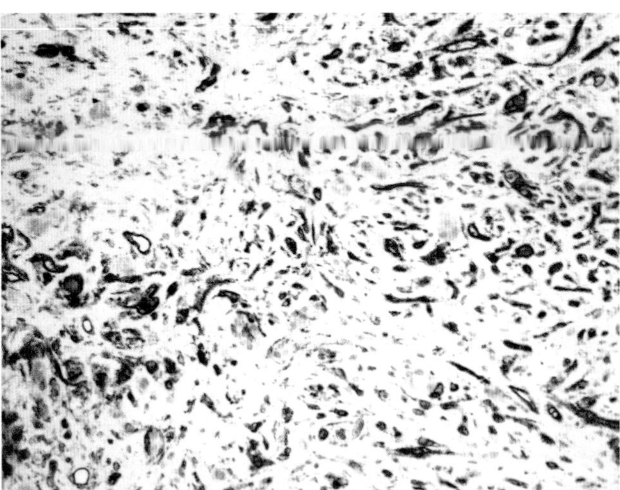

Figure 26.10 Epithelioid hemangioendothelioma. A CD31 highlights the neoplastic cells.

Differential diagnosis

The most important differential diagnosis for epithelioid hemangioendothelioma is adenocarcinoma including cholangiocarcinoma or metastatic adenocarcinoma. Some adenocarcinomas involving the liver can elicit a desmoplastic stroma which mimics epithelioid hemangioendothelioma. Also, adenocarcinoma may be distributed as single cells, abortive glands, or cell clusters. Immunohistochemistry is helpful in resolving the differential diagnosis. Epithelioid hemangioendothelioma is positive for vascular markers unlike adenocarcinoma. As noted above, anomalous cytokeratin expression is common in epithelioid hemangioendothelioma, reinforcing the need to employ a panel of markers. Angiosarcoma has a destructive growth and higher grade cytological atypia than epithelioid hemangioendothelioma. The cells in angiosarcoma are often spindled and form complex anastomosing channels. Some nonneoplastic lesions, such as parenchymal collapse or scar, may mimic hemangioendothelioma because of a fibromyxoid stroma with scattered atypical stromal cells and histiocytes. Careful microscopic examination to identify the characteristic neoplastic epithelioid cells and immunohistochemistry can help to distinguish these two entities.

Prognosis and treatment

The prognosis of epithelioid hemangioendothelioma is better than angiosarcoma,[33,34] and patients can have good long-term outcomes even with metastatic disease.[33,34] Epithelioid hemangioendothelioma is treated with surgical excision or liver transplantation in those cases with unresectable disease.[26] The presence of extrahepatic disease does not preclude surgical intervention.[26]

Angiosarcoma

Definition

Hepatic angiosarcoma is a primary high-grade malignant vascular neoplasm in the liver.

Etiology

Most angiosarcomas develop without a clear etiology.[35] A minor fraction of hepatic angiosarcomas arise in a background of occupational vinyl chloride exposure.[35,36] Thorotrast exposure was historically a risk factor for hepatic angiosarcoma, but is no longer in use.[37]

Clinical features

Hepatic angiosarcoma is the third most common primary liver malignancy, after hepatocellular carcinoma and cholangiocarcinoma, but still only accounts for 2% to 3% of all primary liver malignancies.[38] Angiosarcomas usually arise in middle-aged or elderly adults.[39,40] The clinical presentation of hepatic angiosarcoma is nonspecific. Patients may present with abdominal pain, weight loss, hepatomegaly, liver failure, or thrombocytopenia.[40] Catastrophic intra-abdominal bleeding occurs in about one-fourth of all cases.[38]

Gross findings

Angiosarcomas form large hemorrhagic tumor masses with solid and cystic blood containing areas and ill-defined borders (Fig. 26.11). Satellite masses may be present. It can involve either lobe or the entire liver.

Microscopic findings

Angiosarcoma is a remarkably protean tumor that shows a widely variable appearance from tumor to tumor, and even within a single tumor. Angiosarcoma may display sinusoidal, papillary, cavernous/peliotic, or solid architectural patterns. The cytology also varies widely, from minimal atypia, often with a "hobnail" appearance, to severely anaplastic. Growth along the sinusoids of the hepatic plate, the so-called "sinusoidal pattern" (Fig. 26.12), may be particularly subtle; in such cases, the endothelial cells often show minimal atypia and frequently have spindled morphology. The presence of endothelial cell multilayering is a valuable clue to the diagnosis of angiosarcoma in cases with sinusoidal growth. The cavernous or peliotic pattern of hepatic angiosarcoma may also be quite treacherous because these lesions consist of relatively well-formed, large blood filled spaces lined by malignant endothelial cells with minimal atypia. Angiosarcoma can also purely consist of spindle cells with abundant extracellular matrix that mimics other sarcomas. Occasionally, the solid areas of angiosarcomas can undergo necrosis and cavitation, leaving a cavity filled with blood, fibrin, and necrotic debris that has only small rim of viable malignant cells. Thankfully, many hepatic angiosarcomas are much more obvious, consisting of a proliferation of obviously malignant endothelial cells forming papillary (Fig. 26.13), sieve-like, spindled, or solid formations (Fig. 26.14). Some angiosarcomas may show almost exclusively epithelioid morphology, mimicking carcinoma, mesothelioma, or a high-grade lymphoma (Fig. 26.15). In such cases, the presence of occasional intracytoplasmic lumen formation and the presence of small, peripheral zones of more typical

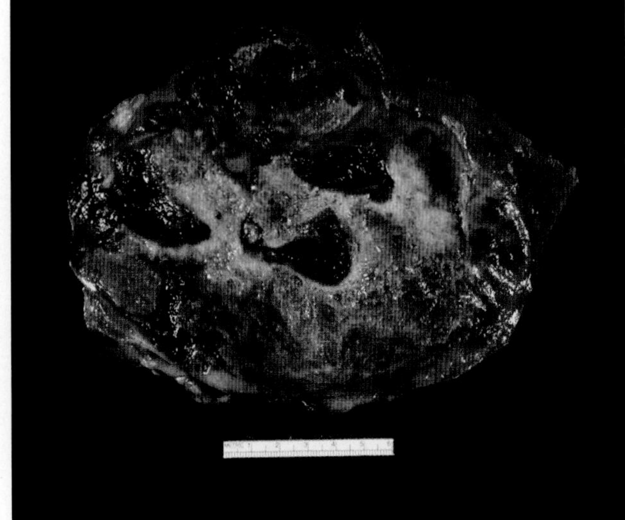

Figure 26.11 Angiosarcoma. The tumor is cystic and hemorrhagic.

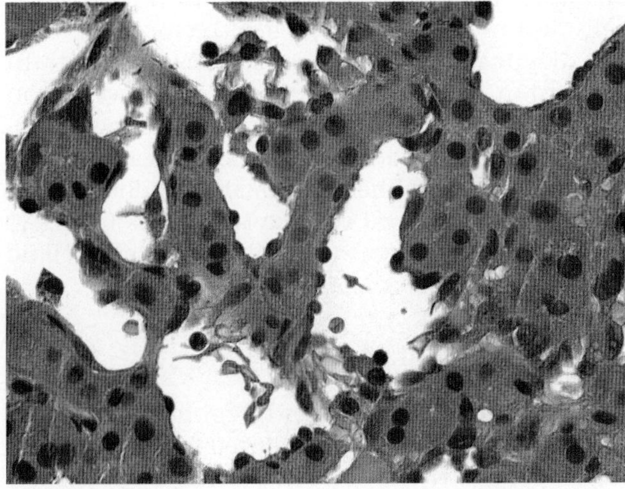

Figure 26.12 Angiosarcoma. A sinusoidal pattern of growth is seen. Note the hobnail appearance of the neoplastic cells and subtle multilayering.

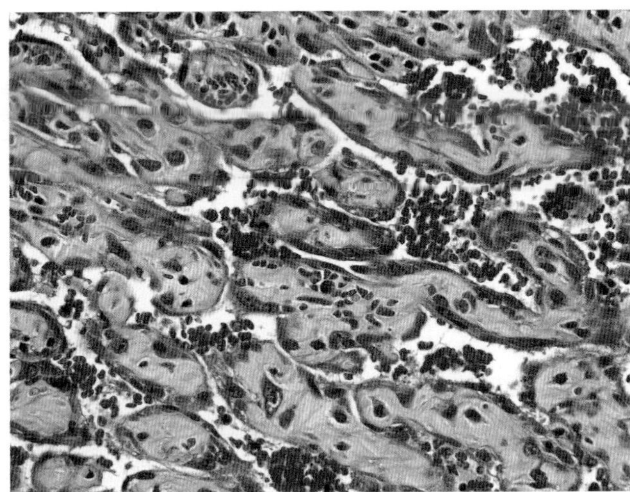

Figure 26.13 Angiosarcoma. The neoplastic cells appear to line collagenous cores creating a papillary appearance.

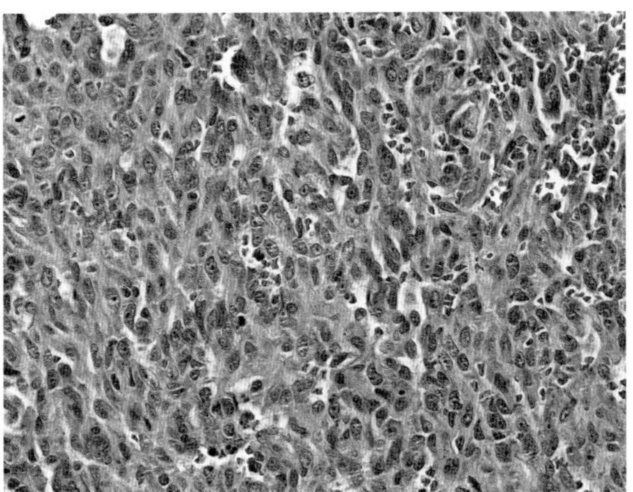

Figure 26.14 Angiosarcoma. The obviously malignant spindle-shaped cells of angiosarcoma.

vasoformative growth are valuable clues to the correct diagnosis. Mitotic figures, including atypical mitotic forms, are usually easily identified in hepatic angiosarcoma, but may on occasion be difficult to identify. Mitotic activity is not required for the diagnosis of angiosarcoma, particularly when infiltrative growth is present.[4]

Hepatic angiosarcoma in children may have Kaposiform areas consisting of spindle cells, sometimes containing PAS-positive intracytoplasmic globules. Thorotrast-associated angiosarcoma may have brown-gray Thorotrast granules, which can be present either free or within macrophages. A precursor lesion consisting of endothelial hypertrophy and hyperplasia has been described in cases related to Thorotrast, vinyl chloride, and arsenic exposure.[41,42]

Immunohistochemical findings

Angiosarcomas are variably positive for vascular markers (CD31, CD34, factor VIII, ERG, and FLI1) (Fig. 26.16). Overall, the frequency of positivity of vascular markers in angiosarcomas is as follows: 40% to 90% of cases are positive for factor VIII, 60% to 90% are positive for CD34, 30% to 100% are positive for CD31, and nearly 100% are positive for ERG and FLI1.[43–46] An important diagnostic pitfall is the expression of cytokeratins.[47] Cytokeratin expression is seen in about 30% to 50% of cases (Fig. 26.17), in particular those showing epithelioid morphology, emphasizing the need to apply a panel of immunohistochemical stains in this differential diagnostic setting. Rare angiosarcomas also express synaptophysin and/or chromogranin, mimicking neuroendocrine tumors.[48]

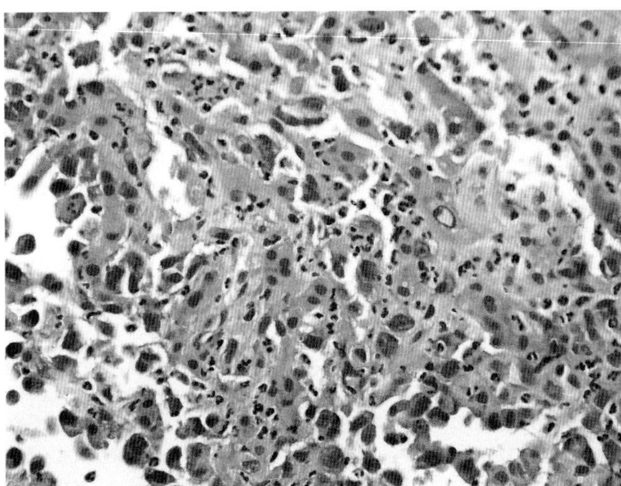

Figure 26.15 Epithelioid angiosarcoma. The tumor cells resemble a poorly differentiated carcinoma.

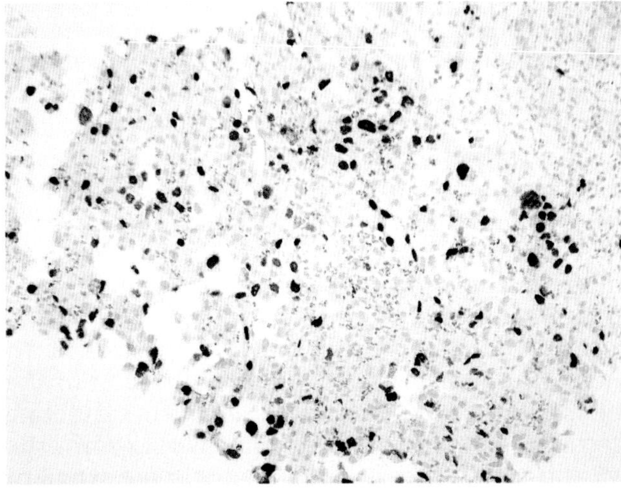

Figure 26.16 Angiosarcoma. An immunostain for ERG is positive.

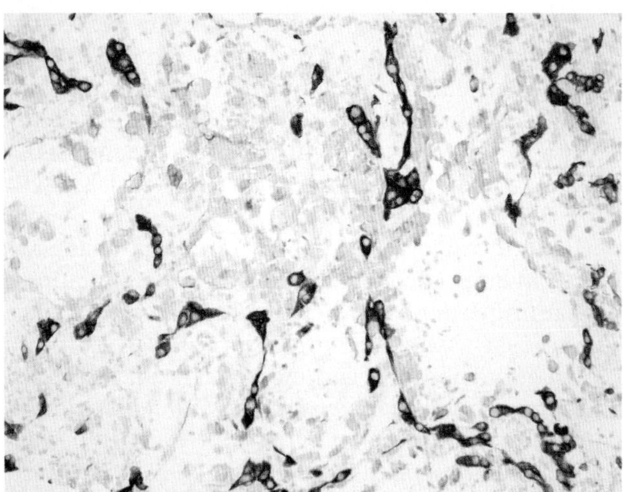

Figure 26.17 Angiosarcoma. An immunostain for CAM 5.2 is positive.

Molecular and special techniques

Recent studies have described recurrent genetic abnormalities in skin and visceral angiosarcomas. Angiosarcomas of the liver have not been specifically studied but the findings of these studies deserve mention. *CIC* mutations or rearrangements have been found in approximately 10% of angiosarcomas,[49] and *PLCG1*, *PTPRB*, and *KDR* mutations have each been noted in another 10%.[49] These alterations are mutually exclusive. Recurrent *NUP160–SLC43A3* fusion genes have been identified in approximately 35% of angiosarcomas.[50] This fusion gene was mutually exclusive of *KDR* mutations. The relevance of these findings to primary hepatic angiosarcomas is unclear at this time.

Differential diagnosis

Hepatic angiosarcoma can mimic poorly differentiated carcinoma.[4] However, as long as angiosarcoma is considered and vascular markers are performed, this distinction should be made without undue difficulty. Epithelioid hemangioendothelioma usually has distinct mucopolysaccharide-rich stroma and has a pushing and not a destructive growth pattern. In contrast, angiosarcoma often has significantly more destructive growth and more striking cytologic atypia.

Angiosarcoma can mimic a simple cyst with hemorrhage or peliosis.[51] Careful attention to the morphology of the lining cells is important on routine sections. Immunohistochemistry will confirm the vascular phenotype and also highlight the extent of the neoplastic proliferation, which may be surprisingly deceptive in peliotic areas.

Some cases of angiosarcoma are characterized by neoplastic cells with minimal atypia that line well-formed vascular spaces, raising consideration for anastomosing hemangioma or cavernous hemangioma. The presence of sinusoidal growth, infiltrative growth around biliary structures, endothelial cell multilayering, and nuclear atypia all point toward angiosarcoma and away from benign diagnoses.[14]

Prognosis and treatment

The prognosis of angiosarcoma is dismal. The median survival rate is 5 to 6 months without treatment.[38] Survival beyond 12 months after diagnosis is unusual.[38,52] Angiosarcomas are treated with a combination of surgical excision and multimodal adjuvant therapy, but they are typically resistance to traditional chemotherapy and radiotherapy.[53]

26.4 TUMORS OF ADIPOSE TISSUE

Lipoma

Definition

A lipoma is a benign neoplasm of mature adipocytes.

Etiology

Lipomas in soft-tissue locations frequently harbor structural rearrangements involving the chromosomal region 12q13-15.[54,55] The most common translocations involve *HMGA2*.[56] A subset of cases reveals *HMGA1* rearrangements.[57,58] Primary hepatic lipomas have not been studied for these molecular genetic events.

Clinical features

Primary hepatic lipomas are uncommon and are discovered incidentally during imaging for other clinical indications.[59] Lipomas are more frequent in patients with hepatic steatosis and obesity.[60]

Gross findings

Hepatic lipomas have a yellow, lobulated solid cut surface and well-defined border.

Microscopic findings

Lipomas are well circumscribed and capsulated lobular tumors. The tumor is composed of mature adipocytes that are cytologically bland (Fig. 26.18). Hemorrhage and fat necrosis are commonly seen. The background liver often shows steatosis.

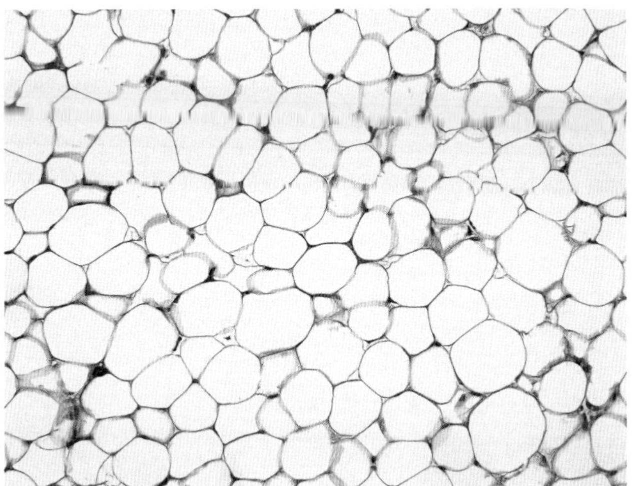

Figure 26.18 Lipoma. Bland appearing adipocytes with central lipid containing vacuoles comprise this hepatic lipoma.

Immunohistochemical findings

Immunohistochemistry is rarely employed in the diagnosis of lipoma because the diagnosis is comfortably and reliably made on routine sections. Nevertheless, lipomas are positive for S100 protein.

Differential diagnosis

The most important considerations are focal fatty change, myelolipoma, and angiomyolipoma. Focal fatty change is not neoplastic but instead represents a multiacinar collection of steatotic hepatocytes. In focal fatty change, portal structures and hepatic plate architecture are intact. Thus, this distinction is comfortably made on routine sections. The bone marrow elements of myelolipoma are not seen in lipoma. Angiomyolipoma is discussed in detail later.

Prognosis and treatment

The prognosis of hepatic lipomas is excellent. Lipomas are cured by simple excision.

Liposarcoma

Primary hepatic liposarcoma is extremely rare.[61] The ages of reported cases can range from 2 to 86 years and it affects men and women equally.[62]

Grossly, liposarcoma is usually a large well-circumscribed lobulated mass with yellow to white cut surface, depending on the proportions of adipose tissue and fibrotic tissue. Areas of fat necrosis are common in larger tumors.

Microscopically, hepatic liposarcomas have the same morphological features to those arising in soft tissue. All subtypes described in soft-tissue liposarcomas have also been reported in primary hepatic liposarcomas. Myxoid/round cell liposarcoma is the most common type occurring in the liver. This type of liposarcoma is characterized by a lobulated hypocellular lesion with a myxoid matrix containing individual bland fusiform or round cells and delicate plexiform capillary vascular network. The cellularity is increased at the periphery. Lipoblasts are usually easy to identify. Well-differentiated liposarcoma is composed of a mature adipose tissue with, scattered large hyperchromatic cells. Dedifferentiated liposarcoma is defined as the presence of transition from a well-differentiated component to any type of nonlipogenic high-grade sarcoma. Pleomorphic and spindle cell liposarcomas have also been reported in the literature.

Immunostains are usually not required for establishing a diagnosis of liposarcoma.

26.5 ANGIOMYOLIPOMA

Definition

Angiomyolipomas are neoplasms composed of morphologically and immunohistochemically distinctive perivascular epithelioid cells and thick-walled blood vessels. These perivascular epithelioid cells may closely resemble smooth muscle or fat, and it was originally mistakenly believed that these lesions represented hamartomas rather than true neoplasms. Angiomyolipomas are members of the perivascular epithelioid cell family of tumors.[63–66]

Etiology

Approximately 5% to 10% of hepatic angiomyolipomas are related to germline inactivation of the tuberous sclerosis-associated gene *TSC2* or less commonly *TSC1*.[67–69] The etiology for the majority of hepatic angiomyolipomas is not completely understood but recent data identified frequent loss of heterozygosity at the *TSC1/TSC2* loci, suggesting these genes and the mTOR pathway are important in sporadic angiomyolipoma as well.[70]

Clinical features

Hepatic angiomyolipomas are uncommon. Many cases are incidentally discovered during imaging for an unrelated clinical indication, but patients may present with abdominal discomfort or malaise.[71] Hepatic angiomyolipomas are most often sporadic and have a modal age of clinical presentation in the fourth to fifth decades.[71,72] There is a female predominance (2:1 to 5:1). Approximately 5% to 10% of cases arise in individuals with tuberous sclerosis, who often manifest other features of that disorder.[67,68]

Gross findings

Angiomyolipomas show a variable appearance, reflecting the relative percentages of lipid-distended and myoid perivascular epithelioid cells. Tumors with abundant lipidization appear more yellow. Hemorrhage and areas of necrosis are common.

Microscopic findings and histological types

Histologically, these tumors consist of a variable admixture of perivascular epithelioid cells showing epithelioid morphology, spindled morphology resembling smooth muscle, lipid-distended cells mimicking adipocytes, and nonneoplastic thick-walled blood vessels. Essentially any combination of these various elements may be present.[72]

Classic angiomyolipomas show triphasic histology including tortuous, thick-walled blood vessels, bundles of spindled (myoid-appearing) cells, and clusters of perivascular epithelioid cells with abundant intracytoplasmic fat (so-called "adipocytes"). However, there is considerable variation in the relative proportion of epithelioid, spindled, and lipid-distended cells[65,66,73] (Figs. 26.19, 26.20, 26.21, and 26.22). This variation can lead to confusion with other neoplasms including lipomas,[74] carcinomas, and smooth muscle tumors.[73,75–77]

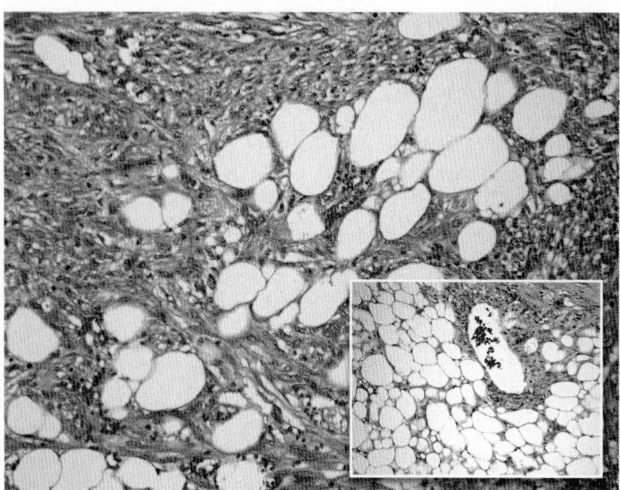

Figure 26.19 Angiomyolipoma. An area of a classic angiomyolipoma is composed of spindled appearing perivascular epithelioid cells and lipid-distended perivascular epithelioid cells. The inset shows the characteristic vessels.

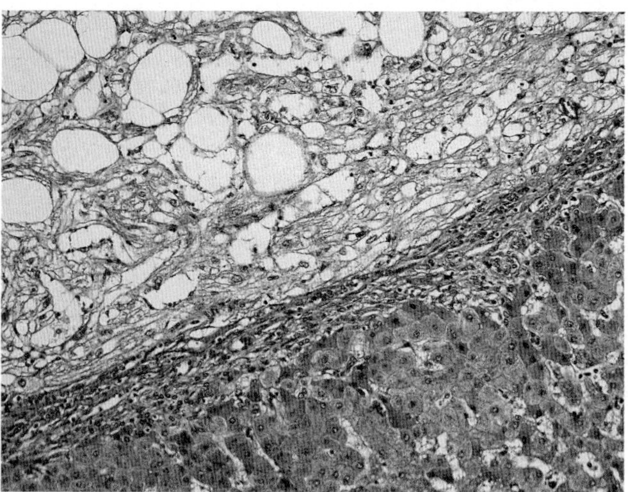

Figure 26.20 Angiomyolipoma. This hepatic angiomyolipoma displays the typical cytologic features of the tumor cells. The cytoplasm of the neoplastic cells is often palely eosinophilic or clear. The perivascular epithelioid cells shown here display lipid accumulation and mimic adipocytes.

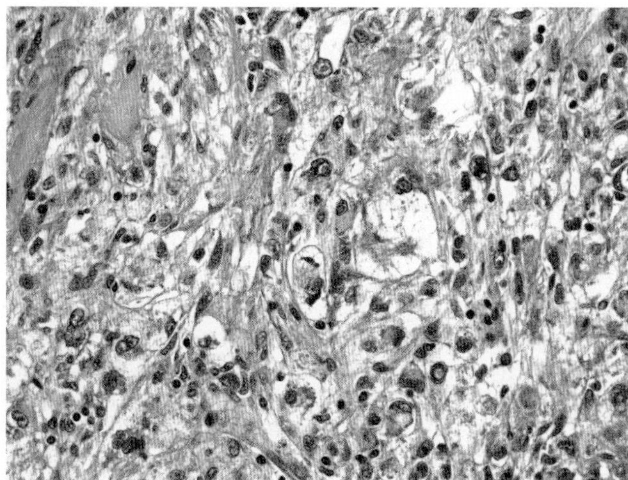

Figure 26.21 Epithelioid angiomyolipoma. In the center of this photomicrograph is a "spider cell." This perivascular epithelioid cells show a clear rim of cytoplasm surrounding a central area of condensed eosinophilia.

Perivascular epithelioid cells, characterized by a perivascular location and at least partially epithelioid morphology, often appear to surround the vascular lumen and replace the smooth muscle and collagen of the vessel, forming distinctive, thick vessel walls. Characteristically, the perivascular epithelioid cells are most epithelioid adjacent to the vessel lumen and become progressively more spindle shaped further away from the vessel lumen.[65,66] Vessels with normal

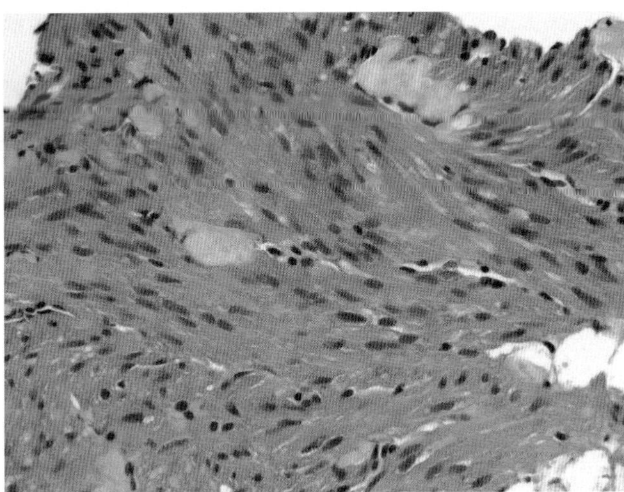

Figure 26.22 Angiomyolipoma. Occasionally, angiomyolipoma may be spindled mimicking a smooth muscle tumor.

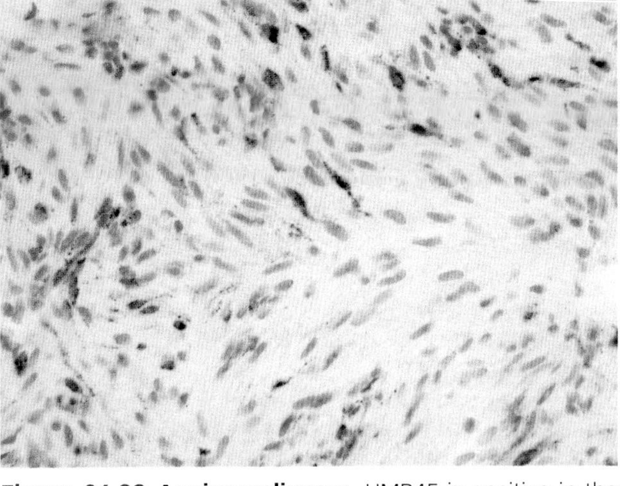

Figure 26.23 Angiomyolipoma. HMB45 is positive in the spindle perivascular epithelioid cells confirming the diagnosis.

smooth muscle walls are also present in angiomyolipomas and most likely represent nonneoplastic host vasculature.

The cytoplasm of perivascular epithelioid cells is clear or slightly eosinophilic, unlike the dense eosinophilia of true smooth muscle cells. As previously mentioned, perivascular epithelioid cells can accumulate large amounts of lipid, mimicking adipocytes or lipoblasts (Fig. 26.20). These are usually found distant from blood vessels.[65,66] Occasionally, perivascular epithelioid cells show a perinuclear zone of condensed eosinophilia, with surrounding cytoplasmic clearing, referred to as "spider cells" (Fig. 26.21). This is a useful diagnostic clue.

The nuclei of perivascular epithelioid cells are typically small, centrally placed, normochromatic, and round to oval nuclei with small nucleoli. Occasional cases of angiomyolipomas may disclose marked nuclear atypia, multiple nuclei, conspicuous mitotic activity, and foci of necrosis. Such cases have been dubbed "atypical angiomyolipomas."[78] Angiomyolipomas may also show almost exclusively epithelioid morphology and are classified as "epithelioid angiomyolipomas."[79] Epithelioid angiomyolipomas can mimic hepatocellular neoplasms closely on routine histologic sections[33,80] and cytology preparations.[81]

Angiomyolipomas frequently display foamy macrophages within the tumor, foci of extramedullary hematopoiesis, lymphoid aggregates, and areas of recent or remote hemorrhage.[33,72] Melanin pigment is rarely seen.[33,72] Tumors showing exclusively epithelioid morphology, high nuclear grade, vascular invasion, conspicuous mitotic activity, and/or necrosis may be more likely to behave in an aggressive manner.[34,69,82]

Immunohistochemical findings

Angiomyolipomas have a distinctive myomelanocytic immunophenotype which can help to confirm the diagnosis.[64,72] HMB-45 (Fig. 26.23), Melan-A, caldesmon, and smooth muscle actin are characteristically positive in the perivascular epithelioid cells of angiomyolipoma. Epithelioid variants may show predominantly expression of melanocytic markers, with limited or absent expression of myoid markers.[83] Desmin expression is uncommon and typically limited in extent.[84]

Differential diagnosis

Angiomyolipoma may mimic hepatocellular adenoma and hepatocellular carcinoma (including the fibrolamellar variant) but angiomyolipoma is typically negative for cytokeratins and is consistently negative for hepatocellular markers, such as HepPar-1 and Arginase. Metastatic melanoma may resemble epithelioid angiomyolipoma histologically and immunohistochemically. Melanoma, though, typically has more conspicuous mitotic activity and more prominent nucleoli, shows robust S100 protein and SOX10 expression, and lacks expression of myoid markers. Although limited S100 protein expression may be seen in epithelioid angiomyolipoma, SOX10 is consistently negative, in our experience. A prior history of melanoma should obviously suggest the diagnosis of metastatic melanoma.

Molecular and special techniques

Less than 10% of hepatic angiomyolipoma will show biallelic loss of function mutations in *TSC1* or *TSC2*.[67] Other cases may show loss of heterozygosity at these loci.[70] Importantly, the *BRAF* p.V600E mutation, which is found in 45% of hepatic metastatic melanoma cases,[85] has not been found in angiomyolipoma.

Treatment and prognosis

Angiomyolipoma is typically cured by excision with negative margins. Angiomyolipoma typically has a good prognosis but reports of malignant angiomyolipomas have been described.[34,69,82] Malignant examples in the liver display epithelioid morphology with high nuclear grade, vascular invasion, frequent mitoses, and/or necrosis.[34,69,82]

Most hepatic angiomyolipomas are sporadic but a minority will be related to tuberous sclerosis.[67] In such cases, there is potential for the patient to present with multiple angiomyolipomas or to synchronously or metachronously develop other tumors associated with tuberous sclerosis. Other tumors associated with tuberous sclerosis include periungal fibroma, subependymal giant cell astrocytoma, cardiac rhabdomyoma, and lymphangioleiomyomatosis.[86]

26.6 INFLAMMATORY MYOFIBROBLASTIC TUMOR

Definition

A neoplasm composed of myofibroblastic cells accompanied by plasma cells and lymphocytes, characterized genetically by oncogenic rearrangements of the *ALK*, *ROS*, *PDGFRβ*, or *NTRK3* genes.[47,87–89] Inflammatory myofibroblastic tumor was formerly grouped with reactive plasma cell-rich processes under the heading Inflammatory pseudotumor.

Etiology

Inflammatory myofibroblastic tumors are caused most commonly by recurrent rearrangement of the *ALK* gene.[89] Alternatively, *ROS1*, *PDGFRβ* rearrangements, or the *ETV6-NTRK3* fusion gene is responsible for tumorigenesis.[47,87,88]

Clinical features

Inflammatory myofibroblastic tumor is a rare neoplasm found in both the liver and other sites. Inflammatory myofibroblastic tumor presents with symptoms referable to a liver mass and not infrequently manifests systemic symptoms of fever and chills.

Gross findings

The macroscopic appearance of inflammatory myofibroblastic tumors is nonspecific. Lesions are often in the region of the porta hepatis but they can develop in any location.

Microscopic findings

Inflammatory myofibroblastic tumors are most often composed of monotonous spindle cells growing in short fascicles (Fig. 26.24), in association with areas of prominent stromal hyalinization. The nuclei of the neoplastic cells are bland appearing, and mitotic figures are not prominent, though these findings do not confirm indolent behavior.[90] The spindled cells are accompanied by a brisk inflammatory infiltrate, which often includes plasma cells (Fig. 26.24) and lymphocytes but may also include neutrophils and eosinophils.[91] Myxoid change and calcifications may be present.[90,91]

Rare cases of epithelioid IMT have been described in the abdomen.[53,92] This variant is usually large at presentation and may be multifocal. Histologically, typical spindle cell areas are seen focally but the predominant neoplastic cells are epithelioid with abundant amphophilic–eosinophilic cytoplasm and large nucleoli. The accompanying reactive inflammatory infiltrate is devoid of plasma cells and instead shows prominent neutrophils and or lymphocytes.[92] Mitotic activity and necrosis are frequent findings in epithelioid inflammatory myofibroblastic tumor, and the clinical course is marked by local recurrence and poor outcome.[53,92]

Immunohistochemical findings

Inflammatory myofibroblastic tumors typically show a "tram-track" pattern of smooth muscle actin expression,

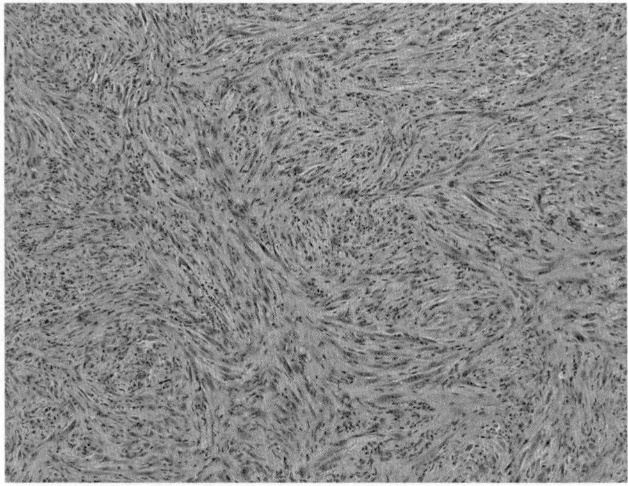

Figure 26.24 Inflammatory myofibroblastic tumor. A classic inflammatory myofibroblastic tumor characterized by spindle cells displaying fascicular growth and accompanied by a lymphoplasmacytic infiltrate.

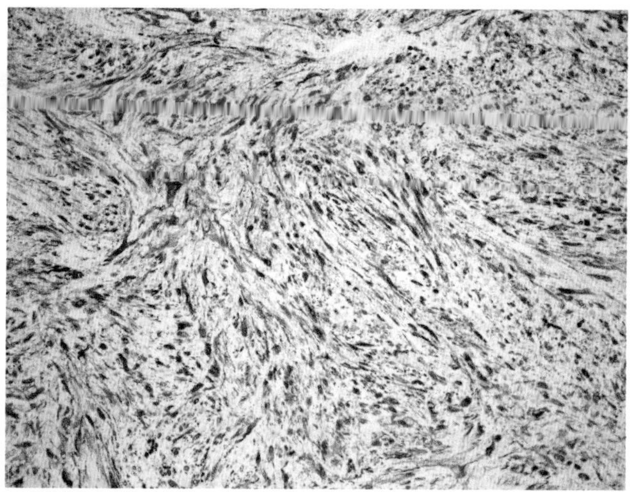

Figure 26.25 Inflammatory myofibroblastic tumor. ALK is strongly positive in this example, confirming the diagnosis.

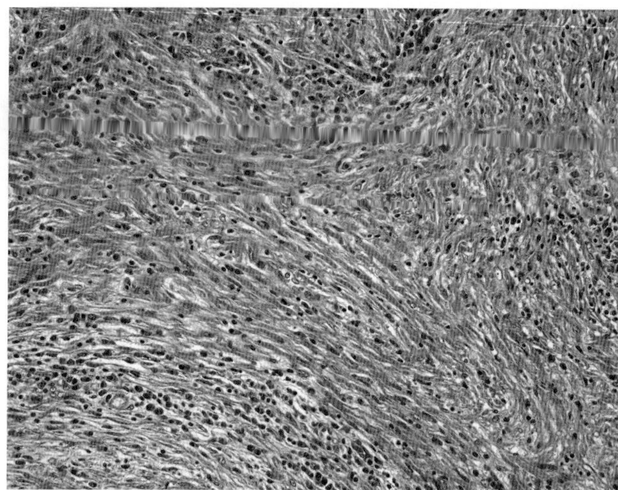

Figure 26.26 Inflammatory pseudotumor. This case of IgG4-related sclerosing cholangitis presenting as a pseudotumor. Note the storiform pattern of fibrosis and marked plasma cell infiltrate.

which confirms a myofibroblastic phenotype. ALK immunohistochemistry, with compatible morphology, typically confirms the diagnosis (Fig. 26.25). ALK expression is usually cytoplasmic but may be nuclear membrane or perinuclear in the epithelioid variant.[92] Approximately 40% to 50% of inflammatory myofibroblastic tumors are ALK negative.[47] They display a myofibroblastic immunophenotype and may show expression of ROS1 instead,[93] if ROS1 is rearranged in the tumor. Cytokeratins, S100 protein, HMB-45, and Melan-A are negative.

Differential diagnosis

The differential diagnosis includes reactive inflammatory pseudotumors such as IgG4-related disease. Most inflammatory pseudotumors have no specific etiology and similarly display a nonspecific appearance characterized by nondescript fibrosis and a mixed inflammatory infiltrate. Granulomas have been reported. In IgG4-related disease, there is characteristically storiform fibrosis, phlebitis, and numerous IgG4-positive plasma cells (Fig. 26.26).

Other differential diagnoses include follicular dendritic cell tumor and metastatic sarcomas. Follicular dendritic tumor (Fig. 26.27) may closely simulate spindle cell inflammatory myofibroblastic tumors but typically contains only small lymphocytes, without plasma cells, and expresses CD21 and CD35 (Fig. 26.28), but not ALK.[94,95]

Many metastatic sarcomas demonstrate spindle cell growth and so can mimic inflammatory myofibroblastic tumors. In most cases, though, the inflammatory infiltrate is not prominent, and the combination of careful histologic review and thorough sampling will allow for recognition of helpful or specific diagnostic features of the metastasis. Also, awareness of an antecedent clinical history is helpful. One important exception is dedifferentiated liposarcoma showing a prominent inflammatory, neutrophil-rich reaction, the so-called "inflammatory variant of malignant fibrous histiocytoma."[96] In such cases, careful evaluation of the tumor mass looking for areas of well-differentiated liposarcoma, and sometimes ancillary molecular cytogenetic studies for *MDM2* amplification, should allow distinction from inflammatory myofibroblastic tumors.[97,98]

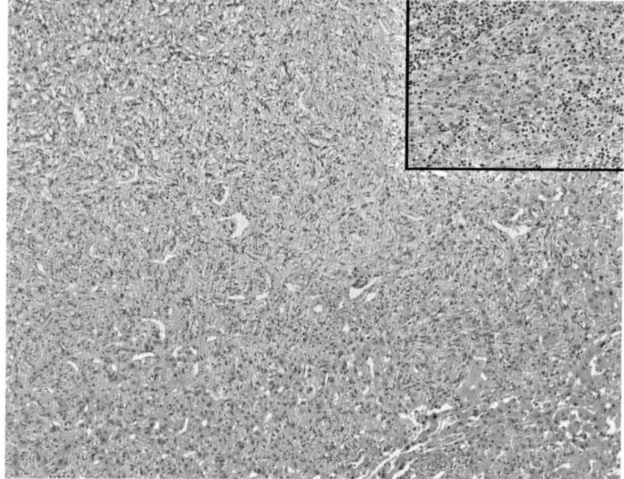

Figure 26.27 Follicular dendritic cell sarcoma. The tumor cells grow in short fascicles and may mimic inflammatory myofibroblastic tumor. Inset: On high magnification, the neoplastic cells are intimately intermixed with lymphocytes.

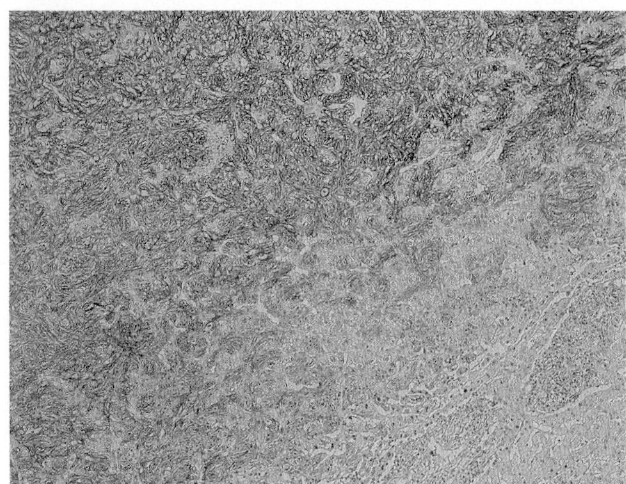

Figure 26.28. Follicular dendritic cell sarcoma. The A CD35 is positive in the tumor cells.

Molecular and special techniques

The *ALK* gene is the most frequently rearranged oncogene in inflammatory myofibroblastic tumors[89] and shows a tendency to rearrange with any of a number of gene partners including *TPM3*, *TPM4*,[99] *CLTC*,[100] *RANBP2*,[101] *CARS*,[102] *ATIC*,[103] and *SEC31L1*.[104] *ALK-CLTC* fusion corresponds to a granular cytoplasmic staining with ALK immunostains, which is believed to be due to *CLTC* encoding the main component of coated cytoplasmic vesicles.[100] The remaining fusion genes give rise to a diffuse cytoplasmic pattern on ALK IHC. *RANBP2* is a large protein at the nuclear pores. *RANBP2-ALK* is the fusion identified in cases of epithelioid inflammatory myofibroblastic tumors which show aggressive behavior.[92] Given the various ALK fusion genes and their varied structure, FISH for *ALK* rearrangement or next generation sequencing assays are used to identify *ALK* fusion genes rather than RT-PCR.

Treatment

Inflammatory myofibroblastic tumors are treated by surgical excision in cases amenable to surgical intervention. Targeted ALK inhibition is another approach which is utilized in cases where oncologic resection is not possible.[105]

Prognosis

The behavior of most inflammatory myofibroblastic tumors is unpredictable. Patients who have an oncologic resection often have a benign clinical course but reports of aggressive behavior are well known.[90,92] Unfortunately, no histologic features can predict which inflammatory myofibroblastic tumors will behave aggressively, with the exception of the epithelioid variant described earlier.[53,92] The overwhelming majority of pediatric inflammatory myofibroblastic tumors behave in a benign fashion.

26.7 SMOOTH MUSCLE TUMORS

Leiomyoma

Primary hepatic leiomyomas are extremely rare[132] and when present are often associated with immunosuppression and Epstein–Barr virus (EBV) infection.[133,134] Such cases are classified as EBV-positive smooth muscle tumors, and EBV-encoded RNA in situ hybridization shows nuclear positivity (Figs. 26.29 and 26.30).

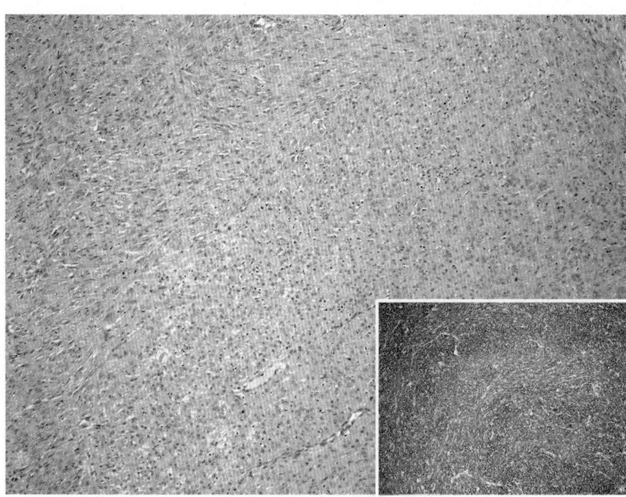

Figure 26.29 Leiomyoma. The bland spindle-shaped tumor cells of this smooth muscle tumor show a fascicular arrangement and dense cytoplasmic eosinophilia. Inset: Smooth muscle actin is strongly positive in the tumor cells.

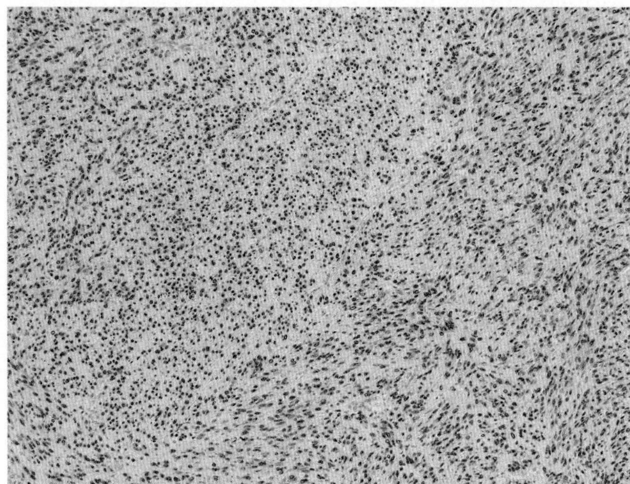

Figure 26.30 Leiomyoma. EBV in situ hybridization shows EBV-encoded RNA (EBER) in virtually all tumor nuclei.

Multifocality is not unusual and does not indicate metastatic disease.[97–99] EBV-associated smooth muscle tumors often show at least partial epithelioid morphology, have bland nuclear features, and frequently elicit a chronic inflammatory cell infiltrate. In general, hepatic leiomyomas have the same morphology as those arising at elsewhere in the body, which are composed of bland spindle cells forming well organized long and short fascicles that are typically intersecting at right angles. The smooth muscle differentiation can be readily recognized by H&E and immunostains. They must be distinguished from primary or metastatic leiomyosarcoma that is discussed in detail in the following section.

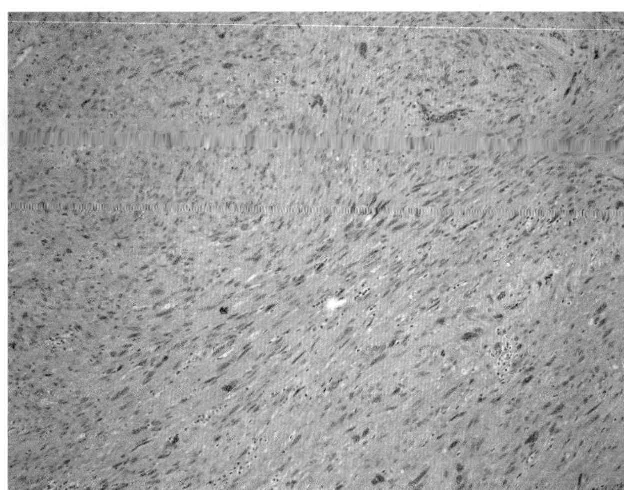

Figure 26.31 Leiomyosarcoma. The tumor shows obviously malignant spindle cells forming fascicles. Expression of smooth muscle markers confirms the diagnosis.

Leiomyosarcoma

Definition

Primary hepatic leiomyosarcomas are malignant tumors that originate from smooth muscle in intrahepatic vascular structures, bile duct muscular wall, or the ligamentum teres. Leiomyosarcoma arising from inferior vena cava is usually subclassified as a distinct entity.

Clinical features

Most leiomyosarcomas involving the liver are metastatic. Primary hepatic leiomyosarcomas are very rare and occur equally in men and women, but those arising in the inferior vena cava are more frequently seen in women. The median age of patients with leiomyosarcoma is at 58 years, but occasional cases have been reported in immunosuppressed children.[106,107] Most cases are asymptomatic, and some may present with a wide spectrum of nonspecific symptoms, such as abdominal pain, weight loss, anorexia, vomiting, jaundice, and rarely present with acute intra-abdominal bleeding secondary to tumor rupture. Tumors arising in the hepatic veins can develop Budd–Chiari syndrome and usually have a worse prognosis.

Gross findings

Primary hepatic leiomyosarcomas are typically solitary and large. They are firm and fleshy with pinkish white color on cut surface. Foci of necrosis and hemorrhage are common.

Microscopic findings

Histologically, hepatic leiomyosarcomas have an identical morphology to those arising in other parts of the body. The tumor is composed of bundles of elongated atypical spindle cells intersecting at right angles (Fig. 26.31). Focal storiform, palisaded, or hemangiopericytoma-like patterns can also be present. The tumor cells contain abundant eosinophilic cytoplasm which may occasionally show hair-like longitudinal striations. The nucleus is usually enlarged, hyperchromatic, atypical, and centrally located, with a blunt-ended or "cigar-shaped" appearance. Focal necrosis and increased mitotic activity (>10 mitoses in 50 high-powered fields) are common. In high-grade leiomyosarcoma, the tumor cells can be highly atypical and pleomorphic and resemble undifferentiated pleomorphic sarcoma.

Immunohistochemical findings

Immunostains for smooth muscle actin and muscle-specific actin are positive in most leiomyosarcomas. H-caldesmon is also positive in the majority of tumors, but desmin positivity ranges from about 50% to nearly 100% of tumors. Of note, none of these markers is entirely specific for smooth muscle neoplasms. Therefore, a panel of several muscle markers should be applied, and positivity of two of these markers is supportive of smooth muscle phenotype. Some tumors are also focally positive for EMA, CD34, keratin, and S-100.

Molecular and special techniques

Little is known about molecular genetic changes in hepatic leiomyosarcomas. Molecular subtypes of leiomyosarcomas with potential therapeutic targets have been proposed by a recent study.[108]

Differential diagnosis

The differential diagnosis typically includes other spindle cell tumors in the liver, either primary or metastatic. Of note, metastatic leiomyosarcoma is more common than primary liver tumors, and this can only be ruled out clinically. Distinguishing leiomyosarcomas from leiomyomas is usually readily achieved by careful morphological review. Compared with benign leiomyomas, leiomyosarcomas show cytological atypia, necrosis, and increased mitotic activity (>10 mitoses in 50 high-powered fields). Metastatic gastrointestinal stromal tumors can show morphological features similar to leiomyosarcoma, but immunohistochemical stains for KIT and DOG-1 can separate these two tumors. High-grade leiomyosarcomas can have an undifferentiated appearance mimicking undifferentiated carcinomas or sarcomas, and careful examination to identify areas with typical smooth muscle differentiation, by both H&E and immunohistochemistry, can be helpful. Inflammatory pseudotumors are reactive myofibroblastic proliferations resembling leiomyosarcomas. The spindle cells in these pseudotumors are usually bland, more basophilic, and randomly distributed, with a dense mixed inflammatory infiltrate in the background.

Prognosis and treatment

The standard therapy is complete surgical resection followed by adjuvant chemotherapy. After complete resection, the 5-year survival can reach 67%.[109]

26.8 MISCELLANEOUS TUMORS

There are a number of other tumor types which rarely arise as primary neoplasms in the liver. Their rarity as primary hepatic lesions limits most of the published literature on them to case reports. These include myelolipoma, paraganglioma, chondroma, glomus tumor, fibrosarcoma, and nerve sheath tumors. The morphological and immunohistochemical features of these rare hepatic tumors are identical to their soft-tissue counterparts. Some tumors are of interest, including undifferentiated pleomorphic sarcoma, solitary fibrous tumor, and inflammatory pseudotumors are discussed later.

Undifferentiated pleomorphic sarcoma

Definition

Undifferentiated pleomorphic sarcoma is a high-grade sarcoma composed of histologically anaplastic mesenchymal cells without a clear line of differentiation.

Etiology

The etiology of undifferentiated pleomorphic sarcoma is unknown.

Clinical features

Undifferentiated pleomorphic sarcoma is a very rare primary hepatic neoplasm. It must be emphasized that this is a diagnosis of exclusion, which should be made only when there is no prior history of a previous extrahepatic malignancy, and only in cases that lack any light microscopic or immunohistochemical evidence of specific differentiation after comprehensive evaluation. Patients often present with features referable to a large hepatic mass.

Gross findings

Undifferentiated pleomorphic sarcoma forms a large solitary mass with a variegated cut surface, reflecting areas of necrosis and hemorrhage interspersed between fleshy areas of viable tumor.

Microscopic findings

Histologically, undifferentiated pleomorphic sarcomas may show a wide variety of nonspecific histologic patterns (Fig. 26.32), similar to its soft-tissue counterpart. Such cases should be closely evaluated for any features that may suggest a more specific diagnosis, including (but not limited to) spindled cells with a myoid appearance (pleomorphic leiomyosarcoma or rhabdomyosarcoma), lipoblasts (pleomorphic liposarcoma), and osteocartilaginous matrix (osteosarcoma). Additionally, such cases should be carefully sampled

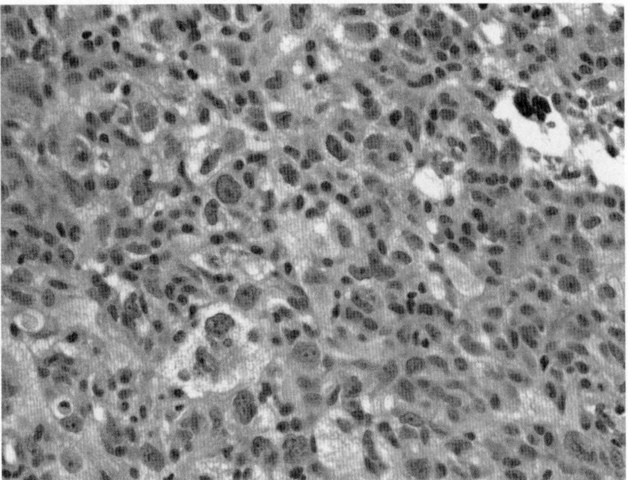

Figure 26.32 Undifferentiated pleomorphic sarcoma. The neoplastic cells appear highly anaplastic and do not have any specific features.

looking for small areas with a more epithelioid appearance, particularly for patients with a history of carcinoma or melanoma elsewhere.

Immunohistochemical findings

By definition, undifferentiated pleomorphic sarcomas lack expression of immunohistochemical markers that might point toward a specific alternative diagnosis. A comprehensive immunohistochemical workup is thus critical to exclude other tumors that enter this differential diagnosis, including undifferentiated carcinoma, malignant melanoma, high-grade gastrointestinal stromal tumors, and other specific high-grade sarcomas including histiocytic and dendritic cell tumors. It should be emphasized that expression of CD68, a nonspecific marker of lysosomes, is by no means indicative of a malignant "fibrohistiocytic" sarcoma.[110,111]

Differential diagnosis

The differential diagnosis of undifferentiated pleomorphic sarcoma is exceptionally broad. A detailed clinical history, diligent sampling, and a comprehensive immunohistochemical panel should allow for the distinction of other anaplastic malignancies from undifferentiated sarcoma.

Prognosis and treatment

The prognosis is dismal. Current chemotherapy and radiation therapy display very limited efficacy. The treatment is complete surgical resection where possible.

Solitary fibrous tumor

Definition

Solitary fibrous tumor is a spindle cell tumor with fibroblastic differentiation, possibly originating from the submesothelial tissue extending from Glisson capsule into the liver.

Etiology

A recurrent gene fusion *NAB2-STAT6* has been identified as the disease driver mutations in solitary fibrous tumors.[112,113] This genetic change results in a chimeric protein that combines the early growth response-binding domain of *NAB2* and the transactivation domain of *STAT6*.

Clinical findings

Primary hepatic solitary fibrous tumors are rare. They typically occur in older adults, with a slight female predominance. The mean age is 55 years, with a wide age range (16 to 84 years).[114,115] Patients may present with a palpable abdominal mass or with mild abdominal discomfort and weight loss. Rare cases are associated with a clinical syndrome of hypoglycemia because of overproduction of insulin-like growth factor 2.[116,117]

Gross findings

Most solitary fibrous tumors are solitary lesions with variable sizes, ranging from 2 to 32 cm. Some solitary fibrous tumors are pedunculated. Rarely, multiple tumors can occur, but possible metastatic disease has to be ruled out clinically. Solitary fibrous tumors have a smooth external surface and firm consistency. On cut surface, the tumors are typically well-circumscribed, unencapsulated, lobulated, and gray-white lesion with a whorled texture.

Microscopic findings

Microscopically, solitary fibrous tumors are characterized by a so-called "patternless pattern" with dense collagenous stroma, irregularly distributed thick-walled "staghorn" vessels, and bland spindle cells (Fig. 26.33). The "patternless pattern" refers to the variable cellularity and histologic appearances within the same tumor. The fibroblast-like spindle cells are bland and uniform and are embedded in dense collagenous stroma (often described as "ropey collagen"). The "staghorn" vessels are also known as hemangiopericytoma-like vessels. At the periphery, the spindle cells can be focally infiltrative with entrapped islands of hepatocytes and bile ducts.

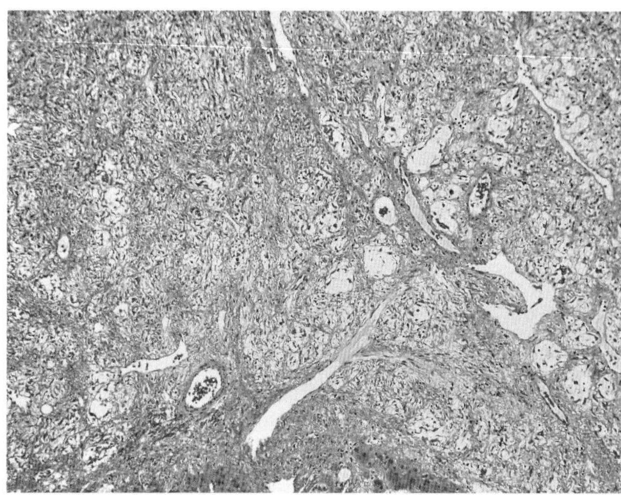

Figure 26.33 Solitary fibrous tumor. The tumor is cytologically bland and shows a pattern less pattern of growth.

About 10% to 15% of solitary fibrous tumors may undergo malignant transformation. However, there are no defined histologic features to distinguish "benign" and "malignant" tumors, i.e., some degree of malignant potential cannot be rule out in any solitary fibrous tumor. Findings that are thought to increase the risk of aggressive behavior include increased mitotic activity (>4 mitoses per 10 high-power fields), tumor necrosis, infiltrative margins, vascular invasion, high cellularity, marked atypia, and large tumor size (>10 cm).[114,117,118]

Immunohistochemical findings

Immunohistochemical detection of nuclear STAT6 is helpful in diagnosing solitary fibrous tumors. Nearly 100% of cases show strong nuclear expression of STAT6.[119,120] Molecular detection of the NAB2-STAT6 fusion is diagnostic. Other commonly used markers for solitary fibrous tumors include CD34, Bcl-2, and CD99, but they are less sensitive and less specific than STAT6. The tumor cells are negative for S100, desmin, KIT, and cytokeratins. Smooth muscle actin is typically negative, but may be weakly positive in some cases.

Differential diagnosis

The differential generally includes other spindle cell tumors identified in the liver. Of note, metastatic tumors are more common than primary liver tumors, and this can only be ruled out clinically. Gastrointestinal stromal tumors are composed of spindle cells in a well-organized pattern. Although some gastrointestinal stromal tumors can be positive for CD34, KIT and/or DOG1 positivity essentially rules out solitary fibrous tumors. Leiomyosarcomas are composed of atypical spindle cells forming fascicles intersecting at right angles. The smooth muscle differentiation usually can be recognized on morphology or by immunostains. Although a hemangiopericytoma-like pattern can be seen in some synovial sarcomas, it typically has a denser cellularity, less stroma, a biphasic pattern, and focal keratin positivity.

Prognosis and treatment

In general, the majority of solitary fibrous tumors are benign. They do not recur either locally or with distant metastases after complete resection. However, about 10% to 15% case may recur and rare cases may recur as high-grade undifferentiated sarcomas, so-called "de-differentiation." Late recurrences can occur up to 20 years after initial diagnosis.[121] A risk stratification model has been proposed based on a large-scale study. The scoring system uses the patient's age, tumor size, and mitotic rate to divide patients into low-, moderate-, and high-risk groups.[118]

Inflammatory pseudotumors

Inflammatory pseudotumor of liver can mimic a hepatic neoplasm in clinical, radiologic, and even histopathologic aspects. A variety of different names have been used to describe this benign mass-forming lesion in liver, including postinflammatory tumor, plasma cell granuloma, xanthogranuloma, inflammatory myofibroblastic lesion, fibroxanthoma, pseudolymphoma, histiocytoma, and IgG4-related pseudotumor.

Hepatic inflammatory pseudotumors are rare. They typically occur in adults between the fourth and seven decades of life with a male predominance.[122,123] The clinical presentations are nonspecific, including fever, abdominal pain, weight loss, jaundice, or an incidental finding of a mass in liver. The etiology is not fully understood but an exaggerated inflammatory response to infection, autoimmune condition, or systemic inflammation has been postulated. Inflammatory pseudotumors usually have a good prognosis. Complete regression may be achieved by conservative treatment including steroids or other anti-inflammatory drugs, and/or antibiotics. Surgical resection may occasionally take place for cases with uncertain diagnosis or local complications.

Most inflammatory pseudotumors within the liver are solitary but they are multiple in about 20% of cases. The sizes can range from <1 cm to >10 cm. They are usually well circumscribed and appear as firm, yellow, or tan white lesions grossly. Microscopically, inflammatory pseudotumors are composed of fibrous tissue, proliferating myofibroblasts, and a plasma cell-rich inflammatory infiltrate (Fig. 26.34). Lymphocytes, neutrophils, macrophages, and eosinophils are also variably present and can sometimes be focally prominent. The bland spindled myofibroblastic cells are intermixed with inflammatory cells, and mitoses are essentially absent to very rare. The collagen deposition is variable with alternative dense and loose areas. Other features, such as xanthogranulomatous inflammation, multinucleated giant cells, prominent lymphoid aggregates, and follicles, can also be seen.

A subset of inflammatory pseudotumors may represent liver involvement of IgG4-related disease (Fig. 26.35). These lesions often involve the hepatic hilum, mimicking cholangiocarcinoma. Microscopically, these inflammatory pseudotumors show characteristic features of IgG4-related systemic diseases in other organs, including dense lymphoplasmacytic infiltration, obliterative phlebitis, storiform fibrosis, and increased IgG4-positive plasma cells (>10/HPF) or

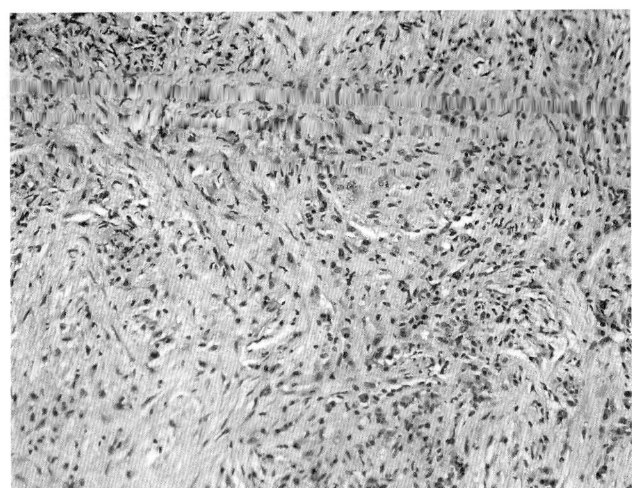

Figure 26.34 Inflammatory pseudotumor. A mass lesion was biopsied and showed fibrous tissue, proliferating myofibroblasts, and chronic inflammation that was rich in plasma cells.

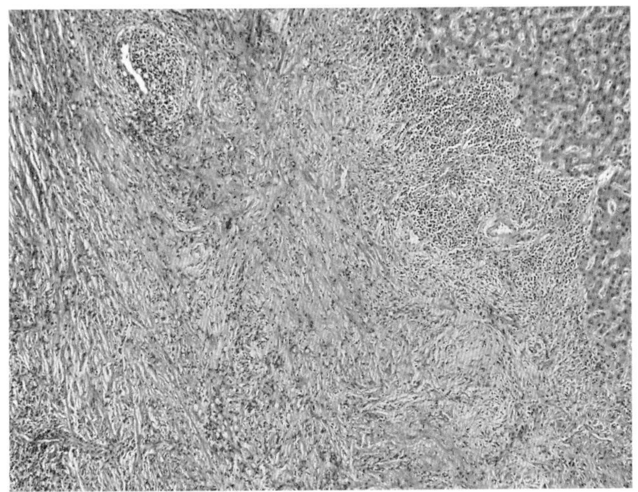

Figure 26.35 Inflammatory pseudotumor. This mass lesion was located in the liver hilum and was concerning on imaging for cholangiocarcinoma. Histologic examination showed storiform fibrosis and chronic inflammation with numerous plasma cells. An IgG 4 stain was positive (see next image).

increased IgG4/IgG positive plasma cell ratio (>40%) (Fig. 26.36).[124]

The diagnosis of inflammatory pseudotumors is always one of exclusion. An organizing abscess or tissue from the edge of liver abscess shows essentially identical morphologic changes, and a possibility of liver abscess should always be included in the differential. Syphilis in liver can also form a mass lesion with very prominent plasma cell infiltrate, and a silver stain or treponema immunostain should be performed to exclude this possibility. The spindled cells in inflammatory pseudotumors are positive for vimentin and smooth muscle actin, while they

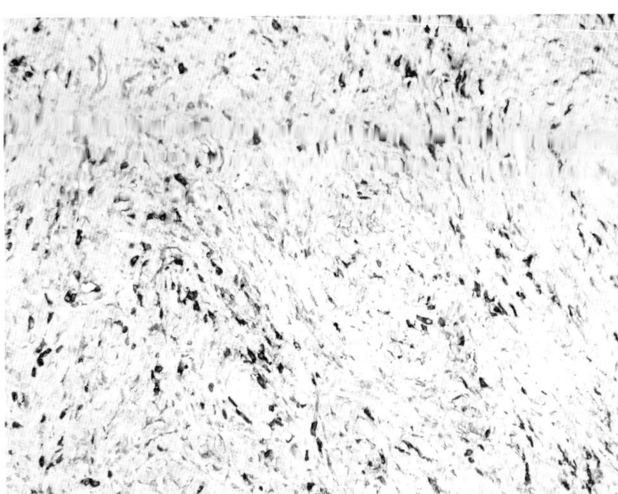

Figure 26.36 Inflammatory pseudotumor, IgG 4. This mass lesion represents IgG4 disease involving the liver.

are negative for ALK which is helpful to rule out inflammatory myofibroblastic tumor. Of note, some inflammatory pseudotumors can show patchy cytokeratin immunostaining[125] and may be mistakenly diagnosed as sarcomatoid carcinoma.

REFERENCES

1. Takahashi T, Kuwao S, Katagiri H, et al. Multiple liver hemangiomas enlargement during long-term steroid therapy for myasthenia gravis. *Dig Dis Sci.* 1998;43(7):1553–1561.
2. Giannitrapani L, Soresi M, La Spada E, et al. Sex hormones and risk of liver tumor. *Ann N Y Acad Sci.* 2006;1089:228–236.
3. Saegusa T, Ito K, Oba N, et al. Enlargement of multiple cavernous hemangioma of the liver in association with pregnancy. *Intern Med.* 1995;34(3):207–211.
4. Bioulac-Sage P, Laumonier H, Laurent C, et al. Benign and malignant vascular tumors of the liver in adults. *Semin Liver Dis.* 2008;28(3):302–314.
5. Ishak KG, Rabin L. Benign tumors of the liver. *Med Clin North Am.* 1975;59(4):995–1013.
6. Farges O, Daradkeh S, Bismuth H. Cavernous hemangiomas of the liver: are there any indications for resection? *World J Surg.* 1995;19(1):19–24.
7. Karhunen PJ. Benign hepatic tumours and tumour like conditions in men. *J Clin Pathol.* 1986;39(2):183–188.
8. Haase VH, Glickman JN, Socolovsky M, et al. Vascular tumors in livers with targeted inactivation of the von Hippel-Lindau tumor suppressor. *Proc Natl Acad Sci U S A.* 2001;98(4):1583–1588.

9. Takahashi K, Iida K, Okimura Y, et al. A novel mutation in the von Hippel-Lindau tumor suppressor gene identified in a Japanese family with pheochromocytoma and hepatic hemangioma. *Intern Med.* 2006;45(5):265–269.
10. Jhaveri KS, Vlachou PA, Guindi M, et al. Association of hepatic hemangiomatosis with giant cavernous hemangioma in the adult population: prevalence, imaging appearance, and relevance. *AJR Am J Roentgenol.* 2011;196(4):809–815.
11. Jhuang JY, Lin LW, Hsieh MS. Adult capillary hemangioma of the liver: case report and literature review. *Kaohsiung J Med Sci.* 2011;27(8):344–347.
12. Lin J, Bigge J, Ulbright TM, et al. Anastomosing hemangioma of the liver and gastrointestinal tract: an unusual variant histologically mimicking angiosarcoma. *Am J Surg Pathol.* 2013;37(11):1761–1765.
13. Montgomery E, Epstein JI. Anastomosing hemangioma of the genitourinary tract: a lesion mimicking angiosarcoma. *Am J Surg Pathol.* 2009;33(9):1364–1369.
14. John I, Folpe AL. Anastomosing hemangiomas arising in unusual locations: a clinicopathologic study of 17 soft tissue cases showing a predilection for the paraspinal region. *Am J Surg Pathol.* 2016;40(8):1084–1089.
15. Gill RM, Buelow B, Mather C, et al. Hepatic small vessel neoplasm, a rare infiltrative vascular neoplasm of uncertain malignant potential. *Hum Pathol.* 2016;54:143–151.
16. Miura JT, Amini A, Schmocker R, et al. Surgical management of hepatic hemangiomas: a multi-institutional experience. *HPB.* 2014;16(10):924–928.
17. Belli G, D'Agostino A, Fantini C, et al. Surgical treatment of giant liver hemangiomas by enucleation using an ultrasonically activated device (USAD). *Hepatogastroenterology.* 2009;56(89):236–239.
18. Asch MJ, Cohen AH, Moore TC. Hepatic and splenic lymphangiomatosis with skeletal involvement: report of a case and review of the literature. *Surgery.* 1974;76(2):334–339.
19. Haratake J, Koide O, Takeshita H. Hepatic lymphangiomatosis: report of two cases, with an immunohistochemical study. *Am J Gastroenterol.* 1992;87(7):906–909.
20. Saltz RK, Kurtz RC, Lightdale CJ, et al. Kaposi's sarcoma. Gastrointestinal involvement correlation with skin findings and immunologic function. *Dig Dis Sci.* 1984;29(9):817–823.
21. Errani C, Zhang L, Sung YS, et al. A novel WWTR1-CAMTA1 gene fusion is a consistent abnormality in epithelioid hemangioendothelioma of different anatomic sites. *Genes Chromosomes Cancer.* 2011;50(8):644–653.
22. Mendlick MR, Nelson M, Pickering D, et al. Translocation t(1;3)(p36.3;q25) is a nonrandom aberration in epithelioid hemangioendothelioma. *Am J Surg Pathol.* 2001;25(5):684–687.
23. Tanas MR, Sboner A, Oliveira AM, et al. Identification of a disease-defining gene fusion in epithelioid hemangioendothelioma. *Sci Transl Med.* 2011;3(98):98ra82.
24. Antonescu CR, Le Loarer F, Mosquera JM, et al. Novel YAP1-TFE3 fusion defines a distinct subset of epithelioid hemangioendothelioma. *Genes Chromosomes Cancer.* 2013;52(8):775–784.
25. Ishak KG, Sesterhenn IA, Goodman ZD, et al. Epithelioid hemangioendothelioma of the liver: a clinicopathologic and follow-up study of 32 cases. *Hum Pathol.* 1984;15(9):839–852.
26. Grotz TE, Nagorney D, Donohue J, et al. Hepatic epithelioid haemangioendothelioma: is transplantation the only treatment option? *HPB.* 2010;12(8):546–553.
27. Eckstein RP, Ravich RB. Epithelioid hemangioendothelioma of the liver. Report of two cases histologically mimicking veno-occlusive disease. *Pathology.* 1986;18(4):459–462.
28. Walsh MM, Hytiroglou P, Thung SN, et al. Epithelioid hemangioendothelioma of the liver mimicking Budd-Chiari syndrome. *Arch Pathol Lab Med.* 1998;122(9):846–848.
29. Makhlouf HR, Ishak KG, Goodman ZD. Epithelioid hemangioendothelioma of the liver: a clinicopathologic study of 137 cases. *Cancer.* 1999;85(3):562–582.
30. Flucke U, Vogels RJ, de Saint Aubain Somerhausen N, et al. Epithelioid Hemangioendothelioma: clinicopathologic, immunhistochemical, and molecular genetic analysis of 39 cases. *Diagn Pathol.* 2014;9:131.
31. Doyle LA, Fletcher CD, Hornick JL. Nuclear expression of CAMTA1 distinguishes epithelioid hemangioendothelioma from histologic mimics. *Am J Surg Pathol.* 2016;40(1):94–102.
32. Shibuya R, Matsuyama A, Shiba E, et al. CAMTA1 is a useful immunohistochemical marker for diagnosing epithelioid haemangioendothelioma. *Histopathology.* 2015;67(6):827–835.
33. Tsui WM, Colombari R, Portmann BC, et al. Hepatic angiomyolipoma: a clinicopathologic study of 30 cases and delineation of unusual morphologic variants. *Am J Surg Pathol.* 1999;23(1):34–48.
34. Nguyen TT, Gorman B, Shields D, et al. Malignant hepatic angiomyolipoma: report of a case and review of literature. *Am J Surg Pathol.* 2008;32(5):793–798.
35. Chaudhary P, Bhadana U, Singh RA, et al. Primary hepatic angiosarcoma. *Eur J Surg Oncol.* 2015;41(9):1137–1143.

36. Elliott P, Kleinschmidt I. Angiosarcoma of the liver in Great Britain in proximity to vinyl chloride sites. *Occup Environ Med*. 1997;54(1):14–18.
37. Lipshutz GS, Brennan TV, Warren RS. Thorotrast-induced liver neoplasia: a collective review. *J Am Coll Surg*. 2002;195(5):713–718.
38. Zheng YW, Zhang XW, Zhang JL, et al. Primary hepatic angiosarcoma and potential treatment options. *J Gastroenterol Hepatol*. 2014;29(5):906–911.
39. Duan XF, Li Q. Primary hepatic angiosarcoma: a retrospective analysis of 6 cases. *J Dig Dis*. 2012;13(7):381–385.
40. Molina E, Hernandez A. Clinical manifestations of primary hepatic angiosarcoma. *Dig Dis Sci*. 2003;48(4):677–682.
41. Mark L, Delmore F, Creech JL, Jr, et al. Clinical and morphologic features of hepatic angiosarcoma in vinyl chloride workers. *Cancer*. 1976;37(1):149–163.
42. Howard RJ, Todd EP, Dietzman RH, et al. Thorotrast-induced endothelial cell sarcoma of liver. *Minn Med*. 1971;54(9):685–688.
43. Meis-Kindblom JM, Kindblom LG. Angiosarcoma of soft tissue: a study of 80 cases. *Am J Surg Pathol*. 1998;22(6):683–697.
44. Rao P, Lahat G, Arnold C, et al. Angiosarcoma: a tissue microarray study with diagnostic implications. *Am J Dermatopathol*. 2013;35(4):432–437.
45. Sullivan HC, Edgar MA, Cohen C, et al. The utility of ERG, CD31 and CD34 in the cytological diagnosis of angiosarcoma: an analysis of 25 cases. *J Clin Pathol*. 2015;68(1):44–50.
46. Wang ZB, Yuan J, Chen W, et al. Transcription factor ERG is a specific and sensitive diagnostic marker for hepatic angiosarcoma. *World J Gastroenterol*. 2014;20(13):3672–3679.
47. Lovly CM, Gupta A, Lipson D, et al. Inflammatory myofibroblastic tumors harbor multiple potentially actionable kinase fusions. *Cancer Discov*. 2014;4(8):889–895.
48. Tessier Cloutier B, Costa FD, Tazelaar HD, et al. Aberrant expression of neuroendocrine markers in angiosarcoma: a potential diagnostic pitfall. *Hum Pathol*. 2014;45(8):1618–1624.
49. Huang SC, Zhang L, Sung YS, et al. Recurrent CIC gene abnormalities in angiosarcomas: a molecular study of 120 cases with concurrent investigation of PLCG1, KDR, MYC, and FLT4 gene alterations. *Am J Surg Pathol*. 2016;40(5):645–655.
50. Shimozono N, Jinnin M, Masuzawa M, et al. NUP160-SLC43A3 is a novel recurrent fusion oncogene in angiosarcoma. *Cancer Res*. 2015;75(21):4458–4465.
51. Kahraman A, Miller M, Baba H, et al. Angiosarcoma of the liver as a rare cause of rapidly progressive liver failure. *Med Klin*. 2006;101(9):746–750.
52. Huang IH, Wu YY, Huang TC, et al. Statistics and outlook of primary hepatic angiosarcoma based on clinical stage. *Oncol Lett*. 2016;11(5):3218–3222.
53. Mandahl N, Heim S, Johansson B, et al. Lipomas have characteristic structural chromosomal rearrangements of 12q13-q14. *Int J Cancer*. 1987;39(6):685–688.
54. Turc-Carel C, Dal Cin P, Boghosian L, et al. Breakpoints in benign lipoma may be at 12q13 or 12q14. *Cancer Genet Cytogenet*. 1988;36(1):131–135.
55. Ashar HR, Fejzo MS, Tkachenko A, et al. Disruption of the architectural factor HMGI-C: DNA-binding AT hook motifs fused in lipomas to distinct transcriptional regulatory domains. *Cell*. 1995;82(1):57–65.
56. Pierantoni GM, Battista S, Pentimalli F, et al. A truncated HMGA1 gene induces proliferation of the 3T3-L1 pre-adipocytic cells: a model of human lipomas. *Carcinogenesis*. 2003;24(12):1861–1869.
57. Wang X, Zamolyi RQ, Zhang H, et al. Fusion of HMGA1 to the LPP/TPRG1 intergenic region in a lipoma identified by mapping paraffin-embedded tissues. *Cancer Genet Cytogenet*. 2010;196(1):64–67.
58. Bruneton JN, Kerboul P, Drouillard J, et al. Hepatic lipomas: ultrasound and computed tomographic findings. *Gastrointest Radiol*. 1987;12(4):299–303.
59. Martin-Benitez G, Marti-Bonmati L, Barber C, et al. Hepatic lipomas and steatosis: an association beyond chance. *Eur J Radiol*. 2012;81(4):e491–494.
60. Binesh F, Akhavan A, Kargar S, et al. Primary liposarcoma of liver: a rare case and literature review. *BMJ Case Rep*. 2012;2012.
61. Nelson V, Fernandes NF, Woolf GM, et al. Primary liposarcoma of the liver: a case report and review of literature. *Arch Pathol Lab Med*. 2001;125(3):410–412.
62. Bonetti F, Pea M, Martignoni G, et al. Clear cell ("sugar") tumor of the lung is a lesion strictly related to angiomyolipoma--the concept of a family of lesions characterized by the presence of the perivascular epithelioid cells (PEC). *Pathology*. 1994;26(3):230–236.
63. Martignoni G, Pea M, Reghellin D, et al. PEComas: the past, the present and the future. *Virchows Arch*. 2008;452(2):119–132.
64. Folpe AL, Kwiatkowski DJ. Perivascular epithelioid cell neoplasms: pathology and pathogenesis. *Hum Pathol*. 2010;41(1):1–15.
65. Thway K, Fisher C. PEComa: morphology and genetics of a complex tumor family. *Ann Diagn Pathol*. 2015;19(5):359–368.
66. Black ME, Hedgire SS, Camposano S, et al. Hepatic manifestations of tuberous sclerosis complex: a genotypic and phenotypic analysis. *Clin Genet*. 2012;82(6):552–557.

67. Ben Hamida F, Gorsane I, Gharbi C, et al. Renal manifestations in tuberous sclerosis. *Rev Med Interne*. 2006;27(11):836–842.
68. Liu J, Zhang CW, Hong DF, et al. Primary hepatic epithelioid angiomyolipoma: a malignant potential tumor which should be recognized. *World J Gastroenterol*. 2016;22(20):4908–4917.
69. Huang SC, Chuang HC, Chen TD, et al. Alterations of the mTOR pathway in hepatic angiomyolipoma with emphasis on the epithelioid variant and loss of heterogeneity of TSC1/TSC2. *Histopathology*. 2015;66(5):695–705.
70. Yang X, Li A, Wu M. Hepatic angiomyolipoma: clinical, imaging and pathological features in 178 cases. *Med Oncol*. 2013;30(1):416.
71. Nonomura A, Enomoto Y, Takeda M, et al. Angiomyolipoma of the liver: a reappraisal of morphological features and delineation of new characteristic histological features from the clinicopathological findings of 55 tumours in 47 patients. *Histopathology*. 2012;61(5):863–880.
72. Folpe AL, Mentzel T, Lehr HA, et al. Perivascular epithelioid cell neoplasms of soft tissue and gynecologic origin: a clinicopathologic study of 26 cases and review of the literature. *Am J Surg Pathol*. 2005;29(12):1558–1575.
73. Nonomura A, Mizukami Y, Shimizu K, et al. Angiomyolipoma mimicking true lipoma of the liver: report of two cases. *Pathol Int*. 1996;46(3):221–227.
74. Fadare O. Perivascular epithelioid cell tumors (PEComas) and smooth muscle tumors of the uterus. *Am J Surg Pathol*. 2007;31(9):1454–1455; author reply 5–6.
75. Simpson KW, Albores-Saavedra J. HMB-45 reactivity in conventional uterine leiomyosarcomas. *Am J Surg Pathol*. 2007;31(1):95–98.
76. Nonomura A, Minato H, Kurumaya H. Angiomyolipoma predominantly composed of smooth muscle cells: problems in histological diagnosis. *Histopathology*. 1998;33(1):20–27.
77. Delgado R, de Leon Bojorge B, Albores-Saavedra J. Atypical angiomyolipoma of the kidney: a distinct morphologic variant that is easily confused with a variety of malignant neoplasms. *Cancer*. 1998;83(8):1581–1592.
78. Eble JN, Amin MB, Young RH. Epithelioid angiomyolipoma of the kidney: a report of five cases with a prominent and diagnostically confusing epithelioid smooth muscle component. *Am J Surg Pathol*. 1997;21(10):1123–1130.
79. Zhong DR, Ji XL. Hepatic angiomyolipoma-misdiagnosis as hepatocellular carcinoma: a report of 14 cases. *World J Gastroenterol*. 2000;6(4):608–612.
80. Xie L, Jessurun J, Manivel JC, et al. Hepatic epithelioid angiomyolipoma with trabecular growth pattern: a mimic of hepatocellular carcinoma on fine needle aspiration cytology. *Diagn Cytopathol*. 2012;40(7):639–650.
81. Parfitt JR, Bella AJ, Izawa JI, et al. Malignant neoplasm of perivascular epithelioid cells of the liver. *Arch Pathol Lab Med*. 2006;130(8):1219–1222.
82. Makhlouf HR, Ishak KG, Shekar R, et al. Melanoma markers in angiomyolipoma of the liver and kidney: a comparative study. *Arch Pathol Lab Med*. 2002;126(1):49–55.
83. Hornick JL, Fletcher CD. PEComa: what do we know so far? *Histopathology*. 2006;48(1):75–82.
84. Colombino M, Capone M, Lissia A, et al. BRAF/NRAS mutation frequencies among primary tumors and metastases in patients with melanoma. *J Clin Oncol*. 2012;30(20):2522–2529.
85. Curatolo P, Moavero R, Roberto D, et al. Genotype/phenotype correlations in tuberous sclerosis complex. *Semin Pediatr Neurol*. 2015;22(4):259–273.
86. Yamamoto H, Yoshida A, Taguchi K, et al. ALK, ROS1 and NTRK3 gene rearrangements in inflammatory myofibroblastic tumors. *Histopathology*. 2016;69(1):72–83.
87. Alassiri AH, Ali RH, Shen Y, et al. ETV6-NTRK3 is expressed in a subset of ALK-negative inflammatory myofibroblastic tumors. *Am J Surg Pathol*. 2016;40(8):1051–1061.
88. Griffin CA, Hawkins AL, Dvorak C, et al. Recurrent involvement of 2p23 in inflammatory myofibroblastic tumors. *Cancer Res*. 1999;59(12):2776–2780.
89. Coffin CM, Hornick JL, Fletcher CD. Inflammatory myofibroblastic tumor: comparison of clinicopathologic, histologic, and immunohistochemical features including ALK expression in atypical and aggressive cases. *Am J Surg Pathol*. 2007;31(4):509–520.
90. Coffin CM, Watterson J, Priest JR, et al. Extrapulmonary inflammatory myofibroblastic tumor (inflammatory pseudotumor). A clinicopathologic and immunohistochemical study of 84 cases. *Am J Surg Pathol*. 1995;19(8):859–872.
91. Marino-Enriquez A, Wang WL, Roy A, et al. Epithelioid inflammatory myofibroblastic sarcoma: an aggressive intra-abdominal variant of inflammatory myofibroblastic tumor with nuclear membrane or perinuclear ALK. *Am J Surg Pathol*. 2011;35(1):135–144.
92. Li J, Yin WH, Takeuchi K, et al. Inflammatory myofibroblastic tumor with RANBP2 and ALK gene rearrangement: a report of two cases and literature review. *Diagn Pathol*. 2013;8:147.
93. Hornick JL, Sholl LM, Dal Cin P, et al. Expression of ROS1 predicts ROS1 gene rearrangement in

inflammatory myofibroblastic tumors. *Mod Pathol.* 2015;28(5):732–739.

94. Chen TC, Kuo TT, Ng KF. Follicular dendritic cell tumor of the liver: a clinicopathologic and Epstein-Barr virus study of two cases. *Mod Pathol* 2001;14(4):354–360.
95. Perez-Ordonez B, Rosai J. Follicular dendritic cell tumor: review of the entity. *Semin Diagn Pathol.* 1998;15(2):144–154.
96. Lucas DR, Shukla A, Thomas DG, et al. Dedifferentiated liposarcoma with inflammatory myofibroblastic tumor-like features. *Am J Surg Pathol.* 2010;34(6):844–851.
97. Sirvent N, Coindre JM, Maire G, et al. Detection of MDM2-CDK4 amplification by fluorescence in situ hybridization in 200 paraffin-embedded tumor samples: utility in diagnosing adipocytic lesions and comparison with immunohistochemistry and real-time PCR. *Am J Surg Pathol.* 2007;31(10):1476–1489.
98. Binh MB, Sastre-Garau X, Guillou L, et al. MDM2 and CDK4 immunostainings are useful adjuncts in diagnosing well-differentiated and dedifferentiated liposarcoma subtypes: a comparative analysis of 559 soft tissue neoplasms with genetic data. *Am J Surg Pathol.* 2005;29(10):1340–1347.
99. Lawrence B, Perez-Atayde A, Hibbard MK, et al. TPM3-ALK and TPM4-ALK oncogenes in inflammatory myofibroblastic tumors. *Am J Pathol.* 2000;157(2):377–384.
100. Bridge JA, Kanamori M, Ma Z, et al. Fusion of the ALK gene to the clathrin heavy chain gene, CLTC, in inflammatory myofibroblastic tumor. *Am J Pathol.* 2001;159(2):411–415.
101. Ma Z, Hill DA, Collins MH, et al. Fusion of ALK to the Ran-binding protein 2 (RANBP2) gene in inflammatory myofibroblastic tumor. *Genes Chromosomes Cancer.* 2003;37(1):98–105.
102. Cools J, Wlodarska I, Somers R, et al. Identification of novel fusion partners of ALK, the anaplastic lymphoma kinase, in anaplastic large-cell lymphoma and inflammatory myofibroblastic tumor. *Genes Chromosomes Cancer.* 2002;34(4):354–362.
103. Debiec-Rychter M, Marynen P, Hagemeijer A, et al. ALK-ATIC fusion in urinary bladder inflammatory myofibroblastic tumor. *Genes Chromosomes Cancer.* 2003;38(2):187–190.
104. Panagopoulos I, Nilsson T, Domanski HA, et al. Fusion of the SEC31L1 and ALK genes in an inflammatory myofibroblastic tumor. *Int J Cancer.* 2006;118(5):1181–1186.
105. Butrynski JE, D'Adamo DR, Hornick JL, et al. Crizotinib in ALK-rearranged inflammatory myofibroblastic tumor. *N Engl J Med.* 2010;363(18):1727–1733.
106. Shamseddine A, Faraj W, Mukherji D, et al. Unusually young age distribution of primary hepatic leiomyosarcoma: case series and review of the adult literature. *World J Surg Oncol.* 2010;8:56.
107. Chi M, Dudek AZ, Wind KP. Primary hepatic leiomyosarcoma in adults: analysis of prognostic factors. *Onkologie.* 2012;35(4):210–214.
108. Guo X, Jo VY, Mills AM, et al. Clinically relevant molecular subtypes in leiomyosarcoma. *Clin Cancer Res.* 2015;21(15):3501–3511.
109. Weitz J, Klimstra DS, Cymes K, et al. Management of primary liver sarcomas. *Cancer.* 2007;109(7):1391–1396.
110. Ye MF, Zheng S, Xu JH, et al. Primary hepatic malignant fibrous histiocytoma: a case report and review of the literature. *Histol Histopathol.* 2007;22(12):1337–1342.
111. Li YR, Akbari E, Tretiakova MS, et al. Primary hepatic malignant fibrous histiocytoma: clinicopathologic characteristics and prognostic value of ezrin expression. *Am J Surg Pathol.* 2008;32(8):1144–1158.
112. Robinson DR, Wu YM, Kalyana-Sundaram S, et al. Identification of recurrent NAB2-STAT6 gene fusions in solitary fibrous tumor by integrative sequencing. *Nat Genet.* 2013;45(2):180–185.
113. Barthelmess S, Geddert H, Boltze C, et al. Solitary fibrous tumors/hemangiopericytomas with different variants of the NAB2-STAT6 gene fusion are characterized by specific histomorphology and distinct clinicopathological features. *Am J Pathol.* 2014;184(4):1209–1218.
114. Moran CA, Ishak KG, Goodman ZD. Solitary fibrous tumor of the liver: a clinicopathologic and immunohistochemical study of nine cases. *Ann Diagn Pathol.* 1998;2(1):19–24.
115. Perini MV, Herman P, D'Albuquerque LA, et al. Solitary fibrous tumor of the liver: report of a rare case and review of the literature. *Int J Surg.* 2008;6(5):396–399.
116. Fama F, Le Bouc Y, Barrande G, et al. Solitary fibrous tumour of the liver with IGF-II-related hypoglycaemia. A case report. *Langenbecks Arch Surg.* 2008;393(4):611–616.
117. Chan G, Horton PJ, Thyssen S, et al. Malignant transformation of a solitary fibrous tumor of the liver and intractable hypoglycemia. *J Hepatobiliary Pancreat Surg.* 2007;14(6):595–599.
118. Demicco EG, Park MS, Araujo DM, et al. Solitary fibrous tumor: a clinicopathological study of 110 cases and proposed risk assessment model. *Mod Pathol.* 2012;25(9):1298–1306.
119. Doyle LA, Vivero M, Fletcher CD, et al. Nuclear expression of STAT6 distinguishes solitary fibrous tumor from histologic mimics. *Mod Pathol.* 2014;27(3):390–395.

120. Vogels RJ, Vlenterie M, Versleijen-Jonkers YM, et al. Solitary fibrous tumor – clinicopathologic, immunohistochemical and molecular analysis of 28 cases. *Diagn Pathol.* 2014;9:224.
121. Baldi GG, Stacchiotti S, Mauro V, et al. Solitary fibrous tumor of all sites: outcome of late recurrences in 14 patients. *Clin Sarcoma Res.* 2013;3:4.
122. Schmid A, Janig D, Bohuszlavizki A, et al. Inflammatory pseudotumor of the liver presenting as incidentaloma: report of a case and review of the literature. *Hepatogastroenterology.* 1996;43(10):1009–1014.
123. Park JY, Choi MS, Lim YS, et al. Clinical features, image findings, and prognosis of inflammatory pseudotumor of the liver: a multicenter experience of 45 cases. *Gut Liver.* 2014;8(1):58–63.
124. Zen Y, Fujii T, Sato Y, et al. Pathological classification of hepatic inflammatory pseudotumor with respect to IgG4-related disease. *Mod Pathol.* 2007;20(8):884–894.
125. Tang L, Lai EC, Cong WM, et al. Inflammatory myofibroblastic tumor of the liver: a cohort study. *World J Surg.* 2010;34(2):309–313.

27 Benign hepatocellular tumors

Dora Lam-Himlin, MD

27.1 FOCAL NODULAR HYPERPLASIA

Definition

Focal nodular hyperplasia is a benign hyperplastic reactive lesion composed of nodules of hepatocytes separated by fibrotic bands in a noncirrhotic liver. Other historical names for focal nodular hyperplasia include solitary hyperplastic nodule, hepatic hamartoma, focal cirrhosis, hamartomatous cholangiohepatoma, and hepatic pseudotumor.

Clinical features

Focal nodular hyperplasia is the second most common benign lesion of the liver after hemangioma. It represents up to 86% of nonhemangiomatous benign lesions and occurs 3 to 10 times more frequently than hepatic adenomas.[1–3] Although focal nodular hyperplasia is seen in both sexes throughout the age spectrum, these lesions are 10 times more common in women, with 75% occurring in young women between the ages of 20 and 50 years (median 41 years).[4] Less commonly, they are seen in children and adolescents, where they comprise up to 2% of all hepatic lesions in children.[5]

Focal nodular hyperplasia is usually solitary, although multiple nodules have been reported in 20% to 30% of cases.[6] Most cases are asymptomatic and discovered incidentally at the time of surgery, on unrelated imaging studies, or at autopsy. Patients who do report symptoms describe abdominal discomfort, pain, or a palpable mass.[6,7] Focal nodular hyperplasia can be evaluated by computed tomography or magnetic resonance imaging because imaging studies show highly characteristic features and are diagnostic in 90% of cases.[8,9] In these cases, a biopsy is usually unnecessary for diagnosis. Unlike hepatic adenomas, focal nodular hyperplasias do not carry any risk for malignant transformation and they only rarely present with acute infarction, necrosis, or hemorrhage.[10,11]

Etiology

Focal nodular hyperplasias are the result of parenchymal hyperplasia in response to increased blood flow and arterial shunting, usually as a result of vascular malformations.[12] In fact, 23% of patients with focal nodular hyperplasia have associated hemangiomas.[13] The relationship between these lesions and vascular shunting is further supported by the presence of focal nodular hyperplasia lesions in patients with hereditary hemorrhagic telangiectasia (Osler–Weber–Rendu disease)[14] as well as hemihypertrophy and vascular malformations (Klippel–Trénaunay–Weber syndrome).[15]

A tenuous relationship between oral contraceptives and focal nodular hyperplasia has been reported,[16] but the data arguing against a causal relationship are strong. For example, focal nodular hyperplasias occur in men and children who do not use oral contraceptives.[17] Furthermore, focal nodular hyperplasia was first described in the early 1900s, long before the advent of oral contraceptives, and its incidence has remained steady after the introduction of oral contraceptives in the 1960s.[18,19] This observation is in sharp contrast to the dramatic rise in the incidence of hepatic adenomas in the same time period.[19] Although likely not causal, estrogens may play a role in the growth of focal nodular hyperplasia because there have been reports of focal nodular hyperplasia enlarging in the setting of oral contraceptives or pregnancy.[16]

In the pediatric population, focal nodular hyperplasias are often preceded by chemotherapy for malignancies of other organs and typically occur many years after the treatment.

Gross findings

By definition, the background liver is noncirrhotic. The lesions are usually solitary (80% to 95%), well demarcated, without a capsule, and can occasionally be pedunculated.[6] They are found more commonly in the right lobe and are usually <5 cm in diameter, with only 3% larger than 10 cm; rare reports describe focal nodular hyperplasias as large as 19 cm.[6,20] On cut section, the lesions are lobulated and have a firm rubbery texture. They may be lighter in color than the surrounding liver. A characteristic finding is the presence of a central stellate scar, or multiple scars, with radiating fibrous bands separating lobules of parenchyma (Fig. 27.1), imparting the "spoke and wheel" architecture commonly seen on imaging studies. Smaller lesions, particularly those that are <3 cm, may lack this characteristic scar, which is seen in 62% of lesions overall.[6,21]

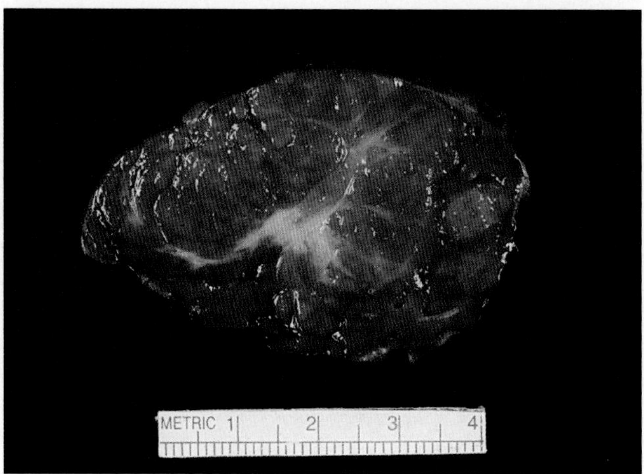

Figure 27.1 Focal nodular hyperplasia. On gross examination, the cut section shows pale fibrous bands separating the hepatic parenchyma into lobules with a central scar.

Microscopic findings

Histologically, focal nodular hyperplasias are well demarcated but unencapsulated lesions composed of benign hepatocytes with characteristic fibrous bands radiating from a central scar-like area (Figs. 27.2 and 27.3). These fibrous bands can encompass cords or nodules of hepatic parenchyma, resulting in the appearance of focal cirrhosis, a potential pitfall in needle biopsy specimens. However, the scar-like tissue within focal nodular hyperplasia nodules does not contain true portal tracts, but instead contains abnormal large feeder arteries that may have medial hypertrophy and intimal fibrosis (Fig. 27.4), at times even occluding the lumen. The native bile ducts are replaced by a prominent bile ductular proliferation traveling along the edge of the fibrous septae (Fig. 27.5). These characteristics may be less developed in smaller lesions, instead appearing more like bridging fibrosis than focal cirrhosis.

The hepatocytes within the lesion are essentially indistinguishable from those in the background noncirrhotic parenchyma and show no cytological or architectural atypia. However, the poor bile drainage in these lesions can result in cholate stasis, copper deposition, feathery degeneration of hepatocytes, and

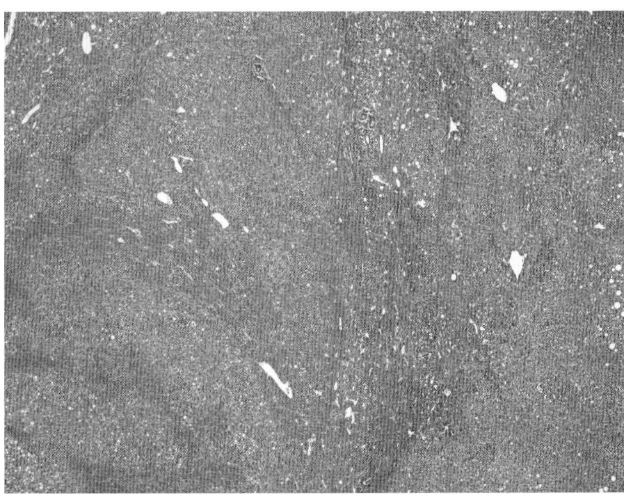

Figure 27.2 Focal nodular hyperplasia. The lesion is seen to the left of this photo, with radiating fibrous bands. Although the lesion is unencapsulated, the edge of the lesion can be well demarcated due to a fibrous rim or the presence of ductular proliferation.

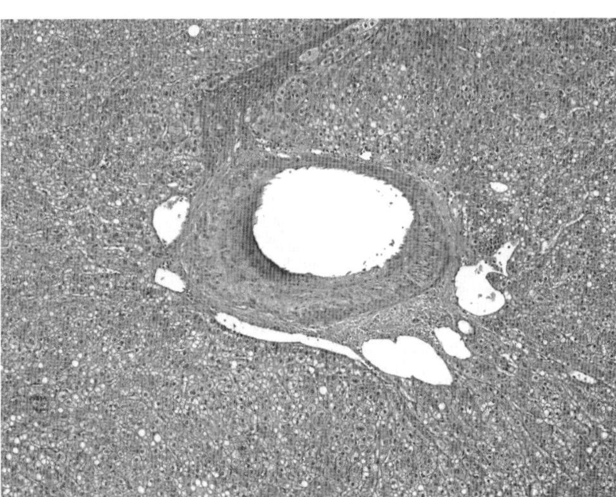

Figure 27.4 Focal nodular hyperplasia. The scar-like tissue within these lesions contain abnormal large arteries, some of which may have medial hypertrophy, such as seen in this eccentric artery.

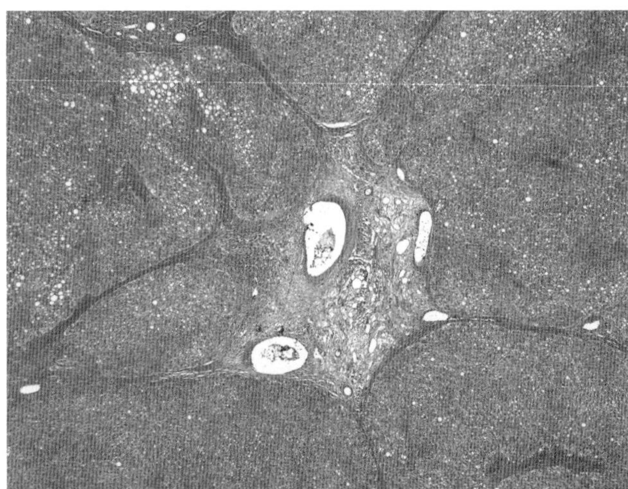

Figure 27.3 Focal nodular hyperplasia. The central stellate scar with radiating "spoke in wheel" fibrous bands is a highly characteristic feature, although may be absent in smaller lesions.

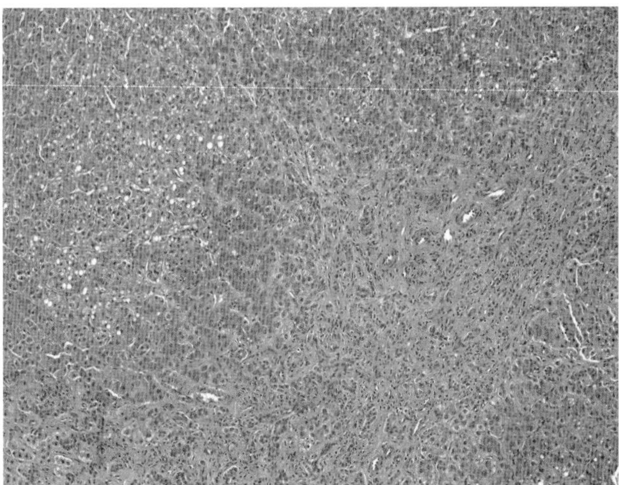

Figure 27.5 Focal nodular hyperplasia. Native bile ducts are replaced by prominent bile ductular proliferation traveling along the edge of the fibrous septae or at the periphery of the lesion.

Mallory hyaline accumulation in areas adjacent to the fibrous bands. Hepatocytes within the focal nodular hyperplasia can also show steatosis, and lymphocytic inflammation may be found in the fibrous bands.

Immunohistochemical findings

Because most diagnoses of focal nodular hyperplasias can be made on radiologic examination, excision or biopsy occurs only when radiologic features are atypical and the diagnosis is unclear, such as in smaller lesions that do not exhibit classic stellate scars. The lack of classic features can also prove diagnostically challenging for pathologists, and special stains or immunohistochemistry can aid in the diagnosis. Glutamine synthetase, a surrogate marker for β-catenin activation, is perhaps the most useful immunostain in the diagnosis of focal nodular hyperplasias. One study demonstrated an increase in confident diagnosis to 90% of cases with the addition of this immunostain, as compared with only 50% of cases using morphology alone.[22] Glutamine synthetase results in a "map-like" pattern of staining in 90% of focal nodular hyperplasias (Fig. 27.6), with strong cytoplasmic reactivity in central areas, contrasted by broad geographic areas of nonreactive hepatocytes near the fibrous bands.[22] By comparison, the normal liver shows glutamine synthetase staining limited to the few hepatocytes directly adjacent to the central vein. This map-like staining quality can be useful in differentiating focal nodular hyperplasias from hepatic adenoma (see section Differential Diagnosis). Other immunostains commonly used to subtype hepatic adenomas include liver fatty acid-binding protein (L-FABP), β-catenin, serum amyloid A, and C-reactive protein. In focal nodular hyperplasias, immunostains for L-FABP show normal retained expression, β-catenin is nonreactive for nuclear expression (but shows normal cytoplasmic or membranous reactivity), and serum amyloid A and C-reactive protein are negative for strong and diffuse staining, though patchy staining can be seen in some cases of focal nodular hyperplasias.[23]

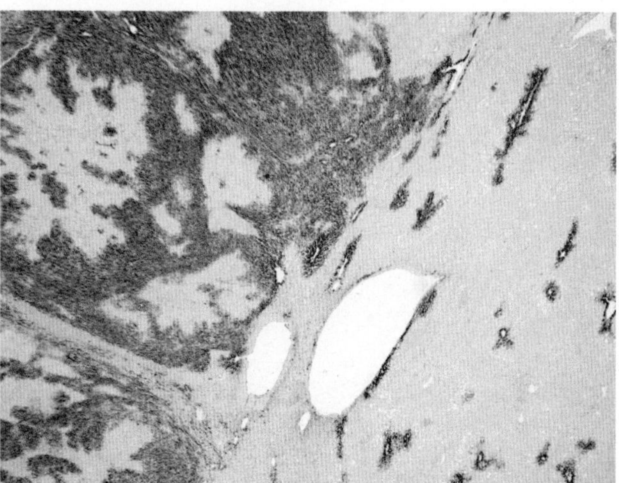

Figure 27.6 Focal nodular hyperplasia. Glutamine synthetase immunostain shows broad bands of hepatocyte staining in a geographic map-like pattern in the lesional tissue (left), whereas the nonneoplastic liver (right) shows only peri-central-venular staining.

Other stains commonly used in the evaluation of liver biopsies include reticulin, which will highlight a normal reticulin framework with cell plates 1 to 2 hepatocytes in width, and copper stains such as Rhodamine, which can highlight copper accumulation in hepatocytes adjacent to the fibrous bands, a result of impaired bile drainage. Copper is not specific for focal nodular hyperplasia, as it is also positive in some inflammatory adenomas and hepatocellular carcinomas.

Cytology findings

In the setting of a noncirrhotic patient, the diagnosis of focal nodular hyperplasia can be suggested if hepatocytes are accompanied by bile duct epithelium and, sometimes, by fibrous tissue. The presence of bile duct epithelium essentially rules out adenomas and hepatocellular carcinomas.

Differential diagnosis

The differential diagnoses for focal nodular hyperplasia include benign reactive changes, such as cirrhosis and mass effect. The differential can also include hepatocellular carcinoma, fibrolamellar carcinoma, and inflammatory hepatic adenomas, which will be covered in a later section. The use of glutamine synthetase immunostain can be very helpful in this differential.

When clinical and radiologic history is unavailable, the presence of fibrous bands and bile ductular proliferation may raise the possibility of cirrhosis as a morphologic consideration. However, the absence of normal portal tracts and the presence of large abnormal blood vessels with thickened walls should alert one to the possibility of a focal nodular hyperplasia. A glutamine synthetase immunostain with map-like reactivity can confirm the diagnosis of focal nodular hyperplasia.

Likewise, if a targeted needle biopsy fails to sample a mass lesion, but instead samples the adjacent reactive/hyperplastic parenchyma, one may see fibrous bands, bile ductular proliferation, and periportal cholate stasis, all changes resembling focal nodular hyperplasia. However, the presence of native bile ducts within true portal tracts should steer one away from a diagnosis of focal nodular hyperplasia. As noted before, glutamine synthetase immunostains will show a map-like staining pattern in focal nodular hyperplasia, whereas the normal liver parenchyma will show reactivity in only a small rim of hepatocytes surrounding the central vein.

In both cirrhosis and mass effect changes, a vascular shunt can result in reactive hyperplastic areas that resemble focal nodular hyperplasia. Despite the histologic similarities, these lesions are best regarded as "focal nodular hyperplasia-like" lesions rather than true focal nodular hyperplasia.

Fibrolamellar carcinomas can be associated with a focal nodular hyperplasia-like change at their periphery, and the frequent finding of a central scar in fibrolamellar carcinoma may cause confusion radiologically.[24,25] However, the histologic differentiation should be uncomplicated. Although fibrolamellar carcinoma can have areas of scar and fibrosis, the similarities end there. Hepatocytes in fibrolamellar carcinoma are atypical and enlarged with abundant eosinophilic cytoplasm and nuclei containing prominent nucleoli—features never seen in focal nodular hyperplasia.

The steatohepatitic variant of hepatocellular carcinoma might also be a consideration in cases where a focal nodular hyperplasia shows fat plus extensive cholate stasis, resulting in feathery degeneration and Mallory hyaline. However, as mentioned above, focal nodular hyperplasia lacks the cytological and architectural atypia seen in hepatocellular carcinoma. Focal nodular hyperplasias do not show nuclear pleomorphism, prominent nucleoli, widened cell plates, or disruption of the reticulin network. Immunostains can help with this differential diagnosis because glutamine synthetase will show the characteristic map-like reactivity in focal nodular hyperplasia. Another potentially helpful immunostain, Glypican-3 (further discussed in the following chapter on Malignant hepatocellular tumors) is positive in the many hepatocellular carcinoma but is negative in focal nodular hyperplasia. Table 27.1 highlights the main histologic features and staining patterns of the lesions covered in this chapter and provides a comparison with hepatocellular carcinoma.

Focal nodular hyperplasia-like lesions

Cirrhotic livers can develop vascular shunts that lead to nodular lesions that histologically look like focal nodular hyperplasias and show similar staining characteristics.[26] In cirrhotic livers, these lesions are called focal nodular hyperplasia-like lesions. They are found more commonly in individuals who have undergone chemoembolization for liver tumors.[27]

Treatment

Focal nodular hyperplasia lesions are typically stable, although some lesions may become smaller over time,[28] and others have enlarged in the setting of oral contraceptive use or pregnancy.[16] Regardless, in contrast to hepatic adenomas, focal nodular hyperplasia lesions do not carry much risk for infarction, necrosis, or hemorrhage and have no risk for malignant transformation.[6,7,29] Patients are managed conservatively. If a diagnosis remains unclear following biopsy, follow-up studies at 3 and 6 months are often sufficient to confirm the stability of the lesion and its benign nature, after which long-term follow-up may not be required. Surgery is reserved for rare symptomatic lesions or lesions with atypical features that cannot be distinguished from malignancy. Oral contraceptives and other estrogen containing preparations need not be discontinued, although follow-up imaging study in 6 to 12 months is reasonable. Small focal nodular hyperplasias do not appear to pose a significant risk to a successful pregnancy, although larger focal nodular hyperplasia (>8 cm) may require close observation and resection.[30,31]

27.2 HEPATIC ADENOMA

Definition

Hepatic adenoma, also known as hepatocellular adenoma and liver cell adenoma, is a benign neoplasm composed of hepatocytes.

Clinical features

Hepatic adenomas are typically solitary lesions that arise more commonly in the right lobe of the liver and can range in size from 1 to 30 cm. Patients may be asymptomatic, have mild abdominal discomfort, or present acutely with tumor rupture and hemorrhage.[32] Larger lesions are more likely to present with symptoms such as abdominal pain,[33] and lesions >5 cm have higher risk of bleeding—a sequela which is accompanied by sudden severe pain and hypotension. On physical examination, an abdominal mass can be identified in up to 30% of patients, whereas hepatomegaly is present in approximately 25%. Elevations in liver function tests are rare, but elevations of alkaline phosphatase and jaundice have been described, presumably reflecting compression of intrahepatic bile ducts by an enlarging tumor. γ glutamyl transpeptidase (GGT) may be elevated, particularly in patients with intratumoral bleeding or multiple adenomas. α fetoprotein is normal except in some cases of malignant transformation. Whereas up to half of patients can have multiple adenomas,[32] about 10% to 15% of

Table 27.1 Key histologic features and staining patterns of benign hepatocellular neoplasms with comparison to hepatocellular carcinoma

Tumor	Subtype, if applicable	Key histologic features	Glutamine synthetase	Fatty acid-binding protein (L-FABP)	C-reactive protein (CRP)	Serum amyloid A	β-Catenin (nuclear localization)	Glypican 3
FNH		Central stellate fibrous scar, ductular proliferation, thickened-wall abnormal arteries, bland hepatocytes	++ (90%) map-like pattern	Retained	– or patchy	– or patchy	–	–
Adenoma	HNF1α-inactivated adenoma	Absence of bile ducts, naked arteries, bland hepatocytes, no cyto-architectural atypia or mitoses	– (1% may show diffuse staining)	Lost	–	–	–	–
	Inflammatory hepatic adenoma	Typical adenoma features, plus: chronic inflammatory cells, ductular proliferation mimicking portal areas, dilated sinusoids and congestion, frequently fatty	– (10% may show diffuse staining)	Retained	+	+	–	–
	β-catenin-activated adenoma	Typical adenoma features, plus: may show mild cytologic atypia	++ (strong, diffuse cytoplasmic reactivity	Retained	–	–	++	–
	Unclassified adenoma	Typical adenoma features	–	Retained	–	–	–	–
	Pigmented adenoma	Typical adenoma features, plus: cytoplasmic pigment deposition distinctive from background liver	± (if present, diffuse)	±	±	±	±	–
	Atypical adenoma	Typical adenoma features, plus any of the following: older male, background liver disease, cytologic atypia, pseudoacinar formation, nodule-in-nodule appearance, focal reticulin loss	± (if present, diffuse)	±	±	±	±	–
Hepatocellular carcinoma		Absence of bile ducts, naked arteries, pseudoacinar formation, thickened cell plates, cytologic atypia, loss of reticulin	± (20% may show diffuse staining)	20% show loss	50% positive	20% positive	30% positive	75%–90% positive
Macroregenerative nodule		Cirrhotic backdrop, true portal tracts with bile ducts, bland hepatocytes, no cyto-architectural atypia	– (normal central perivenular reactivity)	Retained	–	–	–	–

patients have 10 or more lesions—a condition called hepatic adenomatosis.[34]

Hepatic adenomatosis

Hepatic adenomatosis is defined formally by the presence of 10 or more adenomas in the liver. Originally, hepatic adenomatosis was thought to be a genetically distinct entity from cases with a single or few hepatic adenomas, but this is no longer generally thought to be true. Early definitions excluded cases arising in glycogen storage diseases, or in the setting of steroid use, or that improved upon steroid withdrawal. Hepatic adenomatosis in some studies has a more equal distribution in men and women, and cases typically show elevation of alkaline phosphatase and GGT levels.[35,36] Currently, hepatic adenomatosis is no longer considered to be distinct entity.[37]

Hepatic adenomatosis can be associated with congenital or acquired abnormalities of hepatic vasculature (e.g., congenital absence of portal vein, portal venous thrombosis with cavernous transformation, or intrahepatic portosystemic shunts).[38] Lesions in adenomatosis appear to have a higher rate of hemorrhage when compared with traditional hepatic adenomas (62% vs. 26% in one study),[36] in particular those >4 cm and subcapsular in location. The adenomas found in hepatic adenomatosis may be of any subtype, including inflammatory, hepatocyte nuclear factor 1 α (HNF1α) inactivated, β-catenin activated, or unclassified.[39] In some cases of adenomatosis, subclassification can show a mixture of separate inflammatory adenomas, β-catenin-activated adenomas, and inflammatory adenomas with secondary β-catenin activation. Malignant transformation has been well documented.[38,39]

Demographics

Hepatic adenomas are uncommon tumors, with 85% of cases occurring in young to middle-aged women with a history of oral contraceptive use.[40–42] The annual incidence is 30 to 40 per million in long-term users (>2 years), compared with 1 per million in women who have never used oral contraceptives.[42,43] Hepatic adenomas were rarely reported before the advent of oral contraceptives in the 1960s, and subsequent studies have shown that dose and duration of hormonal therapy directly correlates with the size, number, and frequency of bleeding in these tumors.[41,42,44–48] Regression of adenomas has been observed after discontinuation of oral contraceptive, with recurrence during readministration or pregnancy.[49,50] The current formulations of low-dose estrogen oral contraceptive have led to a reduction in tumor incidence, but tumor development is not limited to oral contraceptive use because any population receiving estrogen for medical purposes can develop adenomas.

Exogenous androgen and anabolic steroid administration have also been associated with development of hepatic adenomas. Androgens may be used in the treatment of impotence, Fanconi syndrome, and muscle mass development for body builders and transsexuals. Similar to oral contraceptives, androgens predispose to multiple adenomas that frequently regress after discontinuation.[51–54]

Patients with glycogen storage diseases, particularly Types I and III, are also at risk for the development of hepatic adenomas. The incidence is up to 51% with Type I and 25% with Type III glycogen storage disease, and the hepatic adenomas tend to be multiple, more common in males, and occur before the age of 20 years.[55–58] Adenomas occurring in glycogen storage disease Type IV have also been reported.[59]

Other associated conditions have also been reported, such as familial adenomatous polyposis, polycystic ovary syndrome, Peutz–Jeghers syndrome, and patients taking the antiepileptic medications carbamazepine and valproate.[60,61] Fatty liver disease, either from the metabolic syndrome or alcohol use, is common in the background livers of inflammatory adenomas.

Etiology

Although the association with estrogen therapy is well documented, the mechanism by which this contributes to the development of hepatic adenomas is incompletely understood. Some authors postulate that estrogens cause direct transformation of hepatocytes via steroid receptors, but immunohistochemical staining for estrogen, progesterone, and androgen receptors have shown reactivity in less than a third of patients.[62,63] Similarly, the mechanism by which anabolic androgen use and glycogen storage diseases promote the development of hepatic adenomas is unknown.

Gross findings

Tumors are well circumscribed, although not encapsulated, and they arise in noncirrhotic livers (Fig. 27.7). Hepatic adenomas can be single or multiple, and the majority range from 5 to 15 cm, with rare adenomas as large as 30 cm.[20] The cut surface ranges from soft to dense in texture, and the color may be yellow-tan to brown, with or without hemorrhage and cystic change. Areas of necrosis may leave scarring, but adenomas lack the conspicuous central scars that are seen in focal nodular hyperplasia.

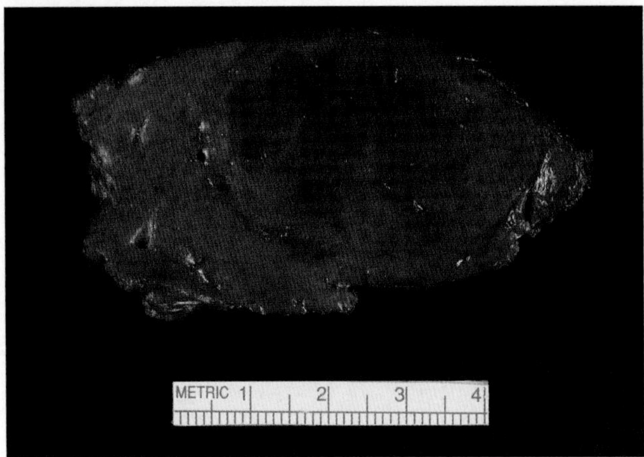

Figure 27.7 Hepatic adenoma. Grossly, a well-circumscribed noncapsulated mass within noncirrhotic liver.

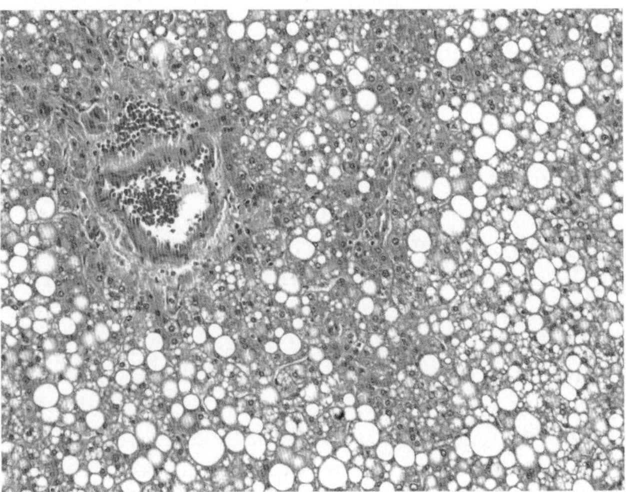

Figure 27.8 Hepatic adenoma. Hepatic adenomas lack portal tracts and isolated naked arteries are a hallmark of this lesion.

Microscopic findings

Hepatic adenomas arise in noncirrhotic livers and can be clearly demarcated from the background liver or show an imperceptible border with the nontumoral liver. In some cases, the mass lesion can compress adjacent vessels and connective tissue, resulting in a fibrous rim, but hepatic adenomas do not have a true capsule. Other adenomas can be barely perceptible because their edges blend in closely with the background liver. These cases can prove challenging to identify. In patients with inflammatory adenomas, the background liver can have fatty change because these patients frequently have an increased body mass index. Similarly, adenomas arising in patients with glycogen storage diseases can show background liver alterations such as glycogen accumulation and fibrosis.

Hepatic adenomas, although sometimes difficult to distinguish from the background liver, can be identified by their lack of portal tracts and the presence of isolated naked arteries (Fig. 27.8). The tumor cells are cytologically bland hepatocytes that are essentially identical to the hepatocytes found in the background liver, showing no atypia or mitotic activity. Androgen-associated adenomas are the exception because they can show mild cytological atypia and features such as cholestasis and pseudoacini. Fatty change can also be seen in hepatic adenomas (Fig. 27.9), but is characterized by steatosis only, without evidence of steatohepatitis, Mallory hyaline, ballooning degeneration, or subsinusoidal fibrosis. These latter features should raise suspicion for the steatohepatitic variant of hepatocellular carcinoma. Some hepatic adenomas, particularly the inflammatory or telangiectatic variant, demonstrate congestion, hemorrhage, and focal necrosis.

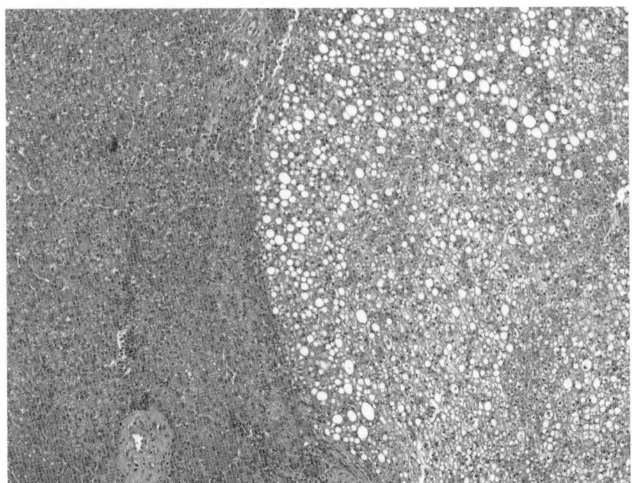

Figure 27.9 Hepatic adenoma with fatty change. In this example, the fatty change is limited to the lesion (right) and shows a sharp demarcation with the background nonneoplastic parenchyma (left). Despite the abundant fatty change, there should be no evidence of steatohepatitis, associated Mallory hyaline, ballooning degeneration or subsinusoidal fibrosis, which would raise suspicion for steatohepatitic variant of HCC.

When histologic features are typical, a diagnosis may be rendered with confidence. However, biopsy specimens can be challenging to interpret because needle biopsies only represent a small sample of the lesion. Consequently, if the clinical or histologic features are atypical, one might use the term "well-differentiated hepatocellular neoplasm" with an explanatory note describing the diagnostic challenge and giving a differential diagnosis of hepatic adenoma with atypical features or a well-differentiated hepatocellular carcinoma. In these cases, conclusive classification may require excision of the specimen.

Immunohistochemical findings

Immunohistochemistry is used for two purposes with hepatic adenomas. First, stains are used to make the diagnosis of hepatic adenoma. Second, after a diagnosis of hepatic adenoma is made, then an additional round of immunostains is used for subtyping the adenoma. However, the stains used in subtyping (see later) have no role in determining whether a tumor is an adenoma or carcinoma.

All hepatic adenomas have intact reticulin networks. A reticulin stain will highlight a retained network comparable with that of the normal background liver, with cell plates 1 to 2 hepatocytes in width. Approach fatty tumors with caution, however, because areas of fatty change may show occasional foci of reticulin loss that should not be over interpreted as evidence of hepatocellular carcinoma. Similarly, focal areas of reticulin disruption may be seen in areas of necrosis or hemorrhage and, again, should not be interpreted as indicating malignancy.

Immunohistochemically, hepatic adenomas are positive for HepPar1 and Arginase-1 and are nonreactive for Glypican-3. CD34, an immunostain that shows strong and diffuse sinusoidal reactivity in hepatocellular carcinomas, may show patchy reactivity within hepatic adenomas, but shows diffuse reactivity in a third of inflammatory adenomas.[64] As such, the CD34 stain may be useful to help distinguish the lesion from background hepatic parenchyma, but is not discriminatory for hepatocellular carcinoma. The Ki-67 proliferation index is low (<1% to 2%) in hepatic adenomas. As with other lesions, Ki-67 should be interpreted in areas away from tumor necrosis and inflammation, which may falsely elevate the overall proliferative index.

The immunostains used for subclassification of hepatic adenomas are further described in the following sections.

Histological subtypes

There are four main subtypes of hepatic adenomas, which can be differentiated based on morphology, immunohistochemistry, and molecular findings.[65–69] Table 27.2 summarizes the histologic and immunophenotypic features of these subtypes. As noted above, attempts at subtyping adenomas should only be performed after one makes an unequivocal diagnosis of hepatic adenoma. For instance, there is no utility in adenoma subtyping if the diagnosis is unclear and a lesion is best considered a "well-differentiated hepatocellular neoplasm" with hepatocellular carcinoma in the differential diagnosis, there is no utility in adenoma subtyping. The function of subtyping adenomas is to provide additional prognostic information and to

Table 27.2 Hepatic adenoma subtypes and their features

	Type 1 HNF1α inactivated	Type 2 Inflammatory	Type 3 β-Catenin activated	Type 4 Unclassified
Histologic features				
Fatty change	±	±	±	±
Pseudoportal tract	–	+	–	–
Inflammation	–	+	–	–
Telangiectasia	–	+	–	–
Atypia	–	–/rare	±	±
Immunostaining characteristics				
L-Fatty acid-binding protein (L-FABP)	Lost	Retained	Retained	Retained
β-Catenin (nuclear staining)	–	– (very rare positive)	++	–
Glutamine synthetase (strong diffuse cytoplasmic)	1% positive	10% positive	++	–
C-reactive protein	–	+	–	–
Serum amyloid A	–	+	–	–

guide follow-up and treatment. As such, attempts at subtyping should be performed on needle biopsies.

Hepatic adenomas with HNF1α inactivation

Thirty to 50% of hepatic adenomas have inactivation of HNF1α, a transcription factor thought to control regulatory networks important in the differentiation of endocrine β cells. This can be the result of either sporadic mutations or germline mutations in the *HNF1α* gene, a homeobox gene found on chromosome 12. Germline mutations are responsible for maturity onset diabetes of the young 3 (MODY 3). Patients with MODY 3 often develop diabetes before age 25 and develop hepatic adenomatosis.

Histologically, this subtype shows classic features of hepatic adenoma and also commonly shows diffuse steatosis (Fig. 27.10). As noted previously, adenomas with steatosis typically lack features of steatohepatitis, the presence of which should raise suspicion for the steatohepatitic variant of hepatocellular carcinoma. By definition, this subset of adenoma shows loss of L-FABP by immunohistochemistry (Fig. 27.11). Rarely (1%), these adenomas may also show nuclear localization of β-catenin or diffuse glutamine synthetase reactivity.

Inflammatory hepatic adenomas

Inflammatory adenomas, previously termed telangiectatic adenomas, represent 35% to 65% of hepatic adenomas and are associated with alcohol consumption or an increased body mass index. As might be expected, the background liver often shows features of fatty liver disease.

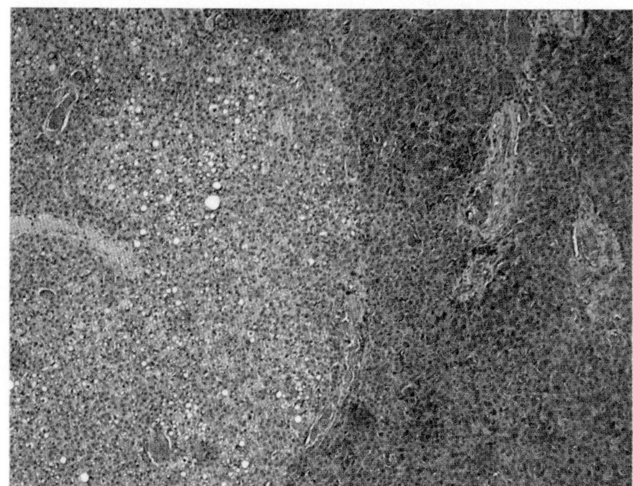

Figure 27.11 Hepatic adenoma with HNF1α inactivation. An immunostain for fatty acid-binding protein (L-FABP) shows loss of staining in the neoplasm (left), whereas cytoplasmic staining is retained (normal) in the nonneoplastic liver (right).

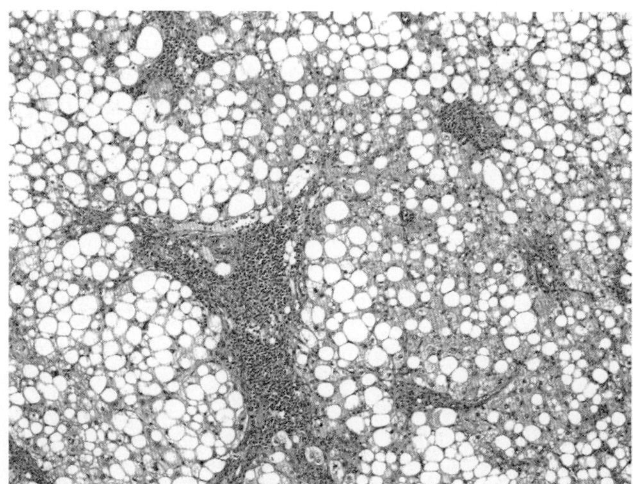

Figure 27.12 Inflammatory hepatic adenoma. This inflammatory adenoma has a background of fat accumulation. Pockets of inflammation are present in areas that resemble portal tracts.

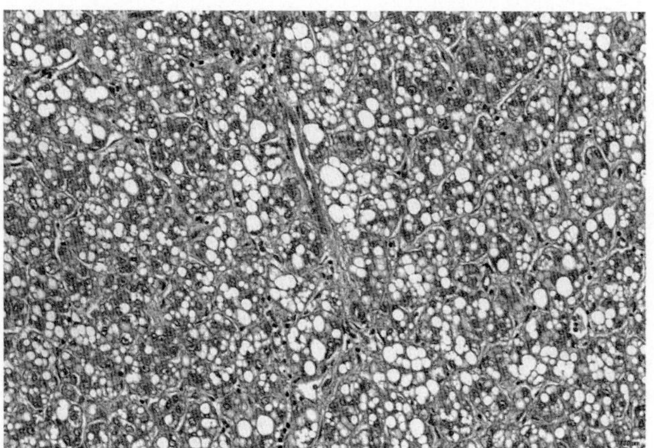

Figure 27.10 Hepatic adenoma with HNF1α inactivation. Histologically, these lesions show classic features of hepatic adenoma and may also show diffuse steatosis.

Histologically, these tumors show classic features of hepatic adenoma, but have several additional distinctive features. For example, inflammatory adenomas have a chronic inflammatory infiltrate, predominantly lymphocytic, that is usually located in areas that at first glance resemble portal tracts (Figs. 27.12, 27.13, and 27.14). However, closer examination shows that these areas lack true bile ducts and are instead composed of connective tissue, small arteries, and bile ductular proliferation (Figs. 27. and 27.15). Unless careful attention is given, one could easily mistake these areas for portal tracts and miss the adenomatous lesion entirely. As reflected by its previous name of

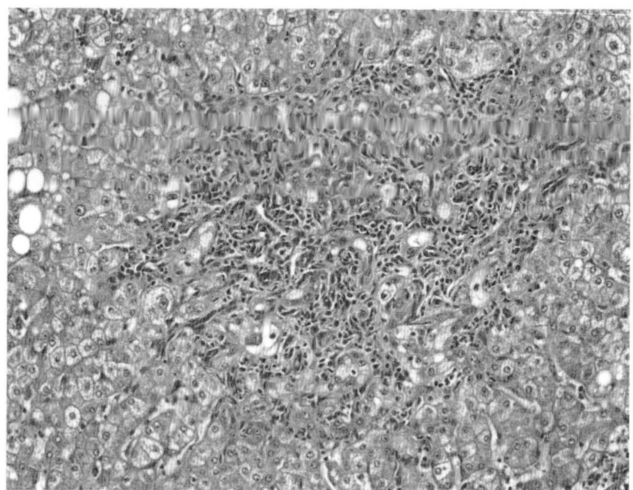

Figure 27.13 Inflammatory hepatic adenoma. The inflammatory infiltrate is predominantly lymphocytic and frequently found in areas that resemble portal tracts, but lack bile ducts.

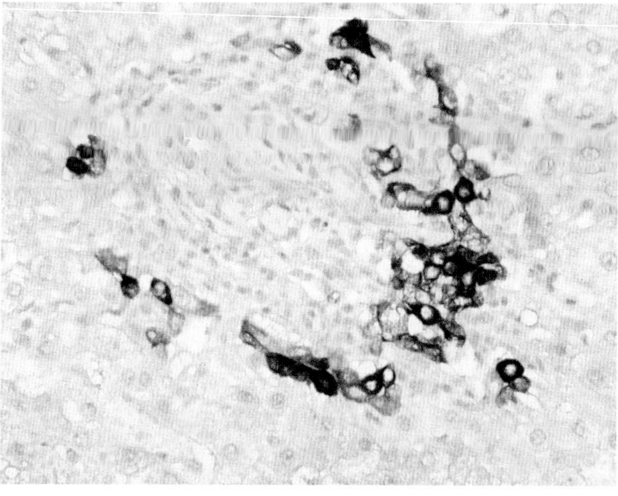

Figure 27.15 Inflammatory hepatic adenoma. A cytokeratin 7 immunostain highlights the pseudoportal tracts which contain ductular proliferation and lack a native bile duct.

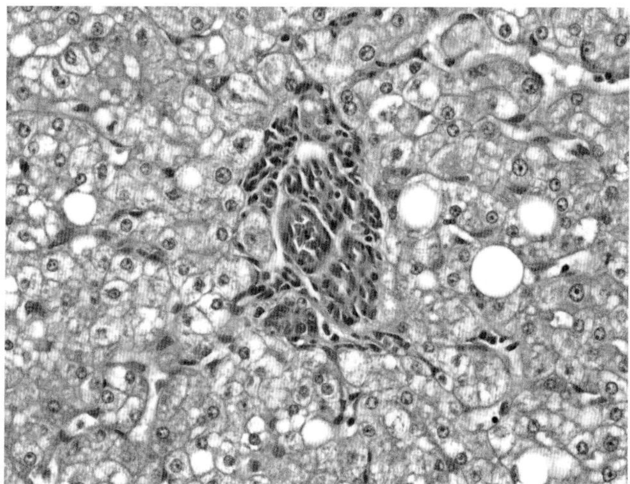

Figure 27.14 Inflammatory hepatic adenoma. The pseudoportal tracts are composed of connective tissue, small arteries, and ductular proliferation.

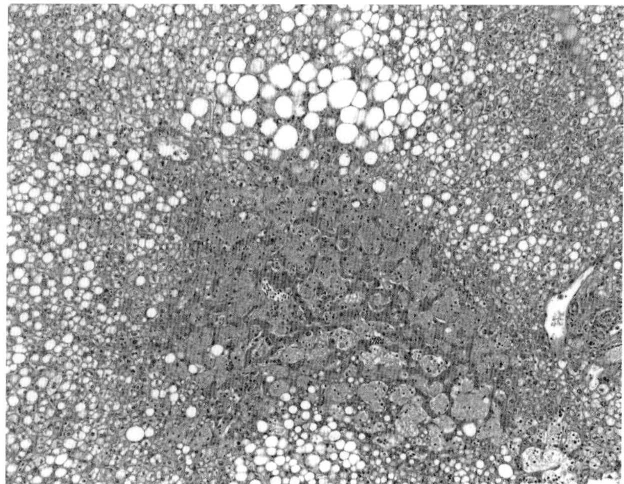

Figure 27.16 Inflammatory hepatic adenoma. As reflected in its previous name "telangiectatic adenoma," these lesions contain areas of dilated and congested sinusoids.

telangiectatic adenoma, these inflammatory adenomas can also contain areas of dilated and congested sinusoids (Fig. 27.16). Combine the faux portal tracts with a telangiectatic backdrop in a needle biopsy, and one could conceivably interpret the findings as passive congestion rather than an adenomatous lesion (Fig. 26.17). An increased risk of hemorrhage is associated with this subtype of adenoma.

Immunostains for C-reactive protein and/or serum amyloid A (also called hepatic amyloid A in some medical centers) identify these lesions as inflammatory subtype (Figs. 27.18, 27.19, 27.20, and 27.21). As mentioned previously, subtyping of adenomas should only be attempted after a solid diagnosis of adenoma has been made lest the immunostains lead one astray. For example, in the case of C-reactive protein and serum amyloid A, these markers can be reactive in nonneoplastic inflamed or congested liver tissue, a potential diagnostic pitfall. In addition, C-reactive protein and serum amyloid A are positive in a subset of hepatocellular carcinomas.[70] Inflammatory adenomas do not show loss of L-FABP reactivity, as is seen in HNF1α-inactivated adenomas, but β-catenin activation can be seen in 10% of cases based on diffuse glutamine synthetase reactivity.

β-Catenin-activated adenomas

β-Catenin-activated adenomas represented 10% to 15% of hepatic adenomas in early studies, but are now less than 5% in more recent series.[71] They are found more frequently in men. Histologically, these lesions do not show any special features, but they are

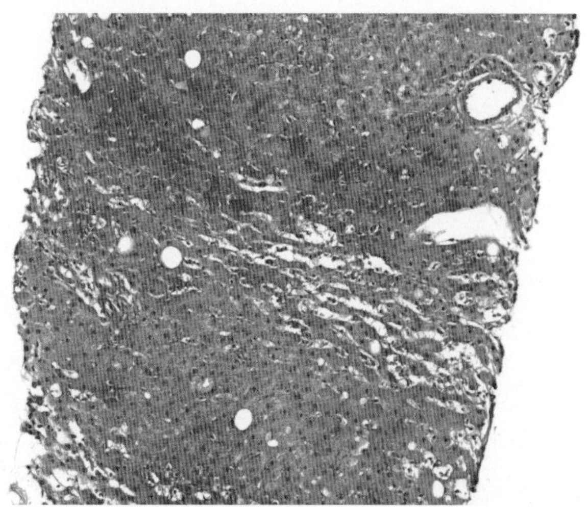

Figure 27.17 Inflammatory hepatic adenoma. Needle biopsies may be challenging to interpret because superficial review shows congestion. However, the presence of a naked artery (top right) should alert one to the diagnosis of inflammatory hepatic adenoma.

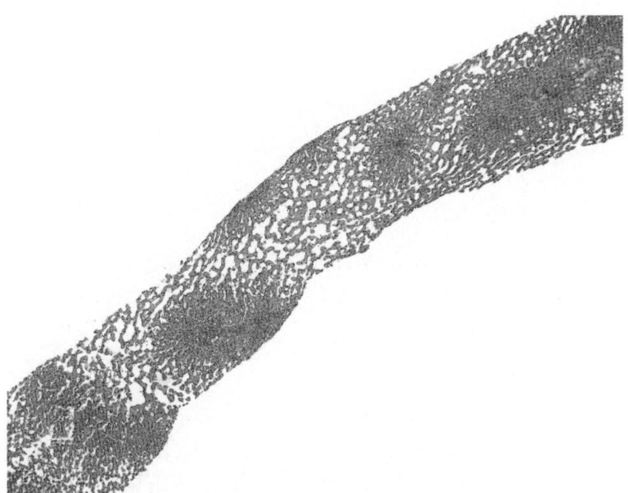

Figure 27.18 Inflammatory hepatic adenoma. At low magnification, another needle biopsy at shows markedly dilated sinusoids and portal-tract-like areas with chronic inflammation.

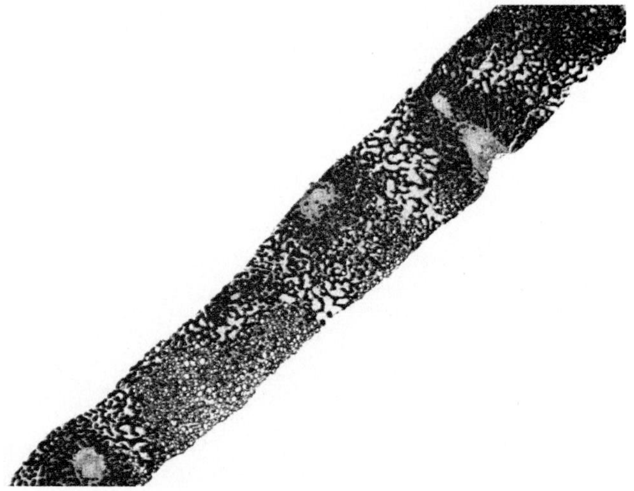

Figure 27.19 Inflammatory hepatic adenoma. C-reactive protein immunostain shows strong and diffuse reactivity in the lesion seen in the previous figure.

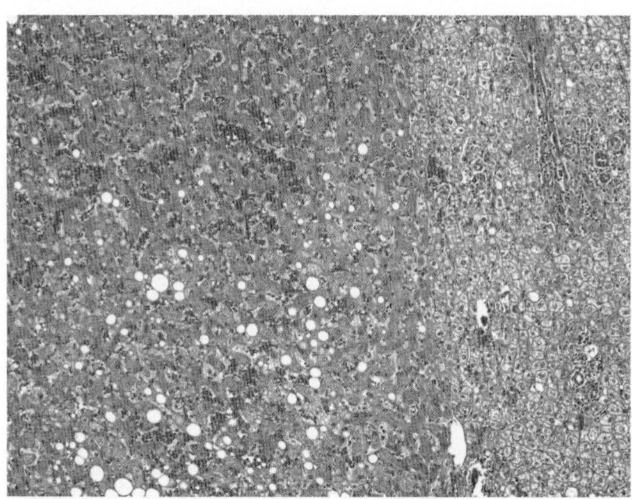

Figure 27.20 Inflammatory hepatic adenoma. The border of these lesions can be imperceptible from the nonneoplastic background liver.

more likely to show cytological atypia. Immunohistochemistry will show strong and diffuse cytoplasmic reactivity for glutamine synthetase and/or nuclear reactivity of β-catenin (Figs. 27.22 and 27.23). Recall that map-like reactivity of glutamine synthetase is seen in focal nodular hyperplasia, whereas isolated Zone 3 reactivity is seen in nonneoplastic liver. Thus, only strong and diffuse cytoplasmic reactivity should be interpreted as supportive of β-catenin activation. By comparison, β-catenin nuclear reactivity may be sparse and patchy. Any strong and convincing nuclear positivity is sufficient to call the stain positive. Owing to the sparse nature of β-catenin nuclear reactivity, concurrent use of glutamine synthetase is recommended because this stain is more likely to pick up β-catenin activation. Background membranous or cytoplasmic reactivity is seen in normal tissues and should not be interpreted as positive.

These β-catenin-activated adenomas are reported to have a higher risk of transformation to malignancy, particularly those also showing cytological atypia. As with all adenomas, staining for subtyping should only be performed following a definitive diagnosis of adenoma because they do not distinguish adenomas from carcinoma. For example, diffuse glutamine synthetase staining and β-catenin nuclear staining is found in about 20% of hepatocellular carcinomas. It is worth reiterating that none of the stains used for subtyping adenomas will discriminate a hepatic

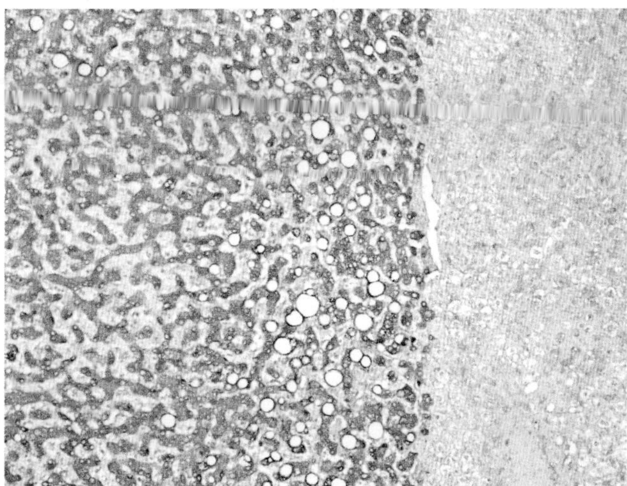

Figure 27.21 Inflammatory hepatic adenoma. A C-reactive protein immunostain highlights a sharp demarcation between the adenoma (left) and nonneoplastic liver parenchyma (right) in the lesion seen in the previous figure.

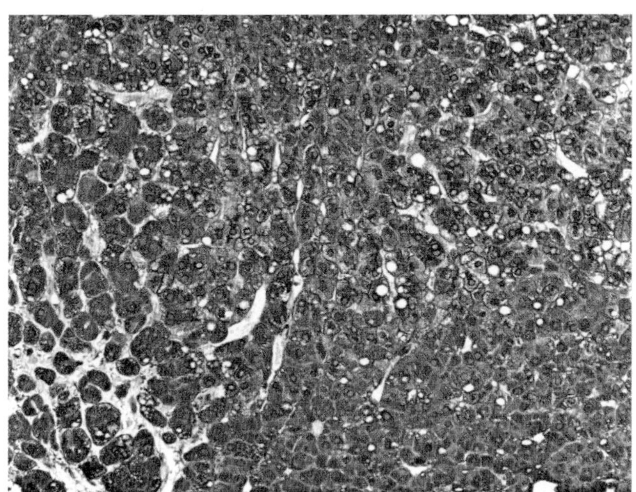

Figure 27.22 β-Catenin-activated adenoma. Glutamine synthetase acts as a surrogate marker for β-catenin activation and is seen as strong and diffuse cytoplasmic staining in these adenomas.

adenoma from other lesions such as hepatocellular carcinoma.

Secondary β-catenin activation can also be seen in otherwise typical HNF1α-inactivated adenomas (~1%) and inflammatory adenomas (~10%). In these cases, the adenomas are classified as either HNF1α-inactivated adenomas or inflammatory adenomas, with note made of secondary β-catenin activation.

Unclassified adenomas

A small subset of adenomas (5% to 10%) remains unclassified after immunostains have been performed. These lesions show typical H&E features of adenoma,

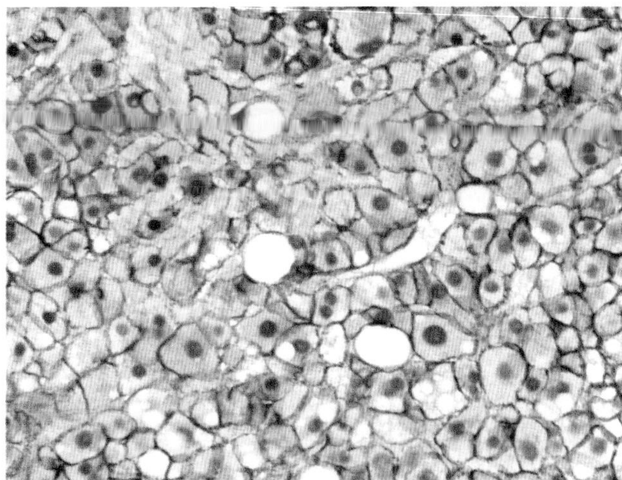

Figure 27.23 β-Catenin-activated adenoma. β-Catenin immunostain is considered positive when at least 5% of cells show nuclear reactivity.

but lack reactivity with β-catenin (nuclear), C-reactive protein, and serum amyloid A, while retaining L-FABP reactivity. These lesions are simply referred to as "hepatic adenoma, unclassified."

Pigmented adenomas

Pigmented adenomas are an uncommon type of adenoma found in both men and women, and are characterized by prominent cytoplasmic pigment within the tumor hepatocytes. This pigment has been identified as lipofuschin ultrastructurally and is negative for iron stains. Although many adenomas can show very mild lipofuschin accumulation, only adenomas with pronounced pigment accumulation, distinctive from the background liver, should be considered true pigmented adenomas (Fig. 27.24).

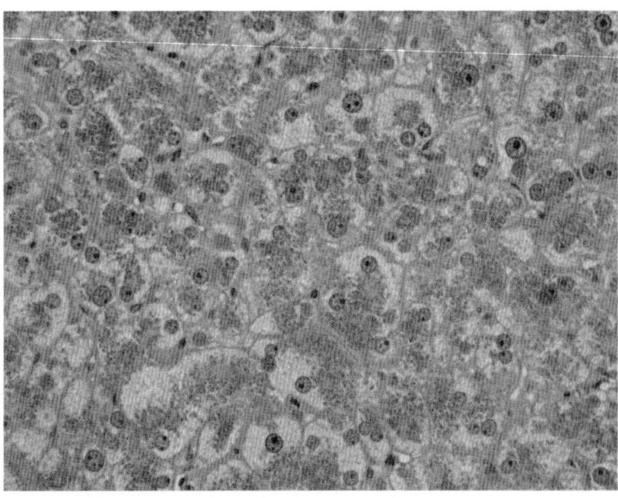

Figure 27.24 Pigmented adenoma. The adenoma shows abundant cytoplasmic lipofuschin pigments.

In patients with multiple adenomas, only one or a few of the adenomas may show pigmented change, a feature that some authors cite as evidence for additional genetic changes beyond that which caused the adenomatosis. These pigmented lesions represent a heterogeneous group of adenomas with the most common subtype being HNF1α-inactivated adenoma.[72] Pigmented adenomas are at increased risk for malignant transformation.[72,73]

Androgen-related adenomas

Most androgen-related adenomas develop in men (2/3), often in association with androgen use for building muscle mass. The adenomas can be multifocal. Mild nuclear atypia and pseudogland formation are common in androgen adenomas. Most have sufficient atypia that they are classified as atypical adenomas (see later). There is an increased risk for malignant transformation, and hepatocellular carcinoma should be thoroughly excluded in each case.

When subtyped, androgen-associated adenomas are most commonly β-catenin mutated (~50%), inflammatory adenomas (~20%), unclassified (~20%), or HNF1α inactivated (~10%).[74] Most of the inflammatory adenomas and the HNF1α-inactivated adenomas show secondary β-catenin activation, either by β-catenin nuclear accumulation or by strong and diffuse glutamine synthetase staining.

Myxoid hepatic adenomas

Myxoid hepatic adenomas are rare, making up less than 1% of all hepatic adenomas. The tumors are radiologically distinct, showing marked T2 hyperintensity with thin internal septations. The tumors also show heterogeneous enhancement on arterial phase imaging and more homogeneous enhancement on delayed phase.[75]

Myxoid hepatic adenomas show characteristic histological findings,[76] with abundant myxoid material distending the sinusoids (Fig. 27.25). The adenomas show no loss of reticulin and no cytological atypia. The myxoid material is Alcian blue positive and can be weakly mucicarmine positive, but should not be mistaken for a mixed biliary and hepatic tumor. Most cases show loss of L-FABP by immunohistochemistry and some, but not all, show *HNF1α* mutations. Although data are limited, some cases have been associated with malignant transformation to hepatocellular carcinoma. Given the loss of L-FABP staining, these tumors might be a subtype of HNF1α-inactivated adenomas. However, more data are needed before determining the best classification. In any case, the myxoid change is an atypical finding that suggests an increased risk for malignancy.

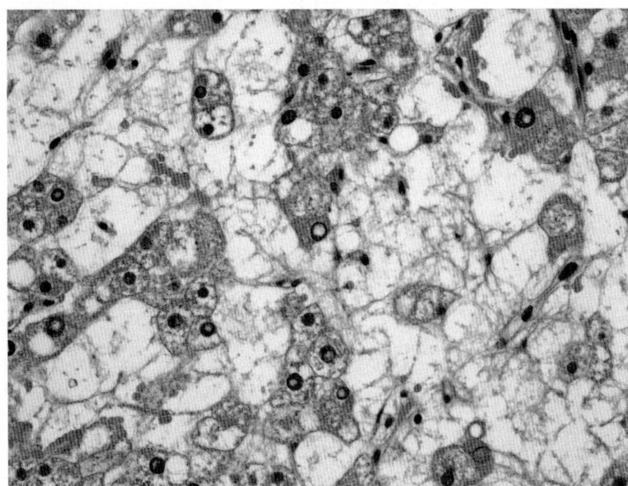

Figure 27.25 Myxoid adenoma. The sinusoids of the adenoma are distended by loose, flocculent, myxoid material.

Atypical adenoma

Some adenomas show atypical features that are concerning for malignancy but are insufficient for a diagnosis of hepatocellular carcinoma. These features might include unusual clinical findings, such as an adenoma in an older male or in the presence of background liver disease. Some lesions show cyto-architectural atypia such as nuclear pleomorphism, cytoplasmic inclusions, mitotic activity, pseudogland formation, nodule-in-nodule appearance, or equivocal, focal reticulin loss. Diffuse glutamine synthetase reactivity or nuclear β-catenin expression can be seen in either β-catenin-activated hepatic adenomas or in up to 30% of hepatocellular carcinomas, and is not discriminatory. A lesion in this category can be called atypical adenoma or hepatocellular neoplasm of uncertain malignant potential.[77] Clinical management of these lesions includes close clinical follow-up or resection with clear margins.

Adenoma-like nodules in cirrhotic livers

Cirrhotic livers can rarely have nodules that have histological features of an inflammatory adenoma.[78] These nodules can also be positive for C-reactive protein and/or serum amyloid A and can have mutations that are typical for inflammatory adenomas.[79] Some authors have suggested calling these lesions hepatic adenomas. However, such an approach is premature because the natural history of these lesions in cirrhotic livers is unknown. Certainly, making a diagnosis of hepatic adenoma on a needle biopsy in a cirrhotic liver cannot be encouraged at this point.

Cytology findings

A diagnosis of hepatic adenoma is very challenging with fine needle aspiration and lesions in the liver typically undergo core needle biopsy. Fine needle aspiration specimens show large three-dimensional and cohesive clusters of benign hepatocytes that appear essentially normal with smooth nuclear membranes.[80] The absence of biliary epithelial cells supports a diagnosis of hepatic adenoma.

Differential diagnosis

Hepatocellular carcinoma

Most hepatic adenomas can be differentiated from hepatocellular carcinoma, but this task can be more challenging when the hepatocellular carcinomas are well differentiated. Table 27.3 highlights key differentiating features of hepatic adenoma and hepatocellular carcinoma. The background liver in cases of hepatic adenomas shows no evidence for advanced fibrosis or cirrhosis. Other key differentiating features in favor of hepatic adenoma include: retained normal reticulin framework, lack of cytological atypia, absence of mitotic activity, and low proliferation index by Ki-67 immunostain (<1% to 2%). Typical hepatic adenomas do not show cholestasis or pseudoacinar growth, and despite the predilection for fatty change in adenomas, there should not be features of steatohepatitis, such as ballooning degeneration, Mallory hyaline, or perisinusoidal fibrosis. Features of steatohepatitis are more likely seen in the steatohepatitic variant of hepatocellular carcinoma. Rarely, focal nodular hyperplasias can also show steatohepatitis-like changes if the background liver shows steatohepatitis.

Table 27.3 Differentiating features of hepatic adenoma and hepatocellular carcinoma

	Hepatic adenoma	Hepatocellular carcinoma
Histologic features		
Background cirrhosis	–	+ (80%)
Aberrant naked vessels	+	+
Cytological atypia	– (except for androgen adenomas)	+
Pseudoacinar formation	– (rarely +)	±
Fatty change	±	±
Steatohepatitic features (ballooning degeneration, Mallory-Denk bodies)	–	±
Cholestasis	– (rarely +)	±
Necrosis	– (rarely +)	±
Mitoses	–	±
Staining characteristics		
Reticulin	Intact	Disrupted
Glutamine synthetase (strong diffuse cytoplasmic staining)	± (seen in β-catenin mutated adenomas; about 15% of all adenomas)	± (seen in 20%)
Glypican-3	–	+ (50%–90%)
Arginase	+	+ (90%)
HepPar-1	+ (inflammatory adenomas can show areas of HepPar-1 loss)	+ (90%)
CD34 (sinusoidal staining)	± (patchy)	+ (diffuse)
Ki-67 proliferation index	<2%	++ Variable

The reticulin stain is a key tool for separating adenomas from hepatocellular carcinoma. Adenomas show a retained reticulin network, whereas hepatocellular carcinomas show disruption or focal loss of the reticulin network. As mentioned previously, steatosis and areas of hemorrhage or necrosis may show disruption of reticulin staining and this can be a pitfall in interpretation. This can be avoided by focusing evaluation of the reticulin stain on those areas of the tumor that are not fatty and do not show hemorrhage/necrosis.

Glypican 3 immunoreactivity is found in 75% to 90% of hepatocellular carcinomas and is negative in hepatic adenomas.[81,82] However, lesions expressing glypican 3 are typically higher grade tumors and can already be distinguished from adenomas by H&E stain. By contrast, well-differentiated hepatocellular carcinomas have a lower frequency of glypican 3 sensitivity (~50%), and thus a negative stain may not be informative.

Focal nodular hyperplasia

In a noncirrhotic liver, the top differential diagnosis for hepatic adenoma is focal nodular hyperplasia. Although, radiologic features can often differentiate these two tumors in many cases, this is not always possible, especially with smaller lesions or those with atypical imaging features.

Both types of lesions show bland hepatocytes without cytological atypia, contain intact reticulin networks, and contain abnormal arteries. However, focal nodular hyperplasias are more nodular and commonly have fibrous bands radiating from a central scar. Unpaired arteries are typically absent or may be rarely seen in periportal regions in focal nodular hyperplasia, which are more likely due to tangential cuts rather than a neoplastic process.

Inflammatory adenomas can be particularly challenging to differentiate from focal nodular hyperplasia because both lesions contain inflammation and ductular proliferation. The most useful distinguishing feature in these cases is the nodularity of focal nodular hyperplasia, with bands of fibrosis surrounding benign nodules of hepatocytes. The fibrous bands usually show a mild ductular proliferation and sometimes show large vessels with eccentrically thickened walls. In addition, glutamine synthetase immunohistochemistry is also very helpful and will show a map-like pattern of reactivity in focal nodular hyperplasia and a perivenular pattern in hepatic adenomas. A diffuse pattern of glutamine synthetase is seen in 5% to 10% of inflammatory adenomas that are also β-catenin activated, but is never seen in focal nodular hyperplasia. Additionally, inflammatory adenomas will typically show strong and diffuse immunoreactivity for serum amyloid A and C-reactive protein, whereas these stains are negative or show patchy staining in focal nodular hyperplasias.

A small number of cases remain difficult to classify as a result of small sample size. In addition, some cases show atypical staining patterns, making interpretation challenging. For example, up to 15% of focal nodular hyperplasias can be reactive for serum amyloid A, and 10% of focal nodular hyperplasias show a pseudo-map-like staining pattern, instead of the characteristic map-like staining pattern.[83] This pseudo-map-like pattern is seen as thin bands of cytoplasmic staining at the periphery of the lesion as compared with the more characteristic wide geographic areas of strong cytoplasmic staining with sparing of periseptal hepatocytes. Similarly, 15% of inflammatory adenomas show this pseudo-map-like staining pattern.[83]

Other parenchymal changes

On needle biopsies, the hepatic parenchyma adjacent to a mass lesion can show features mimicking inflammatory adenomas, such as portal expansion with inflammation, bile ductular proliferation, and sinusoidal dilatation. Similarly, venous outflow impairment can result in dilation and congestion of the sinusoids resulting in peliosis-like areas found in inflammatory adenomas. In both cases, the reactive parenchyma contains true portal tracts with native bile ducts, whereas inflammatory adenomas have pseudoportal tracts without native bile ducts. Naked vessels are also a feature seen in adenomas and are absent in most nonneoplastic liver tissue. In challenging cases, immunohistochemical stains may be helpful.

Treatment

The management of asymptomatic patients who are taking oral contraceptives is controversial. In patients with small (<5 cm) lesions, discontinuation of oral contraceptives and close observation with repeat imaging at 6 months is suggested.[84] Complete regression of tumor has been documented after discontinuing steroid medications.[50] However, even after discontinuation of steroid medications, growth, rupture, and malignant transformation (despite a decrease in size of the adenoma) have been documented.[46] As a result, other authors recommend resection of all adenomas regardless of size, if technically feasible.[85]

The current management guidelines for hepatic adenomas are based mainly on tumor size, patient gender, and to a lesser degree on histologic subtype. Surgical resection is generally recommended for symptomatic patients and adenomas greater than 5 cm in size, because of the risk of hemorrhage, rupture, and malignant transformation. Hepatic adenomas in males are also generally referred for surgery because of a higher risk for malignancy (up to 50% risk in some studies). Inflammatory adenomas are often treated by surgery because of a modestly increased risk for bleeding. However, much of this increased risk for bleeding appears to be a function of tumor size, and tumors larger than 5 cm would be typically managed by surgery anyway.

Surgical options include enucleation, resection, and rarely liver transplantation. Liver transplantation is reserved for patients in whom surgical resection is not possible due to tumor size/location, and those with a heavy burden of adenomatosis. The risk of malignancy is not strongly related to the number of lesions, so liver transplantation is not indicated solely on the basis of multiple adenomas.[32]

Prognosis

Hepatic adenomas, in contrast to focal nodular hyperplasias, carry a risk of bleeding and malignant transformation. Hemorrhage is reported in 20% to 25% of adenomas and can rarely result in rupture and hemoperitoneum.[32,66,86] Patients who present with abdominal pain and hypotension as a result of intraperitoneal bleeding from a ruptured adenoma have a mortality of up to 20%.[42] Such patients should undergo surgery for definitive resection and control of hemorrhage; the use of presurgical selective arterial embolization coils and particulate matter may improve outcomes.

Based on the data from resection specimens, the risk of malignant transformation into hepatocellular carcinoma is 5% to 10%,[87] and this risk increases with increasing tumor size.[32] Some studies also suggest that β-catenin-activated adenomas have an increased risk for malignancy,[65,88] although not all studies have replicated this finding.[32]

27.3 MACROREGENERATIVE NODULE

Definition

A macroregenerative nodule is a benign hepatocellular nodule caused by multiacinar regenerative growth in cirrhotic livers or livers undergoing significant regrowth following massive necrosis. The larger size of the macroregenerative nodule causes it to stand out conspicuously from background cirrhotic nodules, but histologically it is otherwise identical to the background liver. Other outdated names that have fallen out of favor include adenomatous hyperplasia and cirrhotic pseudotumor. The term regenerative nodule may also be used.

Demographics

About a quarter of cirrhotic livers contain macroregenerative nodules. Livers undergoing regenerative changes following parenchymal loss, such as in fulminant viral hepatitis or autoimmune hepatitis, may contain macroregenerative nodules in the absence of cirrhosis. Other liver diseases that can develop macroregenerative nodules in the absence of cirrhosis include severe vascular disease.

Etiology

Macroregenerative nodules are the result of regenerative hepatic growth in the setting of cirrhosis, necrosis, or vascular disease.

Gross findings

Macroregenerative nodules may be single or multiple and are found in a backdrop of cirrhotic liver. These lesions stand out as larger nodules, usually measuring larger than 10 mm and rarely exceed 5 cm. Their cut surface resembles that of the background liver in color and texture, but may also be bile stained.

Microscopic findings

Macroregenerative nodules are composed of benign hepatocytes with normal architecture and intact portal tracts (Fig. 27.26). The hepatocytes are bland, show no atypia, and are identical to those found in the background liver. Mitoses are rare, but may be seen during regeneration following necrosis.

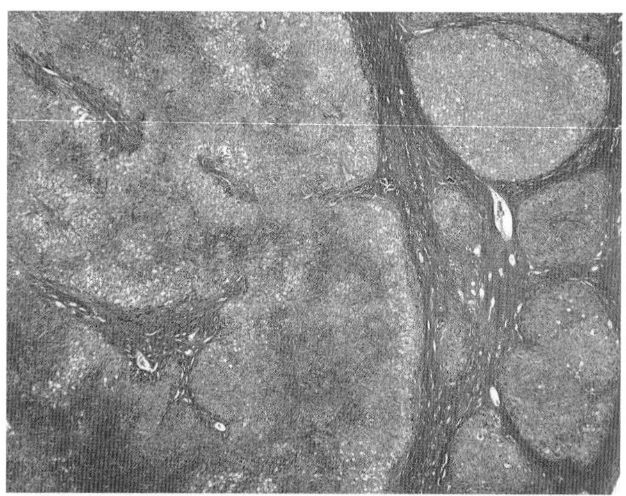

Figure 27.26 Macroregenerative nodule. These lesions stand out as larger nodules in a background of cirrhotic nodules. They contain portal tracts and bland hepatocytes that show no atypia, and are identical to that found in the background liver.

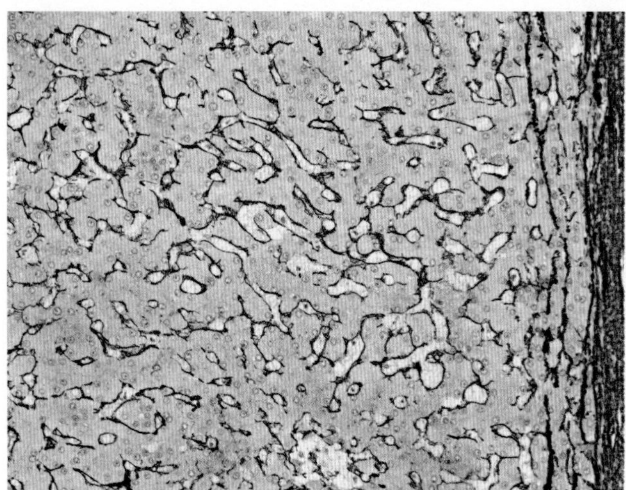

Figure 27.27 Macroregenerative nodule. A reticulin stain highlights a normal reticulin framework with cell plates no more than 1 to 2 hepatocytes in width.

Immunohistochemical findings

A reticulin stain will show no evidence of reticulin loss and will highlight the reticulin framework surrounding the cell plates, which are no more than 1 to 2 hepatocytes in width (Fig. 27.27). Staining for glutamine synthetase will highlight Zone 3 hepatocytes, as expected in benign liver. Glypican 3, β-catenin, HSP-70, C-reactive protein, and serum amyloid A will be nonreactive or show normal staining patterns. There is no loss of L-FABP reactivity, and CD34 should be negative in the sinusoids.

Differential diagnosis

The main differential diagnosis for macroregenerative nodules is the dysplastic nodule. The distinction between these two lesions can only be made histologically because the lesions appear identical grossly. Immunostains are not helpful to distinguish the two, so one must rely on H&E features. In contrast to macroregenerative nodules which are bland and contain no atypia, dysplastic nodules show atypical features, which can include cytological atypia (small cell change or large cell change), architectural atypia (psuedoglands), and nodule-in-nodule growth.

REFERENCES

1. John TG, Greig JD, Crosbie JL, et al. Superior staging of liver tumors with laparoscopy and laparoscopic ultrasound. *Ann Surg.* 1994;220:711–719.
2. Cherqui D, Mathieu D, Zafrani ES, et al. Focal nodular hyperplasia and hepatocellular adenoma in women. Current data. *Gastroenterol Clin Biol.* 1997;21:929–935.
3. Karhunen PJ, Penttila A, Liesto K, et al. Occurrence of benign hepatocellular tumors in alcoholic men. *Acta Pathol Microbiolt Immunol Scand.* 1986;94:141–147.
4. Wanless IR, Mawdsley C, Adams R. On the pathogenesis of focal nodular hyperplasia of the liver. *Hepatology.* 1985;5:1194–1200.
5. Reymond D, Plaschkes J, Luthy AR, et al. Focal nodular hyperplasia of the liver in children: review of follow-up and outcome. *J Pediatr Surg.* 1995;30:1590–1593.
6. Nguyen BN, Flejou JF, Terris B, et al. Focal nodular hyperplasia of the liver: a comprehensive pathologic study of 305 lesions and recognition of new histologic forms. *Am J Surg Pathol.* 1999;23:1441–1454.
7. Cherqui D, Rahmouni A, Charlotte F, et al. Management of focal nodular hyperplasia and hepatocellular adenoma in young women: a series of 41 patients with clinical, radiological, and pathological correlations. *Hepatology.* 1995;22:1674–1681.
8. Tranquart F, Correas JM, Ladam Marcus V, et al. Real-time contrast-enhanced ultrasound in the evaluation of focal liver lesions: diagnostic efficacy and economical issues from a French multicentric study. *J Radiol.* 2009;90:109–122.
9. Zech CJ, Grazioli L, Breuer J, et al. Diagnostic performance and description of morphological features of focal nodular hyperplasia in Gd-EOB-DTPA-enhanced liver magnetic resonance imaging: results of a multicenter trial. *Invest Radiol.* 2008;43:504–511.
10. Brunt EM, Flye MW. Infarction in focal nodular hyperplasia of the liver. A case report. *Am J Clin Pathol.* 1991;95:503–506.
11. Lee MJ, Saini S, Hamm B, et al. Focal nodular hyperplasia of the liver: MR findings in 35 proved cases. *AJR Am J Roentgenol.* 1991;156:317–320.
12. Paradis V, Benzekri A, Dargere D, et al. Telangiectatic focal nodular hyperplasia: a variant of hepatocellular adenoma. *Gastroenterology.* 2004;126:1323–1329.
13. Mathieu D, Zafrani ES, Anglade MC, et al. Association of focal nodular hyperplasia and hepatic hemangioma. *Gastroenterology.* 1989;97:154–157.
14. Wanless IR, Gryfe A. Nodular transformation of the liver in hereditary hemorrhagic telangiectasia. *Arch Pathol Lab Med.* 1986;110:331–335.
15. Haber M, Reuben A, Burrell M, et al. Multiple focal nodular hyperplasia of the liver associated with hemihypertrophy and vascular malformations. *Gastroenterology.* 1995;108:1256–1262.
16. Scott LD, Katz AR, Duke JH, et al. Oral contraceptives, pregnancy, and focal nodular hyperplasia of the liver. *JAMA.* 1984;251:1461–1463.

17. Geders JM, Haque S, Tesi RJ, et al. A young man with a solitary hepatic mass. *Hepatology*. 1995;22:655–659.
18. Fechner RE. Benign hepatic lesions and orally administered contraceptives. A report of seven cases and a critical analysis of the literature. *Hum Pathol*. 1977;8:255–268.
19. Ishak KG. Hepatic neoplasms associated with contraceptive and anabolic steroids. *Recent Results Cancer Res*. 1979;66:73–128.
20. Craig JR, Peters RL, Edmondson HA, ed. *Tumors of the Liver and Intrahepatic Bile Ducts*. Vol 26. Washington, DC: Armed Forces Institute of Pathology; 1989:280 pp.
21. Bertin C, Egels S, Wagner M, et al. Contrast-enhanced ultrasound of focal nodular hyperplasia: a matter of size. *Eur Radiol*. 2014;24:2561–2571.
22. Bioulac-Sage P, Cubel G, Taouji S, et al. Immunohistochemical markers on needle biopsies are helpful for the diagnosis of focal nodular hyperplasia and hepatocellular adenoma subtypes. *Am J Surg Pathol*. 2012;36:1691–1699.
23. Bioulac-Sage P, Cubel G, Balabaud C, et al. Revisiting the pathology of resected benign hepatocellular nodules using new immunohistochemical markers. *Semin Liver Dis*. 2011;31:91–103.
24. Imkie M, Myers SA, Li Y, et al. Fibrolamellar hepatocellular carcinoma arising in a background of focal nodular hyperplasia: a report of 2 cases. *J Reprod Med*. 2005;50:633–637.
25. Hamrick-Turner JE, Shipkey FH, Cranston PE. Fibrolamellar hepatocellular carcinoma: MR appearance mimicking focal nodular hyperplasia. *J Comput Assist Tomogr*. 1994;18:301–304.
26. Quaglia A, Tibballs J, Grasso A, et al. Focal nodular hyperplasia-like areas in cirrhosis. *Histopathology*. 2003;42:14–21.
27. Libbrecht L, Cassiman D, Verslype C, et al. Clinicopathological features of focal nodular hyperplasia-like nodules in 130 cirrhotic explant livers. *Am J Gastroenterol*. 2006;101:2341–2346.
28. Di Stasi M, Caturelli E, De Sio I, et al. Natural history of focal nodular hyperplasia of the liver: an ultrasound study. *J Clin Ultrasound*. 1996;24:345–350.
29. Wanless IR. Nodular regenerative hyperplasia, dysplasia, and hepatocellular carcinoma. *Am J Gastroenterol*. 1996;91:836–837.
30. Mathieu D, Kobeiter H, Maison P, et al. Oral contraceptive use and focal nodular hyperplasia of the liver. *Gastroenterology*. 2000;118:560–564.
31. Weimann A, Mossinger M, Fronhoff K, et al. Pregnancy in women with observed focal nodular hyperplasia of the liver. *Lancet*. 1998;351:1251–1252.
32. Dokmak S, Paradis V, Vilgrain V, et al. A single-center surgical experience of 122 patients with single and multiple hepatocellular adenomas. *Gastroenterology*. 2009;137:1698–1705.
33. Grazioli L, Federle MP, Brancatelli G, et al. Hepatic adenomas: imaging and pathologic findings. *Radiographics*. 2001;21:877–892; discussion 92–94.
34. Greaves WO, Bhattacharya B. Hepatic adenomatosis. *Arch Pathol Lab Med*. 2008;132:1951–1955.
35. Flejou JF, Barge J, Menu Y, et al. Liver adenomatosis. An entity distinct from liver adenoma? *Gastroenterology*. 1985;89:1132–1138.
36. Ribeiro A, Burgart LJ, Nagorney DM, et al. Management of liver adenomatosis: results with a conservative surgical approach. *Liver Transpl Surg*. 1998;4:388–398.
37. Frulio N, Chiche L, Bioulac-Sage P, et al. Hepatocellular adenomatosis: what should the term stand for! *Clin Res Hepatol Gastroenterol*. 2014;38:132–136.
38. Grazioli L, Federle MP, Ichikawa T, et al. Liver adenomatosis: clinical, histopathologic, and imaging findings in 15 patients. *Radiology*. 2000;216:395–402.
39. Chiche L, David A, Adam R, et al. Liver transplantation for adenomatosis: European experience. *Liver Transpl*. 2016;22:516–526.
40. Baum JK, Bookstein JJ, Holtz F, et al. Possible association between benign hepatomas and oral contraceptives. *Lancet*. 1973;2:926–929.
41. Edmondson HA, Henderson B, Benton B. Liver-cell adenomas associated with use of oral contraceptives. *N Engl J Med*. 1976;294:470–472.
42. Rooks JB, Ory HW, Ishak KG, et al. Epidemiology of hepatocellular adenoma. The role of oral contraceptive use. *JAMA*. 1979;242:644–648.
43. Reddy KR, Schiff ER. Approach to a liver mass. *Semin Liver Dis*. 1993;13:423–435.
44. Nime F, Pickren JW, Vana J, et al. The histology of liver tumors in oral contraceptive users observed during a national survey by the American College of Surgeons Commission on Cancer. *Cancer*. 1979;44:1481–1489.
45. Rosenberg L. The risk of liver neoplasia in relation to combined oral contraceptive use. *Contraception*. 1991;43:643–652.
46. Shortell CK, Schwartz SI. Hepatic adenoma and focal nodular hyperplasia. *Surg Gynecol Obstet*. 1991;173:426–431.
47. Meissner K. Hemorrhage caused by ruptured liver cell adenoma following long-term oral contraceptives: a case report. *Hepato-gastroenterology*. 1998;45:224–225.
48. Klatskin G. Hepatic tumors: possible relationship to use of oral contraceptives. *Gastroenterology*. 1977;73:386–394.

49. Aseni P, Sansalone CV, Sammartino C, et al. Rapid disappearance of hepatic adenoma after contraceptive withdrawal. *J Clin Gastroenterol.* 2001;33:234–236.
50. Edmondson HA, Reynolds TB, Henderson B, et al. Regression of liver cell adenomas associated with oral contraceptives. *Ann Intern Med.* 1977;86:180–182.
51. Nakao A, Sakagami K, Nakata Y, et al. Multiple hepatic adenomas caused by long-term administration of androgenic steroids for aplastic anemia in association with familial adenomatous polyposis. *J Gastroenterol.* 2000;35:557–562.
52. Resnick MB, Kozakewich HP, Perez-Atayde AR. Hepatic adenoma in the pediatric age group. Clinicopathological observations and assessment of cell proliferative activity. *Am J Surg Pathol.* 1995;19:1181–1190.
53. Touraine RL, Bertrand Y, Foray P, et al. Hepatic tumours during androgen therapy in Fanconi anaemia. *Eur J Pediatr.* 1993;152:691–693.
54. Coombes GB, Reiser J, Paradinas FJ, et al. An androgen-associated hepatic adenoma in a trans-sexual. *Br J Surg.* 1978;65:869–870.
55. Fujiyama S, Sato K, Sakai M, et al. A case of type Ia glycogen storage disease complicated by hepatic adenoma. *Hepato-gastroenterology.* 1990;37:432–435.
56. Labrune P, Trioche P, Duvaltier I, et al. Hepatocellular adenomas in glycogen storage disease type I and III: a series of 43 patients and review of the literature. *J Pediatr Gastroenterol Nutr.* 1997;24:276–279.
57. Leese T, Farges O, Bismuth H. Liver cell adenomas. A 12-year surgical experience from a specialist hepato-biliary unit. *Ann Surg.* 1988;208:558–564.
58. Talente GM, Coleman RA, Alter C, et al. Glycogen storage disease in adults. *Ann Internal Med.* 1994;120:218–226.
59. Alshak NS, Cocjin J, Podesta L, et al. Hepatocellular adenoma in glycogen storage disease type IV. *Arch Pathol Lab Med.* 1994;118:88–91.
60. Toso C, Rubbia-Brandt L, Negro F, et al. Hepatocellular adenoma and polycystic ovary syndrome. *Liver Int.* 2003;23:35–37.
61. Bioulac-Sage P, Balabaud C, Zucman-Rossi J. Focal nodular hyperplasia, hepatocellular adenomas: past, present, future. *Gastroenterol Clin Biol.* 2010;34:355–358.
62. Cohen C, Lawson D, DeRose PB. Sex and androgenic steroid receptor expression in hepatic adenomas. *Hum Pathol.* 1998;29:1428–1432.
63. Masood S, West AB, Barwick KW. Expression of steroid hormone receptors in benign hepatic tumors. An immunocytochemical study. *Arch Pathol Lab Med.* 1992;116:1355–1359.
64. Bellamy CO, Maxwell RS, Prost S, et al. The value of immunophenotyping hepatocellular adenomas: consecutive resections at one UK centre. *Histopathology.* 2013;62:431–445.
65. Bioulac-Sage P, Rebouissou S, Thomas C, et al. Hepatocellular adenoma subtype classification using molecular markers and immunohistochemistry. *Hepatology.* 2007;46:740–748.
66. Bioulac-Sage P, Balabaud C, Zucman-Rossi J. Subtype classification of hepatocellular adenoma. *Digestive Surg.* 2010;27:39–45.
67. Rebouissou S, Bioulac-Sage P, Zucman-Rossi J. Molecular pathogenesis of focal nodular hyperplasia and hepatocellular adenoma. *J Hepatol.* 2008;48:163–170.
68. Zucman-Rossi J, Jeannot E, Nhieu JT, et al. Genotype-phenotype correlation in hepatocellular adenoma: new classification and relationship with HCC. *Hepatology* 2006;43:515–524.
69. van Aalten SM, Verheij J, Terkivatan T, et al. Validation of a liver adenoma classification system in a tertiary referral centre: implications for clinical practice. *J Hepatol.* 2011;55:120–125.
70. Liu L, Shah SS, Naini BV, et al. Immunostains used to subtype hepatic adenomas do not distinguish hepatic adenomas from hepatocellular carcinomas. *Am J Surg Pathol.* 2016;40:1062–1069.
71. Shafizadeh N, Genrich G, Ferrell L, et al. Hepatocellular adenomas in a large community population, 2000 to 2010: reclassification per current World Health Organization classification and results of long-term follow-up. *Hum Pathol.* 2014;45:976–983.
72. Mounajjed T, Yasir S, Aleff PA, et al. Pigmented hepatocellular adenomas have a high risk of atypia and malignancy. *Mod Pathol.* 2015;28:1265–1274.
73. Masuda T, Beppu T, Ikeda K, et al. Pigmented hepatocellular adenoma: report of a case. *Surg Today.* 2011;41:881–883.
74. Gupta S, Naini BV, Munoz R, et al. Hepatocellular neoplasms arising in association with androgen use. *Am J Surg Pathol.* 2016;40:454–461.
75. Young JT, Kurup AN, Graham RP, et al. Myxoid hepatocellular neoplasms: imaging appearance of a unique mucinous tumor variant. *Abdom Radiol.* 2016;41:2115–2122.
76. Salaria SN, Graham RP, Aishima S, et al. Primary hepatic tumors with myxoid change: morphologically unique hepatic adenomas and hepatocellular carcinomas. *Am J Surg Pathol.* 2015;39:318–324.
77. Bedossa P, Burt AD, Brunt EM, et al. Well-differentiated hepatocellular neoplasm of uncertain malignant potential: proposal for a new diagnostic category. *Hum Pathol.* 2014;45:658–660.

78. Sasaki M, Yoneda N, Kitamura S, et al. A serum amyloid A-positive hepatocellular neoplasm arising in alcoholic cirrhosis; a previously unrecognized type of inflammatory hepatocellular tumor. *Mod Pathol*. 2012;25:1584–1593.
79. Calderaro J, Nault JC, Balabaud C, et al. Inflammatory hepatocellular adenomas developed in the setting of chronic liver disease and cirrhosis. *Mod Pathol*. 2016;29:43–50.
80. Tao LC. Oral contraceptive-associated liver cell adenoma and hepatocellular carcinoma. Cytomorphology and mechanism of malignant transformation. *Cancer*. 1991;68:341–347.
81. Coston WM, Loera S, Lau SK, et al. Distinction of hepatocellular carcinoma from benign hepatic mimickers using Glypican-3 and CD34 immunohistochemistry. *Am J Surg Pathol*. 2008;32:433–444.
82. Libbrecht L, Severi T, Cassiman D, et al. Glypican-3 expression distinguishes small hepatocellular carcinomas from cirrhosis, dysplastic nodules, and focal nodular hyperplasia-like nodules. *Am J Surg Pathol*. 2006;30:1405–1411.
83. Joseph NM, Ferrell LD, Jain D, et al. Diagnostic utility and limitations of glutamine synthetase and serum amyloid-associated protein immunohistochemistry in the distinction of focal nodular hyperplasia and inflammatory hepatocellular adenoma. *Mod Pathol*. 2014;27:62–72.
84. Sherlock S. Hepatic reactions to drugs. *Gut*. 1979;20:634–648.
85. Foster JH, Berman MM. The malignant transformation of liver cell adenomas. *Arch Surg*. 1994;129:712–717.
86. Bioulac-Sage P, Blanc JF, Rebouissou S, et al. Genotype phenotype classification of hepatocellular adenoma. *World J Gastroenterol*. 2007;13:2649–2654.
87. Micchelli ST, Vivekanandan P, Boitnott JK, et al. Malignant transformation of hepatic adenomas. *Mod Pathol*. 2008;21:491–497.
88. Bioulac-Sage P, Laumonier H, Couchy G, et al. Hepatocellular adenoma management and phenotypic classification: the Bordeaux experience. *Hepatology*. 2009;50:481–489.

28 Hepatocellular carcinoma

Michael S. Torbenson, MD

28.1 DEFINITIONS AND TERMINOLOGY

Hepatocellular carcinoma is defined as a malignant epithelial tumor that (1) originates in the liver, (2) is differentiated toward hepatocytes as its primary line of differentiation, and (3) is not a hepatoblastoma.

In addition to this basic definition, there are several commonly used terms that focus on small tumors. These terms are primarily used in research studies and in clinical management algorithms, but are worth knowing as a pathologist.

Small hepatocellular carcinoma

By definition, this refers to any hepatocellular carcinoma that is less than 2 cm in greatest dimension. In research studies, small hepatocellular carcinomas that arise in cirrhotic livers, and are either well or moderately differentiated, are further divided into early hepatocellular carcinomas versus progressed hepatocellular carcinomas.

Early hepatocellular carcinoma

By definition, these carcinomas are less than 2 cm in greatest dimension. They arise in cirrhotic livers and have ill-defined borders on gross examination. On histologic examination, the carcinoma is well differentiated and has residual portal tracts within the tumor, suggesting it arose out of a high-grade dysplastic nodule. Less commonly used terms that are synonyms include *vaguely nodular hepatocellular carcinoma* or *small hepatocellular carcinoma with indistinct margins*.

Progressed hepatocellular carcinoma

By definition, these carcinomas are less than 2 cm in greatest dimension. They arise in cirrhotic livers and have distinct margins on gross examination. These carcinomas are well to moderately differentiated and are more likely than early hepatocellular carcinomas to have angiolymphatic invasion.

28.2 CLINICAL FEATURES

Risk factors, noncirrhotic livers

About 20% of hepatocellular carcinomas develop in noncirrhotic livers. Of these, the background livers are clinically and histologically within normal limits in 50% of cases. However, in the remaining 50% of cases, there is evidence for chronic hepatitis, and many have mild fibrosis. Etiologies include chronic hepatitis B,[1] chronic hepatitis C,[2] genetic iron overload,[3] fatty liver disease,[4,5] chronic vascular disease,[6–8] or malignant transformation of hepatic adenomas.[9]

Risk factors, cirrhotic livers

Most hepatocellular carcinomas (80%) develop in cirrhotic livers. The most frequent overall causes of cirrhosis (chronic hepatitis B, chronic hepatitis C, and alcohol abuse) are also the most frequent causes of hepatocellular carcinoma. Chronic hepatitis B is the most common risk for hepatocellular carcinoma in most countries in Asia. Chronic hepatitis C is the most common risk factor in the United States, much of Europe, and Japan. The new and potent antiviral drugs targeting hepatitis C and hepatitis B greatly reduce the risks for both cirrhosis and cancer. However, successful suppression or clearance of these viruses only reduces and does not eliminate the risk of hepatocellular carcinoma.[10,11] Fatty liver disease is also a key risk factor, including both alcohol and metabolic syndrome driven fatty liver disease. Both of these are independent risk factors and can also be cofactors when present with other diseases such as chronic viral hepatitis. Aflatoxin B1 exposure is an important risk factor for hepatocellular carcinoma, particularly with chronic exposure. Aflatoxin B1 is produced by *Aspergillus*, a fungus that grows on food stored in warm, damp conditions.[12] This risk factor is best documented in cases from Africa. Finally, hepatic iron accumulation is a cofactor for the development of hepatocellular carcinoma in cirrhotic livers, even when the underlying liver disease is not genetic hemochromatosis.[13]

Although cirrhosis from any cause is a key risk factor for hepatocellular carcinoma, the risk is not equitably distributed. For example, the 5-year cumulative incidences for hepatocellular carcinoma in one study was as follows: hereditary hemochromatosis (21%), chronic hepatitis C (17%), chronic hepatitis B virus (10%), and biliary cirrhosis (5%).[14]

Signs and symptoms

Hepatocellular carcinomas are commonly identified in asymptomatic individuals who are being screened because they have cirrhosis. Even in individuals that do have clinical signs or symptoms, the findings are nonspecific, such as vague abdominal pain, fatigue, anorexia, and weight loss.[15]

A dramatic but rare presentation is rupture of the hepatocellular carcinoma with hemoperitoneum.[16] This presentation has a worse prognosis. The frequency of rupture in untreated tumors depends on the size of the tumor: larger tumors are more likely to rupture. The frequency varies considerably in untreated individuals, being as high as 15% in parts of Asia and Africa, but considerably lower in the West, with frequencies of about 2%.[16–18] In addition to spontaneous cases, rupture can also occur as a consequence of transarterial chemoembolization (TACE), with a frequency of about 0.5%.[19]

Demographics

Hepatocellular carcinoma can develop in the pediatric population, but almost all cases present after the age of 5. The most common risk factors are chronic hepatitis B, glycogen storage disease, and tyrosinemia; however, there are many others (Table 28.1).

In adults, hepatocellular carcinomas are generally divided into those that occur in cirrhotic livers (80%) and those that occur in noncirrhotic livers (20%). For hepatocellular carcinomas arising in cirrhotic livers, the incidence begins to rise around age 40 and peaks at approximately age 62 years. Men are at greater risk than women, about 8:1. In contrast, hepatocellular carcinomas in noncirrhotic livers develop later, with about 40% of individuals age 70 or older.[15,20,21] There is still a male predominance, but it is much less striking at about 1.5:1. The prognosis is better overall, even though the hepatocellular carcinomas in noncirrhotic livers tend to be larger than in cirrhotic livers.[21]

Table 28.1 Etiologies for hepatocellular carcinoma in the pediatric population

Clinical setting	Comment and/or reference
Chronic viral hepatitis	
Hepatitis B	Cirrhotic and noncirrhotic livers[264]
Hepatitis C	Very rare, cirrhotic livers[265]
Inherited diseases	
Tyrosinemia type 1	Livers are typically cirrhotic[266–268]
Arginase deficiency	Noncirrhotic liver[269]
Wilson disease	Cirrhotic liver[270]
PFIC 1 (*ATP8B1* mutation)	Ref.[270]
PFIC 2 (*ABCB11* mutation; BSEP deficiency)	Cirrhotic and noncirrhotic livers[267,271,272]
PFIC 3 (*ABCB4* mutation; MDR3 deficiency)	Ref.[273]
Tight-junction protein 2 deficiency	Cirrhotic livers[274]
Glycogen storage diseases	Types 1a,[275] IV,[267,276] and VI[275]
Other	
Alagille syndrome	Ref.[280]
Biliary Atresia	Refs.[267,279]
Cardiac cirrhosis	Ref.[277]
Congenital absence of portal vein	Ref.[278]
Prolonged TPN therapy	Noncirrhotic liver[281]
Radiation therapy for Wilm tumor	Noncirrhotic liver[283]
Turner syndrome	Refs.[278,282]

Table 28.2 Serum markers of hepatocellular carcinoma

Marker	Commonly used cutoff	Sensitivity (%)	Specificity (%)
AFP	400 ng/mL	35	95
AFP-L3	10%	40	95
DCP	7.5 ng/mL	75	70

28.3 SERUM FINDINGS

There are several useful serum markers for hepatocellular carcinoma: α-fetoprotein (AFP), lens culinaris agglutinin-reactive AFP (AFP-L3), and des-γ-carboxy-prothrombin (DCP) (Table 28.2). Although current management guidelines do not recommend their use in screening programs, they find considerable clinical use as diagnostic and follow-up markers. All of these markers have prognostic value, with positive testing indicating a worse prognosis.[22]

28.4 SPREAD AND METASTASES

Metastatic disease is found in 40% of individuals at the time of first presentation, with the most common sites being the lungs (50%), bones (30%), abdominal lymph nodes (30%), and adrenal glands (10%).[23,24] Peritoneal spread (carcinomatosis) is uncommon at presentation but can develop in time, with autopsy studies showing focal (6%) or diffuse (3%) peritoneum spread.[25]

Needle track seeding

Hepatocellular carcinoma can rarely spread along needle tracks after biopsies or after ablation therapies. Subcapsular and high-grade hepatocellular carcinomas are the most likely to cause needle tract seeding and most tumor deposits develop within 6 months.[26,27] The older literature demonstrated a frequency of tumor seeding of approximately 2.5%,[28] leading some authors to advocate against using biopsies to diagnose hepatocellular carcinoma. However, tumor seeding is readily treated and does not reduce life expectancy.[26] In addition, there is no evidence that pretransplant biopsy of a hepatocellular carcinoma reduces post-transplant survival.[29] In addition to being readily treated, more recent and larger studies show the risk of seeding is actually 10× lower than previous thought, at approximately 0.25%.[27] Finally, the increased use of more sophisticated biopsy methods, such as the coaxial technique, brings the risk of seeding down to essentially 0%.[30]

Table 28.3 AJCC staging system (8th Edition)

Tumor	Definition	Note
TX	Primary tumor cannot be assessed	
T0	No primary tumor identified	
T1a	Solitary tumor that is ≤ 2 cm	The tumor can be negative or positive for vascular invasion.
T1b	Solitary tumor > 2 cm but without vascular invasion	
T2	Solitary tumor that is > 2 cm with vascular invasion; or multiple tumors with no tumor > 5 cm	
T3	At least two tumors with at least one that is >5 cm	Tumors can be with or without vascular invasion
T4	Direct invasion of any organ, except gallbladder; Or, perforation of the visceral peritoneum; Or tumor involving a major branch of the portal vein (including right or left branches, but not the smaller branches); Or tumor involving the right, left, or middle hepatic veins	Tumors can be single or multiple

From Amin MB, et al. *AJCC Cancer Staging Manual*. 8th ed. New York: Springer; 2017. © American Joint Committee on Cancer.

Staging

Hepatocellular carcinomas are staged for both clinical management decisions and for prognosis. After resection or transplantation, the AJCC system is commonly used to provide a traditional tumor stage based on tumor variables (Table 28.3). In addition to this tumor-based staging system, other systems are commonly used to decide if patients are candidates for surgery and to guide therapy in those patients who have unresectable tumors. To help guide therapy, patients are classified using the underlying liver function (e.g., Child–Pugh score) or physiologic reserve (e.g., performance status). The Barcelona Clinic Liver Cancer (BCLC) staging system incorporates tumor variables, underlying liver function and overall health status to classify patients into different stages, with each stage linked to recommended therapies. Stage 0 and stage A tumors are candidates for surgery with curative intent. Stage B tumors are not resectable and instead are treated with transarterial chemoembolization (TACE) or ablation therapy. Stage C tumors are treated with sorafenib, whereas Stage D tumors are treated by best supportive care.

28.5 TREATMENT MODALITIES

Surgery

The preferred treatment for solitary or small numbers of tumors in individuals with well-preserved liver function is surgical resection with curative intent.[31] Anatomical resections are performed whenever possible. In general, liver function is considered adequate for surgery when bilirubin levels are normal and the hepatic venous pressure gradient is less than or equal to 10 mmHg and/or the platelet count is greater than 100,000. In some individuals, surgery is not possible even with adequate liver reserve because of comorbid conditions such as heart disease.

Ablation

Ablation therapy is used for small tumors (less than 3 cm) that are unresectable because of their location or because the patient has other serious comorbid conditions. Ablation methods include radiofrequency ablation (RFA) and ETOH injection. In general, radiofrequency ablation is preferred over ETOH injection because radiofrequency ablation has both a lower recurrence rate and better overall survival. However, ETOH injection is still used in cases where the anatomic location of the tumor precludes radiofrequency ablation therapy. Radiofrequency ablation can also be combined with transarterial chemoembolization for locoregional therapy.[32,33] In addition to use as primary therapy for unresectable hepatocellular carcinomas, radiofrequency ablation is also used to downstage tumors >3 cm, either as bridge to transplantation or to surgery.[34] The use of radiofrequency ablation as primary therapy in tumors larger than 3 cm is controversial.[35]

Transarterial chemoembolization

Transarterial chemoembolization or transarterial radioembolization therapy is used for tumors that are (1) unresectable and (2) in patients who are not candidates for ablative therapy and (3) in patients who do not have metastatic disease. Contraindications to transarterial chemoembolization are primarily Child–Pugh C cirrhosis or portal vein invasion, whereas relative contraindications are benign portal vein thrombosis or bilirubin levels greater than 3 mg/dL.[35] Transarterial chemoembolization leads to improved

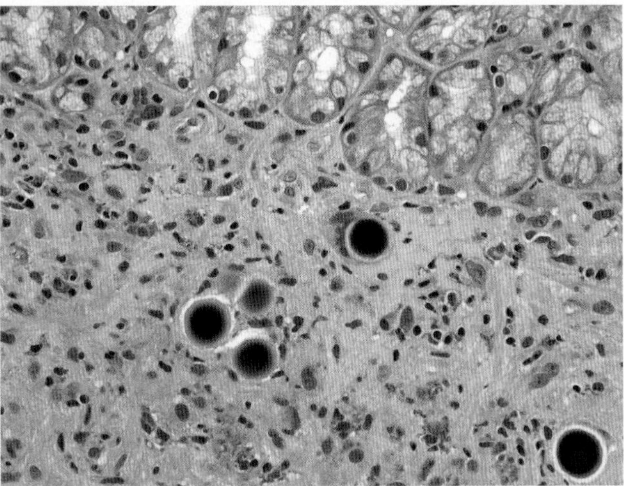

Figure 28.1 Y90 beads. These beads escaped from the liver and lodged in the stomach.

survival compared to nontreatment groups,[36] but is not curative. Transarterial chemoembolization is also used as a bridge to downstage tumors in hopes of making them resectable, or as a bridge to transplantation. In the transarterial chemoembolization procedure, microsphere beads are loaded with chemotherapy agents and injected into the branch(es) of the hepatic artery that are feeding the hepatocellular carcinoma. Radioembolization is quite similar, but the microspheres are loaded with Yttrium-90, which delivers high levels of local radiation. Of note, there is a relatively high frequency of complications following transarterial chemoembolization because the beads can spread outside the tumor, injuring the nonneoplastic liver. Transarterial chemoembolization is followed by acute hepatic decompensation in up to 20% of individuals, which is irreversible in about 3% of cases.[35] Transarterial embolization beads can also spread to other organs, such as the stomach (Fig. 28.1), leading to ischemic injury.

Systemic chemotherapy

Systemic chemotherapy is used when other therapies are contraindicated, mostly in the setting of portal vein invasion or metastatic disease. Sorafenib is the only therapy widely used outside the setting of specific clinical trials. The SHARP trial[37] is widely considered a landmark study in hepatocellular carcinoma therapy. The multicenter SHARP trial showed that sorafenib was superior to placebo for individuals with hepatocellular carcinoma and Child A cirrhosis, with a better median overall survival (11 versus 8 months). Although this improvement is clearly modest, it has led to renewed efforts to improve systemic chemotherapy for hepatocellular carcinoma.

28.6 PROGNOSIS

The median survival after a diagnosis of hepatocellular carcinoma is between 10 and 18 months.[38–40] There are many clinical and pathologic factors that influence prognosis, but none are as important as whether the tumor can be resected, with successful resection providing a 5-year overall survival ranging from 25% to 80%.[41] Other important prognostic findings include clinical factors such as patient age, gender, underlying liver disease, and overall physiologic status. Tumor variables that strongly influence survival include tumor size, tumor grade, and microvascular invasion. Portal vein invasion and metastatic disease indicate a poor prognosis.

Tumor subtypes also have prognostic significance. Hepatocellular carcinomas subtypes with a better prognosis, compared to conventional hepatocellular carcinoma, are clear cell hepatocellular carcinoma and lymphocyte-rich hepatocellular carcinoma. Subtypes with a worse prognosis are combined cholangiocarcinoma-hepatocellular carcinoma, combined neuroendocrine carcinoma-hepatocellular carcinoma, cirrhotomimetic hepatocellular carcinoma, sarcomatoid hepatocellular carcinoma, granulocyte colony stimulating factor (GCSF) producing hepatocellular carcinoma, and carcinosarcoma.

After successful surgery, approximately 60% of individuals will have tumor recurrences, with most recurrent disease located in the liver.[42,43] The tumor recurrences represent the original tumor clone in two-thirds of cases, presumably from micrometastases that were not removed at the time of the original surgery. The remaining one-third of recurrent hepatocellular carcinomas result from a second independent primary, only seen in individuals with a background of severe chronic liver disease, usually with cirrhosis.[44,45]

Angiolymphatic invasion

Vascular invasion predicts tumor recurrence after TACE,[46] after resection,[47,48] and after liver transplantation.[49] Vascular invasion is divided into macrovascular and microvascular invasion. For clinical care, macrovascular invasion is defined as tumor involving blood vessels that are large enough to be recognized by imaging or by gross examination. Macrovascular invasion almost exclusively involves either the portal venous system or the central veins/vena cava,[50] whereas the hepatic arteries are almost never involved. The frequency of macrovascular invasion is between 5% and 30%. Macrovascular invasion can be a contraindication to resection so is more commonly identified in imaging-based studies or in autopsy studies than in surgical pathology specimens.

Microvascular invasion is evident only on histologic examination and has a frequency of about 30%, with a range of 15% to 60%.[51] The wide range in the frequency results from small studies that can lead to skewed results and from varying sectioning protocols (finding vascular invasion is to some degree a function of the number of sections taken). Sections taken from the tumor—nontumor interface are generally the most productive for finding vascular invasion. Portal vein invasion is 10× more common than central vein invasion,[52] whereas hepatic artery invasion is hardly ever found. When there is invasion of the hepatic arteries, the tumor is generally very aggressive and the prognosis is poor.

In most cases, the vascular invasion is fairly obvious, but there can diagnostic challenges. For clinical care, an endothelial lining should be present to make the diagnosis of vascular invasion. Retraction artifact can sometimes mimic lymphatic or venous invasion, but will lack an endothelial lining. In many cases, the vascular invasion leads to a distended vessel, with sides molded around the tumor thrombus. Fibrin or an organized blood clot can occasionally be associated with the vascular invasion, but they are not necessary for the diagnosis. In contrast, the presence of rare individual tumor cells, or even small clusters of tumor cells, are counted as sectioning artifacts and not vascular invasion when they are floating freely in an otherwise empty vascular lumen.

28.7 PRECURSOR LESIONS TO HEPATOCELLULAR CARCINOMA

Overview

Putative precursor lesions to hepatocellular carcinoma can be microscopic or macroscopic findings, most of which occur in cirrhotic livers. No convincing precursor lesion has been found in noncirrhotic human livers, other than hepatic adenomas.

Glycogen storing foci

Although glycogen storing foci have been considered possible precursor lesions,[53,54] the data on this point does not strongly support a major role for these lesions as precursors to hepatocellular carcinoma. Glycogen storing foci are composed of hepatocytes with more glycogen than the background liver. They are easily identified at low power, standing out from the background liver as well-circumscribed clusters of clear cells (Fig. 28.2). Although the genetic changes are not well studied, the data to date indicates they are polyclonal.[55] In hepatocellular carcinoma resection specimens, they are found in the background liver

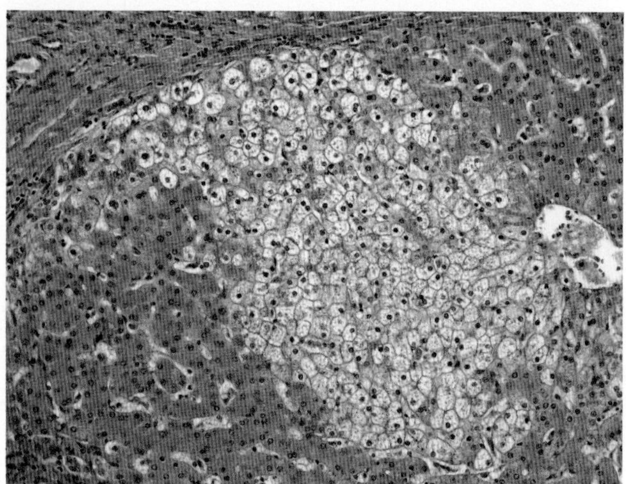

Figure 28.2 Glycogen storing foci. A distinct cluster of hepatocytes with clear cell change stand out at low power from the background liver.

sections of cirrhotic (10%) and noncirrhotic (20%) livers, but the likelihood for any role as a precursor for hepatocellular carcinoma is diminished by their also being found in similar frequencies in the background liver sections of specimens resected for metastatic carcinoma (20%).[56] In some cases, glycogen storing foci will have intermediate hepatocytes that stain positive for CK7.[57]

Small cell change

Small cell change, also known as *small cell dysplasia*, is defined as clusters of hepatocytes with reduced cytoplasm and mild nuclear hyperchromasia, but otherwise normal nuclear and cytoplasmic cytology (Fig. 28.3). Their increased N:C ratio causes them stand out at low-power magnification. Consistent with their role as a precursor for hepatocellular carcinomas, small cell change in cirrhotic livers can be clonal,[55] have chromosomal damage, and telomere shortening.[58–60]

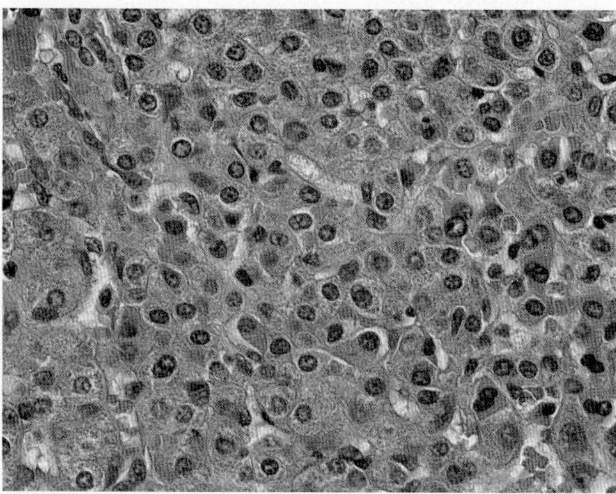

Figure 28.3 Small cell change. The hepatocytes show small cell change, with an increased N:C ratio and mild nuclear hyperchromasia.

Large cell change

Hepatocytes with large cell change have large and hyperchromatic nuclei that stand out at low power, but retain a normal or nearly normal N:C ratio (Fig. 28.4). Large cell change was previously known as large cell dysplasia, with the named changed in order to reflect a more nuanced understanding of this lesion. Large cell change appears to be genetically heterogeneous, with data showing DNA damage, especially in cirrhotic livers.[61] Large cell change is also associated with hepatitis B related cirrhosis[62] and with cholestatic changes.[63]

The frequency of large cell change increases with the frequency of hepatocellular carcinoma in cirrhotic livers, but data suggests large cell change results from cellular senescence, designed to eliminate hepatocytes with DNA damage because hepatocytes with large cell change show increased apoptosis and decreased cell cycling.[61,64] Even if large cell change is not a direct precursor to hepatocellular carcinoma, it does indicate liver parenchyma with widespread DNA damage and thus is associated with an increased risk for a subsequent diagnosis of hepatocellular carcinoma.[65,66] Large cell change can rarely be found in noncirrhotic livers. This change has not been well studied, but is largely thought to be senescent in nature.

Macroregenerative nodule

Macroregenerative nodules are defined as cirrhotic nodules that are at least 10 mm in diameter and

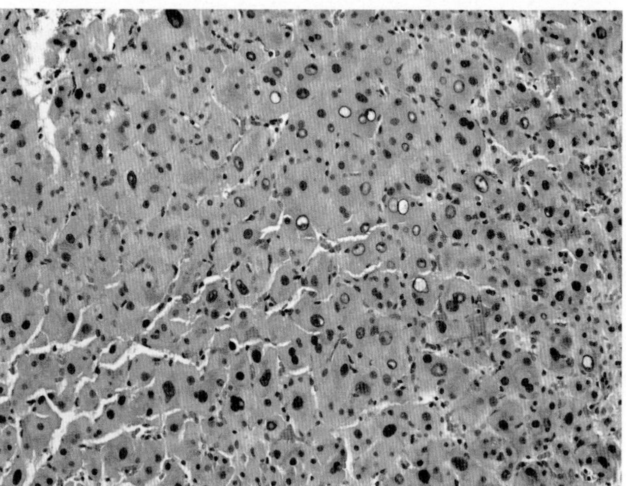

Figure 28.4 Large cell change. Scattered hepatocytes show large atypical nuclei, but overall have a preserved N:C ratio.

most stand out from the background liver because of differences in color or texture or because they bulge out from the cut surface more than other cirrhotic nodules. The vast majority of macroregenerative nodules develop in cirrhotic livers, being found in 15% to 30% of cases.[71,72] Macroregenerative nodules are multifocal in about two-thirds of cases.[77] Macroregenerative nodules average 12 mm in diameter and almost all are between 10 and 20 mm.[71,72] As an exception, macroregenerative nodules in cases of biliary cirrhosis, especially extrahepatic biliary atresia, can get a lot bigger, often in the 5 to 7 cm range.

The core concept of a macroregenerative nodule is rather simple: a cirrhotic nodule that stands out on gross examination (see above), yet shows no or minimal cytologic atypia. The hepatocytes in the macroregenerative nodule should look cytologically like the hepatocytes in the rest of the liver. Patchy large cell change is acceptable when the background liver shows similar changes. There should be no small cell change or other cytologic atypia. Macroregenerative nodules also have scattered portal tracts (Fig. 28.5). They have no reticulin loss, are glypican 3–negative, and their proliferative rate is the same as the background liver.[73] Imaging studies are limited in many cases by the lack of histologic confirmation, but do suggest a low risk of malignant transformation with long term follow-up.[74] Macroregenerative nodules can be challenging to reliably separate from low-grade dysplastic nodules, especially on biopsy specimens.

Large regenerative nodules can rarely develop in noncirrhotic livers following a severe hepatic injury that leads to large areas of panacinar collapse,[75] for example after fulminant autoimmune hepatitis. When the surviving hepatocytes regenerate, they can from large benign regenerative nodules that can suggest carcinoma on imaging studies and on gross examination.

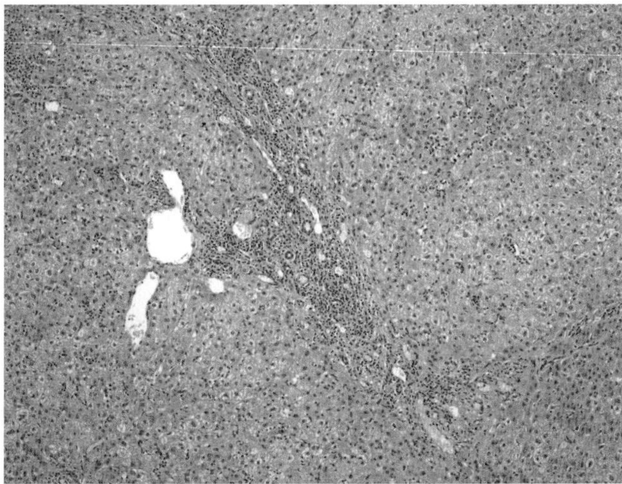

Figure 28.5 Macroregenerative nodule. Portal tracts are present throughout the macroregenerative nodule.

Dysplastic nodules

Dysplastic nodules are found only in cirrhotic livers and are the most widely accepted precursor lesions for hepatocellular carcinoma. Based on histologic findings, they are further classified into low- and high-grade dysplastic nodules (Table 28.4).

The core concept of a dysplastic nodule is straightforward: dysplastic nodules show more cytologic and/or architectural atypia than cirrhotic nodules in the background liver, but do not have the full histologic features of malignancy. In practice, there are nodules that show only minimal and somewhat equivocal atypia, making them hard to classify as a large regenerative nodule versus a low-grade dysplastic nodules.

Natural history

Dysplastic nodules are associated with increased risk for hepatocellular carcinoma. Although many of the dysplastic nodules will disappear over time, others will progress to hepatocellular carcinoma. In addition, dysplastic nodules serve as a general marker of increased hepatocellular carcinoma risk for the liver as a whole. Overall, about 10% of low-grade dysplastic

Table 28.4 High-grade versus low-grade dysplastic nodules

Finding	Low-grade dysplastic nodule	High-grade dysplastic nodule
Cytology		
Large cell change	May be present	May be present
Small cell change	Absent	May be present
Nuclear hyperchromasia	Absent to mild	Usually mild
Overall nuclear atypia	Minimal to mild	Usually mild
Architectural changes		
Portal tracts	Several to many	Few to none
Lobular arterioles	Few	Many
Psuedoglands[a]	Absent	May be present
Nodule-in-nodule	Absent	May be present

[a]Assuming a noncholestatic liver.

nodules and 30% of high-grade dysplastic nodules will progress to hepatocellular carcinoma within 2 to 3 years.[74,76,77] During a 2-year study interval, an additional 25% of individuals developed hepatocellular carcinoma outside of the dysplastic nodule in one study.[76]

Histologic findings

In terms of cytologic atypia, dysplastic nodules can show either large cell or small cell change. In terms of architectural findings, dysplastic nodules retain portal tracts, which are found in essentially all low-grade dysplastic nodules and many high-grade dysplastic nodules. The architectural atypia in dysplastic nodules can include pseudogland formation (less helpful in cholestatic livers), vague nodule-in-nodule growth, or increased lobular arterioles. The finding of increased lobular arteries can be accompanied by strong and diffuse staining of the sinusoids with CD34. However, this pattern of CD34 staining is also found in some ordinary cirrhotic nodules. Dysplastic nodules will show a retained reticulin pattern. Mitotic figures are rare or absent and Ki-67 proliferation is often similar to the background liver or minimally elevated. Immunostains are negative for AFP and β-catenin nuclear accumulation. Most dysplastic nodules are either negative for glypican 3 or show patchy staining. Nodules that show strong and diffuse glypican 3 staining suggest hepatocellular carcinoma. Likewise, strong and diffuse staining for glutamine synthetase favors hepatocellular carcinoma. Immunostains for heat-shock protein 70 are not widely available, but positivity in a nodule also favors hepatocellular carcinoma.[78] Dysplastic nodules are further divided into low- and high-grade dysplastic nodules (Figs. 28.6 and 28.7). Low-grade dysplastic nodules have mild dysplasia but clearly show more atypia than the background liver. High-grade dysplastic nodules have sufficient atypia that they would qualify in most cases for well-differentiated hepatocellular carcinoma if they had convincing reticulin loss (Table 28.4). Classifying dysplastic nodules as low grade or high grade can be challenging on needle biopsy specimens, but works reasonably well in resection specimens.

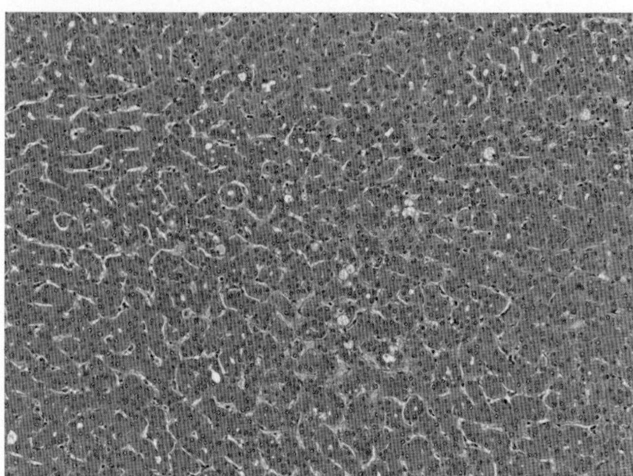

Figure 28.6 Dysplastic nodule, low grade. The hepatocytes show a slight increase in N:C ratio and patchy foci of psuedoglandular architecture.

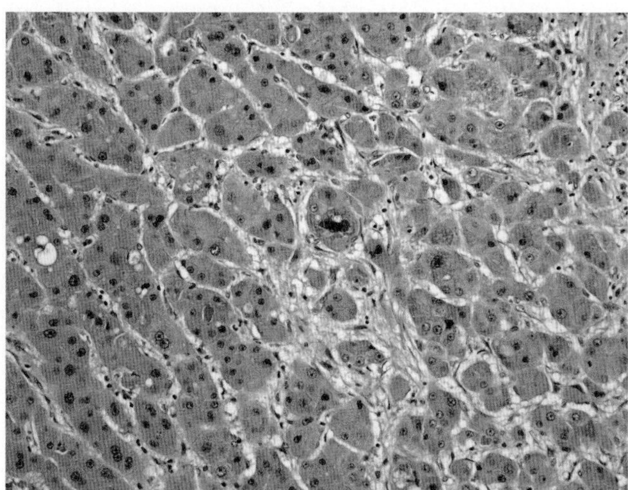

Figure 28.7 Dysplastic nodule, high grade. This nodule shows significant nuclear pleomorphism and pseudogland formation.

Differential

The differential for a low-grade dysplastic nodule is a macroregenerative nodule. In most cases, comparison to the background liver is sufficient to make a diagnosis because low-grade dysplastic nodules will have cytologic and architectural changes that are not present to the same degree in the background liver. Inevitably, there are nodules with just a smidgen more atypia than the background liver, making them hard to classify. One reasonable approach is show these cases to a colleague; if you're both still uncertain if there is enough atypia for a dysplastic nodule, call it a macroregenerative nodule.

The differential for a high-grade dysplastic nodule is primarily a well-differentiated hepatocellular carcinoma. High-grade dysplastic nodules can have similar levels of cytologic atypia to that of a well-differentiate hepatocellular carcinoma, but they will not have definite loss of reticulin, easily identified mitotic figures, or a significantly increased Ki-67 proliferative rate compared to the background liver. Almost all high-grade dysplastic nodules have retained portal structures, so their absence favors hepatocellular carcinoma. Dysplastic nodules are negative for nuclear accumulation of β-catenin and lack AFP expression. Unfortunately, neither marker is very sensitive for the diagnosis of hepatocellular carcinoma, but they can

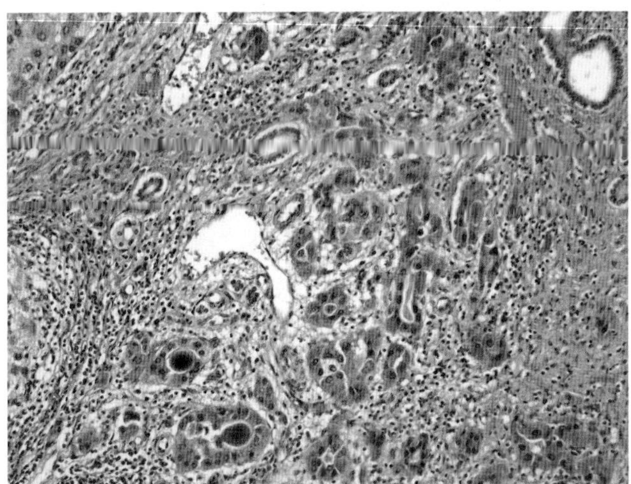

Figure 28.8 Stromal invasion. The hepatocellular carcinoma invades into this portal tract.

be helpful when positive. As noted above, strong and diffuse staining for glypican 3 or glutamine synthetase also favors hepatocellular carcinoma.

Stromal invasion, when present, is consistent with hepatocellular carcinoma.[79–81] Stromal invasion is defined as malignant cells invading the stroma of portal tracts or fibrous bands (Fig. 28.8). Stromal invasion is very helpful when present, but is very challenging to confidently identify in biopsies. Overall, stromal invasion is most frequently seen in moderately to poorly differentiated hepatocellular carcinomas, in which cases a dysplastic nodule is unlikely to be in your differential. The use of CK7 or CK19 immunostains can improve detection of stromal invasion, because a ductular reaction (highlighted by the keratin stains) is typically absent at the edges of hepatocellular carcinomas with stromal invasion, but present at the edges of high-grade dysplastic nodules.[82] Nonetheless, CK7 and CK19 staining patterns do not map perfectly with stromal invasion and the criteria of stromal invasion remains sufficiently challenging to implement on needle biopsy that it is not widely employed to make this distinction. In essentially all cases, the cytologic and immunohistochemic findings are sufficient to make the appropriate diagnosis without stromal invasion.

Management

Formal clinical management guidelines of small hepatocellular lesions are based more on lesion size and imaging findings because many are not biopsied, but in general dysplastic nodules are followed radiographically every 6 months until they either disappear or enlarge. If they enlarge, biopsies are helpful to determine if hepatocellular carcinoma has developed. Some centers treat high-grade dysplastic nodules with ablation therapies.[83,84]

Focal nodular-like hyperplasia

Cirrhotic livers have many vascular shunts and sometimes these can lead to nodules that look and stain-like focal nodular hyperplasias.[67,68] To separate them from conventional focal nodular hyperplasias, they are called focal nodular hyperplasia-like lesions. They do not have neoplastic potential.[69] In keeping with vascular shunting as their etiology, these lesions are more common after chemoembolization and in individuals with esophageal varices.[69] However, this lesion does not appear to be identical to typical focal nodular hyperplasia based on transcriptome profiling.[70]

28.8 HEPATOCELLULAR CARCINOMA

Gross findings

The gross findings of hepatocellular carcinoma are important for staging and for guiding sampling for sections. The gross description should comment on the number of tumors, their size(s), the margin status (distance to closest margin) the percent of tumor necrosis (estimated to the nearest 10%), and the presence or absence of gross vascular invasion.

Most hepatocellular carcinomas are soft and bulge out from the cut surface of the liver, a helpful finding when grossing in a cirrhotic liver explant. Hepatocellular carcinomas also frequently have different colors than the background liver. Some hepatocellular carcinomas have a capsule of inflamed fibrotic tissue.

Hepatocellular carcinomas can be further classified into one of four growth patterns on gross examination: (1) a single distinct tumor nodule; (2) a large dominant nodule and multiple smaller "satellite" nodules, usually within 2 cm of the dominant nodule, a pattern that results from local spread of the large dominant nodule; (3) multiple distinct tumor nodules that are sufficiently distant from each other that they would not fit for satellite tumors, a pattern that reflects a field effect, with foci of independent hepatocellular carcinomas; (4) numerous small tumor nodules that are about the same size as a cirrhotic nodule, usually with 30 or more nodules, a pattern called diffuse" or "cirrhotomimetic." The tumor burden with this last pattern is always greater than recognized on imaging studies and often by gross examination, with the extent of tumor only evident with histologic examination.

As another gross finding, up to 4% of hepatocellular carcinomas are pedunculated, protruding from the surface of the liver.[85] Pedunculated hepatocellular carcinomas can mimic metastatic disease to the adrenal gland on imaging studies,[86] but the gross findings are otherwise typical of hepatocellular carcinoma. In addition, tumors with this growth pattern do not have any unique histologic findings.[87] Clinically, some studies have suggested pedunculated tumors have a better prognosis, but overall the data is limited and this growth pattern is not entirely convincing as an independent prognostic factor.[85,88]

The optimal number of sections needed to evaluate a hepatocellular carcinoma specimen has not been well defined, but the standard of care is generally regarded as at least one section per cm of tumor. Some pathologists put two or three or more mini-sections into a single cassette, cleverly counting them toward the total section count, an approach that does not always seem to be within the spirit of striving for the best possible patient care. Tumor grade and microscopic vascular invasion are key prognostic findings, ones that depend on reasonably thorough sampling. The tumor–nontumor interface should be well sampled, being high yield for identifying vascular invasion.

Sections from the background liver are used to examine for ongoing liver disease and to determine the fibrosis stage. Sections should be taken as far away from the hepatocellular carcinoma as possible because the liver near the edge of the tumor commonly shows significant inflammation and fibrosis. The surgical resection margin section is often taken separate from the background liver section because the surgical margin commonly shows cautery effect.

Microscopic findings

Diagnosis

Hepatocellular carcinomas are diagnosed when significant cytologic and/or architectural atypia is identified. These architectural and cytologic abnormalities are often easiest to see by examining the hematoxylin and eosin (H&E) at low-power magnification, looking for populations of cells that look different from the background liver. These cytologic and architectural changes serve two functions. First, they can separate tumor from the nontumor background liver. Second, they are used to distinguish benign hepatic tumors from hepatocellular carcinoma. None are perfectly sensitive or specific, so they need to be used together and are typically supplemented with immunohistochemical stains.

Architectural changes

Neither benign nor malignant hepatic neoplasms have normal portal tracts. Some hepatocellular carcinomas and fibrolamellar carcinomas will have entrapped normal portal tracts, mostly at the edge of the tumor, but the lack of true portal tracts is an important finding supporting a diagnosis of neoplasm. Some tumors can also have fibrous septae with vascular structures, but true portal tracts are absent. A second useful architectural feature is small arteries located in the hepatic lobules (Fig. 28.9). In the normal liver, arterioles are present only in the portal tracts, but hepatic neoplasms frequently show small arterioles in the hepatic lobules. As a caveat, aberrant lobular arteries are not diagnostic of a neoplasm, also being found when nontumor liver parenchyma shows vascular flow abnormalities, including portal and hepatic vein flow obstruction in nonfibrotic livers (Fig. 28.10) and cirrhosis from many different causes, especially when there is widespread central vein sclerosis, for example with alcohol related cirrhosis. A third useful architectural finding is abnormal hepatic cord organization. In the nonneoplastic liver, the hepatic cords or plates have a regular organization and are

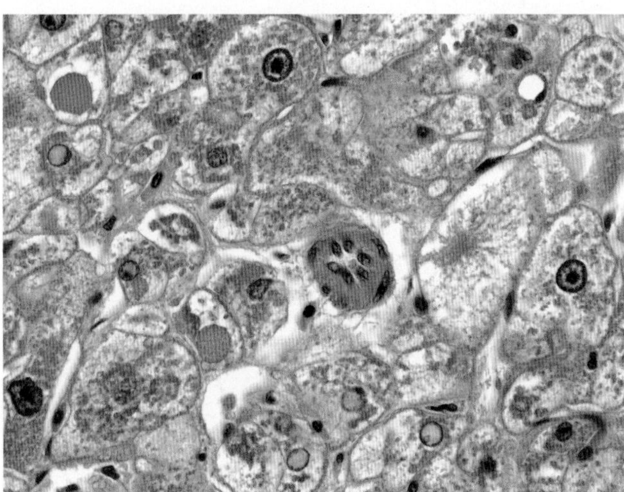

Figure 28.9 Hepatocellular carcinoma, abnormal lobular artery. This finding is also called a naked artery.

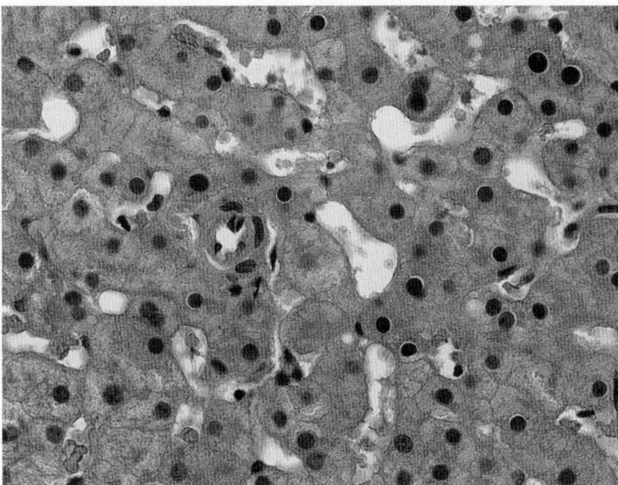

Figure 28.10 Aberrant arteriole in nontumor liver. A small lobular arteriole in seen in this case with a long-standing portal vein thrombosis.

one to two cells in thickness. In contrast, neoplasms will have abnormal growth patterns, such as plate thickening and pseudoacinar structures. The reticulin stain is discussed below and is a key method used to identify abnormal plate organization.

Cytologic changes

Cytologic atypia includes nuclear and cytoplasmic changes. Cytologic atypia varies a lot between hepatocellular carcinomas, forming the basis for determining tumor grade. Nuclear changes consist largely of prominent nucleoli, variable amounts of hyperchromasia, membrane irregularities (Fig. 28.11), nuclear size variation, and rarely multinucleation (Fig. 28.12). One area with some uncertainty are cases with focal cytologic atypia similar to large cell change (larger hyperchromatic nuclei with a normal N:C ratio) in a tumor that would otherwise qualify for a hepatic adenoma. Some pathologists consider these to be "degenerative changes" acceptable within a hepatic adenoma, but many pathologists do not. At this point, data on this specific point is limited, but such tumors are best considered as atypical adenomas at a minimum.

Cytoplasmic changes include reduced volume, often accompanied by increased basophilia. Although an increased N:C ratio is common in hepatocellular carcinoma, this finding is not universal and some carcinomas retain abundant pink cytoplasm. Other cytoplasmic changes include heavy lipofuschin deposits (Fig. 28.13), hyaline bodies (Fig. 28.14), pale

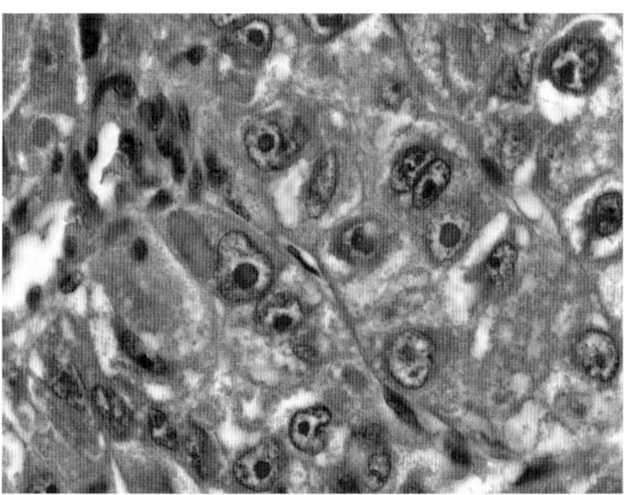

Figure 28.11 Hepatocellular carcinoma, nuclear abnormalities. The tumor cells show nuclear pleomorphism with prominent nucleoli.

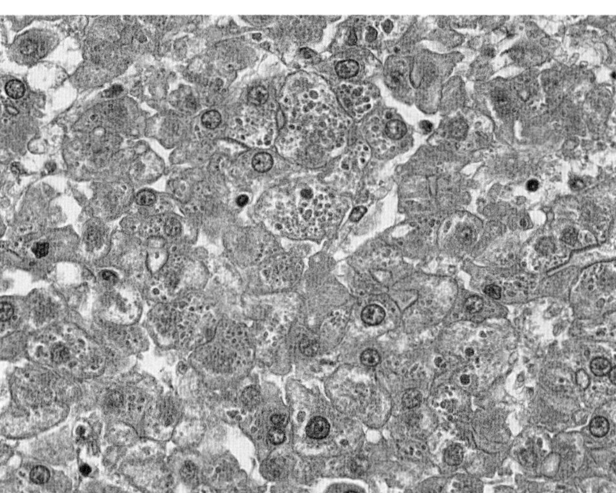

Figure 28.13 Hepatocellular carcinoma, lipofuschin. The tumor cells have abundant lipofuschin.

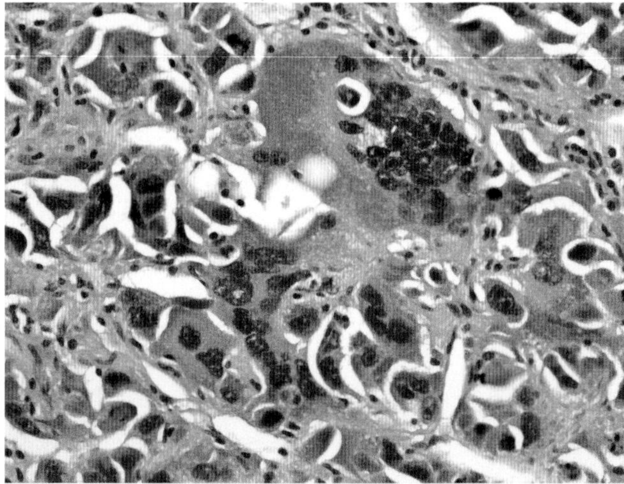

Figure 28.12 Hepatocellular carcinoma, multinucleation. Many of the tumor cells are multinucleated.

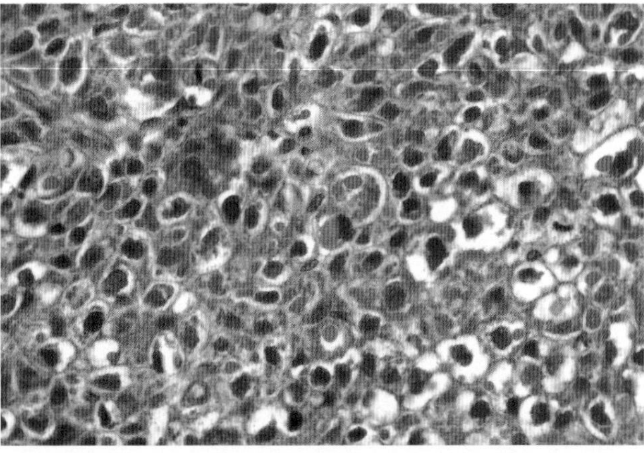

Figure 28.14 Hepatocellular carcinoma, hyaline bodies. This image is from a subtumor in a clear cell hepatocellular carcinoma that had high-grade cytology and numerous hyaline bodies, whereas the background tumor did not.

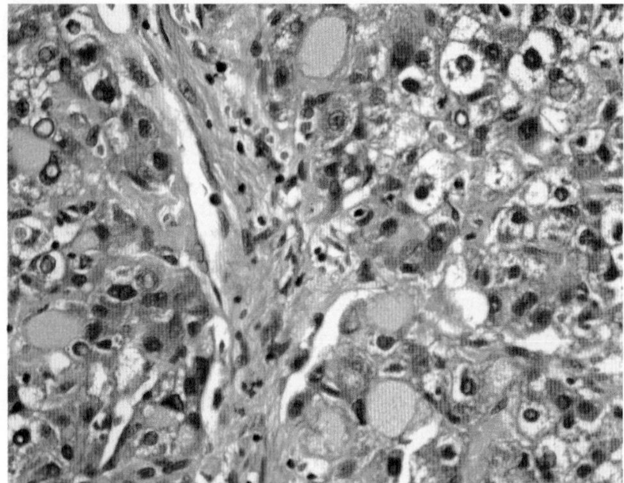

Figure 28.15 Pale bodies in a conventional hepatocellular carcinoma.

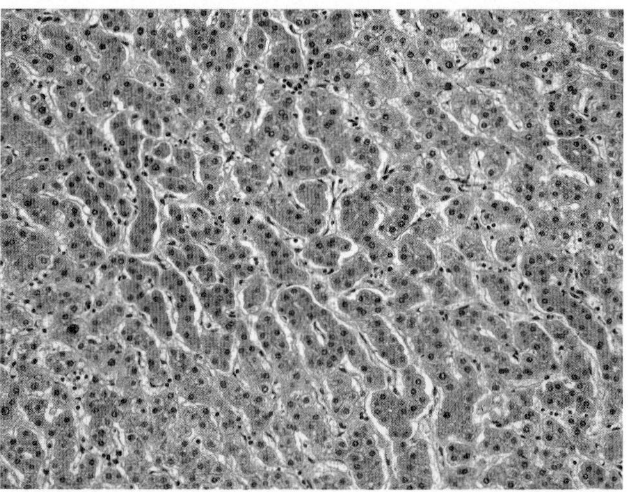

Figure 28.17 Hepatocellular carcinoma, trabecular growth pattern.

bodies (Fig. 28.15), or Mallory–Denk bodies (Fig. 28.16). Hepatocellular carcinomas with hyaline bodies appear to have a worse prognosis, but there are no known clinical correlates for Mallory–Denk bodies or pale bodies. Hepatocellular carcinoma can also show abundant glycogen accumulation, steatosis, or cholestasis, making them stand out from the background liver.

Growth patterns

These are the four major histologic growth patterns found in hepatocellular carcinomas (Figs. 28.17, 28.18, 28.19, and 28.20)[89]: trabecular (70%), solid (also known as compact, 20%), pseudoglandular (also known as pseudoacinar, 10%), and macrotrabecular (1%). All are defined by the H&E findings without use of special stains. Growth patterns are not the same as hepatocellular carcinoma subtypes,

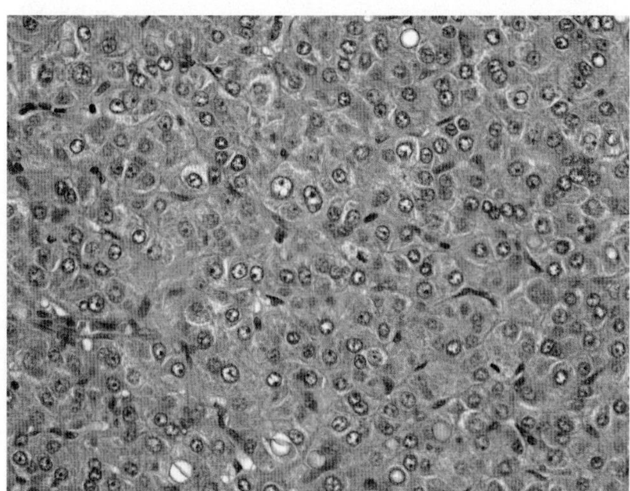

Figure 28.18 Hepatocellular carcinoma, solid growth pattern.

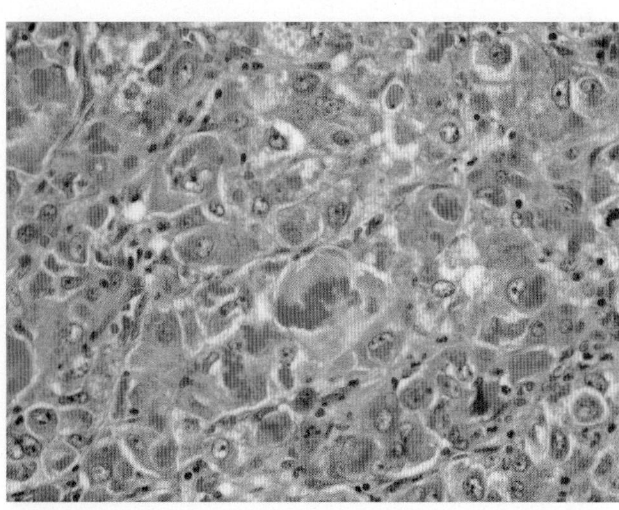

Figure 28.16 Hepatocellular carcinoma, Mallory–Denk bodies.

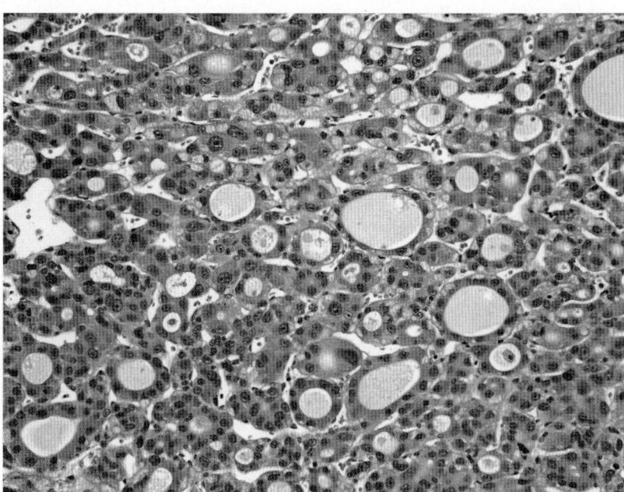

Figure 28.19 Hepatocellular carcinoma, psuedoglandular growth pattern.

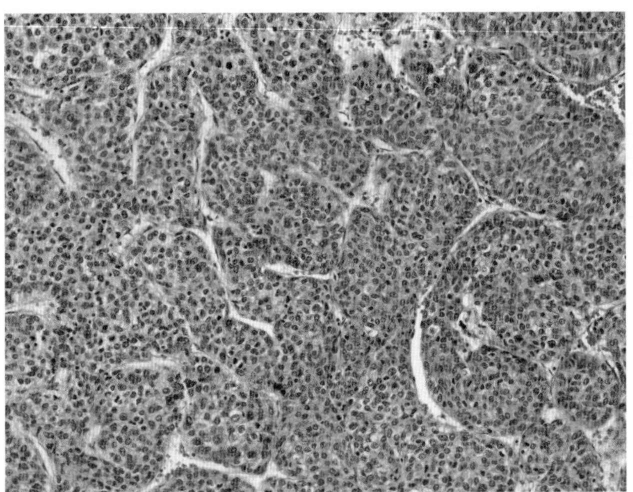

Figure 28.20 **Hepatocellular carcinoma, macrotrabecular growth pattern.**

which are described in their own section below. In fact, any of the growth patterns can be found in any of the hepatocellular carcinoma subtypes.

The solid growth pattern is just like it sounds: solid sheets of cells with no definite trabecular, pseudoacinar, or macrotrabecular growth. The trabecular variant has trabeculae of variable thickness, but less than 10 cells. In contrast, the macrotrabecular pattern is defined by trabeculae at least 10 cells in thickness on average. In the pseudoglandular pattern, the tumor cells form small gland- or rosette-like structures. In some cases, the psuedoglands are considerably large, often being filled with thin, granular material, a pattern of growth sometimes called acinar or pseudocyst of follicle-like (Fig. 28.21). Additional changes can accompany any of the above growth patterns. These include bile accumulation (Fig. 28.22), peliosis-like areas (Fig. 28.23), or clusters of benign macrophages in the tumor sinusoids (Fig. 28.24).

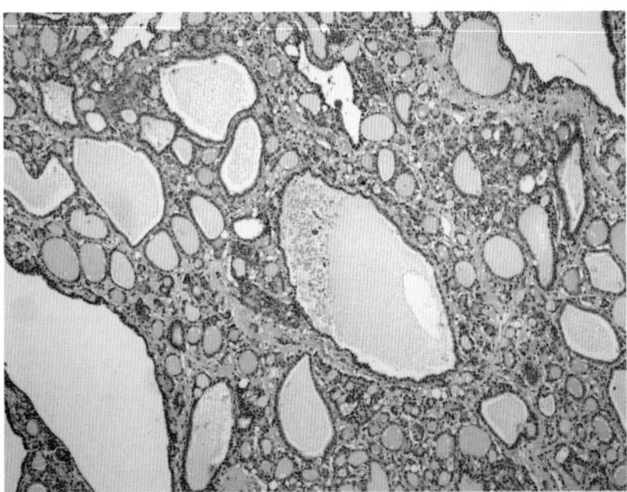

Figure 28.21 **Hepatocellular carcinoma, large pseudocyst.**

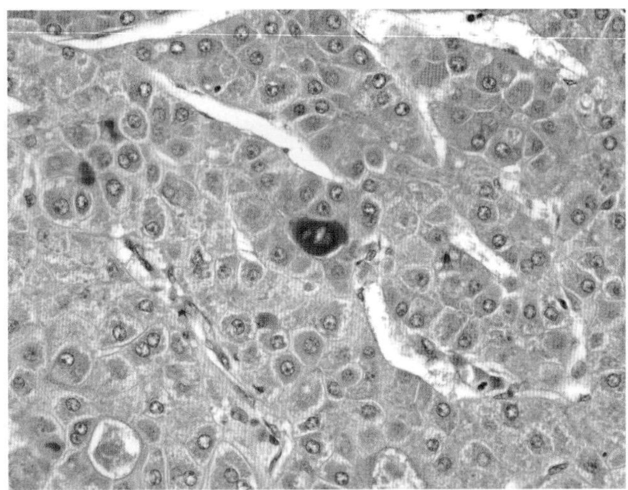

Figure 28.22 **Hepatocellular carcinoma with bile.**

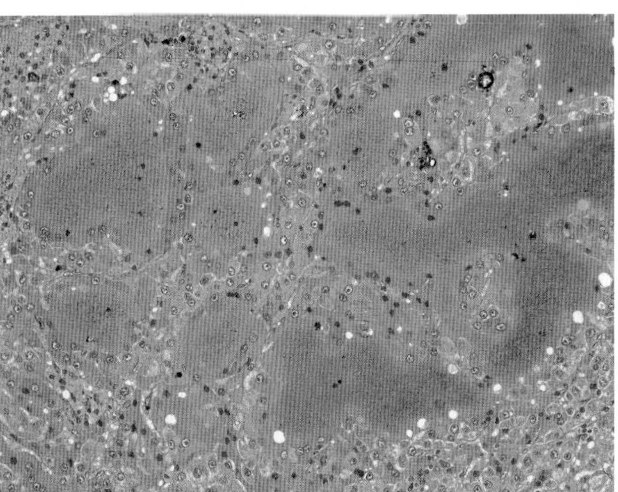

Figure 28.23 **Hepatocellular carcinoma, peliosis-like changes.**

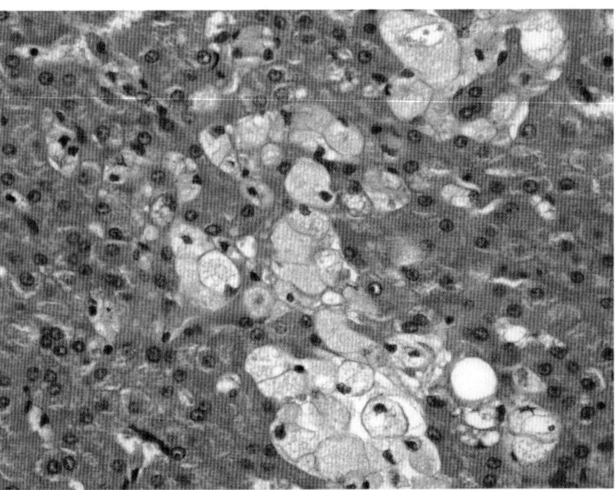

Figure 28.24 **Hepatocellular carcinoma, macrophages in sinusoids.** Benign macrophages are seen within the tumor sinusoids.

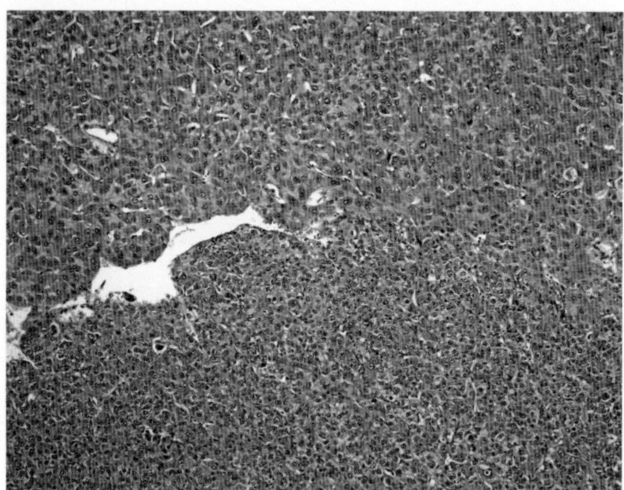

Figure 28.25 Hepatocellular carcinoma, nodule within nodule. This hepatocellular carcinoma (**top**) had a distinct nodule within it that shows higher grade cytology (**bottom**).

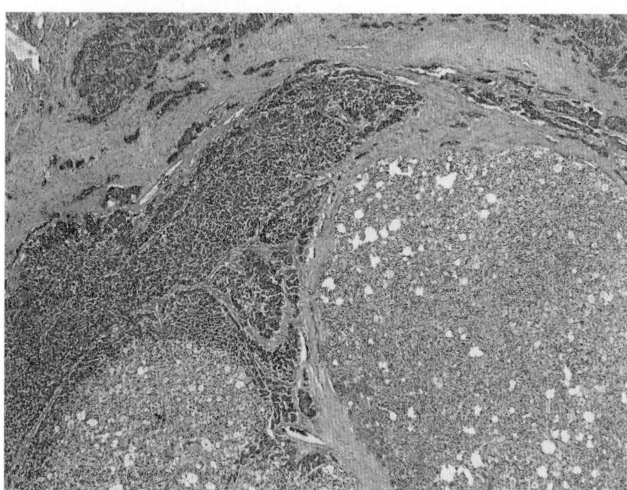

Figure 28.26 Hepatocellular carcinoma, multiple morphologies. The nodules are adjacent to each other and show distinctly different morphologies.

The above patterns are straightforwardly defined, but not always so straightforward to apply. In some cases, compressed trabeculae can resemble a solid growth pattern. Likewise, the macrotrabecular pattern can also show areas of more compressed growth that resembles a solid growth pattern. In addition, about 50% of resection specimens have mixed patterns, most commonly trabecular plus one or two others. Finally, the results will vary, sometimes considerably, depending on the cutoff used to score a growth pattern as being present. Most studies use the reasonable cutoff of 5% but others use higher or lower cutoffs.

These growth patterns are significant for several reasons. First, familiarity with them can be useful when making a diagnosis of hepatocellular carcinoma. For example, recognizing the pseudoacinar growth pattern can help avoid a misdiagnosis of cholangiocarcinoma or combined hepatocellular-cholangiocarcinoma. Secondly, the macrotrabecular pattern has a worse prognosis when compared to the solid growth pattern.[90] In particular, macrotrabecular hepatocellular carcinomas with small basophilic tumor cells are typically AFP-positive and have extensive angiolymphatic invasion.

Some hepatocellular carcinomas show a nodule-in-nodule growth pattern, with a main tumor mass showing one morphology and within it morphologically distinct nodule(s) with higher grade cytology that represent emergence of a more aggressive tumor clone (Fig. 28.25). These higher grade nodules often show some morphologic similarities to the larger, lower grade nodule. In addition to this pattern, other hepatocellular carcinomas don't show a dominant nodule with emergence of a higher grade nodule, but instead show multiple adjacent nodules that have distinctly different morphologies (Fig. 28.26) often with the same overall cytologic grade, a finding of uncertain molecular genesis, but one that possibly reflects genomic instability.

Histologic grading

Tumor grade is a strong predictor of overall patient survival and disease free survival. This prognostic power is seen after resections in cirrhotic livers,[47,91] noncirrhotic livers,[48] and after liver transplantation.[47,49] Many (one-third) of hepatocellular carcinomas have two or more nuclear grades. In these cases, the predominant tumor grade and the worse tumor grade should be reported. The worse grade tends to drive prognosis.[92] Tumor grade correlates with tumor size and with angiolymphatic invasion, but has independent prognostic value in most multivariate studies.

The modified Edmondson-Steiner grading system (Table 28.5) is frequently used in research studies.[89]

Table 28.5 Modified Edmondson–Steiner grading system for hepatocellular carcinoma

Grade	Criteria
1	Abundant cytoplasm; minimal nuclear atypia
2	Mild nuclear atypia with prominent nucleoli, hyperchromasia, and nuclear irregularity
3	Moderate nuclear atypia with greater hyperchromasia and nuclear irregularity
4	Marked nuclear pleomorphism, marked hyperchromasia, and anaplastic giant cells

In clinical practice, and many research studies, a three-tier system is used: well differentiated, moderately differentiated, and poorly differentiated (Table 28.6). In addition, some pathologists will use additional categories of very well differentiated and undifferentiated (Table 28.6 and Figs. 28.27, 28.28, 28.29, 28.30, and 28.31).

Table 28.6 Grading hepatocellular carcinomas

Grade	Criteria
Very well differentiated	• Adenoma-like on H&E • Minimal to no nuclear atypia • N:C ratio is normal • Diagnosis based on patchy reticulin loss or abnormal immunostain findings
Well-differentiated	• Hepatic differentiation is readily evident on H&E • Mild nuclear atypia • N:C ratio is normal or increased • Additional stains needed to prove malignancy in most cases
Moderately differentiated	• Clearly malignant on H&E • Overall morphology strongly suggests hepatocellular origin • Moderate nuclear atypia • N:C ratio increased almost always • Stains are helpful to confirm hepatocyte differentiation
Poorly differentiated	• Clearly malignant on H&E • H&E morphology consistent with a range of poorly differentiated carcinomas • Marked nuclear atypia, or moderate nuclear atypia but minimal tumor cytoplasm with very high N:C ratio • Immunostains needed to confirm hepatocellular differentiation
Undifferentiated	• No morphologic features of hepatic differentiation or glandular differentiation on the H&E • Stains are needed to prove the neoplasm is epithelial • H&E differential includes lymphoma, melanoma, or mesenchymal tumors • Keratin-positive, but keratin-negative for hepatic markers such as HepPar1, Arginase, and glypican 3 • Metastatic disease excluded by immunostains, imaging, and clinical findings

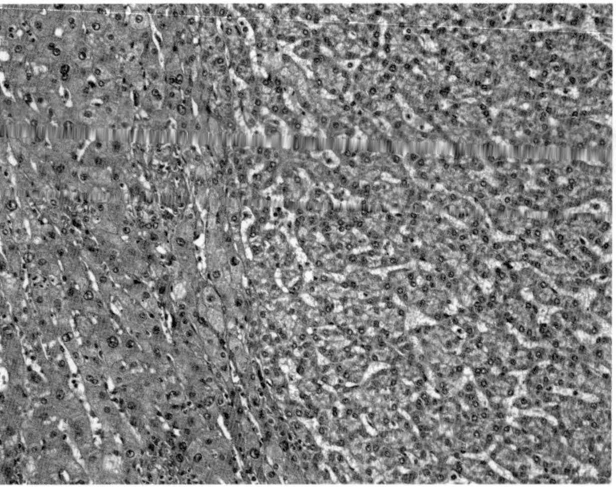

Figure 28.27 Hepatocellular carcinoma, very well differentiated. This hepatocellular carcinoma (**right**, with normal liver on the **left**) cannot be distinguished from an adenoma without special stains.

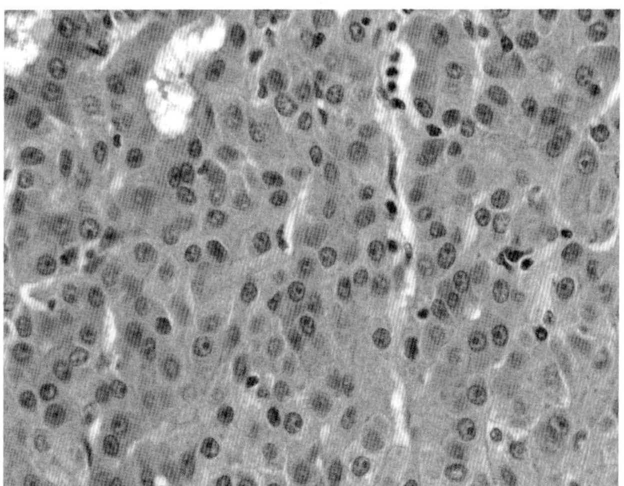

Figure 28.28 Hepatocellular carcinoma, well differentiated. The tumor cells have plenty of cytoplasm, and there is only mild nuclear atypia. Note, however, that the tumor nuclei lack the regular, orderly spacing of benign proliferations.

Changes after chemoembolization therapy

Chemoembolization or ablation therapy is used to treat hepatocellular carcinomas localized to the liver, both as primary therapy in unresectable tumors and to shrink tumors, allowing surgery in previously unresectable tumors. Not surprisingly, chemoembolization or ablation therapy can affect both the gross and microscopic findings.

Treated tumors are staged in the same fashion as nontreated tumors. The percent necrosis should be estimated to the nearest 10% using the gross and/or histologic findings. The percent necrosis after TACE

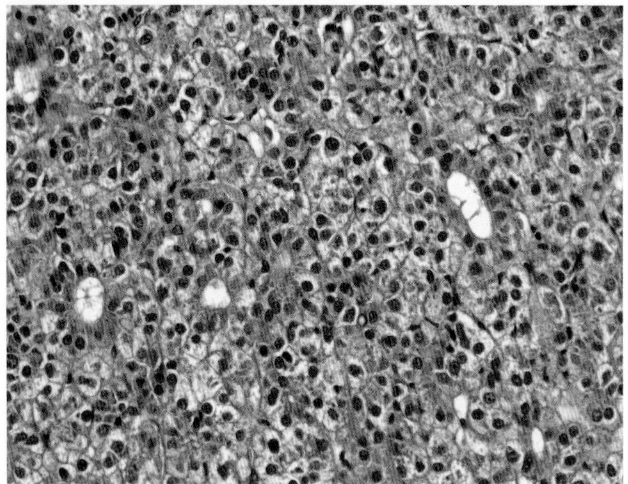

Figure 28.29 Hepatocellular carcinoma, moderately differentiated. The tumor morphology strongly suggests hepatic differentiation and the tumor is clearly malignant.

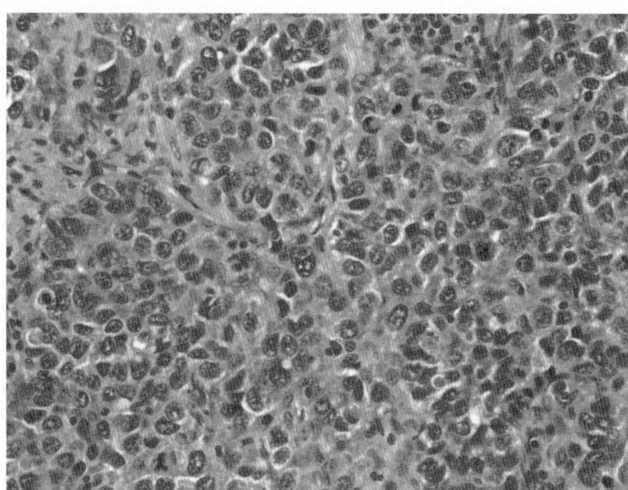

Figure 28.31 Hepatocellular carcinoma, poorly differentiated. This tumor has scant basophilic cytoplasm with large pleomorphic nuclei.

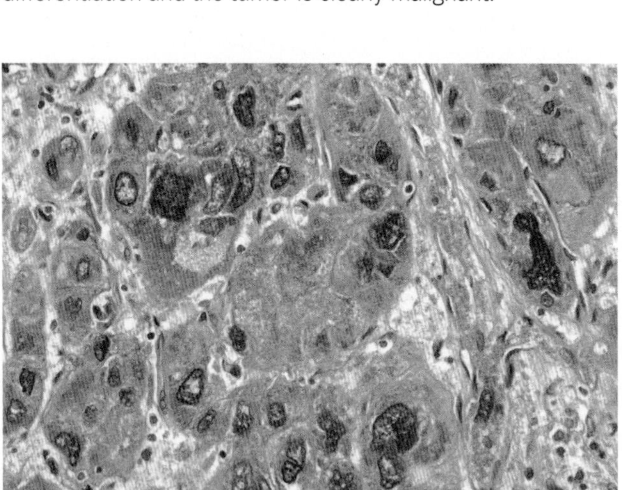

Figure 28.30 Hepatocellular carcinoma, poorly differentiated. There is striking nuclear atypia. Immunostains demonstrated hepatic differentiation. Imaging studies reported no other tumor sites.

ranges from 0% to 100%, with an average of 50% to 70% necrosis in those tumors with necrosis.[46,93,94] About 30% of tumors are completely necrotic.[46] Hepatocellular carcinomas with strong and diffuse CD34 staining and negative VEGF staining appear to be more resistant to TACE.[95] There is no reliable way to distinguish necrosis that resulted from treatment versus spontaneous tumor necrosis and all necrosis is included in the estimate.

Treatment can lead to other histologic changes, such as intratumoral inflammation and intratumoral fibrosis. Treated tumors are also more likely to express CK19 and have areas with biliary and/or spindled cell morphology.[96,97] The potential effect of treatment on tumor grade has not been well studied, but one study found a higher tumor grade in TACE-treated hepatocellular carcinomas.[98] This same study also found an increase in multinucleated tumor cells and cytoplasmic hyaline inclusions following treatment.[98] Embolic beads can be found in the tumor and in the adjacent nontumor liver. Embolic beads can also escape the liver, leading to damage to other organs, in particular the stomach (Fig. 28.1).

Immunohistochemical stains and special stains

Immunohistochemical stains are used to (1) decide if a well-differentiated hepatic tumor is benign or malignant (Table 28.7) and (2) decide if a clearly malignant tumor is hepatocellular carcinoma (Table 28.8).

The differential for a well-differentiated hepatic tumor depends in part on the background liver. In noncirrhotic livers, the differential is focal nodular hyperplasia, hepatic adenoma, and hepatocellular carcinoma. In a cirrhotic liver, the differential is focal nodular hyperplasia-like lesion, macroregenerative nodule, dysplastic nodule, and hepatocellular carcinoma. Of note, some nodules in cirrhotic livers can express CRP or SAA,[99,100] but at this point the term hepatic adenoma for these nodules is hard to justify, both because it leads to unnecessary confusion for the clinical team and because there is no evidence that such lesions behave clinically like an adenoma.

A wide variety of immunostains can be used when evaluating poorly differentiated tumors. Some of the more commonly used stains are shown in Table 28.9 along with the frequency of positive staining in hepatocellular carcinomas.

Table 28.7 Stains used to distinguish benign from malignant hepatic lesions

Stains	Comment
Reticulin	• Rarely (<1%), well-differentiated hepatocellular carcinomas will have no obvious reticulin loss
Ki-67	• To be helpful, staining should be significantly higher than background liver • Of note, not all hepatocellular carcinomas will have a higher proliferative rate
CD34	• Not widely used as there are better stains • Strong diffuse staining is commonly but not always found in hepatocellular carcinoma. Also, some hepatic adenomas can show strong and diffuse CD34 staining
Glypican 3	• Positive in about 50% of well-differentiated hepatocellular carcinomas • Also stains lipofuschin and benign hepatocytes with significant inflammation • Focal staining also found in some dysplastic nodules
α-Fetoprotein	• Positive in about one-third of all hepatocellular carcinomas
Glutamine synthetase	• Diffuse and strong positive in about 50% of hepatocellular carcinomas • β-Catenin inactivated adenoma also diffuse positive

Table 28.8 Stains used to demonstrate hepatocellular differentiation

Stains	Comment
Arginase 1	• Positive in 90% of hepatocellular carcinomas • Negative tumors cluster at both ends of differentiation: well and poorly differentiated can both be negative
HepPar1	• Positive in 90% of hepatocellular carcinomas • Negative cases are usually poorly differentiated
Glypican 3	• Positive in 80%–90% of hepatocellular carcinomas • Performs poorly in well-differentiated hepatocellular carcinomas, where only 50% are positive
In situ hybridization for albumin	• Positive in >95% of hepatocellular carcinomas • Positive in 80%–95% of cholangiocarcinomas
Polyclonal CEA (canalicular pattern)	• Positive in 60%–80% of hepatocellular carcinomas • Canalicular staining indicates hepatic differentiation • Membranous or cytoplasmic staining is compatible with hepatocellular carcinoma but not specific • There are better stains as this one tends to be challenging to interpret in poorly differentiated carcinomas
CD10 (canalicular pattern)	• Performance is similar to polyclonal CEA
α-Fetoprotein	• Positive in about one-third of hepatocellular carcinomas • Can be useful in poorly differentiated tumors, which may lose expression of other markers such as HepPar and Arginase

None of these stains are 100% specific and they are best used in combination with clinical findings and H&E morphology

Universal rules governing the use of immunohistochemistry

Four fundamental, immutable laws govern the use of immunohistochemistry in tumors.

Law 1. *All special stains should be interpreted in conjunction with the H&E findings.* For example, if a tumor's morphology is inconsistent with hepatocellular carcinoma, immunostain findings will not change that. Cross checking positive immunostains with the H&E is also important to avoid mistaking the positive staining of entrapped hepatocytes for positive staining of a tumor.

Law 2. *The sensitivity and specificity of immunostains invariably get worse as more studies are published.* The first one is (almost) always the best, but the sensitivity and specificity will fall as more data accumulates. This is because the performances of stains depend on a variety of factors including those specific to laboratory methods and those that reflect biology, such as the strong correlation that can be seen between stain sensitivity and tumor grade, underlying liver disease, and/or tumor subtype. For these

Table 28.9 Frequency of positive staining for nonhepatocellular markers in hepatocellular carcinoma

Immunostain	Approximate frequency	Comments
Epithelial markers		
CAM5.2	>99%	
Cytokeratin AE1/AE3	10%	
CK19	15%	Positive tumors have a worse prognosis. Positive cases typically coexpress CK7
CK7	30%	Hepatocellular carcinomas that are cholestatic or occur in younger individuals (<40) are positive in the majority of cases
CK20	10%	Positive cases typically coexpress CK7
CK5/6	1%	
EMA	5%	
Stains for site of origin		
CDX2	5%	Staining is often focal in hepatocellular carcinoma. Also, 20%–30% of cholangiocarcinomas are CDX2-positive
TTF1	0%	TTF1 can show cytoplasmic staining with some antibodies, but not nuclear staining
Napsin		
PAX8	0%	Limited data
SALL4	45%	May be a marker of "stem cellness"
Villin	30%	Staining is typically strong and cytoplasmic and can have a membranous accentuation
GCDFP-15	0%	
Mammaglobin	0%	
Mesothelioma markers		
Moc31	35%	Usually patchy. Strong diffuse staining is seen in many cholangiocarcinomas
WT1	>80%	
Calretinin	0%	Limited data
D2-40	0%	Limited data
Stains used to subtype hepatic adenomas		
LFABP	20%	Stain is positive in normal liver; lost staining is informative
CRP	50%	Should be strong and fairly diffuse to be informative; some clones show considerable background staining
SAA	15%	
β-Catenin (nuclear)	30%	Can be very patchy
Glutamine synthetase	50%	Should be strong and diffuse to be informative
Other markers		
CD117 (Kit)	70%	
CD138	65%	Nonneoplastic hepatocytes are also positive. Membranous staining is seen in both tumor and nontumor
Vimentin	10%	About 10% of conventional hepatocellular carcinomas are positive. Sarcomatoid hepatocellular carcinomas are positive

reasons, most expert liver pathologists will choose from a panel of top performing stains because a wisely chosen panel of stains will help mitigate individual weaknesses of different immunostains.

Law 3. *If there is a discrepancy between the morphology and immunohistochemical findings, additional studies must be performed.* Examples of additional studies include submitting more sections on resection specimens, repeating discrepant stains, and performing an additional round of immunostains that focuses on clarify the differential(s) raised by the discrepant findings.

Law 4. *A difficult case is the wrong time to first use a stain with which you're not familiar.* The temptation can be very strong to use an unfamiliar stain in the hopes of getting yourself out of a diagnostic jam. However, this often leads to diagnostic misadventures. If you cannot resist temptation, at a minimum, the results of unfamiliar stains should be reviewed (not just verbally, but actually reviewed) by somebody with skill in interpreting the stain.

Reticulin stain

Normal hepatocytes are organized in thin plates/cords, with each hepatocyte touching reticulin on one of their borders. Reticulin loss is used to support a diagnosis of malignancy. Of note, poor quality or "light" reticulin stains can show artifactual reticulin loss that mimics hepatocellular carcinoma. When available on the same section, the nonneoplastic liver should be carefully examined to ensure that the staining in the background liver is strong and crisp, with each hepatocyte clearly touching the reticulin framework. If this is not the case, then the stain should be repeated.

In hepatocellular carcinoma, groups of hepatocytes will not be touching the reticulin framework on any of their cell membranes (Figs. 28.32 and 28.33). The reticulin loss in hepatocellular carcinomas will vary from patchy loss to near total loss. However, focal equivocal reticulin loss as an isolated finding is insufficient for a diagnosis of hepatocellular carcinoma. In addition, benign hepatocytes with macrovesicular steatosis commonly show patchy loss of reticulin that can mimic hepatocellular carcinoma, especially when the steatosis is marked (Fig. 28.34).[101,102] In this situation, it is best to focus on areas of the tumor with little or no steatosis. If this is not possible because of extensive fatty change, then the reticulin loss should be substantial and widespread to be informative.

A small percentage of well-differentiated hepatocellular carcinomas (less than 1%) do not have reticulin loss[103,104] (Fig. 28.35) and the final diagnosis relies on

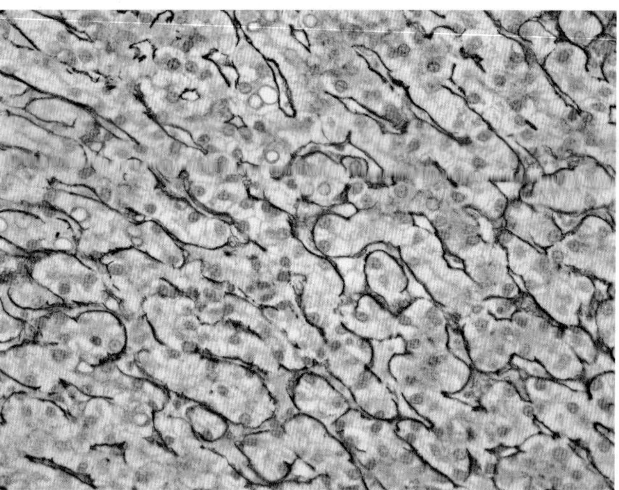

Figure 28.32 Reticulin, nonneoplastic liver. A normal reticulin pattern is seen, with every hepatocyte touching reticulin on one of its borders.

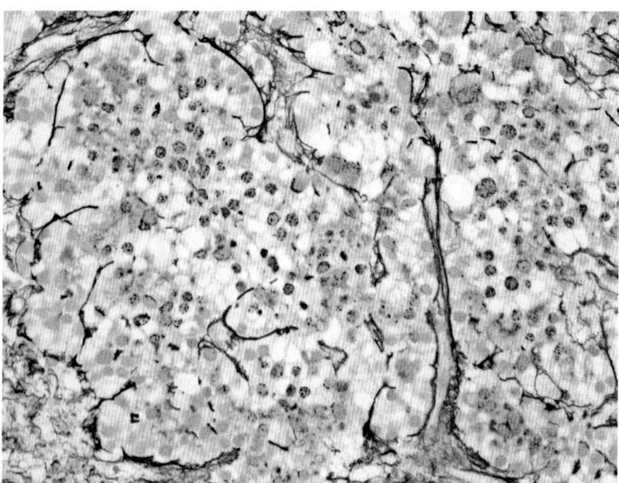

Figure 28.33 Reticulin, hepatocellular carcinoma There is patchy but extensive loss of reticulin.

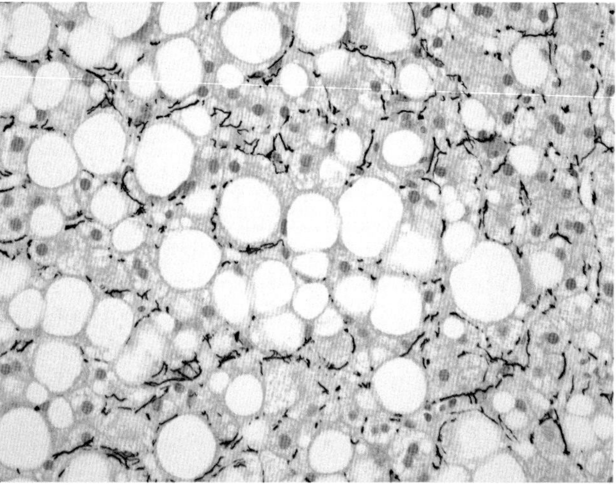

Figure 28.34 Reticulin, nonneoplastic liver with fatty change. This is a medical liver biopsy, with no tumor, but the areas of fatty change show reduced reticulin.

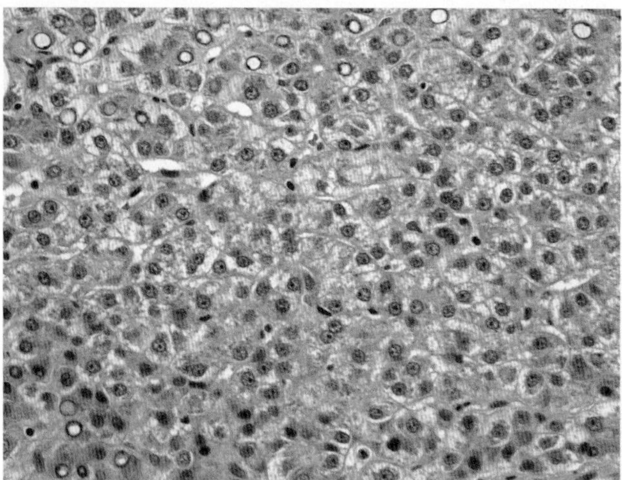

Figure 28.35 Hepatocellular carcinoma with no reticulin loss. Although rare, some hepatocellular carcinomas will show no reticulin loss, as seen in this biopsy specimen. Perhaps the full resection would have shown reticulin loss.

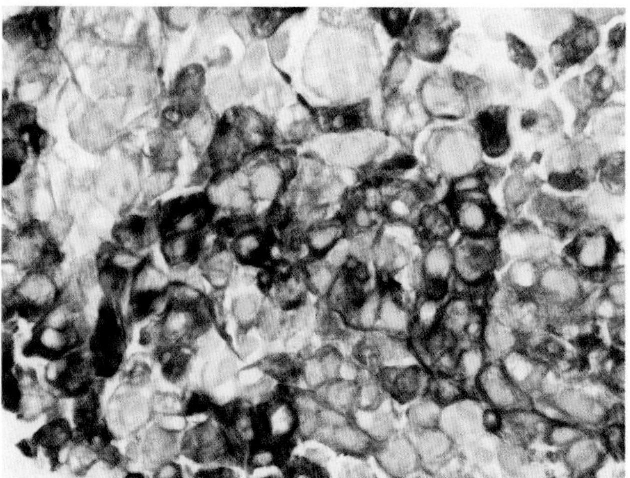

Figure 28.36 Hepatocellular carcinoma, CK20. Five percent of hepatocellular carcinomas can be CK20-positive.

other findings such as cytologic atypia, increased proliferation rates, and/or strong expression of AFP or glypican 3. Many but not all of these cases have dense intratumoral fibrosis.

CD34

In the normal liver, CD34 stains the zone 1 sinusoids. In contrast, many hepatocellular carcinomas will show strong and diffuse staining of all of the sinusoids,[105] reflecting the increased arterial blood flow in the tumor. However, this finding is not very sensitive and not very specific, which limits the usefulness of this stain. For example, hepatocellular carcinomas at both ends of the differentiation spectrum (well and poorly differentiated) often lack this staining pattern.[106] On the other hand, both hepatic adenomas and focal nodular hyperplasias can sometimes have a strong and diffuse staining pattern.[106–109]

Ki-67

Ki-67 stains can be helpful when evaluating a well-differentiated tumor, though a set cutoff should not be relied upon. Instead, Ki-67 is interpreted by comparing the background nonneoplastic liver on the same stained section as the tumor. If there is no nonneoplastic liver on the section, the stain is considerably less useful, except for when the results are very high, such as greater than 20%.

Cytokeratin stains

Hepatocellular carcinomas are positive for a number of different keratins. Keratin stains are generally not used to differentiate hepatocellular carcinoma from benign hepatic lesions or to distinguish hepatocellular carcinoma from metastatic disease. However, keratin stains are commonly used when working up moderately to poorly differentiated carcinomas of uncertain lineage. Almost all hepatocellular carcinomas are positive for CK8, CK18, and CAM5.2. Almost all hepatocellular carcinomas are negative for CK 5/6.[110] Fifteen percent of hepatocellular carcinomas are positive for CK AE1/3.[111]Thirty percent of hepatocellular carcinomas are positive for CK7[112,113] and 5% are positive for CK20 (Fig. 28.36). Fifteen percent of hepatocellular carcinomas are positive for CK19 and this indicates a worse prognosis.[112–114] Both CK20 and CK19 expression are typically found in hepatocellular carcinomas that also express CK7.[112,113]

pCEA and CD10

Both of these stains are considered positive when they show a canalicular pattern of staining. Their sensitivities for hepatocellular carcinoma are about 60% (CD10) and 75% (pCEA). In addition to the canalicular staining pattern, both markers can show cytoplasmic or membranous staining. In fact, one-third of hepatocellular carcinomas with canalicular staining also have "noncanalicular" staining of the cytoplasm and/or cell membrane, which is acceptable as being consistent with hepatic differentiation, as long as the canalicular staining is convincing. An additional 10% to 15% of hepatocellular carcinomas show only membranous or cytoplasmic staining without canalicular staining, a nonspecific pattern also seen with some metastatic carcinomas.

Both CD10 and pCEA perform best with well-differentiated and moderately differentiated hepatocellular carcinomas. Both perform poorly with poorly differentiated hepatocellular carcinomas. In addition, the canalicular staining pattern is often focal and equivocal in moderately and poorly differentiated tumors, contributing more confusion than clarity to the diagnosis.

α-Fetoprotein

AFP is a cytoplasmic stain. Only one-third of hepatocellular carcinomas are positive,[115] a sensitivity sufficiently low that its usefulness as a routine stain is limited. The stain also tends to have a high background, further discouraging its use. However, the stain can sometimes be helpful in very poorly differentiated hepatocellular carcinomas that are negative or equivocal for other markers of hepatic differentiation.

HepPar1

HepPar1 is directed against carbamoyl phosphate synthetase 1, a mitochondrial protein in the urea cycle,[116] leading to a strong granular staining pattern of the cytoplasm.[117,118] Benign hepatocytes are strongly and diffusely positive, whereas staining in tumors can be strong and diffuse or patchy. Patchy staining is acceptable as evidence of hepatic differentiation, though care must be taken to not mistake the staining of entrapped benign hepatocytes for the staining of tumor cells. The sensitivity is about 90%, with excellent performance in well-differentiated and moderately differentiated hepatocellular carcinomas and a drop off in sensitivity for poorly differentiated tumors.

In terms of specificity, HepPar1 stains a number of tumors from other sites,[119] the most common being gastric adenocarcinomas (up to 40%), ovarian clear cell and ovarian mucinous carcinoma (up to 35% each), adrenal cortical carcinoma (up to 15%), lung adenocarcinoma (up to 15%), cholangiocarcinoma (up to 10%), and neuroendocrine carcinoma (up to 10%). Fortunately, in most cases this is not a big problem because these carcinomas do not typically look like hepatocellular carcinoma on the H&E. A bigger challenge can be small biopsies of metastatic ovarian clear cell carcinomas, neuroendocrine carcinomas, or adrenal cortical carcinomas. Even in these settings, most cases are successfully managed by (1) incorporating the clinical and imaging findings and (2) a panel of immunostains to both rule in hepatocellular carcinoma and rule out potential mimics, choosing the panel based on the clinical, radiologic, or morphologic findings.

Glypican 3

Normal hepatocytes do not express glypican 3, though patchy staining can be seen in the setting of marked inflammation.[120] Glypican 3 is a cytoplasmic stain. Hepatocellular carcinomas often show diffuse or patchy staining. Glypican 3 stains many other tumors, so compatible morphology is necessary for the stain to indicate hepatic differentiation.[121] Glypican 3 has a sensitivity of about 90%. In contrast to most markers of hepatic differentiation, glypican 3 performs better in poorly differentiated hepatocellular carcinomas than it does in well-differentiated tumors, with only 50% of well-differentiated hepatocellular carcinomas staining positive. Hepatocellular carcinomas arising in noncirrhotic livers are less frequently positive than those arising in cirrhotic livers.[122] Of note, glypican 3 stains lipofuschin. Both benign and malignant hepatocytes can accumulate lipofuschin, so the H&E stain needs to be double checked to make sure that positive glypican 3 staining is not because of lipofuschin deposition. Finally, both macroregenerative nodules and dysplastic nodules can be focally glypican 3–positive.[122] On the other hand, strong and diffuse staining in a well-differentiated hepatic nodule in a cirrhotic liver is most consistent with hepatocellular carcinoma.

Arginase 1

Arginase 1 is a cytoplasmic and/or nuclear stain that is positive in benign and malignant hepatocytes.[123] Arginase is a urea cycle enzyme, explaining the cytoplasmic staining, but less so the nuclear staining. The overall sensitivity is about 90%. Arginase 1 can be negative in well-differentiated hepatocellular carcinomas (5%), but performs better than HepPar1 in poorly differentiated hepatocellular carcinomas. Arginase is more specific than HepPar1 and glypican 3, but other tumors can be Arginase-positive, including cholangiocarcinomas and metastatic carcinomas from the breast, pancreas, and colon.[124–126] Both Arginase 1 and HepPar1 are positive in hepatoid carcinomas from other sites.[127]

Albumin in situ hybridization

In situ hybridization for albumin shows cytoplasmic staining. The stain is sensitive and reasonably specific, but other carcinomas can also be positive, including many hepatoid adenocarcinomas,[127] many acinar cell carcinomas of the pancreas,[128,129] and occasional neuroendocrine tumors and adenocarcinomas of the lung (Figs. 28.37 and 28.38), breast, and gallbladder. Cholangiocarcinomas, are also frequently positive (reported range, 75% to 95%).[128,130] For these reasons, correlation with clinical and imaging findings and H&E morphology is necessary when interpreting the stain. The sole basis for a hepatocellular carcinoma diagnosis should not be positive in situ hybridization for albumin. Likewise, the sole basis

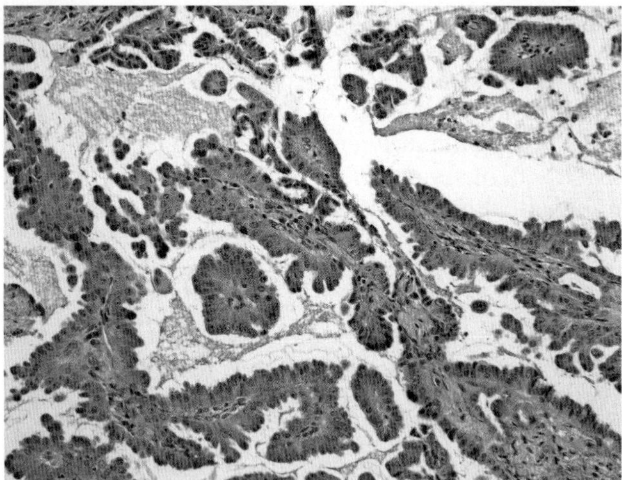

Figure 28.37 Papillary lung adenocarcinoma.

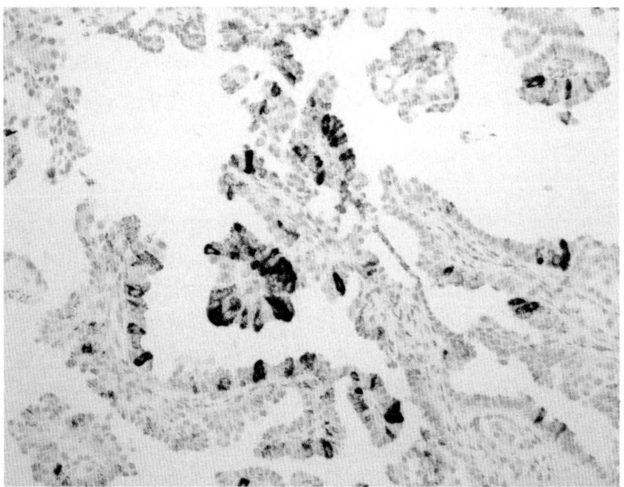

Figure 28.38 Papillary lung adenocarcinoma. An albumin in situ hybridization stain is positive; same case as above.

for a cholangiocarcinoma diagnosis should not be positive in situ hybridization for albumin in a gland forming carcinoma.

Molecular and other special techniques

Molecular methods do not currently play a role in diagnosis, other than for fibrolamellar carcinoma[131] and they also play no role in prognosis. It is not the case that molecular findings have no diagnostic and prognostic information per se, but rather that they contain less clinically useful information than that available through routine surgical pathology methods. However, this area of research is still in its infancy and this may change in time. For example, in other organs, molecular findings help guide therapy for cancer and this will likely develop for hepatocellular carcinoma in time.

Differential diagnosis

The differential for hepatocellular carcinoma depends primarily on two factors: (1) the degree of differentiation and (2) the presence or absence of cirrhosis in the background liver. When deciding between a benign versus malignant process, features that favor malignancy include cytologic atypia, pseudoglands, and cholestasis on H&E, with the exception of androgen related adenomas, which can show mild cytologic atypia, cholestatic changes, and psuedoglands. Hyaline inclusions and a nodule-in-nodule growth pattern strongly suggest hepatocellular carcinoma. Readily identified mitotic figures and a Ki-67 proliferative rate that is clearly above the background liver also favor malignancy. Convincing reticulin loss indicates malignancy, with the caveat of fatty areas of the tumor. Malignancy is strongly favored when there is more than focal glypican 3 staining or any AFP staining.

The differential for well-differentiated hepatic nodules in cirrhotic livers is essentially that of macroregenerative nodules, dysplastic nodules, or well-differentiated hepatocellular carcinoma. In contrast to hepatocellular carcinoma, both macroregenerative nodules and dysplastic nodules typically contain portal tracts and show no reticulin loss. They have low proliferative rates and lack mitotic figures. Cytologic atypia is absent or mild and focal in macroregenerative but is more evident in dysplastic nodules. Glypican 3 can be focally positive in some high-grade dysplastic nodules, but should not be strong and diffuse. AFP should be negative. β-Catenin staining is negative for nuclear accumulation and glutamine synthetase staining is patchy, without a strong and diffuse staining pattern. Of note, some nodules in cirrhotic livers can stain positive for CRP or SAA and can have some morphologic features of an inflammatory adenomas.[99,100] However, these should not be called hepatic adenomas in clinical practice, especially on biopsy specimens, because the natural history of these CRP/SAA-positive cirrhotic nodules is unclear. In this regard, their shared activation of a pathway does not make them the same tumor as a hepatic adenoma.

The great majority of well-differentiated hepatocellular tumors are confidently classified as benign or malignant, even on biopsy material, after full histologic evaluation and incorporation of the clinical and imaging findings. However, biopsy specimens rarely show tumors that straddle the histologic dividing line between benign and malignant, being well differentiated but with more atypia than is comfortable for a diagnosis of hepatic adenoma. A reasonable approach in this setting is to use the term *well-differentiated hepatocellular neoplasm* in the diagnostic line and then provide a prioritized differential in the note/

comment section of the pathology report, indicating the atypical features and degree of concern for hepatocellular carcinoma. Additional possible approaches in non-cirrhotic livers are to use the terms atypical hepatic adenoma or hepatocellular tumors of uncertain malignant potential (HUMP), along with an explanatory note.[132] These cases should be clinically followed with care and resection should be considered.

28.9 HISTOLOGIC SUBTYPES

About 35% of all hepatocellular carcinomas can be classified as unique histologic subtypes (Table 28.10). All but one of these subtypes occurs in both cirrhotic and noncirrhotic livers, the one exception being fibrolamellar carcinoma, which develops only in noncirrhotic livers. Hepatocellular carcinoma subtypes have been defined primarily for two reasons: (1) to improve understanding of the biology of hepatocellular carcinomas and (2) to aide in tumor recognition and diagnosis in surgical pathology. Currently, the subtypes do not otherwise impact clinical management, though this seems likely to change over time.

Histologic subtypes are different than molecular subtypes. Molecular subtypes are defined solely on the basis of mutation patterns, epigenetic changes, or patterns of gene expression, without regards to morphology. To date, histologic subtypes of hepatocellular carcinoma have overall been more robust entities than molecular subtypes. In time, its anticipated that molecular findings will be fully incorporated into morphologic hepatocellular carcinoma subtyping.

Histologic subtypes are defined by the four features listed below.[133] These four different features are almost never equally well developed when a subtype is first defined, but are developed over time.

1. Unique H&E histologic findings that are consistently and reproducibly present.
2. Unique results from immunostains or other special studies that can confirm the H&E morphology.
3. Unique clinical correlates.
4. Unique molecular findings.

Of note, hepatocellular carcinoma subtypes are different than growth patterns. Growth patterns are defined solely by the architectural patterns found in hepatocellular carcinomas on H&E stains. There are four main growth patterns: trabecular, solid, pseudoglandular, and macrotrabecular. Any of the four different growth patterns can be found in any given hepatocellular carcinoma subtype.

Table 28.10 Hepatocellular carcinoma subtypes

Subtype	Frequency in surgical pathology specimens[a]	Prognosis[b]
Steatohepatitic	20%	Similar
Clear cell	7%	Better
Scirrhous	4%	Similar to better
Cirrhotomimetic	1%	Worse
Combined hepatocellular-cholangiocarcinoma	1%	Worse
Fibrolamellar carcinoma	1%	Similar to better
Combined hepatocellular and neuroendocrine	<1%	Worse
GCSF producing	<1%	Worse
Sarcomatoid	<1%	Worse
Carcinosarcoma	<1%	Worse
Lymphocyte rich	<1%	Better

[a]The frequencies of the more aggressive subtypes are routinely higher in autopsy studies.
[b]Compared to conventional hepatocellular carcinoma.

Carcinosarcoma

The frequency is less than 1%. The prognosis is worse than conventional hepatocellular carcinoma.[134] Carcinosarcomas have both a malignant epithelial component and a malignant mesenchymal component (Fig. 28.39). The epithelial component is usually either cholangiocarcinoma or hepatocellular carcinoma, but in rare cases both a hepatocellular and glandular component can be present.[135] The following discussion will focus on cases with hepatocellular carcinoma as the epithelial component of the carcinosarcoma. The sarcomatous component should show morphologic or immunohistochemical evidence of mesenchymal differentiation, such as differentiation toward leiomyosarcoma, rhabdomyosarcoma, chondrosarcoma, fibrosarcoma, or osteosarcoma.[136–138] Some carcinosarcomas can also secrete GCSF and have numerous intratumoral neutrophils.[137] Although molecular data is sparse, in one study both components shared a TP53 mutation but then had additional component-specific mutations, with PIK3CA mutations in the hepatocellular carcinoma component and FGFR3 mutations in the sarcoma component.[139]

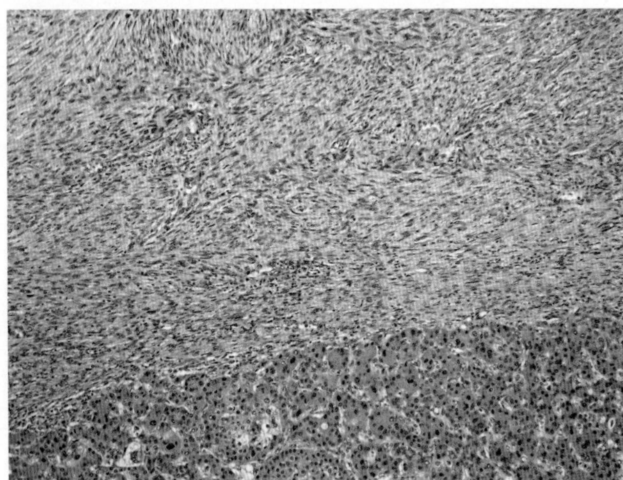

Figure 28.39 Carcinosarcoma. A component of fibrosarcoma (top) is seen in this carcinosarcoma. The bottom of the image shows the hepatocellular carcinoma component.

The main differential is a sarcomatoid hepatocellular carcinoma because both have a malignant hepatocellular carcinoma component and both have a spindle cell component. They are differentiated by the spindle cell component using both cytologic findings and immunostains. If the spindle cell component shows definite evidence for mesenchymal lineage by either morphology or by immunohistochemistry and is keratin-negative, then the tumor is classified as a carcinosarcoma. In contrast, if the spindle cell component lacks differentiation toward a specific mesenchymal lineage and is keratin-positive, then the term *sarcomatoid hepatocellular carcinoma* is used. In addition, the spindle cell component in a sarcomatoid hepatocellular carcinoma may show focal staining for markers of hepatic differentiation. The immunostain findings in some cases can be a bit mixed, in which case the relative strength of staining can be helpful. For example, strong and diffuse keratin staining with only focal weak smooth actin staining would favor a sarcomatoid hepatocellular carcinoma. Also, if the nuclear cytology is similar in both the epithelial and mesenchymal component, then sarcomatoid hepatocellular carcinoma is favored. In resection specimens, additional blocks often help clarify the diagnosis. Sharing the case with a colleague with a focused interest/expertise in sarcomas can also be helpful. Small transition zones between the carcinoma and sarcomatous component can be found in both sarcomatous hepatocellular carcinomas and hepatic carcinosarcomas and do not clearly separate these entities

Hepatoblastomas are theoretically in the differential because they also can have mesenchymal components. However, the ages of the patients are very different. Case reports have proposed the diagnosis of hepatoblastoma for rare adult tumors, but most of the case reports are unconvincing. In addition, the epithelial components in hepatoblastomas typically show fetal or embryonal growth patterns that are not present in adult tumors. Underlying liver disease is common in carcinosarcomas but not in hepatoblastomas.

Carcinosarcoma with osteoclast-like giant cells

The frequency is less than 1% and the prognosis is worse than conventional hepatocellular carcinoma.[140] Carcinosarcoma with osteoclast-like giant cells is distinct from the carcinosarcomas described above. The hepatocellular carcinoma component can vary from well to poorly differentiated and is overall similar to that seen in carcinosarcomas. The epithelial and the mesenchymal components can be admixed or distinct but adjacent nodules. In either case, the transition between the two components is often abrupt. The sarcomatous component shows the following triad of findings[141–145]:

- Sheets of mononuclear, plump to spindled tumor cells (Fig. 28.40). These tumor cells outnumber the multinucleated giant cells and are negative for keratins, markers of hepatic differentiation, and markers of specific mesenchymal linage differentiation.
- Scattered amongst the mononuclear cells are benign osteoclast-like giant cells. These giant cells have up to 30 nuclei and stain strongly for CD68 (Fig. 28.41) and other markers of osteoclast-like differentiation.[140–142]

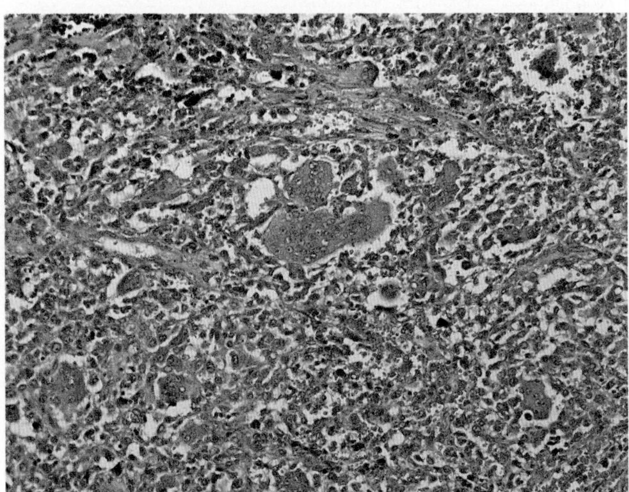

Figure 28.40 Carcinosarcoma with osteoclast-like giant cells. The sarcomatous component is composed of mononuclear tumor cells, but they are admixed with benign osteoclast-like giant cells. Hemosiderin deposits are also evident.

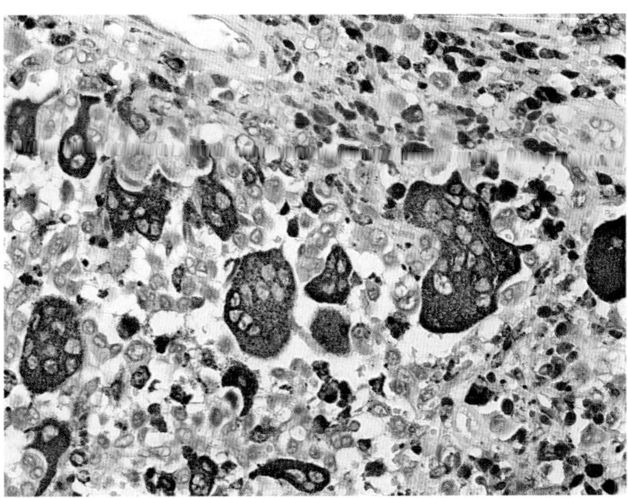

Figure 28.41 Carcinosarcoma with osteoclast-like giant cells. The osteoclast-like giant cells are strongly CD68-positive.

- The tumor also shows extensive hemorrhage, cystic change, and necrosis. These changes are most evident in resection specimens and can be absent in small biopsies. Also, the hemorrhage also commonly leads to numerous pigment laden macrophages (Fig. 28.40). Metastases from these tumors can also show the osteoclast-like giant cells.[146,147]

A hepatocellular carcinoma component is required and should be confirmed by immunostains because the epithelial component can be a cholangiocarcinoma in some cases. Likewise, carcinosarcoma with osteoclast-like giant cells can arise in other organs and metastasize to the liver. Finally, rarely there can be primary tumors of the liver that consist entirely of a carcinoma with osteoclast-like giant cells, without a hepatocellular or cholangiocarcinoma or sarcomatous component.

Cirrhotomimetic hepatocellular carcinoma

The frequency is less than 1% in surgical specimens, though it can be as high as 10% in autopsy studies[148] and imaging studies.[149] The prognosis is worse than conventional hepatocellular carcinoma.[150] Although successful liver transplantation has been reported,[151,152] these tumors tend to behave aggressively, with early recurrences in the liver and distant metastases. The tumor also behaves aggressively after resection, though cases with lower total tumor burden tend to do better.[152] Some studies have found an association with a younger age at presentation and chronic hepatitis B as the underlying liver disease.[153]

Synonyms and partial synonyms include diffuse hepatocellular carcinoma, infiltrative hepatocellular carcinoma, diffuse infiltrative hepatocellular carcinoma, and cirrhosis-like hepatocellular carcinoma, but these terms are used quite differently by different authors and different specialties, so considerable care is required when reading the literature because the materials and methods sections have to be carefully checked to figure out what type of tumors were included in the study.

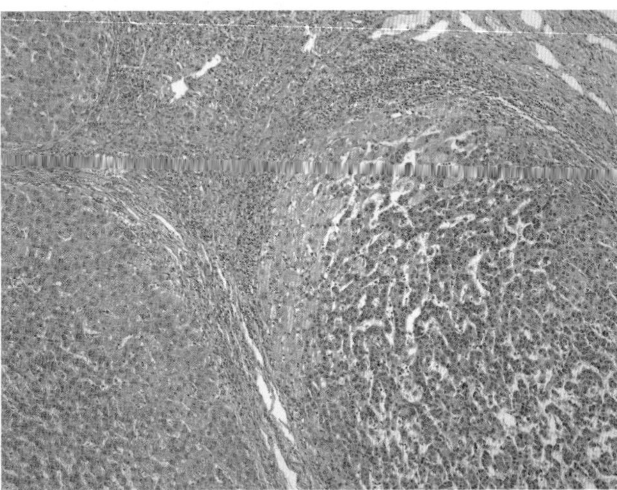

Figure 28.42 Hepatocellular carcinoma, cirrhotomimetic. This subtype of hepatocellular carcinoma is defined by its growth pattern. The tumor grows as numerous small nodules that are the same size as cirrhotic nodules.

This subtype of hepatocellular carcinoma is the only one defined by gross findings. The tumor grows as numerous small nodules that are similar in size and gross appearance to the nodules in the background cirrhotic liver (Fig. 28.42). Because the hepatocellular carcinoma so closely resembles the background cirrhotic liver, the tumor burden is invariably underestimated, often substantially, on both imaging and gross findings. Almost all cirrhotomimetic hepatocellular carcinomas arise in cirrhotic livers, but rarely an identical growth pattern is observed in noncirrhotic livers, with numerous small tumor nodules spread throughout the liver (Fig. 28.43).

In many cases, the tumor nodules coalesce to form a larger ill-defined mass, a finding that is consistent with the cirrhotomimetic variant of hepatocellular carcinoma. However, this pattern has to be distinguished from a conventional hepatocellular carcinoma with a few satellite nodules. In most cases, this is not much of an issue. However, in some cases the term cirrhotomimetic carcinoma has been inappropriately applied to conventional hepatocellular carcinomas that have a dominant nodule and scattered small satellite nodules, only because the satellite nodules were not evident on imaging studies, but this finding alone does not indicate the cirrhotomimetic subtype. In general, the satellite nodules in conventional

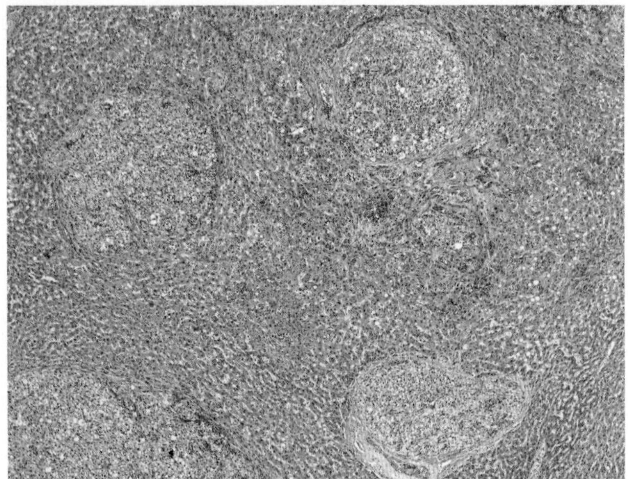

Figure 28.43 Hepatocellular carcinoma, cirrhotomimetic. The background liver is noncirrhotic, but the tumor has spread throughout the liver as small nodules.

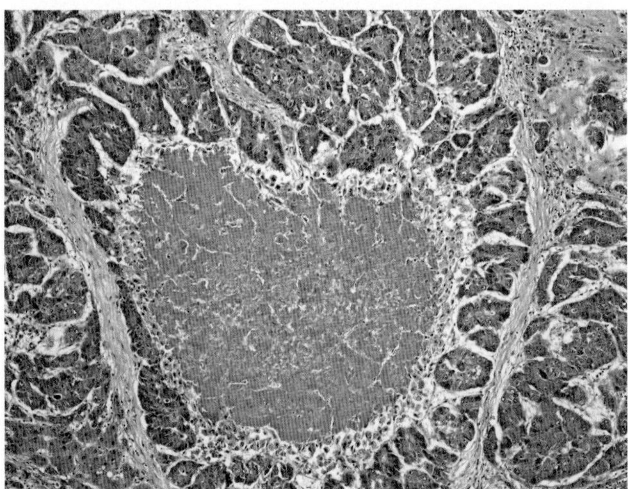

Figure 28.44 Hepatocellular carcinoma, cirrhotomimetic. In this case, many of the small tumor nodules showed central ischemic type necrosis.

hepatocellular carcinomas are found in close proximity to the dominant nodule, typically within a few centimeters. In contrast, the nodules in cirrhotomimetic hepatocellular carcinoma are more widely dispersed and more evenly distributed throughout hepatic lobe/liver, even if there is an area of tumor coalescence. In almost all cases of cirrhotomimetic hepatocellular carcinoma, there are greater than 30 small cirrhosis-like nodules of tumor. In contrast, the satellite nodules in conventional hepatocellular carcinomas are less than 5 in 90% of cases and less than 10 in almost 100% of cases. The explanation for the distinctive growth pattern in cirrhotomimetic hepatocellular carcinomas is unclear. Autopsy studies suggest this growth pattern results from early tumor spread to the large hilar portal vein branches, leading to subsequent seeding of the rest of the liver.[149,150] However, the full explanation is likely more nuanced and presumably reflects tumor specific genetic changes because many cases of hepatocellular carcinoma involve the hilar branches of the portal veins yet do not have a cirrhotomimetic growth pattern.

On microscopic examination, the tumors are typically moderately to poorly differentiated and can show solid, trabecular, or pseudoglandular growth patterns. The tumors can show clear cell change, fatty change, and bile production. Although data is limited, clear cell change has been associated with a better prognosis.[152] Even if there is enough clear cell change to reach the threshold of clear cell carcinoma subtype, the tumors are classified as cirrhotomimetic. Interestingly, the tumor nodules are often not arterialized like conventional hepatocellular carcinoma and can central necrosis despite their small size (Fig. 28.44). Some sections can show scattered tumorlets of a few dozen cells growing in the center of nonneoplastic cirrhotic nodules (Fig. 28.45). The background livers in many cases also show moderate to marked iron accumulation, but there is insufficient data to know if this is related to *HFE* mutations or a secondary finding. The cirrhotomimetic subtype of hepatocellular carcinoma is positive for the conventional markers of hepatic differentiation.

Clear cell hepatocellular carcinoma

The frequency of clear cell hepatocellular carcinoma is approximately 7%, but the frequency varies depending on the strictness of the definition.[154] Clear cell hepatocellular carcinomas have better prognosis than conventional hepatocellular carcinoma.[155–157] As correlates of their better prognosis, clear cell

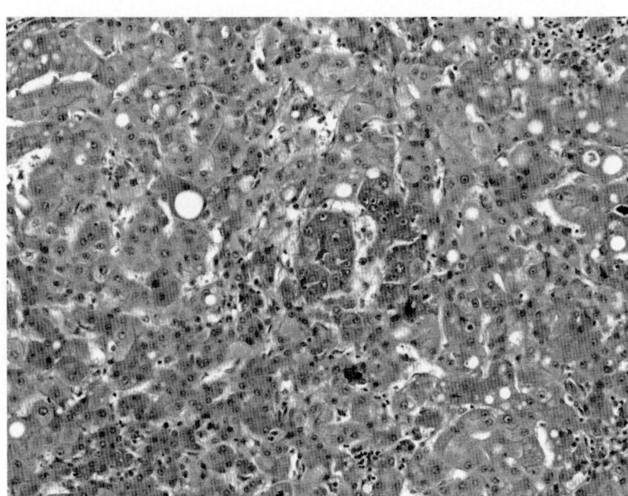

Figure 28.45 Hepatocellular carcinoma, cirrhotomimetic, tumorlet. A small cluster of tumor cells can be seen.

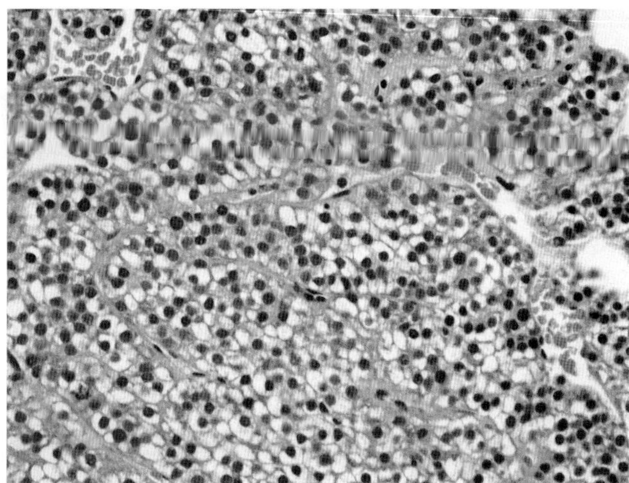

Figure 28.46 Hepatocellular carcinoma, clear cell. The tumor cells have abundant clear cytoplasm in this moderately differentiated hepatocellular carcinoma.

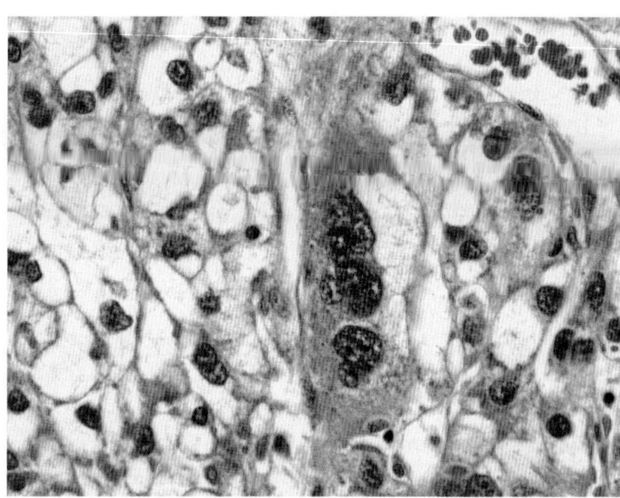

Figure 28.47 Hepatocellular carcinoma, clear cell with high-grade cytology. Abundant clear cytoplasm is seen, but this tumor shows higher grade nuclear cytology.

hepatocellular carcinomas tend to be smaller,[156,157] better differentiated,[156] and have lower rates of vascular invasion.[155–157]

The basic notion of clear cell hepatocellular carcinoma is straightforward: a hepatocellular carcinoma composed principally of tumor cells with abundant clear cytoplasm. However, classification challenges result when cases have tumor cells with and without abundant clear cytoplasm, requiring a threshold definition. A minimum requirement of at least 50% clear cells should be used, but a more pure group of tumors is achieved using the criteria of at least 80% of cells having clear cell change. Finally, some cases will show multiple morphologies, with adjacent but well-delineated nodules showing different histologic patterns. Although data is sparse, it is generally considered that the more aggressive histologic pattern in these cases will drive prognosis. Thus, these cases should not be classified as clear cell hepatocellular carcinoma, but instead as hepatocellular carcinomas with multiple morphologies

The most distinctive feature of clear cell hepatocellular carcinomas are their abundant clear cytoplasm (Fig. 28.46). Most cases are well or moderately differentiated, though a subset of cases show high-grade nuclear cytology despite their abundant clear cytoplasm (Fig. 28.47). Steatosis is also common, being found in about a third of cases,[158] and can be focal or more diffuse and abundant. Most clear cell hepatocellular carcinomas show a trabecular or solid growth pattern, but pseudoacinar or macrotrabecular growth patterns can be occasionally found. Rare cases have a cirrhotomimetic growth pattern.[152,159]

Clear cell hepatocellular carcinomas are positive for HepPar1, Arginase 1, and albumin in situ hybridization. As a potential diagnostic pitfall, about 35% of clear cell carcinomas of the ovary can be HepPar1-positive,[119] so additional stains may be needed in some cases. In contrast, clear cell carcinomas of the kidney are HepPar1-negative.[160] The differential includes hepatocellular carcinomas with clear cell change that results from diffuse lipid accumulation (see section on lipid-rich hepatocellular carcinoma, under provisional subtypes).[161,162] These cases are very rare, but should not be classified as clear cell hepatocellular carcinomas. The high power morphologic findings are distinctive enough to separate these two entities in most cases, but PAS stains can be used as needed, showing strong positivity in clear cell hepatocellular carcinomas. The differential can also include benign adrenal rests and epithelioid angiomyolipomas, which can sometimes show a clear cell type change.

Combined hepatocellular carcinoma-cholangiocarcinoma

The frequency of combined hepatocellular carcinoma-cholangiocarcinomas is about 1%.[163–166] The prognosis is worse than conventional hepatocellular carcinoma. Synonyms include biphenotypic hepatocellular carcinoma-cholangiocarcinoma and mixed hepatocellular carcinoma and cholangiocarcinoma. The term *collision tumor* is discouraged.

Overall, the risk factors for combined hepatocellular carcinoma-cholangiocarcinoma are similar to those of conventional hepatocellular carcinoma. However, combined hepatocellular carcinoma-cholangiocarcinomas differ in their serologic findings because both serum CA-19-9 levels (from the cholangiocarcinoma component) and serum AFP levels (from the hepatocellular carcinoma component) are elevated in about 50% of cases.[167] The cholangiocarcinoma component is a major driver of prognosis, which can be indirectly measured by the CA19-9 levels.[164,168] In fact, a dose-effect curve has been reported with higher CA19-9 levels associated with worse prognosis.[164] Hilar lymph node dissection should be considered in cases where the diagnosis of a combined tumor is known prior to or at the time of surgery because the frequency of lymph node disease is higher than convention hepatocellular carcinomas. As one example, one study found the frequency of regional lymph node metastases was 2% for conventional hepatocellular carcinomas, 13% for combined hepatocellular carcinoma-cholangiocarcinomas, and 21% for cholangiocarcinomas.[169]

These tumors develop in both cirrhotic and noncirrhotic livers[164] and share the same general risk factors as hepatocellular carcinoma. Combined hepatocellular carcinoma-cholangiocarcinomas can be multifocal (20% of cases) or unifocal.[165,169–171] However, a diagnosis of combined hepatocellular carcinoma-cholangiocarcinoma requires that both components are in one nodule or in immediately adjacent nodules. In contrast, cases are classified as double primaries when the liver shows both cholangiocarcinoma and hepatocellular carcinoma but in clearly separate nodules with intervening normal liver.

Combined hepatocellular carcinoma-cholangiocarcinomas have two distinct morphologies evident on the H&E (Fig. 28.48), one of hepatocellular carcinoma and one of cholangiocarcinoma. In fact, preoperative biopsies frequently misdiagnose these tumors as either hepatocellular carcinomas or cholangiocarcinomas based on which component was sampled.[172] The two components are found as adjacent nodules or areas within the same tumor, sometimes with a transition zone. In surgical pathology reports of resection specimens, it is helpful to convey the percent of each component because some cases are predominately hepatocellular carcinoma with only a small focus of cholangiocarcinoma, whereas others are predominately cholangiocarcinoma with only a small focus of hepatocellular carcinoma. Immunostains are used to confirm the H&E impression. The hepatocellular carcinoma component is positive for typical markers of hepatocellular differentiation such as HepPar1 (Fig. 28.49), Arginase 1, and glypican 3. The cholangiocarcinoma component is positive for biliary type keratins, such as CK19, and negative for markers of hepatocellular differentiation. Mucin production can be present but is not needed in the cholangiocarcinoma component.

The most important pitfall in making a diagnosis of combined hepatocellular carcinoma-cholangiocarcinoma is basing the diagnosis on immunostain findings, without having morphologic correlates. For example, an otherwise conventional hepatocellular carcinoma should not be classified as combined hepatocellular carcinoma-cholangiocarcinoma because of positive CK7 or CK19 staining. Likewise, HepPar1 or glypican 3 or Arginase staining in an otherwise typical cholangiocarcinoma should not be called a combined tumor.

Combined hepatocellular carcinoma-cholangiocarcinomas have a prognosis that falls in between that of cholangiocarcinoma and hepatocellular carcinoma.[173,174,178] Compared to conventional hepatocellular carcinoma, they have a higher risk for recurrence after resection[172] and liver transplantation.[175] They are staged in the AJCC

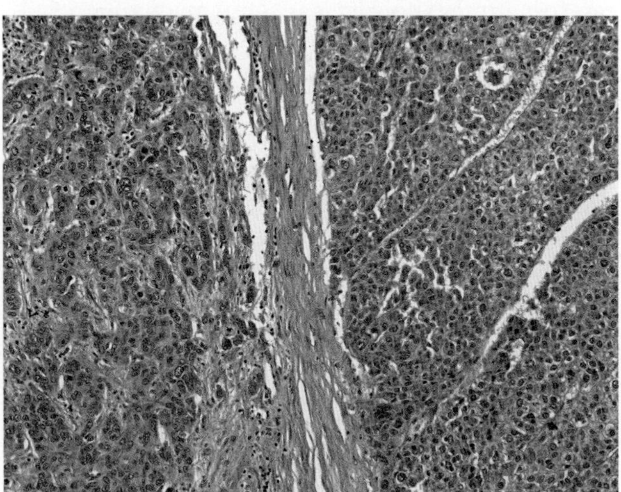

Figure 28.48 Combined hepatocellular-cholangiocarcinoma. The cholangiocarcinoma component is evident on the left of the image, the hepatocellular carcinoma component on the right.

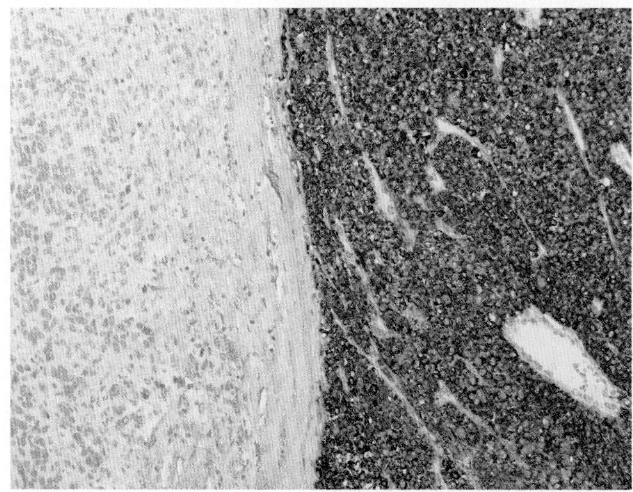

Figure 28.49 Combined hepatocellular-cholangiocarcinoma. HepPar1 stains only the hepatitic component (same case as above).

system using the cholangiocarcinoma protocol. At a practical level, the cholangiocarcinoma component drives prognosis, so using the cholangiocarcinoma staging system is not unreasonable. However, they are biologically distinct from cholangiocarcinomas, so it seems reasonable to hope for a unique staging system in the future, one that would better capture their unique histologic findings.

Double primary carcinomas

Double primary carcinomas have two physically separated nodules, one of hepatocellular and one of cholangiocarcinoma, with intervening nonneoplastic hepatic parenchyma. They should not be classified as combined hepatocellular carcinoma-cholangiocarcinoma and should be graded and staged separately. The cholangiocarcinoma component tends to drive the prognosis.[176] The largest study to date, with over 14,000 primary liver tumors, found the frequency of double primary carcinomas to be 0.2%.[176]

Combined hepatocellular carcinoma-cholangiocarcinoma with stem cell features

The 2010 World Health Organization (WHO) classification of liver tumors[177] created a separate section for tumors called combined hepatocellular carcinoma-cholangiocarcinomas with stem cell features. This category was originally designed to capture cases that had the classic morphology of conventional combined hepatocellular carcinoma-cholangiocarcinomas, but also had additional morphologic findings or immunostain findings that suggested stem cellness. These stem cell like findings could be found in either or both of the epithelial components. However, this approach did not work well because the term combined hepatocellular carcinoma-cholangiocarcinomas with stem cell features rather quickly was applied to conventional hepatocellular carcinomas that had some features of stem cellness, but were not combined tumors. The same thing happened with cholangiocarcinomas. This sequence of events did have the value of highlighting that stem cell–like features could be found in hepatocellular carcinomas, cholangiocarcinomas, and combined tumors, but the categories will need to be refined to be useful.

The literature on this topic is still interesting and has value, but it can be hard to figure out exactly what types of tumors were studied in some papers. Although the 2010 WHO classification system is challenging to apply in its current form, the core features of the different subtypes are interesting (Table 28.11) and (Figs. 28.50, 28.51, and 28.52). As a brief summary, there are three subtypes called typical subtype, intermediate-cell subtype, and cholangiocellular subtype. The stem cell–like features in the first two are associated with areas of hepatic differentiation, whereas the third subtype (cholangiocellular) is associated with areas of cholangiocarcinoma differentiation. All of the subtypes share in common the frequent finding of dense intratumoral fibrosis.

Table 28.11 2010 WHO-based definitions for combined hepatocellular-cholangiocarcinoma with stem cell features

Subtype	H&E and immunohistochemical features
Typical	Core histology: The edge of the hepatocellular carcinoma component has areas with a peripheral rim of smaller cells with a high nuclear to cytoplasmic ratio and hyperchromatic nuclei. Stains: The hepatocellular carcinoma component is positive for usual markers of hepatocellular differentiation. The peripheral cells can be positive for CK7 and CK19 and often for CD56, c-Kit, and EpCAM.
Intermediate cell	Core histology: The stem cell–like areas are usually associated with the hepatocellular carcinoma component and show small oval cells with mild to focally moderate cytologic atypia. These stem cell–like areas can be hard to classify as hepatic or biliary on morphology, but are positive for hepatic markers. Stains: Coexpression of markers of hepatocellular and biliary differentiation, e.g., HepPar1, CK19, and CEA. c-Kit expression is common. Mucicarmine is negative.
Cholangiolocellular	Core histology: This morphology is often associated with areas of conventional cholangiocarcinoma growth. In the areas of stem cell–like growth, the tumor cells are small with a high nuclear to cytoplasmic ratio but only mild cytologic atypia and a branching, anastomosing cord-like pattern of growth. Small tubular structures can be seen. Stains: Tumor cells are positive for CK19, CK7, CD56, c-Kit, and EpCAM but negative for makers of hepatic differentiation (e.g., HepPar and Arginase).

From Bosman F, Carneiro F, Hruban RH, et al. *WHO Classification of Tumors of the Digestive System*. Lyon: IARC; 2010.

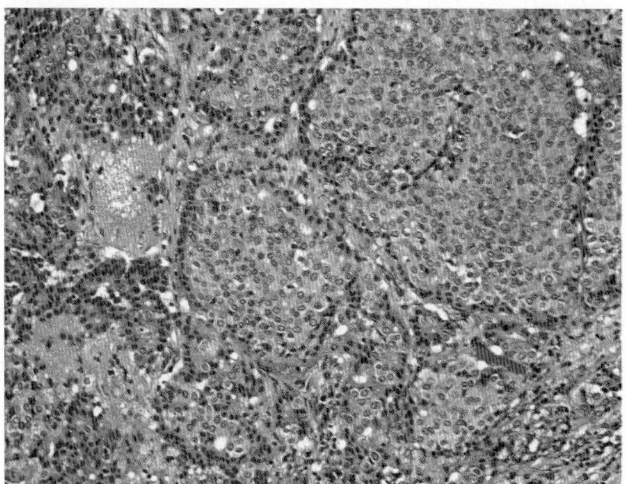

Figure 28.50 Combined hepatocellular-cholangiocarcinoma, with stem cell features. Subtype 1 (typical subtype) shows nests of conventional hepatocellular carcinoma tumor cells surrounded by a thin rim of smaller more basophilic cells.

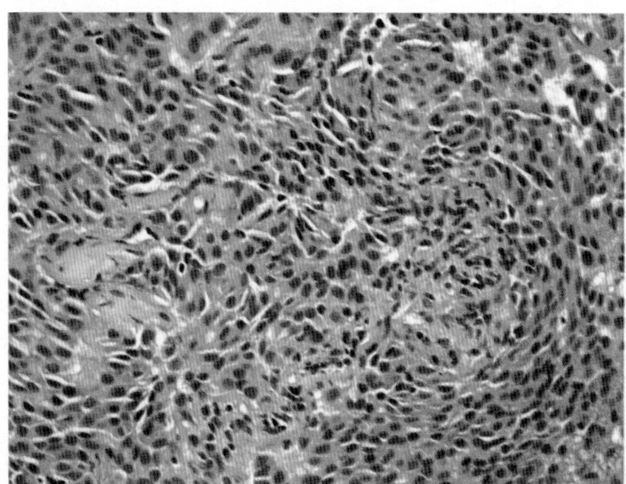

Figure 28.51 Combined hepatocellular-cholangiocarcinoma, with stem cell features. Subtype 2 (intermediate cell subtype) is composed of small basophilic cells that are difficult to classify based on morphology, but stain with hepatic markers.

Combined hepatocellular and neuroendocrine carcinoma

Combined hepatocellular and neuroendocrine carcinomas are rare, with a frequency of less than 1%. Their prognosis is not entirely clear because of their rarity but the weight of the data suggests a worse prognosis. This tumor is well described by its name: there is a morphologic component of hepatocellular carcinoma and a morphologic component of neuroendocrine carcinoma. These two components are recognizable on the H&E, but are typically intermingled.

In contrast, if there are two clearly separate nodules of tumor with intervening normal hepatic parenchyma,

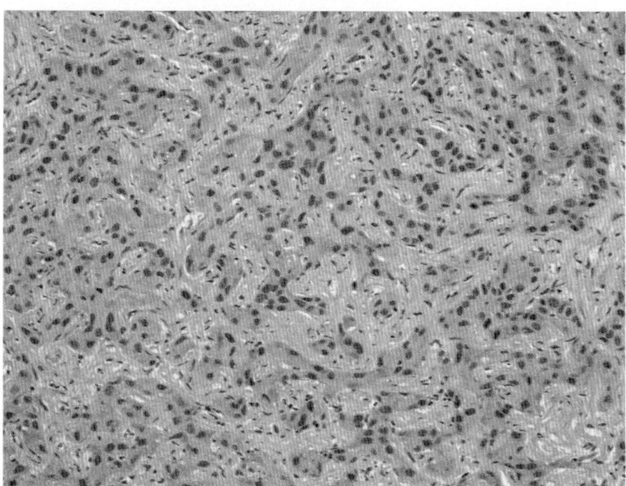

Figure 28.52 Combined hepatocellular-cholangiocarcinoma, with stem cell features. Subtype 3 (cholangiolocellular subtype) looks and stains like a cholangiocarcinoma.

then they are classified as separate primaries. If the two nodules are immediately adjacent, then the classification is that of a combined tumor. Two independent morphologies are required for this tumor subtype. It is a mistake to classify a case as combined hepatocellular carcinoma-neuroendocrine carcinoma based solely on immunostains in a monomorphic tumor, such as a focal synaptophysin or CD56 staining in a conventional hepatocellular or focal HepPar1 or glypican 3 staining in a neuroendocrine carcinoma.

Combined hepatocellular and neuroendocrine carcinoma can develop in cirrhotic and noncirrhotic livers[179,180] and there is no strong association with any specific underlying liver disease. The hepatocellular carcinoma component shows conventional morphology, is usually well to moderately differentiated, and stains in an ordinary fashion with markers of hepatic differentiation. Rare cases can also show sarcomatoid differentiation.[181] The neuroendocrine component is usually found within the sinusoids of the hepatocellular carcinoma component and most commonly has a small cell morphology (Fig. 28.53), though a large cell morphology can also be seen. The neuroendocrine component will stain for neuroendocrine markers such as synaptophysin or chromogranin. The relative proportion of hepatocellular carcinoma versus neuroendocrine carcinoma will vary case by case, but most are primarily composed of the hepatocellular component. However, metastatic disease is often purely neuroendocrine carcinoma.

Fibrolamellar carcinoma

Fibrolamellar carcinomas make up about 1% of hepatocellular carcinomas.[182–185] Their prognosis is similar to perhaps slightly better when compared to

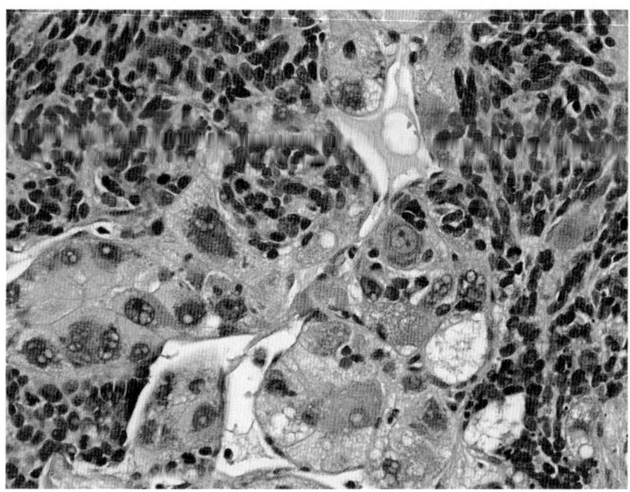

Figure 28.53 Combined hepatocellular-neuroendocrine carcinoma. The sinusoids of this moderately-differentiated hepatocellular carcinoma have nests of small cell neuroendocrine carcinoma.

conventional hepatocellular carcinomas that develop in noncirrhotic livers. Fibrolamellar carcinomas are defined by characteristic histologic findings plus confirmatory tests. The tumor is composed of large eosinophilic cells with prominent nucleoli and typically shows striking intratumoral fibrosis. Although the diagnosis on H&E seems straightforward, there are many cases that have histologic overlap with conventional hepatocellular carcinomas and the H&E impression should be confirmed by immunostains (CD68, CK7 coexpression) or by molecular tests, which can include DNA-based testing for the deletion leading to the DNAJB1-PRKACA fusion transcript, or RNA testing for the fusion transcript itself. The *DNAJB1-PRKACA* microdeletion is a defining feature of this tumor, found in nearly all cases, with the exception of rare cases developing in the Carney Syndrome.

Clinical features

Fibrolamellar carcinomas occur throughout the world, but there is insufficient epidemiologic to determine if there is any geographic or ethnic association. In the United States, no differences in the frequency of fibrolamellar carcinoma was found between white, black, Hispanic, or Asian populations.[183] The gender distribution is about equal,[183,185,186] without the male predominance seen in conventional hepatocellular carcinomas. Fibrolamellar carcinomas occur in younger individuals, with 50% of cases presenting between the ages of 17 and 30 years and 80% between the ages of 10 and 35 years.[187] Nonetheless, conventional hepatocellular carcinomas are still the most common liver cancer in children and young adults, accounting for 60% to 80% of cases.[56,182,188–190] The cause of fibrolamellar carcinoma is unknown. The background livers are essentially normal by light microscopy.[56]

Serum findings

In about 5% of cases, serum AFP levels can be mildly elevated,[186,191,192] typically less than 100 ng/ML, but this is a nonspecific finding. Serum AFP levels are essentially never greater than 200 ng/ML and immunohistochemistry for AFP is consistently negative. In contrast, serum levels of PIVKA-II, also known as DCP, are commonly elevated in fibrolamellar carcinomas.[193] Other elevated serum proteins include the vitamin B12 binding protein transcobalamin1[194,195] and neurotensin.[196] However, none of these serum markers are sufficiently sensitive or specific to be broadly useful for clinical care.

Gross findings

Fibrolamellar carcinomas are unifocal in 80% to 90% of cases.[197] Even when there are multifocal tumors, one nodule is typically dominant, with adjacent smaller satellite nodules, and there is no evidence for a "field effect" with multiple independent tumors. Fibrolamellar carcinomas tend to be large, commonly measuring 10 cm or more in greatest dimension (Fig. 28.54). A central scar is found in about two-thirds of cases, especially the larger ones. Gross vascular invasion is seen in up to 25% of cases.[198]

Microscopic findings

The tumor cells in fibrolamellar carcinomas are large, polygonal-shaped, and have abundant eosinophilic cytoplasm that is rich in mitochondria and lysosomes. The tumor nuclei often have vesiculated chromatin and large nucleoli (Fig. 28.55). Fibrolamellar carcinomas

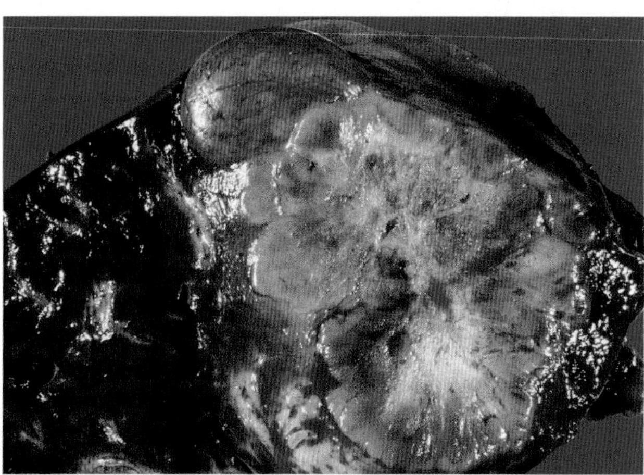

Figure 28.54 Fibrolamellar carcinoma. On gross examination, the tumor is yellow and has a central scar.

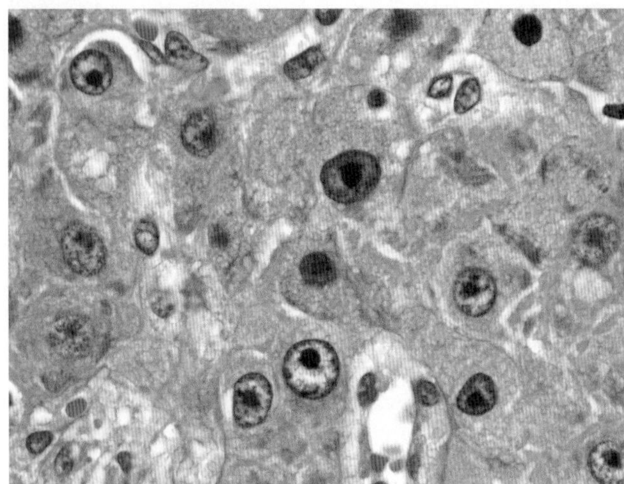

Figure 28.55 Fibrolamellar carcinoma. The tumor cells have abundant cytoplasm and prominent nucleoli.

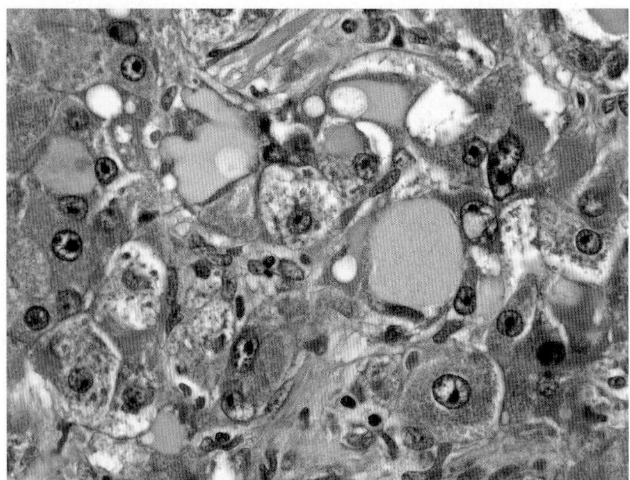

Figure 28.57 Fibrolamellar carcinoma. Pale bodies can be seen within the tumor cell cytoplasm. This finding is not specific for fibrolamellar carcinoma.

also show striking intratumoral fibrosis, with collagen that is often deposited in parallel bands (Fig. 28.56). In other cases, the collagen is deposited in a more haphazard pattern. In some of the larger tumors, the center can become densely sclerotic and have few if any residual tumor cells. Also of note, the fibrosis in fibrolamellar carcinomas can be heterogeneous and about 10% of cases will show areas with a solid pattern of growth containing little or no fibrosis. The cytologic features in these solid areas are that of ordinary fibrolamellar carcinoma and molecular studies confirm the presence of the typical DNAJB-PRKACA fusion.[131] This pattern is acceptable as fibrolamellar carcinoma and should not be called mixed conventional and fibrolamellar carcinoma.

Other common but nonspecific histologic findings include pales bodies, pink bodies, intratumoral cholestasis, and variably dilated psuedoglands (Figs. 28.57, 28.58, and 28.59). The frequency of pale bodies and hyaline bodies isn't well established, but pale bodies are found in about 70% of cases and hyaline bodies in about 50% of cases, though the frequency for both is probably higher if they are specifically searched for. Small psuedoglands are common in fibrolamellar carcinoma and appear to result from dilated bile canaliculi. In some cases, the psuedoglands are much larger and produce mucinous material that is Alcian blue–positive and often weakly to moderately positive on mucicarmine.[199] Despite the mucin production, these cases should not be called combined cholangiocarcinoma-fibrolamellar carcinomas.

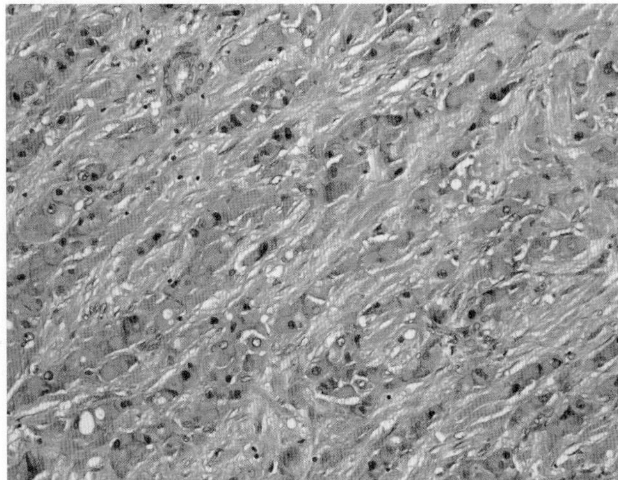

Figure 28.56 Fibrolamellar carcinoma. Intratumoral fibrosis is striking in this case and the fibrotic bands tend to run parallel to each other.

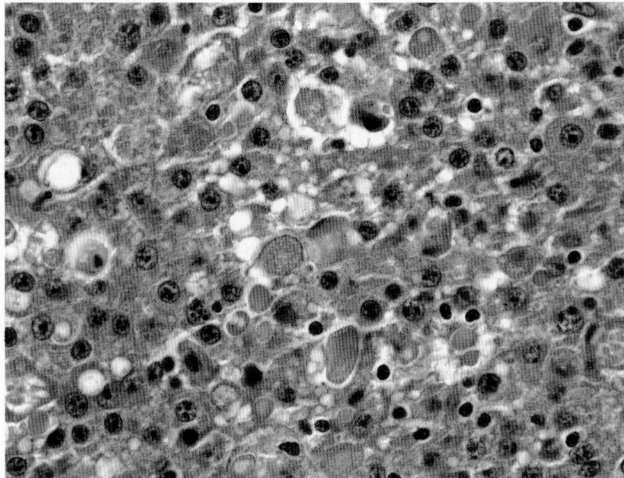

Figure 28.58 Fibrolamellar carcinoma. Hyaline or pink bodies can be seen within the tumor cell cytoplasm. This finding is not specific for fibrolamellar carcinoma.

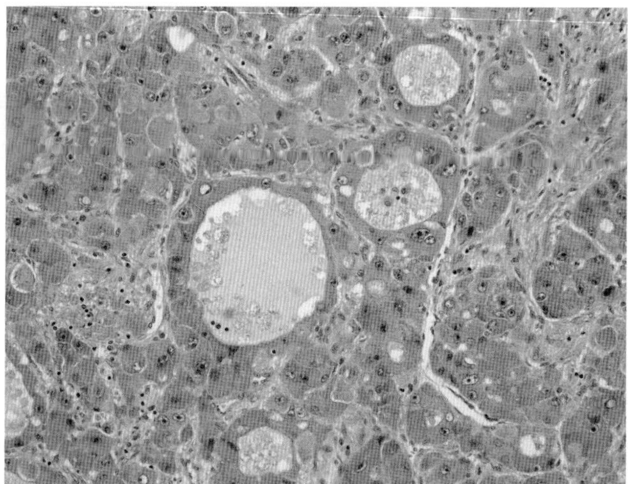

Figure 28.59 Fibrolamellar carcinoma. Pseudoglands are common in fibrolamellar carcinoma.

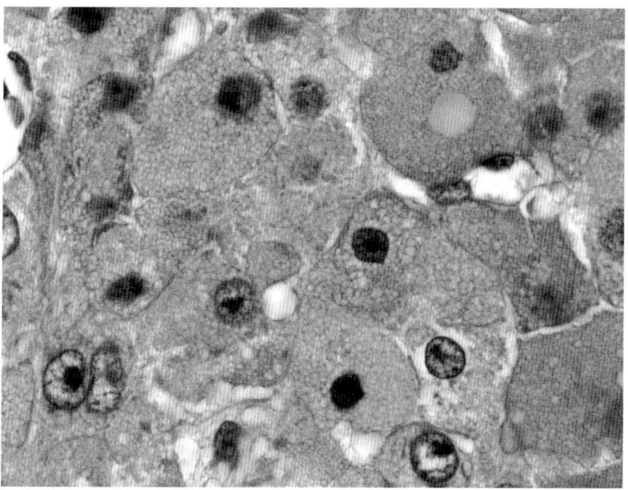

Figure 28.60 Fibrolamellar carcinoma. A cluster of tumor cells show what appears to be microvesicular steatosis.

Other histologic findings in fibrolamellar carcinomas include microcalcifications, macrovesicular steatosis, and scattered single tumor cells that have a distinctive "bubbly" cytoplasm of microvesicular steatosis (Fig. 28.60). Rarely, tumors can show focal areas of intense lymphocytic inflammation (Fig. 28.61).

Association with other tumors

Rarely, type 1 hepatic adenomas with LFABP loss can be associated with fibrolamellar carcinoma (Figs. 28.62 and 28.63).[187,200–202] Fibrolamellar carcinomas can also induce a secondary, reactive nodular hyperplasia at their periphery (Fig. 28.64) that resembles focal nodular hyperplasia and stains with a "map-like" pattern with glutamine synthetase. However, true focal nodular hyperplasias do not give rise to fibrolamellar carcinomas and they do not share any genetic or etiologic associations.

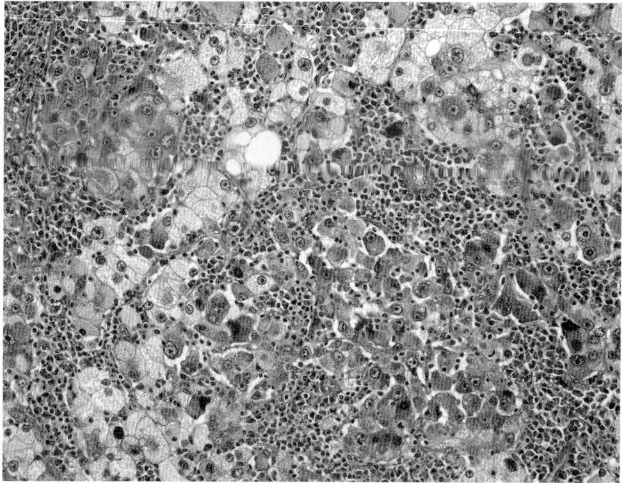

Figure 28.61 Fibrolamellar carcinoma. Dense lymphocytic inflammation was present focally in this case.

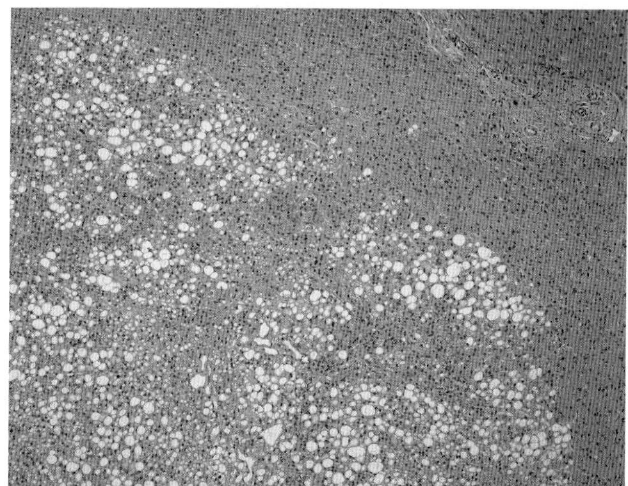

Figure 28.62 Fibrolamellar carcinoma and hepatic adenoma. Both tumors were present in this liver resection specimen. This image shows the hepatic adenoma, which shows fatty change, and the background liver, which does not.

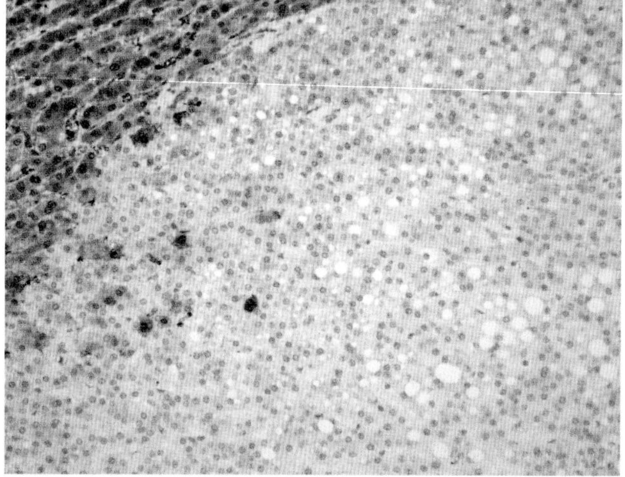

Figure 28.63 Fibrolamellar carcinoma and hepatic adenoma. The adenoma shows loss of LFABP expression (same case as the preceding image).

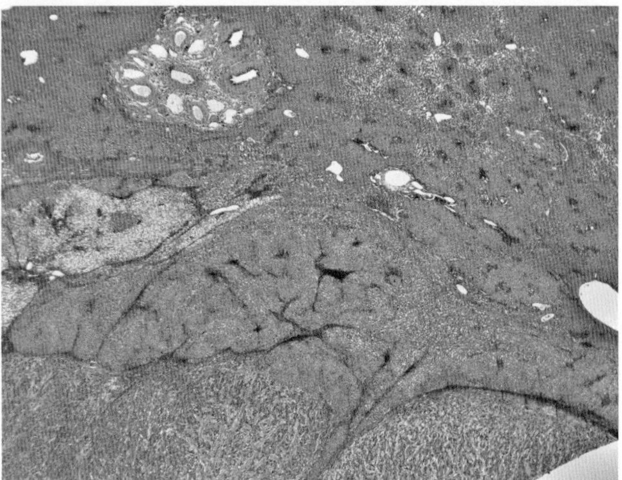

Figure 28.64 Fibrolamellar carcinoma. The fibrolamellar carcinoma is at the bottom and the typical noncirrhotic liver is on top. In between is a distinctive rim of reactive benign hepatic tissue that looks and stains like focal nodular hyperplasia.

Rare fibrolamellar carcinomas acquire additional mutations that lead to the development of a distinct nodule of conventional appearing hepatocellular carcinoma growing in the midst of the fibrolamellar carcinoma (Fig. 28.65).[203] These cases represent tumor progression and not mixed tumors.

Grading

Fibrolamellar carcinomas in general lack the range of differentiation seen in ordinary hepatocellular carcinomas and almost all tumors are moderately differentiated. Rarely, multinucleated tumor cells can be found with higher grade nuclear cytology.

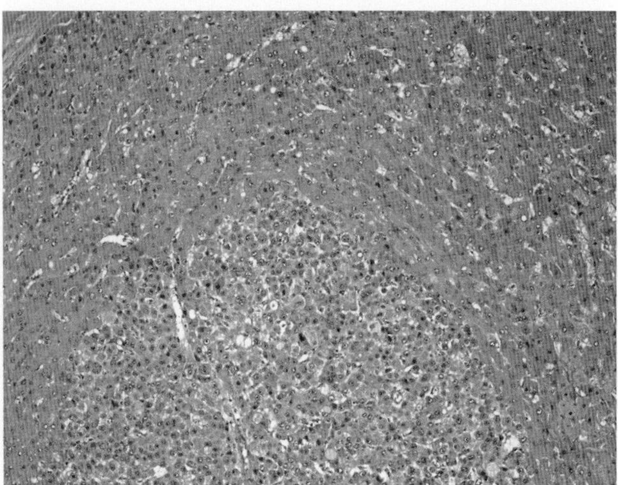

Figure 28.65 Fibrolamellar carcinoma. This fibrolamellar carcinoma has a nodule within that showed dedifferentiation, resembling conventional hepatocellular carcinoma.

Immunohistochemical findings

Fibrolamellar carcinomas are positive for markers of hepatic differentiation, such as HepPar1, Arginase, and albumin in situ hybridization. Glypican 3 is positive in about 50% of cases. Immunostains for AFP are negative. The vast majority of fibrolamellar carcinomas are negative for chromogranin and synaptophysin by immunohistochemistry.[204,205] When combined with morphology, the coexpression of CD68 (KP-1 clone) and CK7 is very specific for fibrolamellar carcinoma. Both CK7 and CD68 staining can be patchy, but they still perform very well on biopsy material. Tumors that do not coexpress CK7 or CD68 are most likely not fibrolamellar carcinoma. When using these stains, it is important to make sure that the internal controls are brightly positive, confirming a robust stain performance (CK7 is positive in benign bile ducts and CD68 is positive in Kupffer cells within the tumor and nontumor tissue).

Diagnostic approach

The distinctive H&E findings in fibrolamellar carcinoma suggest the diagnosis should be pretty easy to make. However, experience has shown this is not always the case. Many cases seen in consultation as possible fibrolamellar carcinomas are not and some published cases are suspect. It turns out that the H&E findings of fibrolamellar carcinoma are reasonably sensitive but they are not as specific. A subset of conventional hepatocellular carcinomas can closely mimic fibrolamellar carcinoma (Fig. 28.66). Thus, it is important to confirm the H&E impression of fibrolamellar carcinoma with additional studies.

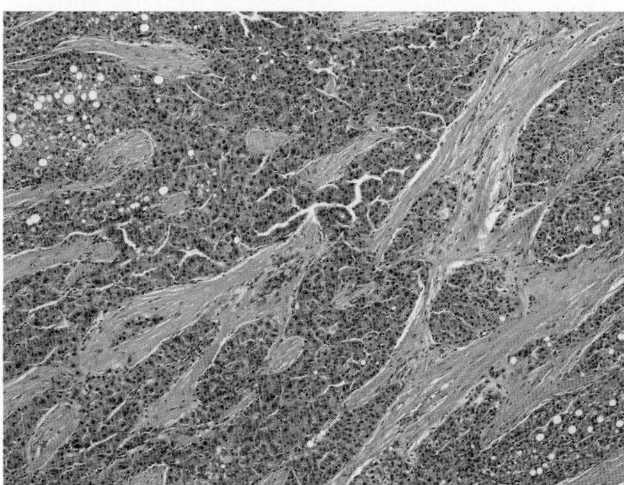

Figure 28.66 Hepatocellular carcinoma, mimicking fibrolamellar carcinoma. The intratumoral fibrosis in this scirrhous hepatocellular carcinoma, as well as the morphology, mimics fibrolamellar carcinoma.

Molecular methods are excellent tools to confirm a diagnosis of fibrolamellar carcinoma and are preferred, when available. They have the advantage of direct detection of the genetic lesion. When molecular testing is not available, a useful approach is to confirm the H&E findings by co-expression of CK7 and CD68 (KP-1 clone). Of note, both molecular testing or immunostains for CK7 and CD68 are best employed when the histologic findings are consistent with fibrolamellar carcinoma. There is no need to test conventional hepatocellular carcinomas solely because they occur in children.

Molecular findings

Fibrolamellar carcinomas are characterized by activation of protein kinase A. In essentially all sporadic cases, this results from a microdeletion on chromosome 19[206] that leads to a fusion transcript between the *DNA-JB1* gene and the *PRKACA* gene. *PRKACA* encodes one of the catalytic units of a protein called protein kinase A. This genetic lesion can be detected by RT-PCR for the fusion transcript or by FISH, which detects the DNA deletion that leads to the fusion transcript. Of note, in paraffin embedded tissues, RT-PCR has the disadvantage of a higher rate of false-negative testing secondary to RNA degradation, giving advantages to FISH as routine diagnostic tool.

Rare cases, less than 1% of fibrolamellar carcinomas, also develop in the setting of the Carney complex, where germline mutations are present in the regulatory unit PRKAR1A and second hit mutations also lead to activation of protein kinase A. These cases are typically negative for the microdeletion on chromosome 19.

Differential diagnosis

Some scirrhous hepatocellular carcinomas have areas that can closely mimic fibrolamellar carcinomas, including large eosinophilic cells and intratumoral fibrosis. In resection specimens, this is usually not a problem because other more typical areas of scirrhous hepatocellular carcinoma are present. In challenging cases, immunostains for CD68 and CK7 and/or molecular testing will clarify the diagnosis. The differential diagnosis can also include conventional hepatocellular carcinomas. In fact, a small subset of cases show essentially identical cytologic findings to fibrolamellar carcinoma, with big pink cells and prominent nucleoli, the cytologic hallmarks of fibrolamellar carcinoma. On biopsy specimens, this can be a particular challenge and immunostains or molecular confirmation are strongly recommended to confirm a diagnosis of fibrolamellar carcinoma. In resection specimens, examination of other sections can help clarify the diagnosis. Finally, a subset of neuroendocrine carcinomas metastatic to the liver can closely mimic fibrolamellar carcinoma. These diagnostic pitfalls can all be resolved by careful attention to clinical and histologic findings, coupled with additional testing such as immunostains for CD68 and CK7 and/or molecular testing.

When evaluating difficult cases, there are additional findings that make a diagnosis of fibrolamellar carcinoma unlikely. Tumors are most likely not fibrolamellar carcinoma if they are associated with high serum AFP levels, for example, more than 200 IU/L, or are positive for AFP by immunohistochemistry. A diagnosis of fibrolamellar carcinoma is probably wrong if there is advanced fibrosis in sections of the background liver. Finally, a diagnosis of fibrolamellar carcinomas should be approached very cautiously, and certainly requires confirmation by immunostains or molecular testing, in individuals younger than 5 years or older than 60 years.

Spread and metastases

Distant metastatic disease is found in about 30% of individuals at presentation,[192] with a metastatic pattern that is largely similar to conventional hepatocellular carcinoma, with frequent lung and adrenal gland metastases. Peritoneal disease, such as abdominal carcinomatosis, is found at presentation in approximately 10% to 15% of individuals,[186] whereas lymph nodes are positive in approximately two-thirds of individuals at initial presentation.[186,192,207]

Staging

Fibrolamellar carcinomas are staged using the same staging system as conventional hepatocellular carcinoma. However, the current pathology tumor stages do not strongly predict disease free survival,[207] suggesting the potential value of a staging system specifically designed for fibrolamellar carcinoma. Vascular invasion is present in 50% to 75% of resection specimens.[188,198,207,208] There are several findings that are not part of the current staging system but are anecdotally associated with a worse prognosis: perineural invasion and direct spread into the soft tissue of the liver hilum.

Prognosis

The overall prognosis is similar to that seen in conventional hepatocellular carcinomas without underlying liver disease,[205,209] although some studies suggest fibrolamellar carcinoma may have still have a very modest survival benefit in this setting.[198,210,211] The single most important prognostic finding for fibrolamellar carcinoma is whether or not the tumor can be resected, which improves the median 5-year survival from 0% to 75%.[185,189,192,207,208] In resection specimens, the key prognostic findings are regional lymph node disease and angiolymphatic invasion.[192,197] Following complete resection, there is disease recurrent in 70% to 80% of individuals,[197] commonly involving the lungs (40% of cases) or peritoneum.[212,213]

Granulocyte colony stimulating factor producing hepatocellular carcinoma

The frequency is much less than 1%.[137,214–219] Most of the cases are found in older individuals and the prognosis is poor.[137,214,215,217] The basic criterion for this tumor is a definite hepatocellular carcinoma that produces GCSF. Individuals typically present with markedly elevated peripheral white blood cell counts, elevated serum IL-6 levels[137,214,215,217] and elevated serum CRP levels.[137,214–217] This subtype is also called GCSF secreting hepatocellular carcinoma.

Most cases are poorly differentiated and focal areas of sarcomatoid dedifferentiation are common.[137,214,215,217] The production of GCSF by the tumor leads to dense neutrophil infiltrates within the tumor sinusoids (Fig. 28.67), though the neutrophilia can be absent in sarcomatoid areas. The GCSF is produced by the hepatocellular carcinoma component in most cases,[137,216,218] but can be produced by the sarcomatoid component,[214,215] or by both components.[217]

There are two main diagnostic pitfalls. First, treated conventional hepatocellular carcinomas can sometimes show areas of necrosis and intense neutrophilia, but these changes are typically focal and the serological findings of true GCSF hepatocellular carcinomas will not be present. Secondly, GCSF can also be produced by cholangiocarcinomas[220] and metastatic carcinomas,[221] so the diagnosis of hepatocellular carcinoma has to be secured by morphology and immunostains.

Lymphocyte-rich hepatocellular carcinoma and lymphoepithelioma-like hepatocellular carcinoma

Lymphocyte-rich hepatocellular carcinomas are rare, with a frequency of less than 1%. The prognosis is better than for conventional hepatocellular carcinomas.[222–225] Both lymphocyte-rich hepatocellular carcinomas and lymphoepithelioma-like hepatocellular carcinomas have striking lymphocytic infiltrates, but they differ in that the epithelial component is well to moderately differentiated in lymphocyte-rich hepatocellular carcinomas versus poorly differentiated in lymphoepithelioma-like hepatocellular carcinomas. In both, the lymphocytic infiltrates should be diffuse and striking on the H&E stains, with the number of lymphocytes being greater than the number of tumor cells in most fields. Of note, hepatocellular carcinomas with dense but focal areas of inflammation do not qualify and neither do hepatocellular carcinomas with a more generalized but mild lymphocytosis.

Lymphocyte-rich hepatocellular carcinomas (Fig. 28.68) have no strong etiologic associations and they can be found in both cirrhotic and noncirrhotic livers.[222,223,225] The distinctive lymphocytic infiltrates do not result from microsatellite instability.[225] Essentially all lymphoepithelioma-like hepatocellular carcinomas and lymphocyte-rich hepatocellular carcinomas are EBV-negative by in situ hybridization.[223,225–228] This stands in contrast to lymphoepithelioma-like carcinomas in other organs, which are often EBV-positive, including cholangiocarcinoma.[229] Low levels of EBV DNA

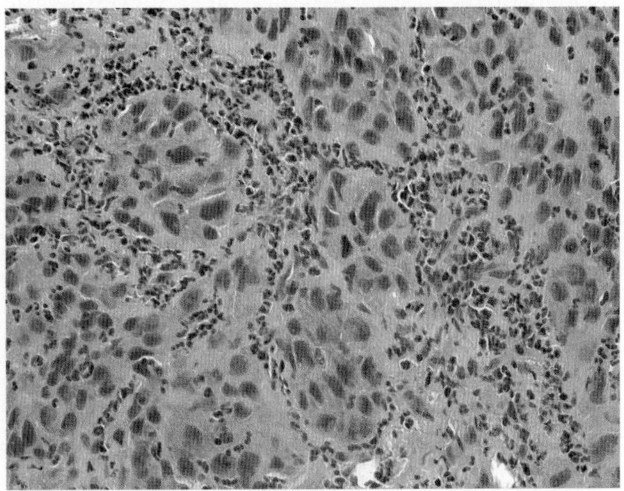

Figure 28.67 Hepatocellular carcinoma, granulocyte colony stimulating factor producing. The tumor was characterized by numerous infiltrating neutrophils.

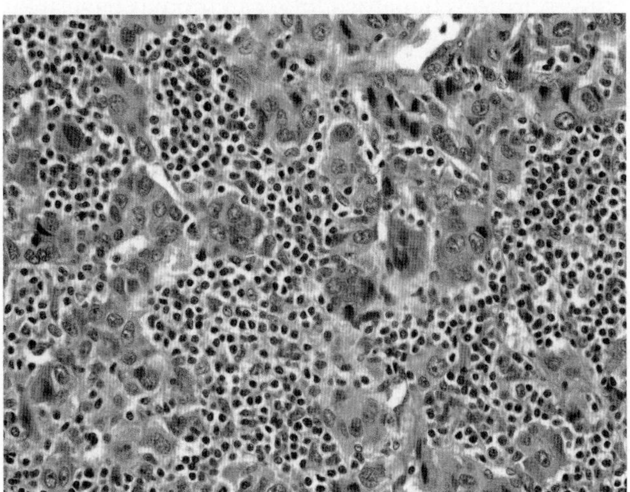

Figure 28.68 Hepatocellular carcinoma, lymphocyte rich. The tumor infiltrating lymphocytes are a dominant part of the histology, outnumbering the tumor cells.

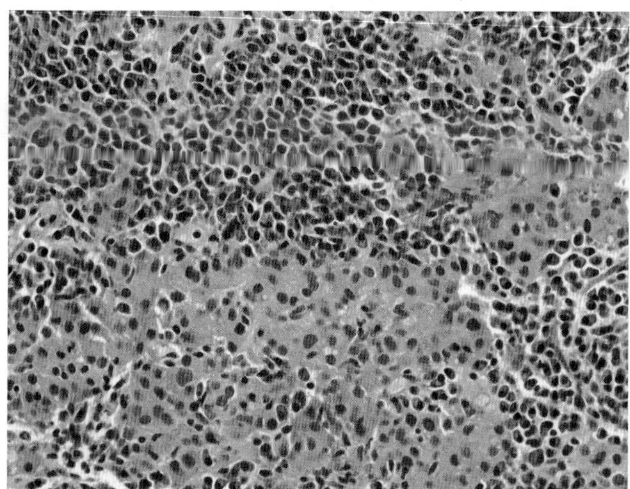

Figure 28.69 Hepatocellular carcinoma, lymphocyte rich. The tumor infiltration was plasma cell rich in this case

can be detected by PCR in both lymphoepithelioma-like hepatocellular carcinomas[229] and conventional hepatocellular carcinomas[230] and does not by itself support a role for EBV in tumorigenesis.

Most tumors are unifocal but multifocal cases have been reported, with tumor nodules showing the same lymphocyte-rich morphology.[227] The hepatocellular component is typically moderately differentiated with a solid or trabecular growth pattern, often with occasional scattered pale bodies. Routine markers of hepatic differentiation such as Arginase and HepPar1 are positive. The inflammatory cells are mostly T lymphocytes with scattered germinal centers containing B cells.[222,225,227] Plasma cells are usually sparse but rarely can be prominent (Fig. 28.69).

Lymphoepithelioma-like hepatocellular carcinomas are poorly differentiated by definition (Fig. 28.70). In some cases, the epithelial cells can be hard to see on H&E, appearing as ragged sheets of epithelial cells largely obscured by the dense lymphocyte infiltrates. Cholangiocarcinomas and metastatic disease can have similar findings, so immunostains should be used to prove hepatic differentiation. It is unclear if lymphoepithelioma-like hepatocellular carcinomas and lymphocyte-rich hepatocellular carcinomas are the same basic tumor, with the latter being a high-grade version of the former, but a reasonable approach is to keep these entities separate at this point. Many authors have not done so, using the terms somewhat interchangeably, limiting the value of the already scant literature on these rare tumors.

Sarcomatoid hepatocellular carcinoma

Sarcomatoid hepatocellular carcinomas are rare, making up less than 1% of hepatocellular carcinomas in surgical pathology specimens. In autopsy studies, the frequency is as high as 9% because these studies are enriched for advanced stage tumors.[231] Chemoembolization therapy can also induce sarcomatoid changes.[231] The prognosis is worse than conventional hepatocellular carcinoma.

Sarcomatoid hepatocellular carcinomas have components of both conventional hepatocellular carcinoma as well as a spindle cell component (Fig. 28.71). The spindle cell component can range from 1% to 80% of the tumor, but in most cases is the minor component.[232] The spindle cell component clearly stands out from the epithelial component but retains at least focal keratin positivity. The spindle cell component should have no evidence for specific mesenchymal differentiation by morphology or by immunostains. In contrast, the spindle cell component

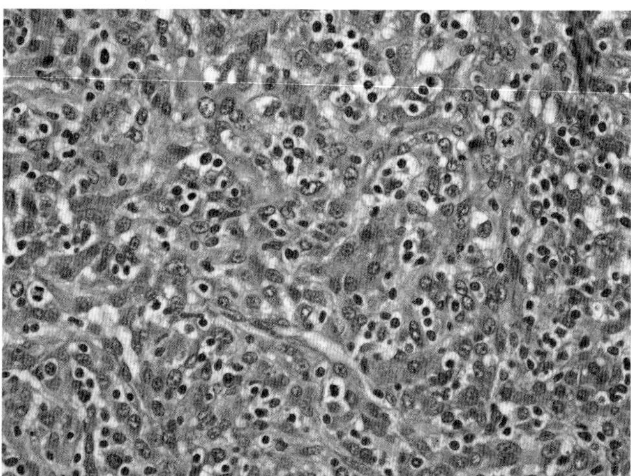

Figure 28.70 Lymphoepithelioma-like hepatocellular carcinomas. The tumor is poorly differentiated, with ragged sheets of epithelial cells that are difficult to see on the H&E.

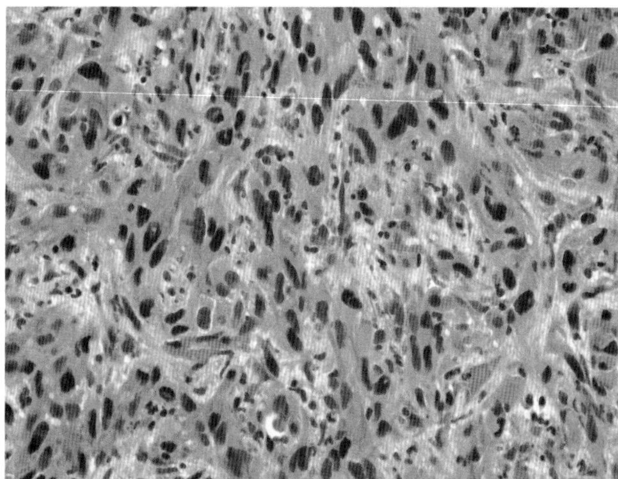

Figure 28.71 Hepatocellular carcinoma, sarcomatoid. This hepatocellular carcinoma had a central nodule with spindle cell growth.

in carcinosarcomas show evidence of lineage differentiation and are keratin-negative. Finally, rare cases of primary liver carcinoma show a spindle cell morphology and coexpress vimentin and keratin, but are not associated with a conventional hepatocellular component or cholangiocarcinoma component on H&E and lack expression of hepatic markers. These cases do not have convincing evidence for hepatic differentiation and so should not be called sarcomatoid hepatocellular carcinoma. Instead, the best approach is to use the term sarcomatoid carcinoma of the liver, with an explanatory note.

Sarcomatoid hepatocellular carcinomas arise in both cirrhotic and noncirrhotic livers.[233] They can be unifocal or multifocal.[234] The hepatocellular carcinoma component is sometimes moderately differentiated but most commonly is poorly differentiated. The hepatocellular component stains with the usual markers of hepatic differentiation.[234,235] In most cases, the spindle cell component is negative for hepatic markers, but occasional cases are positive.[234] The sarcomatoid component is vimentin-positive and keratin-positive.[233–236]

Scirrhous hepatocellular carcinoma

The frequency of scirrhous hepatocellular carcinoma is about 5%.[237–240] The prognosis has not been entirely sorted out, but is similar to[237,238] or better than[239,241] typical hepatocellular carcinoma. This subtype is defined by intratumoral fibrosis. The fibrosis in most cases is fairly diffuse, but should involve at least 50% of the tumor. The fibrosis also tends to be dense, making up at least 25% of the surface area in most low-power fields. In some cases, particularly with larger tumors, the central areas of the tumor can be densely sclerotic with few tumor cells.

Scirrhous hepatocellular carcinomas are often located beneath the liver capsule and are most common found in noncirrhotic livers.[238,242,243] The tumors are only rarely encapsulated and often are composed of clusters of adjacent smaller subnodules. Most scirrhous hepatocellular carcinomas are well to moderately differentiated (Fig. 28.72). The tumor is typically composed of thin trabeculae with a fibrous stroma, though the trabeculae can also be thicker and more bulbous. Cytoplasmic inclusions are common, including hyaline bodies and pale bodies.[239] The tumor cells can also show fatty change or clear cell change.[239] Despite the clear cell change and or fatty change, these cases are classified as scirrhous hepatocellular carcinomas. Entrapped intratumoral portal tracts are common within the tumor.[239]

The scirrhous subtype of hepatocellular carcinoma has several immunohistochemical findings that differ from conventional hepatocellular carcinoma. First, reticulin stains in some cases will not have convincing reticulin loss, in which case the diagnosis of malignancy rests on cytology, increased cell proliferation and or aberrant expression of proteins such as glypican 3. Secondly, this variant commonly has focal or absent expression of HepPar1 (only about 40% to 60% of cases are positive).[237,241,244,245] Overall, Arginase is a more sensitive marker of hepatic differentiation, staining 85% of cases.[245] Glypican 3 is also positive in about 80% of cases.[245]

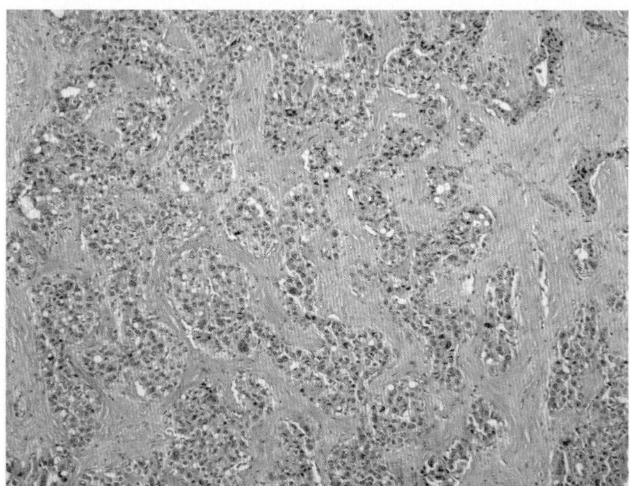

Figure 28.72 Hepatocellular carcinoma, scirrhous subtype. Thin trabeculae or tumor cells are growing in a dense desmoplastic background.

The differential includes primarily fibrolamellar carcinoma, cholangiocarcinoma, or metastatic disease. Both fibrolamellar carcinoma and scirrhous hepatocellular carcinoma can be CK7-positive,[237] but only fibrolamellar carcinomas consistently express CD68.[246,247] Molecular testing for fibrolamellar carcinoma is also very helpful in this situation.[131] Markers of hepatic differentiation will exclude cholangiocarcinoma and metastatic disease.

Steatohepatitic hepatocellular carcinoma

This subtype of hepatocellular carcinoma is the most frequent, making about 20% of cases in published series.[248–250] The prognosis is similar to conventional hepatocellular carcinoma.[248,249] This variant shows steatohepatitis within the tumor parenchyma, with macrovesicular steatosis, lymphocytic inflammation, balloon cells, Mallory–Denk bodies, and pericellular fibrosis (Figs. 28.73 and 28.74).[248,251] The presence of steatosis alone in a hepatocellular carcinoma doesn't meet the minimal findings needed for this subtype. Most steatohepatitic hepatocellular carcinomas are well to moderately differentiated. Not all of the features of steatohepatitis need to be present in every

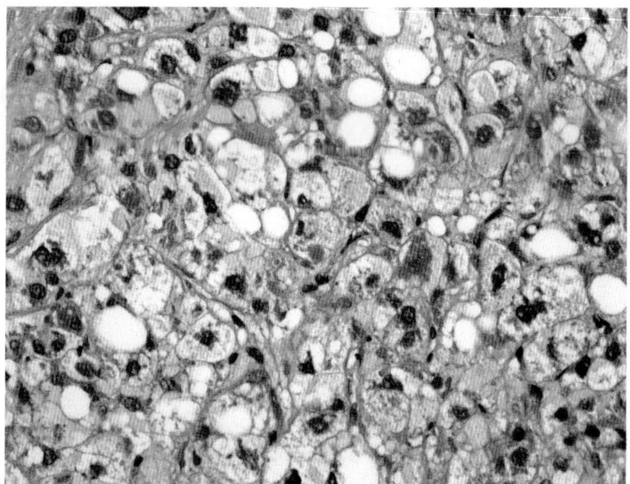

Figure 28.73 Hepatocellular carcinoma, steatohepatitic subtype. This tumor shows macrovesicular steatosis, ballooned hepatocytes, and Mallory–Denk bodies.

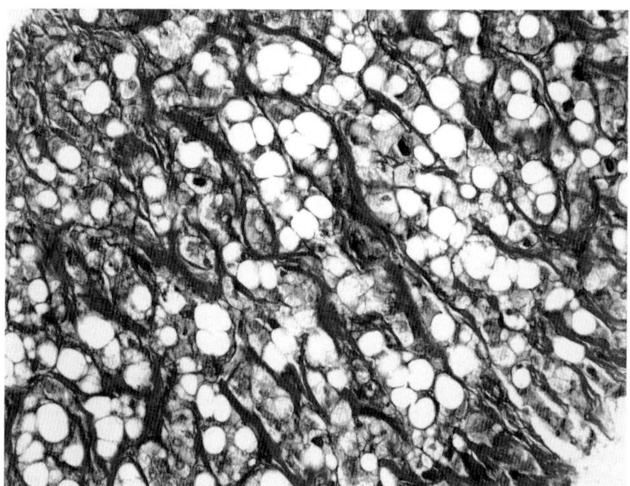

Figure 28.74 Hepatocellular carcinoma, steatohepatitic subtype. The intratumoral fibrosis is highlighted by a trichrome stain (same case as above).

case, but there should be macrovesicular steatosis (at least 5%), active injury (lymphocytic inflammation, ballooned tumor cells), and usually some degree of intratumoral fibrosis. When the percent of steatosis is low, it should be widely distributed. The intratumoral fibrosis can be inconspicuous on the H&E, but highlighted by a trichrome stain. In addition, the steatohepatitic changes should be a dominant part of the histology and not a focal finding: a cutoff of 50% of the tumor area is a reasonable approach.[248,251]

Steatohepatitic hepatocellular carcinomas are strongly associated with the metabolic syndrome or with chronic ETOH use. The background nonneoplastic liver usually shows steatosis or steatohepatitis[248–250] and the changes within the tumor reflect the same broad changes seen in the background liver. However, the steatohepatitic variant of hepatocellular carcinoma in rare cases is found in livers that have no fatty change in the nonneoplastic parenchyma.[252] In these cases, the steatohepatitic morphology presumably represents tumor specific mutations or epigenetic changes and not tumor response to an overall systemic condition (metabolic syndrome or ETOH).

The steatohepatitic variant stains like a conventional hepatocellular carcinoma for markers of hepatic differentiation. Molecular studies have found that the steatohepatitic variant of hepatocellular carcinoma is less likely to have activation of the β-catenin pathway, with fewer β-catenin mutations, and is less likely to have strong and diffuse glutamine synthesis staining.[253]

The diagnosis can be challenging because the steatohepatitic features are similar to that seen in medical liver biopsies and the tumor can be missed. The correct diagnosis is made by recognizing the architectural and cytologic atypia, increased cell proliferation, and loss of reticulin. Focal nodular hyperplasia can occasionally can show steatohepatitic changes and should also be excluded.[254]

Provisional subtypes of hepatocellular carcinoma

The following subtypes are categorized as provisional because published data is limited to a few papers.

Chromophobe hepatocellular carcinoma

Chromophobe hepatocellular carcinomas are characterized by tumor cells with amphophilic to eosinophilic cytoplasm. The tumor has a solid or trabecular growth pattern in most cases and larger tumors commonly have scattered small cystic spaces that are filled with a thin serum-like substance (Fig. 28.75). The nuclear cytology is distinctive because most tumor cells have bland nuclear changes, but scattered throughout the tumor are cells with more striking nuclear pleomorphism (Fig. 28.76). At the molecular level, chromophobe hepatocellular carcinoma is strongly associated with alternative lengthening of telomeres (ALT),[133] where tumor cells maintain their telomeres by a telomerase-independent mechanism that involves homologous recombination of the telomeres.[255] In other organs, ALT is associated with mutations that lead to loss of nuclear expression of ATRX or DAXX, but this is not the case in hepatocellular carcinomas and the mutations leading to the ALT phenotype are not known.

Lipid-rich hepatocellular carcinoma

Lipid-rich hepatocellular carcinomas have clear cytoplasm at low power and are commonly confused with clear cell hepatocellular carcinomas. However, on higher power examination, the tumor cells in

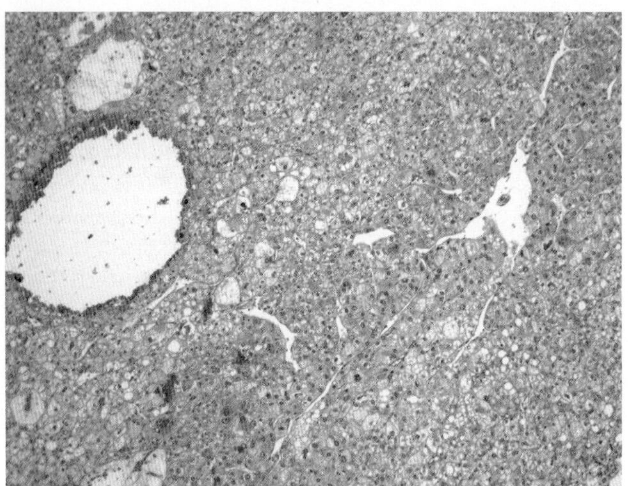

Figure 28.75 Hepatocellular carcinoma, chromophobe subtype. Irregular cyst-like spaces are seen in this case.

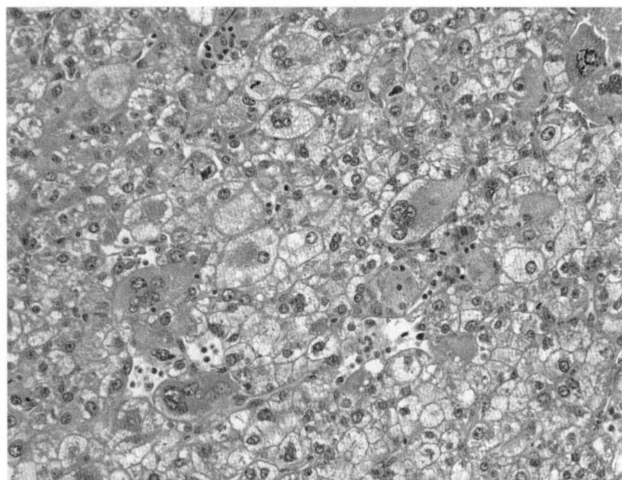

Figure 28.76 Hepatocellular carcinoma, chromophobe subtype. The tumor nuclei are generally bland, but scattered cells have striking nuclear anaplasia.

lipid-rich hepatocellular carcinomas are filled with numerous tiny droplets of fat, similar to the changes seen in microvesicular steatosis (Fig. 28.77). To qualify for this subtype, the microvesicular steatosis should be diffuse and the predominant pattern, though occasional larger droplets of fat are acceptable. Small foci of microvesicular steatosis can also sometimes be seen in the steatohepatitic subtype of hepatocellular carcinoma, but the predominant patterns between these two subtypes are distinct.

Almost all cases are well differentiated, which can be a particular challenge on fine needle aspirates because the findings can resemble benign fatty liver disease.[256] The clinical and morphologic findings correlates are not clear because of limited data, but in one case report the background liver showed nonalcoholic fatty liver disease and advanced fibrosis.[162]

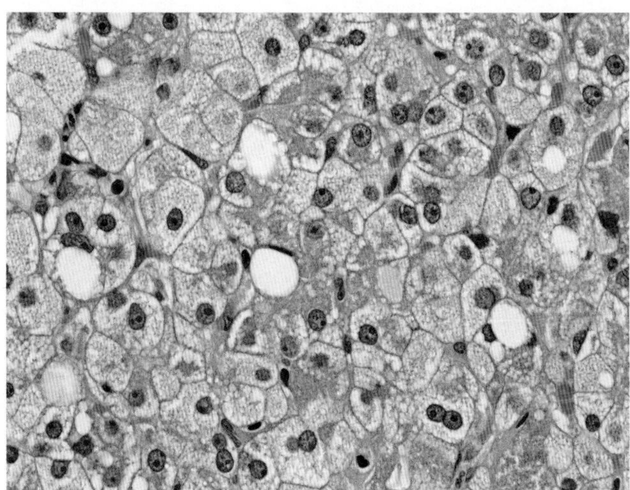

Figure 28.77 Hepatocellular carcinoma, lipid-rich subtype. The cytoplasm is filled with numerous small droplets of fat. These changes can mimic clear cell hepatocellular carcinoma on low power and, for this reason, are commonly misclassified as clear cell hepatocellular carcinoma.

Other metastatic carcinomas can show a similar lipid-rich pattern, so hepatic differentiation needs to be demonstrated by immunostains. Anecdotally, some of these cases are HepPar1-negative, so other markers such as Arginase are a good choice. Adrenal glands adherent to the liver or adrenal rest tumors can also enter the differential[257] and are excluded by immunostains.

Myxoid hepatocellular carcinoma

Myxoid hepatocellular carcinomas are typically well to moderately differentiated and have a trabecular growth pattern. Clear cell change can also be seen.[258] The tumor cells stain strongly with HepPar1 and Arginase and are negative for CDX2 and CK19. In addition, they typically show loss of LFABP staining and are strongly and diffusely positive for glutamine synthetase.[259] There is no gland formation but the trabeculae are spread apart by myxoid material within the sinusoids (Fig. 28.78). The myxoid material is Alcian blue–positive. Depending on the strength of the stain, mucicarmine can also be weakly to moderately positive. The overall pattern resembles the myxoid changes seen in some chromophobe renal carcinomas, but the explanation for the myxoid deposits in myxoid hepatocellular carcinomas remains unclear. There is no strong evidence for degenerative changes. Despite the myxoid material and often some mucicarmine staining, there is no true gland formation and these tumors should not be classified as cholangiocarcinoma. Finally, some hepatic adenomas can show similar myxoid changes as well as LFABP loss and glutamine synthetase staining, so the tumor needs to be fully

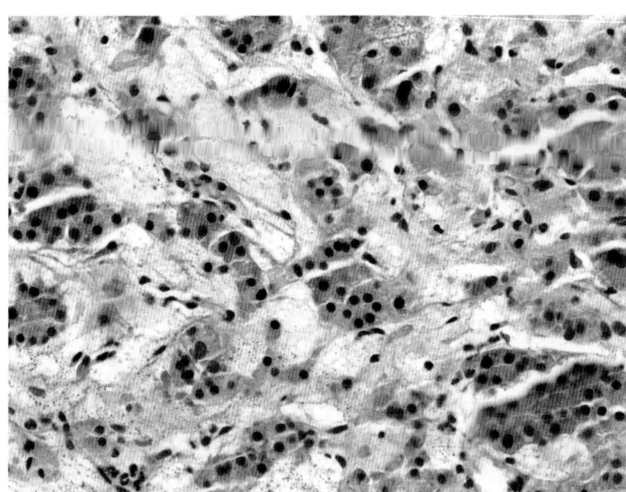

Figure 28.78 Hepatocellular carcinoma, myxoid subtype. The tumor sinusoids contain abundant myxoid material.

worked up to prove hepatocellular carcinoma. Distinct radiologic findings have also been reported.[260]

Hepatocellular carcinoma with syncytial giant cells

This variant has been proposed in a case report, so data is quite limited. The hepatocellular carcinoma was well differentiated but had numerous syncytial multinucleated giant cells, similar to those seen in infantile giant cell hepatitis, but not like the bizarre and very atypical multinucleated giant cells that can be found in poorly differentiated hepatocellular carcinomas.[261] The case report also describes foci of smaller, less differentiated nests of tumor cells in a desmoplastic background. The tumor was HepPar1 positive and negative for CK7 and CK19.

Transitional liver cell tumor

Hepatocellular carcinomas in older children and adolescents can sometimes have focal areas that resemble the fetal or embryonal growth patterns of hepatoblastoma.[262] The term transitional liver cell tumor has been proposed for these cases. These foci can be somewhat subjective, making it challenging to distinguish these cases from conventional hepatocellular carcinoma. These tumors behave clinically like hepatocellular carcinomas and there is no evidence for a prognostic difference between this subtype and conventional hepatocellular carcinoma. Serum AFP levels are typically elevated. One case was identified in the setting of Li-Fraumeni syndrome.[263]

The proposed explanations for transitional cell liver tumors include "maturation" of a pure fetal hepatoblastoma, changes secondary to preoperative chemotherapy, or intrinsic genetic changes enriched in hepatocellular carcinomas arising in this young age group. Of note, the macrotrabecular growth pattern is found in conventional hepatocellular carcinomas and does not suggest a transitional liver cell tumor by itself.

REFERENCES

1. Wang Q, Luan W, Villanueva GA, et al. Clinical prognostic variables in young patients (under 40 years) with hepatitis B virus-associated hepatocellular carcinoma. *J Dig Dis.* 2012;13(4):214–218.
2. Yeh MM, Daniel HD, Torbenson M. Hepatitis C-associated hepatocellular carcinomas in non-cirrhotic livers. *Mod Pathol.* 2010;23(2):276–283.
3. von Delius S, Lersch C, Schulte-Frohlinde E, et al. Hepatocellular carcinoma associated with hereditary hemochromatosis occurring in non-cirrhotic liver. *Z Gastroenterol.* 2006;44(1):39–42.
4. Baffy G, Brunt EM, Caldwell SH. Hepatocellular carcinoma in non-alcoholic fatty liver disease: an emerging menace. *J Hepatol.* 2012;56(6):1384–1391.
5. Alexander J, Torbenson M, Wu TT, et al. Nonalcoholic fatty liver disease contributes to hepatocellular carcinoma in non-cirrhotic liver: a clinical and pathological study. *J Gastroenterol Hepatol.* 2013;28(5):848–854.
6. Benedict M, Rodriguez-Davalos M, Emre S, et al. Congenital extrahepatic portosystemic shunt (abernethy malformation type Ib) with associated hepatocellular carcinoma: case report and literature review. *Pediatr Dev Pathol.* 2016.
7. Sharma VK, Ranade PR, Marar S, et al. Long-term clinical outcome of Budd-Chiari syndrome in children after radiological intervention. *Eur J Gastroenterol Hepatol.* 2016;28(5):567–575.
8. Dang X, Li L, Li S, et al. Studies on Budd-chiari syndrome complicated with hepatocellular carcinoma: most patients without inferior vena cava obstruction. *Int J Clin Exp Med.* 2015;8(6):9071–9078.
9. Micchelli ST, Vivekanandan P, Boitnott JK, et al. Malignant transformation of hepatic adenomas. *Mod Pathol.* 2008;21(4):491–497.
10. Hirakawa M, Ikeda K, Arase Y, et al. Hepatocarcinogenesis following HCV RNA eradication by interferon in chronic hepatitis patients. *Intern Med.* 2008;47(19):1637–1643.
11. Tokita H, Fukui H, Tanaka A, et al. Risk factors for the development of hepatocellular carcinoma among patients with chronic hepatitis C who achieved a sustained virological response to

interferon therapy. *J Gastroenterol Hepatol.* 2005;20(5):752–758.
12. Kew MC. Aflatoxins as a cause of hepatocellular carcinoma. *J Gastrointestin Liver Dis.* 2013;22(3):305–310.
13. Ko C, Siddaiah N, Berger J, et al. Prevalence of hepatic iron overload and association with hepatocellular cancer in end-stage liver disease: results from the National Hemochromatosis Transplant Registry. *Liver Int.* 2007;27(10):1394–1401.
14. Fattovich G, Stroffolini T, Zagni I, et al. Hepatocellular carcinoma in cirrhosis: incidence and risk factors. *Gastroenterology*. 2004;127(5 suppl 1):S35–50.
15. Dorfman JD, Schulik R, Choti MA, et al. Differences in characteristics of patients with and without known risk factors for hepatocellular carcinoma in the United States. *World J Gastroenterol.* 2007;13(5):781–784.
16. Chedid AD, Klein PW, Tiburi MF, et al. Spontaneous rupture of hepatocellular carcinoma with haemoperitoneum: a rare condition in Western countries. *HPB*. 2001;3(3):227–230.
17. Vivarelli M, Cavallari A, Bellusci R, et al. Ruptured hepatocellular carcinoma: an important cause of spontaneous haemoperitoneum in Italy. *Eur J Surg.* 1995;161(12):881–886.
18. Lai EC, Lau WY. Spontaneous rupture of hepatocellular carcinoma: a systematic review. *Arch Surg*. 2006;141(2):191–198.
19. Battula N, Srinivasan P, Madanur M, et al. Ruptured hepatocellular carcinoma following chemoembolization: a western experience. *Hepatobiliary Pancreat Dis Int.* 2007;6(1): 49–51.
20. Martin RC, 2nd, Loehle J, Scoggins CR, et al. Kentucky hepatoma: epidemiologic variant or same problem in a different region? *Arch Surg.* 2007;142(5):431–436; discussion 436–437.
21. van Meer S, an Erpecum KJ, Sprengers D, et al. Hepatocellular carcinoma in cirrhotic versus noncirrhotic livers: results from a large cohort in the Netherlands. *Eur J Gastroenterol Hepatol.* 2016;28(3):352–359.
22. Toyoda H, Kumada T, Tada T, et al. Tumor markers for hepatocellular carcinoma: simple and significant predictors of outcome in patients with HCC. *Liver Cancer.* 2015;4(2):126–136.
23. Katyal S, Oliver JH 3rd, Peterson MS, et al. Extrahepatic metastases of hepatocellular carcinoma. *Radiology*. 2000;216(3):698–703.
24. Aino H, Sumie S, Niizeki T, et al. Clinical characteristics and prognostic factors for advanced hepatocellular carcinoma with extrahepatic metastasis. *Mol Clin Oncol.* 2014;2(3):393–398.
25. Matsukuma S, Sato K. Peritoneal seeding of hepatocellular carcinoma: clinicopathological characteristics of 17 autopsy cases. *Pathol Int.* 2011;61(6):356–362.
26. Mullhaupt B, Durand F, Roskams T, et al. Is tumor biopsy necessary? *Liver Transpl.* 2011;17(suppl 2):S14–25.
27. Chen Q-w, Cheng C-s, Chen H, et al. Effectiveness and complications of ultrasound guided fine needle aspiration for primary liver cancer in a Chinese population with serum alpha-fetoprotein levels </=200 ng/ml—a study based on 4,312 patients. *PLoS One*. 2014;9(8):e101536.
28. Silva MA, Hegab B, Hyde C, et al. Needle track seeding following biopsy of liver lesions in the diagnosis of hepatocellular cancer: a systematic review and meta-analysis. *Gut*. 2008;57(11):1592–1596.
29. Jain D. Tissue diagnosis of hepatocellular carcinoma. *J Clin Exp Hepatol.* 2014;4(suppl 3):S67–73.
30. Maturen KE, Nghiem HV, Marrero JA, et al. Lack of tumor seeding of hepatocellular carcinoma after percutaneous needle biopsy using coaxial cutting needle technique. *AJR Am J Roentgenol.* 2006;187(5):1184–1187.
31. Guo W, He X, Li Z, et al. Combination of transarterial chemoembolization (TACE) and radiofrequency ablation (RFA) vs. surgical resection (SR) on survival outcome of early hepatocellular carcinoma: a meta-analysis. *Hepatogastroenterology*. 2015;62(139):710–714.
32. Iezzi R, Pompili M, Posa A, et al. Combined locoregional treatment of patients with hepatocellular carcinoma: state of the art. *World J Gastroenterol.* 2016;22(6):1935–1942.
33. Wang Y, Hu Y, Ren M, et al. Efficacy and safety of radiofrequency ablation and transcatheter arterial chemoembolization for treatment of hepatocellular carcinoma: a meta-analysis. *Hepatol Res*. 2016;46(1):58–71.
34. Parikh ND, Waljee AK, Singal AG. Downstaging hepatocellular carcinoma: a systematic review and pooled analysis. *Liver Transpl.* 2015;21(9):1142–1152.
35. Fong ZV, Tanabe KK. The clinical management of hepatocellular carcinoma in the United States, Europe, and Asia: a comprehensive and evidence-based comparison and review. *Cancer.* 2014;120(18):2824–2838.
36. Llovet JM, Real MI, Montaña X, et al. Arterial embolisation or chemoembolisation versus symptomatic treatment in patients with unresectable hepatocellular carcinoma: a randomised controlled trial. *Lancet.* 2002;359(9319):1734–1739.
37. Llovet JM, Ricci S, Mazzaferro V, et al. Sorafenib in advanced hepatocellular carcinoma. *N Engl J Med.* 2008;359(4):378–390.

38. Greten TF, Papendorf F, Bleck JS, et al. Survival rate in patients with hepatocellular carcinoma: a retrospective analysis of 389 patients. *Br J Cancer*. 2005;92(10):1862–1868.
39. op den Winkel M, Nagel D, Sappl J, et al. Prognosis of patients with hepatocellular carcinoma. Validation and ranking of established staging-systems in a large western HCC-cohort. *PLoS One*. 2012;7(10):e45066.
40. Tandon P, Garcia-Tsao G. Prognostic indicators in hepatocellular carcinoma: a systematic review of 72 studies. *Liver Int*. 2009;29(4):502–510.
41. Earl TM, Chapman WC. Hepatocellular carcinoma: resection versus transplantation. *Semin Liver Dis*. 2013;33(3):282–292.
42. Tabrizian P, Jibara G, Shrager B, et al. Recurrence of hepatocellular cancer after resection: patterns, treatments, and prognosis. *Ann Surg*. 2015;261(5):947–955.
43. Lee SY, Konstantinidis IT, Eaton AA, et al. Predicting recurrence patterns after resection of hepatocellular cancer. *HPB*. 2014;16(10):943–953.
44. Li Q, Wang J, Juzi JT, et al. Clonality analysis for multicentric origin and intrahepatic metastasis in recurrent and primary hepatocellular carcinoma. *J Gastrointest Surg*. 2008;12(9):1540–1547.
45. Ng IO, Guan XY, Poon RT, et al. Determination of the molecular relationship between multiple tumour nodules in hepatocellular carcinoma differentiates multicentric origin from intrahepatic metastasis. *J Pathol*. 2003;199(3):345–353.
46. Vasuri F, Malvi D, Rosini F, et al. Revisiting the role of pathological analysis in transarterial chemoembolization-treated hepatocellular carcinoma after transplantation. *World J Gastroenterol*. 2014;20(37):13538–13545.
47. Benckert C, Jonas S, Thelen A, et al. Liver transplantation for hepatocellular carcinoma in cirrhosis: prognostic parameters. *Transplant Proc*. 2005;37(4):1693–1694.
48. Lang H, Sotiropoulos GC, Brokalaki EI, et al. Survival and recurrence rates after resection for hepatocellular carcinoma in noncirrhotic livers. *J Am Coll Surg*. 2007;205(1):27–36.
49. Jonas S, Bechstein WO, Steinmüller T, et al. Vascular invasion and histopathologic grading determine outcome after liver transplantation for hepatocellular carcinoma in cirrhosis. *Hepatology*. 2001;33(5):1080–1086.
50. Pesi B, Ferrero A, Grazi GL, et al. Liver resection with thrombectomy as a treatment of hepatocellular carcinoma with major vascular invasion: results from a retrospective multicentric study. *Am J Surg*. 2015;210(1):35–44.
51. Rodriguez-Peralvarez M, Luong TV, Andreana L, et al. A systematic review of microvascular invasion in hepatocellular carcinoma: diagnostic and prognostic variability. *Ann Surg Oncol*. 2013;20(1):325–339.
52. Ohashi M, Wakai T, Korita PV, et al. Histological evaluation of intracapsular venous invasion for discrimination between portal and hepatic venous invasion in hepatocellular carcinoma. *J Gastroenterol Hepatol*. 2010;25(1):143–149.
53. Su Q, Zerban H, Otto G, et al. Cytokeratin expression is reduced in glycogenotic clear hepatocytes but increased in ground-glass cells in chronic human and woodchuck hepadnaviral infection. *Hepatology*. 1998;28(2):347–359.
54. Su Q, Benner A, Hofmann WJ, et al. Human hepatic preneoplasia: phenotypes and proliferation kinetics of foci and nodules of altered hepatocytes and their relationship to liver cell dysplasia. *Virchows Arch*. 1997;431(6):391–406.
55. Gong L, Li YH, Su Q, et al. Clonality of nodular lesions in liver cirrhosis and chromosomal abnormalities in monoclonal nodules of altered hepatocytes. *Histopathology*. 2010;56(5):589–599.
56. Klein WM, Molmenti EP, Colombani PM, et al. Primary liver carcinoma arising in people younger than 30 years. *Am J Clin Pathol*. 2005;124(4):512–518.
57. Libbrecht L, Desmet V, Van Damme B, et al. The immunohistochemical phenotype of dysplastic foci in human liver: correlation with putative progenitor cells. *J Hepatol*. 2000;33(1):76–84.
58. Park YN. Update on precursor and early lesions of hepatocellular carcinomas. *Arch Pathol Lab Med*. 2011;135(6):704–715.
59. Marchio A, Terris B, Meddeb M, et al. Chromosomal abnormalities in liver cell dysplasia detected by comparative genomic hybridisation. *Mol Pathol*. 2001;54(4):270–274.
60. Plentz RR, Park YN, Lechel A, et al. Telomere shortening and inactivation of cell cycle checkpoints characterize human hepatocarcinogenesis. *Hepatology*. 2007;45(4):968–976.
61. El-Sayed SS, El-Sadany M, Tabll AA, et al. DNA ploidy and liver cell dysplasia in liver biopsies from patients with liver cirrhosis. *Can J Gastroenterol*. 2004;18(2):87–91.
62. Le Bail B, Bernard PH, Carles J, et al. Prevalence of liver cell dysplasia and association with HCC in a series of 100 cirrhotic liver explants. *J Hepatol*. 1997;27(5):835–842.
63. Natarajan S, Theise ND, Thung SN, et al. Large-cell change of hepatocytes in cirrhosis may represent a reaction to prolonged cholestasis. *Am J Surg Pathol*. 1997;21(3):312–318.
64. Lee RG, Tsamandas AC, Demetris AJ. Large cell change (liver cell dysplasia) and hepatocellular

carcinoma in cirrhosis: matched case-control study, pathological analysis, and pathogenetic hypothesis. *Hepatology*. 1997;26(6):1415–1422.
65. Koo JS, Kim H, Park BK, et al. Predictive value of liver cell dysplasia for development of hepatocellular carcinoma in patients with chronic hepatitis B. *J Clin Gastroenterol*. 2008;42(6):738–743.
66. Libbrecht L, Craninx M, Nevens F, et al. Predictive value of liver cell dysplasia for development of hepatocellular carcinoma in patients with non-cirrhotic and cirrhotic chronic viral hepatitis. *Histopathology*. 2001;39(1):66–73.
67. Quaglia A, Tibballs J, Grasso A, et al. Focal nodular hyperplasia-like areas in cirrhosis. *Histopathology*. 2003;42(1):14–21.
68. Nakashima O, Kurogi M, Yamaguchi R, et al. Unique hypervascular nodules in alcoholic liver cirrhosis: identical to focal nodular hyperplasia-like nodules? *J Hepatol*. 2004;41(6):992–998.
69. Libbrecht L, Cassiman D, Verslype C, et al. Clinicopathological features of focal nodular hyperplasia-like nodules in 130 cirrhotic explant livers. *Am J Gastroenterol*. 2006;101(10):2341–2346.
70. Rebouissou S, Couchy G, Libbrecht L, et al. The beta-catenin pathway is activated in focal nodular hyperplasia but not in cirrhotic FNH-like nodules. *J Hepatol*. 2008;49(1):61–71.
71. Furuya K, Nakamura M, Yamamoto Y, et al. Macroregenerative nodule of the liver. A clinicopathologic study of 345 autopsy cases of chronic liver disease. *Cancer*. 1988;61(1):99–105.
72. Hytiroglou P, Theise ND, Schwartz M, et al. Macroregenerative nodules in a series of adult cirrhotic liver explants: issues of classification and nomenclature. *Hepatology*. 1995;21(3):703–708.
73. Theise ND, Marcelin K, Goldfischer M, et al. Low proliferative activity in macroregenerative nodules: evidence for an alternate hypothesis concerning human hepatocarcinogenesis. *Liver*. 1996;16(2):134–139.
74. Sato T, Kondo F, Ebara M, et al. Natural history of large regenerative nodules and dysplastic nodules in liver cirrhosis: 28-year follow-up study. *Hepatol Int*. 2015;9(2):330–336.
75. Kim H, Park YN. Massive hepatic necrosis with large regenerative nodules. *Korean J Hepatol*. 2010;16(3):334–337.
76. Seki S, Sakaguchi H, Kitada T, et al. Outcomes of dysplastic nodules in human cirrhotic liver: a clinicopathological study. *Clin Cancer Res*. 2000;6(9):3469–3473.
77. Iavarone M, Manini MA, Sangiovanni A, et al. Contrast-enhanced computed tomography and ultrasound-guided liver biopsy to diagnose dysplastic liver nodules in cirrhosis. *Dig Liver Dis*. 2013;45(1):43–49.
78. Nguyen TB, Roncalli M, Di Tommaso L, et al. Combined use of heat-shock protein 70 and glutamine synthetase is useful in the distinction of typical hepatocellular adenoma from atypical hepatocellular neoplasms and well-differentiated hepatocellular carcinoma. *Mod Pathol*. 2016;29(3):283–292.
79. Nakano M, Saito A, Yamamoto M, et al. Stromal and blood vessel wall invasion in well-differentiated hepatocellular carcinoma. *Liver*. 1997;17(1):41–46.
80. Kojiro M, Roskams T. Early hepatocellular carcinoma and dysplastic nodules. *Semin Liver Dis*. 2005;25(2):133–142.
81. Kondo F. Assessment of stromal invasion for correct histological diagnosis of early hepatocellular carcinoma. *Int J Hepatol*. 2011;2011:241652.
82. Park YN, Kojiro M, Di Tommaso L, et al. Ductular reaction is helpful in defining early stromal invasion, small hepatocellular carcinomas, and dysplastic nodules. *Cancer*. 2007;109(5):915–923.
83. Kim SH, Lim HK, Kim MJ, et al. Radiofrequency ablation of high-grade dysplastic nodules in chronic liver disease: comparison with well-differentiated hepatocellular carcinoma based on long-term results. *Eur Radiol*. 2008;18(4):814–821.
84. Cho YK, Wook Chung J, Kim Y, et al. Radiofrequency ablation of high-grade dysplastic nodules. *Hepatology*. 2011;54(6):2005–2011.
85. Yeh CN, Lee WC, Jeng LB, et al. Pedunculated hepatocellular carcinoma: clinicopathologic study of 18 surgically resected cases. *World J Surg*. 2002;26(9):1133–1138.
86. M Mashfiqul MM, Tan YM, Thng CH, et al. Pedunculated HCC or adrenal metastasis: a diagnostic conundrum. *Singapore Med J*. 2007;48(2):e50–52.
87. Anthony PP, James K. Pedunculated hepatocellular carcinoma. Is it an entity? *Histopathology*. 1987;11(4):403–414.
88. Horie Y, Shigoku A, Tanaka H, et al. Prognosis for pedunculated hepatocellular carcinoma. *Oncology*. 1999;57(1):23–28.
89. Nzeako UC, Goodman ZD, Ishak KG. Comparison of tumor pathology with duration of survival of North American patients with hepatocellular carcinoma. *Cancer*. 1995;76(4):579–588.
90. Lauwers GY, Terris B, Balis UJ, et al. Prognostic histologic indicators of curatively resected hepatocellular carcinomas: a multi-institutional analysis of 425 patients with definition of a histologic prognostic index. *Am J Surg Pathol*. 2002;26(1):25–34.
91. Zhou L, Rui JA, Wang SB, et al. Outcomes and prognostic factors of cirrhotic patients with hepatocellular carcinoma after radical major hepatectomy. *World J Surg*. 2007;31(9):1782–1787.

92. Han DH, Choi GH, Kim KS, et al. Prognostic significance of the worst grade in hepatocellular carcinoma with heterogeneous histologic grades of differentiation. *J Gastroenterol Hepatol* 2013;28(8):1384–1390.
93. Cotoi CG, Khorsandi SE, Pleşea IE, et al. Histological aspects of post-TACE hepatocellular carcinoma. *Rom J Morphol Embryol.* 2012;53(3 suppl):677–682.
94. Herber S, Biesterfeld S, Franz U, et al. Correlation of multislice CT and histomorphology in HCC following TACE: predictors of outcome. *Cardiovasc Intervent Radiol.* 2008;31(4):768–777.
95. Sciarra A, Ronot M, Di Tommaso L, et al. TRIP: a pathological score for transarterial chemoembolization resistance individualized prediction in hepatocellular carcinoma. *Liver Int.* 2015;35(11):2466–2473.
96. Lai JP, Conley A, Knudsen BS, et al. Hypoxia after transarterial chemoembolization may trigger a progenitor cell phenotype in hepatocellular carcinoma. *Histopathology.* 2015;67(4):442–450.
97. Zen C, Zen Y, Mitry RR, et al. Mixed phenotype hepatocellular carcinoma after transarterial chemoembolization and liver transplantation. *Liver Transpl.* 2011;17(8):943–954.
98. Nishihara Y, Aishima S, Kuroda Y, et al. Biliary phenotype of hepatocellular carcinoma after preoperative transcatheter arterial chemoembolization. *J Gastroenterol Hepatol.* 2008;23(12):1860–1868.
99. Sasaki M, Yoneda N, Kitamura S, et al. A serum amyloid A-positive hepatocellular neoplasm arising in alcoholic cirrhosis: a previously unrecognized type of inflammatory hepatocellular tumor. *Mod Pathol.* 2012;25(12):1584–1593.
100. Calderaro J, Nault JC, Balabaud C, et al. Inflammatory hepatocellular adenomas developed in the setting of chronic liver disease and cirrhosis. *Mod Pathol.* 2016;29(1):43–50.
101. Singhi AD, Jain D, Kakar S, et al. Reticulin loss in benign fatty liver: an important diagnostic pitfall when considering a diagnosis of hepatocellular carcinoma. *Am J Surg Pathol.* 2012;36(5): 710–715.
102. Bergman S, Graeme-Cook F, Pitman MB. The usefulness of the reticulin stain in the differential diagnosis of liver nodules on fine-needle aspiration biopsy cell block preparations. *Mod Pathol.* 1997;10(12):1258–1264.
103. Hong H, Patonay B, Finley J. Unusual reticulin staining pattern in well-differentiated hepatocellular carcinoma. *Diagn Pathol.* 2011;6:15.
104. Wilkens L, Becker T, Schlegelberger B, et al. Preserved reticulin network in a case of hepatocellular carcinoma. *Histopathology.* 2006;48(7):876–878.
105. Ruck P, Xiao JC, Kaiserling E. Immunoreactivity of sinusoids in hepatocellular carcinoma. An immunohistochemical study using lectin UEA-1 and antibodies against endothelial markers, including CD34. *Arch Pathol Lab Med.* 1995;119(2):173–178.
106. Coston WM, Loera S, Lau SK, et al. Distinction of hepatocellular carcinoma from benign hepatic mimickers using Glypican-3 and CD34 immunohistochemistry. *Am J Surg Pathol.* 2008;32(3):433–444.
107. Ahmad I, Iyer A, Marginean CE, et al. Diagnostic use of cytokeratins, CD34, and neuronal cell adhesion molecule staining in focal nodular hyperplasia and hepatic adenoma. *Hum Pathol.* 2009;40(5): 726–734.
108. Kong CS, Appenzeller M, Ferrell LD. Utility of CD34 reactivity in evaluating focal nodular hepatocellular lesions sampled by fine needle aspiration biopsy. *Acta Cytol.* 2000;44(2):218–222.
109. Bellamy CO, Maxwell RS, Prost S, et al. The value of immunophenotyping hepatocellular adenomas: consecutive resections at one UK centre. *Histopathology.* 2013;62(3):431–445.
110. Vlasoff DM, Baschinsky DY, Frankel WL. Cytokeratin 5/6 immunostaining in hepatobiliary and pancreatic neoplasms. *Appl Immunohistochem Mol Morphol.* 2002;10(2):147–151.
111. Christensen WN, Boitnott JK, Kuhajda FP. Immunoperoxidase staining as a diagnostic aid for hepatocellular carcinoma. *Mod Pathol.* 1989;2(1):8–12.
112. Durnez A, Verslype C, Nevens F, et al. The clinicopathological and prognostic relevance of cytokeratin 7 and 19 expression in hepatocellular carcinoma. A possible progenitor cell origin. *Histopathology.* 2006;49(2):138–151.
113. Uenishi T, Kubo S, Yamamoto T, et al. Cytokeratin 19 expression in hepatocellular carcinoma predicts early postoperative recurrence. *Cancer Sci.* 2003;94(10):851–857.
114. Kim H, Choi GH, Na DC, et al. Human hepatocellular carcinomas with "Stemness"-related marker expression: keratin 19 expression and a poor prognosis. *Hepatology.* 2011;54(5):1707–1717.
115. Torbenson M, Kannangai R, Abraham S, et al. Concurrent evaluation of p53, beta-catenin, and alpha-fetoprotein expression in human hepatocellular carcinoma. *Am J Clin Pathol.* 2004;122(3):377–382.
116. Butler SL, Dong H, Cardona D, et al. The antigen for Hep Par 1 antibody is the urea cycle enzyme carbamoyl phosphate synthetase 1. *Lab Invest.* 2008;88(1):78–88.
117. Wennerberg AE, Nalesnik MA, Coleman WB. Hepatocyte paraffin 1: a monoclonal antibody that reacts with hepatocytes and can be used for

differential diagnosis of hepatic tumors. *Am J Pathol.* 1993;143(4):1050–1054.

118. Chan ES, Yeh MM. The use of immunohistochemistry in liver tumors. *Clin Liver Dis.* 2010;14(4):687–703.
119. Fan Z, van de Rijn M, Montgomery K, et al. Hep par 1 antibody stain for the differential diagnosis of hepatocellular carcinoma: 676 tumors tested using tissue microarrays and conventional tissue sections. *Mod Pathol.* 2003;16(2):137–144.
120. Abdul-Al HM, Makhlouf HR, Wang G, et al. Glypican-3 expression in benign liver tissue with active hepatitis C: implications for the diagnosis of hepatocellular carcinoma. *Hum Pathol.* 2008;39(2):209–212.
121. Mounajjed T, Zhang L, Wu TT. Glypican-3 expression in gastrointestinal and pancreatic epithelial neoplasms. *Hum Pathol.* 2013;44(4):542–550.
122. Shafizadeh N, Ferrell LD, Kakar S. Utility and limitations of glypican-3 expression for the diagnosis of hepatocellular carcinoma at both ends of the differentiation spectrum. *Mod Pathol.* 2008;21(8):1011–1018.
123. Yan BC, Gong C, Song J, et al. Arginase-1: a new immunohistochemical marker of hepatocytes and hepatocellular neoplasms. *Am J Surg Pathol.* 2010;34(8):1147–1154.
124. Radwan NA, Ahmed NS. The diagnostic value of arginase-1 immunostaining in differentiating hepatocellular carcinoma from metastatic carcinoma and cholangiocarcinoma as compared to HepPar-1. *Diagn Pathol.* 2012;7:149.
125. Fujiwara M, Kwok S, Yano H, et al. Arginase-1 is a more sensitive marker of hepatic differentiation than HepPar-1 and glypican-3 in fine-needle aspiration biopsies. *Cancer Cytopathol.* 2012;120(4):230–237.
126. Geramizadeh B, Seirfar N. Diagnostic value of arginase-1 and glypican-3 in differential diagnosis of hepatocellular carcinoma, cholangiocarcinoma and metastatic carcinoma of liver. *Hepat Mon.* 2015;15(7):e30336.
127. Chandan VS, Shah SS, Torbenson MS, et al. Arginase-1 is frequently positive in hepatoid adenocarcinomas. *Hum Pathol.* 2016;55:11–16.
128. Terris B, Hergli I, Lin-Marq N, et al. Letter to the editor with regard to the article entitled: "branched chain in situ hybridization for albumin as a marker of hepatocellular differentiation". *Am J Surg Pathol.* 2015;39(8):1156–1157.
129. Askan G, Deshpande V, Klimstra DS, et al. Expression of markers of hepatocellular differentiation in pancreatic acinar cell neoplasms: a potential diagnostic pitfall. *Am J Clin Pathol.* 2016;146(2):163–169.
130. Ferrone CR, Ting DT, Shahid M, et al. The ability to diagnose intrahepatic cholangiocarcinoma definitively using novel branched DNA-enhanced albumin RNA in situ hybridization technology. *Ann Surg Oncol.* 2016;23(1):290–296.
131. Graham RP, Jin L, Knutson DL, et al. DNAJB1-PRKACA is specific for fibrolamellar carcinoma. *Mod Pathol.* 2015.
132. Bedossa P, Burt AD, Brunt EM, et al. Well-differentiated hepatocellular neoplasm of uncertain malignant potential: proposal for a new diagnostic category. *Hum Pathol.* 2014;45(3):658–660.
133. Wood LD, Heaphy CM, Daniel HD, et al. Chromophobe hepatocellular carcinoma with abrupt anaplasia: a proposal for a new subtype of hepatocellular carcinoma with unique morphological and molecular features. *Mod Pathol.* 2013;26(12):1586–1593.
134. Lu J, Zhang J, Xiong XZ, et al. Primary hepatic sarcomatoid carcinoma: clinical features and prognosis of 28 resected cases. *J Cancer Res Clin Oncol.* 2014;140(6):1027–1035.
135. Goto H, Tanaka A, Kondo F, et al. Carcinosarcoma of the liver. *Intern Med.* 2010;49(23):2577–2582.
136. Lao XM, Chen DY, Zhang YQ, et al. Primary carcinosarcoma of the liver: clinicopathologic features of 5 cases and a review of the literature. *Am J Surg Pathol.* 2007;31(6):817–826.
137. Aita K, Seki K. Carcinosarcoma of the liver producing granulocyte-colony stimulating factor. *Pathol Int.* 2006;56(7):413–419.
138. Xiang S, Chen YF, Guan Y, et al. Primary combined hepatocellular-cholangiocellular sarcoma: an unusual case. *World J Gastroenterol.* 2015;21(23):7335–7342.
139. Luchini C, Capelli P, Fassan M, et al. Next-generation histopathologic diagnosis: a lesson from a hepatic carcinosarcoma. *J Clin Oncol.* 2014;32(17):e63–66.
140. Dioscoridi L, Bisogni D, Freschi G. Hepatocellular carcinoma with osteoclast-like giant cells: report of the seventh case in the literature. *Case Rep Surg.* 2015;2015:836105.
141. Lee KB. Sarcomatoid hepatocellular carcinoma with mixed osteoclast-like giant cells and chondroid differentiation. *Clin Mol Hepatol.* 2014;20(3):313–316.
142. Kuwano H, Sonoda T, Hashimoto H, et al. Hepatocellular carcinoma with osteoclast-like giant cells. *Cancer.* 1984;54(5):837–842.
143. Hood DL, Bauer TW, Leibel SA, et al. Hepatic giant cell carcinoma. An ultrastructural and immunohistochemical study. *Am J Clin Pathol.* 1990;93(1):111–116.

144. Sasaki A, Yokoyama S, Nakayama I, et al. Sarcomatoid hepatocellular carcinoma with osteoclast-like giant cells: case report and immunohistochemical observations. *Pathol Int.* 1997;47(5):318–324.
145. Tanahashi C, Nagae H, Nukaya T, et al. Combined hepatocellular carcinoma and osteoclast-like giant cell tumor of the liver: possible clue to histogenesis. *Pathol Int.* 2009;59(11):813–816.
146. Dahm HH. Immunohistochemical evaluation of a sarcomatoid hepatocellular carcinoma with osteoclastlike giant cells. *Diagn Pathol.* 2015;10:40.
147. Ikeda T, Seki S, Maki M, et al. Hepatocellular carcinoma with osteoclast-like giant cells: possibility of osteoclastogenesis by hepatocyte-derived cells. *Pathol Int.* 2003;53(7):450–456.
148. Yuki K, Hirohashi S, Sakamoto M, et al. Growth and spread of hepatocellular carcinoma. A review of 240 consecutive autopsy cases. *Cancer.* 1990;66(10):2174–2179.
149. Kanematsu M, Semelka RC, Leonardou P, et al. Hepatocellular carcinoma of diffuse type: MR imaging findings and clinical manifestations. *J Magn Reson Imaging.* 2003;18(2):189–195.
150. Okuda K, Noguchi T, Kubo Y, et al. A clinical and pathological study of diffuse type hepatocellular carcinoma. *Liver.* 1981;1(4):280–289.
151. Han YS, Choi DL, Park JB. Cirrhotomimetic type hepatocellular carcinoma diagnosed after liver transplantation--eighteen months of follow-up: a case report. *Transplant Proc.* 2008;40(8): 2835–2836.
152. Clayton EF, Malik S, Bonnel A, et al. Liver transplantation and cirrhotomimetic hepatocellular carcinoma: classification and outcomes. *Liver Transpl.* 2014;20(7):765–774.
153. Myung SJ, Yoon JH, Kim KM, et al. Diffuse infiltrative hepatocellular carcinomas in a hepatitis B-endemic area: diagnostic and therapeutic impediments. *Hepatogastroenterology.* 2006;53(68):266–270.
154. Emile JF, Lemoine A, Azoulay D, et al. Histological, genomic and clinical heterogeneity of clear cell hepatocellular carcinoma. *Histopathology.* 2001;38(3):225–231.
155. Liu Z, Ma W, Li H, et al. Clinicopathological and prognostic features of primary clear cell carcinoma of the liver. *Hepatol Res.* 2008;38(3):291–299.
156. Li T, Fan J, Qin LX, et al. Risk factors, prognosis, and management of early and late intrahepatic recurrence after resection of primary clear cell carcinoma of the liver. *Ann Surg Oncol.* 2011;18(7):1955–1963.
157. Xu W, Ge P, Liao W, et al. Edmondson grade predicts survival of patients with primary clear cell carcinoma of liver after curative resection: a retrospective study with long-term follow-up. *Asia Pac J Clin Oncol.* 2016. doi:10.1111/ajco.12494.
158. Yang SH, Watanabe J, Nakashima O, et al. Clinicopathologic study on clear cell hepatocellular carcinoma. *Pathol Int.* 1996;46(7):503–509.
159. Buchanan TF, Jr, Huvos AG. Clear-cell carcinoma of the liver. A clinicopathologic study of 13 patients. *Am J Clin Pathol.* 1974;61(4):529–539.
160. Murakata LA, Ishak KG, Nzeako UC. Clear cell carcinoma of the liver: a comparative immunohistochemical study with renal clear cell carcinoma. *Mod Pathol.* 2000;13(8):874–881.
161. Noro T, Gotohda N, Kojima M, et al. Hepatocellular carcinoma with foamy histiocyte-like appearance: a deceptively clear cell carcinoma appearing variant. *Case Rep Gastroenterol.* 2010;4(2):286–292.
162. Orikasa H, Ohyama R, Tsuka N, et al. Lipid-rich clear-cell hepatocellular carcinoma arising in non-alcoholic steatohepatitis in a patient with diabetes mellitus. *J Submicrosc Cytol Pathol.* 2001;33(1–2):195–200.
163. Garancini M, Goffredo P, Pagni F, et al. Combined hepatocellular-cholangiocarcinoma: a population-level analysis of an uncommon primary liver tumor. *Liver Transpl.* 2014;20(8):952–959.
164. Chu KJ, Lu CD, Dong H, et al. Hepatitis B virus-related combined hepatocellular-cholangiocarcinoma: clinicopathological and prognostic analysis of 390 cases. *Eur J Gastroenterol Hepatol.* 2014;26(2):192–199.
165. Groeschl RT, Turaga KK, Gamblin TC. Transplantation versus resection for patients with combined hepatocellular carcinoma-cholangiocarcinoma. *J Surg Oncol.* 2013;107(6):608–612.
166. Wang J, Wang F, Kessinger A. Outcome of combined hepatocellular and cholangiocarcinoma of the liver. *J Oncol.* 2010;2010.
167. Li R, Yang D, Tang CL, et al. Combined hepatocellular carcinoma and cholangiocarcinoma (biphenotypic) tumors: clinical characteristics, imaging features of contrast-enhanced ultrasound and computed tomography. *BMC Cancer.* 2016;16(1):158.
168. Kim KH, Lee SG, Park EH, et al. Surgical treatments and prognoses of patients with combined hepatocellular carcinoma and cholangiocarcinoma. *Ann Surg Oncol.* 2009;16(3):623–629.
169. Yin X, Zhang BH, Qiu SJ, et al. Combined hepatocellular carcinoma and cholangiocarcinoma: clinical features, treatment modalities, and prognosis. *Ann Surg Oncol.* 2012;19(9):2869–2876.
170. Kim SH, Park YN, Lim JH, et al. Characteristics of combined hepatocelluar-cholangiocarcinoma and comparison with intrahepatic cholangiocarcinoma. *Eur J Surg Oncol.* 2014;40(8):976–981.

171. Song S, Moon HH, Lee S, et al. Comparison between resection and transplantation in combined hepatocellular and cholangiocarcinoma. *Transplant Proc*. 2013;45(8):3041–3046.
172. Yap AQ, Chen CL, Yong CC, et al. Clinicopathological factors impact the survival outcome following the resection of combined hepatocellular carcinoma and cholangiocarcinoma. *Surg Oncol*. 2013;22(1):55–60.
173. Yeh MM. Pathology of combined hepatocellular-cholangiocarcinoma. *J Gastroenterol Hepatol*. 2010;25(9):1485–1492.
174. Lee JH, Chung GE, Yu SJ, et al. Long-term prognosis of combined hepatocellular and cholangiocarcinoma after curative resection comparison with hepatocellular carcinoma and cholangiocarcinoma. *J Clin Gastroenterol*. 2011;45(1):69–75.
175. Park YH, Hwang S, Ahn CS, et al. Long-term outcome of liver transplantation for combined hepatocellular carcinoma and cholangiocarcinoma. *Transplant Proc*. 2013;45(8):3038–3040.
176. Cao J, Huang L, Liu C, et al. Double primary hepatic cancer (hepatocellular carcinoma and intrahepatic cholangiocarcinoma) in a single patient: a clinicopathologic study of 35 resected cases. *J Gastroenterol Hepatol*. 2013;28(6):1025–1031.
177. Bosman F, Carneiro F, Hruban RH, et al. *WHO Classification of Tumors of the Digestive System*. Lyon: IARC; 2010.
178. Yoon YI, Hwang S, Lee YJ, et al. Postresection outcomes of combined hepatocellular carcinoma-cholangiocarcinoma, hepatocellular carcinoma and intrahepatic cholangiocarcinoma. *J Gastrointest Surg*. 2016;20(2):411–420.
179. Yang CS, Wen MC, Jan YJ, et al. Combined primary neuroendocrine carcinoma and hepatocellular carcinoma of the liver. *J Chin Med Assoc*. 2009;72(8):430–433.
180. Yamaguchi R, Nakashima O, Ogata T, et al. Hepatocellular carcinoma with an unusual neuroendocrine component. *Pathol Int*. 2004;54(11):861–865.
181. Nakanishi C, Sato K, Ito Y, et al. Combined hepatocellular carcinoma and neuroendocrine carcinoma with sarcomatous change of the liver after transarterial chemoembolization. *Hepatol Res*. 2012;42(11):1141–1145.
182. Niederle IM, Wörns MA, Koch S, et al. Clinicopathologic features and prognosis of young patients with hepatocellular carcinoma in a large German cohort. *J Clin Gastroenterol*. 2012;46(9):775–778.
183. Eggert T, McGlynn KA, Duffy A, et al. Fibrolamellar hepatocellular carcinoma in the USA, 2000-2010: a detailed report on frequency, treatment and outcome based on the Surveillance, Epidemiology, and End Results database. *United European Gastroenterol J*. 2013;1(5):351–357.
184. Kaczynski J, Gustavsson B, Hansson G, et al. Fibrolamellar hepatic carcinoma in an area with a low incidence of primary liver cancer: a retrospective study. *Eur J Surg*. 1996;162(5):367–371.
185. El-Serag HB, Davila JA. Is fibrolamellar carcinoma different from hepatocellular carcinoma? A US population-based study. *Hepatology*. 2004;39(3):798–803.
186. Ang CS, Kelley RK, Choti MA, et al. Clinicopathologic characteristics and survival outcomes of patients with fibrolamellar carcinoma: data from the fibrolamellar carcinoma consortium. *Gastrointest Cancer Res*. 2013;6(1):3–9.
187. Torbenson M. Fibrolamellar carcinoma: 2012 update. *Scientifica*. 2012;2012:15.
188. Farhi DC, Shikes RH, Murari PJ, et al. Hepatocellular carcinoma in young people. *Cancer*. 1983;52(8):1516–1525.
189. Katzenstein HM, Krailo MD, Malogolowkin MH, et al. Fibrolamellar hepatocellular carcinoma in children and adolescents. *Cancer*. 2003;97(8):2006–2012.
190. Allan BJ, Wang B, Davis JS, et al. A review of 218 pediatric cases of hepatocellular carcinoma. *J Pediatr Surg*. 2014;49(1):166–171; discussion 171.
191. Maniaci V, Davidson BR, Rolles K, et al. Fibrolamellar hepatocellular carcinoma: prolonged survival with multimodality therapy. *Eur J Surg Oncol*. 2009;35(6):617–621.
192. Darcy DG, Malek MM, Kobos R, et al. Prognostic factors in fibrolamellar hepatocellular carcinoma in young people. *J Pediatr Surg*. 2015;50(1):153–156.
193. Meriggi F, Forni E. Surgical therapy of hepatic fibrolamellar carcinoma. *Ann Ital Chir*. 2007;78(1):53–58.
194. Lildballe DL, Nguyen KQ, Poulsen SS, et al. Haptocorrin as marker of disease progression in fibrolamellar hepatocellular carcinoma. *Eur J Surg Oncol*. 2011;37(1):72–79.
195. Wheeler K, Pritchard J, Luck W, et al. Transcobalamin I as a "marker" for fibrolamellar hepatoma. *Med Pediatr Oncol*. 1986;14(4):227–229.
196. Soreide O, Czerniak A, Bradpiece H, et al. Characteristics of fibrolamellar hepatocellular carcinoma. A study of nine cases and a review of the literature. *Am J Surg*. 1986;151(4):518–523.
197. Herman P, Chagas AL, Perini MV, et al. Surgical treatment of fibrolamellar hepatocellular carcinoma: an underestimated malignant tumor? *Hepatobiliary Pancreat Dis Int*. 2014;13(6):618–621.
198. Pinna AD, Iwatsuki S, Lee RG, et al. Treatment of fibrolamellar hepatoma with subtotal hepatectomy or transplantation. *Hepatology*. 1997;26(4):877–883.

199. Goodman ZD, Ishak KG, Langloss JM, et al. Combined hepatocellular-cholangiocarcinoma. A histologic and immunohistochemical study. *Cancer*. 1985;55(1):124–135.
200. LeBrun DP, Silver MM, Freedman MH, et al. Fibrolamellar carcinoma of the liver in a patient with Fanconi anemia. *Hum Pathol*. 1991;22(4):396–398.
201. Terracciano LM, Tornillo L, Avoledo P, et al. Fibrolamellar hepatocellular carcinoma occurring 5 years after hepatocellular adenoma in a 14-year-old girl: a case report with comparative genomic hybridization analysis. *Arch Pathol Lab Med*. 2004;128(2):222–226.
202. Graham RP, Terracciano LM, Meves A, et al. Hepatic adenomas with synchronous or metachronous fibrolamellar carcinomas: both are characterized by LFABP loss. *Mod Pathol*. 2016;29(6):607–615.
203. Seitz G, Zimmermann A, Friess H, et al. Adult-type hepatocellular carcinoma in the center of a fibrolamellar hepatocellular carcinoma. *Hum Pathol*. 2002;33(7):765–769.
204. Ward SC, Huang J, Tickoo SK, et al. Fibrolamellar carcinoma of the liver exhibits immunohistochemical evidence of both hepatocyte and bile duct differentiation. *Mod Pathol*. 2010;23(9):1180–1190.
205. Kakar S, Burgart LJ, Batts KP, et al. Clinicopathologic features and survival in fibrolamellar carcinoma: comparison with conventional hepatocellular carcinoma with and without cirrhosis. *Mod Pathol*. 2005;18(11):1417–1423.
206. Honeyman JN, Simon EP, Robine N, et al. Detection of a recurrent DNAJB1-PRKACA chimeric transcript in fibrolamellar hepatocellular carcinoma. *Science*. 2014;343(6174):1010–1014.
207. Kaseb AO, Shama M, Sahin IH, et al. Prognostic indicators and treatment outcome in 94 cases of fibrolamellar hepatocellular carcinoma. *Oncology*. 2013;85(4):197–203.
208. Stipa F, Yoon SS, Liau KH, et al. Outcome of patients with fibrolamellar hepatocellular carcinoma. *Cancer*. 2006;106(6):1331–1338.
209. Njei B, Konjeti VR, Ditah I. Prognosis of patients with fibrolamellar hepatocellular carcinoma versus conventional hepatocellular carcinoma: a systematic review and meta-analysis. *Gastrointest Cancer Res*. 2014;7(2):49–54.
210. Houben KW, McCall JL. Liver transplantation for hepatocellular carcinoma in patients without underlying liver disease: a systematic review. *Liver Transpl Surg*. 1999;5(2):91–95.
211. Mayo SC, Mavros MN, Nathan H, et al. Treatment and prognosis of patients with fibrolamellar hepatocellular carcinoma: a national perspective. *J Am Coll Surg*. 2014;218(2):196–205.
212. Groeschl RT, Miura JT, Wong RK, et al. Multi-institutional analysis of recurrence and survival after hepatectomy for fibrolamellar carcinoma. *J Surg Oncol*. 2014;110(4): 412–415.
213. Do RK, McErlean A, Ang CS, et al. CT and MRI of primary and metastatic fibrolamellar carcinoma: a case series of 37 patients. *Br J Radiol*. 2014;87(1040):20140024.
214. Kohno M, Shirabe K, Mano Y, et al. Granulocyte colony-stimulating-factor-producing hepatocellular carcinoma with extensive sarcomatous changes: report of a case. *Surg Today*. 2012;43(4):439–445.
215. Amano H, Itamoto T, Emoto K, et al. Granulocyte colony-stimulating factor-producing combined hepatocellular/cholangiocellular carcinoma with sarcomatous change. *J Gastroenterol*. 2005;40(12):1158–1159.
216. Joshita S, Nakazawa K, Koike S, et al. A case of granulocyte-colony stimulating factor-producing hepatocellular carcinoma confirmed by immunohistochemistry. *J Korean Med Sci*. 2010;25(3):476–480.
217. Araki K, Kishihara F, Takahashi K, et al. Hepatocellular carcinoma producing a granulocyte colony-stimulating factor: report of a resected case with a literature review. *Liver Int*. 2007;27(5):716–721.
218. Yamamoto S, Takashima S, Ogawa H, et al. Granulocyte-colony-stimulating-factor-producing hepatocellular carcinoma. *J Gastroenterol*. 1999;34(5):640–644.
219. Snyder RA, Liu E, Merchant NB. Granulocyte colony stimulating factor secreting hepatocellular carcinoma. *Am Surg*. 2012;78(7):821–822.
220. Takenaka M, Akiba J, Kawaguchi T, et al. Intrahepatic cholangiocarcinoma with sarcomatous change producing granulocyte-colony stimulating factor. *Pathol Int*. 2013;63(4):233–235.
221. Shimakawa T, Asaka S, Usuda A, et al. Granulocyte-colony stimulating factor (G-CSF)-producing esophageal squamous cell carcinoma: a case report. *Int Surg*. 2014;99(3):280–285.
222. Wada Y, Nakashima O, Kutami R, et al. Clinicopathological study on hepatocellular carcinoma with lymphocytic infiltration. *Hepatology*. 1998;27(2):407–414.
223. Emile JF, Adam R, Sebagh M, et al. Hepatocellular carcinoma with lymphoid stroma: a tumour with good prognosis after liver transplantation. *Histopathology*. 2000;37(6):523–529.
224. Park HS, Jang KY, Kim YK, et al. Hepatocellular carcinoma with massive lymphoid infiltration: a regressing phenomenon? *Pathol Res Pract*. 2009;205(9):648–652.

225. Chan AW, Tong JH, Pan Y, et al. Lymphoepithelioma-like hepatocellular carcinoma: an uncommon variant of hepatocellular carcinoma with favorable outcome. *Am J Surg Pathol.* 2015;39(3):304–312.
226. Chen CJ, Jeng LB, Huang SF. Lymphoepithelioma-like hepatocellular carcinoma. *Chang Gung Med J.* 2007;30(2):172–177.
227. Patel KR, Liu TC, Vaccharajani N, et al. Characterization of inflammatory (lymphoepithelioma-like) hepatocellular carcinoma: a study of 8 cases. *Arch Pathol Lab Med.* 2014;138(9):1193–1202.
228. Nemolato S, Fanni D, Naccarato AG, et al. Lymphoepitelioma-like hepatocellular carcinoma: a case report and a review of the literature. *World J Gastroenterol.* 2008;14(29):4694–4696.
229. Si MW, Thorson JA, Lauwers GY, et al. Hepatocellular lymphoepithelioma-like carcinoma associated with epstein barr virus: a hitherto unrecognized entity. *Diagn Mol Pathol.* 2004;13(3):183–189.
230. Li W, Wu B-A, Zeng Y-M, et al. Epstein-Barr virus in hepatocellular carcinogenesis. *World J Gastroenterol.* 2004;10(23):3409–3413.
231. Kojiro M, Sugihara S, Kakizoe S, et al. Hepatocellular carcinoma with sarcomatous change: a special reference to the relationship with anticancer therapy. *Cancer Chemother Pharmacol.* 1989;23(suppl):S4–8.
232. Nishi H, Taguchi K, Asayama Y, et al. Sarcomatous hepatocellular carcinoma: a special reference to ordinary hepatocellular carcinoma. *J Gastroenterol Hepatol.* 2003;18(4):415–423.
233. Giunchi F, Vasuri F, Baldin P, et al. Primary liver sarcomatous carcinoma: report of two cases and review of the literature. *Pathol Res Pract.* 2013;209(4):249–254.
234. Wang QB, Cui BK, Weng JM, et al. Clinicopathological characteristics and outcome of primary sarcomatoid carcinoma and carcinosarcoma of the liver. *J Gastrointest Surg.* 2012;16(9):1715–1726.
235. Kakizoe S, Kojiro M, Nakashima T. Hepatocellular carcinoma with sarcomatous change. Clinicopathologic and immunohistochemical studies of 14 autopsy cases. *Cancer.* 1987;59(2):310–316.
236. Oda Y, Katsuda S, Nakanishi I. An autopsy case of hepatic sarcomatoid tumor: immunohistochemical comparison with a sarcomatous component of hepatocellular carcinoma. *Pathol Int.* 1994;44(3):230–236.
237. Matsuura S, Aishima S, Taguchi K, et al. "Scirrhous" type hepatocellular carcinomas: a special reference to expression of cytokeratin 7 and hepatocyte paraffin 1. *Histopathology.* 2005;47(4):382–390.
238. Lee JH, Choi MS, Gwak GY, et al. Clinicopathologic characteristics and long-term prognosis of scirrhous hepatocellular carcinoma. *Dig Dis Sci.* 2012;57(6):1698–1707.
239. Kurogi M, Nakashima O, Miyaaki H, et al. Clinicopathological study of scirrhous hepatocellular carcinoma. *J Gastroenterol Hepatol.* 2006;21(9):1470–1477.
240. Sooklim K, Sriplung H, Piratvisuth T. Histologic subtypes of hepatocellular carcinoma in the southern Thai population. *Asian Pac J Cancer Prev.* 2003;4(4):302–306.
241. Sugiki T, Yamamoto M, Taka K, et al. Specific characteristics of scirrhous hepatocellular carcinoma. *Hepatogastroenterology.* 2009;56(93):1086–1089.
242. Fujii T, Zen Y, Harada K, et al. Participation of liver cancer stem/progenitor cells in tumorigenesis of scirrhous hepatocellular carcinoma--human and cell culture study. *Hum Pathol.* 2008;39(8):1185–1196.
243. Kim GJ, Rhee H, Yoo JE, et al. Increased expression of CCN2, epithelial membrane antigen, and fibroblast activation protein in hepatocellular carcinoma with fibrous stroma showing aggressive behavior. *PLoS One.* 2014;9(8):e105094.
244. Sugiki T, Yamamoto M, Aruga A, et al. Immunohistological evaluation of single small hepatocellular carcinoma with negative staining of monoclonal antibody hepatocyte paraffin 1. *J Surg Oncol.* 2004;88(2):104–107.
245. Krings G, Ramachandran R, Jain D, et al. Immunohistochemical pitfalls and the importance of glypican 3 and arginase in the diagnosis of scirrhous hepatocellular carcinoma. *Mod Pathol.* 2013;26(6):782–791.
246. Limaiem F, Bouraoui S, Sboui M, et al. Fibrolamellar carcinoma versus scirrhous hepatocellular carcinoma: diagnostic usefulness of CD68. *Acta Gastroenterol.* 2015;78(4):393–398.
247. Ross HM, Daniel HD, Vivekanandan P, et al. Fibrolamellar carcinomas are positive for CD68. *Mod Pathol.* 2011;24(3):390–395.
248. Salomao M, Remotti H, Vaughan R, et al. The steatohepatitic variant of hepatocellular carcinoma and its association with underlying steatohepatitis. *Hum Pathol.* 2012;43(5):737–746.
249. Shibahara J, Ando S, Sakamoto Y, et al. Hepatocellular carcinoma with steatohepatitic features: a clinicopathological study of Japanese patients. *Histopathology.* 2014;64(7):951–962.
250. Jain D, Nayak NC, Kumaran V, et al. Steatohepatitic hepatocellular carcinoma, a morphologic indicator of associated metabolic risk factors: a study from India. *Arch Pathol Lab Med.* 2013;137(7):961–966.

251. Salomao M, Yu WM, Brown RS Jr, et al. Steatohepatitic hepatocellular carcinoma (SH-HCC): a distinctive histological variant of HCC in hepatitis C virus-related cirrhosis with associated NAFLD/NASH. *Am J Surg Pathol*. 2010;34(11):1630–1636.
252. Yeh MM, Liu Y, Torbenson M. Steatohepatitic variant of hepatocellular carcinoma in the absence of metabolic syndrome or background steatosis: a clinical, pathological, and genetic study. *Hum Pathol*. 2015;46(11):1769–1775.
253. Ando S, Shibahara J, Hayashi A, et al. beta-catenin alteration is rare in hepatocellular carcinoma with steatohepatitic features: immunohistochemical and mutational study. *Virchows Arch*. 2015;467(5):535–542.
254. Deniz K, Moreira RK, Yeh MM, et al. Steatohepatitis-like changes in focal nodular hyperplasia, a finding not to be confused with steatohepatitic variant of hepatocellular carcinoma. *Lab Invest*. 2014;94:418A–419A.
255. Heaphy CM, Subhawong AP, Hong SM, et al. Prevalence of the alternative lengthening of telomeres telomere maintenance mechanism in human cancer subtypes. *Am J Pathol*. 2011;179(4):1608–1615.
256. Mitchell CM, Sturgis CD. Lipid-rich hepatocellular carcinoma in fine-needle aspiration biopsy. *Diagn Cytopathol*. 2009;37(1):36–37.
257. Sugiyama T, Tajiri T, Hiraiwa, S, et al. Hepatic adrenal rest tumor: diagnostic pitfall and proposed algorithms to prevent misdiagnosis as lipid-rich hepatocellular carcinoma. *Pathol Int*. 2015;65(2):95–99.
258. Fukuda T, Ohnishi Y, Miyazaki Y, et al. Clear cell hepatocellular carcinoma with abundant myxoid stroma. *Acta Pathol Jpn*. 1992;42(12):897–903.
259. Salaria SN, Graham RP, Aishima S, et al. Primary hepatic tumors with myxoid change: morphologically unique hepatic adenomas and hepatocellular carcinomas. *Am J Surg Pathol*. 2015;39(3):318–324.
260. Young JT, Kurup AN, Graham RP, et al. Myxoid hepatocellular neoplasms: imaging appearance of a unique mucinous tumor variant. *Abdom Radiol*. 2016;41(11):2115–2122.
261. Atra A, Al-Asiri R, Wali S, et al. Hepatocellular carcinoma, syncytial giant cell: a novel variant in children: a case report. *Ann Diagn Pathol*. 2007;11(1):61–63.
262. Prokurat A, Kluge P, Kościesza A, et al. Transitional liver cell tumors (TLCT) in older children and adolescents: a novel group of aggressive hepatic tumors expressing beta-catenin. *Med Pediatr Oncol*. 2002;39(5):510–518.
263. Yoshida GJ, Fuchimoto Y, Osumi T, et al. Li-Fraumeni syndrome with simultaneous osteosarcoma and liver cancer: increased expression of a CD44 variant isoform after chemotherapy. *BMC Cancer*. 2012;12:444.
264. Lanier AP, Holck P, Ehrsam Day G, et al. Childhood cancer among Alaska Natives. *Pediatrics*. 2003;112(5):e396.
265. Gonzalez-Peralta RP, Langham MR Jr, Andres JM, et al. Hepatocellular carcinoma in 2 young adolescents with chronic hepatitis C. *J Pediatr Gastroenterol Nutr*. 2009;48(5):630–635.
266. van Ginkel WG, Gouw AS, van der Jagt EJ, et al. Hepatocellular carcinoma in tyrosinemia type 1 without clear increase of AFP. *Pediatrics*. 2015;135(3):e749–752.
267. Romano F, Stroppa P, Bravi M, et al. Favorable outcome of primary liver transplantation in children with cirrhosis and hepatocellular carcinoma. *Pediatr Transplant*. 2011;15(6):573–579.
268. Bahador A, Dehghani SM, Geramizadeh B, et al. Liver transplant for children with hepatocellular carcinoma and hereditary tyrosinemia type 1. *Exp Clin Transplant*. 2015;13(4):329–332.
269. Schlune A, Vom Dahl S, Häussinger D, et al. Hyperargininemia due to arginase I deficiency: the original patients and their natural history, and a review of the literature. *Amino Acids*. 2015;47(9):1751–1762.
270. Yu SB, Kim HY, Eo H, et al. Clinical characteristics and prognosis of pediatric hepatocellular carcinoma. *World J Surg*. 2006;30(1):43–50.
271. Vilarinho S, Erson-Omay EZ, Harmanci AS, et al. Paediatric hepatocellular carcinoma due to somatic CTNNB1 and NFE2L2 mutations in the setting of inherited bi-allelic ABCB11 mutations. *J Hepatol*. 2014;61(5):1178–1183.
272. Knisely AS, Strautnieks SS, Meier Y, et al. Hepatocellular carcinoma in ten children under five years of age with bile salt export pump deficiency. *Hepatology*. 2006;44(2):478–486.
273. Vij M, Safwan M, Shanmugam NP, et al. Liver pathology in severe multidrug resistant 3 protein deficiency: a series of 10 pediatric cases. *Ann Diagn Pathol*. 2015.
274. Zhou S, Hertel PM, Finegold MJ, et al. Hepatocellular carcinoma associated with tight-junction protein 2 deficiency. *Hepatology*. 2015.
275. Manzia TM, Angelico R, Toti L, et al. Glycogen storage disease type Ia and VI associated with hepatocellular carcinoma: two case reports. *Transplant Proc*. 2011;43(4):1181–1183.
276. de Moor RA, Schweizer JJ, van Hoek B, et al. Hepatocellular carcinoma in glycogen storage disease type IV. *Arch Dis Child*. 2000;82(6):479–480.
277. Yamada K, Shinmoto H, Kawamura Y, et al. Transarterial embolization for pediatric

hepatocellular carcinoma with cardiac cirrhosis. *Pediatr Int*. 2015;57(4):766–770.

278. Morotti RA, Killackey M, Shneider BL, et al. Hepatocellular carcinoma and congenital absence of the portal vein in a child receiving growth hormone therapy for turner syndrome. *Semin Liver Dis*. 2007;27(4):427–431.
279. Kim JM, Lee S-K, Kwon CHD, et al. Hepatocellular carcinoma in an infant with biliary atresia younger than 1 year. *J Pediatr Surg*. 2012;47(4):819–821.
280. Bhadri VA, Stormon MO, Arbuckle S, et al. Hepatocellular carcinoma in children with Alagille syndrome. *J Pediatr Gastroenterol Nutr*. 2005;41(5):676–678.
281. Patterson K, Kapur SP, Chandra RS. Hepatocellular carcinoma in a noncirrhotic infant after prolonged parenteral nutrition. *J Pediatr*. 1985;106(5):797–800.
282. Zhao X, Wang Z, Cao L, et al. Hyperfibrinogenemia and prolonged clotting times in a Turner syndrome patient with hepatocellular carcinoma. *Blood Coagul Fibrinolysis*. 2010;21(5):398–405.
283. Lack EE, Neave C, Vawter GF. Hepatocellular carcinoma. Review of 32 cases in childhood and adolescence. *Cancer*. 1983;52(8):1510–1515.

29

Benign and malignant biliary tumors

Murli Krishna, MD

29.1 INTRODUCTION

Biliary neoplasms and tumor like lesions form a diverse group of lesions in the liver, and include tumors with characteristics similar to those in the extrahepatic biliary tract, pancreas, and upper gastrointestinal tract. Primary intrahepatic biliary malignancies are far less common than metastases and should be evaluated with awareness of the clinical context, presence or absence of precursor lesions, and morphologic variability. This chapter discusses the clinicopathologic aspects of intrahepatic biliary neoplasms (Table 29.1) and selected non-neoplastic biliary lesions.

29.2 CILIATED HEPATIC FOREGUT CYST

Ciliated hepatic foregut cyst is a rare benign cystic lesion that represents a developmental anomaly. Although rare, the number of reported cases has increased dramatically in the past few decades, presumably reflecting increased detection by imaging.[1] The cyst is usually an incidental finding in adults, but they are also well described in children.[2] They

Table 29.1 Biliary epithelial neoplasms of liver
Bile duct adenoma
Serous microcystic adenoma
Biliary adenofibroma
Biliary intraepithelial neoplasia
Intraductal papillary neoplasm
Mucinous cystic neoplasm
Intrahepatic cholangiocarcinoma
Intraductal papillary neoplasm with invasive carcinoma
Mucinous cystic neoplasm with invasive carcinoma

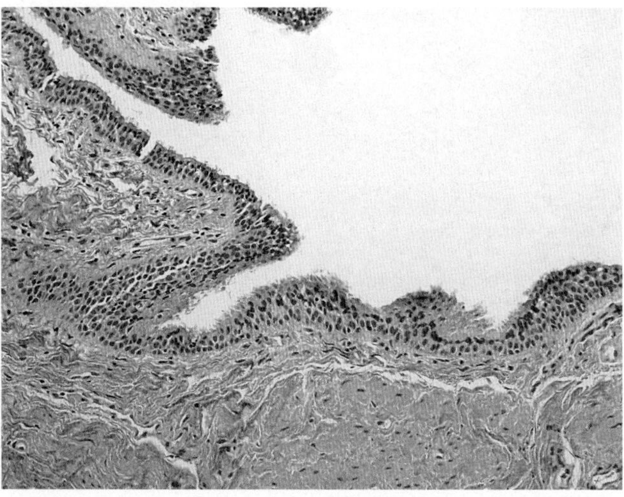

Figure 29.1 Ciliated hepatic foregut cyst, lined by a ciliated and stratified columnar epithelium with smooth muscle and fibrosis in the wall.

are isolated findings that are not associated with other developmental abnormalities. Rarely, there can be elevated serum CA19-9 levels.[3]

Ciliated hepatic foregut cyst usually presents as solitary unilocular lesions with an average size of 7 cm and a range from subcentimeter to 19 cm.[2,3] Most are located in segment IV of the liver.[3] The cyst contains either clear fluid or mucoid material. Biliary communication has been observed in rare cases.[2]

There are two characteristic findings (Fig. 29.1). First, the cyst is lined by a ciliated, pseudostratified columnar epithelium. Second, the wall of the cyst contains smooth muscle that tends to be somewhat ill defined, growing in bundles that surround all or parts of the cyst. There can be one or two layers of smooth muscle, but a myenteric plexus is absent. In addition, there can be a thin layer of connective tissue between the muscle and an outermost later of fibrous tissue. Not all these layers in the cyst wall (smooth muscle, loose connective tissue, fibrous capsule) are seen in every case. The epithelium can occasionally show goblet cells or squamous metaplasia. The cyst fluid may contain high levels of carcinoembryonic antigen (CEA) and CA19-9, with the lining epithelium also staining positive for CEA and CA19-9 on immunohistochemistry.[4]

There is a risk for carcinoma, with about 5% of all cases reported to date having undergone malignant transformation.[5] Squamous cell carcinomas are the most common malignancy.

29.3 SOLITARY BILE DUCT CYST

Solitary bile duct cysts are also known as simple biliary cysts. The cysts are unilocular and lined by a single layer of cuboidal to flattened biliary epithelium. The wall of the cyst is made of fibrous tissue with no muscle or ovarian-type stroma. The etiology of the cyst is unknown, and most are incidental findings in middle-aged women, with about a 10:1 female predominance.

Solitary bile duct cysts are usually single unilocular cysts, although rarely multiple cysts can be seen within the same liver, sometimes in

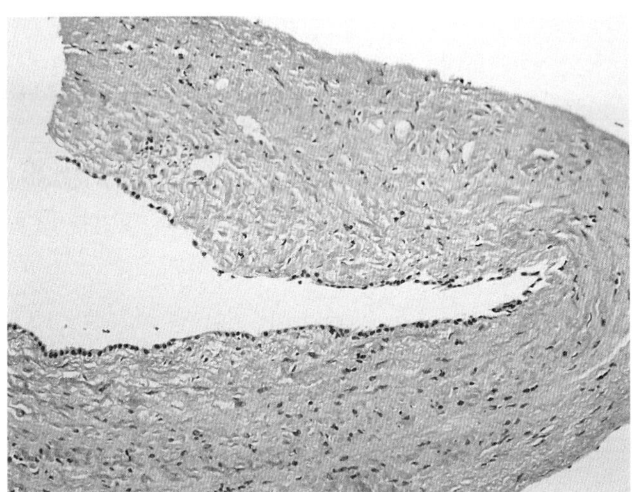

Figure 29.2 Solitary bile duct cyst, lined by a single layer of cuboidal epithelium with fibrotic wall.

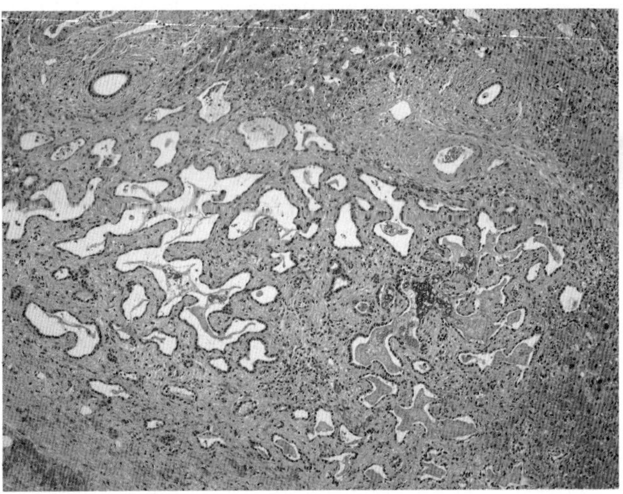

Figure 29.3 Bile duct hamartoma (von Meyenburg complex), showing anastomosing bile duct structures with open lumens, bile plugs, and fibrotic stroma

a small cluster. The cysts are filled with thin, clear to bilious fluid, and may be complicated by hemorrhage. The cyst lining is usually smooth and without septa. If septae are present, they are usually located at the periphery of the cyst.

The epithelial lining in solitary bile duct cysts is cuboidal to flat, resembling biliary epithelium, and often shows extensive denudation (Fig. 29.2). In the areas of epithelial denudation, the cyst wall may show fibrin and mild chronic inflammation. Occasionally, there is more extensive erosion and granulation tissue reaction. In larger cysts, various types of metaplasia may be present such as intestinal, pyloric, or squamous metaplasia.

The diagnosis is usually straightforward, but differential diagnostic considerations may include mucinous cystic neoplasms and mesothelial cysts. Mucinous cystic neoplasms are lined by mucinous epithelium and have ovarian-type stroma in the cyst wall. However, in both of these cysts the diagnostic findings can be obscured by epithelial denudation and inflammation of the cyst wall, so extensive sampling is often needed. In difficult cases, the most helpful stains are for mucin, estrogen receptor, and progesterone receptor, which are positive in mucinous cystic neoplasms but negative in simple biliary cysts. Although mesothelial cyst lining can mimic bile duct cysts on hematoxylin and eosin (H&E), they are usually subcapsular, very small, and stain for markers of mesothelial differentiation, such as calretinin.

29.4 BILE DUCT HAMARTOMA

Bile duct hamartomas are also called *von Meyenburg complexes* and are small benign lesions composed of interanastomosing bile ducts.

Despite being designated as a hamartoma, most sporadic cases are acquired lesions. Overall, bile duct hamartomas are more commonly found in cirrhotic livers than in noncirrhotic livers. Within cirrhotic livers, they are most commonly seen in cases of chronic hepatitis C and alcohol-related liver disease. The malignant potential of these lesions is very low, but there have been reports of cholangiocarcinomas that arose from or adjacent to von Meyenburg complexes.[6]

Bile duct hamartomas are most commonly encountered by surgeons while doing abdominal surgery for cancers of other organs. In this setting, biopsies are often submitted for frozen section to rule out metastatic disease. The diagnosis in most cases is readily made because of the lack of cytological atypia and the distinctive histological findings, as discussed below.

Bile duct hamartomas can be single or multiple, and most and usually measure less than 1 cm in size. Histologically, they are composed of bile duct structures that grow in an irregular inter-anastomosing fashion. The duct structures have open lumens, often contain bile, and are associated with either a myxoid or fibrotic stroma (Fig. 29.3). Bile duct hamartomas are distinct from bile duct adenomas, although the distinction is mostly academic, with relatively modest clinical relevance. Bile duct adenomas tend to have small, round, gland-like, or tubular structures, with small to absent lumens, and no luminal bile.

29.5 BILE DUCT ADENOMA

Bile duct adenoma is a benign lesion that is composed of small compactly arranged ducts within a fibrous stroma. It is often an incidental lesion, but can be clinically significant because it may grossly resemble

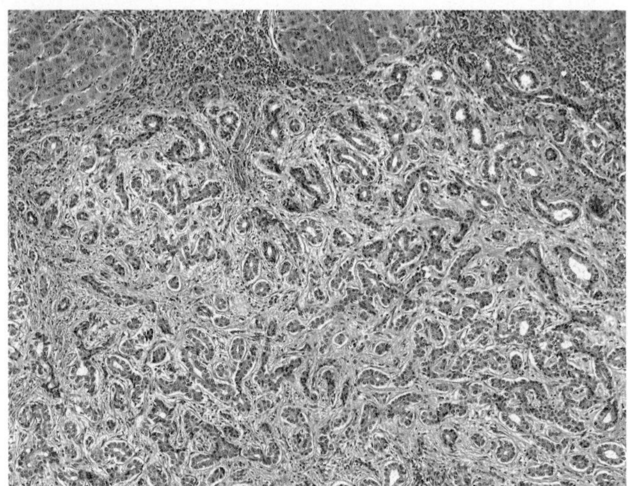

Figure 29.4 Bile duct adenoma. The lesion is well circumscribed, and the proliferating ducts lack cytologic atypia.

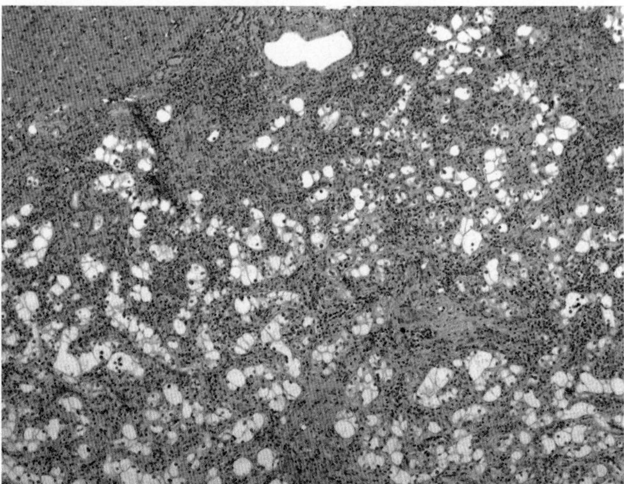

Figure 29.5 Clear cell bile duct adenoma. Small nests of bland clear cells without recognizable lumens.

a metastasis. In this setting, bile duct adenomas are often submitted intraoperatively for frozen section evaluation.

Most bile duct adenomas are diagnosed in middle-aged patients, with men slightly more often affected than women. Grossly, bile duct adenomas are well circumscribed, firm, white lesions that are commonly seen in a subcapsular location. Most measure less than 1 cm in size. Histologically, the proliferating ducts are small and form tubules, embedded in a variably desmoplastic stroma.[8] The ducts are lined by a single layer of cuboidal epithelial cells that lack atypia (Fig. 29.4). The well-delineated margin and absence of atypia distinguishes this lesion from carcinoma. Bile duct adenomas have also been called *peribiliary gland hamartomas* in the past, implying that it is a nonneoplastic lesion. However, the distinctive morphological features are now considered to represent a neoplastic proliferation. In addition, a recent study found *BRAF* V600E mutations in 53% of these lesions, further indicating that these are true neoplasms.[9] A common differential diagnostic consideration for the bile duct adenoma is the bile duct hamartoma. The latter is usually smaller, associated with portal tracts and characterized by the presence of dilated inter-anastamosing ducts; the duct lumens often contain bile or proteinaceous debris. Similar to bile duct hamartomas bile duct adenomas have a very low proliferative rate of about 2% on Ki-67 immunostaining.[7]

29.6 CLEAR CELL BILE DUCT ADENOMA

Clear cell bile duct adenoma is a rare but distinctive subtype of bile duct adenoma.[10] They are generally small, usually about 1 cm, though a larger example of about 3 cm has also been reported.[11] The cells grow in small nests and cords, often with no visible lumen (Fig 29.5). There can be mild nuclear atypia. Clear cell bile duct adenomas are often less well circumscribed than typical bile duct adenomas and often show extension into the adjacent hepatic parenchyma. In some cases, preexisting bile ducts in portal tracts appear to be colonized by the lesional cells. Mild chronic inflammation can also be found in the lesion, even if not present in the background liver. Although data is limited by the rarity of these tumors, clear cell bile duct adenomas have a low proliferative rate by Ki-67 immunostain.

The differential diagnoses include clear cell carcinomas, including clear cell cholangiocarcinoma, clear cell hepatocellular carcinoma, and metastatic clear cell carcinoma. Clear cell bile duct adenomas stain with typical biliary markers, whereas markers of hepatic differentiation are negative. In contrast to clear cell cholangiocarcinomas, only mild cytological atypia is present and the proliferative rate is low. Clear cell bile duct adenomas can be positive for p53,[10] and this finding should not be interpreted in isolation as evidence for malignancy. Metastatic clear cell carcinomas typically are larger, show more atypia, and often show necrosis. Clinical context and immunohistochemical findings are important in excluding metastatic clear cell carcinomas.

29.7 BILIARY ADENOFIBROMA

Biliary adenofibromas are rare neoplasms with some similarities to bile duct hamartomas but are larger, often show epithelial atypia, and can be associated with frank carcinoma.[12–15] Histologically, these lesions are characterized by a tubulocystic biliary epithelial proliferation with prominent fibrotic stroma (Fig. 29.6).

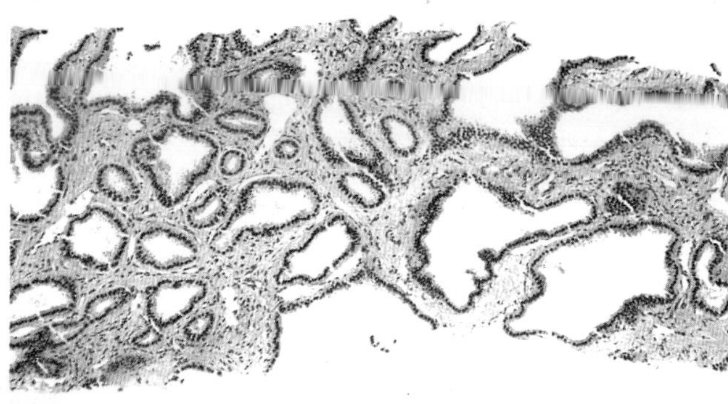

Figure 29.6 Biliary adenofibroma. Tubulocystic structures lined by bland biliary epithelium within fibrotic stroma.

There is no mucin production and the epithelium stains like typical biliary epithelium. Relatively few cases have been reported in literature, and the clinicopathologic characteristics are not well defined. Although some cases can be indolent, there is a clear association with malignancy. Complete excision with follow-up is recommended.

29.8 SEROUS MICROCYSTIC ADENOMA

The serous microcystic adenoma is an exceedingly rare benign multiloculated cystic tumor of the liver. Histologically, it resembles its pancreatic counterpart, where it is more common. The locules are lined by a single layer of bland cuboidal epithelial cells with clear cytoplasm containing glycogen. They do not contain the ovarian-type stroma characteristic of mucinous cystic neoplasm[16] (Fig. 29.7). Serous microcystic adenomas have a benign course. The differential diagnoses include other clear cell lesions such as metastatic renal cell carcinoma with cystic features. Rare histologically bland appearing serous cystadenocarcinomas of the pancreas can metastasize to the liver, so correlation with imaging studies of the pancreas is important.

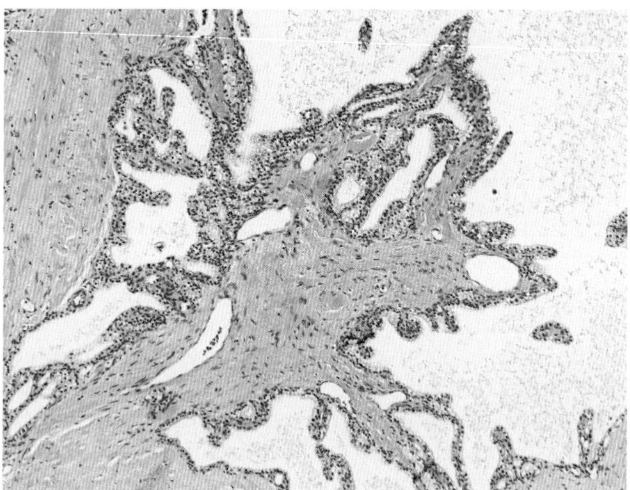

Figure 29.7 Serous microcystic adenoma. The locules are lined by low cuboidal epithelium with clear cytoplasm.

29.9 MUCINOUS CYSTIC NEOPLASM

Definition and etiology

Mucinous cystic neoplasm is a rare cystic neoplasm composed of variably mucinous epithelium associated with ovarian-type stroma, occurring almost exclusively in women. They occur mostly in the liver, with very rare cases reported in the extrahepatic biliary ducts and gallbladder. The etiology of these tumors is not known; however, an origin from peribiliary glands and underlying hormonal factors have been suggested in its pathogenesis.[17]

Epidemiology and clinical features

Mucinous cystic neoplasms are rare, accounting for less than 5% of cystic lesions of the liver, and these are seen almost exclusively in women. Benign mucinous cystic neoplasms usually present in the fifth decade, whereas mucinous cystic neoplasms associated with invasive carcinoma tend to present about a decade older. The most common symptoms include abdominal fullness and discomfort because of the mass, symptoms of biliary obstruction, ascending cholangitis, or even cyst rupture. Rarely, these tumors are discovered as an incidental radiographic finding.[17]

Serum CA19-9 can be elevated, especially if there is associated carcinoma; however, this marker does not reliably distinguish between benign and malignant tumors. Imaging studies reveal a multiloculated cyst with internal septations. Malignancy can be suggested by mural nodules or by irregular cyst wall thickening. The presence of multiloculation contrasts with simple biliary hepatic cysts, which are much more common than mucinous cystic neoplasms.[16–18]

Gross findings

Grossly the lesions are typically multiseptated cysts filled with variably mucoid or hemorrhagic fluid. There is no communication between the mucinous cystic neoplasms and the bile ducts. Mural nodules or papillary areas are uncommon, but these should be generously sampled for microscopic examination to evaluate for malignancy. These tumors can grow large, with reports of tumors approaching 30 cm. Approximately, two-thirds of tumors are within the left lobe.[19,20]

Microscopic findings

The cells lining the cyst wall and locules range from columnar mucinous cells to low cuboidal cells without mucin, resembling biliary epithelium. Intestinal-type goblet cells may be present. In most cases, the cytologic atypia is minimal to absent. The defining histologic feature is the presence of ovarian-type stroma underlying the epithelium (Fig. 29.8). The lining epithelium is immunoreactive for CK7 and CK19 in cases with a biliary phenotype, and CK20 and CDX2 in cases with an intestinal phenotype. The stroma is commonly immunoreactive for estrogen and progesterone receptors, and variably for inhibin. Although immunostaining is not necessary for diagnosis when the ovarian-type stroma is obvious, in many cases the stroma is fibrotic, attenuated, or equivocal, and immunohistochemistry is beneficial.[20] Secondary changes may be present, such as hemorrhage and granulation tissue reaction, and the subepithelial stroma may contain areas of dense collagen.

Practically, as is true for grading intraductal papillary mucinous neoplasms and biliaryintraepithelial neoplasia, classifying dysplasia in mucinous cystic neoplasms into low- and high-grade dysplasia is more reproducible for pathologists and clinically more useful. Some authors also recognize a category of moderate dysplasia; however, this terminology is currently not used in the World Health Organization (WHO) classification.[19] Invasive adenocarcinoma arising in mucinous cystic neoplasms usually has tubular or tubulopapillary morphology. The role of fine-needle aspiration cytology for diagnosing mucinous cystic neoplasms is limited because of scant cellular yield and the risk of pleural and peritoneal dissemination.

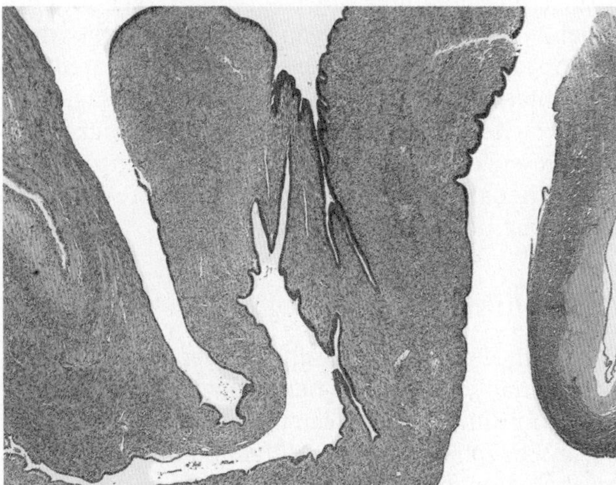

Figure 29.8 Mucinous cystic neoplasm, characterized by mucinous lining epithelium and ovarian-type stroma. Foci of stromal hyalinization are present.

Intraoperative frozen section analysis is often used to distinguish between nonneoplastic and neoplastic cystic masses, with the aim of complete resection for neoplasms. Cystic lesions often show extensive degenerative changes including denudation of the epithelium, making this distinction difficult. In such cases, the presence of ovarian-type stroma indicates a mucinous cystic neoplasm.

Differential diagnosis

The most common differential diagnostic considerations are other cystic lesions of the liver and include intraductal papillary neoplasms, bile duct cysts, ciliated foregut cysts, peribiliary cysts and cystic endometriosis. An important distinction with these lesions is the presence of ovarian-type stroma in mucinous cystic neoplasms. Additionally, intraductal papillary neoplasms generally show a greater degree of papillary epithelial proliferation. Bile duct cysts show simple cuboidal epithelial lining. Ciliated foregut cysts are lined by ciliated epithelium and often have smooth muscle in their wall. Peribiliary cysts are small cysts, usually multifocal, located in the perihilar region closely associated with large bile ducts and lined by cuboidal epithelium.

Endometriosis shows hemorrhagic material in the lumen instead of mucin. Histologically, endometriosis shows cysts lined by glandular epithelium with underlying endometrial stroma, which tends to be less densely cellular than the ovarian stroma of mucinous cystic neoplasms. Hemorrhage can be seen along with numerous hemosiderin-laden macrophages. The endometrial epithelium can be flattened to pseudostratified, but is non-mucinous. The stroma in endometriosis is positive for CD10, whereas both the epithelium and stroma are positive for estrogen and progesterone receptors. In contrast, the epithelium of mucinous cystic neoplasms is negative for estrogen and progesterone receptors.

Treatment and prognosis

Complete surgical resection of mucinous cystic neoplasms is the optimal treatment. Tumor recurrence is common in patients with subtotal resection.[16] Malignant transformation in untreated cases is estimated to occur in up to 32% of cases. Prognosis after complete resection is excellent in the absence of carcinoma. Cystadenocarcinomas arising from mucinous cystic neoplasms appear to have a better prognosis than pure cholangiocarcinomas, emphasizing the importance of this distinction.[19,21–23]

29.10 INTRADUCTAL BILIARY LESIONS

Definitions

Two types of biliary intraductal lesions are recognized as precursor lesions for adenocarcinomas of the biliary tree: (1) biliary intraepithelial neoplasia (BilIN), a flat or micropapillary lesion that is seen only microscopically, and (2) intraductal papillary neoplasms, a radiographically and grossly recognizable lesion.[24,25] The predisposing risk factors for both lesions are similar to those for cholangiocarcinoma.

Biliary intraepithelial neoplasia

BilINs are characterized by dysplastic change in the biliary epithelial cells, without forming a mass lesion, similar to pancreatic intraepithelial neoplasia (PanIN). The bile ducts are of normal caliber or may be dilated because of another primary cause such as hepatolithiasis. BilINs are largely seen in livers resected or explanted for an underlying chronic disease (such as primary sclerosing cholangitis) or as a noninvasive component associated with cholangiocarcinoma. The epithelium can be flat or show a micropapillary growth pattern. The lesion has been classically graded as BilIN-1, BilIN-2, and BilIN-3, corresponding to mild, moderate, and severe dysplasia/carcinoma in situ respectively. In practice, it is often preferable to classify the dysplasia as low grade (mild to moderate dysplasia) and high grade (severe dysplasia/carcinoma in situ) (Figs. 29.9, 29.10, and 29.11). Such a two-tiered classification is easier, clinically more meaningful, and follows a similar approach for noninvasive neoplasms at other sites (e.g., cervix, urinary bladder, prostate, gastrointestinal tract).[24,26] In one study of liver explants from patients with primary sclerosing cholangitis, BilIN was seen in 83% and 36% of cases with and without cholangiocarcinoma, respectively.[27] Other major risk factors are hepatitis C cirrhosis and alcoholic cirrhosis.[28]

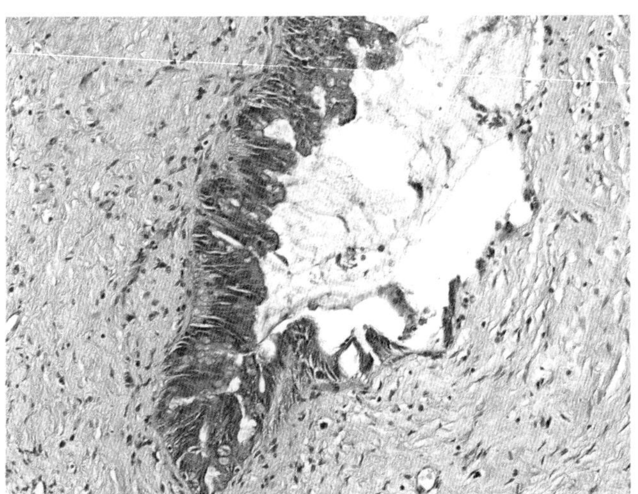

Figure 29.9 Low-grade biliary intraepithelial neoplasia, intestinal type with micropapillary features.

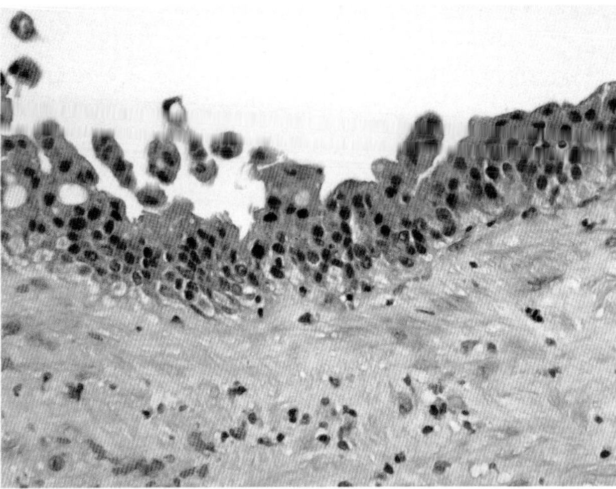

Figure 29.10 High-grade biliary intraepithelial lesion, predominantly flat type with early micropapillary changes.

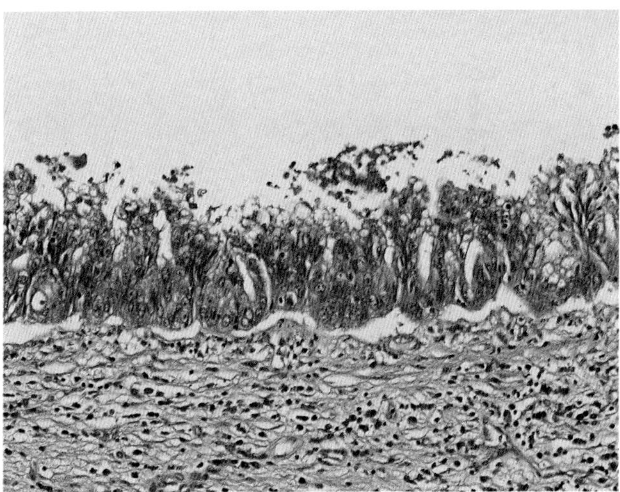

Figure 29.11 High-grade biliary intraepithelial lesion with micropapillary features.

Intraductal papillary neoplasm

Definition and etiology

Intraductal papillary neoplasms of the bile duct resemble the intraductal papillary mucinous neoplasms in the pancreas and are characterized by a neoplastic papillary intraductal epithelial proliferation, with dilatation of the ducts (Fig. 29.12). This category of neoplasm includes lesions previously designated as intraductal papilloma, biliary papillomatosis, and

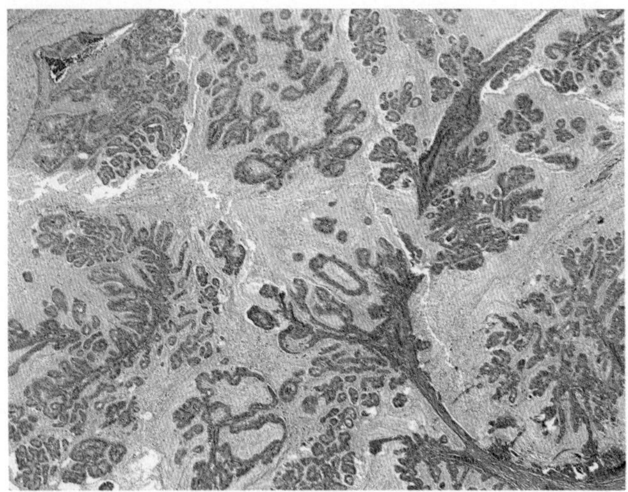

Figure 29.12 Intraductal papillary neoplasm. Characteristic arborizing intraductal papillary proliferation is present.

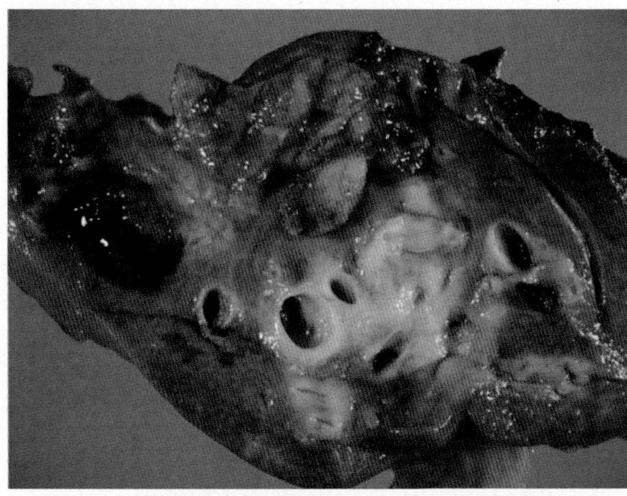

Figure 29.13 Intraductal papillary neoplasm. Fleshy tumor growth is present in the duct lumen (**upper left**), associated with obstructive duct changes and fibrosis more proximally.

noninvasive papillary carcinoma of the bile duct. Although similar to the pancreatic lesion, biliary intraductal papillary neoplasms are less often mucinous, and therefore the term *mucinous* is not used for this entity.

Epidemiology and clinical features

Intraductal papillary neoplasms are uncommon lesions, accounting for 10% to 15% of bile duct tumors. They occur in adults, with a male predominance, and median age of 60 to 70 years.[25] Clinical presenting symptoms include jaundice, fever, and abdominal pain. Some patients can have hepatomegaly.

Imaging and gross findings

On imaging studies the ducts are dilated and can show filling defects. Gross examination of resected specimens show fusiform or cystically dilated ducts that are variably filled with fleshy or villiform growths arising from the wall (Fig. 29.13). The larger perihilar and extrahepatic ducts are more commonly involved than intrahepatic ducts, and the lesions may be multifocal. Involvement of large ducts in the liver corresponds to the intraductal growth pattern of intrahepatic cholangiocarcinoma.[24,26]

Microscopic findings

Based on the type of epithelium, intraductal papillary neoplasms can be histologically divided into pancreaticobiliary, intestinal, gastric, and oncocytic subtypes, listed in decreasing order of frequency, with rare lesions that are unclassifiable. The prognostic significance of subtyping is currently unclear. Invasive adenocarcinomas arising from the pancreaticobiliary subtype of intraductal papillary neoplasm usually shows a tubulopapillary growth pattern, whereas the intestinal subtype is associated with mucinous carcinoma.[24,29]

The grading of intraductal papillary neoplasms is similar to that used for BilINs and intraductal papillary mucinous neoplasms in the pancreas. Mild to moderate dysplasia is classified as low grade, and severe dysplasia/carcinoma in situ as high grade.[26] The reported prevalence of invasive carcinoma arising in intraductal papillary neoplasms ranges from 31% to 74%.[25,30]

The main differential diagnosis for intraductal papillary neoplasm is a mucinous cystic neoplasm, especially if a predominantly cystic mass is present. Unlike intraductal papillary neoplasms, mucinous cystic neoplasms show ovarian-type stroma and do not communicate with bile the ducts (Table 29.2).

There is general consensus that a size of 1 cm should be used as a criterion for designating a lesion as an intraductal papillary neoplasm. In the biliary tree, a lesion greater than 1 cm is classified as an intraductal papillary neoplasm, whereas a similar lesion in the pancreas is classified as an intraductal papillary mucinous neoplasm. In both organs, smaller lesions that are seen only on microscopy are classified differently, being called BilIN in the bile ducts and PanIN in the pancreas.[24] Although some lesions may be difficult to classify, it is important to note that both are precursor lesions with potential for neoplastic progression and multifocality.

Table 29.2 Clinicopathologic characteristics of precursor biliary lesions

	BilIN	IPN	MCN
Age	Variable	Sixth decade	Fifth decade
Sex predilection	M > F	M > F	F, rare in M
Location	Intra- or extrahepatic	Intra- or extrahepatic	Mostly intrahepatic
Mass lesion	Absent	Dilated duct or cyst	Multiloculated cyst
Ovarian-type stroma	Absent	Absent	Present
Communication with ducts	Present	Present	Absent
Microarchitecture	Flat or micropapillary	Papillary or tubulopapillary	Variable

Abbreviations: BilIN: biliary intraepithelial neoplasia; IPN: intraductal papillary neoplasm; MCN: mucinous cystic neoplasm.

Cytology

Brush cytology and biopsies are commonly performed for strictures and filling defects involving the extrahepatic ducts. Lesional cells may be mucinous or nonmucinous and are arranged in sheets or papillary groups with variable atypia.[31,32] Specimens are also commonly submitted for molecular analysis for biliary tract malignancy using fluorescence in situ hybridization.[33]

Immunohistochemistry

Immunohistochemistry for mucin subtypes, CK7/20, and CDX-2 can be helpful in subclassification of the epithelium in intraductal papillary neoplasms, but it is not commonly used in clinical practice.

Molecular features of precursor lesions

Both BilIN and intraductal papillary neoplasms evolve through a stepwise neoplastic progression, from low-grade through high-grade noninvasive lesions to invasive adenocarcinoma, with similar molecular alterations. *KRAS* mutations are common in low-grade lesions, and higher grade lesions show nuclear p53 expression, loss of SMAD4, and inactivation of p16.[30]

Treatment and prognosis

BilINs are usually diagnosed as secondary noninvasive components of cholangiocarcinoma, or as a finding in predisposing underlying biliary conditions such as primary sclerosing cholangitis, hepatolithiasis, and Caroli disease. Chronic hepatitis and alcoholic cirrhosis are also known risk factors. BilINs are usually incidental findings in surgical resection specimens and do not change management. In those rare instances when BilINs are sampled on needle biopsy specimens, the management focuses on regular imaging surveillance for cholangiocarcinoma.

Intraductal papillary neoplasm is treated by surgical resection as clinically indicated, based on symptomatology and risk of malignancy. The risk of malignancy is significantly higher in biliary intraductal papillary neoplasms compared to pancreatic intraductal papillary mucinous neoplasms. The extent of invasive tumor correlates with prognosis. Invasive papillary or mucinous carcinomas have a better prognosis compared to other types. Compared to noninvasive intraductal papillary neoplasms, the presence of invasive carcinoma reduces the 5-year survival from more than 90% to approximately 50%.[30]

Intraoperative frozen sections are commonly used to evaluate margins. In some centers, the surgeons may attempt additional resection if the initial margin is involved by high-grade BilIN or intraductal papillary neoplasm; however, involvement of the margin by high-grade dysplasia may not impact overall survival.[34]

29.11 INTRAHEPATIC CHOLANGIOCARCINOMAS

Definition

Intrahepatic cholangiocarcinoma is a malignant neoplasm of the biliary epithelium arising in any portion of the biliary system within the liver. Carcinomas arising in extrahepatic bile ducts are further divided into perihilar and distal bile duct carcinomas, with the separating anatomic landmark being the insertion of the cystic duct. Perihilar carcinomas involving the confluence of right and left hepatic ducts are commonly referred to as *Klatskin tumors*. In practice, it may not be possible to establish with certainty whether a tumor originated from the intrahepatic bile ducts or the extrahepatic perihilar ducts.[35,36] The focus of this chapter is intrahepatic cholangiocarcinoma.

Epidemiology

Intrahepatic cholangiocarcinomas represent approximately 2% of all malignancies and 10% to 20% of primary malignancies of the liver (after hepatocellular carcinoma).[37] The incidence of intrahepatic cholangiocarcinoma varies geographically, with the highest incidence reported in Asia, where it accounts for up to 30% of primary liver malignancies. This high risk is a result of biliary parasitic infestations. In northeastern Thailand, the reported incidence is 96/100,000. In contrast, the incidence in the United States is approximately 1/100,000 population, with estimated 5,000 cases diagnosed annually.

The incidence of cholangiocarcinoma increases with age, and most cases are diagnosed in individuals over the age of 60 years.[38–40] There is also a slight male predominance. In most developed countries, the incidence of intrahepatic cholangiocarcinoma has been rising over the past two decades, not only because of improved diagnostic methods, but also because of an increase in risk factors, such as chronic liver disease. In the United States, intrahepatic cholangiocarcinomas have increased by more than 160% over this time period and now represent approximately 40% of all biliary tract carcinomas, whereas the incidence of hilar and distal cholangiocarcinomas has been decreasing.

Etiology and risk factors

There are several well-recognized risk factors associated with the development intrahepatic cholangiocarcinoma (Table 29.3). In Asian countries, infestation with liver flukes (*Clonorchis sinensis* and *Ophisthorchis viverrini*) is a strong risk factor. In Western countries, primary sclerosing cholangitis is a major risk factor, with 5% to 15% patients developing cholangiocarcinoma, usually within the first few years after diagnosis. Other risk factors include fibropolycystic liver diseases, hepatolithiasis, chronic hepatitis, and cirrhosis from any cause. Most of these risk factors share in common chronic inflammation of the bile ducts. Lynch syndrome (hereditary nonpolyposis colorectal cancer) patients are also at increased risk of developing intrahepatic cholangiocarcinoma because of underlying genomic instability. Thorotrast is a radiographic agent that was banned in the 1960s for its carcinogenic role. A clear association exists between Thorotrast and cholangiocarcinoma, with malignancy developing decades after exposure. A majority of intrahepatic cholangiocarcinoma patients, however, have no recognizable risk factors and no precursor lesions.[41–45]

Table 29.3 Risk factors for development of cholangiocarcinoma
Liver fluke infestations
Ophisthorchis viverinii
Clonorchis sinensis
Primary sclerosing cholangitis
Chronic hepatitis and cirrhosis
Hepatitis B
Hepatitis C
Alcoholic liver disease
Fibropolycystic liver disease
Toxins
Thorotrast
Diaoxin
Vinyl chloride

Clinical features

The clinical presentation of intrahepatic cholangiocarcinoma depends on the location of the tumor within the liver. Peripheral tumors may be asymptomatic and detected incidentally. These tumors usually attain a larger size and often present with symptoms related to metastatic disease. Patients can also present with nonspecific symptoms such as abdominal pain and weight loss. Tumors involving the larger intrahepatic ducts can lead to biliary strictures with the development of biliary obstruction symptoms. The imaging characteristics of intrahepatic cholangiocarcinoma depend on the location and growth pattern of the tumors, ranging from mass lesions to tumors in large ducts with enhancing mural nodules.

The serum markers elevated in intrahepatic cholangiocarcinoma include carbohydrate antigen 19-9 (CA19-9), 125 (CA125), and CEA. Of these, CA19-9 is the most helpful, especially if levels are increasing over time.[46]

Gross findings

Although cirrhosis from any cause is a risk factor for intrahepatic cholangiocarcinoma, most tumors develop in a background of noncirrhotic livers. Based on the growth pattern, intrahepatic cholangiocarcinomas are grossly classified into mass-forming tumors, periductal infiltrating tumors, and intraductal tumors[47] (Figs. 29.14 and 29.15). The intraductal pattern corresponds to carcinoma arising in intraductal papillary neoplasm.

These growth patterns correlate with prognosis, but combined patterns are not uncommon. Tumors with a periductal infiltrating growth pattern have the

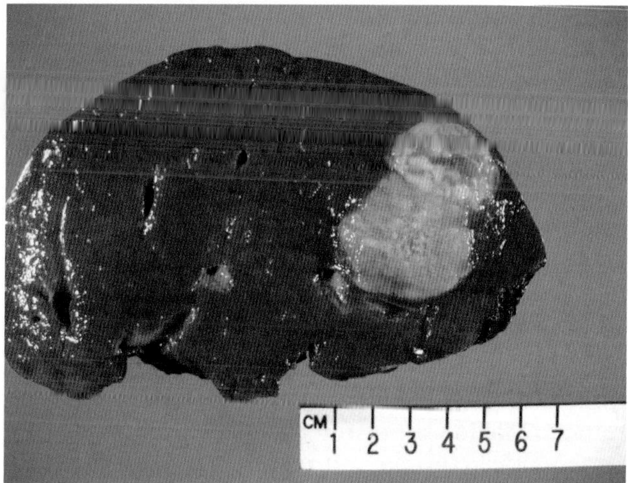

Figure 29.14 Intrahepatic cholangiocarcinoma with a mass-forming pattern and areas of necrosis.

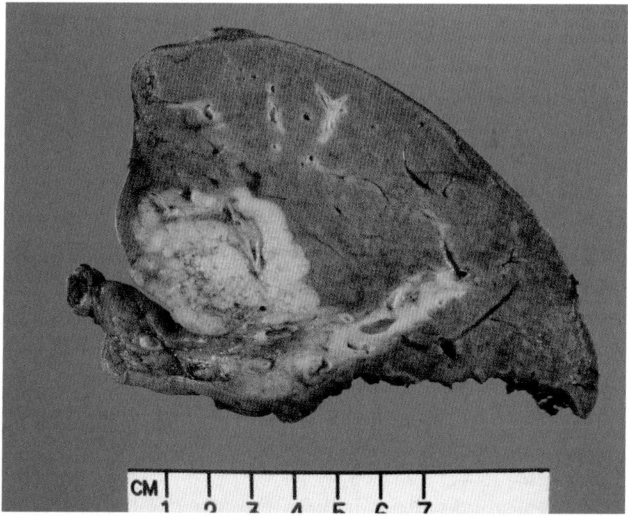

Figure 29.15 Intrahepatic cholangiocarcinoma with combined mass-forming and periductal infiltrating patterns.

worst prognosis, whereas intraductal tumors have the best prognosis. Intrahepatic cholangiocarcinoma arising from the peripheral bile ducts and ductules are generally mass-forming. Tumors located close to the hilum are more variable and can show an intraductal component with dilated ducts, or form a stricture or a mass. Tumors are multicentric in as many as 40% of cases, which often raises the possibility of metastases from a nonhepatic primary.[48] Most tumors are densely fibrotic, appearing white and firm.

Microscopic findings

Most cholangiocarcinomas show variably desmoplastic stroma (Fig. 29.16). The predominant growth pattern is tubular/glandular, with less common patterns including papillary, trabecular, solid, and cholangiolar, the latter characterized by thin arborizing cords of tumor cells. A mixture of patterns is not uncommon. Mucin is often present, a feature helpful in distinguishing these tumors from the pseudoacinar pattern of hepatocellular carcinoma. Rarely, abundant extracellular mucin (colloid pattern) or signet ring cell differentiation may be seen. Squamous, clear cell, and sarcomatoid differentiation can be present, usually as a minor component within the tumor (Figs. 29.17, 29.18, and 29.19). Rare cases of small cell intrahepatic cholangiocarcinomas have been reported; however, metastasis should be excluded by a thorough clinical evaluation and immunostain studies.[44–46]

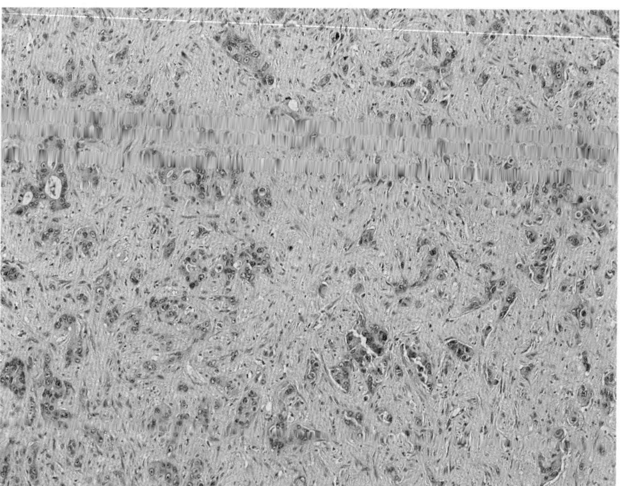

Figure 29.16 Cholangiocarcinoma, poorly differentiated, with a characteristic desmoplastic stroma and areas of acinar pattern.

Intrahepatic cholangiocarcinoma are graded based on the extent of gland formation into a four-tiered system: well differentiated (>95% gland formation), moderately differentiated (50% to 95%), poorly differentiated (5% to 49%), and undifferentiated tumors (<5%).

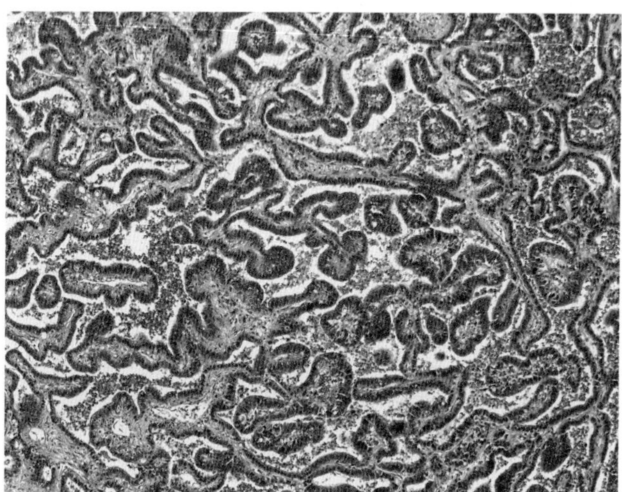

Figure 29.17 Cholangiocarcinoma, papillary pattern.

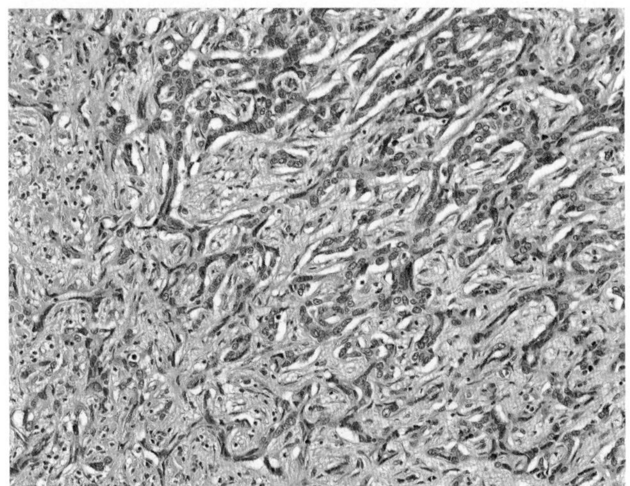

Figure 29.18 Cholangiocarcinoma, cholangiolar pattern.

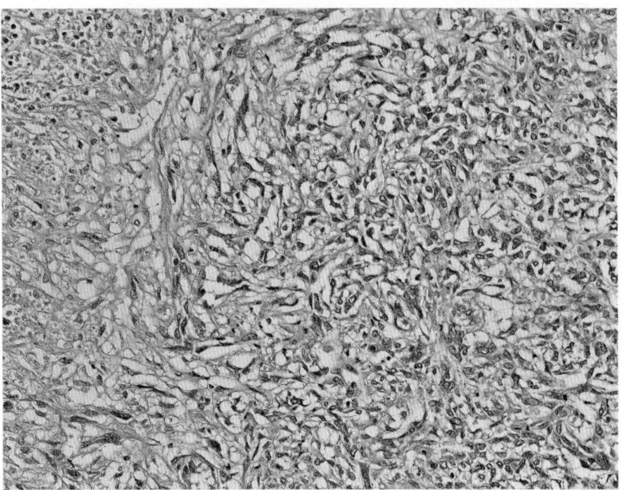

Figure 29.19 Cholangiocarcinoma, sarcomatoid type with necrosis.

A noninvasive component (precursor lesion) may be present, either as BilIN or as intraductal papillary neoplasm. In general, intrahepatic cholangiocarcinomas are slow growing, locally invasive tumors with a propensity for vascular and perineural invasion.

Immunohistochemistry

No pathognomonic immunohistochemical staining is currently available to specifically confirm biliary epithelial differentiation. However, a panel of immunostains can support the diagnosis of intrahepatic cholangiocarcinoma in the appropriate clinical context. Biliary carcinomas in general share immunohistochemical features with pancreatic and upper gastrointestinal tract carcinomas and are often positive either for CK7 (peripheral tumors) or for CK7 and CK20 (hilar tumors). Overall, 10% to 40% of cholangiocarcinomas are positive for CK20,[49,50] in particular hilar tumors.[51] Although staining for CK20 is usually not as diffuse as in colon carcinomas, there can be significant overlap. Further confounding CK20 interpretation, some right-sided colon carcinomas can be CK20 negative.[52–54] In fact, colon carcinomas that are microsatellite unstable because of defective DNA mismatch repair (microsatellite instability [MSI]–high tumors) can show reduced expression of CK20 and CDX2 and positive staining for CK7.[52–54]

CK19 is also positive in 70% to 80% of cases, whereas MOC31 is positive in approximately 90% of cases.[55] CDX2 is positive in about 50%, with hilar tumors more likely to stain positive than peripheral tumors. Making the distinction between intrahepatic cholangiocarcinoma and metastatic carcinomas requires clinical correlation and the use of additional immunostains specific for other primary sites. Of note, TTF-1 nuclear staining in an adenocarcinoma should not be used in isolation as a marker of lung adenocarcinoma because TTF-1 is positive in 50% of extrahepatic biliary carcinomas.[56]

For tumors in which combined hepatocellular-cholangiocarcinoma is being considered, use of hepatocyte-lineage markers (e.g., HepPar-1, Arginase) can be used to support hepatocellular differentiation; however, these tumors are classified primarily on the basis of morphology because separate morphological components of both hepatocellular carcinoma and cholangiocarcinoma are required for a diagnosis. Immunostains are then used to confirm the distinct hepatic and biliary differentiation.

Cytology

The cytologic findings in intrahepatic cholangiocarcinomas reflect the cell type and differentiation. Thus, in the majority of cases, the fine-needle aspiration smears show typical features of adenocarcinoma. Well-differentiated carcinomas show a honeycomb cytoarchitecture with or without mucin. With higher grade carcinomas there is increasing crowding, hyperchromasia, nucleolar prominence, and pleomorphism. Squamous, sarcomatoid, or other unusual features on cytologic preparations require appropriate evaluation for a broader differential diagnosis.[57]

Molecular findings

Understanding of the molecular pathogenesis of intrahepatic cholangiocarcinoma is not as well developed as it is in some other cancers such as colonic carcinoma. A subset of intrahepatic cholangiocarcinomas are thought to progress from normal, through noninvasive dysplastic epithelium (BilIN and intraductal papillary neoplasm), to frankly invasive tumors. The process involves multiple cytokines (such as interleukin-6 and nitric oxide), and complex molecular alterations involving multiple genetic pathways, including p53, β catenin, isocitrate dehydrogenase, ErbB2, KRAS, CDKN2B, and fibroblast growth factor receptor (see Chapter 23 for molecular pathology of liver tumors). There is growing utilization of molecular analysis by next-generation sequencing to identify genes and pathways for clinically helpful targeted therapies.

Differential diagnosis

Differential diagnostic considerations include benign biliary lesions and other primary or metastatic malignancies. Bile duct adenomas are circumscribed lesions that are typically small, without infiltration into the surround hepatic parenchyma. Von Meyenburg complexes are also small lesions, usually a few millimeters in size and subcapsular. These lesions may also contain a desmoplastic stroma, but they lack significant atypia. Reactive bile ductular proliferations may be exuberant and concerning for carcinoma, especially in the presence of inflammation and reactive atypia. The proliferation is usually secondary to a nearby lesion or occurs as a regenerative process in the setting of localized or diffuse parenchymal loss.

Metastatic adenocarcinomas, which are more common than primary liver tumors, may present a diagnostic dilemma. Clinical correlation and an appropriate panel of immunohistochemical stains should be used in this setting. The presence of a noninvasive intraductal component may also be helpful. However, metastatic carcinoma can also involve the biliary tree, mimicking cholangiocarcinoma. Immunohistochemistry can be useful in distinguishing hepatocellular carcinoma with a pseudoacinar pattern from cholangiocarcinoma. Epithelioid hemangioendothelioma and epithelioid angiosarcoma can be distinguished from cholangiocarcinoma by using vascular markers such as CD31, Fli-1, ERG, CD34, and Factor VIII.

Challenging bile duct lesions

Some bile duct lesions can be challenging to classify as benign or malignant. Although most cholangiocarcinomas are large and most bile duct adenomas and hamartomas are small, there are many exceptions. Histological findings that can help make this distinction include architectural features, cytological findings, and proliferative rate. None of these are diagnostic in isolation, but when used together, these can allow appropriate classification of most cases.

Bile ductular reactions can sometimes be striking, raising the possibility of a cholangiocarcioma. Ductular reactions are found at the periphery of portal tracts or cirrhotic nodules. Even when there are large areas of proliferation, the cytology of a ductular reaction is bland. The cytology of ductular cells in the areas of brisk ductular reactions is the same as found in other clearly benign areas of the specimen that show milder ductular reactions.

Atypical architectural findings that would favor malignancy include luminal necrotic debris and "incomplete glands," where a gland does not appear to be lined by epithelial cells around its entire circumference. Cytological atypia can be very helpful in diagnosing malignancy, particularly when it is striking; however, some cholangiocarcinomas are very well differentiated, showing bland cytologic features. Ki-67 immunostains can be helpful because cholangiocarcinomas show increased proliferation, whereas proliferation is absent or minimal in a bile duct adenoma or hamartoma. Immunostains for p53 are potentially helpful because strong and diffuse staining favors malignancy. However, most cases that have strong and diffuse p53 staining are morphologically malignant.

A ductular reaction can also have a high Ki-67 proliferative rate when there is a history of recent substantial parenchymal injury/collapse. In this situation, the ductular reaction tends to retain a lobular pattern at low-power examination. Also, the proliferating ductules in this setting are often iron-positive, and residual portal tracts and small islands of hepatocytes are commonly found.

Treatment and prognosis

Partial liver resection (lobectomy or segmentectomy) is the most suitable option for intrahepatic cholangiocarcinoma in carefully selected patients. Overall, approximately 30% of patients present with resectable disease. After resection, the reported median survival is 12 to 28 months, and most centers report 5-year survival between 20% and 60%. The presence of a positive surgical margin is associated with a prognosis similar to untreated patients, and adjuvant therapy confers limited survival benefit.[58–60]

For patients who are not operative candidates, nonsurgical ablative treatments have been used, including external beam radiation and targeted percutaneous and transarterial procedures. Chemotherapy has yielded limited success, with gemcitabine, cisplatin, and 5-fluorouracil–based regimens used most commonly. More recently, there have been a growing number of clinical trials using targeted therapies, including inhibitors for epidermal growth factor receptor, fibroblast growth factor receptor, tyrosine kinase, vascular endothelial growth factor, and cyclooxygenase-2. Results from these trials will determine the future role of targeted therapies for cholangiocarcinoma.[61]

Long-term survival for cholangiocarcinoma remains dismal, especially for carcinomas that are mass-forming or periductal infiltrative types. Tumors with a predominantly intraductal growth and mucinous differentiation are associated with better prognosis, whereas those with squamous or sarcomatoid differentiation have a worse prognosis.

Liver transplantation is currently an option for carefully selected patients with perihilar carcinomas after neoadjuvant chemoradiation, but is generally not an option for peripheral intrahepatic cholangiocarcinoma.[62,63] The 5-year survival after transplantation is 72%.[64]

29.12 COMBINED HEPATOCELLULAR-CHOLANGIOCARCINOMA

Combined hepatocellular-cholangiocarcinomas are tumors with unequivocal biphenotypic differentiation, containing mixed elements of both hepatocellular carcinoma and cholangiocarcinoma (also see Chapter 28). This terminology is not used when the liver contains separate masses of hepatocellular carcinoma and cholangiocarcinoma with intervening benign liver. Combined tumors are rare, comprising <1% of primary liver carcinomas. The gross appearance of these tumors depends on the extent of each component, but it is more commonly similar to hepatocellular carcinoma. Both components are morphologically evident, but this may be confirmed by appropriate immunohistochemistry (Fig. 29.20). Many mixed carcinomas show areas of intermediate morphology at the interface between the two components. Prognosis of these tumors is worse than for pure hepatocellular carcinoma. For treatment, staging and prognosis these tumors are considered more similar to cholangiocarcinomas.[65]

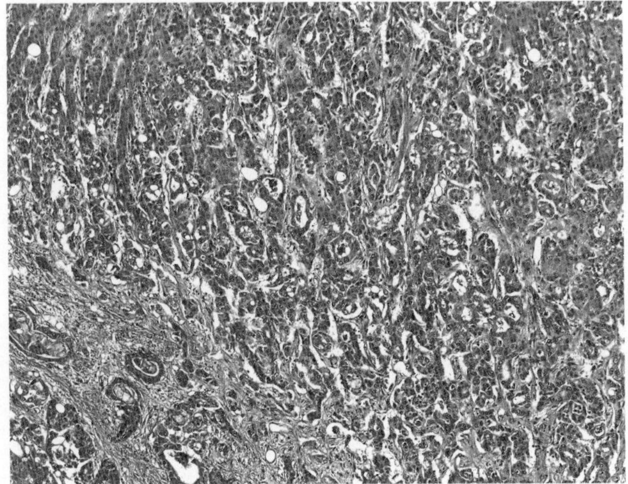

Figure 29.20 Combined hepatocellular-cholangiocarcinoma. Both components are intermixed and morphologically recognizable.

29.13 OTHER TUMORS

Although not biliary carcinomas, several other types of primary liver carcinoma have been reported that show pancreatic differentiation. These carcinomas are very rare but can show features identical to that of acinar cell carcinoma of the pancreas.[66,67] Very rare solid pseudopapillary neoplasms primary to the liver have also been reported.[68,69] In both tumors, the morphologic and staining characteristics are similar to the corresponding tumors of the pancreas. Of course, a pancreatic primary has to be carefully excluded before making a diagnosis of either of these as primary tumors in the liver.

REFERENCES

1. Jakowski JD, Lucas JG, Seth S, et al. Ciliated hepatic foregut cyst: a rare but increasingly reported liver cyst. *Ann Diagn Pathol.* 2004;8:342–346.
2. Fujita AW, Steelman CK, Abramowsky CR, et al. Ciliated hepatic foregut cyst: four case reports with a review of the literature. *Pediatr Dev Pathol.* 2011;14:418–421.
3. Bishop KC, Perrino CM, Ruzinova MB, et al. Ciliated hepatic foregut cyst: a report of 6 cases and a review of the English literature. *Diagn Pathol.* 2015;10:81.
4. Ben Ari Z, Cohen-Ezra O, Weidenfeld J, et al. Ciliated hepatic foregut cyst with high intra-cystic carbohydrate antigen 19-9 level. *World J Gastroenterol.* 2014;20:16355–16358.
5. Wilson JM, Groeschl R, George B, et al. Ciliated hepatic cyst leading to squamous cell carcinoma of the liver – a case report and review of the literature. *Int J Surg Case Rep.* 2013;4:972–975.
6. Jain D, Ahrens W, Finkelstein S. Molecular evidence for the neoplastic potential of hepatic Von-Meyenburg complexes. *Appl Immunohistochem Mol Morphol.* 2010;18:166–171.
7. Tsokos CG, Krings G, Yilmaz F, et al. Proliferative index facilitates distinction between benign biliary lesions and intrahepatic cholangiocarcinoma. *Hum Pathol.* 2016;57:61–67.
8. Allaire GS, Rabin L, Ishak KG, et al. Bile duct adenoma. A study of 152 cases. *Am J Surg Pathol.* 1988;12:708–715.
9. Pujals A, Bioulac-Sage P, Castain C, et al. BRAF V600E mutational status in bile duct adenomas and hamartomas. *Histopathology.* 2015;67:562–567.
10. Albores-Saavedra J, Hoang MP, Murakata LA, et al. Atypical bile duct adenoma, clear cell type: a previously undescribed tumor of the liver. *Am J Surg Pathol.* 2001;25:956–960.
11. Wu WW, Gu M, Lu D. Cytopathologic, histopathologic, and immunohistochemical features

of intrahepatic clear cell bile duct adenoma: a case report and review of the literature. *Case Rep Pathol.* 2014;2014:874826.

12. Tsui WM, Loo KT, Chow LT, et al. Biliary adenofibroma. A heretofore unrecognized benign biliary tumor of the liver. *Am J Surg Pathol.* 1993;17:186–192.
13. Varnholt H, Vauthey JN, Dal Cin P, et al. Biliary adenofibroma: a rare neoplasm of bile duct origin with an indolent behavior. *Am J Surg Pathol.* 2003;27:693–698.
14. Nguyen NT, Harring TR, Holley L, et al. Biliary adenofibroma with carcinoma in situ: a rare case report. *Case Rep Hepatol.* 2012;2012:793963.
15. Akin O, Coskun M. Biliary adenofibroma with malignant transformation and pulmonary metastases: CT findings. *AJR Am J Roentgenol.* 2002;179:280–281.
16. Devaney K, Goodman ZD, Ishak KG. Hepatobiliary cystadenoma and cystadenocarcinoma. A light microscopic and immunohistochemical study of 70 patients. Am J Surg Pathol. 1994;18:1078–1091.
17. Williamson JM, Rees JR, Pope I, et al. Hepatobiliary cystadenomas. *Ann R Coll Surg Engl.* 2013;95: 507–510.
18. Buetow PC, Buck JL, Pantongrag-Brown L, et al. Biliary cystadenoma and cystadenocarcinoma: clinical-imaging-pathologic correlations with emphasis on the importance of ovarian stroma. *Radiology.* 1995;196:805–810.
19. Zen Y, Pedica F, Patcha VR, et al. Mucinous cystic neoplasms of the liver: a clinicopathological study and comparison with intraductal papillary neoplasms of the bile duct. *Mod Pathol.* 2011;24:1079–1089.
20. Albores-Saavedra J, Cordova-Ramon JC, Chable-Montero F, et al. Cystadenomas of the liver and extrahepatic bile ducts: morphologic and immunohistochemical characterization of the biliary and intestinal variants. *Ann Diagn Pathol.* 2015;19:124–129.
21. Ishak KG, Willis GW, Cummins SD, et al. Biliary cystadenoma and cystadenocarcinoma: report of 14 cases and review of the literature. *Cancer.* 1977;39:322–338.
22. Kim K, Choi J, Park Y, et al. Biliary cystadenoma of the liver. *J Hepatobiliary Pancreat Surg.* 1998;5:348–352.
23. Ratti F, Ferla F, Paganelli M, et al. Biliary cystadenoma: short- and long-term outcome after radical hepatic resection. *Updates Surg* 2012;64:13–18.
24. Adsay V, Mino-Kenudson M, Furukawa T, et al. Pathologic evaluation and reporting of intraductal papillary mucinous neoplasms of the pancreas and other tumoral intraepithelial neoplasms of pancreatobiliary tract: recommendations of verona consensus meeting. *Ann Surg.* 2016;263:162–177.
25. Kloppel G, Adsay V, Konukiewitz B, et al. Precancerous lesions of the biliary tree. *Best Pract Res Clin Gastroenterol.* 2013;27:285–297.
26. Basturk O, Hong SM, Wood LD, et al. A revised classification system and recommendations from the baltimore consensus meeting for neoplastic precursor lesions in the pancreas. *Am J Surg Pathol.* 2015;39:1730–1741.
27. Lewis JT, Talwalkar JA, Rosen CB, et al. Precancerous bile duct pathology in end-stage primary sclerosing cholangitis, with and without cholangiocarcinoma. *Am J Surg Pathol.* 2010;34:27–34.
28. Torbenson M, Yeh MM, Abraham SC. Bile duct dysplasia in the setting of chronic hepatitis C and alcohol cirrhosis. *Am J Surg Pathol.* 2007;31:1410–1413.
29. Kim KM, Lee JK, Shin JU, et al. Clinicopathologic features of intraductal papillary neoplasm of the bile duct according to histologic subtype. *Am J Gastroenterol.* 2012;107:118–125.
30. Serra S. Precursor neoplastic lesions of the biliary tract. *J Clin Pathol.* 2014;67:875–882.
31. Gupta M, Pai RR, Dileep D, et al. Role of biliary tract cytology in the evaluation of extrahepatic cholestatic jaundice. *J Cytol.* 2013;30:162–168.
32. Smoczynski M, Jablonska A, Matyskiel A, et al. Routine brush cytology and fluorescence in situ hybridization for assessment of pancreatobiliary strictures. *Gastrointest Endosc.* 2012;75:65–73.
33. Fritcher EG, Kipp BR, Halling KC, et al. A multivariable model using advanced cytologic methods for the evaluation of indeterminate pancreatobiliary strictures. *Gastroenterology.* 2009;136:2180–2186.
34. Matthaei H, Lingohr P, Strasser A, et al. Biliary intraepithelial neoplasia (BilIN) is frequently found in surgical margins of biliary tract cancer resection specimens but has no clinical implications. *Virchows Arch.* 2015;466:133–141.
35. Nakanuma Y, Sato Y, Harada K, et al. Pathological classification of intrahepatic cholangiocarcinoma based on a new concept. *World J Hepatol.* 2010;2:419–427.
36. Washington MK, Berlin J, Branton PA, et al. Protocol for the examination of specimens from patients with carcinoma of the intrahepatic bile ducts. *Arch Pathol Lab Med.* 2010;134:e14–18.
37. Ustundag Y, Bayraktar Y. Cholangiocarcinoma: a compact review of the literature. *World J Gastroenterol.* 2008;14:6458–6466.
38. Patel T. Increasing incidence and mortality of primary intrahepatic cholangiocarcinoma in the United States. *Hepatology.* 2001;33:1353–1357.
39. Shaib YH, Davila JA, McGlynn K, et al. Rising incidence of intrahepatic cholangiocarcinoma in the United States: a true increase? *J Hepatol.* 2004;40:472–477.
40. Blechacz B, Gores GJ. Cholangiocarcinoma: advances in pathogenesis, diagnosis, and treatment. *Hepatology.* 2008;48:308–321.

41. Lazaridis KN, Gores GJ. Primary sclerosing cholangitis and cholangiocarcinoma. *Semin Liver Dis*. 2006;26:42–51.
42. Welzel TM, Graubard BI, El-Serag HB, et al. Risk factors for intrahepatic and extrahepatic cholangiocarcinoma in the United States: a population-based case-control study. *Clin Gastroenterol Hepatol*. 2007;5:1221–1228.
43. Koornstra JJ, Mourits MJ, Sijmons RH, et al. Management of extracolonic tumours in patients with Lynch syndrome. *Lancet Oncol*. 2009;10:400–408.
44. Cai Y, Cheng N, Ye H, et al. The current management of cholangiocarcinoma: a comparison of current guidelines. *Biosci Trends*. 2016;10:92–102.
45. Aarnio M. Clinicopathological features and management of cancers in lynch syndrome. *Patholog Res Int*. 2012;2012:350309.
46. Levy C, Lymp J, Angulo P, et al. The value of serum CA 19-9 in predicting cholangiocarcinomas in patients with primary sclerosing cholangitis. *Dig Dis Sci*. 2005;50:1734–1740.
47. Hirohashi K, Uenishi T, Kubo S, et al. Macroscopic types of intrahepatic cholangiocarcinoma: clinicopathologic features and surgical outcomes. *Hepatogastroenterology*. 2002;49:326–329.
48. Suzuki M, Takahashi T, Ouchi K, et al. The development and extension of hepatohilar bile duct carcinoma. A three-dimensional tumor mapping in the intrahepatic biliary tree visualized with the aid of a graphics computer system. *Cancer*. 1989;64:658–666.
49. Chu PG, Schwarz RE, Lau SK, et al. Immunohistochemical staining in the diagnosis of pancreatobiliary and ampulla of Vater adenocarcinoma: application of CDX2, CK17, MUC1, and MUC2. *Am J Surg Pathol*. 2005;29:359–367.
50. Maeda T, Kajiyama K, Adachi E, et al. The expression of cytokeratins 7, 19, and 20 in primary and metastatic carcinomas of the liver. *Mod Pathol*. 1996;9:901–909.
51. Shimonishi T, Miyazaki K, Nakanuma Y. Cytokeratin profile relates to histological subtypes and intrahepatic location of intrahepatic cholangiocarcinoma and primary sites of metastatic adenocarcinoma of liver. *Histopathology*. 2000;37:55–63.
52. Hinoi T, Tani M, Lucas PC, et al. Loss of CDX2 expression and microsatellite instability are prominent features of large cell minimally differentiated carcinomas of the colon. *Am J Pathol*. 2001;159:2239–2248.
53. McGregor DK, Wu TT, Rashid A, et al. Reduced expression of cytokeratin 20 in colorectal carcinomas with high levels of microsatellite instability. *Am J Surg Pathol*. 2004;28:712–718.
54. Gurzu S, Jung I. Aberrant pattern of the cytokeratin 7/cytokeratin 20 immunophenotype in colorectal adenocarcinomas with BRAF mutations. *Pathol Res Pract*. 2012;208:163–166.
55. Chan ES, Yeh MM. The use of immunohistochemistry in liver tumors. *Clin Liver Dis*. 2010;14:687–703.
56. Surrey LF, Frank R, Zhang PJ, et al. TTF-1 and Napsin-A are expressed in a subset of cholangiocarcinomas arising from the gallbladder and hepatic ducts: continued caveats for utilization of immunohistochemistry panels. *Am J Surg Pathol*. 2014;38:224–227.
57. Conrad R, Castelino-Prabhu S, Cobb C, et al. Cytopathologic diagnosis of liver mass lesions. *J Gastrointest Oncol*. 2013;4:53–61.
58. Lee SY, Cherqui D. Operative management of cholangiocarcinoma. *Semin Liver Dis*. 2013;33:248–261.
59. Ohtsuka M, Ito H, Kimura F, et al. Results of surgical treatment for intrahepatic cholangiocarcinoma and clinicopathological factors influencing survival. *Br J Surg*. 2002;89:1525–1531.
60. DeOliveira ML, Cunningham SC, Cameron JL, et al. Cholangiocarcinoma: thirty-one-year experience with 564 patients at a single institution. *Ann Surg*. 2007;245:755–762.
61. Ross JS, Wang K, Gay L, et al. New routes to targeted therapy of intrahepatic cholangiocarcinomas revealed by next-generation sequencing. *Oncologist*. 2014;19:235–242.
62. Blechacz BR, Gores GJ. Cholangiocarcinoma. *Clin Liver Dis*. 2008;12:131–150, ix.
63. Heimbach JK, Gores GJ, Haddock MG, et al. Liver transplantation for unresectable perihilar cholangiocarcinoma. *Semin Liver Dis*. 2004;24:201–207.
64. Rea DJ, Rosen CB, Nagorney DM, et al. Transplantation for cholangiocarcinoma: when and for whom? *Surg Oncol Clin N Am*. 2009;18: 325–337, ix.
65. Akiba J, Nakashima O, Hattori S, et al. Clinicopathologic analysis of combined hepatocellular-cholangiocarcinoma according to the latest WHO classification. *Am J Surg Pathol*. 2013;37:496–505.
66. Wildgruber M, Rummeny EJ, Gaa J. Primary acinar cell carcinoma of the liver. *Rofo*. 2013;185:572–573.
67. Agaimy A, Kaiser A, Becker K, et al. Pancreatic-type acinar cell carcinoma of the liver: a clinicopathologic study of four patients. *Mod Pathol*. 2011;24:1620–1626.
68. Thai E, Dalla Valle R, Silini EM. Primary solid papillary tumor of the liver. *Pathol Res Pract*. 2012;208:250–253.
69. Kim YI, Kim ST, Lee GK, et al. Papillary cystic tumor of the liver. A case report with ultrastructural observation. *Cancer*. 1990;65:2740–2746.

30

Hematopathology and the liver

Michael S. Torbenson, Ellen D. McPhail

30.1 OVERVIEW

The liver can be involved by reactive lymphoid hyperplasia and by various hematological malignancies. The appropriate diagnosis can be very challenging and often requires careful correlation with clinical, imaging, and laboratory findings. Leukemia represents secondary involvement of the liver, while lymphomas can be either primary or secondary to the liver. Most primary lymphomas of the liver are non-Hodgkin lymphoma, and about two-thirds are first diagnosed at liver biopsy.[1] The most common primary B-cell lymphoma of the liver is diffuse large B-cell lymphoma (approximately 75% of cases), followed by marginal zone lymphoma (approximately 20%).[2–5] About 5% of primary hepatic lymphomas are Burkitt lymphoma,[2,4] with the remaining entities all contributing 1% or less.

30.2 REACTIVE HEMATOLOGICAL DISORDERS

Hematological disorders of many different types are associated with vascular flow changes to the liver, even if the disease itself does not directly involve the liver. The frequency and types of changes are variable, depending on the hematological disease, but include portal venopathy, nodular regenerative hyperplasia, and veno-occlusive disease. Each of these entities is considered in more detail in their respective chapters. Amyloid deposition is another important process that can result from hematological disorders.

Reactive conditions

The most common reactive hematopoietic conditions found in liver biopsies are extramedullary hematopoiesis, Kupffer cell hyperplasia, and the hemophagocytic syndrome. Extramedullary hematopoiesis can include myeloid precursors, red blood cell precursors, and/or megakaryocytes (Fig. 30.1). Extramedullary hematopoiesis is not a disease entity per se, but instead is a secondary manifestation of both benign and malignant conditions. In infants and children, extramedullary hematopoiesis is commonly found in a variety of liver diseases, but in particular cholestatic diseases. Even in adults, cholestatic liver disease can occasionally be accompanied by mild extramedullary hematopoiesis. Extramedullary hematopoiesis can also be found in

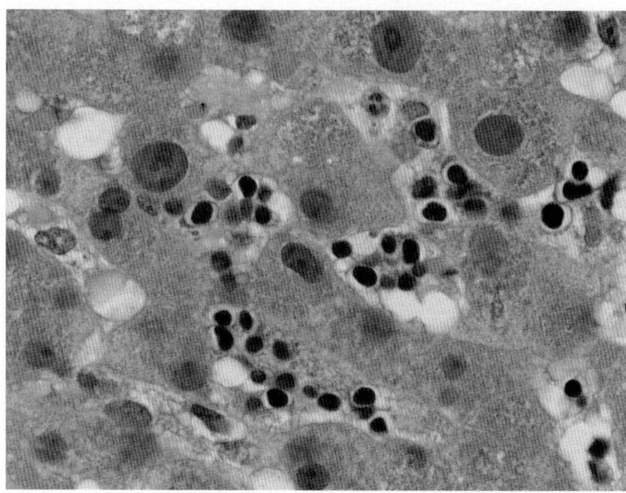

Figure 30.1 Extramedullary hematopoiesis. Red blood cell precursors are seen in the sinusoids.

diseases with impaired red blood cell synthesis, including the chronic hemolytic anemias and hemoglobinopathies. Finally, extramedullary hematopoiesis can result from malignant conditions involving the bone marrow, such as chronic myeloproliferative neoplasms or myelophthisic processes such as lymphomas or carcinomas.

Kupffer cell hyperplasia

Generalized Kupffer cell hyperplasia is a common secondary event in cholestatic conditions and with marked hepatitis. Kupffer cell hyperplasia outside of these settings is most commonly seen with acute viral hepatitis, such as cytomegalovirus (CMV) or Epstein–Barr virus (EBV), and can be accompanied by hemophagocytosis. When hemophagocytosis is prominent, a diagnosis of hemophagocytic syndrome should be considered. In one study, 1.6% of sequential nontumor liver biopsies showed Kupffer cell hyperplasia with hemophagocytosis.[6] The hemophagocytic syndrome results from uncontrolled macrophage activation and is seen as either as a primary (familial) disease or as a secondary disease.

Secondary hemophagocytic syndrome

The secondary hemophagocytic syndrome can be seen with many different underlying disease conditions (Table 30.1), but most can be categorized as infections, malignancies, autoimmune conditions, or drug effects. The histological findings will vary, depending on the underlying disease conditions, but all share the findings of Kupffer cell hyperplasia and hemophagocytosis (Fig. 30.2). The hemophagocytosis should be convincing because Kupffer cell hyperplasia without hemophagocytosis is also common in many different inflammatory and cholestatic diseases of the liver.

The list of infections associated with the secondary hemophagocytic syndrome is very long and seems to grow ever longer, including both infections passed from human to human as well as many zoonotic infections.[7] Overall, EBV and CMV are the most common triggers in nonimmunosuppressed patients. In immunosuppressed patients, a

Table 30.1 Secondary Kupffer cell hyperplasia and hemophagocytosis[6,90]

Associations
Malignancies B-cell lymphoma T-cell lymphoma Hodgkin lymphoma Myeloproliferative disorders
Infections CMV EBV Varicella–zoster (chickenpox) HHV8 Tuberculosis *E. coli* Shigella Nocardiosis Coxiellaburnetii (Q fever) Rickettsia conorii (Mediterranean spotted fever)
Autoimmune diseases Crohn disease Rheumatoid arthritis Ankylosing spondylitis Dermatomyositis Sarcoidosis CVID Castleman disease
Still disease
Drug Effects

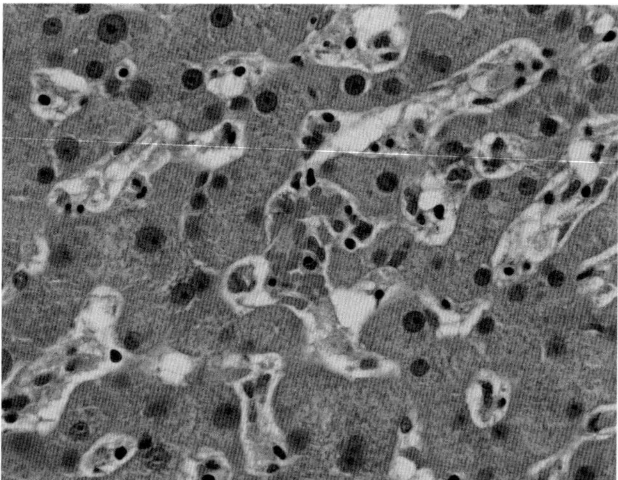

Figure 30.2 **Kupffer cell hyperplasia with hemophagocytosis**. The Kupffer cells are very prominent and some have phagocytized red blood cells.

much wider range of infectious associations are found. In fact, the frequency of secondary hemophagocytic syndrome on liver biopsy is particularly high with HIV infection, up to 8%.[6] In most HIV cases, an infectious trigger is eventually identified and can be viral or bacterial.

Overall, about one-third of individuals with secondary Kupffer cell hyperplasia and hemophagocytosis on liver biopsy will have additional findings that fulfill the criteria for the complete hemophagocytic syndrome (Table 30.2).[6] Nonetheless, cases that don't fulfill the full criteria typically have some of the findings seen in Table 30.2 and overall there appears to be a continuum, with the full hemophagocytic syndrome at the severe end. Secondary hemophagocytic syndromes are generally managed through treatment of the underlying disease process.

Familial hemophagocytic lymphohistiocytosis

Familial hemophagocytic lymphohistiocytosis typically affects children less than 2 years of age. Familial hemophagocytic lymphohistiocytosis is rapidly fatal if untreated by immunosuppression and bone marrow transplant. Familial hemophagocytic lymphohistiocytosis can result from mutations in a number of different genes that impair the function of T-cells and NK-cells, including *PRF1* (encode perforin), *UNC13D*, *STXBP2*, and *STX11*. Overall, genetic mutations are found in about 65% of cases, with the remaining presumably having mutations in unknown genes. The diagnosis is made either by identifying mutations or by clinical criteria employed in clinical trials (Table 30.2). Because not all affected individuals will meet these criteria, in particular at first presentation, a modified set of criteria has been suggested for routine clinical care (Table 30.3).

Familial hemophagocytic lymphohistiocytosis is typically associated with hepatomegaly and liver dysfunction that ranges from mild to severe. Histologically, there can be several different patterns of injury, but common to all of these patterns are the core findings of hemophagocytosis, bile duct lymphocytosis and injury, and significant endothelialitis.[8] In addition to phagocytosis of red blood cells, phagocytosis of leukocytes can be observed.

Some cases show a chronic hepatitis pattern, with portal tract infiltrates that in most cases are moderate to marked.[8,9] The inflammation is predominantly lymphocytic with varying numbers of histiocytes. Plasma cells, eosinophils, and neutrophils are rare. Almost all cases show bile duct lymphocytosis and injury. In addition, endothelialitis is present in almost all cases and can involve the central veins or the portal veins. In some cases, the phlebitis can be marked, with necrosis of the vein and surrounding parenchyma. The lobules can show mild zone 1 macrovesicular steatosis. The sinusoidal lymphohistiocytic infiltrates can be striking, resembling a leukemic infiltrate, or

Table 30.2 Criteria for Hemophagocytic Lymphohistiocytosis. Five of Eight Are Needed for a Diagnosis

	Criteria	Comments
1	Prolonged fever	>100.4°F (38.5°C)
2	Splenomegaly	
3	Cytopenias affecting at least two of three lineages in the peripheral blood	Hemoglobin<9 g/100 mL (in infants <4 weeks: hemoglobin<10 g/100 mL) Platelets <100 × 10^9/L Neutrophils <1 × 10^9/L
4	Hypertriglyceridemia and/or hypofibrinogenemia	Hypertriglyceridemia: fasting, greater than or equal to 265 mg/100 mL Hypofibrinogenemia: ≤150 mg/100 mL
5	Hemophagocytosis	Bone marrow, spleen lymph nodes, liver
6	Low or absent natural killer cell activity	
7	Ferritin ≥ 500 ng/mL	Some prefer a criteria of >3,000 ng/mL or a rapidly rising serum ferritin
8	Soluble CD25 (soluble IL-2 receptor)	Two standard deviations above age adjusted laboratory normals

Reprinted by permission from Macmillan Publishers Ltd: Jordan MB, Filipovich AH. Hematopoietic cell transplantation for hemophagocytic lymphohistiocytosis: a journey of a thousand miles begins with a single (big) step. *Bone Marrow Transplant*. 2008;42:433–7.

Table 30.3 Modified criteria for hemophagocytic lymphohistiocytosis

	Criteria	Comments
Clinical findings		
1	Fever	≥38.5°C
2	Splenomegaly	
3	Cytopenias	hemoglobin <9 g/dL (for infants <4 weeks, hemoglobin <10 g/dL) Platelets <100,000/μL Absolute neutrophil count <1,000/μL
4	Hepatitis	
Immune markers		
1	Hemophagocytosis	Note that hemophagocytosis is NOT required for the diagnosis
2	Increased ferritin	At least >500 ng/mL; >3,000 ng/mL is concerning; >10,000 ng/mL is highly suggestive
3	Increased soluble CD25 (soluble IL-2 receptor)	
4	Absent or very decreased NK cell function	

A diagnosis requires three of four clinical findings and one of four immune markers [92]

can be more subtle and patchy. Hemophagocytosis is universally present.

A second major pattern, found in about 25% of cases, is that of giant cell hepatitis, which histologically can be essentially identical to idiopathic neonatal giant cell hepatitis. Both show similar lobular cholestatic changes and giant cell transformation of hepatocytes. However, idiopathic neonatal giant cell hepatitis typically lacks the endothelialitis and hemophagocytosis seen in familial hemophagocytic lymphohistiocytosis. Also, the lymphohistiocytic infiltrates are denser in most cases of familial hemophagocytic lymphohistiocytosis than they are in idiopathic neonatal giant cell hepatitis. Nonetheless, some cases have sufficient overlap that correlation with the clinical and laboratory findings are needed to clarify the diagnosis.

In a third pattern, the histiocytic component is sufficiently prominent to suggest a storage disease.[8] The histiocytic cells in the sinusoids have abundant cytoplasm that takes on an eosinophilic color, making them hard to distinguish from hepatocytes. Also, the histiocytic inflammation can fill the terminal hepatic venules in a subset of cases, suggesting a veno-occlusive injury.

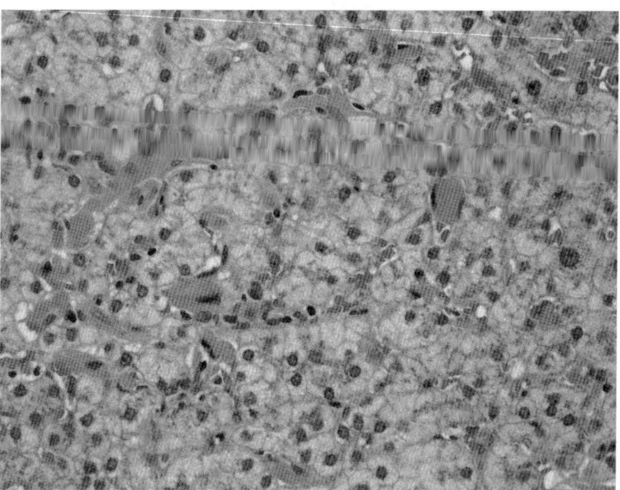

Figure 30.3 Crystal storing histiocytosis. The Kupffer cells have dense, eosinophilic inclusions.

Crystal storing histiocytosis

Crystal storing histiocytosis is a rare condition where the Kupffer cells of the liver are enlarged and distended with pink, chunky material (Fig. 30.3). On high-power examination, striations can be found in many cases (Fig. 30.4). One study found that crystals also involved

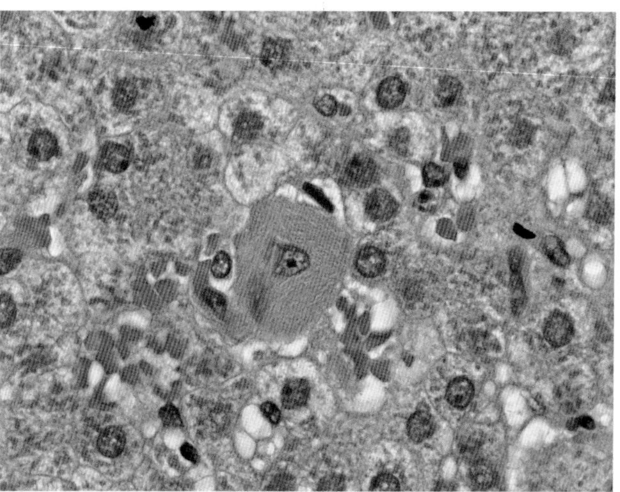

Figure 30.4 Crystal storing histiocytosis. Striations can be seen in some cases under high magnification.

the hepatocytes.[10] The material in most cases represents kappa immunoglobulin light chain, but rarely other material has been reported, including clofazimine crystals, cysteine, and silica.[11] In most cases, there is a history of multiple myeloma, lymphoplasmacytic lymphoma, or monoclonal gammopathy of undetermined significance.[11] The deposits in crystal storing histiocytosis are commonly not limited to the liver, and involve multiple organs. Overall, the bone marrow, liver, lymph nodes, spleen, and kidney are the most commonly affected sites.[11]

Rosai–Dorfman disease

Rosai–Dorfman disease is also known as sinus histiocytosis with massive lymphadenopathy and is a histiocytic disorder of unknown etiology. Overall, the disease appears to be more common in children than adults. Most individuals are immunocompetent and the male to female is about equal. The clinical findings at presentation are variable, but can include fever, weight loss, lymphadenopathy, and elevated liver enzymes.[12] Coexisting lymphomas in other organ systems have also been reported.[13,14] The disease only rarely involves the liver, and when it does, it is typically part of systemic disease. Other organs commonly involved by Rosai–Dorfman disease include the lymph nodes, skin, and upper respiratory tract. The disease course is quite variable: there can be spontaneous resolution, but rare cases can lead to death.

On liver biopsy, Rosai–Dorfman disease not only typically involves primarily the portal tracts (Fig. 30.5) but also has patchy infiltrates in the lobules. Rarely, a mass lesion in the liver is found.[15] The infiltrates can resemble ordinary hepatitis, with admixed lymphocytes, plasma cells, and eosinophils that largely

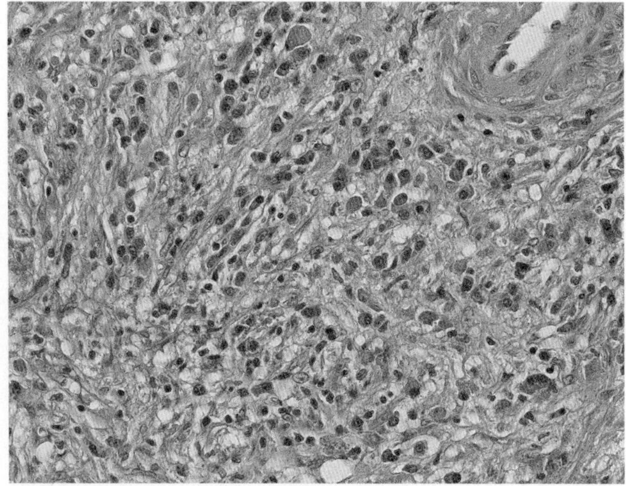

Figure 30.5 Rosai–Dorfman disease. The portal tracts show a dense infiltrate of macrophages, lymphocytes, and plasma cells.

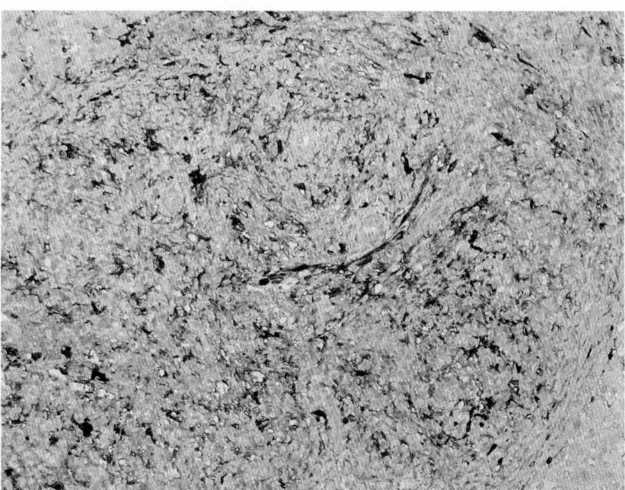

Figure 30.6 Rosai–Dorfman disease, S100. The histiocytes are strongly S100-positive.

obscure the histiocytic infiltrates. In other cases, the histiocytes are more evident and can even be granulomatous.[15] The histiocytes may have mild nuclear irregularities. Their cytoplasm is typically moderate to abundant and a clear or a pale, eosinophilic color. Emperipolesis is common. Bile duct damage is often found and can be striking. In many cases, the portal veins can be atrophic or absent in the affected portal tracts. The abnormal histiocytes stain strongly with S-100 (Fig. 30.6) and CD68 but are negative for CD1a.

Castleman disease (angiofollicular hyperplasia)

Definition

Castleman disease is a benign disease characterized by follicular hyperplasia and regressively transformed germinal centers.

Clinical findings

Castleman disease can involve the liver parenchyma or the hilar lymph nodes.[16] Imaging studies often suggest hepatocellular carcinoma.[17–19] Clinically, Castleman disease is commonly divided into localized versus multicentric disease. In some classification systems, Castleman disease is further divided into those cases that are human herpesvirus 8 (HHV8) positive or negative. Unicentric Castleman disease commonly presents in younger adults as a localized mass, typically involving the mediastinum, but without systemic symptoms. Most of these cases are classified histologically as the hyaline vascular type.

Multicentric disease has a more aggressive clinical course and is treated with systemic therapies. Most of these cases are classified histologically as plasma cell Castleman disease. Multicentric disease is often associated with systemic signs and symptoms, including generalized lymphadenopathy, fevers, night sweats, weight loss, and fatigue. Affected individuals often have anemia and hypergammaglobulinemia. Some individuals with the plasma cell variant of Castleman disease will have the POEMS (polyneuropathy, organomegaly, endocrinopathy, monoclonal protein, and skin lesions) syndrome. HHV8 infections are more common in the plasma cell variant, often in the setting of HIV infection, solid organ transplantation, or other immunosuppressed conditions.

Gross findings

Not all lesions are grossly visible. When they are, the lesions are often subcapsular, soft, and tan-yellow. Most are less than 2 cm in size.

Microscopic findings

The core histological pattern is that of florid lymphoid hyperplasia, including follicles with regressively transformed germinal centers and increased vascularity in the interfollicular spaces. Four histological types have been recognized: hyaline vascular type, plasma cell type, mixed type, and plasmablastic type.

The hyaline vascular type is the most common, tends to be localized, has few symptoms, and has a good prognosis. Histologically, hyaline vascular Castleman disease tends to involve the portal tracts, showing lymphoid hyperplasia with regressively transformed germinal centers. The regressively transformed germinal centers are depleted of lymphocytes and composed mostly of follicular dendritic cells, giving the center a hyalinized appearance. These regressed germinal centers are often surrounded by an expanded mantle zone with concentric rings of lymphocytes, a finding that has been described as an "onion skin" appearance. Finding multiple regressively transformed germinal centers within a single mantle zone is essentially pathognomonic for Castleman disease. The interfollicular areas are hypervascular. Sometimes the blood vessels from the hypervascular interfollicular region penetrate the regressively transformed germinal centers at right angles, leading to a "lollipop" appearance.

Plasma cell Castleman disease is more likely to cause symptoms and to be multicentric, thus is more commonly encountered in liver specimens. Plasma cell Castleman disease also shows follicular lymphoid hyperplasia but has significantly fewer regressively transformed germinal centers than the hyaline vascular type. In addition, the interfollicular space and subcapsular sinuses may have sheets of plasma cells.

The mixed subtype shows areas of both hyaline vascular and plasma cell types. HHV8-positive multicentric Castleman disease, a rare disease with an aggressive clinical course, contains plasma cells with a plasmablastic appearance.

Other findings

Castleman disease, in particular with multicentric disease and the plasma cell subtype, can be associated with other patterns of liver injury, even if the liver is not directly involved by the Castleman disease. These changes fall largely into the category of vascular abnormalities, including Budd–Chiari syndrome,[20] nonspecific sinusoidal dilatation,[21,22] peliosis hepatis,[23–25] and nodular regenerative hyperplasia.[24] Hepatic amyloid deposition, usually AA type, has also been well described.[26–28] Regression of the AA amyloid deposits has been observed following successful treatment of the Castleman disease.[29]

In most cases the background liver shows no underlying disease, though a case has been reported in the setting of cirrhosis.[30] Hilar lymph node involvement can lead to secondary bile duct obstruction.[31]

Differential diagnosis

The florid lymphoid hyperplasia seen in Castleman disease can mimic both reactive lymphoid hyperplasia as well as B-cell lymphomas, including follicular lymphoma and mantle cell lymphoma. Identifying the regressed germinal centers, including multiple regressively transformed germinal centers within a single mantle zone, and vascular hyperplasia in the interfollicular spaces will separate Castleman disease from reactive lymphoid hyperplasia. In addition, sheets of plasma cells in the subcapsular sinuses are characteristic of the plasma cell type of Castleman disease. Finally, HHV8 positivity in the setting of HIV infection favors Castleman disease. The typical histology of Castleman disease can differentiate it from B-cell lymphomas, but immunohistochemistry can be very helpful in difficult cases.

Reactive lymphoid hyperplasia

Definition

A small, benign, well-circumscribed nodule of reactive lymphoid follicles.

Clinical findings

Reactive lymphoid hyperplasia is also called *pseudolymphoma* and *nodular lymphoid lesion* of the liver. The term pseudolymphoma is perhaps best avoided, as the term can be confusing to clinical colleagues. The lesion is very rare, with about 50 cases reported in the literature.

Reactive lymphoid hyperplasia is commonly misdiagnosed as hepatocellular carcinoma, cholangiocarcinoma, or metastatic disease on imaging studies. The mean age at presentation is approximately 55 years, range 15 to 85 years, and there is an 8 to 1 female predominance.[32] Reactive lymphoid hyperplasia also occurs in other organs, such as the lung, skin, and gastrointestinal tract. However, in most reported cases, reactive lymphoid hyperplasia of the liver is restricted to the liver and there is no multiorgan disease. The etiology of reactive lymphoid hyperplasia is unclear, but at least in part appears to result from a localized immunological response to various infection antigens, neoplastic antigens, or autoimmune antigens. Reactive lymphoid hyperplasia is seen most commonly in either the setting of malignancies in other organ systems (most commonly the stomach or kidney) or in a variety of autoimmune conditions, some that are systemic, such as common variable immunodeficiency (CVID), and others that are hepatic, such as primary biliary cirrhosis.

Gross findings

The lesion(s) can be single (80%) or multifocal (20%). When multifocal, cases to date have had either two or three lesions. The lesions are well circumscribed, yellow, and soft to firm. Many have a subcapsular location and almost all reported lesions are 2 cm or less in size. The largest case reported to date measured 5.5 cm.[33]

Histology findings

Histologically, reactive lymphoid hyperplasia is composed of a well circumscribed cluster of reactive lymphoid follicles. The follicles have polarized germinal centers that contain a mixture of centroblasts and centrocytes with admixed tingible-body macrophages. The germinal centers are surrounded by reactive mantles and the follicles lack the back-to-back arrangement seen in follicular lymphoma. They are nonclonal by immunohistochemical or polymerase chain reaction (PCR) studies.

Rare cases can have prominent histiocytic infiltration within the lesion or have focal areas of granulomatous inflammation.[34] In some cases, there can be microcalcifications.[33] Reactive bile ductules are common at the interface with the background liver and rare cases can have psuedocapsules of compressed fibrotic tissue.[33] Although lesions are generally well circumscribed, the portal tracts adjacent to the lesions can show increased chronic inflammation. The background liver is either normal or shows changes of underlying disease, such as chronic viral hepatitis or primary biliary cirrhosis. When there is underlying liver disease, the changes in the background liver are typical for that disease, with no unusual features.

Differential

The differential includes Castleman disease, but reactive lymphoid hyperplasia lacks the regressed germinal centers and the interfollicular vascular hyperplasia. One reported case of reactive lymphoid hyperplasia had interfollicular plasma cells,[35] but most cases lack the sheets of plasma cells in the interfollicular spaces and subcapsular sinuses that are typical of the plasma cell variant of Castleman disease. Lymphoma can be excluded by immunostains and molecular testing, with the differential primarily that of follicular lymphoma, mantle cell lymphoma, and marginal zone lymphoma.

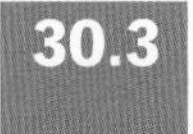

30.3 MALIGNANT LYMPHOMA: GENERAL CLINICAL AND PATHOLOGIC FINDINGS

Definition

Lymphomas and leukemias are neoplastic proliferations arising from cell types within the hematopoietic system.

Gross findings

The gross findings with liver involvement vary considerably depending on the type of lymphoma or leukemia. A subset of lymphomas and most leukemias show diffuse sinusoidal infiltration of the liver.[36,37] In these cases, imaging studies commonly show hepatomegaly, but either no mass lesion or only ill-defined lesions on ultrasound and other imaging techniques. Individuals with this pattern of disease presentation also commonly have elevated liver enzymes and the biopsy can be performed to evaluate for potential causes of acute hepatitis. In contrast, mass-forming lymphomas are commonly hypoechoic on ultrasound. Computed tomography (CT) studies frequently show hypodense lesions without enhancement, mimicking carcinoma.[2] Primary hepatic lymphomas can be solitary or multifocal and occasionally cystic, mimicking an abscess.[2,38] On gross examination, mass-forming primary lymphomas are classically soft, gray-white to yellow, and well circumscribed (Fig. 30.7). Necrosis, hemorrhage, and cystic degeneration can also be found. The background livers tend to be noncirrhotic.

Clinical findings

The clinical findings depend in part on the type of malignancy. The term *B symptoms* classically refers

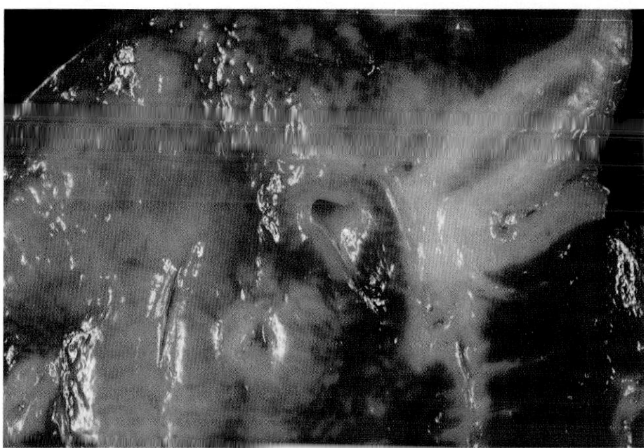

Figure 30.7 Lymphoma, gross. This follicular lymphoma grew as a solid, white, fleshy mass.

to drenching night sweats, fevers, and unintentional weight loss of at least 10 lbs. These systemic symptoms are generally associated with more advanced or aggressive lymphomas and are a negative prognostic finding.

Histological findings, general approach

Lymphomas of the liver are divided into Hodgkin and non-Hodgkin types, and the non-Hodgkin category is further subclassified into B- and T-cell types. The diagnosis can usually be established based on morphology and routine immunohistochemistry, although sometimes molecular genetics and/or interphase FISH studies must be employed. Pan-B-cell markers include CD19, CD20, CD22, CD79a, and PAX-5, and pan-T-cell markers include CD2, CD3, CD5, and CD7. Of these, starting with CD20 and CD3 is a common and practical approach. Useful plasma cell markers include MUM1 and CD138, although hepatocytes and bile ducts will also be positive for CD138, and B-cells and T-cells may be positive for MUM1. Light chain restriction of B-cells and/or plasma cells can be evaluated using immunostains for kappa and lambda immunoglobulin light chains. Histiocyte markers include CD68 and CD163, among others. If classical Hodgkin lymphoma is in the differential diagnosis, helpful immunostains include CD3, CD20, CD15, CD30, CD45, and PAX-5.

Lymphomas differ in their general patterns of liver involvement.[1,39] Although there are exceptions, these general patterns provide a useful starting point when evaluating a case (Table 30.4).

Table 30.4 Patterns of growth in the liver

Portal tract predominant	Sinusoidal predominant	Mass lesion predominant
CLL/SLL	Peripheral T-cell lymphoma, NOS	Diffuse large B-cell lymphoma
Hodgkin lymphoma	Hepatosplenic T-cell lymphoma	Burkitt lymphoma
Marginal zone lymphoma	Hairy cell leukemia	Anaplastic large cell lymphoma
Mantle cell lymphoma	B lymphoblastic leukemia/lymphoma	
Follicular lymphoma		
T-Cell/histiocyte-rich large B-cell lymphoma		

Differential, general considerations

The histological differential typically depends on the degree of tumor differentiation and on the presence or absence of a mass lesion, but overall falls into four different categories.

1. Well differentiated mass lesion: When there is a mass lesion composed of well differentiated cells, the differential tends to be that of malignant lymphoma, inflammatory pseudotumor, Castleman disease, or benign reactive lymphoid hyperplasia.
2. Poorly differentiated mass lesion: In contrast, when there is a mass lesion composed of poorly differentiated, cytologically atypical cells, the differential is primarily that of malignant lymphoma versus carcinoma, follicular dendritic cell sarcoma or other sarcomas, or melanoma, a differential that can usually be resolved by immunohistochemistry and/or molecular studies.
3. Sinusoidal pattern: When there is no mass lesion, the differential depends on the location of the infiltrates. With predominantly sinusoidal disease, the differential is that of hepatitis versus lymphoma/leukemia.
4. Portal-based pattern: With no mass lesion and predominantly portal-based disease, the differential includes chronic hepatitis with prominent lymphoid aggregates/follicles, B-cell lymphomas, and classical Hodgkin lymphoma.

These four general scenarios are discussed next. In the first setting, a mass-forming lesion can have a differential of a reactive condition, such as inflammatory pseudotumor, Castleman disease, or reactive lymphoid hyperplasia, versus malignant lymphoma.

Most inflammatory pseudotumors can be separated from lymphomas by their mixed inflammatory infiltrates, which are composed primarily of T lymphocytes with scattered B-cell aggregates, and prominent admixed plasma cells. These inflammatory changes are seen against a backdrop of spindled myofibroblasts and variably dense collagenous deposits. Many inflammatory pseudotumors have inflammation and sclerosis of central veins, though these areas may not be sampled in biopsy material. Classical Hodgkin lymphoma and B-cell lymphomas such as T-cell/histiocyte-rich large B-cell lymphoma should be carefully ruled out by histologic review and immunohistochemistry if necessary, although these disorders typically present as portal-based disease rather than a mass lesion. The differential diagnosis also includes Castleman disease (see discussion above).

In the second setting, the hematoxylin and eosin (H&E) findings are clearly malignant and the differential is typically large cell lymphoma (usually diffuse large B-cell lymphoma) versus sarcoma, a poorly differentiated carcinoma, or melanoma. Immunohistochemistry will lead to the correct diagnosis in most cases. Burkitt lymphoma can also present as a mass lesion, although other large cell lymphomas, such as anaplastic large cell lymphoma, are rare in the liver. Of note, one immunostain pitfall is that a subset of diffuse large B-cell lymphomas can be p63-positive. Also, B-cell lymphomas that have been previously treated with rituximab may recur as CD20-negative B-cell lymphomas. As another diagnostic pitfall, lymphocyte-rich hepatocellular carcinomas have dense sinusoidal infiltrates of lymphocytes that can be mistaken for lymphoma. However, the lymphocytes are primarily cytologically bland T-cells with scattered small aggregates of B-cells and occasional lymphoid follicles. The hepatocytes will show architectural and cytological atypia.

In the third setting, with a sinusoidal pattern of disease, important clues to possible malignancy include lymphocytes that have either too much cytoplasm or show significant nuclear atypia. Another finding that suggests malignancy is unusually dense sinusoidal cellularity with relatively little hepatocyte injury. Atypical patterns of lobular necrosis can also be an important observation, as necrosis in the setting of marked hepatitis tends to begin in zone 3. Zone 1 predominant necrosis or nonzonal necrosis (outside the setting of panacinar necrosis) are unusual for the hepatotropic viruses (A, B, C, E), autoimmune hepatitis, or drug induced hepatitis and such cases benefit from workup to exclude lymphoma. Infarct-like coagulative necrosis in the setting of marked inflammation also can be seen with lymphomas.

In the fourth setting, liver specimens show no mass lesions, but on histological examination there are lymphoid infiltrates predominantly in the portal tracts. The differential is primarily chronic hepatitis (e.g., viral, autoimmune, etc.) versus a B-cell lymphoma, such as a small B-cell lymphoma or T-cell/histiocyte-rich large B-cell lymphoma, versus classical Hodgkin lymphoma. Because many primary B-cell lymphomas arise in the setting of chronic viral hepatitis, positive viral serology does not rule out lymphoma. The lymphoid aggregates in chronic viral hepatitis tend to be scattered and small and involve medium-sized and larger sized portal tracts. For this reason, diffuse portal tract involvement, or unusually large aggregates, can be important clues to a diagnosis of lymphoma. Cytological monotony or cytological atypia can also suggest a diagnosis of lymphoma. Challenging cases often show borderline findings on H&E, with only mild atypia. Most borderline cases are classified as benign on further work up, but a subset are lymphoma and borderline cases benefit from further evaluation.

30.4 DIFFUSE LARGE B-CELL LYMPHOMA

Diffuse large B-cell lymphomas are the most common primary lymphoma of the liver, making up 50% to 90% of cases in most case series.[40–42] They typically involve the liver as radiologically and grossly visible mass lesions. Diffuse large B-cell lymphomas are composed of B-cells growing in diffuse sheets. The neoplasms are called large B-cell lymphomas because the tumor cells are more than twice the size of a normal lymphocyte and have nuclei that are larger in size than the nucleus of a normal macrophage or normal endothelial cell. Most diffuse large B-cell lymphomas arise de novo, but some can result from transformation of a small B-cell lymphoma, such as CLL/SLL or follicular lymphoma.

Clinical findings

Chronic hepatitis C and immunosuppression are two well established risk factors for diffuse large B-cell lymphoma primary to the liver.[2] Lymphomas arising in the setting of immunosuppression are more likely to be EBV-associated. Overall, there is a wide age range at presentation, but most are older individuals, with a median age in the seventh decade at diagnosis.

Microscopic findings

About 80% of diffuse large B-cell lymphomas are mass-forming lesions, with sheets of neoplastic cells and destruction of the underlying hepatic architecture (Fig. 30.8). There can be vascular involvement (Fig. 30.9),

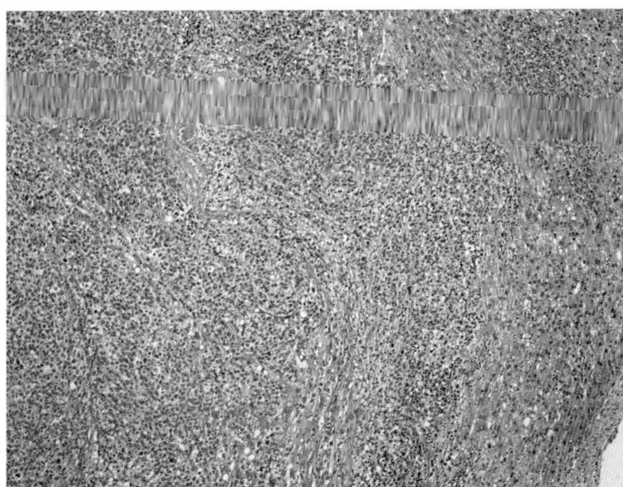

Figure 30.8 Diffuse large B-cell lymphoma. A sheet-like pattern of growth is seen with effacement of the underlying hepatic architecture.

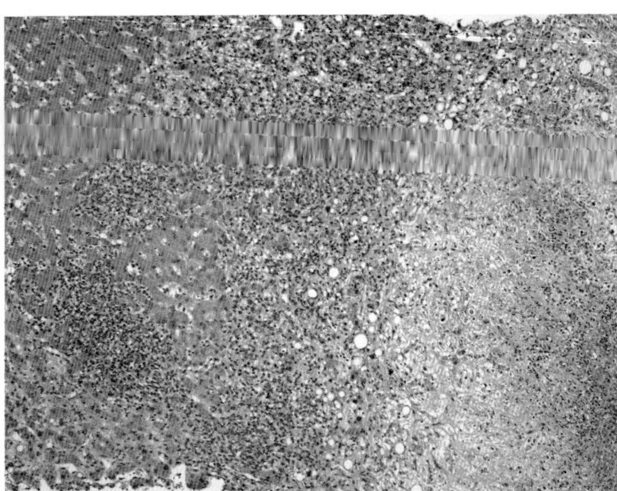

Figure 30.10 Diffuse large B-cell lymphoma. Much of the center of the lymphoma is necrotic. Based on radiological findings, the working diagnosis was an abscess at the time of biopsy.

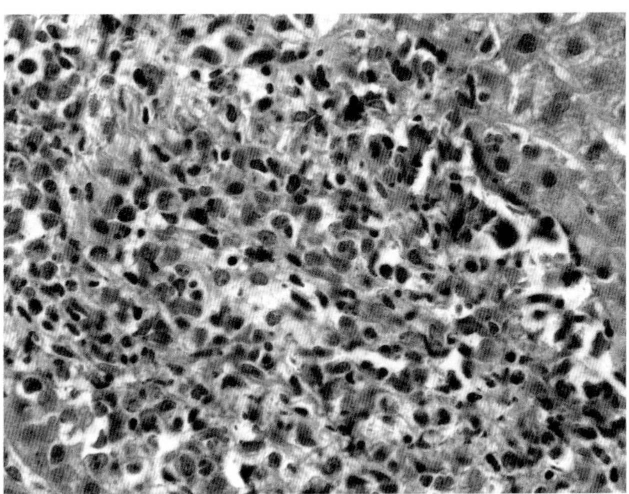

Figure 30.9 Diffuse large B-cell lymphoma. The lymphoma involves a central vein.

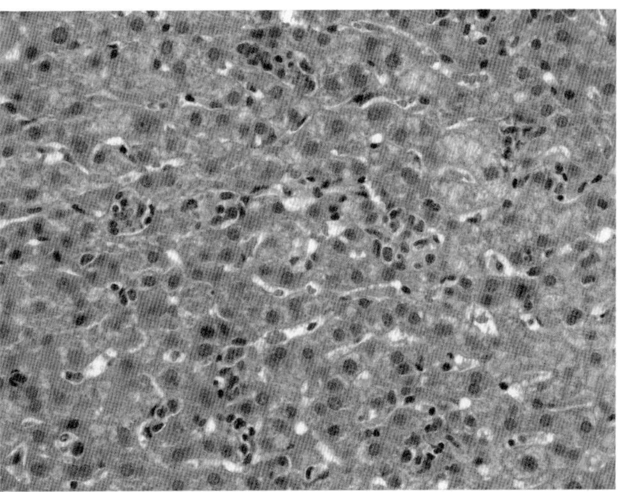

Figure 30.11 Diffuse large B-cell lymphoma. In this case, there are sinusoidal infiltrates.

often associated with necrosis (Fig. 30.10). Some diffuse large B-cell lymphomas are associated with fibrosis, which can mimic the desmoplastic response seen with cholangiocarcinomas and metastatic disease. In a minority of cases, the diffuse large B-cell lymphomas show a portal-based growth pattern, often with tumor infiltrates in the sinusoids (Fig. 30.11), giving a hepatitis-like pattern.[41,44]

Diffuse large B-cell lymphomas have two main cell types, the centroblast and the immunoblast. A centroblast is a B-cell with moderate amounts of basophilic cytoplasm, round to oval nuclei with vesicular chromatin, and one to several nucleoli that are adjacent to the nuclear membrane. In contrast, an immunoblast is a larger cell with abundant basophilic to amphophilic cytoplasm, large oval nucleus with vesicular chromatin and a single centrally located "cherry red" nucleolus. Anaplastic cells, which have marked nuclear pleomorphism, can also be present. Plasmablastic cells, which show eccentrically located nuclei with abundant basophilic cytoplasm, are characteristic of a separate entity known as plasmablastic lymphoma.

General immunohistochemical findings

Diffuse large B-cell lymphomas, not otherwise specified, are positive for pan-B-cell markers, including CD19, CD20, CD22, CD79a, and PAX-5. A CD20 immunostain should always be performed, both because it is a robust B-cell marker and because CD20 expression is a target for monoclonal antibody therapy. Some cases, particularly after monoclonal antibody therapy (e.g., rituximab), can lose expression of CD20 and other B-cell markers, so multiple additional pan B-cell stains may be needed. The neoplastic cells may be positive for the activation marker CD30, but should be negative for CD15. Ki-67 proliferation rate is variable but is often high (>40%).

The Hans algorithm provides prognostic and therapeutic information. The algorithm uses immunostain expression to separate diffuse large B-cell lymphomas into germinal center and nongerminal center subtypes, based on the staining pattern seen with CD10, BCL6, and MUM1 (Figs. 30.12 and 30.13). The Hans algorithm is reasonably simple to use, even for a liver pathologist (Table 30.5). A stain cut-off of 30% or more of the tumor cells is used for scoring a stain as positive. Overall, about 65% of hepatic diffuse large cell B-cell lymphomas are of the nongerminal center type.[1] In general, the germinal center B-cell-like subgroup has a better clinical outcome than those with the nongerminal center B-cell-like subgroup.[44] In addition, it is recommended that immunohistochemistry for BCL2 and MYC be performed on all diffuse large B-cell lymphomas for prognostic purposes, as those that coexpress BCL2 and MYC (so called *double expressors*) tend to have a poorer prognosis than those that do not.[45] Recommended cutoffs for positivity are ≥40% for MYC and >50% for BCL2. Finally, it is recommended that interphase fluorescence in situ hybridization (FISH) for MYC (and additional probes such as BCL2, BCL6, IGH/MYC, IGL/MYC, and IGK/MYC as needed) be performed in all diffuse large B-cell lymphomas to exclude the possibility of a "high-grade B-cell lymphoma with MYC and BCL2 and/or BCL6 translocations" (discussed below).

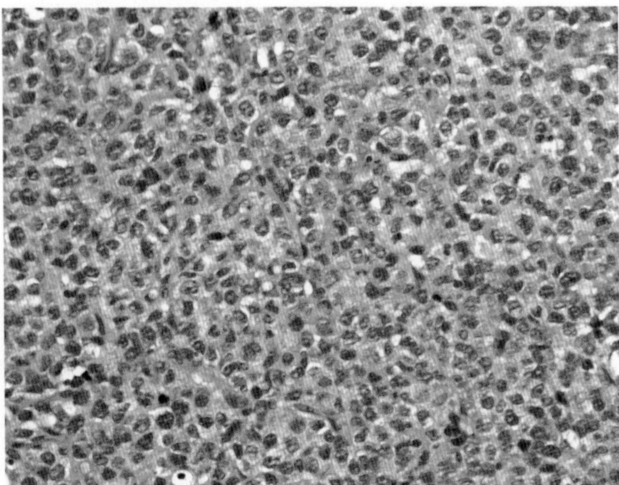

Figure 30.12 Diffuse large B-cell lymphoma. This case presented with a solid tumor mass. Immunostains showed a germinal center B-cell phenotype by the Hans algorithm: CD 10-negative, BCL6-positive, and MUM1-negative.

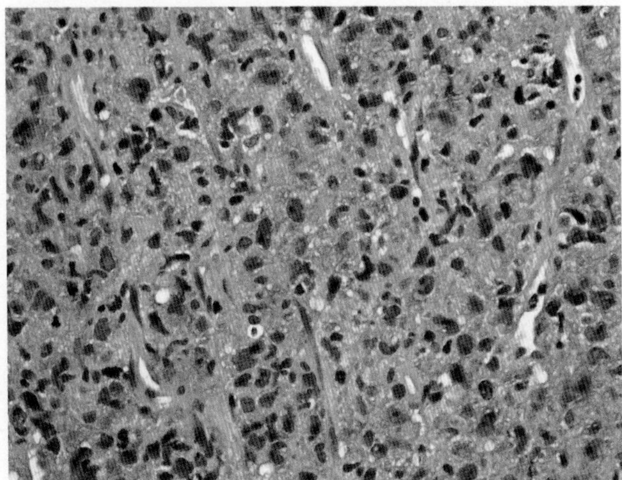

Figure 30.13 Diffuse large B-cell lymphoma. The cells are large with irregular nuclear profiles. Immunostains showed a nongerminal center B-cell phenotype by the Hans algorithm: CD10-negative, BCL6-positive, MUM1-positive.

High-grade B-cell lymphomas

Some lymphomas are very difficult to classify because they have features that overlap with both diffuse large B-cell lymphoma and with Burkitt lymphoma. For example, the histology can fit well enough for Burkitt lymphoma in some areas, but other areas may have more nuclear pleomorphism and cells may express BCL2 and/or MUM-1, or may have a Ki-67 proliferative rate that is less than 95%. These B-cell lymphomas with aggressive histology were referred to in the 2008 World Health Organization (WHO) classification as "B-cell, lymphoma unclassifiable with features intermediate between diffuse large B-cell lymphoma and Burkitt lymphoma." However, it was also recognized that a 5% to 10% of diffuse large B-cell lymphomas and 25% to 40% of B-cell lymphomas with high-grade histologic features have translocations involving MYC and BCL2 and/or BCL6, and that these lymphomas have a much more aggressive clinical course. These lymphomas were informally called "double hit" or "triple hit" lymphomas. To unify these histologic, cytogenetic and prognostic features, the diagnosis of "B-cell lymphoma, unclassifiable, with features intermediate between diffuse large B-cell lymphoma and Burkitt lymphoma" has been replaced by two new diagnostic categories per the revised 2016 WHO classification.[46] Diffuse large B-cell lymphomas and high-grade B-cell lymphomas that have translocations involving MYC and BCL2 and/or BCL6 are referred to as *high-grade B-cell lymphoma with MYC and BCL2 and/or BCL6 translocations*, and, those with high-grade histology but lack MYC and BCL2 and/or BCL6 translocations are referred to as *high grade B-cell lymphoma, not otherwise specified*. The translocations are typically identified by interphase FISH.

Table 30.5 Hans algorithm for sub classifying diffuse large B cell lymphoma

Marker			
CD10-positive	Germinal center B-cell		
CD10-negative	BCL6-negative	MUM1-negative	Non-Germinal center B-cell
CD10-negative	BCL6-positive/negative	MUM1-positive	Non-germinal center B-cell
CD10-negative	BCL6-positive	MUM1-negative	Germinal center B-cell

Most "high-grade B-cell lymphomas with translocations involving MYC and BCL2 and/or BCL6" are of germinal center B-cell phenotype by Hans criteria.[47,48] As some "high-grade B-cell lymphomas with translocations involving MYC and BCL2 and/or BCL6" have the histologic features of diffuse large B-cell lymphoma, many centers routinely perform immunohistochemistry and interphase FISH to exclude this possibility in all newly diagnosed diffuse large B-cell lymphomas[43] as well as in all high-grade B-cell lymphomas.

Other large B-cell lymphomas

ALK-positive large B-cell lymphoma is very rare.[47] Immunostains for ALK typically show granular cytoplasmic staining, though nuclear staining may also be present, with staining patterns correlating with the type of translocation. The tumor cells should be negative for T-cell markers and for T-cell receptor rearrangements. CD45 is expressed in most cases and epithelial membrane antigen (EMA) in nearly all cases. Many of the usual pan-B-cell markers will be negative, but plasma cell markers are often positive, such as CD38 and CD138. CD30 is positive in about 5% of cases. EBV and HHV8 studies should be negative.

The 2008 WHO provisional entity, "EBV-associated diffuse large B-cell lymphoma of the elderly," has been replaced by the diagnosis "EBV-positive diffuse large B-cell lymphoma" in the 2016 revised WHO classification.[46] This change was brought about because it was recognized that EBV+ DLBCL may occur in younger patients, the morphologic spectrum is broader than previously recognized, and clinical outcome may be more favorable than originally thought. T-cell-rich/histiocyte-rich large B-cell lymphoma looks different from other members of the diffuse large B-cell lymphoma family, because most of the cells in the infiltrate are small, reactive T lymphocytes (Fig. 30.14). However, CD20 will highlight large cells scattered throughout the infiltrates. Scattered clusters of histiocytes can also be seen. The large B-cells are sometimes easiest to find by first identifying histiocyte clusters, and then looking nearby. This variant may resemble classical Hodgkin lymphoma, but can be distinguished by immunohistochemistry.

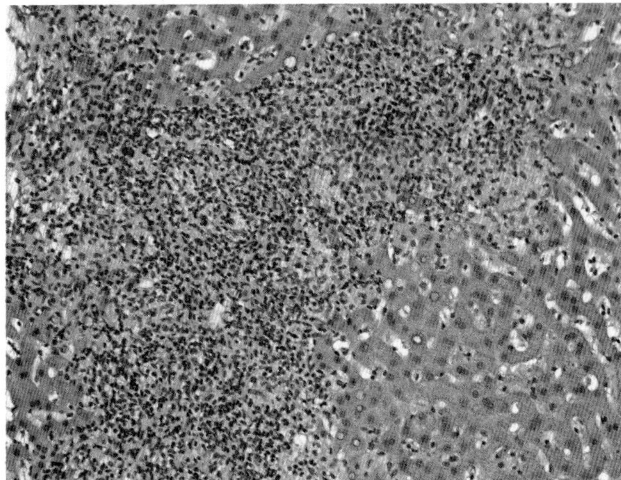

Figure 30.14 T-cell rich/histiocyte-rich large B-cell lymphoma. Most of the infiltrates are small lymhoyctes with scattered clusters of histiocytes.

Differential diagnosis

The differential diagnosis for diffuse large B-cell lymphoma includes other lymphomas, such as classical Hodgkin lymphoma, high-grade B-cell lymphoma, and anaplastic large cell lymphoma, among others, as well as poorly differentiated carcinoma and malignant melanoma. A helpful approach with poorly differentiated cases is to include markers in the first round of immunostains that cover a broad spectrum of keratins as well as multiple B-cell and lymphocyte markers and multiple melanoma markers. One example would be CAM5.2, CKAE1/3, CD3, CD20, CD30, CD45, PAX5, S100, and Melan A. Additional markers could be included based on the morphological findings and results of the first round of immunohistochemical stains.

30.5 BURKITT LYMPHOMA

Burkitt lymphoma is a B-cell lymphoma composed of intermediate-sized malignant B-cells that can present with liver disease. Burkitt lymphoma is an aggressive lymphoma and is seen more frequently in children. The well-known *MYC* translocation at 8q24 is highly characteristic, but not specific.

Clinical findings

Burkitt lymphoma can be endemic, sporadic, or immunodeficiency-associated. The endemic form is found in equatorial Africa in young children and is most commonly associated with EBV infection, less often with malarial infection. Liver involvement is secondary, with the primary disease involving the jaws and facial bones. Individuals with the sporadic form of Burkitt lymphoma can present with bulky disease involving the liver or other organs, or with a leukemic phase. The sporadic form is seen throughout the world and only a small subgroup is associated with EBV infection. Finally, immunodeficiency-associated Burkitt lymphoma is most commonly seen in the setting of HIV infection, with up to 40% associated with EBV infection. Liver involvement is secondary and often not biopsied because of known disease. Therapy for Burkitt lymphoma can lead to the tumor lysis syndrome, with hypocalcemia, hyperkalemia, hyperphosphatemia, and hyperuricemia, all of which results from the rapid death of many tumor cells.

Microscopic findings

Burkitt lymphoma typically presents with bulky, mass forming disease that displaces and destroys the normal liver architecture. The lymphoma is composed of intermediate-sized tumor cells with scant but visible cytoplasm and finely dispersed nuclear chromatin with multiple small nucleoli (Fig. 30.15). There are numerous mitotic figures and apoptotic bodies, along with numerous scattered tingible-body macrophages. The macrophages, when set against the background of a monomorphic population of lymphocytes, give the classic "starry sky" appearance, a pattern most easily recognized in lymph nodes and only rarely seen in the liver.

Immunohistochemical findings

Burkitt lymphomas are positive for pan-B-cell antigens CD19, CD20, CD22, CD79a, and PAX-5. They also coexpress CD10, BCL-6, CD43 and CD38,[47] and are negative for BCL-2. A Ki-67 typically shows nearly a 100% cell proliferation rate.[43,47]

Although *MYC* translocations are not specific, they are characteristic of Burkitt lymphoma. Most

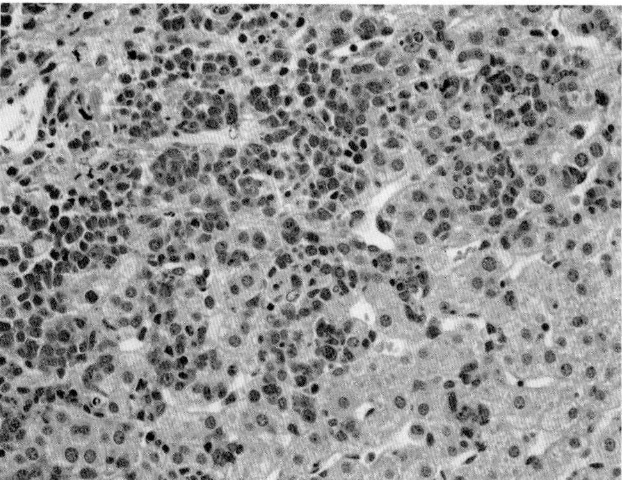

Figure 30.15 Burkitt lymphoma. The tumor cells infiltrate the sinusoids. They have finely dispersed chromatin with multiple small nucleoli.

cases have the classic t(8;14)(q24;q32) translocation, leading to fusion of the *MYC* and *IGH* genes. *MYC* translocations involving the kappa immunoglobulin light chain gene at 2p11 or the lambda immunoglobulin light chain at 22q11 are less common but can be seen in up to 20% of cases. However, MYC translocations involving nonimmunoglobulin genes are rare to absent in Burkitt lymphoma. Most current classification systems require documenting MYC translocations to confirm the diagnosis of Burkitt lymphoma.[47] However, Burkitt lymphomas do not have translocations involving the *BCL2* or *BCL6* genes. Although uncommon, a small number of cases of lymphomas resemble Burkitt lymphoma but lack MYC translocations. Instead, these cases have proximal gains and telomeric losses of chromosome 11q. This lymphoma, termed *Burkitt-like lymphoma with 11q aberration*, is a new provisional entity per the 2016 revised WHO classification.[46]

30.6 MARGINAL ZONE LYMPHOMA

Clinical findings

Extranodal marginal zone lymphomas of mucosa-associated lymphoid tissue, also called mucosa-associated lymphoid tissue (MALT) lymphomas, can be primary to the liver. However, most cases of hepatic marginal zone lymphoma represent secondary liver involvement by nodal marginal zone lymphomas, splenic marginal zone lymphomas or MALT lymphoma arising in another extranodal site, such as the stomach. Risk factors for primary MALT lymphomas of the liver include primary biliary cirrhosis, autoimmune hepatitis, and chronic hepatitis C and B.[3,48]

Microscopic findings

Marginal zone lymphomas are small B-cell lymphomas that have a heterogeneous appearance, being composed of a prominent component of monocytoid lymphocytes, accompanied by small lymphocytes, scattered immunoblasts, and centroblast-like cells. The monocytoid cells are small- to medium-sized, often with fairly abundant, pale cytoplasm. The nuclei have dispersed chromatin and inconspicuous nucleoli. In some cases, the tumor cells can show plasmacytic differentiation (light chain–restricted), although polytypic plasma cells may also be present. Light chain restriction can be demonstrated by immunohistochemical stains for kappa and lambda immunoglobulin light chains. Larger cells, including centroblasts or immunoblasts, make up a minority of the cell population and are typically scattered throughout the lymphoma infiltrates. Marginal zone lymphomas typically show a portal-based pattern of growth (Fig. 30.16). Lymphoepithelial lesions involving the bile ducts can be found, but are not specific for MALT lymphoma. A diagnosis requires exclusion of other small B-cell lymphomas by using immunohistochemistry (Table 30.6).

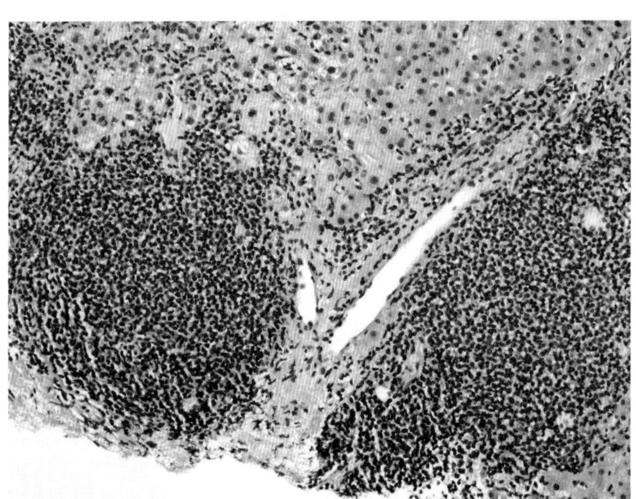

Figure 30.16 Marginal zone lymphoma (MALT Lymphoma). A dense infiltrate of small- to medium-sized lymphocytes is seen within a portal tract.

Immunohistochemical findings

The neoplastic B-cell lymphocytes are positive for pan-B-cell antigens CD19, CD20, CD22, CD79a, and PAX-5. About one-third of cases are CD43-positive. However, the tumor cells are usually negative for CD5 and are also negative for markers that are used to classify other small B-cell lymphomas, such as CD10, CD23, and cyclin D1. They are also typically negative for IgD, in contrast to the B-cells of normal primary follicles.

30.7 MANTLE CELL LYMPHOMA

Microscopic findings

Mantle cell lymphoma is a B-cell lymphoma that typically involves the portal tracts (Fig. 30.17). Most cases are composed of monotonous lymphocytes with small to medium-sized lymphocytes accompanied by scattered epithelioid histiocytes and hyalinized blood vessels. Some cases can undergo blastoid transformation and rare cases can show plasmacytic differentiation.

Immunohistochemical features

The lymphoma cells are positive for the usual pan-B-cell antigens such as CD19, CD20, CD22, CD79a, and PAX-5. The tumor cells also usually coexpress CD5, cyclin D1 (sometimes called BCL1), CD43[49–51] and SOX11, but are negative for CD10 and CD23 (Table 30.6). A t(11;14)(q13;q32) is typically present, which leads to a fusion between the cyclin D1 (*CCND1*) and immunoglobulin heavy chain (*IGH*) genes. This translocation can be detected by interphase FISH in difficult cases,

Table 30.6 Lymphomas composed of small to medium sized B cells with predominant portal tract involvement

Immunohistochemial stain	Follicular (%)	Marginal zone (%)	Mantle cell (%)	CLL/SLL (%)	Lymphoplasmacytic (%)
CD10	90	1	1	0	1
BCL2	90	80	90	95	60
CD43	5	35	90	80	20
CD23	20	10	1	90	10
CD5	<5	20	90	90	5
CyclinD1	0	0	95	0	0

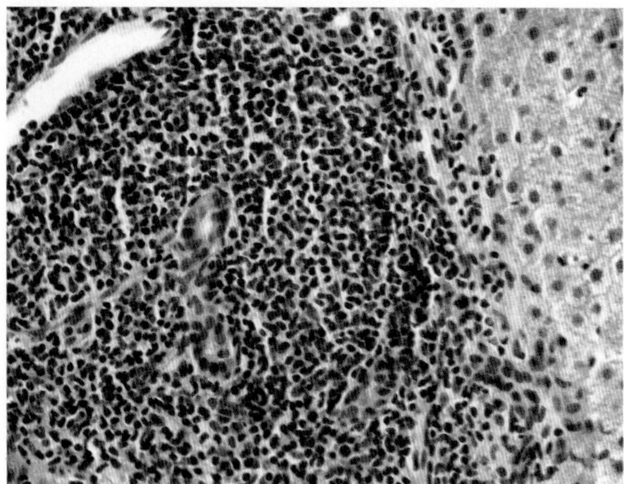

Figure 30.17 Mantle cell lymphoma. The portal tracts are densely infiltrated by monomorphic, small- to medium-sized B-cells. The lymphoma arose in the setting of chronic hepatitis C.

although usually immunohistochemistry for cyclin D1 is sufficient. Rare cases of cyclinD1-negative mantle cell lymphoma have been described, about half of which have translocations involving the CCND2 gene.[52] These cases are typically SOX11-positive.

Differential diagnosis

The differential diagnosis includes other small B-cell lymphomas as well as reactive lymphoid infiltrates. Mantle cell lymphomas may have residual germinal centers and/or may have a nodular growth pattern, but the atypical follicles characteristic of follicular lymphoma are not seen. Proliferation centers, seen in CLL/SLL, are also absent. The neoplastic cells in mantle lymphoma tend to be more uniform in appearance than the cells in marginal zone lymphomas at low power, but often have irregular nuclear contours, somewhat resembling centrocytes at high power. However, immunohistochemistry is necessary to verify the diagnosis of mantle cell lymphoma and exclude other small B-cell lymphomas. This is especially important for the diagnosis of mantle cell lymphoma, as its clinical course is typically more aggressive than that of other small B-cell lymphomas.

30.8 FOLLICULAR LYMPHOMA

Follicular lymphoma typically shows a portal-based infiltration of the liver, with the neoplasm composed of centrocytes (small cleaved B-cells with clumped chromatin and inconspicuous nucleoli) and centroblasts (large noncleaved B-cells with open chromatin and several peripherally located nucleoli), typically with a follicular pattern of growth. The follicular growth pattern can be focal (Fig. 30.18) and is often not apparent on liver biopsy specimens (Fig. 30.19). The neoplastic follicles often lack both tingible-body macrophages as well as the normal polarization of centrocytes and centroblasts into light and dark zones, and the mantle zones are often attenuated.

When there is enough tissue on a biopsy, follicular lymphomas can be graded by calculating the average number of centroblasts per 40× field in a total of ten fields. Lymphomas are graded as follows: grade 1, 0 to 5 centroblasts/hpf; grade 2, 6 to 15 centroblasts/hpf; grade 3A, greater than 15 centroblasts/hpf with centrocytes present; and grade 3B, greater than 15 centroblasts/hpf with solid sheets of centroblasts.[53–55] Follicular lymphomas with grades 3A or 3B tend to behave more aggressively. They also are more likely to progress to diffuse large B-cell lymphoma.[56–68]

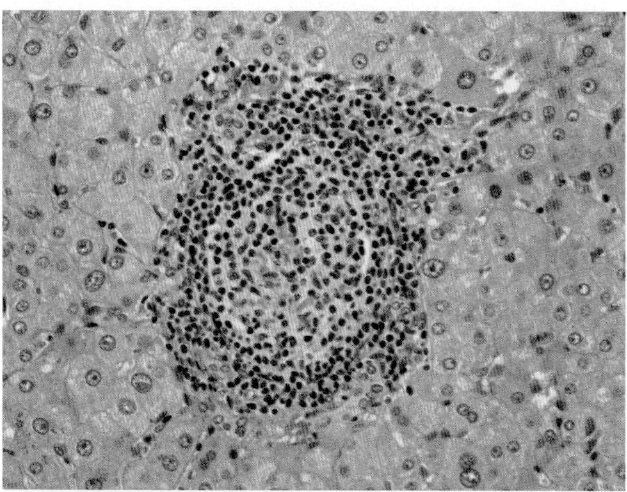

Figure 30.18 Follicular lymphoma. A small follicle is seen in the portal tract.

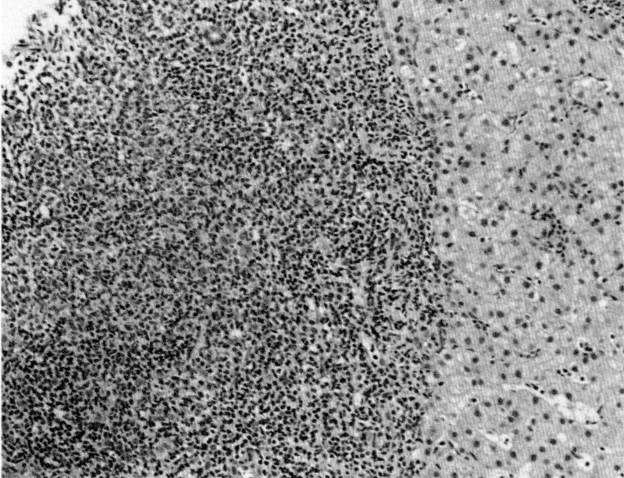

Figure 30.19 Follicular lymphoma. This small B-cell lymphoma arose in the setting of chronic hepatitis C and immunophenotyping was that of a follicular lymphoma.

Immunohistochemical findings

Follicular lymphomas are positive for pan-B-cell markers: CD19, CD20, CD22, CD79a, and PAX-5 and usually coexpress BCL2, BCL6, and CD10. If you're not sure if there is a follicular growth pattern, dendritic cell meshworks can be highlighted with CD21 (preferred) or CD23 immunostains. However, expression of CD10 can be reduced or negative in high-grade follicular lymphomas. Similarly, the tumor cells may lack aberrant expression of BCL2 in 10% of cases overall, but more frequently in grades 3A or 3B. In BCL2-negative cases, clonality can be established either by immunohistochemistry for kappa and lambda immunoglobulin light chains to show light chain restriction or by molecular genetics studies for immunoglobulin gene rearrangements. Interphase FISH to look for a BCL2 gene rearrangement may also be helpful in selected cases. The germinal center B-cells in reactive lymphoid hyperplasia are BCL2-negative. However, BCL2 is still going to be positive in the mantle zones of secondary follicles as well as in primary follicles. Of note, BCL2 positivity is not specific for follicular lymphoma, being present in other low-grade B-cell lymphomas (Table 30.6). Also keep in mind that BCL2 is expressed in normal T-cells.

30.9 CHRONIC LYMPHOCYTIC LEUKEMIA/SMALL LYMPHOCYTIC LYMPHOMA

Chronic lymphocytic leukemia/small lymphocytic lymphomas (CLL/SLL) are B-cell lymphomas composed of small mature lymphocytes that coexpress CD5 and CD23. When mass forming, there can be admixed proliferation centers composed of collections of prolymphocytes and paraimmunoblasts.[69]

Clinical findings

Overall, CLL/SLL is an indolent but incurable neoplasm. The mean age at diagnosis is about 65 years and there is a mild male predominance. Hepatosplenomegaly is often found a presentation, along with generalized lymphadenopathy. The initial diagnosis is only rarely made on liver biopsy.

Occasionally, a diagnosis of diffuse large B-cell lymphoma is made on a liver biopsy in a patient with underlying CLL/SLL (Fig. 30.20). In this setting, the liver biopsy can be prompted by new onset hepatomegaly, as well as other systemic findings such as new onset fever, weight loss, or enlarging lymph nodes. New onset elevations of serum lactate dehydrogenase may be present in about half of cases. Of the diffuse large B-cell lymphomas that arise in CLL/SLL patients,

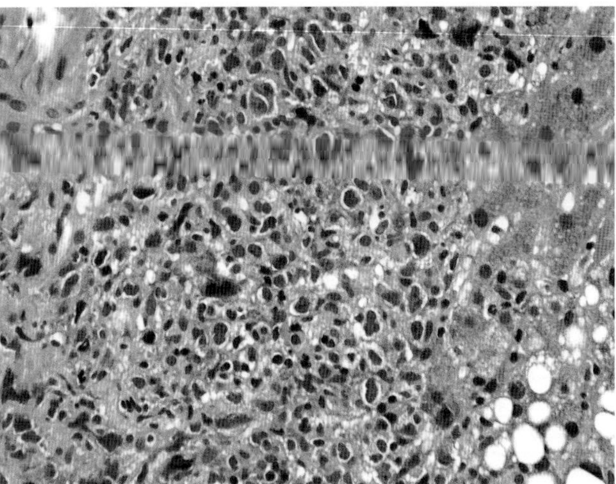

Figure 30.20 Diffuse large B-cell lymphoma. This case arose from Richter transformation of a known chronic lymphocytic leukemia/small lymphocytic lymphoma. By the Hans algorithm, the tumor showed a germinal center B-cell phenotype. The tumor was BCL6, MYC, and BCL2-positive by immunostaining.

about half are transformation of the original CLL/SLL (Richter transformation) and the other half are de novo diffuse large B-cell lymphoma. As the prognosis for the latter group is far more favorable, it is important to look for clonal identity between the original CLL/SLL and the diffuse large B-cell lymphoma by performing molecular genetics studies on both tumors to determine whether the diffuse large B-cell lymphoma is de novo or a Richter transformation. Richter transformation, which occurs in about 5% of CLL/SLL cases, usually manifests as diffuse large B-cell lymphoma, but classical Hodgkin lymphoma and peripheral T-cell lymphoma can also develop.[70,71] The prognosis after transformation is poor, measured in months.

Microscopic findings

Most cases of CLL/SLL are characterized by large nodular aggregates of lymphocytes involving the portal tracts. The lymphocytes are small, with round nuclei, coarsely clumped chromatin, and scant cytoplasm. In some portal tracts, ill-defined pale areas may be found, which correspond to proliferation centers, a finding that is typical of CLL/SLL (Fig. 30.21). In addition to small lymphocytes, proliferation centers contain prolymphocytes and paraimmunoblasts, whose larger size and abundant cytoplasm contribute to the pale color seen at low power. Prolymphocytes are small- to medium-sized cells that have clumped nuclear chromatin and small nucleoli, whereas the paraimmunoblasts are larger cells, with basophilic cytoplasm, somewhat more oval nuclei, dispersed

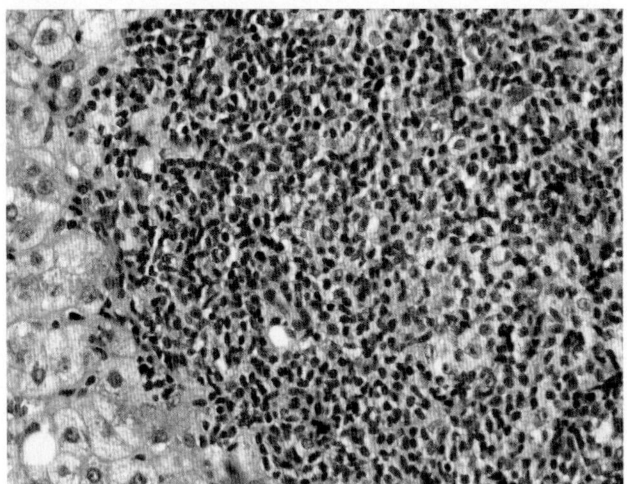

Figure 30.21 Chronic lymphocytic leukemia/small lymphocytic lymphoma. The portal tracts are markedly expanded by small monotonous lymphocytes. The ill-defined pale area in the center is a proliferation center.

chromatin, and a central eosinophilic nucleolus. Although there is often a bit of spillover into the sinusoids, CLL/SLL generally does not show a sinusoidal predominant pattern of growth. However, rare cases can show both portal and sinusoidal growth patterns (Fig. 30.22). Crush artifact is common and can make the diagnosis challenging on small biopsies.

Immunohistochemical findings

The lymphocytes in CLL/SLL are positive for pan-B-cell antigens such as CD19, CD20, CD22, CD79a, and PAX-5. The neoplastic cells also express CD5, CD23, CD43 and LEF1, and are negative for CD10, cyclin D1 and SOX11.[44,68,72,73,78]

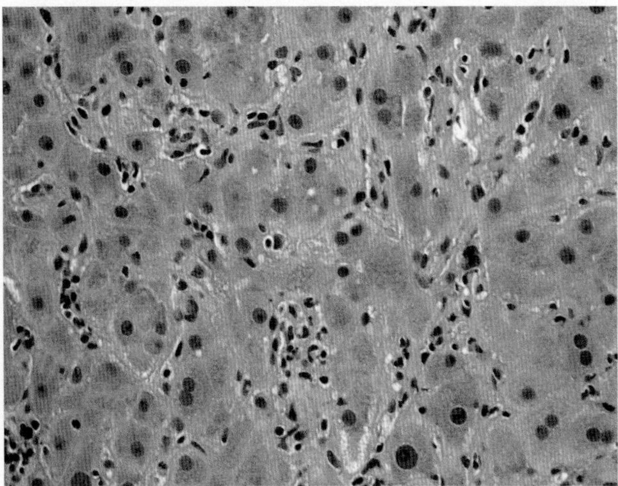

Figure 30.22 Chronic lymphocytic leukemia/small lymphocytic lymphoma. In this case, there was sinusoidal growth in addition to portal tract involvement.

Differential diagnosis

The differential diagnosis includes other small B-cell lymphomas, such as mantle cell lymphoma, lymphoplasmacytic lymphoma, marginal zone lymphoma, and follicular lymphoma (Table 30.6). Proliferation centers strongly favor a diagnosis of CLL/SLL. Mantle cell lymphomas are generally CD23-negative, whereas most CLL/SLLs are CD23-positive. Cyclin D1 is positive in mantle cell lymphomas but not in CLL/SLL. The proliferation centers in CLL/SLL can occasionally show focal cyclin D1 staining, but they are uniformly negative for SOX11.[73] Lymphoplasmacytic lymphomas have marked plasmacytoid differentiation and most are CD5-negative. The neoplastic cells in marginal zone lymphoma tend to have more abundant and pale cytoplasm, and are usually negative for CD5 and CD23. The neoplastic follicles in follicular lymphomas tend to be much better demarcated than the vague borders of proliferation centers. Cleaved cells are easily found in the follicles and interfollicular spaces of follicular lymphoma. Follicular lymphomas are typically CD10-positive and BCL2-positive, but are CD5-negative and CD43-negative.

30.10 POSTTRANSPLANT LYMPHOPROLIFERATIVE DISORDERS

Posttransplant lymphoproliferative disorders develop in transplanted individuals, with either solid organ or bone marrow transplants. Most are EBV-associated. Posttransplant lymphoproliferative disorder (PTLD) involving the liver is most often primary and seen after liver transplantation, but the liver can be secondarily involved when PTLD develops in association with other immunosuppressed conditions. PTLD encompasses a range of lymphoproliferative diseases. At one end of the spectrum are EBV-associated mononucleosis-like polyclonal proliferations. On the other end of the spectrum are aggressive B-cell lymphomas (most common), usually diffuse large B-cell lymphomas or T-cell lymphomas that are essentially identical to those that occur in immunocompetent individuals. Of note, low-grade B-cell lymphomas, such as marginal zone lymphoma, are generally not regarded as PTLD and are classified the same as in the normal host.[69]

There are four types of PTLD in the current classification schema. First, there are early proliferations, mostly mononucleosis-like posttransplant lymphoproliferative disorders, which share significant overlap with EBV hepatitis. Early lesions may also manifest as plasmacytic hyperplasia. The second form is polymorphic PTLD. Polymorphic PTLD can vary considerably in its overall growth pattern, with some showing a sinusoidal growth pattern, some showing mostly portal disease, and others showing large masses. The PTLD infiltrates have a mixture of immature and mature B-cells, with immunoblasts, lymphocytes, and plasma cells. Occasional atypical large cells are acceptable. About 90% of cases are EBV-positive. A key point is that polymorphic PTLD should have no better diagnosis. In other words, the lesion should not meet the criteria for any recognized types of lymphoma. In contrast, monomorphic PTLD (Fig. 30.23) does meet the criteria for one of the recognized lymphomas in immunocompetent individuals, with the exception of low-grade lymphomas, which are simply classified as they would be in an immunocompetent person. Monomorphic PTLD is EBV-positive in 70% to 80% of cases. Finally, the fourth and least common category of PTLD is classical Hodgkin lymphoma-type. Most of these cases are also EBV-positive.

30.11 HODGKIN LYMPHOMA

Hodgkin lymphomas are divided into nodular lymphocyte predominant Hodgkin lymphoma and classical Hodgkin lymphoma. In turn, classic Hodgkin lymphoma has four subtypes: nodular sclerosis (70% of cases), mixed cellularity (20% to 25%), lymphocyte-rich (5%), and lymphocyte-depleted (<1%). Most Hodgkin lymphomas that arise in the liver are classical Hodgkin lymphomas.

Classical Hodgkin lymphoma in the liver typically shows a portal-based growth pattern, but can present as a mass lesion. The infiltrates are often polymorphous and can resemble an inflammatory pseudotumor when they are mass forming. The Hodgkin infiltrates contain mostly reactive small lymphocytes but can have scattered eosinophils and epithelioid histiocytes (Fig. 30.24). Fibrosis can be striking. Classic Hodgkin/Reed–Sternberg cells can also be found in some but not all cases (Fig. 30.25).

Immunohistochemical findings

Hodgkin/Reed–Sternberg cells in classical Hodgkin lymphoma are positive for CD30 and PAX-5, are usually positive for CD15 (75% of cases), and are negative for CD45. They are also typically negative for CD20 and CD79a, although in some cases CD20 and/or CD79a can be weakly/focally positive. Hodgkin/RS cells show membranous staining using CD30 and CD15, but can also show a perinuclear accentuation of the Golgi complex. The Hodgkin/RS cells are positive for EBV (either EBER or EBV LMP) in about 50% of cases overall, most commonly in mixed cellularity classical Hodgkin lymphoma (up to 75% of cases).

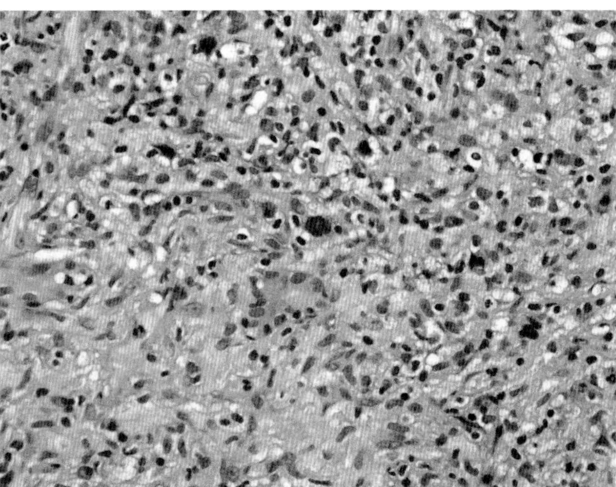

Figure 30.24 Hodgkin lymphoma, classical type. This portal tract has a polymorphous infiltrate including lymphocytes, histiocytes, and scattered esoinophils.

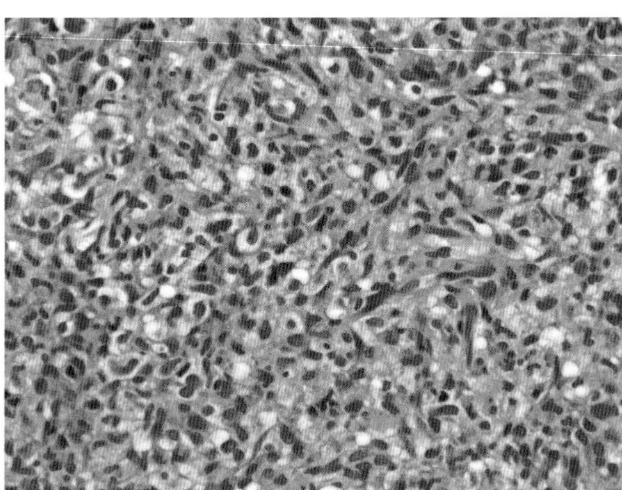

Figure 30.23 Posttransplant lymphoproliferative disorder. A large monomprohic infiltrate is seen in the portal tracts

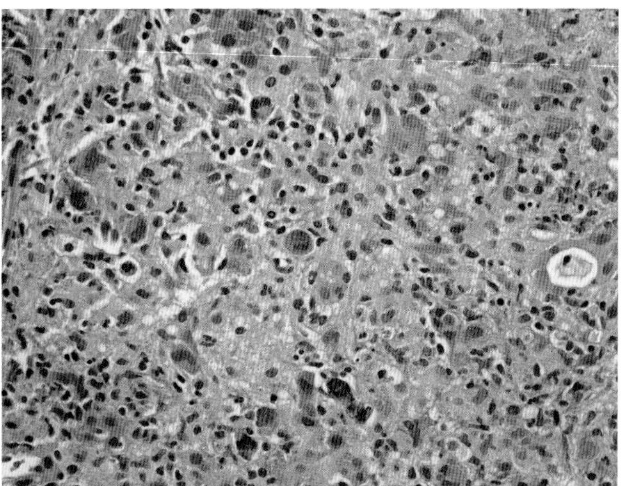

Figure 30.25 Hodgkin lymphoma, classical type. Reed–Sternberg cells are seen.

30.12 ADULT T-CELL LEUKEMIA/ LYMPHOMA

Adult T-cell leukemia/lymphoma is caused by the human T-cell lymphotropic virus type I (HTLV-I) and is found mostly in southwestern Japan, the Caribbean islands, and parts of Central Africa and South America. The disease typically affects adults and is usually systemic, with sinusoidal involvement of the liver and occasionally with portal tract infiltrates. The individual tumor cells can vary widely in morphology, from pleomorphic small cells to anaplastic cells, but in most cases they are medium to large sized. There is significant nuclear atypia, with pleomorphism, coarse chromatin and distinctive but not too prominent nucleoli.

Immunohistochemical findings

The tumor cells are positive for CD2, CD3, and CD5, but usually are negative for CD7. In addition, the tumor cells typically are CD25 and CD4-positive but CD8-negative. The cytotoxic T-cell markers TIA-1 and Granzyme B are negative.

30.13 HEPATOSPLENIC T-CELL LYMPHOMA

Hepatosplenic T-cell lymphoma typically affects young to middle aged men, with a median age at diagnosis of 35 years. Individuals typically have hepatosplenomegaly, but most are without lymphadenopathy or systemic symptoms. However, abnormalities are common in the peripheral blood, including thrombocytopenia, anemia, and leukopenia.

Microscopic findings

Hepatosplenic T-cell lymphomas show a sinusoidal pattern of infiltration (Fig. 30.26), though the portal tracts can also be involved. The tumor cells are larger than normal lymphocytes and often have a thin rim of pale cytoplasm. Overall, nuclear atypia is mild, though scattered more atypical cells can be found in some cases (Fig. 30.27). There is relatively little hepatocyte injury.

Immunohistochemical findings

The neoplastic cells are usually negative for CD4, CD5, and CD8 but positive for CD2, CD3, and CD7. Most cases are classified as γδTCR type and express TCRδ1 but are negative for TCRαβ.[74,75] However, a small subset of cases are of the αβ TCR type.[76,77] Immunostains are positive for TIA-1, but not Granzyme B, consistent with a nonactivated cytotoxic T-cell phenotype. Most cases have an isochromosome 7q.

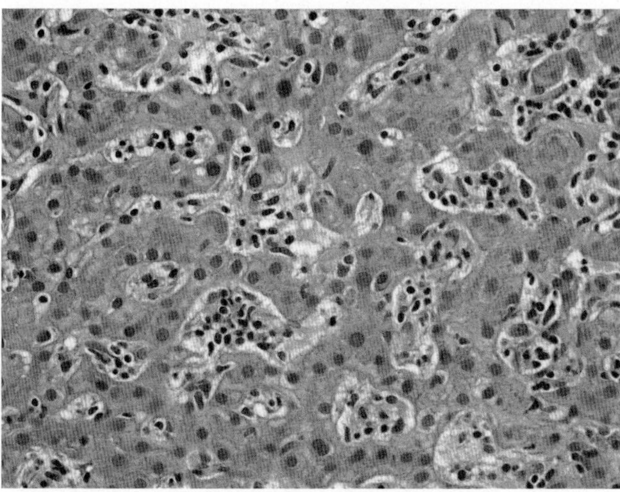

Figure 30.26 Hepatosplenic T-cell lymphoma. The sinusoids are show dense infiltrates of medium-sized lymphocytes.

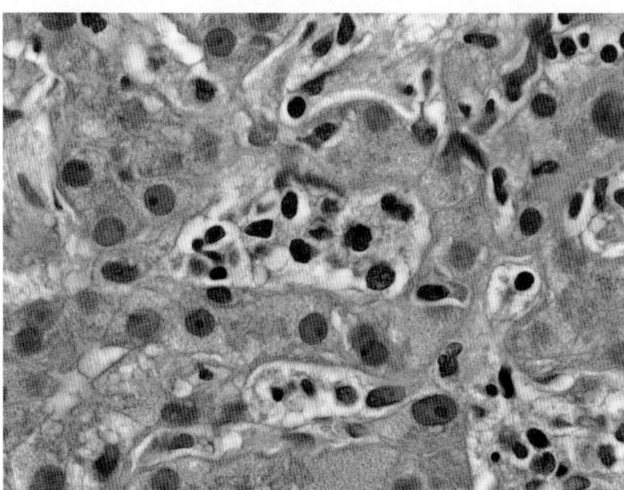

Figure 30.27 Hepatosplenic T-cell lymphoma. On higher power, the lymphocytes have moderate amounts of pale cytoplasm, regular nuclei with loosely condensed chromatin, and small inconspicuous nucleoli.

30.14 ANAPLASTIC LARGE CELL LYMPHOMA

Anaplastic large cell lymphoma is a T-cell lymphoma with a male predominance. The tumor cells express CD30 and are large and pleomorphic. Some have horseshoe-shaped nuclei, a finding called a *hallmark cell* (Fig. 30.28). Four genetic subcategories of anaplastic large cell lymphoma are currently recognized. The first subcategory is ALK-positive and is characterized by ALK expression by immunohistochemistry, corresponding to a rearrangement involving the anaplastic lymphoma kinase (ALK) gene). The other three subcategories are ALK-negative: DUSP22-rearranged, TP63-rearranged, and "triple negative" (negative for ALK, DUSP22, or TP63 rearrangements). The genetic subcategories are important

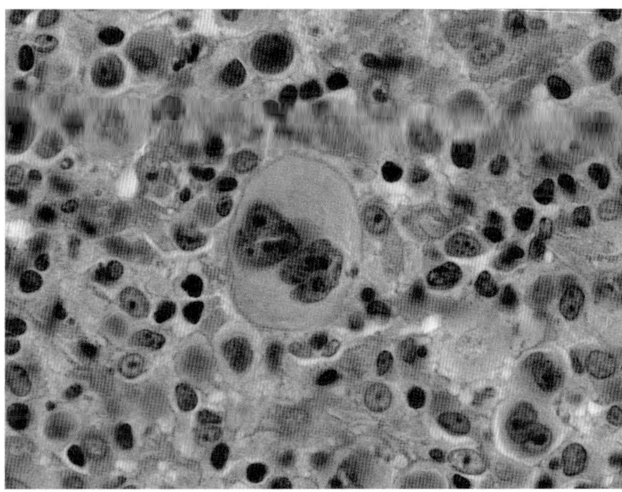

Figure 30.28 Anaplastic large cell lymphoma. "Hallmark" cells are seen, which have eccentric nuclei that are kidney-shaped.

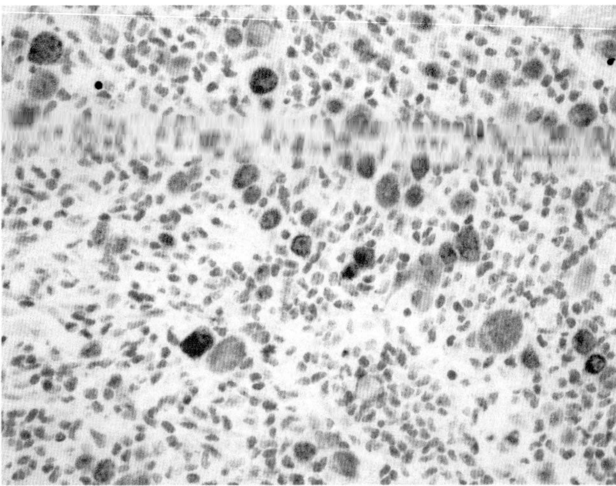

Figure 30.29 Anaplastic large cell lymphoma. The large cells are CD30-positive.

because the ALK-rearranged and DUSP22-rearranged cases tend to have a favorable prognosis, the "triple negative" cases have an intermediate prognosis, and the TP63-rearranged cases tend to have a poor prognosis.[78] ALK-positive cases are most common in younger individuals, often less than 30 years of age, whereas ALK-negative cases are seen in older individuals, most commonly above 40 years of age.

Anaplastic large cell lymphoma can involve the liver with any of the three major growth patterns: mass lesion (most common), portal-based infiltrate, or sinusoidal infiltrates. When growing as a mass lesion, the lymphoma is often destructive with areas of necrosis. In addition to the wide range of growth patterns, anaplastic large cell lymphomas can look very different cytologically. In some cases, the tumor infiltrates are primarily composed of smaller cells (ALK-positive cases), whereas in other case the neoplastic cells are predominantly very large and pleomorphic with abundant cytoplasm. However, in most cases, some cells will show the striking cytological features of hallmark cells: large cells with abundant cytoplasm and eccentrically located nuclei that are horseshoe-shaped or wreath like.

Immunohistochemical findings

Anaplastic large cell lymphoma commonly does not express all of the pan-T-cell antigens. For example, CD3 is negative in about 50% of cases. Overall, CD2, CD3 and CD5 are the most helpful to document lineage. Most cases are CD8-negative and about half are CD4-positive. The tumor cells often express TIA-1 and Granzyme B.[78] CD30 staining is strong and diffuse, with a membranous staining pattern along with staining of the perinuclear Golgi region. The larger cells tend to stain the most strongly for CD30 (Fig. 30.29). Of note, other T-cell lymphomas can show focal CD30 staining, but they will not show the strong diffuse staining seen with anaplastic large cell lymphoma. Most ALK-positive cases show at least focal staining for EMA. The ALK-positive variant of anaplastic large cell lymphoma shows some genotype-phenotype correlation. There is both nuclear and diffuse cytoplasmic staining for ALK with a t(2;5)(p23;q35), correlating with fusion of the *ALK* and *NPM* genes. In contrast, there is diffuse cytoplasmic staining with peripheral enhancement in cases with a t(1;2)(p25;p23), correlating with fusion of the *ALK* and *TPM3* genes. Finally, granular cytoplasmic ALK staining is associated with t(2;17)(p23;q23), correlating with fusion of the *ALK* and *CLTC* genes.

30.15 LEUKEMIAS

Acute leukemias often involve the liver, usually as diffuse hepatomegaly with little or no evidence of hepatic dysfunction. Overall, acute myeloid leukemias tend to diffusely infiltrate the sinusoids (Fig. 30.30), whereas acute lymphoid leukemias tend to involve the portal tracts.[79] Histologically, the liver is infiltrated by myeloblasts or lymphoblasts. Immunostains are needed to positively identify the atypical cells as blasts. Most but not all blasts of both lineages express CD34. Terminal deoxynucleotidyl transferase (TdT) is expressed in most acute lymphoblastic leukemias but may also be positive in a subset of acute myeloid leukemias. By immunohistochemistry, acute myeloid leukemias typically express myeloid markers such as CD13, CD33, CD117, and MPO, and may also express monocytic markers such as CD14, CD68, CD163, and lysozyme. B lymphoblastic leukemia/lymphoma typically expresses CD10, CD19, CD79a, and PAX5, but is often negative for CD20. T lymphoblastic leukemia/lymphoma variably expresses

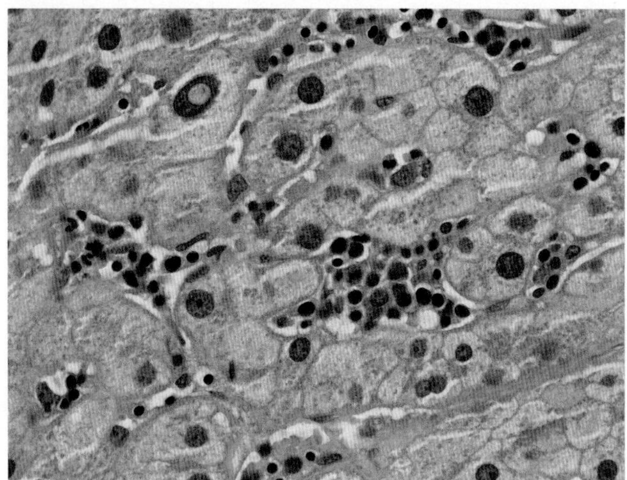

Figure 30.30 Myeloproliferative neoplasm involving the liver. The sinusoids are distended by myeloid precursors.

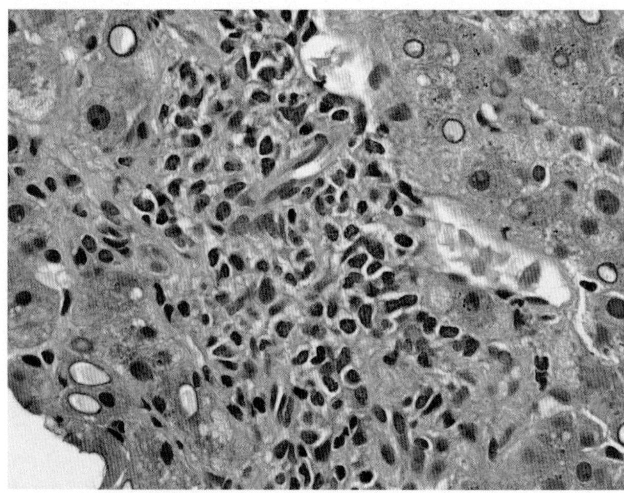

Figure 30.31 Hairy cell leukemia. The neoplastic cells infiltrate the portal tracts.

markers such as CD1a, CD3, CD4, CD5, CD7, and CD8. However, myeloid-lineage markers may be expressed in acute lymphoblastic leukemias and markers typically associated with B- and T-cell lineage may be expressed in acute myeloid leukemias, so it is often prudent to perform extensive immunohistochemical panels if the lineage is unclear. However, a useful starting point may include immunohistochemical stains such as CD3, CD10, CD33, CD34, CD45, CD117, lysozyme, MPO, and TdT.

30.16 HAIRY CELL LEUKEMIA

Hairy cell leukemia is an indolent neoplasm of small mature B-cells that predominately affects middle aged and older men. Hairy cell leukemia shows predominately a sinusoidal growth pattern, but can also involve the portal tracts (Fig. 30.31). The tumor cells are small to medium sized with moderately abundant pale cytoplasm (Fig. 30.32). The nuclei are oval and have inconspicuous nucleoli. The classic "fried-egg" appearance can be seen best in portal infiltrates, but is often hard to appreciate elsewhere. Cases with peliotic-like changes have been described, with pools of red blood cells in dilated sinusoids that are lined by somewhat spindled looking neoplastic cells.[80–82]

Hairy cell leukemia is also positive for the usual pan-B-cell markers of CD19, CD20, CD22, CD79a, and PAX-5. Hairy cell leukemia is positive for CD103 (Fig. 30.33). The tumor cells also express CD25, CD11c, annexin, and tartrate-resistant acid phosphatase, but are negative for both CD5 and CD10. Cyclin D1 can be weakly positive. Hairy cell leukemia has *BRAF* V600E mutations, which can be detected by both molecular methods and immunostains.[83]

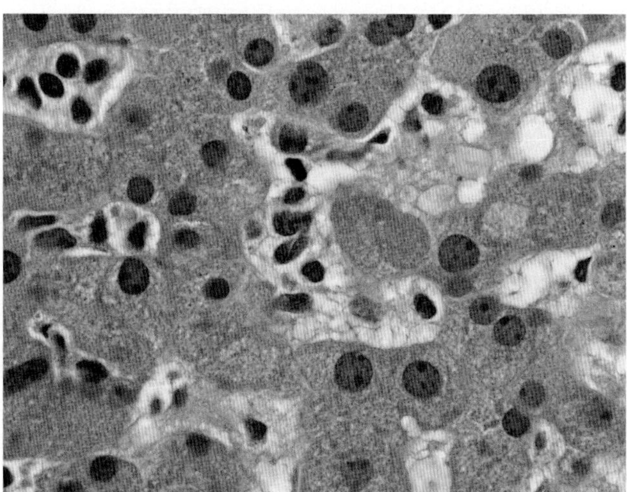

Figure 30.32 Hairy cell leukemia. The tumor cells in the sinusoids have abundant pale cytoplasm.

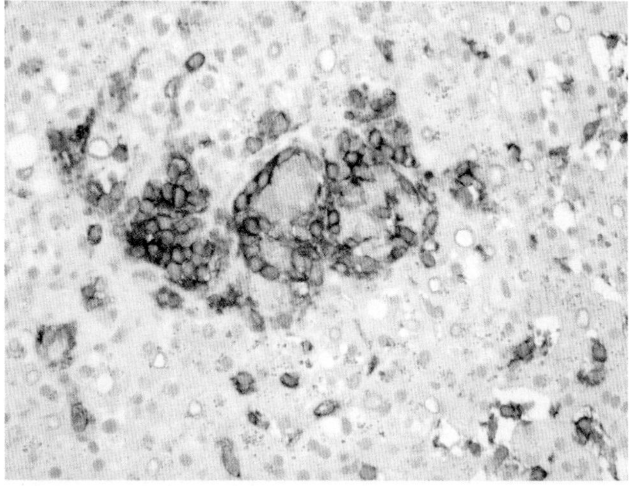

Figure 30.33 Hairy cell leukemia. An immunostain for CD103 is positive.

30.17 LANGERHANS CELL HISTIOCYTOSIS

Langerhans cell histiocytosis typically presents in childhood. Multiple organ involvement is typically present, including the spleen, skin, and bone marrow. Imaging studies of the liver often suggest primary sclerosing cholangitis.

In the liver, Langerhans cell histiocytosis can involve the portal tracts or can diffusely infiltrate the sinusoids, and often does both. In some cases, the Langerhans cells form small clusters in the lobules and portal tracts, suggesting granulomatous disease (Fig. 30.34). Langerhans cell histiocytosis can also form discrete mass lesions that are grossly visible.

The diagnosis can be very subtle and easy to miss when the infiltrates are predominately portal, mimicking an ordinary hepatitis. An important clue is the subtle but distinctive cytology of Langerhans cells, which are oval in shape, and have moderately abundant amphophilic cytoplasm. In some cases, the cytoplasm can appear more vacuolated (Fig. 30.35). Overall, there is minimal to mild nuclear atypia, but the nuclei characteristically have a "coffee bean" morphology, meaning they can be grooved and lobulated. However, this finding is often not as distinctive in the liver as it is in other organs. Another clue to the diagnosis can be a polymorphous infiltrate, which is typical of Langerhans cell histiocytosis, showing scattered single and small clusters of Langerhans cells in a background of abundant eosinophils and scattered neutrophils, lymphocytes, and ordinary histiocytes (Fig. 30.36). Mitotic activity can be brisk. Finally, bile duct damage can also be an important clue, as some cases of Langerhans cell histiocytosis have striking bile duct infiltration and damage, mimicking primary sclerosing cholangitis.

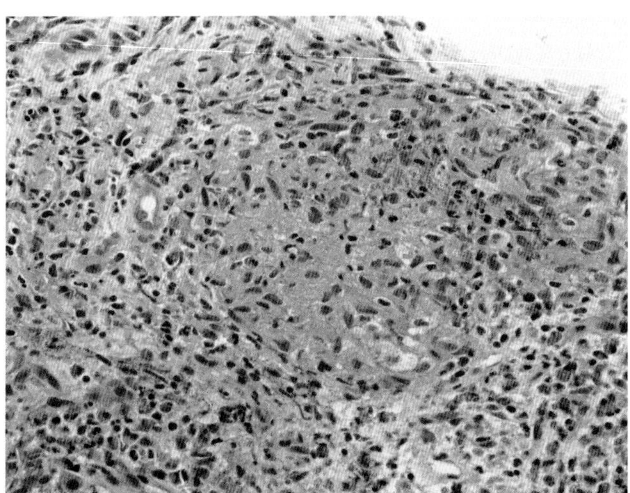

Figure 30.34 Langerhans cell histiocytosis. The granulomatous and eosinophil-rich inflammation initially mimicked a drug reaction.

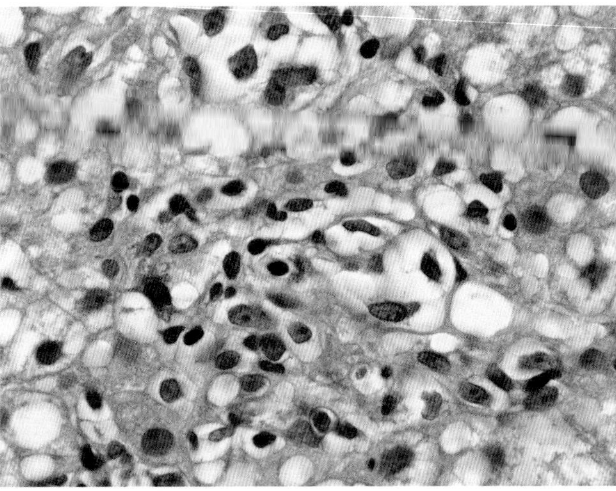

Figure 30.35 Langerhans cell histiocytosis. The Langerhans cells have moderately abundant vacuolated cytoplasm. The nuclei are kidney bean–shaped.

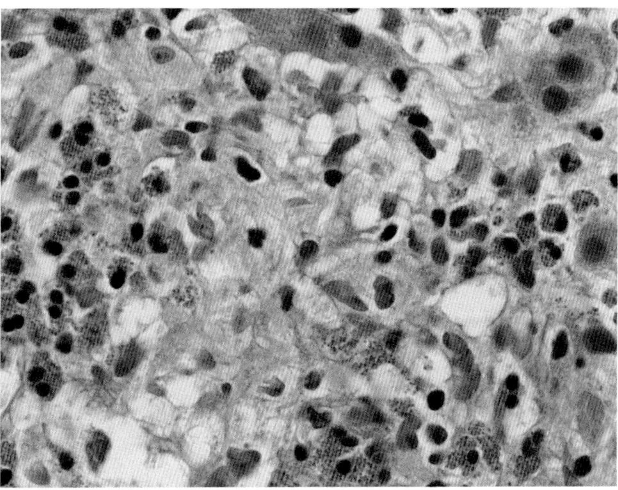

Figure 30.36 Langerhans cell histiocytosis. The Langerhan cells are admixed with numerous eosinophils.

Immunohistochemical findings

Immunostains are positive for CD1a, langerin, and S100. Electron microscopy is only rarely performed, but shows Birbeck granules.

30.18 FOLLICULAR DENDRITIC CELL SARCOMA

Most follicular dendritic cell sarcomas that involve the liver are mass forming and are classified as the inflammatory pseudotumor-like variant because of their close resemblance to inflammatory pseudotumors on H&E. There is a female predominance and most reported cases come from Asia. Histologically, the tumor is composed of spindled to ovoid cells with admixed lymphoplasmacytic inflammation (Fig. 30.37). The spindled cells can grow in sheets, whorls, or have a storiform pattern. Some of the spindle cells can show multinucleation. Follicular dendritic cell sarcomas often have fibrinoid deposits in vessels. Necrosis and hemorrhage can be seen in some cases (Fig. 30.38).

Immunohistochemical findings

Follicular dendritic cell sarcomas, inflammatory pseudotumor-like variant, are positive for markers of follicular differentiation, including CD21, CD23, and CD35. The tumor cells are positive for Epstein–Barr early RNA (EBER) (by in situ hybridization technique) and/or EBV LMP.

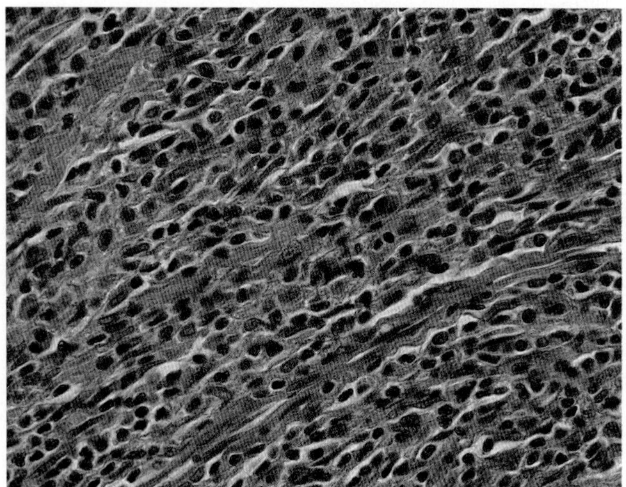

Figure 30.37 Follicular dendritic cell sarcoma. Biopsy of a mass lesion showed a lymphocyte-rich spindle cell proliferation.

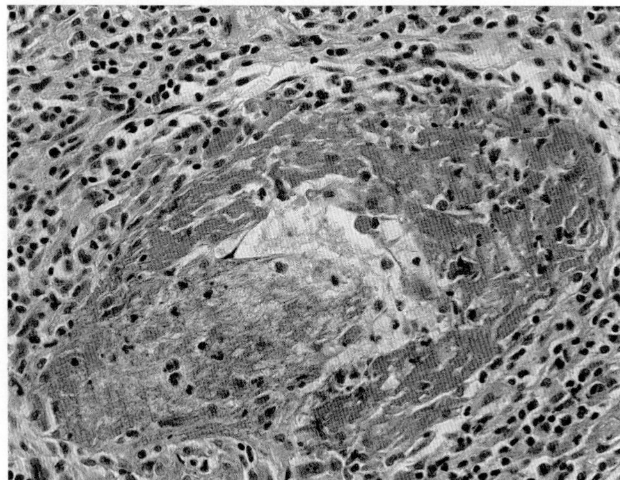

Figure 30.38 Follicular dendritic cell sarcoma. This vessel within the tumor shows inflammatory-type changes and fibrinoid material.

30.19 MASTOCYTOSIS

Systemic mastocytosis can involve the liver and often the diagnosis is first made on the liver biopsy. Hepatomegaly and/or splenomegaly is present in about 50% of individuals. The serum alkaline phosphatase is predominately elevated. Aspartate aminotransferase (AST) and alanine aminotransferase (ALT) levels are normal in most cases, but can be mildly elevated. Clinical findings at presentation can include cholestasis and suggest biliary obstruction.[84,85] About 10% of individuals can present with or later develop ascites.[86] Rarely, individuals can present with a discrete mast cell tumor.[87]

The portal tract and the sinusoids can both be involved and the findings can be very subtle. In some cases, the liver biopsy can look almost normal on low power.[86] In most cases, there are clear portal tract infiltrates (Fig. 30.39) and the first impression is commonly that of a chronic hepatitis. Bile duct injury can also be seen (Fig. 30.40). Mast cells will be admixed with other cells, including lymphocytes, eosinophils, and histiocytes. The mast cells can blend into this background inflammation, but tend to larger and have more cytoplasm (Fig. 30.41). Extramedullary hematopoiesis is found frequently, up to 50% of cases in some studies.[86]

A variety of other secondary changes can also be seen. For example, the lobules show macrovesicular steatosis in about one-third of cases.[86] Mast cell disease of the liver can also be associated with portal venopathy and nodular regenerative hyperplasia.[86] Veno-occlusive disease has been reported.[86] Some cases can have mild portal fibrosis and or mild sinusoidal fibrosis, but advanced fibrosis is uncommon and the ascites seen in most individuals appears to be secondary to portal venopathy and or veno-occlusive disease and not cirrhosis.[86,88]

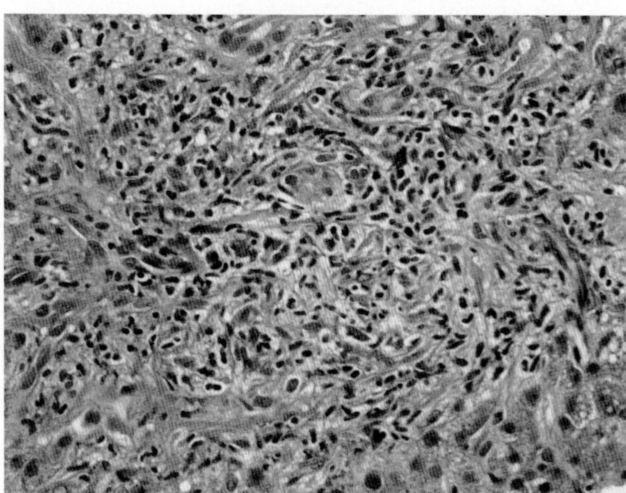

Figure 30.39 Mast cell disease. The portal tract is involved by mast cell disease.

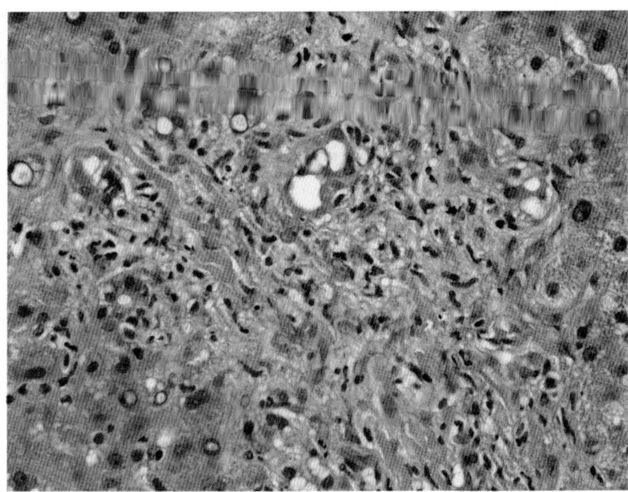

Figure 30.40 Mast cell disease. The mast cell infiltrates are associated with bile duct injury.

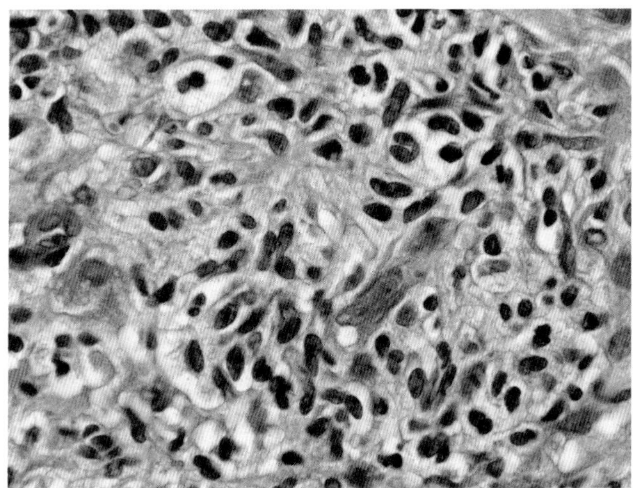

Figure 30.41 Mast cell disease. The mast cell infiltrates have moderately abundant clear cytoplasm.

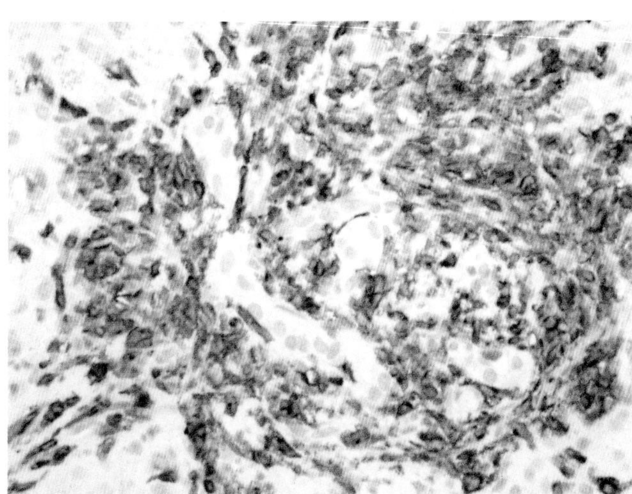

Figure 30.42 Mast cell disease. The mast cell infiltrates are CKIT-positive.

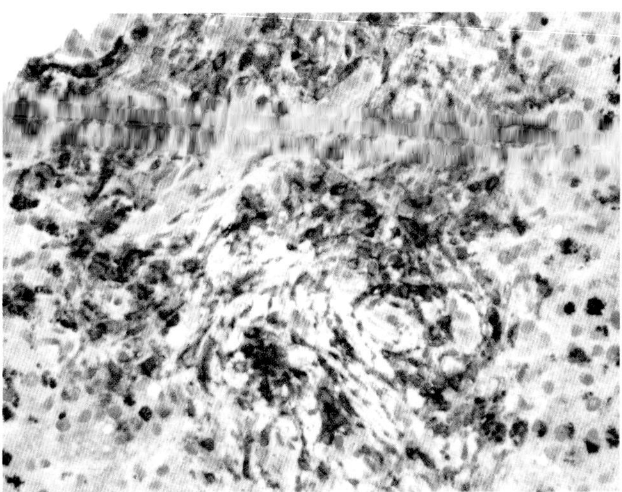

Figure 30.43 Mast cell disease. The mast cell infiltrates are CD25-positive.

Immunohistochemical findings

The mast cells are CD117 and tryptase positive (Fig. 30.42) and show coexpression of CD25 (Fig. 30.43). CD2 can also be positive. In addition, mast cells are positive for CD68,[89] an important potential diagnostic pitfall as mast cells can look a lot like macrophages.

REFERENCES

1. Loddenkemper C, Longerich T, Hummel M, et al. Frequency and diagnostic patterns of lymphomas in liver biopsies with respect to the WHO classification. *Virchows Arch*. 2007;450:493–502.
2. Bronowicki JP, Bineau C, Feugier P, et al. Primary lymphoma of the liver: clinical-pathological features and relationship with HCV infection in French patients. *Hepatology*. 2003;37:781–787.
3. Kikuma K, Watanabe J, Oshiro Y, et al. Etiological factors in primary hepatic B-cell lymphoma. *Virchows Arch*. 2012;460:379–387.
4. Swadley MJ, Deliu M, Mosunjac MB, et al. Primary and secondary hepatic lymphomas diagnosed by image-guided fine-needle aspiration: a retrospective study of clinical and cytomorphologic findings. *Am J Clin Pathol*. 2014;141:119–127.
5. Eom DW, Huh JR, Kang YK, et al. Clinicopathological features of eight Korean cases of primary hepatic lymphoma. *Pathol Int*. 2004;54:830–836.
6. Prendki V, Stirnemann J, Lemoine M, et al. Prevalence and clinical significance of Kupffer cell hyperplasia with hemophagocytosis in liver biopsies. *Am J Surg Pathol*. 2011;35:337–345.
7. Cascio A, Pernice LM, Barberi G, et al. Secondary hemophagocytic lymphohistiocytosis in zoonoses.

A systematic review. *Eur Rev Med Pharmacol Sci.* 2012;16:1324–1337.
8. Chen JH, Fleming MD, Pinkus GS, et al. Pathology of the liver in familial hemophagocytic lymphohistiocytosis. *Am J Surg Pathol.* 2010;34:852–867.
9. Ost A, Nilsson-Ardnor S, Henter JI. Autopsy findings in 27 children with haemophagocytic lymphohistiocytosis. *Histopathology.* 1998;32:310–316.
10. Papla B, Spolnik P, Rzenno E, et al. Generalized crystal-storing histiocytosis as a presentation of multiple myeloma: a case with a possible pro-aggregation defect in the immunoglobulin heavy chain. *Virchows Arch.* 2004;445:83–89.
11. Dogan S, Barnes L, Cruz-Vetrano WP. Crystal-storing histiocytosis: report of a case, review of the literature (80 cases) and a proposed classification. *Head Neck Pathol.* 2012;6:111–120.
12. Krok KL, Torbenson MS, Schulick RD, et al. Lymphadenopathy, elevated liver function tests and weight loss in a 68-year-old man. *J Dig Dis.* 2007;8:103–106.
13. Di Tommaso L, Rahal D, Bossi P, et al. Hepatic Rosai-Dorfman disease with coincidental lymphoma: report of a case. *Int J Surg Pathol.* 2010;18:540–543.
14. Llamas-Velasco M, Cannata J, Dominguez I, et al. Coexistence of Langerhans cell histiocytosis, Rosai-Dorfman disease and splenic lymphoma with fatal outcome after rapid development of histiocytic sarcoma of the liver. *J Cutan Pathol.* 2012;39:1125–1130.
15. Lauwers GY, Perez-Atayde A, Dorfman RF, et al. The digestive system manifestations of Rosai-Dorfman disease (sinus histiocytosis with massive lymphadenopathy): review of 11 cases. *Hum Pathol.* 2000;31:380–385.
16. Karami H, Sahebpour AA, Ghasemi M, et al. Hyaline vascular-type Castleman's disease in the hilum of liver: a case report. *Cases J.* 2010;3:74.
17. Jang SY, Kim BH, Kim JH, et al. A case of Castleman's disease mimicking a hepatocellular carcinoma: a case report and review of literature. *Korean J Gastroenterol.* 2012;59:53–57.
18. Dong A, Dong H, Zuo C. Castleman disease of the porta hepatis mimicking exophytic hepatocellular carcinoma on CT, MRI, and FDG PET/CT. *Clin Nucl Med.* 2014;39:e69–72.
19. Cirillo RL, Jr, Vitellas KM, Deyoung BR, et al. Castleman disease mimicking a hepatic neoplasm. *Clin Imaging.* 1998;22:124–129.
20. Song K, Li M. Budd-Chiari syndrome, a rare complication of multicentric Castleman disease: a case report. *Oncol Lett.* 2015;9:2153–2156.
21. Curciarello J, Castelletto R, Barbero R, et al. Hepatic sinusoidal dilatation associated to giant lymph node hyperplasia (Castleman's): a new case in a patient with periorbital xanthelasmas and history of celiac disease. *J Clin Gastroenterol.* 1998;27:76–78.
22. Kakar S, Kamath PS, Burgart LJ. Sinusoidal dilatation and congestion in liver biopsy: is it always due to venous outflow impairment? *Arch Pathol Lab Med.* 2004;128:901–904.
23. Saritas U, Ustundag Y, Isitan G, et al. Abdominal Castleman disease with mixed histopathology in a patient with iron deficiency anemia, growth retardation and peliosis hepatis. *Am J Med Sci.* 2006;331:51–54.
24. Molina T, Delmer A, Le Tourneau A, et al. Hepatic lesions of vascular origin in multicentric Castleman's disease, plasma cell type: report of one case with peliosis hepatis and another with perisinusoidal fibrosis and nodular regenerative hyperplasia. *Pathol Res Pract.* 1995;191: 1159–1164.
25. Sherman D, Ramsay B, Theodorou NA, et al. Reversible plane xanthoma, vasculitis, and peliosis hepatis in giant lymph node hyperplasia (Castleman's disease): a case report and review of the cutaneous manifestations of giant lymph node hyperplasia. *J Am Acad Dermatol.* 1992;26:105–109.
26. Gaduputi V, Tariq H, Badipatla K, et al. Systemic reactive amyloidosis associated with Castleman's disease. *Case Rep Gastroenterol.* 2013;7:476–481.
27. Yamagata N, Fujio J, Hirai R, et al. Marked hepatomegaly due to AA type amyloidosis in a case with Castleman's disease. *Int J Hematol.* 2006;84:70–73.
28. Ordi J, Grau JM, Junque A, et al. Secondary (AA) amyloidosis associated with Castleman's disease. Report of two cases and review of the literature. *Am J Clin Pathol.* 1993;100:394–397.
29. Shimojima Y, Takei Y, Tazawa K, et al. Histopathological regression of systemic AA amyloidosis after surgical treatment of a localized Castleman's disease. *Amyloid.* 2006;13:184–186.
30. Baruch Y, Ben-Arie Y, Kerner H, et al. Giant lymph node hyperplasia (Castleman's disease): a clinical study of eight patients. *Postgrad Med J.* 1991;67:366–370.
31. Mura G, Tauceri F, Feri M, et al. Report of two cases of Castleman's Disease: a case of benign localized disease and a case of fast progressive multicentric disease. *Acta Biomed.* 2011;82:77–81.
32. Yang CT, Liu KL, Lin MC, et al. Pseudolymphoma of the liver: report of a case and review of the literature. *Asian J Surg.* 2017;40(1):74–80.
33. Zen Y, Fujii T, Nakanuma Y. Hepatic pseudolymphoma: a clinicopathological study of

five cases and review of the literature. *Mod Pathol.* 2010;23:[illegible]

34. Park HS, Jang KY, Kim YK, et al. Histiocyte-rich reactive lymphoid hyperplasia of the liver: unusual morphologic features. *J Korean Med Sci.* 2008;23:156–160.
35. Kwon YK, Jha RC, Etesami K, et al. Pseudolymphoma (reactive lymphoid hyperplasia) of the liver: a clinical challenge. *World J Hepatol.* 2015;7:2696–2702.
36. Rich NE, Sanders C, Hughes RS, et al. Malignant infiltration of the liver presenting as acute liver failure. *Clin Gastroenterol Hepatol.* 2015;13:1025–1028.
37. Allison KH, Fligner CL, Parks WT. Radiographically occult, diffuse intrasinusoidal hepatic metastases from primary breast carcinomas: a clinicopathologic study of 3 autopsy cases. *Arch Pathol Lab Med.* 2004;128:1418–1423.
38. Valladolid G, Adams LL, Weisenberg E, et al. Primary hepatic lymphoma presenting as an isolated solitary hepatic cyst. *J Clin Oncol.* 2013;31:e21–23.
39. Baumhoer D, Tzankov A, Dirnhofer S, et al. Patterns of liver infiltration in lymphoproliferative disease. *Histopathology.* 2008;53:81–90.
40. Lei KI. Primary non-Hodgkin's lymphoma of the liver. *Leuk Lymphoma.* 1998;29:293–299.
41. Ohsawa M, Aozasa K, Horiuchi K, et al. Malignant lymphoma of the liver. Report of five cases and review of the literature. *Dig Dis Sci.* 1992;37:1105–1109.
42. Scoazec JY, Degott C, Brousse N, et al. Non-Hodgkin's lymphoma presenting as a primary tumor of the liver: presentation, diagnosis and outcome in eight patients. *Hepatology.* 1991;13:870–875.
43. Schmidt MT, Huang Q, Alkan S. Aggressive B-cell lymphomas: a review and practical approach for the practicing pathologist. *Adv Anat Pathol.* 2015;22:168–180.
44. Hans CP, Weisenburger DD, Greiner TC, et al. Confirmation of the molecular classification of diffuse large B-cell lymphoma by immunohistochemistry using a tissue microarray. *Blood.* 2004;103:275–282.
45. Hu S, Xu-Monette ZY, Tzankov A, et al. MYC/BCL2 protein coexpression contributes to the inferior survival of activated B-cell subtype of diffuse large B-cell lymphoma and demonstrates high-risk gene expression signatures: a report from The International DLBCL Rituximab-CHOP Consortium Program. *Blood.* 2013;121:4021–4031; quiz 250.
46. Swerdlow SH, Campo E, Pileri SA, et al. The 2016 revision of the World Health Organization classification of lymphoid neoplasms. *Blood.* 2016;127:2375–2390.
47. O'Malley DP, Auerbach A, Weiss LM. Practical applications in immunohistochemistry: evaluation of diffuse large B-cell lymphoma and related large B-cell lymphomas. *Arch Pathol Lab Med.* 2015;139:1094–1107.
48. Takeshima F, Kunisaki M, Aritomi T, et al. Hepatic mucosa-associated lymphoid tissue lymphoma and hepatocellular carcinoma in a patient with hepatitis B virus infection. *J Clin Gastroenterol.* 2004;38:823–826.
49. Swerdlow SH, Yang WI, Zukerberg LR, et al. Expression of cyclin D1 protein in centrocytic/mantle cell lymphomas with and without rearrangement of the BCL1/cyclin D1 gene. *Hum Pathol.* 1995;26:999–1004.
50. Zukerberg LR, Yang WI, Arnold A, et al. Cyclin D1 expression in non-Hodgkin's lymphomas. Detection by immunohistochemistry. *Am J Clin Pathol.* 1995;103:756–760.
51. Yang WI, Zukerberg LR, Motokura T, et al. Cyclin D1 (Bcl-1, PRAD1) protein expression in low-grade B-cell lymphomas and reactive hyperplasia. *Am J Pathol.* 1994;145:86–96.
52. Salaverria I, Royo C, Carvajal-Cuenca A, et al. CCND2 rearrangements are the most frequent genetic events in cyclin D1(-) mantle cell lymphoma. *Blood.* 2013;121:1394–1402.
53. Jaffe ES. *Pathology and Genetics of Tumours of Haematopoietic and Lymphoid Tissues.* IARC Press: Lyon; Washington, DC; 2001.
54. Mann RB, Berard CW. Criteria for the cytologic subclassification of follicular lymphomas: a proposed alternative method. *Hematol Oncol.* 1983;1:187–192.
55. Nathwani BN, Metter GE, Miller TP, et al. What should be the morphologic criteria for the subdivision of follicular lymphomas? *Blood.* 1986;68:837–845.
56. Gallagher CJ, Gregory WM, Jones AE, et al. Follicular lymphoma: prognostic factors for response and survival. *J Clin Oncol.* 1986;4:1470–1480.
57. Anderson JR, Vose JM, Bierman PJ, et al. Clinical features and prognosis of follicular large-cell lymphoma: a report from the Nebraska Lymphoma Study Group. *J Clin Oncol.* 1993;11:218–224.
58. Anderson T, Bender RA, Fisher RI, et al. Combination chemotherapy in non-Hodgkin's lymphoma: results of long-term followup. *Cancer Treat Rep.* 1977;61:1057–1066.
59. National Cancer Institute sponsored study of classifications of non-Hodgkin's lymphomas: summary and description of a working formulation

for clinical usage. The Non-Hodgkin's Lymphoma Pathologic Classification Project. *Cancer.* 1982;49:2112–2135.

60. Bartlett NL, Rizeq M, Dorfman RF, et al. Follicular large-cell lymphoma: intermediate or low grade? *J Clin Oncol.* 1994;12:1349–1357.
61. Glick JH, Barnes JM, Ezdinli EZ, et al. Nodular mixed lymphoma: results of a randomized trial failing to confirm prolonged disease-free survival with COPP chemotherapy. *Blood.* 1981;58:920–925.
62. Glick JH, McFadden E, Costello W, et al. Nodular histiocytic lymphoma: factors influencing prognosis and implications for aggressive chemotherapy. *Cancer.* 1982;49:840–845.
63. Jones SE, Fuks Z, Bull M, et al. Non-Hodgkin's lymphomas. IV. Clinicopathologic correlation in 405 cases. *Cancer.* 1973;31:806–823.
64. Kantarjian HM, McLaughlin P, Fuller LM, et al. Follicular large cell lymphoma: analysis and prognostic factors in 62 patients. *J Clin Oncol.* 1984;2:811–819.
65. Longo DL, Young RC, Hubbard SM, et al. Prolonged initial remission in patients with nodular mixed lymphoma. *Ann Intern Med.* 1984;100:651–656.
66. Martin AR, Weisenburger DD, Chan WC, et al. Prognostic value of cellular proliferation and histologic grade in follicular lymphoma. *Blood.* 1995;85:3671–3678.
67. McLaughlin P, Fuller LM, Velasquez WS, et al. Stage III follicular lymphoma: durable remissions with a combined chemotherapy-radiotherapy regimen. *J Clin Oncol.* 1987;5:867–874.
68. Hicks EB, Rappaport H, Winter WJ. Follicular lymphoma; a re-evaluation of its position in the scheme of malignant lymphoma, based on a survey of 253 cases. *Cancer.* 1956;9:792–821.
69. Swerdlow SH, International Agency for Research on Cancer, World Health Organization. *WHO Classification of Tumours of Haematopoietic and Lymphoid Tissues.* 4th ed. International Agency for Research on Cancer: Lyon, France; 2008.
70. Reddy N, Thompson-Arildsen MA. Hodgkin's lymphoma: Richter's transformation of chronic lymphocytic leukemia involving the liver. *J Clin Oncol.* 2010;28:e543–544.
71. Tsimberidou AM, Keating MJ. Richter syndrome: biology, incidence, and therapeutic strategies. *Cancer.* 2005;103:216–228.
72. Menter T, Dirnhofer S, Tzankov A. LEF1: a highly specific marker for the diagnosis of chronic lymphocytic B cell leukaemia/small lymphocytic B cell lymphoma. *J Clin Pathol.* 2015;68:473–478.
73. Gradowski JF, Sargent RL, Craig FE, et al. Chronic lymphocytic leukemia/small lymphocytic lymphoma with cyclin D1 positive proliferation centers do not have CCND1 translocations or gains and lack SOX11 expression. *Am J Clin Pathol.* 2012;138:132–139.
74. Belhadj K, Reyes F, Farcet JP, et al. Hepatosplenic gammadelta T-cell lymphoma is a rare clinicopathologic entity with poor outcome: report on a series of 21 patients. *Blood.* 2003;102:4261–4269.
75. Przybylski GK, Wu H, Macon WR, et al. Hepatosplenic and subcutaneous panniculitis-like gamma/delta T cell lymphomas are derived from different Vdelta subsets of gamma/delta T lymphocytes. *J Mol Diagn.* 2000;2:11–19.
76. Suarez F, Wlodarska I, Rigal-Huguet F, et al. Hepatosplenic alphabeta T-cell lymphoma: an unusual case with clinical, histologic, and cytogenetic features of gammadelta hepatosplenic T-cell lymphoma. *Am J Surg Pathol.* 2000;24:1027–1032.
77. Macon WR, Levy NB, Kurtin PJ, et al. Hepatosplenic alphabeta T-cell lymphomas: a report of 14 cases and comparison with hepatosplenic gammadelta T-cell lymphomas. *Am J Surg Pathol.* 2001;25:285–296.
78. Parrilla Castellar ER, Jaffe ES, Said JW, et al. ALK-negative anaplastic large cell lymphoma is a genetically heterogeneous disease with widely disparate clinical outcomes. *Blood.* 2014;124:1473–1480.
79. Sternberg SS, Mills SE, Carter D. *Sternberg's Diagnostic Surgical Pathology.* 5th ed. Wolters Kluwer Lippincott Williams & Wilkins: Philadelphia, PA; 2010.
80. Roquet ML, Zafrani ES, Farcet JP, et al. Histopathological lesions of the liver in hairy cell leukemia: a report of 14 cases. *Hepatology.* 1985;5:496–500.
81. Bethel KJ, Sharpe RW. Pathology of hairy-cell leukaemia. *Best Pract Res Clin Haematol.* 2003;16:15–31.
82. Sharpe RW, Bethel KJ. Hairy cell leukemia: diagnostic pathology. *Hematol Oncol Clin North Am.* 2006;20:1023–1049.
83. Turakhia S, Lanigan C, Hamadeh F, et al. Immunohistochemistry for BRAF V600E in the differential diagnosis of hairy cell leukemia vs other splenic B-cell lymphomas. *Am J Clin Pathol.* 2015;144:87–93.
84. Safyan EL, Veerabagu MP, Swerdlow SH, et al. Intrahepatic cholestasis due to systemic mastocytosis: a case report and review of literature. *Am J Gastroenterol.* 1997;92:1197–1200.
85. Baron TH, Koehler RE, Rodgers WH, et al. Mast cell cholangiopathy: another cause of sclerosing cholangitis. *Gastroenterology.* 1995;109:1677–1681.
86. Mican JM, Di Bisceglie AM, Fong TL, et al. Hepatic involvement in mastocytosis: clinicopathologic

correlations in 41 cases. *Hepatology*. 1998;27:1163–1170.

87. Schwaab J, Horny HP, Jonescheit J, et al. Mast cell sarcoma mimicking metastatic colon carcinoma. *Ann Hematol*. 2014;93:1067–1069.
88. Horny HP, Kaiserling E, Campbell M, et al. Liver findings in generalized mastocytosis. A clinicopathologic study. *Cancer*. 1989;63:532–538.
89. Li WV, Kapadia SB, Sonmez-Alpan E, et al. Immunohistochemical characterization of mast cell disease in paraffin sections using tryptase, CD68, myeloperoxidase, lysozyme, and CD20 antibodies. *Mod Pathol*. 1996;9:982–988.
90. Lecronier M, Prendki V, Gerin M, et al. Q fever and Mediterranean spotted fever associated with hemophagocytic syndrome: case study and literature review. *Int J Infect Dis*. 2013;17:e629–633.
91. Jordan MB, Filipovich AH. Hematopoietic cell transplantation for hemophagocytic lymphohistiocytosis: a journey of a thousand miles begins with a single (big) step. *Bone Marrow Transplant*. 2008;42:433–437.
92. Filipovich AH. Hemophagocytic lymphohistiocytosis (HLH) and related disorders. *Hematology Am Soc Hematol Educ Program*. 2009:127–131.

31

Metastatic tumors in the liver

Lizhi Zhang, MD

31.1 INTRODUCTION

The liver is one of the most common organs involved by metastases. In fact, metastatic tumors are the most common malignant neoplasms of the liver. Distinguishing metastatic tumors from primary hepatic tumors and determining their origins are of importance for clinical management. Liver biopsies play two main roles. First, in patients with known primaries, liver biopsies can confirm metastatic disease. Second, in metastatic disease of unknown primary, histological and immunostain findings can help identify the likely site of origin, always being interpreted in the context of clinical, serological, and imaging findings.

31.2 DEFINITION

Metastatic tumors are malignant neoplasms that originate from an extrahepatic organs and spread to the liver by angiolymphatic dissemination or direct extension.

31.3 CLINICAL FEATURES

Most patients with liver metastases present with symptoms and signs related to their primary disease. Most individuals present with nonspecific findings, such as abdominal pain, jaundice, ascites, or weight loss. Metastatic functioning neuroendocrine tumors can present with carcinoid syndrome, which typically develops only after there are liver metastases. In other cases of metastatic disease, patients are completely asymptomatic and liver metastasis is an incidental finding.

Overall, approximately 60% of all primary tumors that metastasize will eventually involve the liver.[1] Carcinomas and melanomas are more likely than sarcomas to metastasize to the liver in adults. Autopsy studies show that the most common carcinomas metastatic to the liver are as follows: colorectal, breast, lung, pancreas, neuroendocrine tumor, stomach, and cervix.[2] By contrast, the liver metastases in children are most likely to be from neuroblastoma, Wilms tumor, or sarcomas.[3] However, these patterns are largely autopsy based and may not be the same as seen in surgical pathology biopsy specimens because most surgical pathology specimens are from cases where the primary tumor is unknown or uncertain based on clinical and imaging evaluations.

31.4 LABORATORY FINDINGS

Liver transaminases and alkaline phosphatase levels are often nonspecifically elevated in patients with liver metastases. However, serum tumor markers can provide some guidance for the possible sites of origin (Table 31.1), though none has sufficient sensitivity or specificity to replace imaging and histological studies. Of note, additional useful markers are likely to be discovered as molecular-based studies mature.

31.5 GENERAL APPROACH TO WORK UP

Working up a liver tumor of unknown origin is the art of pathology. A pathologist must use a logical approach that combines clinical information, morphological features, immunophenotype, and other special stains or techniques to reach a correct diagnosis. Good communication with clinicians and radiologists can obtain useful information regarding the nature of the liver tumor. Although immunohistochemistry has become essential and is readily available, a pathologist must follow a step-by-step approach to avoid underusing or overusing immunohistochemistry.

Primary versus metastatic tumor

The first step is to determine if a liver malignancy is primary or metastatic. The most common primary malignant tumors of the liver are hepatocellular carcinoma and cholangiocarcinoma. When clinical history of known cancer in other organs is available, an accurate diagnosis can be reached with no or very few immunostains. For example, when a liver biopsy from a patient with a known history of colorectal adenocarcinoma reveals an adenocarcinoma with columnar cells and dirty necrosis, then the diagnosis can be achieved based on hematoxylin and eosin (H&E) with few (e.g., CDX2) or no stains.

Other helpful clues come from imaging studies. The presence of numerous hepatic lesions, for example, greater than five, favors metastatic disease. In contrast, the presence of a single hepatic tumor without identifiable lesions elsewhere in the body is more common in primary liver carcinoma. The presence of advanced fibrosis or cirrhosis also favors a primary liver neoplasm, although metastatic tumors can rarely be seen in cirrhotic livers.

Carcinoma versus nonepithelial lineage tumor

Immunostains are key tools for determining epithelial versus nonepithelial differentiation, but morphological examination on the H&E sections is still essential. In addition, morphology needs be taken into account when interpreting immunostaining results because tumors can aberrantly express epithelial markers. For example, epithelioid hemangioendothelioma can be positive for CK7 and can be misdiagnosed as a poorly differentiated adenocarcinoma if morphology and other immunostain findings are not taken into account.

If a tumor is poorly differentiated or undifferentiated, and no useful clinical information is available, then immunostains play a central role in working up the tumor. Immunostains are first used to determine the basic lineage of the neoplasm. Examples of useful stains include stains for carcinoma (EMA, pancytokerin, Oscar keratin, cytokeratin AE1/AE3,

Table 31.1 Commonly used serum tumor markers

Serum tumor markers	Primary associated tumors	Additional associated tumors
α-Fetoprotein (AFP)	Hepatocellular carcinoma, embryonal cell carcinoma, and yolk sac tumor	Cholangiocarcinoma, hepatoid carcinoma, some acinar cell carcinomas
Beta unit of human chorionic gonadotropin (β-hCG)	Choriocarcinoma, embryonal cell carcinoma, and gestational trophoblastic disease	Rare GI carcinomas
Calcitonin	Medullary thyroid carcinoma;	Carcinomas of lung, liver, and kidneys
CA15-3	Breast carcinoma	Other carcinomas
CA19-9	Pancreatobiliary adenocarcinoma	Colorectal, gastric, and esophageal adenocarcinoma
CA125	Ovarian carcinoma	Carcinomas of endometrium, fallopian tube, breast, lung, esophagus, stomach, liver, and pancreas
Carcinoembryonic antigen (CEA)	Colorectal carcinoma	Carcinomas of breast, lung, stomach, pancreas, bladder, medullary thyroid, head and neck, cervix, and liver
Chromogranin A (CgA)	Pheochromocytoma, neuroblastoma	Small cell carcinoma and neuroendocrine tumors
Des-gamma-carboxyprothrombin (DCP)	Hepatocellular carcinoma	
Gastrin	Gastrin producing neuroendocrine tumor (gastrinoma), most arising in the duodenum or pancreas	
Glucagon	Glucagonoma	
Insulin	Insulinoma	
Metanephrines	Pheochromocytoma	Neuroblastoma and ganglioneuromas
Neuron-specific enolase (NSE)	Small cell carcinoma	Neuroblastoma, pheochromocytoma, and neuroendocrine tumors
Pancreatic polypeptide	Pancreatic polypeptide producing neuroendocrine tumor, most arising in the pancreas	
Prostate-specific antigen (PSA)	Prostate carcinoma	
Serotonin	Neuroendocrine tumor	
Squamous cell carcinoma antigen	Squamous cell carcinoma of the cervix, lung, and head and neck	
Vasoactive intestinal polypeptide (VIP)	VIP producing neuroendocrine tumor, most arising in the pancreas	

and Cam5.2), sarcoma (desmin, smooth muscle actin, CD34, and KIT), melanoma (S100, Melan-A, HMB-45, SOX 10, MiTF, and tyrosinase), and lymphoma (CD3, CD20, and CD45). Other stains for rare entities include germ cell tumor markers (PLAP, Oct4, α-fetoprotein [AFP], SALL4, and human chorionic gonadotropin [hCG]), plasmacytoma (CD138 and MUM1), and rhabdoid tumor or epithelioid sarcoma (INI1). Of note, it is often important to use multiple markers because poorly differentiated malignancies may have focal expression or lose expression of some lineage markers. Once the broad lineage of the tumor has been determined, more specific immunostains can be performed for further tumor subclassification. Commonly used immunostain markers are listed in Table 31.2; however, none of immunostaining markers is perfect for a specific entity and there are many pitfalls when interpreting immunostaining results.

Adenocarcinoma versus other types of carcinoma

Once a carcinoma has been identified, the specific type of carcinoma needs to be determined based on both morphology and immunophenotype. If gland formation and/or mucin production are identified, a diagnosis of adenocarcinoma can be established. If a carcinoma shows other morphological features typical for a neoplasm, such as keratinization for squamous cell carcinoma or organoid growth pattern and neuroendocrine nuclear features for neuroendocrine tumor, then specific immunostains can be used to confirm the diagnosis. Otherwise, if the tumor is poorly differentiated or the morphological features are nonspecific, a broad immunostain panel for different types of carcinoma should be considered. Commonly used markers include the following: hepatocellular carcinoma (HepPar-1, arginase, glypican-3, polyclonal CEA, CD10,

Table 31.2 Commonly used tumor origin markers and some pitfalls for primary and metastatic tumors of the liver

Tumors	Tumor lineage markers	Aberrantly expressed markers and pitfalls
Adrenal cortical neoplasm	Melan-A, inhibin, calretinin	
Angiomyolipoma	HMB-45, SMA	
Angiosarcoma	ERG, CD31, CD34, Fli-1, factor VIII	Synaptophysin, cytokeratin
Breast carcinoma	GATA3, ER, GCDFP-15, mammoglobin	S100
Cholangiocarcinoma	CK7, CK20 (variable), CDX2 (variable), VHL	CK20 and CDX2 positivity is more common in hilar and extrahepatic tumors; TTF-1 positive in 50% extrahepatic tumors
Choriocarcinoma	β-hCG, CD10	
Colorectal and appendiceal carcinoma	CDX2, CK20, SATB2, villin	MSI-high tumors with reduced staining for CK20 and CK7 positivity
Embryonal carcinoma	SALL4, OCT4, CD30, SOX2	
Endocervical adenocarcinoma	PAX8, p16, CEA, loss of PAX2	
Endometrial adenocarcinoma	PAX8/PAX2, ER	
Epithelioid hemangioendothelioma	ERG, CD31, CD34, Fli-1, factor VIII	Keratin
Epithelioid sarcoma	Loss INI-1, keratin, CD34	
Gastrointestinal stromal tumor	KIT, DOG1	CD34 (60%), SMA (30%)
Hepatocellular carcinoma	Arginase, glypican-3, HepPar-1, Albumin-ISH, CD10 or polyclonal CEA (canalicular pattern)	MOC31 (35%), CDX2 (5%), CK19 (15%)
Leiomyosarcoma	SMA, MSA, caldesmon	
Lung adenocarcinoma	TTF1, Napsin	
Melanoma	S100, Melan-A, HMB-45, MiTF, SOX10, tyrosinase	KIT, cytokeratin, synaptophysin
Mesothelioma	Calretinin, WT1, D2-40, CK5/6,	GATA-3 (50%)

(continued)

Table 31.2 Commonly used tumor origin markers and some pitfalls for primary and metastatic tumors of the liver *(continued)*

Tumors	Tumor lineage markers	Aberrantly expressed markers and pitfalls
Neuroendocrine tumor	Chromogranin, synaptophysin, CD56, NSE	
Ovarian clear cell carcinoma	PAX8, VHL, CEA	
Ovarian serous carcinoma	PAX8, ER, WT1, p53	
Pancreatic acinar cell carcinoma	Trypsin, α_1-antitrypsin	Glypican-3 (60%); if >30% positive for NET markers, classified as mixed acinar-neuroendocrine carcinoma
Pancreatic ductal adenocarcinoma	MUC5AC, S100P, CDX2 (variable)	Loss of SMAD4 (50%), but also in some cholangiocarcinomas and ampullary carcinoma; monomorphic anaplastic carcinoma loss INI-1
Pancreatic neuroendocrine tumor	Islet-1, PAX8, PDX1	Trypsin (focal), CK19 and KIT positivity indicating aggressive behavior
Prostate adenocarcinoma	PSA, PSAP, ERG, NKX3.1	Chromogranin and synaptophysin after hormone therapy
Renal cell carcinoma, clear cell type	PAX8/PAX2, RCC, VHL, CD10	Napsin (75%)
Renal cell carcinoma, chromophobe type	PAX8, KIT	GATA-3 (50%)
Renal cell carcinoma, papillary type	PAX8/PAX2, RCC	Napsin (30%)
Small intestinal adenocarcinoma	CK7, CK20 (variable), CDX2 (variable)	HepPar-1 (60%)
Solid pseudopapillary tumor	Nuclear β-catenin, PR, CD10	
Solitary fibrous tumor	CD34, Stat6	
Squamous cell carcinoma	p40, CK5/6, p63, desmocollin-3	HPV positivity suggests cervical or oropharynx primary; GATA3 is positive 80% of skin squamous cell carcinomas, 30% of cervical, and 20% of lung/larynx; glypican 3 (20%)
Thyroid papillary or follicular neoplasm	TTF1, PAX8, thyroglobulin	
Thymoma	PAX8, p63, CD5	
Thyroid medullary carcinoma	Calcitonin, TTF1, CEA	
Translocational RCC	TFE3	
Urothelial carcinoma	GATA3, Uroplakin, p40, CK5/6, CK903, p63	
Yolk sac tumor	SALL4, glypican-3, AFP	

and albumin in situ hybridization); squamous cell or urothelial carcinoma (CK5/6, CK903, p40, GATA-3, and p63); neuroendocrine tumors including small cell carcinoma (synaptophysin and chromogranin); mesothelioma (calretinin, WT-1, and D2-40); acinar cell carcinoma (trypsin and Periodic acid-Schiff [PAS]). After a diagnosis of adenocarcinoma is established, a combination of CK7/CK20 can be used with other organ specific markers for lung, gastrointestinal, breast, prostate, or other origins. Different CK7/CK20 staining patterns can provide useful clues for determining tumor origin and deciding second round of immunostain work up (Table 31.3). Of note, there are no organ specific markers for squamous cell carcinoma. In addition, adenocarcinoma arising in upper gastrointestinal tract or pancreatobiliary tract can have similar morphology and immunophenotype.

31.6 GROSS FINDINGS

Most liver metastases are multifocal and involve both lobes of the liver. Scattered nodules with varying sizes are present throughout the hepatic parenchyma. Metastasis less commonly presents as a solitary hepatic lesion. Metastatic tumors are typically seen in noncirrhotic livers, although metastases can occur in cirrhotic livers with a low frequency. Gross features are generally nonspecific, but some findings may suggest certain types of tumors. For instance, melanomas may be black or brown in color. Mucinous adenocarcinomas may have abundant mucin with a gelatinous glistening appearance. Squamous cell carcinomas may be white and granular. Colorectal carcinoma may have an umbilicated appearance. Fibrous capsules are rarely seen in metastases, except for a few colorectal carcinomas.

Most liver metastases are solid masses, but cystic changes may occur due to necrosis. Besides forming masses or nodules, poorly differentiated adenocarcinomas can also diffusely involve the liver sinusoids, causing hepatomegaly with no grossly visible lesion.

31.7 MICROSCOPIC FINDINGS

Morphological clues to determine tumor differentiation lineage

Careful H&E examination is a key step that has not been replaced by immunostains. Often, features identified on H&E sections can provide strong evidence suggesting tumor differentiation and can direct the use of immunostains. For instance, bile production is essentially diagnostic of hepatocelluar differentiation and in most cases, although hepatoid carcinoma from other organs can also produce bile.[4] Glandular differentiation or mucin production indicates an adenocarcinoma. A mucicarmine stain can help to identify mucin production when it is focal or not evident on H&E. True glandular differentiation must be separated from psuedoglands, which are commonly present in hepatocellular carcinoma, fibrolamellar

Table 31.3 General CK7 and CK20 staining patterns

Staining patterns	Tumors predominantly with this pattern	Variable tumors with this pattern
$CK7^+/CK20^+$	Urothelial carcinoma Ovarian mucinous carcinoma Endocervical adenocarcinoma Small intestinal adenocarcinoma	Pancreatic adenocarcinoma Cholangiocarcinoma Gastric adenocarcinoma
$CK7^+/CK20^-$	Ductal and lobular breast carcinoma Malignant mesothelioma Endometrial adenocarcinoma Ovarian serous and endometrioid carcinoma Pulmonary adenocarcinoma Salivary gland neoplasm Thyroid neoplasm	Squamous cell carcinoma Pancreatic adenocarcinoma Cholangiocarcinoma Gastric adenocarcinoma Small intestinal adenocarcinoma
$CK7^-/CK20^+$	Colorectal adenocarcinoma Appendiceal adenocarcinoma Appendiceal goblet cell carcinoid Merkel cell carcinoma	Gastric adenocarcinoma Cholangiocarcinoma
$CK7^-/CK20^-$	Hepatocellular carcinoma Prostatic adenocarcinoma Renal cell carcinoma Small cell carcinoma Neuroendocrine tumor Germ cell tumor Adrenal cortical tumor Squamous cell carcinoma Epithelioid sarcoma	Malignant mesothelioma Thyroid neoplasm Thymoma

carcinoma, neuroendocrine tumors, and acinar cell carcinomas (Figs. 31.1 and 31.2). Squamous differentiation is characterized by keratinization with squamous pearl formation, large cells with glassy eosinophilic cytoplasm, distinct cell borders, and intercellular bridge (Fig. 31.3). If a glandular component is identified in addition to squamous differentiation, a diagnosis of adenosquamous carcinoma is made.

Tumor growth patterns are also important clues to the differential diagnosis. Neuroendocrine tumors often have an organoid pattern similar to that seen in primary tumors (Fig. 31.4). A prominent trabecular growth pattern is also common in neuroendocrine tumors. Acinar structures suggest acinar cell carcinoma or neuroendocrine tumors. When tumor cells form anastomosing channels, a vascular neoplasm should be considered.

Nuclear features can also provide clues for the tumor origin. Uniform nuclei with finely stippled chromatin without conspicuous nucleoli typically suggest a neuroendocrine tumor (Fig. 31.4). Small cell carcinoma is characterized by nuclear molding, smudgy chromatin, and inconspicuous nucleoli, often with crush artifact (Fig. 31.5). Unusually large eosinophilic nucleoli can be seen in melanoma and prostate carcinoma. Nuclear grooves suggest a solid pseudopapillary tumor, papillary thyroid carcinoma, or granulosa cell tumor. Irregular and elongated nuclei with prominent nuclear grooves and folds are suggestive of Langerhans cell histiocytosis.

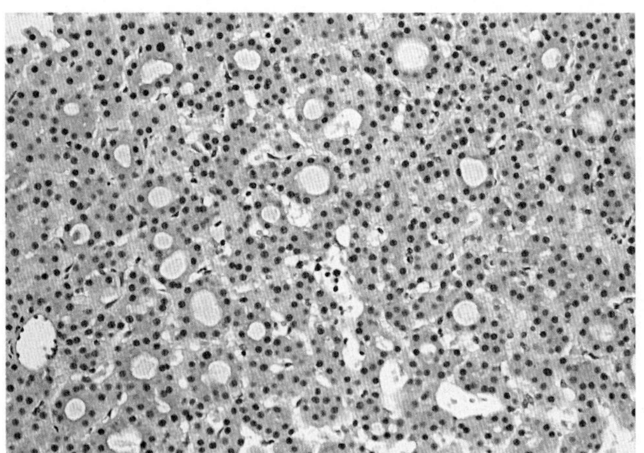

Figure 31.1 Hepatocellular carcinoma. Pseudoglands and bile production in hepatocellular carcinoma.

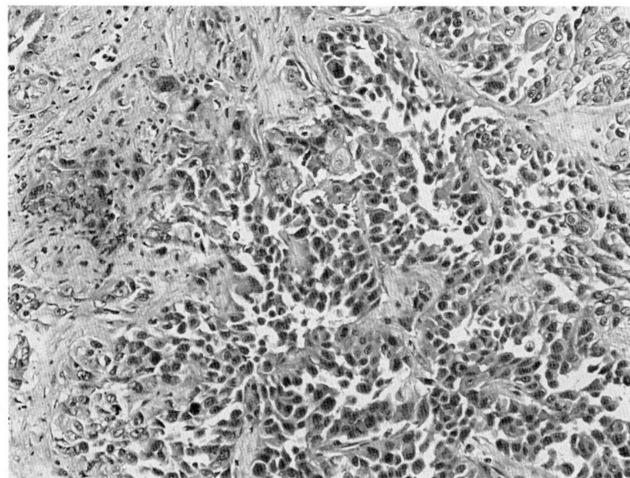

Figure 31.3 Squamous cell carcinoma. Single cell keratinization in squamous cell carcinoma.

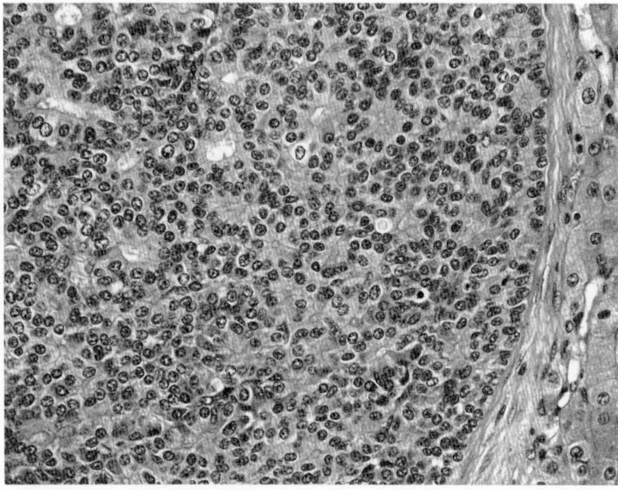

Figure 31.2 Neuroendocrine tumor. Pseudoacinar formation in neuroendocrine tumor.

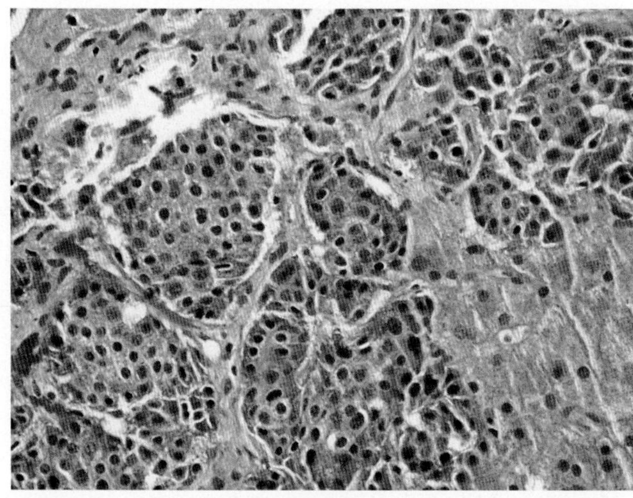

Figure 31.4 Neuroendocrine tumor. Organoid growth pattern with "salt-and-pepper" chromatin pattern without conspicuous nucleoli typically seen in neuroendocrine tumor.

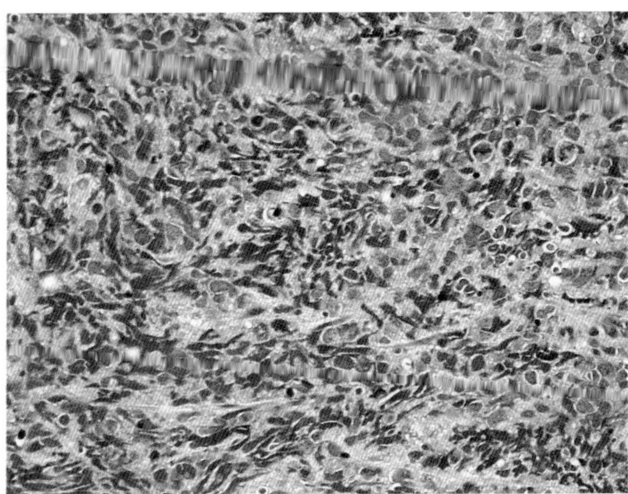

Figure 31.5 Small cell carcinoma. Nuclear features of small cell carcinoma.

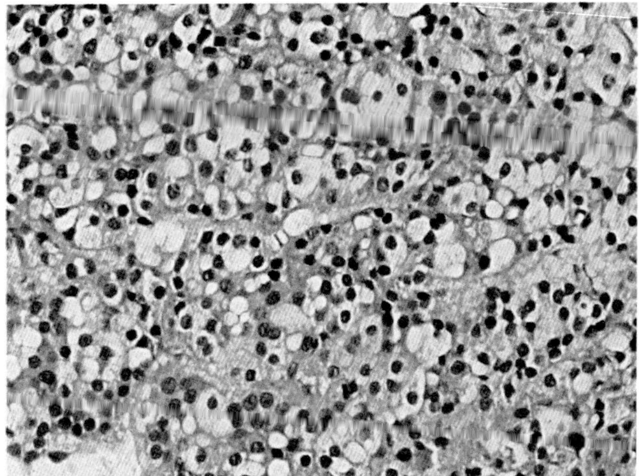

Figure 31.7 Metastatic adrenal cortical carcinoma. Lipid-rich tumor cells.

Eosinophilic hyaline inclusions can be seen in a group of tumors, including solid pseudopapillary tumors (Fig. 31.6), embryonal sarcomas, and rare angiosarcomas. Steatosis is most commonly seen in hepatocellular carcinoma, but other carcinomas can also show fatty change, usually with a microvesicular pattern of steatosis, including adrenal cortical carcinomas (Fig. 31.7) and solid pseudopapillary tumors of the pancreas. The differential for metastatic clear cell carcinoma includes renal cell carcinoma, clear cell neuroendocrine tumor, clear cell acinar cell carcinoma, and adrenal cortical carcinoma. A rhabdoid or plasmacytoid morphology can be seen with tumors of several different lineages, including carcinoma, melanoma, gastrointestinal stromal tumor, plasmacytoma, and anaplastic large cell lymphoma. As part of this, SMARCB1/INI-1 immunostains are important to rule out poorly differentiated rhabdoid tumors, which can be either primary to the liver or metastatic. Spindle cell tumors suggest sarcoma, but sarcomatoid carcinomas have to be excluded by immunostains. The differential for nonepithelial spindle cell tumors includes solitary fibrous tumors (Fig. 31.8), gastrointestinal stromal tumor (Fig. 31.9), leiomyosarcoma (Fig. 31.10), inflammatory myofibroblastic tumor, angiosarcoma, Kaposi sarcoma, follicular dendritic cell sarcoma, or melanoma.

Distinguishing hepatocellular carcinoma from its mimickers

Metastatic tumors that can most closely mimic hepatocellular carcinoma include neuroendocrine tumors,

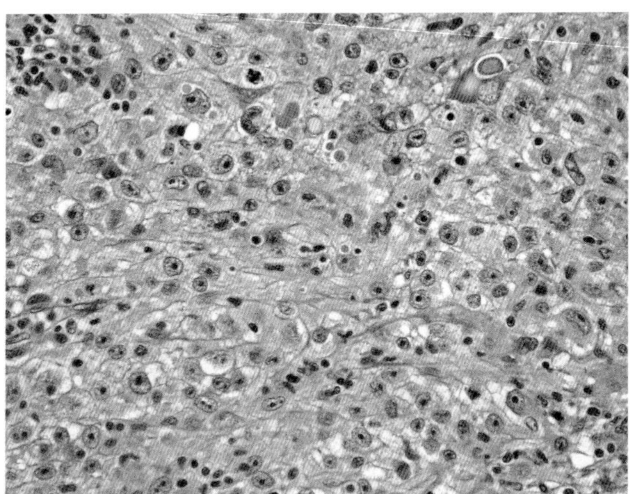

Figure 31.6 Pancreatic solid pseudopapillary tumor. Eosinophilic globules in metastatic pancreatic solid pseudopapillary tumor.

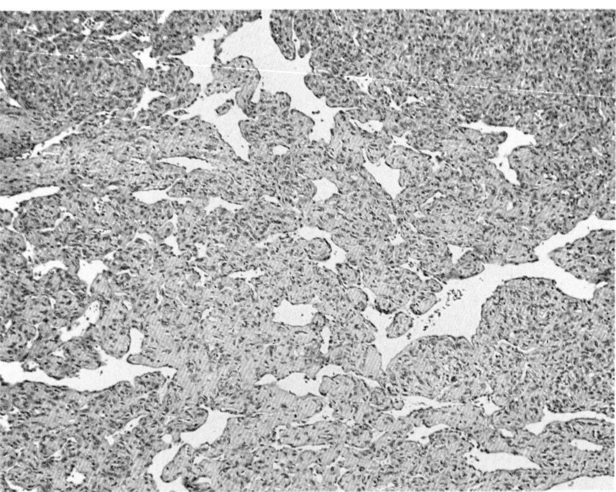

Figure 31.8 Metastatic solid fibrous tumor. Bland spindle cells and "staghorn" vascular pattern.

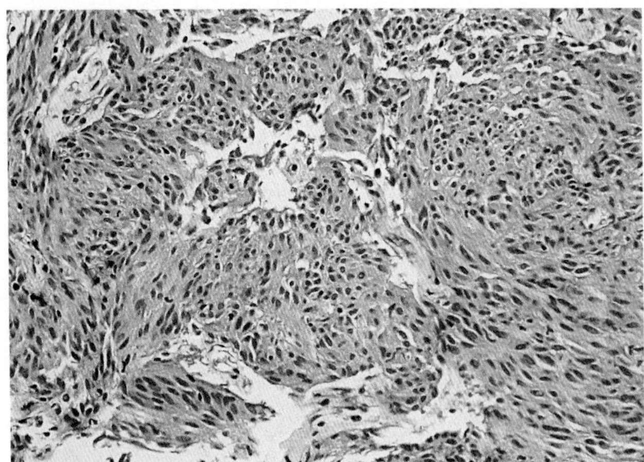

Figure 31.9 Metastatic gastrointestinal stromal tumor. Spindle cell type.

A rare dilemma can be to distinguish primary hepatocellular carcinoma from metastatic hepatoid carcinoma. The most common sites of origin for metastatic hepatoid carcinomas are the stomach, pancreas, and lung. Patients can have elevated serum AFP levels and the tumor can morphological be consistent with hepatocellular carcinoma. Metastatic hepatoid carcinomas can be positive for any of the hepatic markers (HepPar-1, glypican 3, arginase, or albumin in situ hybridization), so none of these will distinguish metastatic from primary disease (Figs. 31.11 and 31.12). Likewise, other proposed markers to separate these two entities (SALL4, MOC31, CK19) have not stood the test of time and are not clinically helpful. Clues

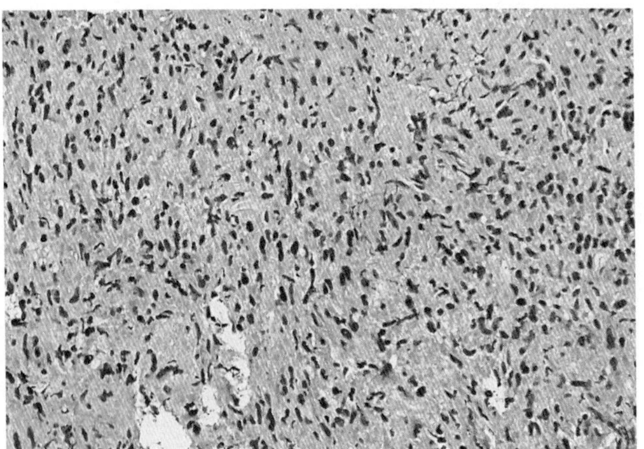

Figure 31.10 Metastatic leiomyosarcoma.

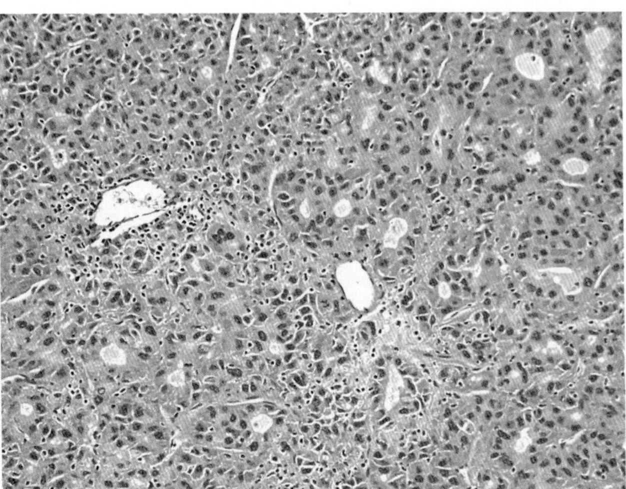

Figure 31.11 Metastatic hepatoid carcinoma from adrenal gland. The tumor composed of epithelioid cells forming broad trabecula and pseudoacini, mimicking hepatocellular carcinoma.

renal cell carcinomas, acinar cell carcinoma, adrenal cortical carcinomas, melanoma, and epithelioid angiomyolipomas. Hepatocellular carcinoma is usually excluded by a panel of multiple hepatocellular markers, such as HepPar-1, arginase, glypican-3, and albumin in situ hybridization. Polyclonal carcinoembryonic antigen (CEA) and CD10 are older markers of hepatic differentiation that depend on identifying a canalicular staining pattern but are not widely used anymore because newer stains have better performance characteristics. In our practice, we typically start with HepPar-1 and/or arginase if the morphological impression is a well to moderately differentiated hepatocellular carcinoma. Positive staining for one of them can usually confirm the diagnosis in morphologically consistent well or moderately differentiated hepatocellular carcinomas. If the immunostains are negative, then tests for other markers including glypican-3 and albumin in situ hybridization are used. Additional stains are used to exclude other tumors depending on the morphology and the clinical findings.

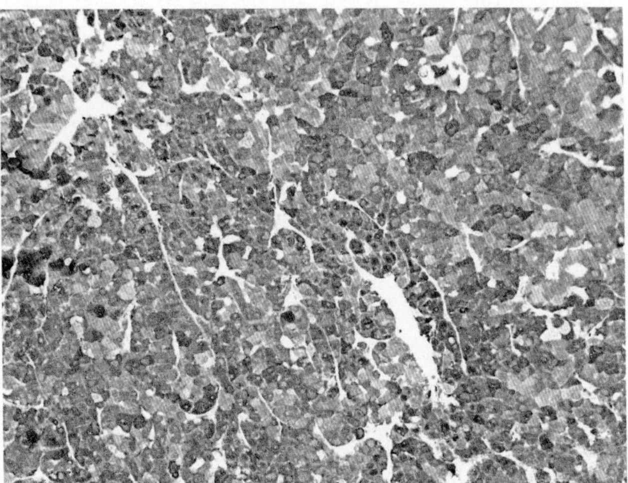

Figure 31.12 Metastatic hepatoid carcinoma, arginase immunostain. The tumor is diffusely positive.

to the possibility of metastatic hepatoid carcinoma include tumors showing only focal areas of hepatic differentiation on H&E, histories of mass lesions in other organs such as the upper gastrointestinal tract, pancreas, or lung, and atypical immunophenotypes. Examples of immunophenotypes that are atypical for hepatocellular carcinoma include strong and diffuse TTF1 nuclear staining or strong and diffuse CDX2 staining. Of note, other nonhepatoid carcinomas may also be positive for hepatic markers (HepPar-1, glypican 3, arginase, or albumin in situ hybridization), but if they do not have hepatoid morphology, then they are not classified as hepatoid carcinomas.

Distinguishing cholangiocarcinoma from metastatic adenocarcinoma

Cholangiocarcinomas have various growth patterns that morphologically overlap with adenocarcinoma arising from other organs, especially from extrahepatic bile ducts, the upper gastrointestinal tract, or pancreas. So far, there are no immunostaining markers specific for cholangiocarcinoma, although some potential markers have been reported, including albumin in situ hybridization, ANXA1, ANXA10, S100P, and pVHL.[5–7] Therefore, the diagnosis of a primary cholangiocarcinoma relies on the combination of morphology and immunophenotype, plus imaging and other clinical information to exclude other primary sites.

There are several clues that favor cholangiocarcinoma over metastatic disease. Although only rarely present, the presence of precursor lesions suggests a primary cholangiocarcinoma. There are several possible precursor lesions including biliary intraepithelial neoplasia (BilIN) (Fig. 31.13). However, an important caveat is that some metastatic adenocarcinomas, such as colorectal carcinoma, can extend into and grow along the bile ducts, a finding known as *cancerization of the bile ducts*.[8] Intraductal papillary neoplasms of bile duct are also precursor lesions. A third precursor lesion is mucinous cystic neoplasms. More information is available in Chapter 29.

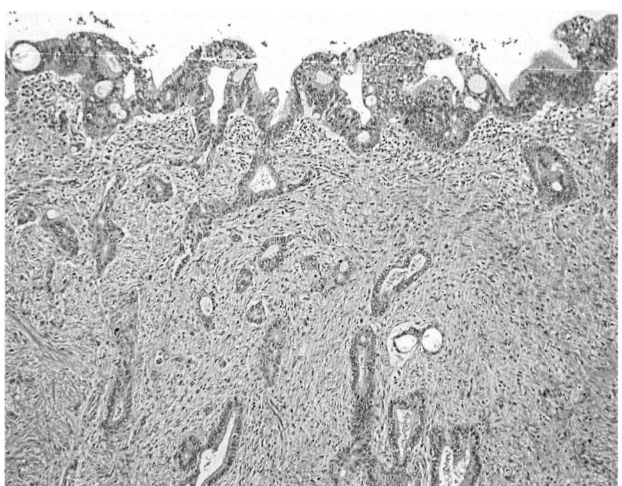

Figure 31.13 Biliary intraepithelial neoplasia. There is high-grade dysplasia (BilIN3) associated with invasive cholangiocarcinoma.

A second clue to a likely diagnosis of cholangiocarcinoma is the presence of diffuse dense intratumoral fibrosis. Although this finding is not sensitive or specific, most cholangiocarcinomas are associated with dense fibrosis. Cirrhosis is an important risk factor for cholangiocarcinoma,[9] so adenocarcinoma in the background of cirrhosis favors cholangiocarcinoma. Finally, when other clinical risk factors for cholangiocarcinoma are known, such as a history of primary sclerosing cholangitis, hepatobiliary flukes, or hepatolithiasis, this also suggests cholangiocarcinoma over metastatic disease.

There are no specific immunostain markers for cholangiocarcinoma. Most cholangiocarcinomas are positive for CK7 (85% to 95%) and CK19 (90%), and negative or only focally positive for CK20. Hilar cholangiocarcinomas are more likely to be CK20-positive and to have stronger and more diffuse staining. Also, 30% to 50% of cholangiocarcinomas can be positive for CDX2, especially hilar tumors.[10] Albumin in situ hybridization is positive in about 80% of cholangiocarcinomas, but it is not entirely specific, because adenocarcinomas from other organs can be positive, including the lung and pancreas. Also of note, TTF1 can be positive in 50% of extrahepatic cholangiocarcinomas.[11] Finally, 5% to 10% cholangiocarcinomas can express glypican-3 and/or HepPar-1,[11,12] but usually focal.

Given the nonspecific morphological and immunostain features of cholangiocarcinoma, a typical approach for biopsy specimens of an adenocarcinoma that is CK7-positive and negative for other specific lineage markers is to indicate the presence of adenocarcinoma with a differential diagnosis that includes cholangiocarcinoma, pancreatic ductal adenocarcinoma, or adenocarcinoma from an upper gastrointestinal location. The histology needs to be correlated with clinical findings, imaging studies, and endoscopic findings.

31.8 SPECIFIC TUMORS METASTASIZING TO LIVER

Colorectal adenocarcinoma

Colorectal adenocarcinoma is one of the most common carcinomas that metastasize to the liver. Overall, 20% of individuals with colorectal adenocarcinoma have

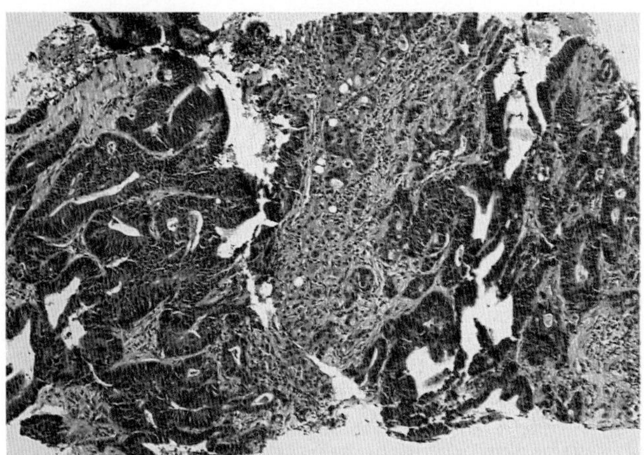

Figure 31.14 Metastatic colorectal adenocarcinoma. Columnar epithelium forming glands with dirty necrosis.

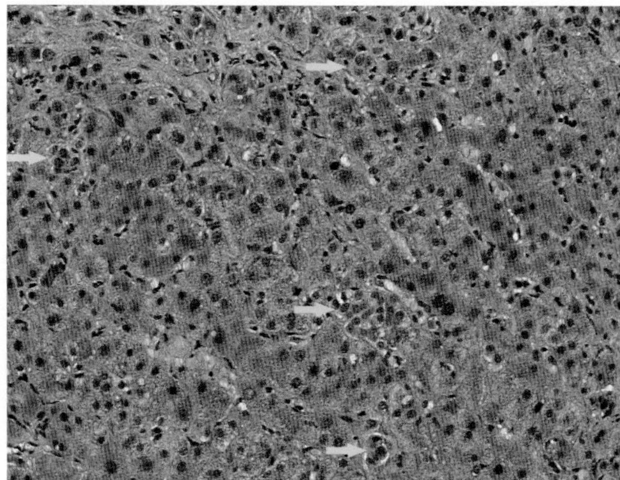

Figure 31.15 Metastatic breast carcinoma. Note small clusters and single tumor cells in sinusoids (*arrows*).

liver metastases at the time of diagnosis and another 50% will develop metastatic liver disease during the course of their disease.[13] Histologically, most metastatic colorectal adenocarcinoma are recognized by their tall columnar tumor cells with pencil-shaped nuclei, large-sized gland formation, and characteristic dirty necrosis inside the glandular lumens (Fig. 31.14). However, some cases lack the classic appearance and a panel of immunostains can help make the diagnosis. Most colorectal adenocarcinomas are strongly and diffusely positive for CK20 and CDX2, and negative for CK7. Of note, colorectal adenocarcinomas associated with microsatellite instability (microsatellite instability [MSI]-high tumors), which usually arise in right colon, may show a different immunophenotype than that of the classic pattern. These MSI-high tumors often show reduced expression of CK20 and CDX2, with increased expression of CK7.[14,15] Identifying loss of DNA mismatch repair enzymes in these tumors by immunostaining for MLH1, MSH2, MSH6, and PMS2 may support a colon primary, as microsatellite instability is more common in colorectal adenocarcinomas. But this does not provide a definitive diagnosis because microsatellite instability can rarely occur in other types of carcinomas, including intrahepatic cholangiocarcinoma.[16,17]

Breast adenocarcinoma

Breast carcinoma metastasizing to liver can present with a wide-spectrum of morphology. A typical panel of immunostains to evaluate for breast carcinoma includes CK7, CK20, estrogen receptor, gross cystic fluid protein-15 (GCDFP-15), mammaglobin, and GATA-3. Progesterone receptor immunostaining is generally not useful because it has poor sensitivity and specificity.[18] Breast carcinomas are usually CK7-positive and CK20-negative. Estrogen receptor positivity is generally seen in about 70% of breast ductal carcinomas and almost all lobular carcinomas, but estrogen receptor is not very specific and can be seen in other tumors. Mammaglobin and GCDFP-15 are more specific markers of breast carcinoma but with lower sensitivity (Figs. 31.15 and 31.16). Cholangiocarcinomas are generally negative for mammaglobin and GCDFP-15.[19] GATA-3 is expressed in over 90% metastatic breast carcinoma and is particularly useful for triple-negative tumors[20] because those tumors are likely to be negative for mammaglobin and GCDFP-15.[21] However, the specificity of GATA-3 is problematic because its expression has been detected in a variety of tumors including squamous or urothelial carcinoma, mesothelioma, salivary gland tumor, and pancreatic ductal carcinomas.[22]

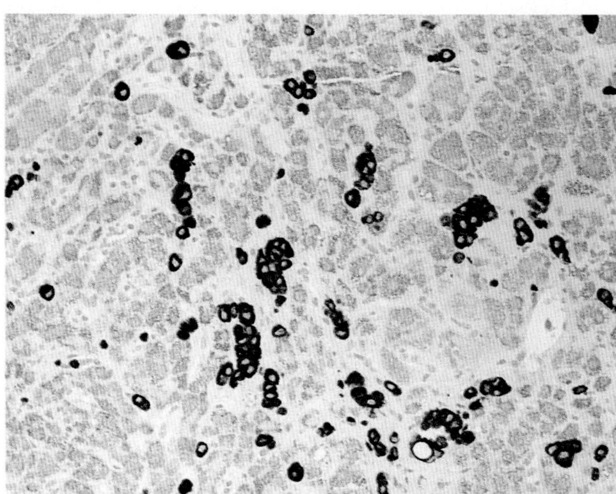

Figure 31.16 Metastatic breast carcinoma, mammaglobin immunostain. The tumor cells are positive.

Lung adenocarcinoma

Both small cell carcinoma and adenocarcinoma of the lung frequently metastasize to the liver. By combining clinical and imaging studies with the histology findings, a diagnosis of metastatic lung adenocarcinoma can be readily made. Lung adenocarcinoma is typically positive for CK7, TTF-1, and Napsin-A (Figs. 31.17 and 31.18). However, an important caveat is that about one third of extrahepatic cholangiocarcinomas and gall bladder adenocarcinomas are positive for nuclear TTF1 and about 10% are Napsin-A positive.[18]

Neuroendocrine tumors/carcinoma

Almost all neuroendocrine tumors in the liver are metastatic. The reported frequency of neuroendocrine tumors primary to the liver is <0.1% of neuroendocrine tumors involving the liver.[23] The diagnosis of a primary liver neuroendocrine tumor is based on excluding tumors from other sites by endoscopy and imaging, but even then the diagnosis remains controversial as the primary tumors outside the liver can be small and hard to detect. The most common primary sites of neuroendocrine tumors are the gastrointestinal tract, pancreas, and lung. The majority of neuroendocrine tumors (about 85%) with no primary site identified on imaging studies arise in the small bowel, in particular the ileum.[24] Neuroendocrine tumors arising in the gut may lead to the carcinoid syndrome after metastasizing to the liver.

Most metastatic neuroendocrine tumors are cytologically well differentiated, composed of monotonous small to medium round cells with finely granular cytoplasm, small or inconspicuous nucleoli, and salt and pepper chromatin (Fig. 31.19). Poorly differentiated neuroendocrine carcinomas can also be seen, with marked atypia, numerous mitosis and apoptosis, tumor necrosis, and large or small cell carcinoma features (Fig. 31.20). Neuroendocrine tumors are positive for broad-spectrum keratin immunostains, whereas CK7 and CK20 are negative or only focally positive. Synaptophysin is positive in most neuroendocrine tumors, but 40% of neuroendocrine tumors from the hindgut and 12% from the foregut are chromogranin-negative.[25] Chromogranin also tends to be negative as tumors become less well differentiated.[26] Of note, many nonneuroendocrine tumors can also express synaptophysin and/or chromogranin, including melanoma,[27] treated prostate adenocarcinoma,[28] and pancreatic acinar cell carcinoma. Malignant gastrointestinal neuroectodermal tumors are very rare and are also positive for synaptophysin and CD56.[29] The diagnosis of malignant gastrointestinal neuroectodermal tumor

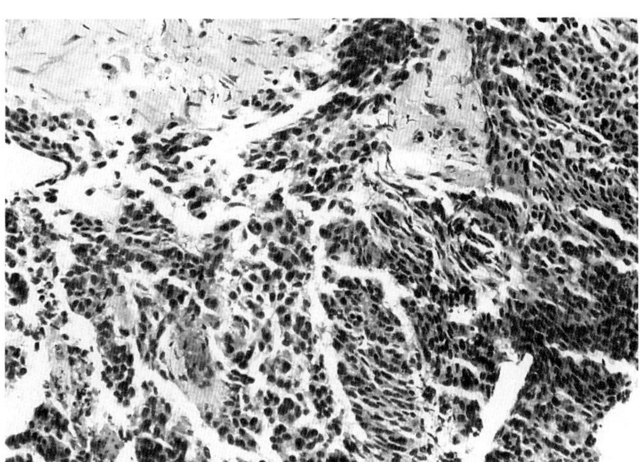

Figure 31.17 Metastatic lung adenocarcinoma. Poorly differentiated non-small cell carcinoma on H&E section.

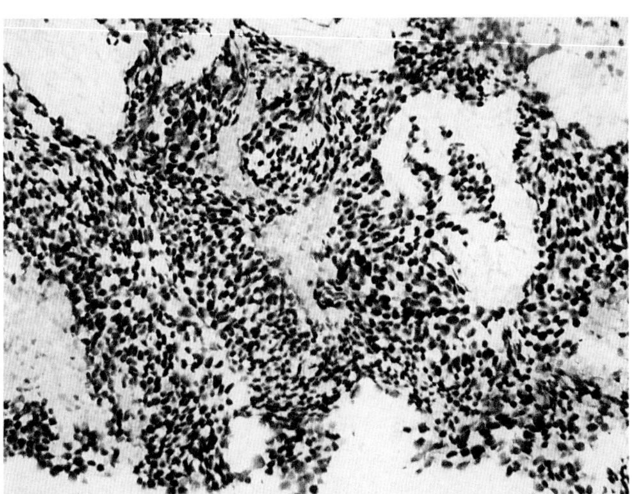

Figure 31.18 Metastatic lung adenocarcinoma. Diffuse nuclear staining of TTF-1.

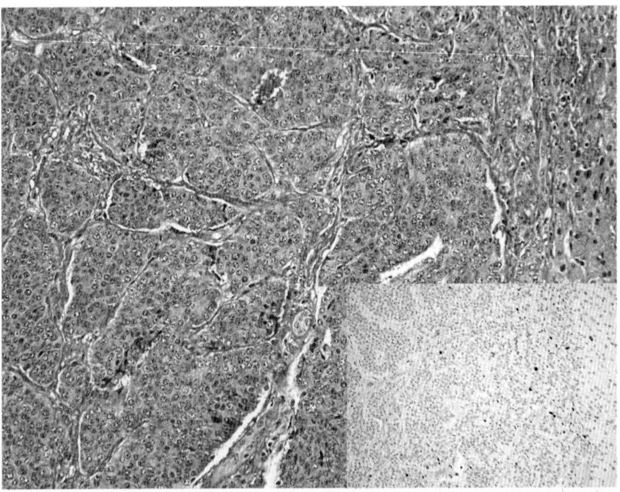

Figure 31.19 Metastatic well-differentiated neuroendocrine tumor. Note the very low Ki-67 index (inset).

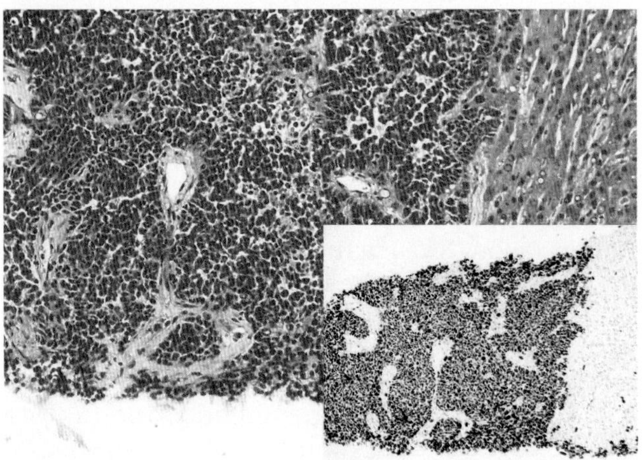

Figure 31.20 Metastatic poorly differentiated neuroendocrine carcinoma. The features are consistent with small cell carcinoma, with nearly 100% Ki-67 index (inset).

can be made using other stains and molecular tests, as these tumors are positive for S100 and SOX10 and *EWSR1* gene rearrangements. For these reasons, the diagnosis of metastatic neuroendocrine tumors should be confirmed by positive staining for synaptophysin and/or chromogranin and also by negative staining for other markers, chosen based on the H&E findings.

Once the diagnosis of metastatic neuroendocrine tumors is established, the site of tumor origin can be suggested by immunostains. Commonly used stains include TTF-1, CDX2, and Islet-1 or Pax8, which cover the most common tumor origins: lung, gastrointestinal, and pancreas, respectively. TTF-1 staining suggests a lung primary in well-differentiated neuroendocrine tumors.[30] Of note, TTF-1 is also positive in thyroid medullary carcinoma, which can rarely metastasize to the liver. Another exemption for TTF-1 is small cell carcinomas, where many tumors are positive, regardless of their origins. Positive staining for CDX2 suggests a gastrointestinal primary. Most neuroendocrine tumors from the appendix and small bowel are positive for CDX2, whereas gastric and colorectal neuroendocrine tumors are less commonly positive. A small subset of pancreatic neuroendocrine tumors are also positive for CDX2, but the staining is usually weak and focal.[31] Islet-1 staining is a sensitive marker for pancreatic neuroendocrine tumors, as over 90% of cases are positive. However, Islet-1 is not a very specific marker, since Islet-1 staining can also be seen in 90% of duodenal neuroendocrine tumors, close to 100% of rectal neuroendocrine tumors, and 40% of colonic neuroendocrine tumors.[32] Pax8 is positive in about 65% of metastatic pancreatic neuroendocrine tumors, but is also not specific. For example, Pax8 is also positive in approximately 80% of rectal neuroendocrine tumors.[33] However, this stain is negative in most ileal neuroendocrine tumors.

Small cell carcinoma

The distinction of small cell carcinoma from non-small cell carcinoma is primarily based on morphology. Small cell carcinoma in the liver has the same morphological and immunostain pattern as they do in any other organ. Tumor cells are small- to medium-sized with scant cytoplasm. The nuclei are small, hyperchromatic with smudgy chromatin, inconspicuous nucleoli, and nuclear molding. There are numerous mitotic and apoptotic cells (Fig. 31.21). The Ki-67 index is typically >90%. Most cases form distinct masses, but rare cases may have diffuse infiltration of the sinusoids with no mass lesions.[34] Metastatic small cell carcinomas can arise from many different organs, though the lungs and gastrointestinal tract are most common. Tumor origin markers such as TTF-1 and CDX2 are not useful in determining the primary site because these stains can be frequently positive regardless of the site of origin.[35]

Carcinoma of Müllerian origin

Adenocarcinomas of Müllerian origin include serous carcinoma (Fig. 31.22), endometrioid carcinoma (Fig. 31.23), mucinous carcinoma, clear cell carcinoma, or mixed Müllerian tumor. The tumors metastasizing to liver share similar histopathologic and immunophenotypic findings to their primaries. High-grade serous carcinoma is the most common type mediatizing to the liver. The highly atypical tumor cells form glandular structures to complex papillary structures to solid sheets of cells. The papillae are usually large, irregularly branching, and highly cellular. Psammoma bodies may be present in varying numbers. The tumor cells are diffusely positive for CK7, WT-1, PAX-8, estrogen

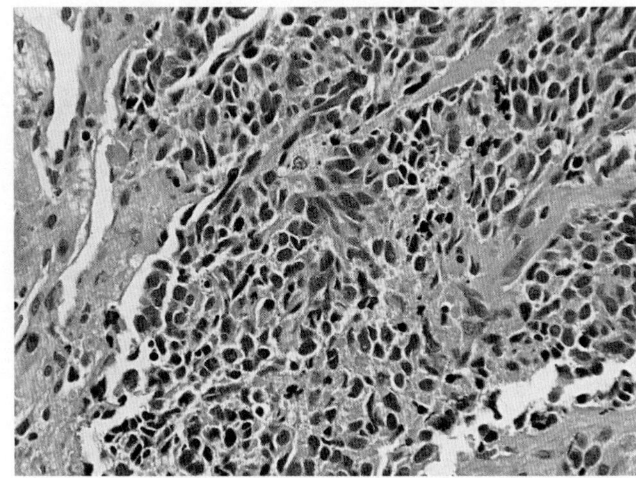

Figure 31.21 Metastatic small cell carcinoma from lung. Note the scant cytoplasm and nuclear features of tumor cells.

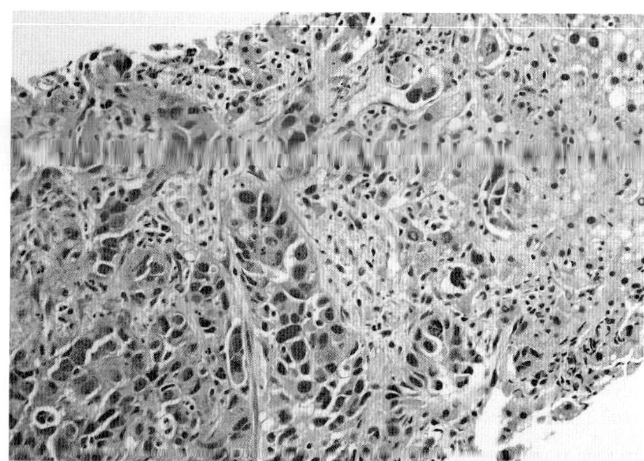

Figure 31.22 Metastatic high-grade serous carcinoma.

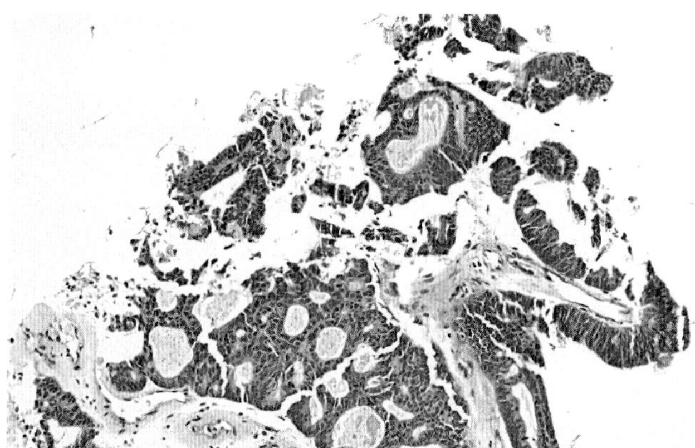

Figure 31.23 Metastatic endometrial carcinoma, endometrioid type.

receptor, p53, and p16. Distinguishing metastatic mucinous carcinoma of Müllerian origin from those arising from gastrointestinal or pancreatobilliary tracts is challenging because they have similar morphology and about 40% of mucinous carcinoma of Müllerian origin can be CDX2-positive.[36] Positive staining for Pax8 can be helpful.

Granulosa cell tumor can rarely present as liver metastasis, often decades after initial resection. Microscopically, granulosa cell tumors are composed of small and bland cuboidal to polygonal cells forming micro- or macrofollicular, trabecular, solid, and insular patterns. Call-Exner bodies are characteristic for this tumor (Fig. 31.24) but are often not seen in biopsies of liver metastases. The tumor nuclei may have a coffee bean appearance with grooves. The tumor is positive for inhibin, smooth muscle actin, and CD99, and some tumors may show dot-like staining pattern for keratin.

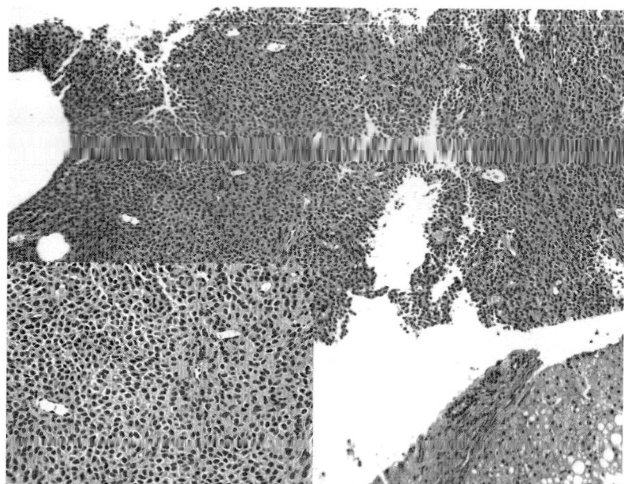

Figure 31.24 Metastatic granulosa cell tumor. Characteristic Call-Exner bodies are seen (inset).

Pancreas carcinoma

Over 50% of patients with pancreatic ductal adenocarcinomas will have liver metastases at the time of diagnosis or with recurrent disease after resection. Well to moderately differentiated pancreatic ductal adenocarcinoma typically shows focal gland formation lined by cuboidal to low columnar cells (Fig. 31.25). Mucin is readily identified in many cases and rarely can be abundant (colloid carcinoma). The poorly differentiated pancreatic ductal adenocarcinomas are similar to any type of poorly differentiated carcinoma, with no strong morphological clue to the tumor origin. If focal squamous differentiation is present, the possibility of metastatic adenosquamous carcinoma or even pancreatoblastoma (Fig. 31.26) has to be raised and careful evaluation to identify glandular, acinar, and neuroendocrine component

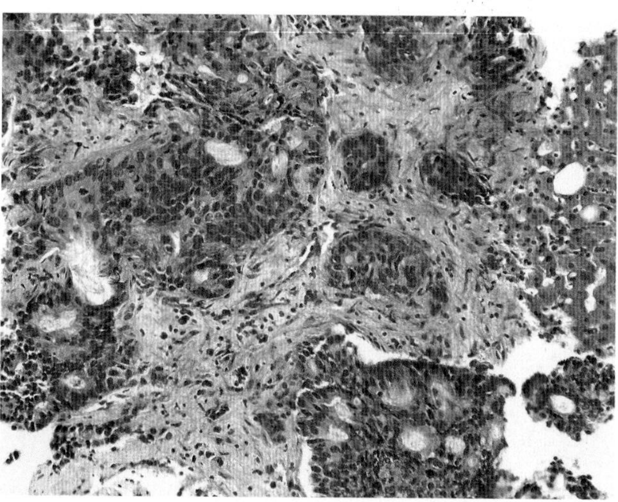

Figure 31.25 Metastatic pancreatic ductal adenocarcinoma.

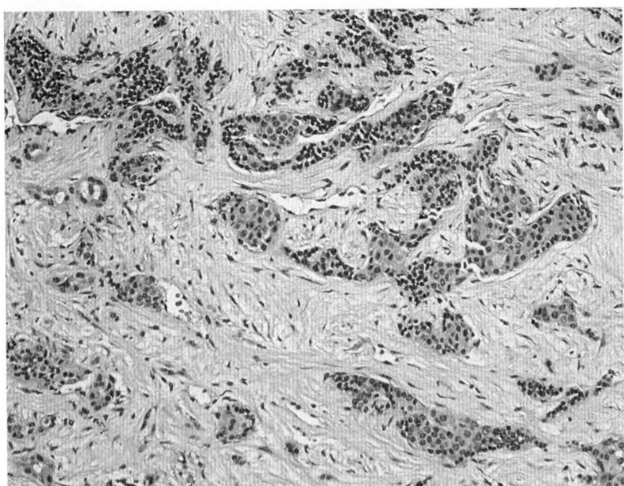

Figure 31.26 Metastatic pancreatoblastoma. Note the squamoid nests, focal glandular differentiation, and round primitive cells.

is necessary. The immunostain profile of pancreatic ductal adenocarcinoma is similar to adenocarcinoma arising in the biliary and upper gastrointestinal tracts. They are typically CK7 and CK19 positive and variably positive for CDX2 and CK20. There is no specific lineage marker for pancreatic ductal adenocarcinoma. SMAD4 staining is lost in about 60% of pancreatic ductal adenocarcinoma, but it is not a tumor lineage marker, as loss of SMAD4 expression can be found in cholangiocarcinomas, carcinomas arising in the ampulla of Vater, and metastatic colorectal carcinoma.[37]

Metastatic pancreas acinar cell carcinomas typically show broad sheets of cells with focal or subtle acinar formation. Immunostains for trypsin or chymotrypsin confirm the diagnosis (Fig. 31.27). However, one pitfall is that neuroendocrine tumors can be focally positive for trypsin and acinar cell carcinomas can be focally positive for synaptophysin and/or chromogranin. Tumor cells with abandon amphophilic granular cytoplasm, prominent nucleoli, acinar structures, and PAS–positive zymogens would favor acinar cell carcinoma. If more than 30% of the cells are positive for each component, a diagnosis of mixed acinar-neuroendocrine carcinoma is made, assuming consistent morphology.[38] Occasionally, hepatocellular carcinoma is also in the differential diagnosis because about 5% of acinar cell carcinomas can be AFP-positive by immunohistochemistry and have elevated serum AFP levels, and about 60% of acinar cell carcinomas are also positive for glypican 3.[39] In these cases, hepatocellular carcinoma can be excluded by using other hepatocyte lineage markers. Of note, very rare acinar cell carcinomas primary to the liver have been reported in the literature,[40,41] but a pancreatic primary has to be carefully excluded before considering a diagnosis of primary acinar cell carcinoma of the liver.

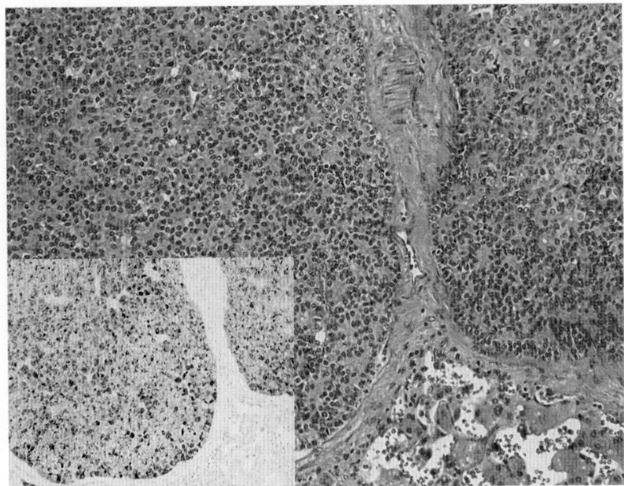

Figure 31.27 Metastatic acinar cell carcinoma (inset, trypsin immunostain).

Pancreas solid pseudopapillary tumors can rarely metastasize to the liver. Pancreas solid pseudopapillary tumors are characterized by solid sheets of polygonal eosinophilic cells with a focal pseudopapillary architecture. Cytoplasmic eosinophilic hyaline globules are often present but are not specific for this entity. Immunostains show strong nuclear staining of β-catenin and positivity for CD10, CD56, progesterone, and patchy staining of keratin. Rare primary solid pseudopapillary tumors to the liver have also been reported,[42] but a pancreatic origin has to be carefully excluded.

Renal cell carcinoma

Clear cell and chromophobe renal cell carcinomas can metastasize to the liver and both can mimic hepatocellular carcinoma. Negative stains for hepatic differentiation (e.g., HepPar-1, arginase), along with positive staining for PAX8, will rule out hepatocellular carcinoma. Chromophobe renal carcinoma is typically composed of compact nests or broad trabeculae of large polygonal cells with abundant eosinophilic cytoplasm, which is a great mimicker of hepatocellular carcinoma. Negative stains for hepatic differentiation along with positive staining for PAX8 and KIT will clarify the diagnosis.

Squamous cell carcinoma and urothelial carcinoma

The morphology of squamous cell carcinoma metastasizing to liver is the same as squamous cell carcinoma anywhere, characterized by nests of large polygonal tumor cells with dense eosinophilic cytoplasm and intercellular bridges. Of note, poorly differentiated nonkeratinizing squamous cell carcinoma can mimic other types of carcinoma such as hepatocellular carcinoma, neuroendocrine tumors, or even small cell carcinoma (Fig. 31.28). A panel of immunostains including p63, p40, and CK5/6 can be used to confirm squamous differentiation. Some high-grade carcinomas can focally express these markers but have morphology that is equivocal for squamous cell carcinoma. In these cases, the terminology of poorly differentiated carcinoma with squamous differentiation is often used, with a differential of squamous cell carcinoma and urothelial carcinoma. Primary squamous cell carcinomas can rarely occur in the liver, either as a cholangiocarcinoma with squamous differentiation, or as a pure squamous cell carcinoma.[43]

Metastatic urothelial carcinomas show cohesive tumor cells forming nests, cords, or trabecular separated by desmoplastic stroma (Fig. 31.29). The immunophenotye overlaps with squamous cell carcinoma (positive for p63, p40, CK5/6). GATA3 can be positive in >90% urothelial carcinoma, but it is fairly nonspecific.[22] Uroplakin III has been shown as a highly specific marker for urothelial carcinoma, but use is limited by its relatively low sensitivity.[44]

Adrenal carcinomas

Both pheochromocytomas and adrenal cortical carcinomas are rare, but the liver is one of the most common sites of metastasis. Adrenal cortical carcinomas can also directly extend to the liver. Adrenal cortical carcinomas can have overlapping features with hepatocellular carcinoma because tumor cells may have abundant eosinophilic cytoplasm and a trabecular growth pattern (Fig. 31.30). Adrenal cortical carcinomas are positive for Melan-A, inhibin, and

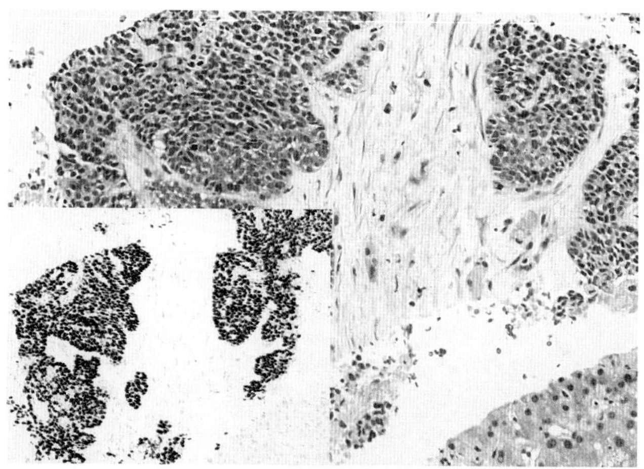

Figure 31.28 Metastatic poorly squamous cell carcinoma. P40 immunostain (inset) confirming squamous cell carcinoma.

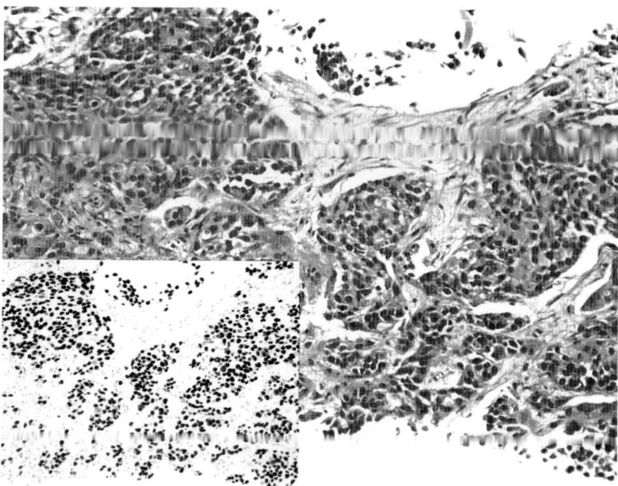

Figure 31.29 Metastatic urothelial carcinoma. P63 immunostain (inset) confirming urothelial carcinoma.

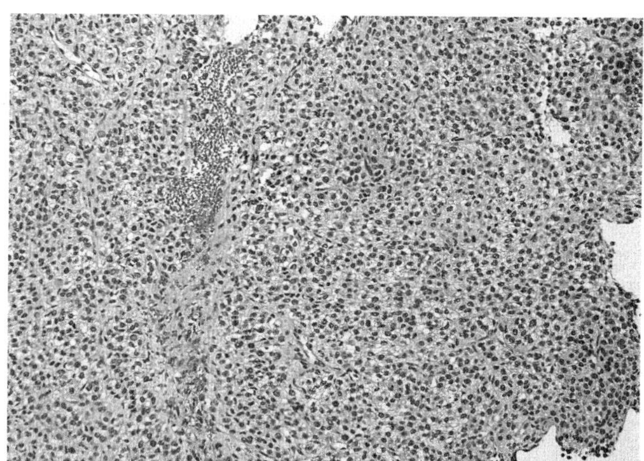

Figure 31.30 Metastatic adrenal cortical adenocarcinoma.

synaptophysin (some cases) and negative for CK7, CK20, chromogranin, and hepatocellular markers. Pheochromocytomas usually have Zellballen pattern, but trabecular or solid patterns can also be seen. The tumor cells may show marked pleomorphism with intracytoplasmic hyaline globules. Pheochromocytomas are positive for chromogranin and synaptophysin but are keratin-negative. S100 stains can highlight sustentacular cells in some cases but is largely negative in metastatic disease.

Prostate adenocarcinoma

Liver metastases are uncommon in individuals with prostate carcinoma. They usually occur late in the course of the disease, are poorly differentiated, and are frequently associated with neuroendocrine features.[28] Metastatic tumors typically show small gland formation with single prominent nucleoli, but they can be poorly differentiated, composed of sheets of

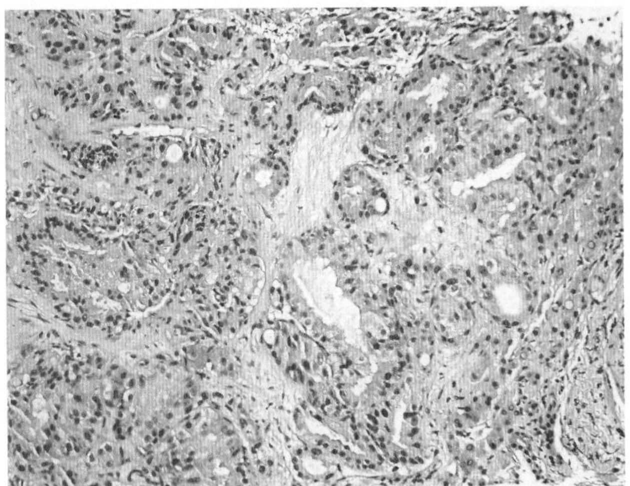

Figure 31.31 Metastatic prostatic adenocarcinoma.

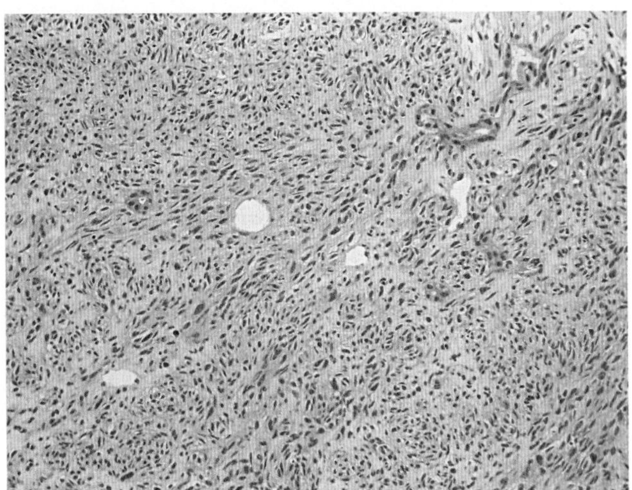

Figure 31.32 Metastatic melanoma. Focal spindle cell morphology is seen.

atypical cells with no gland formation (Fig. 31.31). Immunostains for prostatic differentiation includes PSA and/or prostate-specific acid phosphatase (PSAP). PSA is the most commonly used and most sensitive marker for prostate carcinoma. PSA expression is inversely correlated with tumor differentiation and very poorly differentiated prostate carcinoma tends to be negative for PSA. PSAP is relatively more specific than PSA, but its sensitivity is much lower than PSA. A subset of prostate carcinomas has *TMPRSS2-ERG* gene fusion and nuclear staining with ERG can be seen in about 50% cases. Interestingly, ERG expression tends to be more frequent in metastatic prostate cancer because *TMPRSS2-ERG* rearrangement is more prevalent in metastases.[45] Of note, ERG can be positive in other tumors especially in vascular tumors. Although α-methylacyl-CoA racemase (AMACR) is very useful in distinguishing prostate carcinoma from benign small prostatic glands, its expression is not restricted in prostate at all. Thus, this marker is not useful in identifying metastatic prostate carcinoma. Prostate carcinomas can be negative for both CK7 and CK20, but both stains show an increasing frequency of positivity as the tumors become less well differentiated.[46]

Melanoma

Metastatic melanomas are infrequently seen in liver biopsy specimens and can be challenging to recognize because of their significant morphological variation. Metastatic melanoma cells can appear as monotonous tumors, epithelioid, plasmacytoid, spindle cells, or can be highly pleomorphic. They also can have a wide range of growth patterns, from solid nests or sheets, to diffusely infiltrating the sinusoids (Fig. 31.32). The nuclei are typically large and atypical with intranuclear inclusions and prominent nucleoli. Identifying intracytoplasmic melanin pigments is a helpful feature (Fig. 31.33). However, many metastatic melanomas are nonpigmented or amelanotic. Immunostains for melanoma include S100, Melan-A, and HMB45. MiTF and SOX10 are recently developed markers which also can be helpful.[47,48] If there is a known history of melanoma, a single stain may be enough to confirm a diagnosis. However, a panel with at least three markers is generally ordered to fully exclude melanoma because of varying staining patterns. S100 is still the most sensitive marker for detection of melanoma, although it lacks specificity and up to 4% of melanomas are S100 negative.[49] Spindle cell melanomas tend to be S100-positive, but negative for the other markers. An important diagnostic pitfall is that a subset of melanomas can express nonmelanocytic markers, including keratin, synaptophysin, CD34, CD56, CD10, and smooth muscle actin.[50]

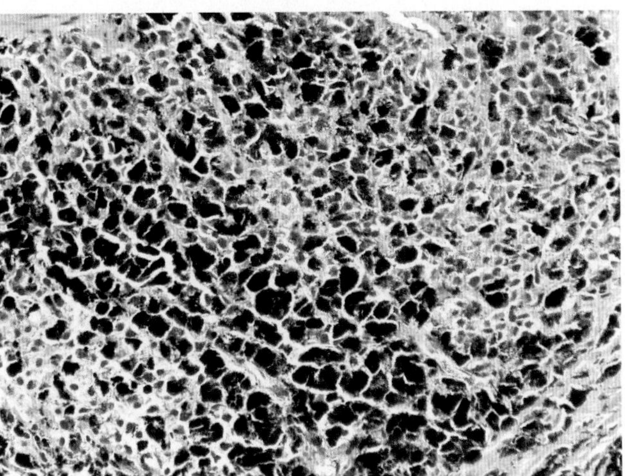

Figure 31.33 Metastatic melanoma. Heavy melanin pigments in metastatic ocular melanoma.

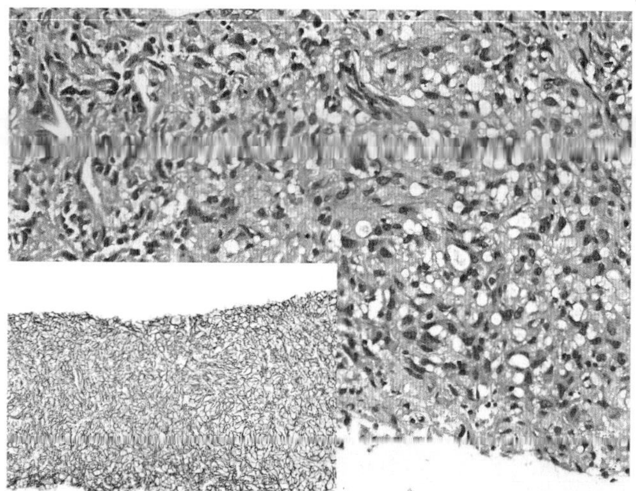

Figure 31.34 Metastatic gastrointestinal stromal tumor. The tumor is positive for DOG1 (inset).

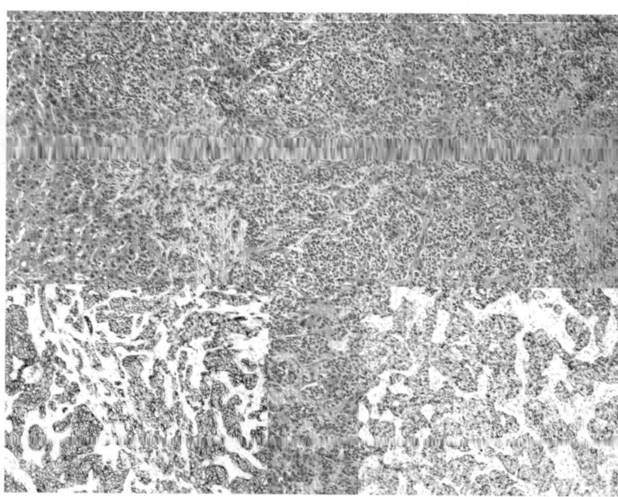

Figure 31.35 Metastatic desmoplastic small round cell tumor. The tumor is positive for CAM5.2 **(left inset)** and dot-like desmin staining **(right inset)**.

Sarcomas

Metastatic sarcomas usually originate from intraabdominal organs, with gastrointestinal stromal tumors and uterine leiomyosarcomas being the two most common sarcomas metastasizing to the liver.[51] Gastrointestinal stromal tumors are typically spindled but also can be epithelioid, myxoid, plasmacytoid, or poorly differentiated. Gastrointestinal stromal tumors are positive for KIT and DOG-1 (Fig. 31.34). A subset of gastrointestinal stromal tumors can coexpress CD34 (70% of cases) and smooth muscle actin (30% of cases). Metastatic leiomyosarcomas are positive for desmin, smooth muscle actin, and caldesmon, whereas negative for KIT and DOG-1. Of note, primary leiomyosarcomas can rarely arise in the liver and extend into the hepatic parenchyma. Clinical history and imaging studies are necessary to rule out this possibility. Other types of sarcomas metastasizing to liver, such as desmoplastic small round cell tumor (Fig. 31.35), rhabdomyosarcoma, liposarcoma, and undifferentiated pleomorphic sarcoma, are exceedingly rare.

31.9 HISTOLOGICAL GRADING

Histological grading is an important factor associated with prognosis, but it is of less value for tumor already metastasizing to liver. Some grading systems for specific cancer types, such as Gleason score for prostatic carcinoma or Nottingham grading for breast carcinoma, are not generally applied for grading such tumors metastasizing in the liver. Carcinomas metastatic to the liver are commonly graded as well, moderately, or poorly differentiated, based on the degree of cytological atypia and evidence for glandular or other differentiation. Neuroendocrine tumors can be graded using the World Health Organization (WHO) classification system by using either mitotic counts or Ki-67 index. Occasionally, neuroendocrine tumors may have higher Ki-67 index (>20%) but still have well-differentiated morphology without large cell or small cell neuroendocrine carcinoma features. This should be stated in pathology reports because of different clinical management between well-differentiated and poorly differentiated neuroendocrine tumors. The term *well-differentiated neuroendocrine tumor with higher proliferative rate* may be used for such tumors.

31.10 MOLECULAR GENETIC FINDINGS

Molecular genetic studies are important tools in modern pathology and have roles in diagnosis and management. Commercial laboratories have also marketed assays for identifying the site of origin for metastatic disease. The test output is typically a list of possible sites of origin with a "percent match" based on gene expression profiling. These tests are likely to be more commonly used in the future as testing platforms and methods are improved, but currently have limited roles in most medical centers.

31.11 PROGNOSIS AND TREATMENT

Liver metastasis indicates advanced-stage disease with a very low possibility for cure of disease. Most individuals are not candidates for surgical treatment, and death typically occurs within 2 years of diagnosis. Even with single metastatic tumors, the median survival is approximately 5 months.[52] However, cryotherapy, arterial chemoembolization, and other regional therapies can benefit some patients, extending survival to approximately 30 months.[53] In addition, select patients with isolated or small numbers of metastases are candidates for metastasectomy.

REFERENCES

1. Budczies J, von Winterfeld M, Klauschen F, et al. The landscape of metastatic progression patterns across major human cancers. *Oncotarget.* 2015;6(1):570–583.
2. Disibio G, French SW. Metastatic patterns of cancers: results from a large autopsy study. *Arch Pathol Lab Med.* 2008;132(6):931–939.
3. Su WT, Rutigliano DN, Gholizadeh M, et al. Hepatic metastasectomy in children. *Cancer.* 2007;109(10):2089–2092.
4. Matsueda K, Yamamoto H, Yoshida Y, et al. Hepatoid carcinoma of the pancreas producing protein induced by vitamin K absence or antagonist II (PIVKA-II) and alpha-fetoprotein (AFP). *J Gastroenterol.* 2006;41(10):1011–1019.
5. Ferrone CR, Ting DT, Shahid M, et al. The ability to diagnose intrahepatic cholangiocarcinoma definitively using novel branched DNA-enhanced albumin RNA in situ hybridization technology. *Ann Surg Oncol.* 2016;23(1):290–296.
6. Padden J, Ahrens M, Kalsch J, et al. Immunohistochemical markers distinguishing cholangiocellular carcinoma (CCC) from pancreatic ductal adenocarcinoma (PDAC) discovered by proteomic analysis of microdissected cells. *Mol Cell Proteomics.* 2016;15(3):1072–1082.
7. Lok T, Chen L, Lin F, et al. Immunohistochemical distinction between intrahepatic cholangiocarcinoma and pancreatic ductal adenocarcinoma. *Hum Pathol.* 2014;45(2):394–400.
8. Estrella JS, Othman ML, Taggart MW, et al. Intrabiliary growth of liver metastases: clinicopathologic features, prevalence, and outcome. *Am J Surg Pathol.* 2013;37(10):1571–1579.
9. Blechacz B, Gores GJ. Cholangiocarcinoma: advances in pathogenesis, diagnosis, and treatment. *Hepatology.* 2008;48(1):308–321.
10. Jinawath A, Akiyama Y, Yuasa Y, et al. Expression of phosphorylated ERK1/2 and homeodomain protein CDX2 in cholangiocarcinoma. *J Cancer Res Clin Oncol.* 2006;132(12):805–810.
11. Ryu HS, Lee K, Shin E, et al. Comparative analysis of immunohistochemical markers for differential diagnosis of hepatocelluar carcinoma and cholangiocarcinoma. *Tumori.* 2012;98(4):478–484.
12. Fan Z, van de Rijn M, Montgomery K, et al. Hep par 1 antibody stain for the differential diagnosis of hepatocellular carcinoma: 676 tumors tested using tissue microarrays and conventional tissue sections. *Mod Pathol.* 2003;16(2):137–144.
13. Adam R, de Gramont A, Figueras J, et al. Managing synchronous liver metastases from colorectal cancer: a multidisciplinary international consensus. *Cancer Treat Rev.* 2015;41(9):729–741.
14. McGregor DK, Wu TT, Rashid A, et al. Reduced expression of cytokeratin 20 in colorectal carcinomas with high levels of microsatellite instability. *Am J Surg Pathol.* 2004;28(6):712–718.
15. Gurzu S, Jung I. Aberrant pattern of the cytokeratin 7/cytokeratin 20 immunophenotype in colorectal adenocarcinomas with BRAF mutations. *Pathol Res Pract.* 2012;208(3):163–166.
16. Liu D, Momoi H, Li L, et al. Microsatellite instability in thorotrast-induced human intrahepatic cholangiocarcinoma. *Int J Cancer.* 2002;102(4):366–371.
17. Liengswangwong U, Karalak A, Morishita Y, et al. Immunohistochemical expression of mismatch repair genes: a screening tool for predicting mutator phenotype in liver fluke infection-associated intrahepatic cholangiocarcinoma. *World J Gastroenterol.* 2006;12(23):3740–3745.
18. Surrey LF, Frank R, Zhang PJ, et al. TTF-1 and Napsin-A are expressed in a subset of cholangiocarcinomas arising from the gallbladder and hepatic ducts: continued caveats for utilization of immunohistochemistry panels. *Am J Surg Pathol.* 2014;38(2):224–227.
19. Bhargava R, Beriwal S, Dabbs DJ. Mammaglobin vs GCDFP-15: an immunohistologic validation survey for sensitivity and specificity. *Am J Clin Pathol.* 2007;127(1):103–113.
20. Cimino-Mathews A, Subhawong AP, Illei PB, et al. GATA3 expression in breast carcinoma: utility in triple-negative, sarcomatoid, and metastatic carcinomas. *Hum Pathol.* 2013;44(7):1341–1349.
21. Lewis GH, Subhawong AP, Nassar H, et al. Relationship between molecular subtype of invasive breast carcinoma and expression of gross cystic disease fluid protein 15 and mammaglobin. *Am J Clin Pathol.* 2011;135(4):587–591.
22. Miettinen M, McCue PA, Sarlomo-Rikala M, et al. GATA3: a multispecific but potentially useful marker in surgical pathology: a systematic analysis of 2500 epithelial and nonepithelial tumors. *Am J Surg Pathol.* 2014;38(1):13–22.
23. Yao JC, Hassan M, Phan A, et al. One hundred years after "carcinoid": epidemiology of and prognostic factors for neuroendocrine tumors in

35,825 cases in the United States. *J Clin Oncol.* 2008;26(18):3063–3072.

24. Bergsland EK, Nakakura EK. Neuroendocrine tumors of unknown primary: is the primary site really not known? *JAMA Surg.* 2014;149(9):889–890.
25. Al-Khafaji B, Noffsinger AE, Miller MA, et al. Immunohistologic analysis of gastrointestinal and pulmonary carcinoid tumors. *Hum Pathol.* 1998;29(9):992–999.
26. Helpap B, Kollermann J. Immunohistochemical analysis of the proliferative activity of neuroendocrine tumors from various organs. Are there indications for a neuroendocrine tumor-carcinoma sequence? *Virchows Arch.* 2001;438(1):86–91.
27. Romano RC, Carter JM, Folpe AL. Aberrant intermediate filament and synaptophysin expression is a frequent event in malignant melanoma: an immunohistochemical study of 73 cases. *Mod Pathol.* 2015;28(8):1033–1042.
28. Pouessel D, Gallet B, Bibeau F, et al. Liver metastases in prostate carcinoma: clinical characteristics and outcome. *BJU Int.* 2007;99(4):807–811.
29. Stockman DL, Miettinen M, Suster S, et al. Malignant gastrointestinal neuroectodermal tumor: clinicopathologic, immunohistochemical, ultrastructural, and molecular analysis of 16 cases with a reappraisal of clear cell sarcoma-like tumors of the gastrointestinal tract. *Am J Surg Pathol.* 2012;36(6):857–868.
30. Agoff SN, Lamps LW, Philip AT, et al. Thyroid transcription factor-1 is expressed in extrapulmonary small cell carcinomas but not in other extrapulmonary neuroendocrine tumors. *Mod Pathol.* 2000;13(3):238–242.
31. Moskaluk CA, Zhang H, Powell SM, et al. Cdx2 protein expression in normal and malignant human tissues: an immunohistochemical survey using tissue microarrays. *Mod Pathol.* 2003;16(9):913–919.
32. Graham RP, Shrestha B, Caron BL, et al. Islet-1 is a sensitive but not entirely specific marker for pancreatic neuroendocrine neoplasms and their metastases. *Am J Surg Pathol.* 2013;37(3):399–405.
33. Sangoi AR, Ohgami RS, Pai RK, et al. PAX8 expression reliably distinguishes pancreatic well-differentiated neuroendocrine tumors from ileal and pulmonary well-differentiated neuroendocrine tumors and pancreatic acinar cell carcinoma. *Mod Pathol.* 2011;24(3):412–424.
34. Sato K, Takeyama Y, Tanaka T, et al. Fulminant hepatic failure and hepatomegaly caused by diffuse liver metastases from small cell lung carcinoma: 2 autopsy cases. *Respir Investig.* 2013;51(2):98–102.
35. Kaufmann O, Dietel M. Expression of thyroid transcription factor-1 in pulmonary and extrapulmonary small cell carcinomas and other neuroendocrine carcinomas of various primary sites. *Histopathology.* 2000;36(5):415–420.
36. Vang R, Gown AM, Wu LS, et al. Immunohistochemical expression of CDX2 in primary ovarian mucinous tumors and metastatic mucinous carcinomas involving the ovary: comparison with CK20 and correlation with coordinate expression of CK7. *Mod Pathol.* 2006;19(11):1421–1428.
37. Liu H, Shi J, Anandan V, et al. Reevaluation and identification of the best immunohistochemical panel (pVHL, Maspin, S100P, IMP-3) for ductal adenocarcinoma of the pancreas. *Arch Pathol Lab Med.* 2012;136(6):601–609.
38. La Rosa S, Adsay V, Albarello L, et al. Clinicopathologic study of 62 acinar cell carcinomas of the pancreas: insights into the morphology and immunophenotype and search for prognostic markers. *Am J Surg Pathol.* 2012;36(12):1782–1795.
39. Mounajjed T, Zhang L, Wu TT. Glypican-3 expression in gastrointestinal and pancreatic epithelial neoplasms. *Hum Pathol.* 2013;44(4):542–550.
40. Wildgruber M, Rummeny EJ, Gaa J. Primary acinar cell carcinoma of the liver. *Rofo.* 2013;185(6):572–573.
41. Agaimy A, Kaiser A, Becker K, et al. Pancreatic-type acinar cell carcinoma of the liver: a clinicopathologic study of four patients. *Mod Pathol.* 2011;24(12):1620–1626.
42. Thai E, Dalla Valle R, Silini EM. Primary solid papillary tumor of the liver. *Pathol Res Pract.* 2012;208(4):250–253.
43. Zhang XF, Du ZQ, Liu XM, et al. Primary squamous cell carcinoma of liver: case series and review of literatures. *Medicine.* 2015;94(28):e868.
44. Kaufmann O, Volmerig J, Dietel M. Uroplakin III is a highly specific and moderately sensitive immunohistochemical marker for primary and metastatic urothelial carcinomas. *Am J Clin Pathol.* 2000;113(5):683–687.
45. Perner S, Svensson MA, Hossain RR, et al. ERG rearrangement metastasis patterns in locally advanced prostate cancer. *Urology.* 2010;75(4):762–767.
46. Goldstein NS. Immunophenotypic characterization of 225 prostate adenocarcinomas with intermediate or high Gleason scores. *Am J Clin Pathol.* 2002;117(3):471–477.
47. Guo R, Franco-Palacios M, Russell M, et al. Micropthalmia transcription factor (MITF) as a diagnostic marker for metastatic melanomas negative for other melanoma markers. *Int J Clin Exp Pathol.* 2013;6(8):1658–1664.
48. Palla B, Su A, Binder S, et al. SOX10 expression distinguishes desmoplastic melanoma from

its histologic mimics. *Am J Dermatopathol.* 2013;35(5):576–581.

49. Aisner DL, Maker A, Rosenberg SA, et al. Loss of S100 antigenicity in metastatic melanoma. *Hum Pathol.* 2005;36(9):1016–1019.
50. Magro CM, Crowson AN, Mihm MC. Unusual variants of malignant melanoma. *Mod Pathol.* 2006;19(suppl 2):S41–70.
51. Stavrou GA, Flemming P, Oldhafer KJ. Liver resection for metastasis due to malignant mesenchymal tumours. *HPB.* 2006;8(2):110–113.
52. Riihimaki M, Thomsen H, Hemminki A, et al. Comparison of survival of patients with metastases from known versus unknown primaries: survival in metastatic cancer. *BMC Cancer.* 2013;13:36.
53. Yan TD, Padang R, Morris DL. Longterm results and prognostic indicators after cryotherapy and hepatic arterial chemotherapy with or without resection for colorectal liver metastases in 224 patients: longterm survival can be achieved in patients with multiple bilateral liver metastases. *J Am Coll Surg.* 2006;202(1):100–111.

INDEX

Note: Page numbers followed by *f* indicate figures; those followed by *t* indicate tabular material.

B

Q

R

T

U

V